Statistics for Clinicians

Ahmed Hassouna

Statistics for Clinicians

How Much Should a Doctor Know?

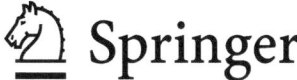 Springer

Ahmed Hassouna ⓘ
Faculty of Medicine
Ain Shams University
Cairo, Egypt

ISBN 978-3-031-20757-0   ISBN 978-3-031-20758-7   (eBook)
https://doi.org/10.1007/978-3-031-20758-7

This Springer imprint is published by the registered company Springer Nature Switzerland AG
The registered company address is: Gewerbestrasse 11, 6330 Cham, Switzerland

To my father, who did his best for us. To my caring mother and aunt Neimat for their pure love and full support. To my wife, sons and daughters. Mohamed, Malak, Tarek, and Farah, who paid the price of my long working hours. To my fellows and students, hoping every one of them finds what he came to look for.

Foreword: The Man and His Dream

If you believe this is a book about the science and practice of statistics, then you have captured only half the truth. A cardiac surgeon carved this book; this is his principal profession. However, his heart and mind were constantly absorbed in the magic world of statistics. If you consider cardiac surgery one of the most demanding medical specialties, you would wonder how he could find the time and energy to produce this work. This is only possible through the power of devotion to your dreams. Professor Hassouna lived through his dream time after time, teaching, preaching, and simplifying the understanding of statistical analysis to students, young investigators, and university scholars.

Statistics is the science of exposing the relationship between assumptions, concepts, observations, and the real world. The arrangement of the book chapters follows the natural flow of statistical analysis from basic concepts to more complex solutions. Moreover, each chapter is assorted with several topics containing the full details the reader needs. Importantly, Chaps. 2 and 3 display in a convenient way how to select the appropriate statistical test and Chap. 4 is a practical guide to sample size calculation. Equally amazing is the unique content of Chap. 7, which describes pitfalls and troubleshooting in statistical analysis. The information in this chapter comes directly from the rich teaching experience of the author and the practical problems met by his students.

Professor Hassouna spent years explaining statistics to a variety of trainees. When he realized that the number of student-years did not rise to his ambitions, he decided to write a book. The book is his gift for communicating with an endless number of interested receivers. Let us hope that you will enjoy and benefit from the numerous pearls enclosed in the pages of this book.

Cairo, Egypt
May 2022

Sherif Eltobgi, MD, FESC, FACC
Professor of cardiology
Cairo University, A long-time colleague
and admirer of Professor Hassouna

Preface: Statistics for Clinicians: How Much Should a Doctor Know?

"Finally, the work is done. Let us look for a statistician to analyze the data." This everyday—apparently benign—phrase jeopardizes any clinical research's credibility for many reasons.

To increase the chance of reaching dependable results, the number of patients necessary for the study has to be calculated before it begins, using well-known mathematical equations and with an acceptable probability of finding what the researcher is looking for. The empirical designation of such a number is the leading cause of missing statistically significant results, known as Type II error or a false-negative study. The question is not just about finding evidence per se, as indicated by a statistically significant P value. It is about evaluating this finding to decide whether it was achieved by a serious researcher who prepared a sufficient sample to find the evidence or was just a matter of good luck.

Data are usually analyzed by the end of the study. However, the conditions necessary for data analysis must be verified before data collection. The type of variable, its distribution, and its expression in a particular mathematical form have to fit the statistical test used for the analysis. The researcher has to choose between pre-planning, a careful match between the data and the statistical test during the preparation of the study, where everything is possible, and reckless decision-making at the end, where a little can be changed. The statistical test must be implanted in fertile land, which should be prepared to receive it. Doing otherwise will only guarantee a poor product.

Common knowledge is that randomization creates comparable groups at the beginning of the study. Any observed differences by the end of the study can then be related to the treatment effect. Unfortunately, many researchers do not appreciate that randomization is just an implant that has to be taken care of throughout the study. Comparability can be easily lost in various situations, such as uncovering blindness, neglecting patients in the placebo group, or any other condition that favors one of the study groups, usually the treatment group. Concluding upon the latter, while it is not, is a false-positive result known as Type I error.

The role of statistics does not end by creating P-values and confidence intervals. I must begin by verifying the conditions of application of the statistical tests used in creating those results. A critical step is a correct interpretation, which needs a clear understanding of the meaning of underlying equations. For example, a statistically non-significant difference between the effects of two treatments does not mean that both treatments are equal because strict equality does not exist in biology; hence, we cannot prove it in the experiment.

Moreover, the need for statistical consultation must include reviewing the manuscript to ensure the use of correct statistical terms in the discussion section. It also should cover answering the statistical queries posed by the editors and the reviewers. Consequently, limiting the statistician's role to data analysis at the end of the study is all wrong. The solution is simple, the researcher has to lead a research team to manage his study from "Protocol to Publisher," with the statistician being a primary indispensable member.

On the other hand, our understanding of biostatistics has to be net and clear. Although we do not need to be involved in every mathematical detail, it would become dangerous not to understand the fundamental idea, assumptions, and, most importantly, the correct interpretation of each statistical analysis we use. It is just like prescribing a treatment to your patient without knowing how it works, when it should be used, and the drawbacks and limitations. The researcher does not have to be involved in the details of complicated statistical equations more than the need of a physician to go into the depth of every complicated biochemical reaction.

The main barrier is the difficulty of gaining statistical knowledge from textbooks, which is the same reason I made this book. My work aims to explain to lay biologists—like me—the basic statistical ideas in our everyday language without distorting knowledge's mathematical and statistical basis. In other words, "Statistics for Clinicians" is not a textbook in biostatistics but a trial to answer the fundamental question raised by every biologist: how much statistics do I need to know? We need basic statistical information to keep in touch with the "exploding" medical knowledge while reading a manuscript or attending a conference. We need it to get more involved, whether as a research team member, as a reviewer, or as a member of an evaluating scientific committee.

I tried to bring the correct statistical reasoning and sound judgment in this book, which is all a biologist need. All statistical tests are actually executed by computer software, which unfortunately does not tell us: which test to use. They point to whether data satisfies the test but rarely put it clearly to the lay researcher. The large amount of statistical information generated by those software packages is sometimes more confusing than informative. Most importantly, the software does not provide a "suggestion" on interpreting the results correctly. I aim to help fellow biologists know which test can be used to answer a specific research question. To ensure that the conditions of application are verified, to interpret the results correctly, and report them fully.

"People never learn anything by being told; they have to find out for themselves (*Paulo Coelho*)." I brought 697 equations; the vast majority can be executed by hand and do not need any statistical background. In order to understand the output of a test, one must know which inputs were introduced in the first place. For example, a researcher who knows the five primary inputs of sample size calculation will be able to reduce the size of his study by manipulating those inputs. In order to be understandable and easily executable, I insisted on using small examples, which were too small to satisfy the conditions of application of some statistical tests. I made my choice to present those user-friendly examples and concomitantly clearly note any limitations. I advise the reader to carefully follow the example to understand this input-output relation. Then, he can continue executing the analysis by the statistical software with confidence and report the results with knowledge.

Prof. Ahmed Hassouna
ChD, MCFCV, DU Microsurgery
Biostatistics Diploma (STARC)
Professor of Cardiothoracic Surgery
Ain-Shams University
Cairo, Egypt

Acknowledgments: The Payoff

I still remember the first lecture by professor Daniel Schwartz (1917–2009) at the center of statistical studies applied in medicine (CESAM) in Paris VI University, Pierre and Marie Curie. It was just 35 years ago, but it never got old; I quote: "In order to understand biostatistics, a biologist must be able to add, subtract, multiply and divide two numbers; this is all that he needs." At that time, everybody just smiled, we thought the great man was exaggerating. I truly believe him as time goes by.

I was supposed to wait three more years to get his course. He saved me the waiting in return for a promise: "to transfer the knowledge to the other side of the world." I have been working on it since then. May his soul rest in peace.

Ahmed Hassouna

Contents

1 Expressing and Analyzing Variability 1
  1.1 Introduction 1
  1.2 Variables: Types, Measurement and Role 2
      1.2.1 Variable Conversion 2
  1.3 Summarizing Data 3
      1.3.1 The Qualitative Variable 4
      1.3.2 The Quantitative Variable 7
      1.3.3 Measures of Central Tendency 7
      1.3.4 Measures of Dispersion 7
  1.4 The Normal Distribution 10
      1.4.1 The Standardized Normal Distribution
           and the Z Score 12
      1.4.2 The Confidence Interval (CI) 15
      1.4.3 Verifying Normality 25
      1.4.4 Normalization of Data 30
  1.5 The P-value 31
      1.5.1 The Primary Risk of Error (α) 31
  1.6 The Null and Alternative Hypothesis 32
      1.6.1 Statistical Significance and the Degree
           of Significance 34
  1.7 Testing Hypothesis 34
      1.7.1 A Simple Parametric Test 34
      1.7.2 Unilateral Study Design 34
      1.7.3 Bilateral Study Design 36
      1.7.4 The Secondary Risk of Error 37
  1.8 Common Indices of Clinical Outcomes 39
      1.8.1 The Risk and the Odds 39
      1.8.2 The Relative Risks and the Odds Ratio 39
      1.8.3 The Hazard Ratio 43
      1.8.4 Relative Risk Increase (RRI) and Relative
           Risk Reduction (RRR) 49
      1.8.5 Absolute Risk Increase (ARI) and Reduction
           (ARR) 50
      1.8.6 Number Needed to Treat Benefit (NNTB)
           and Number Needed to Harm (NNTH) 50
      1.8.7 Calculation of the 95% Confidence Interval
           and Testing Statistical Significance 51

1.9   Diagnostic Accuracy..............................   56
      1.9.1   The Discriminative Measures.................   57
      1.9.2   The Predictive Values   63
      1.9.3   The Likelihood Ratios   66
      1.9.4   Single Indicators of Test Performance   71
      1.9.5   Choosing the Appropriate Diagnostic Test.......   82
      1.9.6   Comparing Two Diagnostic Tests   83
      1.9.7   The Standards for Reporting Diagnostic
              Accuracy (STARD)........................   85
References...   85

2   Bivariate Statistical Analysis...........................   87
    2.1   Choosing a Statistical Test   88
          2.1.1   Independence of Data: Paired Versus
                  Unpaired Tests...........................   89
          2.1.2   Data Distribution: Parametric Versus
                  Distribution-Free Tests.....................   89
    2.2   Consulting Statistical Tables.......................   90
          2.2.1   The Test Statistics   90
          2.2.2   The Degrees of Freedom (Df)   91
          2.2.3   Consulting Individual Tables.................   93
    2.3   Inferences on Two Qualitative Variables   97
          2.3.1   The Unpaired Tests   97
          2.3.2   The Paired Tests 109
    2.4   Inferences on Means and Variances of Normal
          Distribution: The Parametric Tests 114
          2.4.1   The Comparison of Two Means 114
          2.4.2   The Comparison of Two Variances............ 123
          2.4.3   The Comparison of Multiple Means 124
    2.5   Inference on Medians and Other Distributions Than
          Normal: Non-parametric Tests 143
          2.5.1   The Comparison of Two-Groups.............. 143
          2.5.2   The Comparison of Several Groups............ 150
    2.6   Inference on the Relation of Two Quantitative
          Variables..................................... 153
          2.6.1   Correlation.............................. 154
          2.6.2   Regression.............................. 162
    2.7   Inference on Survival Curves 174
          2.7.1   Introduction: Assumptions and Definitions 174
          2.7.2   Kaplan Meier Method 175
          2.7.3   Actuarial Method......................... 181
          2.7.4   Comparison of Survival Curves.............. 183
    2.8   Choosing the Appropriate Bivariate Statistical Test 191
          2.8.1   Introduction............................. 191
          2.8.2   The Unpaired Statistical Tests 193
          2.8.3   The Paired Statistical Tests 194
          2.8.4   The Comparison of Survival Curves 194

2.9 Adjusting Bivariate Analysis: Prognostic Studies 195
    2.9.1 Introduction............................... 195
    2.9.2 Excluding a Qualitative (Reverse) Interaction 197
    2.9.3 Adjusting Two Proportions 200
    2.9.4 Adjusting Two Means 203
    2.9.5 Adjusting Two Quantitative Variables.......... 209
2.10 Measuring Agreement and Testing Reliability 213
    2.10.1 Introduction............................... 213
    2.10.2 Plan of the Analysis 215
    2.10.3 The Qualitative Outcome.................... 218
    2.10.4 The Quantitative Outcome................... 228
References... 244

3 Multivariable Analysis................................. 247
3.1 Introduction 247
3.2 The ANOVA Family 248
    3.2.1 Testing the Main Effects 249
    3.2.2 Testing Interaction Effects of Qualitative
        Variables................................ 251
    3.2.3 Testing Interaction Effects of Quantitative
        Variables: Analysis of Covariance
        (ANCOVA)............................... 254
    3.2.4 Multivariate ANOVA and ANCOVA
        (MANOVA and MANCOVA)................ 271
    3.2.5 Repeated Measures ANOVA (RMANOVA) 277
3.3 General Outlines of Multivariable Models 294
    3.3.1 Indications............................... 294
    3.3.2 Aim of the Model 294
    3.3.3 Selection of Predictors...................... 295
    3.3.4 Model Selection........................... 296
    3.3.5 The Equations and Estimation of Regression
        Coefficients 297
    3.3.6 Evaluation of the Model 298
3.4 Multiple Regression Analysis 299
    3.4.1 Introduction: Simple Versus Multiple Linear
        Regression............................... 300
    3.4.2 The Basic Assumptions 301
    3.4.3 The Example............................. 303
    3.4.4 Designing the Model....................... 305
    3.4.5 Verification of the Assumptions 306
    3.4.6 Model Evaluation 310
    3.4.7 What Should Be Reported.................... 314
    3.4.8 The Case of Multiple Outcome Variables 315
3.5 Binary Logistic Regression Analysis.................. 315
    3.5.1 Introduction: The Linear Versus the Logistic
        Regression............................... 315
    3.5.2 The Basic Assumptions 322
    3.5.3 The Example............................. 323

       3.5.4   Designing the Model 324

       3.5.5   Verification of the Assumptions 324

       3.5.6   Model Evaluation 325

       3.5.7   What Should Be Reported 328

  3.6   Cox Regression Analysis 329

       3.6.1   Introduction: Life Tables Versus Cox
                Regression Analysis. 329

       3.6.2   The Basic Assumptions 330

       3.6.3   The Example 332

       3.6.4   Designing the Model 333

       3.6.5   Verification of the Assumptions 333

       3.6.6   Model Evaluation 335

       3.6.7   What Should Be Reported 336

  References 337

4 **Sample Size Calculation** 339

  4.1   Introduction 339

       4.1.1   Estimation of the Effect Size 340

       4.1.2   Choosing the Risks of Error 341

       4.1.3   The Direction of the Study 342

       4.1.4   Study Specific Factors 343

       4.1.5   Sample Size Calculation 344

  4.2   Comparison of Two Independent Quantitative
       Variables: Student and Mann & Whitney Tests 350

       4.2.1   Effect Size 350

       4.2.2   Sample Size 352

  4.3   Association of Two Independent Binary Variables:
       Chi-Square and Fisher's Exact Tests. 356

       4.3.1   Effect Size 356

       4.3.2   Sample Size 359

  4.4   Categorical and Ordinal Variables: Chi-Square
       Tests of Independence and Goodness of Fit 362

       4.4.1   Effect Size 363

       4.4.2   Sample Size 364

  4.5   Paired Analysis 366

       4.5.1   Paired Student Test 366

       4.5.2   Paired Wilcoxon-Sign-Rank Test 368

       4.5.3   McNemar's Test 370

  4.6   Comparison of Multiple Means: One-Way ANOVA. 372

       4.6.1   Effect Size 372

       4.6.2   Sample Size 375

  4.7   Simple Correlation: Pearson's Correlation
       Coefficient R 377

       4.7.1   Effect Size 378

       4.7.2   Sample Size 378

4.8 Simple Linear Regression 379
    4.8.1 Effect Size 379
    4.8.2 Sample Size 379
4.9 Time to Event 381
    4.9.1 Effect Size 381
    4.9.2 Sample Size 381
4.10 Logistic Regression 384
    4.10.1 Effect Size: Log Odds Ratio 385
    4.10.2 Sample Size 385
4.11 Multiple Regression 387
    4.11.1 Conditional Fixed Factors Model 387
    4.11.2 Unconditional Random Effect Model 389
4.12 Repeated Measures 391
    4.12.1 Repeated Measures ANOVA (RMANOVA) 391
    4.12.2 Friedman Test 395
4.13 Non-inferiority and Equivalence Studies 397
    4.13.1 Comparison of 2 Means 398
    4.13.2 Comparison of Two Proportions 400
    4.13.3 Time to Event Analysis 403
4.14 Diagnostic Accuracy 405
    4.14.1 Sensitivity and Specificity 405
    4.14.2 ROC Analysis 408
4.15 Measuring Agreement 410
    4.15.1 Qualitative Outcome 410
    4.15.2 Quantitative Outcome 411
4.16 Survey Analysis 413
    4.16.1 Introduction 413
    4.16.2 Factors Regulating Sample Size Calculation 413
    4.16.3 Sample Size Calculation 414
References 416

5 The Protocol of a Comparative Clinical Study:
    Statistical Considerations 421
5.1 Background and Rationale 421
5.2 Objectives 421
5.3 Study Design 422
    5.3.1 The Formulation of the Study 422
    5.3.2 Number of Study Groups and Number
          of Effectuated Comparisons 422
    5.3.3 The Classic Parallel Groups Versus Other
          Designs 423
    5.3.4 Design Framework: Superiority, Non-inferiority,
          Equivalence or Pilot Study 423
    5.3.5 Allocation Ratio 423
5.4 Methods 424
    5.4.1 Study Endpoints 424
    5.4.2 Assignment of Interventions 424
    5.4.3 Blinding (Masking) 428

5.5   Study Population and Samples   428
        5.5.1   Study Settings   428
        5.5.2   Inclusion Criteria   428
        5.5.3   Exclusion Criteria   429
        5.5.4   Study Timeline   430
        5.5.5   Follow-Up   430
5.6   Treatments and Interventions   431
        5.6.1   Studied Treatments and Interventions   431
        5.6.2   Associated Treatments and Interventions   432
5.7   Data Management   432
        5.7.1   Data Collection and Storage   432
        5.7.2   Data Monitoring and Auditing   432
5.8   Statistical Methods   433
        5.8.1   Population for the Analysis   433
        5.8.2   Statistical Hypothesis   433
        5.8.3   Statistical Analysis   434
        5.8.4   Sample Size Determination   435
5.9   Study Documentations   437
5.10   Study Ethics   438
5.11   Data Sharing and Publication   438
5.12   Appendices   438
References   438

6   Introduction to Meta-Analysis   441
6.1   Introduction   441
        6.1.1   From Narrative to Systematic Review   441
        6.1.2   Why Do We Need Meta-Analysis?   442
        6.1.3   Types of Meta-Analysis   443
6.2   Stages of Meta-Analysis   444
        6.2.1   Formulation of the Problem   445
        6.2.2   Data Collection   446
        6.2.3   Assessment of Risk of Bias   447
        6.2.4   Choosing the Model   447
        6.2.5   Managing the Effect Size Estimates   449
        6.2.6   Estimation of a Mean Effect Size, Se,
                 95% CI and P Value   452
        6.2.7   Assessment of Heterogeneity   479
        6.2.8   Subgroup Analysis   486
        6.2.9   Meta Regression   498
        6.2.10   Assessment of Publication Bias and Small-Study
                 Effects   503
        6.2.11   Sensitivity Analysis   511
        6.2.12   Reporting Meta-Analysis   513
6.3   Psychometric Meta-Analysis (Hunter and Schmidt)   519
        6.3.1   The Basic Concept   519
        6.3.2   The Bare Bones Meta-Analysis   520
        6.3.3   Meta-Analysis Corrected for All Artifacts   521
References   523

7   Pitfalls and Common Errors.   527
   7.1   Sample Size Calculation   527
       7.1.1   Empower the Study.   527
       7.1.2   Sculpture the Primary Outcome.   528
       7.1.3   Reduce Variability by Ameliorating
             the Study Design.   535
       7.1.4   Prepare the Study to Receive the Selected
             Tests   537
       7.1.5   Account for the Effect of Covariates
             in Multivariable Analysis.   540
       7.1.6   Manage the Secondary Outcomes   540
   7.2   Data Management.   541
       7.2.1   Check on Errors and Data Consistency   541
       7.2.2   Verify Outliers.   541
       7.2.3   Manage Missing Data   541
       7.2.4   Normalizing Data   545
   7.3   Tools of the Analysis   547
       7.3.1   The Statistical Software.   547
       7.3.2   The Complementary Online Calculators   551
   7.4   Data Reporting in a Manuscript   554
       7.4.1   The Introduction   554
       7.4.2   The Material and Methods.   555
       7.4.3   The Results   560
       7.4.4   The Discussion   566
       7.4.5   The Abstract   568
       7.4.6   Common Pitfalls, Misinterpretations,
             and Inadequate Reporting   569
   7.5   The Role of the Statistician.   576
       7.5.1   Include the Statistician in the Research Team   576
       7.5.2   Begin from the Beginning.   577
       7.5.3   The Protocol is not a One-Man Show   577
       7.5.4   Meeting Mid-Way.   578
       7.5.5   Data Management   578
       7.5.6   Statistical Analysis.   579
       7.5.7   Publication.   579
   References.   579

List of Equations.   583

Index   609

List of Figures

Fig. 1.1   Frequency of classes of birth weight in 102 newly born
            babies presented in Table 1.2   5
Fig. 1.2   Frequency% of classes of birth weight in 102 newly
            born babies presented in Table 1.2   5
Fig. 1.3   Frequency polygon of classes of birth weight in 102
            newly born babies presented in Table 1.2   6
Fig. 1.4   Cumulative frequency% of classes of birth weight in
            102 newly born babies presented in Table 1.2   6
Fig. 1.5   Stem and leaf of classes of birth weight in 102 newly
            born babies presented in Table 1.2   7
Fig. 1.6   Box and Whisker plot of a series of 13 observations:
            1, 2, 3, 4, 5, 6, 7, 8, 9, 10, 11, 19, and 20   11
Fig. 1.7   Inverted bell-shaped (Gaussian–Laplace) curve of data
            presented in Table 1.2   12
Fig. 1.8   The standard normal distribution curve showing the
            proportions of values per Z score units   13
Fig. 1.9   The cumulative standardized normal distribution: gives
            the probability of a normal random variable (x) to have a
            standardized value that is smaller than Z. The
            probability for (x) to have a standardized value that is
            equal or larger than Z is calculated by subtracting 1 from
            the value given by the table   14
Fig. 1.10   The standardized normal distribution: gives the
            probability of a normal random variable (x) to have an
            absolute Z value that is smaller than the one given by the
            table. The probability of an equal or larger than Z is
            calculated by subtracting 0.5 from that given by the
            table   14
Fig. 1.11   The 95% interval of confidence (CI) of subjects (mean
            $\pm$ 1.96 Sd) is always larger than the 95% CI of mean
            (mean $\pm$ 1.96 Se). Calculated for data presented in
            Table 1.2   17
Fig. 1.12   Bilateral study design: the primary risk of error is
            equally split between the 2 examined possibilities, 2.5%
            on either side of the centralized 95% interval of
            confidence   20

Fig. 1.13 Unilateral study design: the whole primary risk of error (5%) is confined to the only studied side, shifting the 95% CI to the other side........................... 21

Fig. 1.14 Interpretation of the 95% CI of the bilateral superiority study and the unilateral efficacy study. The CI is statistically significant when it excludes the null......... 22

Fig. 1.15 Interpretation of the unilateral 95% CI of the non-inferiority (NIF) study The CI is statistically significant when it bypasses the null (0) and respects the lower limit of the NIF margin (Δ)............................. 23

Fig. 1.16 Interpretation of the bilateral 90% CI of the equivalence study. The CI is statistically significant when it bypasses the null (0) and respects both NIF margins ($-\Delta$ and $+\Delta$)...................................... 24

Fig. 1.17 The statistically significant bilateral 95% confidence interval (CI) of the superiority study, unilateral 95% CI of the non-inferiority (NIF) study and the bilateral 90% CI of the equivalence study 25

Fig. 1.18 Histogram of birth weight in 50 newly born baby boys showing normal distribution 26

Fig. 1.19 Histogram of birth weight in 52 newly born baby girls showing normal distribution 27

Fig. 1.20 Q–Q plot of birth weight in 50 newly born baby boys showing normal distribution 27

Fig. 1.21 Q–Q plot of birth weight in 52 newly born baby girls showing normal distribution 28

Fig. 1.22 Duration of ICU stay in days in 30 patients: the distribution is positively skewed (right-tailed distribution)....................................... 28

Fig. 1.23 Duration of pregnancy in mothers of 30 live births: the distribution is negatively skewed (left-tailed distribution)....................................... 29

Fig. 1.24 The limit of rejection (α) of a unilateral study design..... 32

Fig. 1.25 Unilateral study design: the relation between the primary risk of error (α) and P value: X1 and X2 are two given data points.............................. 32

Fig. 1.26 Unilateral study design comparing mean systolic blood pressure of patients receiving new antihypertensive treatment to those receiving placebo (control)........... 36

Fig. 1.27 Bilateral study design comparing mean systolic blood pressure of patients receiving new antihypertensive treatment to those receiving active comparator (control)... 37

Fig. 1.28 The relation between the odds and the risk (probability), according to Eq. (1.23)........................... 40

Fig. 1.29 The hazard of cure for patients presented in Table 1.5 ... 44

Fig. 1.30 Cumulative event-free rate (development of bronchial asthmatic attack) in 100 asthmatic patients followed up for ten years 47

Fig. 1.31   The mortality rate in Canadian population (2019) till the
            age of 59 years. Dots represent mortality rates calculated
            for subjects who died before 1 year of age, from
            1–4 years, then every 5 years till the age of 59 years   48
Fig. 1.32   The mortality rate in Canadian population (2019). Dots
            represent mortality rates calculated for subjects who
            died before 1 year of age, from 1 to 4 years, then every
            5 years till the age of 89 years. The last rate represents
            subjects who died at the age of 90 years or after   49
Fig. 1.33   A wishful distribution of health and disease   57
Fig. 1.34   A usual distribution of health and disease.   58
Fig. 1.35   The result of the diagnostic test in a diseased
            population   58
Fig. 1.36   The result of the diagnostic test in the healthy
            population   59
Fig. 1.37   Maximizing sensitivity by moving the cut-off point from
            point 0 towards point A   60
Fig. 1.38   Maximizing specificity by moving the cut-off point from
            point 0 towards point B   61
Fig. 1.39   The distribution of fasting blood sugar in diabetic
            patients and in normal controls. Data are presented
            in Table 1.10.   62
Fig. 1.40   The cumulative distribution of fasting blood sugar in
            diabetic patients and normal controls. FP = false positive
            results: with a cut-off point of 70 mg/dL, 43% (13/30) of
            non-diabetic subjects will be considered as being
            diabetics; FN = false negative: with a cut-off point of
            130 mg/dL, 26% (8/30) of diabetics will be considered
            as being non-diabetic   63
Fig. 1.41   The positive likelihood ratio: true positive/false positive . . .   67
Fig. 1.42   The negative likelihood ratio: false negative/true
            negative   68
Fig. 1.43   Post-test probabilities calculated by Fagan's nomograph
            in; (A) low prevalence population of and, (B) high
            prevalence population of 50%. Positive likelihood
            ratio = 16 and negative likelihood ratio = 0.2. A line
            departing from the pre-test probability on the left of the
            nomograph, passing through the likelihood ratio in the
            middle, lands on the post-test probability on the right
            side of the nomograph   69
Fig. 1.44   The relation between sensitivity (Sn), specificity (Sp)
            and (1 − Sp).   74
Fig. 1.45   Mini ROC plot of data presented in Table 1.14. The dots
            from the 1st to the 11th represent the 11 cut-off points
            figuring in Table 1.14, Sn = sensitivity, Sp = specificity,
            AUC—area under the curve (95% CI)   76
Fig. 1.46   The perfect and the useless ROC plot. A = the perfect
            plot, B = the useless plot, AUC = area under the curve . . .   77

Fig. 1.47   The ROC plot of data presented in Table 1.10 generated
            by SPSS statistical software package, AUC = area under
            the curve (95% CI) 77
Fig. 1.48   The partial AUC of a ROC plot (AUCp) for sensitivity
            $\leq 80\%$ 80
Fig. 1.49   The partial AUC of a ROC plot (AUCp) for sensitivity
            specificity between 80–100%. $AUCp_{min}$ is presented by
            the basal triangular light-shaded area below the
            tangential line of equivalence 81
Fig. 1.50   Youden index 82
Fig. 2.1   The normal versus Student distribution 115
Fig. 2.2   The association between two quantitative variables
            (x and y). Each point on the graph represents the paired
            x and y data 155
Fig. 2.3   Simple correlation: the trend line. Black circles represent
            corresponding 'x' and 'y' values. O–O′ represents the
            trend line that has to pass by the point (m_{xy}), which
            coordinates are the mean of variable (x) and the mean of
            variable (y). The line renders to a minimum the sum of
            squared deviations $[\sum (y - y')^2]$ of those black circles
            calculated parallel to the vertical 'oy' scale; $\sum$ = sum,
            y = individual values of y, y′ = mean value of y 156
Fig. 2.4   Correlation between the duration of surgery and the
            amount of blood loss in ten polytraumatized patients
            (see Table 2.25). Open circles represent paired (x,y)
            data. Dotted horizontal and vertical lines denote mean x
            (duration of surgery) and mean y (amount of blood loss
            in deciliters), respectively. Point m_{xy} = point of leverage
            of the covariance, with the coordinates: mean x, mean y
            (5, 6). Point x1y1 = point that varies from mean x by
            (x1 − mean x)/Sx and from mean y by (y1 − mean y)/
            Sy. Sx = standard deviation of (x), Sy = standard
            deviation of (y) 158
Fig. 2.5   Simple regression of the amount of blood loss (y) on the
            duration of surgery (x) in ten polytraumatized patients.
            Data presented in Table 2.25. P_0 = the slope that
            measures the effect of independent variable (x) on
            outcome (y) 163
Fig. 2.6   Model error under the null hypothesis. Open circles =
            observed amount of blood loss (y1, y2, y3, etc.), solid
            squares = expected amount of blood loss under the null
            hypothesis (mean y = my), E1, E2, E3, etc. = error under
            the null hypothesis = observed − expected values =
            (y1 − my), y2·my), (y3 − my) 166
Fig. 2.7   Model error under the alternative hypothesis. Open
            circles = observed amount of blood loss (y1, y2, y3, etc.),
            solid squares = expected amount of blood loss under the

alternative hypothesis (mean y = my), E1, E2, E3, etc. = error under the null hypothesis = observed − expected values = (y1 − my), y2·my), (y3 − my)................167

Fig. 2.8   Gain in error due to regression. Open circles = observed amount of blood loss (Y), solid square = expected amount of blood loss under the alternative hypothesis (Yfit), solid circle = expected amount of blood loss under the null hypothesis (Ym = mean Y). Error = error under the alternative hypothesis (Y − Yfit), Gain = gain in error due to regression (Yfit − Ym) 168

Fig. 2.9   Checking on independence and homoscedasticity of residuals 172

Fig. 2.10   Checking on normality of residuals. 173

Fig. 2.11   Kaplan–Meier intervals. Data is reported in Table 2.30. There were three intervals, each included between two vertical red lines. Numbers between brackets are the number of patients alive at the beginning of each interval. Vertical blue lines point to the participation times of the five patients. Red horizontal bars are the participation times of the two mortalities (patients II and IV). Blue horizontal bars are the participation times of the three censored cases (patients I, III, and V) 177

Fig. 2.12   Kaplan Meier curve for data reported in Table 2.30. n = numbers of patients living at the beginning of each interval. Rectangles represent censored cases; open circles represent mortalities. Cumulative survival is presented as mean ± standard error % 180

Fig. 2.13   Actuarial survival curve for data reported in Table 2.30. Open circles represent mortalities and "I" represent censored cases, li = number of patients living at the beginning of the interval............................. 183

Fig. 2.14   The Logrank test. Comparison of the survival after resection of lung mesothelioma with (Group A) or without adjuvant therapy (Group B). Data presented in Table 2.33. 187

Fig. 2.15   Unpaired bivariate statistical tests. a = expected values ≥ 5 in ≥ 80% of cells, b = two binomial qualitative variables, c = normal distribution and equality of variance, d = if causality is assumed................. 192

Fig. 2.16   Paired bivariate statistical tests. a = binomial qualitative variable, b = K-class qualitative variable, c = repeated binomial qualitative variable........................ 193

Fig. 2.17   Partial correlation between the duration of surgery and the amount of blood, controlling for the time to hospital transfer for data presented in Table 2.39............... 212

Fig. 2.18   Bland Altman plot of data presented in Table 2.50. 229

Fig. 2.19   Bland Altman plot of log data presented in Table 2.50 ... 231

Fig. 2.20   Line of best fit versus line of agreement for paired data
            acquired with mercury sphygmomanometer A and
            digital manometer C presented in Table 2.50 233
Fig. 2.21   Lin's concordance correlation coefficient of paired data
            presented in Table 2.50: mercury sphygmomanometers
            A and B 235
Fig. 2.22   Lin's concordance correlation coefficient of paired
            data presented in Table 2.9.11. Mercury
            sphygmomanometers A versus digital C 235
Fig. 3.1   One-way ANCOVA: testing linearity on each level
            of the grouping variable. Treatment A = dark circles
            and continuous line, treatment B = gray circles and
            interrupted line, controls = open circles and dotted line,
            R^2 = 0.669, 0.733, and 0.661 257
Fig. 3.2   One-way ANCOVA: testing homoscedasticity of error
            variances within each of the three categories of the
            predictor variable 258
Fig. 3.3   One-way ANCOVA: the analysis flowchart, a = In case
            of a statistically significant factor with >2-class 261
Fig. 3.4   Two-Way ANCOVA: effect of exercise on type of
            treatment received profile plot. Black circles represent
            patients on exercise and open circles represent patients
            not following exercise. 265
Fig. 3.5   Two-Way ANCOVA: effect of type of treatment
            received on exercise profile plot. Black circles represent
            patients treatment A, gray circles represent patients on
            treatment B and open circles represent controls 265
Fig. 3.6   Two-way ANCOVA flow chart. a = number of
            combinations: the product of the number of classes
            of the two categorical preditor variables, b = high
            leverage and enfluencial points, c = adjusted main
            effects can additionally be reported in presence of
            interaction with ordinal effect, d = reported for each
            class of the two categorical predictor variables 270
Fig. 3.7   One-way MANOVA: distribution of outcomes
            (post-treatment HbA1C and CRP) across the categories
            of predictor variable (types of treatment: A, B and
            controls) 273
Fig. 3.8   One-way MANOVA. Verifying linearity of two
            outcomes (Hb A1C and CRP) across the categories
            of one predictor (type of treatment) 274
Fig. 3.9   One-way MANOVA flowchart. a = Levene's test,
            b = Box M test, c = in case of a > 2-class independent
            variable. 278
Fig. 3.10   Two-way repeated measures ANOVA: estimated
            marginal means of time by treatment 282

Fig. 3.11   Two-way repeated measures ANOVA (RMANOVA)
             flowchart. Analysis flowchart. a = a minimum of 3
             repeated measures and 2 conditions or treatments,
             b = the number of combinations is the product of the
             number of repeatitions and the number of conditions,
             c = one-way repeated measures ANOVA (RMANOVA)
             to compare the repeated measures in each class of
             conditions or treatment variables, d = ANOVA or
             Student test to compare conditions or treatment
             variables for each repeated measure 285
Fig. 3.12   Two-way mixed ANOVA. Distribution of outcome
             (INR scores) across the grouping variable (high dose
             versus low-dose warfarin) circles represent outliers,
             numbers represent the order of the case in the list 288
Fig. 3.13   Two-way mixed ANOVA: estimated marginal means of
             three repeated INR measures in patients assigned to high
             dose and low dose warfarin 290
Fig. 3.14   Two-way mixed ANOVA flow chart, a = there is no
             remedy for the violation of this assumption, b = the df of
             F ratio has to be corrected accordingly, c = if the test is
             statistically significant, it is safer to make two separate
             one-way repeated measures ANOVA for each
             categorical predictor 293
Fig. 3.15   Multiple regression analysis: partial regression plot of
             duration of surgery on ICU stay 307
Fig. 3.16   Multiple regression analysis: partial regression plot
             of the amount of blood loss on ICU stay 308
Fig. 3.17   Multiple regression analysis: regression plot of
             unstandardized predictive values on the studentized
             residuals 308
Fig. 3.18   Multiple regression analysis: Histogram with
             superimposed normal curve. 310
Fig. 3.19   Multiple regression analysis: P-P plot 311
Fig. 3.20   Multiple regression analysis flow chart. a = Durbin-
             Watson test, b = individual and collective linearity,
             c = in case of heteroschedacity robust standard error
             regression coefficients are calculated, d = outliers, high
             leverage and influential points. 314
Fig. 3.21   Logistic regression: S-shaped correlation between the
             proportion of myocardial infarction (MI) and the level of
             biomarker of ischemia. 316
Fig. 3.22   Logistic regression analysis: linear correlation between
             the Logit of the proportion of myocardial infarction (MI)
             and the level of biomarker ischemia 317
Fig. 3.23   Logistic regression analysis: transforming the binomial
             values into log odds. Open circles = observed data,
             closed circles = transformed data 317

Fig. 3.24   Logistic regression analysis: projecting the transformed
            log odds values on the logistic curve 319
Fig. 3.25   Logistic regression analysis: the worst fitting line. Open
            circles = observed data, closed circles = data projected
            on the worst fitting line. 321
Fig. 3.26   Logistic regression analysis flowchart. H–L test =
            Hosmer–Lemeshow test 328
Fig. 3.27   Cox regression analysis: the hazard rate and the
            cumulative survival. 330
Fig. 3.28   Cox regression analysis: the Kaplan Meier curves 334
Fig. 3.29   Cox regression analysis flow chart, a = secular trends
            should be maintained (avoided) throughout the analysis . . . 337
Fig. 4.1   The null and the alternative hypothesis of a bilateral
            study. 345
Fig. 4.2   A bilateral study: $\alpha = 5\%$ and 80% power: $Z_{(1 - \alpha /2)} +$
            $Z_{(1 - B)} = 1.96 + 0.84 = 2.8$ 347
Fig. 4.3   Central and non-central F distributions 348
Fig. 4.4   The non-centrality parameter (λ). 349
Fig. 6.1   Flow chart of meta-analysis. a = combines odds ratio,
            risk ratio and risk difference; b = combines odds ratio
            only, preferred with uncommon events observed in
            small equal group 445
Fig. 6.2   Forest plot of meta-analysis I: fixed effect model. ES =
            effect size; n = sample size; Se^2 = variance; W =
            weighting method for effect size = $1/Se^2$; WES =
            weighted effect size = Wx ES; M_{meta} = mean ES of the
            meta-analysis; ΣWES = sum of weighted ES,
            ΣW = sum of weights; Se^2_{meta} = variance of the
            meta-analysis. 454
Fig. 6.3   Forest plot of meta-analysis II: fixed effect model.
            ES = effect size; n = sample size; Se^2 = variance;
            W = weighting method for effect size = $1/Se^2$; WES =
            weighted effect size = Wx ES; M_{meta} = mean ES of the
            meta-analysis; ΣWES = sum of weighted ES,
            ΣW = sum of weights; Se^2_{meta} = variance of the
            meta-analysis. 454
Fig. 6.4   Forest plot of meta-analysis III: fixed effect model. ES =
            effect size; n = sample size; Se^2 = variance; W =
            weighting method for effect size = $1/Se^2$; WES =
            weighted effect size = Wx ES; M_{meta} = mean ES
            of the meta-analysis; ΣWES = sum of weighted ES,
            ΣW = sum of weights; Se^2_{meta} = variance of the
            meta-analysis. 455
Fig. 6.5   Forest plot of meta-analysis III (random-effect model).
            ES = effect size; n = sample size; T^2 = between-study
            variance, Se^2 = within-study variance; W = weighing
            method for effect size = $1/(T^2 + Se^2)$; WES = weighted
            effect size = Wx ES; M_{meta} = mean ES of the meta-

analysis; ΣWES = sum of weighed ES, ΣW = sum of weights, $(Se^2_{meta} + T^2)$ = variance of the meta-analysis ... 456

Fig. 6.6   Forest plot: Pearson's correlation coefficient relating the amount of blood loss and the duration of hospital stay, fixed effect model (FE). Values (95% CI) are presented as normalized Fisher's values. Q = 28.48, df = 4, P < 0.001, I^2 = 85.96%. 461

Fig. 6.7   Forest plot: Pearson's correlation coefficient between the amount of blood loss and the duration of hospital stay, random effect model (RE). Values and 95% CI are presented as normalized Fisher's values. Q = 28.48, df = 4, P < 0.001, I^2 = 85.96%. 462

Fig. 6.8   Forest plot: the row mean difference of hospital stays (95% CI), fixed effect model (FE) Q = 308.7, df = 5, P < 0.001, I^2 = 98.38%. 465

Fig. 6.9   Forest plot: the row mean difference of hospital stay (95% CI), random effect model (RE). Q = 308.7, df = 5, P < 0.001, T^2 = 3.37. I^2 = 98.38% 466

Fig. 6.10   Forest plot: the relative risk of BCG vaccine, fixed effect model (FE). Values (95% CI) are presented in the logarithmic scale, Q = 152.2, df = 12, P < 0.001, I^2 = 92.12% 474

Fig. 6.11   Forest plot: the relative risk of BCG vaccine, random effect model (RE). Values (95% CI) are presented in the logarithmic scale, Q = 152.2, df = 12, P < 0.001, I^2 = 92.12 476

Fig. 6.12   Forest plot: the relative risk of BCG vaccine, subgroup analysis, fixed effect model (FE). Values are presented as relative risk (95% CI). The average relative risk, I^2%, and Q-test P value are calculated independently and presented for each subgroup. 489

Fig. 6.13   Forest plot: the relative risk of BCG vaccine, subgroup analysis, random effect model (RE). Values are presented as relative risk (95% CI). The average relative risk, I^2%, and Q-test P value are calculated independently and presented for each subgroup 494

Fig. 6.14   Meta regression: regressing log relative risk on latitude, fixed effect model 501

Fig. 6.15   Meta regression: regressing log relative risk on latitude, random effects model 502

Fig. 6.16   Funnel plot: **a** the method of precision is sample size, **b** the method of precision is the standard error. 506

Fig. 6.17   Trimming an asymmetrical funnel plot 507

Fig. 6.18   Filling an asymmetrical funnel plot. 508

Fig. 6.19   Egger test: analysis of small-study effects: **a)** the case of a symmetrical funnel plot, **b)** the case of an asymmetrical funnel plot. The thick vertical bar on the y-axis of **(b)** represents the intercept (b_0). 510

Fig. 6.20   Funnel plot: the efficacy of BCG vaccine in preventing
             new cases of tuberculosis, fixed effect model 511
Fig. 6.21   Funnel plot: the efficacy of the BCG vaccine in
             preventing new cases of tuberculosis, random-effects
             model 512
Fig. 6.22   Forrest plot: cumulative meta-analysis. Values
             are presented as relative risk (95% CI) 513
Fig. 6.23   Forest plot: leave one meta-analysis. Values
             are presented as relative risk (95% CI) 514
Fig. 7.1   Variables classified in the increasing natural order
             of expected variability. 529
Fig. 7.2   Sample size calculation: predicting the 95%CI
             of the difference of a future study 534

List of Tables

Table 1.1   Variable conversion: ordinal to quantitative:
            conversion of NYHA functional classes into NYHA
            score.   3
Table 1.2   Distribution of birth weight of 102 newly born babies. . .   4
Table 1.3   Part of SPSS output for skewness and kurtosis
            calculated for different samples   30
Table 1.4   Calculation of the risk and the odds in the treatment
            and the control groups   40
Table 1.5   Relation between the presence of a history of
            rheumatic fever and the development of mitral valve
            stenosis in 100 patients.   41
Table 1.6   The hazard of cure in 200 patients equally randomized
            between treatment and placebo and followed up
            for 5 years period.   44
Table 1.7   The baseline hazard in Cox regression in 200 patients
            equally randomized between treatment and control and
            followed up for three years.   45
Table 1.8   Sudden death after three years in patients with either
            moderate or severe aortic stenosis   50
Table 1.9   Sensitivity versus specificity.   58
Table 1.10 Fasting blood sugar levels in 30 diabetic patients
            and 30 normal controls.   61
Table 1.11 Positive versus negative predictive values   64
Table 1.12 Role of Prevalence in predictive values: comparing
            two sphygmomanometers.   65
Table 1.13 Calculation of post-test probabilities.   68
Table 1.14 Sensitivity and specificity thresholds in a mini-ROC
            plot.   74
Table 2.1   The distribution of hypertension between genders   92
Table 2.2   Chi-Square test goodness of fit: gender distribution
            among 100 newly born babies   97
Table 2.3   Chi-square test of independence: the distribution of
            prosthetic cardiac valve complications among patients
            receiving 3 anticoagulation regimens 100

Table 2.4   Chi-square test of independence: the occurrence of
             complications in patients following antiplatelets B and
             combined therapy C. Data extracted from Table 2.3 101
Table 2.5   Corrected Chi-square test (Yates): the comparison of
             success rates between two prophylactic antibiotic
             regimens. 103
Table 2.6   Chi-square test for trend: the effect of the level of
             hypertension on the occurrence of cerebrovascular
             complications 104
Table 2.7   Chi-square test for trend: calculation of data presented
             in Table 2.6 105
Table 2.8   Fisher's exact test: observed cerebrovascular stroke
             with mono versus dual antiplatelet therapy in high-risk
             patients. 107
Table 2.9   Fisher's exact test: a general contingency two-by-two
             table 107
Table 2.10   Fisher's exact test: expected sets of frequencies
             keeping marginal values of data presented
             in Table 2.8 107
Table 2.11   McNemar-Bowker test: change of the patients'
             symptoms with treatment 110
Table 2.12   Cochran Q test: repeated measurements of depression . . . 112
Table 2.13   Post-hoc analysis of data presented in Table 2.12:
             repeated McNemar's tests. 113
Table 2.14   The unpaired Student's test: extract of IBM-SPSS
             output comparing the fasting blood sugar in two
             groups of patients receiving different oral
             hypoglycemic 120
Table 2.15   Calculation of the paired Student's test 122
Table 2.16   Calculation of the unpaired Student's test. Data
             extracted from Table 2.15 122
Table 2.17   How does ANOVA works? 126
Table 2.18   One-way ANOVA comparing fasting blood sugar
             levels among patients with cirrhosis with and without
             hepatocellular carcinoma and normal controls 129
Table 2.19   A priori contrasts of fasting blood sugar levels among
             patients with cirrhosis with and without hepatocellular
             carcinoma and normal controls. 132
Table 2.20   Post-hoc analysis of fasting blood sugar levels among
             patients with cirrhosis with and without hepatocellular
             carcinoma and normal controls. 133
Table 2.21   Repeated measures ANOVA: repeated dosing of
             warfarin in ten patients presenting with deep vein
             thrombosis (DVT) 139
Table 2.22   Repeated measures ANOVA for data presented in
             Table 2.21: results of correlation and post-hoc student
             tests 142

Table 2.23   Wilcoxon sign rank test: comparison of the durations of pain relief with two analgesics (A and B) in a single group of 10 patients with chronic pain 149

Table 2.24   Friedman's test: repeated measurement of diastolic blood pressure on three occasions 152

Table 2.25   Correlation between the duration of surgery and the total amount of blood loss in ten poly traumatized patients 157

Table 2.26   Spearman's rank test: correlation between duration of surgery and total amount of blood loss in ten poly traumatized patients 161

Table 2.27   Calculation of predicted (y_{fit}) and error sum of squares (SSE) of data presented in Table 2.25 166

Table 2.28   Simple regression: model fit. 168

Table 2.29   Simple regression. Effect of switching predictor and outcome on model coefficients 170

Table 2.30   Survival data of five patients undergoing surgery for mesothelioma 176

Table 2.31   Kaplan Meier analysis of data reported in Table 2.30 . . . 181

Table 2.32   Actuarial analysis of data presented in Table 2.30 182

Table 2.33   Comparison of overall survival after resection of pleural mesothelioma 184

Table 2.34   The Logrank test: comparison of overall survival after resection of pleural mesothelioma 185

Table 2.35   Choosing the appropriate bivariate statistical test (independent groups) 192

Table 2.36   Comparison of the effect of 2 arterial vasodilators (a and b) in patients with intermittent claudication with adjustment on the presence or absence of diabetes mellitus: exclusion of qualitative interaction. 198

Table 2.37   Cochran–Mantel–Haenszel test: Comparison of success of 2 arterial vasodilators in patients with intermittent claudication with adjustment on the presence or absence of diabetes mellitus 201

Table 2.38   Two-Way ANOVA: comparing the effects of two antihypertensive regimens among three hospitals 204

Table 2.39   Partial correlation: correlation between the duration of surgery, the total amount of blood loss and the delay in hospital transfer in ten poly traumatized patients 210

Table 2.40   Accuracy versus precision 214

Table 2.41   Measuring agreement: plan of the analysis. 217

Table 2.42   Cohen Kappa: Measuring agreement between multislice CT (MSCT) and coronary angiography (CA) in patients with in-stent restenosis (ISR) 219

Table 2.43   Role of prevalence and bias between raters in Kappa. Data presented in Table 2.42 220

Table 2.44   Calculation of Kappa Max (K_{max}). Data presented in Table 2.42 221

Table 2.45   Unweighted kappa: 2 clinicians judging on a 3-class
                   categorical variable. 222
Table 2.46   Weighted kappa: 2 clinicians judging on a 3-class
                   categorical variable. 223
Table 2.47   Fleiss Kappa: Measuring agreement between three
                   cardiologists on the best way to manage ten patients
                   with ischemic heart disease: medical therapy,
                   percutaneous angioplasty or surgery. 225
Table 2.48   Fleiss Kappa: SPSS input for data presented in
                   Table 2.47 226
Table 2.49   Extract of SPSS output of overall Fleiss Kappa and
                   Kappa for individual categories of data presented in
                   Table 2.48 227
Table 2.50   Paired measurements of systolic blood pressure in 15
                   patients using two mercury sphygmomanometers A
                   and B and a digital manometer C. 230
Table 2.51   Intraclass correlation coefficient (ICC) models 237
Table 2.52   ANOVA comparing the measurement of blood
                   pressure acquired by two mercury
                   sphygmomanometers in 15 patients. Data presented in
                   Table 2.50 239
Table 2.53   ANOVA comparing the measurement of blood
                   pressure acquired by two mercury
                   sphygmomanometers and a digital manometer in 15
                   patients. Data presented in Table 2.50 240
Table 2.54   Perfect agreement versus total disagreement: a
                   working example 241
Table 2.55   Kendall W test. The results of five raters ranking ten
                   manuscripts 242
Table 3.1   One-Way ANOVA: comparison of the duration of
                   pain relief in hours in two-independent groups of
                   patients receiving different analgesics A and B 250
Table 3.2   One-way ANOVA table: analysis of data presented in
                   Table 3.1 250
Table 3.3   Two-Way ANOVA: comparison of the duration of
                   pain relief in hours per type of analgesic and per
                   gender 251
Table 3.4   Two-way ANOVA table: analysis of data presented in
                   Table 3.3 251
Table 3.5   Two-way ANOVA: comparison of the effects of two
                   antihypertensive regimens in two hospitals. 252
Table 3.6   Two-way ANOVA: analysis of data presented in 2.38
                   and Table 3.5. 253
Table 3.7   One-way ANCOVA: Hb A1C pre-treatment and post-
                   treatment values in three groups of patients receiving
                   treatment A, treatment B or control 255
Table 3.8   One-way ANCOVA: testing interaction between
                   independent variable and covariance 257

Table 3.9   One-way ANOVA: testing group effect 259
Table 3.10   One-way ANCOVA: testing adjusted group effect 259
Table 3.11   One-way ANCOVA: non-adjusted and adjusted means
             of post-treatment Hb A1C 260
Table 3.12   One-way ANCOVA: post hoc-analysis with
             Bonferroni correction 260
Table 3.13   Two-way ANCOVA: testing between-subjects effect   . . . 263
Table 3.14   Two-way ANCOVA: testing adjusted effects 263
Table 3.15   Two-way ANCOVA: non-adjusted and adjusted
             means of post-treatment Hb A1C for factor treatment . . . 267
Table 3.16   Two-way ANCOVA: post hoc-analysis of adjusted
             factor treatment with Bonferroni correction 268
Table 3.17   Two-way ANCOVA: non-adjusted and adjusted
             means of post-treatment Hb A1C for factor exercise 268
Table 3.18   Two-way ANCOVA: estimated adjusted means
             according to treatment and exercise 269
Table 3.19   Two-way ANCOVA: post hoc-analysis of simple
             adjusted effect of factor treatment with Bonferroni
             correction 269
Table 3.20   One-way MANOVA: means of post-treatment
             Hb A1C and CRP for factor treatment 276
Table 3.21   One-way MANOVA: tests of between-subjects
             effects 277
Table 3.22   One-way MANOVA: post hoc-analysis of effect
             treatment on post-treatment Hb A1C and CRP scores
             with Bonferroni correction 277
Table 3.23   Two-way repeated measures ANOVA: the effect
             of low versus high dose warfarin on repeated INR
             measures. 280
Table 3.24   Two-way repeated measures ANOVA: the within-
             subjects effects 283
Table 3.25   Two-way repeated measures ANOVA: estimated
             marginal means of treatment, time and interaction
             of treatment and time 283
Table 3.26   Two-way repeated measures ANOVA: post hoc-
             analysis of effect time with Bonferroni correction
             and paired student test comparing the two levels
             of factor treatment 284
Table 3.27   Two-way mixed ANOVA: repeated INR
             measurements in 30 patients following either low dose
             or high dose warfarin therapy. 287
Table 3.28   Two-way mixed ANOVA: the within-subjects' effects. . . 290
Table 3.29   Two-way mixed ANOVA: estimated means of INR
             and post-hoc analysis with Bonferroni correction 291
Table 3.30   Two-way mixed ANOVA: the between-subjects main
             effect (warfarin dose) 291
Table 3.31   Two-way mixed ANOVA: simple effects of
             within-subject variable 292

Table 3.32   Two-waymixed ANOVA: estimated marginal means
             of INR 292
Table 3.33   Two-way mixed ANOVA: post hoc-analysis of effect
             INR (time) with Bonferroni correction 293
Table 3.34   Common multivariable models. 296
Table 3.35   Outcome of surgery in 60 polytraumatized patients 304
Table 3.36   Multiple regression analysis: results of bivariate
             analysis of the duration of ICU stay in 60
             polytraumatized patients. 306
Table 3.37   Multiple regression analysis: regular versus robust
             standard errors of regression coefficients 309
Table 3.38   Multiple regression analysis: model summary 312
Table 3.39   Multiple regression analysis: ANOVA 312
Table 3.40   Logistic regression analysis: the proportion
             of myocardial infarction (MI), according to the level
             of biomarker of ischemia 316
Table 3.41   Logistic regression analysis: transformation
             of probability (P) into Odds and Logit P 318
Table 3.42   Logisticregression analysis withone discrete predictor . . . 322
Table 3.43   Logistic regression analysis: results of bivariate
             analysis of mortality in 60 polytraumatized patients. 324
Table 3.44   Logistic regression analysis: the coefficients of
             regression. 327
Table 3.45   Logistic regression analysis: the classification tables 327
Table 3.46   Cox proportional regression analysis: the coefficients
             of regression. 336
Table 4.1   Sample size calculation: testing the independence
             between gender and the degree of hypertension 363
Table 4.2   Sample size calculation: the cumulative odds ratio. 364
Table 4.3   Sample size calculation: pain relief following three
             analgesics (one-way ANOVA) 373
Table 4.4   Sample size calculation: comparing sensitivity
             (paired design) 408
Table 4.5   Sample size calculation: Cohen Kappa. 411
Table 5.1   Randomization table (9 elements). 426
Table 6.1   From randomized controlled trials to meta-analysis 442
Table 6.2   The power of meta-analysis: a mini-example 452
Table 6.3   Pearson's correlation coefficient: the duration
             of surgery and the amount of blood loss, fixed effect
             model. 460
Table 6.4   Pearson's correlation coefficient: the duration
             of surgery and the amount of blood loss random effects
             model. 461
Table 6.5   The row mean difference between the durations
             of hospital stay following minimally invasive and
             conventional open-heart surgery, fixed effect model. 463

Table 6.6   The row mean difference between the durations
             of hospital stay following minimally invasive and
             conventional open-heart surgery, random effects
             model 465
Table 6.7   Calculation of the risk and the odds 469
Table 6.8   The relative risk: evaluation of the efficacy of the BCG
             vaccine 471
Table 6.9   The relative risk: evaluation of the efficacy of the BCG
             vaccine, analysis of a fixed effect model 472
Table 6.10   The relative risk: evaluation of the efficacy of the BCG
             vaccine, analysis of a random effects model 475
Table 6.11   The relative risk: evaluation of the efficacy of the BCG
             vaccine, subgroup analysis, fixed effect model 487
Table 6.12   The relative risk: evaluation of the efficacy of the BCG
             vaccine, results of subgroup analysis, fixed effect
             model 488
Table 6.13   The relative risk: evaluation of the efficacy of the BCG
             vaccine, analysis of heterogeneity among subgroups,
             fixed effect model 491
Table 6.14   The relative risk: evaluation of the efficacy of the BCG
             vaccine, subgroup analysis, random effects model,
             assuming separate T^2 492
Table 6.15   The relative risk: evaluation of the efficacy of the BCG
             vaccine, results of subgroup analysis, random effects
             model, assuming separate T^2 493
Table 6.16   The relative risk: evaluation of the efficacy of the BCG
             vaccine, analysis of heterogeneity among subgroups,
             random effects model, assuming separate T^2 495
Table 6.17   The relative risk: evaluation of the efficacy of the BCG
             vaccine, subgroup analysis, random effects model,
             assuming pooled T^2 497
Table 6.18   The relative risk: evaluation of the efficacy of the BCG
             vaccine, results of subgroup analysis, random effects
             model, assuming pooled T^2 497
Table 6.19   The relative risk: evaluation of the efficacy of the BCG
             vaccine, meta regression analysis of a fixed effect
             model 500
Table 6.20   The relative risk: evaluation of the efficacy of the BCG
             vaccine, meta regression analysis of a random effects
             model 501
Table 7.1   Sample size calculation. Evaluation of the role of
             statins in cardiomyopathy 530
Table 7.2   Chi-square test of independence: the comparison
             of the rates of oral anticoagulants-related
             complications in patients following three
             anticoagulation regimens: the input study 538

Table 7.3   Chi-square test of independence: the comparison
            of the rates of oral anticoagulants-related
            complications in patients following three
            anticoagulation regimens: the output study............ 538
Table 7.4   Testing the efficacy of antiplatelet therapy in
            hypertensive patients: subgroup analysis 564

Abstract

Variability is the fundamental rule of biology, and there is no exception up to our knowledge. In order to diagnose and treat our patients, we have to quantify, express, and analyze their variabilities. This chapter outlines variables, distributions, and summaries, emphasizing the most commonly encountered "normal" distribution. We tried to explain in simple but correct terms: the primary and secondary risks of error, study power, basis of testing hypothesis, and P-value. We discussed the meaning, calculations, indications, adequate reporting, and interpretation of the commonly used outcomes indices of clinical studies and standard measurements of diagnostic accuracy. We discussed the odds ratio (OR), relative risk, relative risk increase and reduction, absolute risk increase and reduction, the number needed to treat benefit and harm, and the hazard ratio. Diagnostic measures included the sensitivity, specificity, positive and negative predictive values, likelihood ratios, the area under the ROC curve, the Youden index, and the diagnostic odds ratio. The chapter includes simplified equations, demonstrative examples calculated by hand, and links to online calculators and statistical software.

1.1 Introduction

Life is all about variability. We do not all look the same nor act precisely the same, even under similar conditions. On the individual level, all our biological variables such as our physical signs, hormonal levels and biochemical markers are in a continuous dynamic change. Because of such variability, not everyone who smoked will get lung cancer, and nonsmokers are not immune to the disease. *The disease remains a probability as long as the risk factors do not reflect the entire collection of reasons necessary for its development.* It becomes difficult to analyze and understand those random events and manage our patients systematically and adequately without counting, classifying and analyzing those factors; i.e., without statistics.

We, doctors, do not have the same experience, intelligence, or luck to diagnose and manage our patients equivalently. Statistics permit us to classify, quantify, and evaluate our experiences with an acceptable risk of error. It allows us to express medical information by clinically relevant numerical indices, reflecting the status and progress of our patients. Finally, it allows us to compare our results on a joint scientific background and evaluate and refine patient management. Put it this way, after a sound clinical

© The Author(s), under exclusive license to Springer Nature Switzerland AG 2023
A. Hassouna, *Statistics for Clinicians*,
https://doi.org/10.1007/978-3-031-20758-7_1

relevance, statistics is the valuable tool to assess and improve the three essential elements of our profession; experience, intelligence, and luck.

1.2   Variables: Types, Measurement and Role

Variables are anything we can measure, control, or manipulate in research. They differ in many respects, most notably in the role we give them in the study and the measures they can serve. Concerning roles, we usually as-sign subjects to "groups" based on some pre-existing properties, such as patients receiving treatment versus controls, diabetics versus non-diabetics. For example, if we want to investigate whether the development of wound infection after surgery depends on the patient having diabetes or not, "wound infection" becomes *the dependent variable* because its occurrence will depend upon the presence or absence of diabetes. By deduction, "diabetes" is *the independent variable* because being diabetic is independent of (not caused by) having wound infection. In this context, we usually design clinical studies to investigate whether measured outcomes (disease, morbidity, complications, cure, etc.) depend on the presence of risk factors, type of treatment, the method of investigation, or any other independent variable suspected to influence outcomes.

Concerning measurement, variables are generally *qualitative* (hair color, sex, smoker or not, class I, II, III or IV, etc.) or *quantitative* (height, blood pressure, length of hospital stay, etc.). A more specific classification that depends upon the amount of information the measurement scale provides is to classify variables into nominal, ordinal, interval, and ratio variables. While *nominal* variables allow for only qualitative classification such as hypertensive and normotensive, *ordinal* variables rank the qualitative item in terms of which has less and which has more of the quality, such as mild, moderate, and severe hypertension. Typical examples include rating or measurements scales, such as the Glasgow coma scale, Apgar scale, visual analog scale. The difference between *ratio* and *interval*

variables is the point of origin, which is the absolute zero in the former. In the latter, the point of origin is arbitrary, like temperature, as measured in degrees Fahrenheit or Celsius. Most of our quantitative clinical outcomes are ratio variables, and statistical data analysis procedures rarely distinguish between the interval and ratio properties. We practically analyze variables as being nominal, ordinal, or quantitative.

1.2.1   Variable Conversion

Variable conversion is a standard everyday procedure. We consider one person punctual depending on the number of times he was on schedule, and being reliable depends on the number of times he kept his promise. Changing the quantitative variable (number of times) into a qualitative variable (being punctual, being dependable, or not) is necessary for us to decide; whether to accept the person or how to deal with him? Variable conversion applies to all biology. However, unlike in daily life, where those decisions may sometimes be personal, scientific decisions have to have clear evidence-based rules. For example, a person is considered hypertensive (qualitative variable) when his diastolic blood pressure is above 90 mm Hg (quantitative variable), measured on well-defined occasions. The same applies to describing many qualitative variables, such as diabetes, obesity, and dyslipidemia. Most of our qualitative outcomes are just cut-off points made in a quantitative variable. *Categorization is essential to reach conclusions on whether to treat or not, adopt a management strategy.*

On the other hand, *a significant disadvantage of categorizing numerical data is the loss of information.* For example, a person with a diastolic blood pressure of 89 mm Hg will be considered normotensive. Another patient with higher diastolic blood pressure by 1 mm Hg will be considered hypertensive and treated. Playing the same tune, a patient whose diastolic blood pressure is just 90 mm Hg is viewed as being "as diseased as" someone whose diastolic blood pressure is as high as 120 mm Hg. Breaking down categories into mild, moderate, and severe hypertension will only solve part of the problem. There will still be more or less significant differences between patients in the same subcategory.

On the contrary, *we can achieve better presentation and improve the analysis by converting an ordinal qualitative variable into a quantitative one.* For example, NYHA functional classification (class I, II, III, and IV) is an index of ascending severity of heart disease; patients in class IV are more ill than those in class III, who are sicker than those in class II and so on. However, how much more suffering, ordinal categories cannot tell? Replacing the ranked I, II, III, and IV classes by the respective numbers 1, 2, 3, and 4 needs the approval of the medical community because it will assume that a class II is precisely twice as ill as a patient in class I and so on. Table 1.1 shows the preoperative and postoperative NYHA class of 100 patients in ranking order (columns 1 and 2) then when transformed into numerical values (columns 3 and 4). As shown, the numerical transformation of the ordinal variable gave a straightforward message: patients have improved by about one NYHA class on average (from a mean class of 3.02 to a mean class of 2), which will be hard to visualize from the ranking order in columns 1 and 2. Another advantage is to calculate a standard deviation and standard error (see Sect. 1.3.4), create a 95% confidence interval (see Sect. 1.4.2), and use the "more powerful" parametric tests to assess patients' improvement (See Sect. 2.1.2).

Conversion of a qualitative variable into a score can facilitate data presentation and empower statistical analysis. Transformation of the quantitative variable into distinct categories can help compare clinically distinctive groups and make final decisions but may decrease the study power (see Sect. 1.4).

1.3 Summarizing Data

We need to summarize our data in order to have a "global picture" of collected information, to communicate with each other and with our patients, to analyze results using statistical tests that usually compare those summaries and to take "decisions" about health problems whether in the local (hospital) or general (national) community. Qualitative data are usually summarized as *numbers and percentages*. As example, if in a group of 20 persons we have 4 females and 16 males; the variable "gender" can be simply expressed as: [female gender = 4 (20%)]. This number and (%) combination give all information about gender distribution in the group: we have 4 females who constitute 20% of the total group and by deduction, the number of males will be equal to 16, constituting 80% of the group and, the total number of patients equals 20.

Numbers can be referred to as *frequencies* and hence, percentages can be referred to *relative*

Table 1.1 Variable conversion: ordinal to quantitative: conversion of NYHA functional classes into NYHA score

NYHA class	1—Preoperative class (n = 100)	2—Postoperative class (n = 100)	3—Preoperative score	4—Postoperative score
I	9 (9%)	40 (40%)	$9 \times 1 = 9$	$40 \times 1 = 40$
II	17 (17%)	29 (29%)	$17 \times 2 = 34$	$29 \times 2 = 58$
III	35 (35%)	22 (22%)	$35 \times 3 = 105$	$22 \times 3 = 66$
IV	39 (39%)	9 (9%)	$39 \times 4 = 156$	$9 \times 4 = 36$
Mean	–	–	3.04	2

NYHA class = New York Heart Association functional classification, n = number of patients

Table 1.2 Distribution of birth weight of 102 newly born babies

Birth weight class range[a]	Birth weight class center[a]	Frequency[b]	Relative frequency (%)	Cumulative relative frequency (%)
2000–2200	2100	4	3.9	3.9
2200–2400	2300	5	4.9	8.8
2400–2600	2500	4	3.9	12.7
2600–2800	2700	6	5.9	18.6
2800–3000	2900	12	11.8	30.4
3000–3200	3100	17	16.7	47.1
3200–3400	3300	19	18.6	65.7
3400–3600	3500	15	14.7	80.4
3600–3800	3700	6	5.9	86.3
3800–4000	3900	5	4.9	91.2
4000–4200	4100	4	3.9	95.1
4200–4400	4300	3	2.9	98
4400–4600	4500	2	1.96	100
Total	–	102	100	

[a] = birth weights in g, [b] = number of children

frequencies; which can be either presented in decimals (relative frequency of females = 0.2) or as a percent as shown above (relative frequency of females% = 20%). Quantitate data are usually presented as *mean and standard deviation or median and range*, depending on whether data is following a normal distribution or else. Table 1.2 shows the result of a study performed to analyze the distribution of birth weight in 102 normal babies, as being observed in a local maternity hospital. The results will be used to explain those summary statistics.

1.3.1 The Qualitative Variable

Continuous variables are usually categorized for descriptive purposes, to take decision or to reach a conclusion. As shown in Table 1.2, birth weight was divided into intervals (classes) of 200 g and the resulting 13 classes were tabulated in an ascending ordered category: 2000–2200, 2200–2400, 2400–2600, etc. The first class (2000–2200) included four patients (*frequency*) who represent 4/102 = 0.039 or 3.9% of the total group (*relative frequency = frequency%*). The

second class included 5 patients who represented 5/102 = 0.049 or 4.9% of the total group. In order not to count a patient twice, the upper limit of an interval is usually counted with the next interval; i.e., a baby whose birth weight is 2200 g is counted in the second interval (2200–2400) and not the first.

The *cumulative frequency* is the sum of actual and all previous frequencies, i.e., the cumulative frequency of the second interval = 4 + 5 = 9 patients. The relative cumulative frequency (cumulative frequency%) equals the cumulative frequency/total = 9/102 = 0.088 or 8.8%, in our example. The *cumulative frequency%* is the percent of cases at and below a certain limit, which can be helpful to take cut-offs values decision making. Those measurements are, of course, dependent upon the starting point (2000 g) and class limits (200 g), and hence, both are usually based upon clinical relevance and clear judgment. Frequency (Fig. 1.1) and frequency% (Fig. 1.2) are typically plotted on the y axis, with classes being presented as columns plotted on the x-axis.

We can remove the columns and still present frequency by a polygon running over the tips

Fig. 1.1 Frequency of classes of birth weight in 102 newly born babies presented in Table 1.2

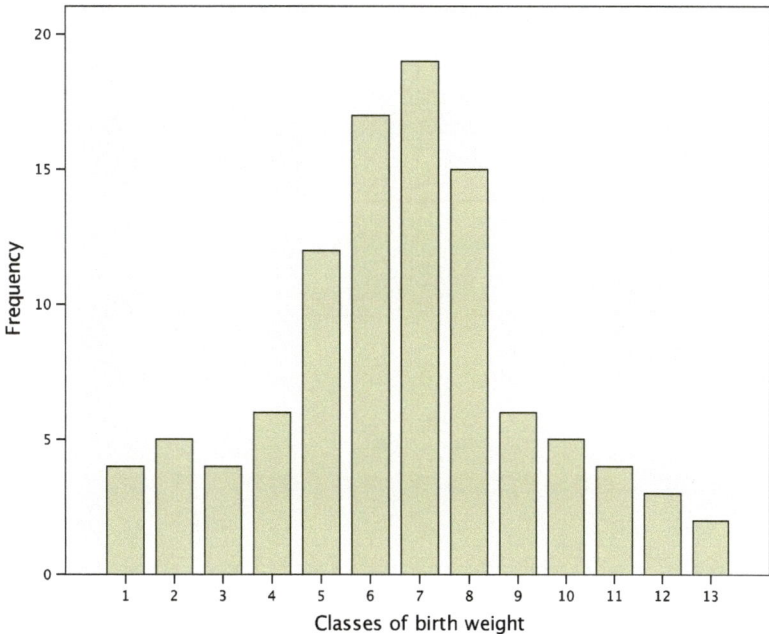

Fig. 1.2 Frequency% of classes of birth weight in 102 newly born babies presented in Table 1.2

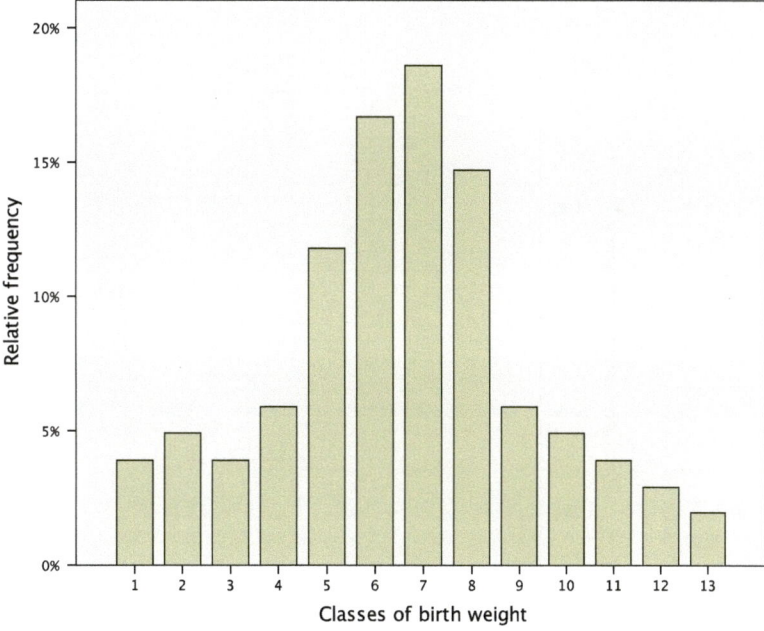

(center) of classes (Fig. 1.3) and cumulative frequency% as a sharp staircase or smooth (dotted) line (Fig. 1.4). In a stem and leaf plot, the numbers themselves replace the columns, where the stem is the first digit of the birth weight and the leaf the trailing digits. The first raw represents the respective birth weights 2090, 2190, 2200, 2300, 2300, 2350, 2400, and 2400 g, having in common the first digit (2) (Fig. 1.5). In addition to the graphic presentation n, a stem and leaf plot

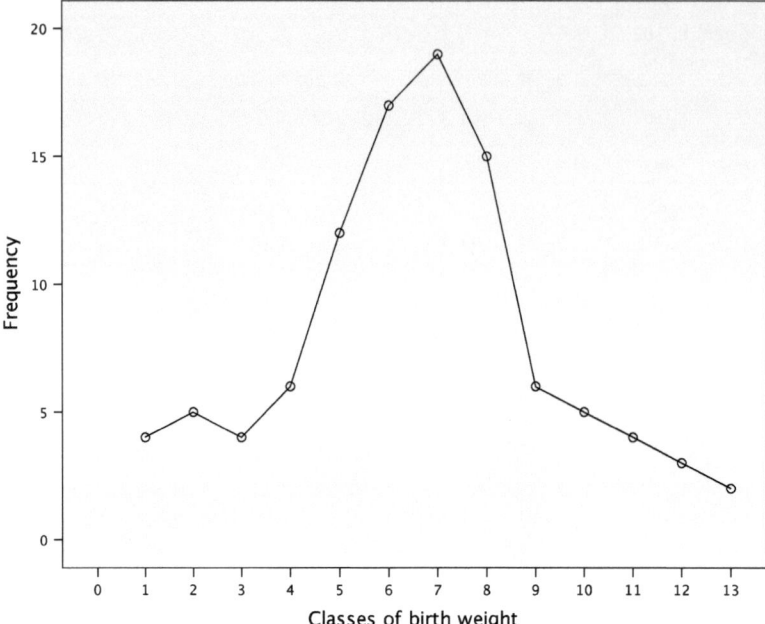

Fig. 1.3 Frequency polygon of classes of birth weight in 102 newly born babies presented in Table 1.2

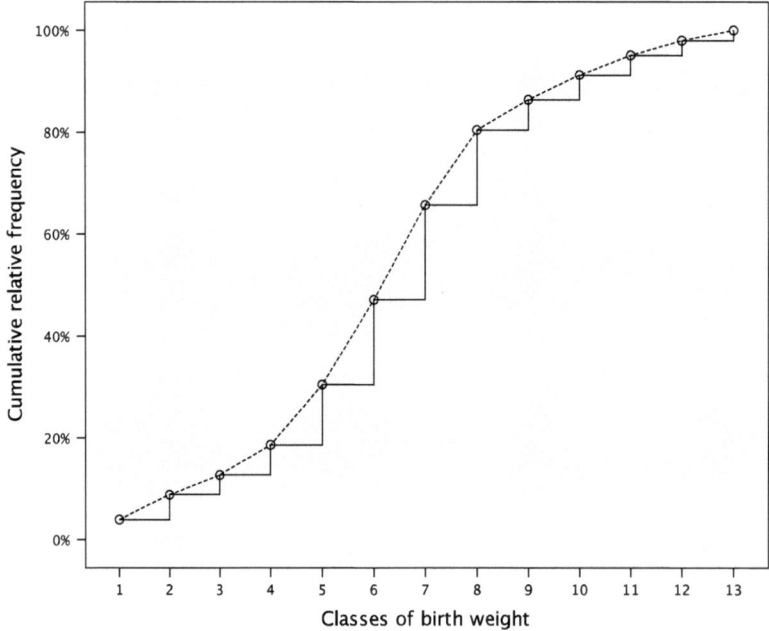

Fig. 1.4 Cumulative frequency% of classes of birth weight in 102 newly born babies presented in Table 1.2

```
birth_weight Stem-and-Leaf Plot

 Frequency    Stem &  Leaf

      4.00       2 .  0111
      5.00       2 .  22333
      4.00       2 .  4455
      6.00       2 .  667777
     12.00       2 .  888888899999
     17.00       3 .  00000111111111111
     19.00       3 .  2222222222222333333
     15.00       3 .  444444444455555
      6.00       3 .  666777
      5.00       3 .  88899
      4.00       4 .  0011
      3.00       4 .  223
      2.00 Extremes    (>=4500)
```

Fig. 1.5 Stem and leaf of classes of birth weight in 102 newly born babies presented in Table 1.2

allows us to observe some characteristics, such as the tendency to prefer some trailing digits to others.

1.3.2 The Quantitative Variable

A quantitative set of data is usually described by its central tendency as well as its dispersion; i.e., values in the center and values on the sides or in the extremes. Measures expressing central tendency include mean and median (see Sect. 1.3.3). Limits of dispersion include standard deviation, standard error mean and interquartile range (see Sect. 1.3.4).

1.3.3 Measures of Central Tendency

The arithmetic mean or average ($\bar{x}$) is referred to as *the mean*, which equals the sum ($\sum$) of individual values (x_i) divided by their number (n) "Eq. (1.1)".

$$\bar{x} = \frac{\sum x_i}{n} \qquad (1.1)$$

To execute calculations by hand, let us take a small example of 2 groups of patients, each composed of 3 men. The age of group (a) patients is 49, 50, and 51 years, while group (b) is: 1, 50, and 99 years. Although the mean age of both groups equals 50 [(49 + 50 + 51)/3

= (99 + 50 + 1)/3 = 50], yet no one can consider that those 2 groups are comparable as regarding age. *The mean alone is not only meaningless, but it can be misleading.* Our example gave the false impression that both groups are comparable for having the same mean and did hide the more important information, i.e., the homogeneity of the group (a) and the extreme heterogeneity of group (b) patients. The mean should always be coupled with a measurement of variability or dispersion of individual values. Another measure of central tendency is *the median*, simply the value in the middle (center) of the series. In the example shown above, the mean is the median value, but this is not a rule, of course. In the series: 1, 1, 3, 4, and 11; the mean is four, but the median value is three, and *the mode*, the value with the highest percentage is 1.

1.3.4 Measures of Dispersion

1.3.4.1 The Variance (S^2)

Our example clearly shows that the three patients in group (a) are dispersed around their mean value (50) by one year, on average. We can calculate this dispersion by subtracting each value (x_i) from the mean ($\bar{x}$), summing those results, and taking the average. *However, statisticians have encountered two technical difficulties using this direct and straightforward approach to calculate an average difference around the mean value* [1]. In every set of data, some of the values are larger than the mean, while others are smaller, resulting in negative and positive differences. *Summing positive and negative values will end by losing part of the differences (variability) that we wanted to express in the first place.* We forward an extreme example, where the calculated variability of the group (a) will be lost "Eq. (1.2)":

$$\sum(x_i - \bar{x}) = (49 - 50) + (50 - 50) + (51 - 50)$$
$$= 0$$

$$(1.2)$$

We can overcome the problem of losing differences by squaring the differences before summing them and then un-squaring the sum later. The sum of squared differences can be abbreviated to *sum of squares or simply (SS)* "Eqs. (1.3) and (1.4)":

$$SS = \sum(x_i - \bar{x})^2 \qquad (1.3)$$

$$SS = (49 - 50)^2 + (49 - 50)^2 + (49 - 50)^2 = 2$$
$$(1.4)$$

Now that we have gotten rid of the signs, let us calculate the mean variability: the variance (S^2). Although the mean of any sum of values is calculated by dividing the sum of values by the sample size, the mean variability is calculated by dividing the sum of values by the sample size minus one, which also needs some explanation. Let us look at the equation above; the second patient whose age was equal to the mean (50 years) did not contribute to the sum of squares, which is 2, simply because the difference between his age and the mean was zero. As we designed the variance to describe the variations around the mean, this patient did not vary from the mean. Consequently, a more appropriate average can be achieved by subtracting 1 (this patient) from the number of values in the denominator (n). The value (n − 1) represents the number (the degree) of patients who were free to vary from the mean, which is why it is called *the degree of freedom (df)*. In every

sample, one or more of the values will be the mean itself or something very near to the mean and hence, will not vary from the mean; i.e., will not share in the formation of SS.

The correction was suggested, not only on the basis of this observation but after computing the variance with repeated samples. *It was clear that variability is dependent upon sample size.* The small samples cannot describe the population well, and their variability (S^2) is always more significant (larger) than that of the population. To express the true (higher) variability inherent in small samples, Bessel has suggested a remedy to this bias by subtracting the constant (1) from any sample size, given a higher pitch for smaller samples [2] "Eq. (1.5)". The variance of our small example equals 1 [SS/(df − 1) = 2/(3–1)]. As the sample size increases, the value of subtracting (1) from (n) decreases systematically, and the population variance is then calculated as SS/n. Let us see how Bessel correction works and suppose that we have five samples with different sizes: three, 30, 100, 1000, and 100,000 patients. We know that the larger the sample, the smaller its variability will be. The variability of a huge sample of 100,000 patients can be considered equal to that of the population. Consequently, we do not need to make any corrections in calculating the variance of the huge sample.

On the contrary, we need to make a harsh correction to the tiny sample of three patients, and as the sample grows in size, the correction has to be more and more gentle. Removing (1) from the small sample of three patients is very crude as we removed 33% of the denominator of the equation, which will significantly correct the variance. Removing (1) from 30 cases will have a minor effect as we did remove only 3%. As the sample grows, removing the same constant (1) will have a minor effect until it becomes negligible with the colossal sample (0.00001%). We believe that such a sample closely matches the population, and hence, it does not need to be corrected.

$$S^2 = \frac{SS}{n-1} = \frac{SS}{df} \qquad (1.5)$$

Let us calculate the average variability within-group (b). Unsurprisingly, the variance equals 2401, meaning that the amount of variation (differences) within-group (b) patients is 2401 times that found between patients in group (a). This example shows you how much we would have been misled by just relaying on the mean of the two groups without coupling a measurement of variability (dispersion) to this mean (a measure of central tendency).

1.3.4.2   Standard Deviation (Sd)

While the "infamous" variance (S^2) is how statisticians precisely calculate variability, it rarely appears in the medical literature for a couple of reasons. First, it can confuse biologists by its squared scale: what does "1 year^2" mean? It means nothing to us; remember that we have squared the differences to protect them from canceling each other during summation. Second, as we have protected our results from being canceled, it will be more practical *to restore variability into the original (standard) scale of individual values* by taking the square root of the variance, which is nothing but the standard deviation. *The standard deviation* (Sd) describes the variability of individual (personal) values around their mean in the regular (standard) scale of values and not in the squared scale of the variance "Eq. (1.6)". Now, we can summarize the factor age in both groups by coupling both information: the mean and the standard deviation: ($\bar{x}$) ± Sd. We can describe the age of group (a) patients as: 50 ± 1 years; meaning that their mean age is 50 years and that the age of individual patients varies by about (1) year, on the average. The heterogeneity of group (b) patients becomes quite evident; for having the same mean as the group (a), but the age of individual patients widely varies (±) around the mean value by as much as 49 years (square root of 2401).

$$Sd = \sqrt{S^2} \qquad (1.6)$$

1.3.4.3   Standard Error of Mean (Se)

Any research aims to understand and hopefully to manipulate what is happening in the population. We cannot bring the population to the study room, but we can take samples, hoping that what we will find in those samples is a reasonable estimate of what happens in the population. We calculate the mean ($\bar{x}$) and standard deviation (Sd) of a study hoping that they will be reasonable estimates of their corresponding values in the population, which are the grand or true mean (u) and sigma or the standard deviation of the population (σ). As no two studies will ever give the exact estimates, the standard error of the mean (SEM) or simply the standard error (Se) was designed to describe the variability (the distance) between the mean "observed" in each study and the "expected" mean of the population. Consequently, each study will have its own Se [3].

One cannot know where the true mean is? Is it larger or smaller than (u), is it more positive or more negative? We do not know? We know that the more we include patients, the more the study will become representative of the population. Hence, the variability (the distance) between the research and the population is inversely proportional to sample size (n). The second question is what other factors make the study more representative of the population and influence this representativeness (distance)? Of course, it cannot be the mean, as we have just shown how misleading it can be. It can neither be any of the individual values of the study. Returning to our example, the variance (S^2) represented each study group and made a clear cut-off point between them? But how does the variance affect representativeness? The smaller is the variance, the more the study is representative of the population, and hence, variance is directly proportional to the distance (variability) between the research and the population. The equation is simple: the distance (variability) between the study and the population is equal to the quantity (S^2/n). Now, remember that variance is in a squared scale, and hence, this quantity should be un-squared, as we did before when we extracted the standard deviation out of the variance "Eq. (1.7)". The resultant is *the standard error of the mean (SEM) or simply the standard error (Se), representing the distance (variability) between the mean of any study and the population's mean.* Returning to our example, the (Se) of group (a) patients is equal to 0.58, compared to as much as 28.3 for group (b) patients. Now, we can compare variability between groups (studies, manuscripts dealing with the same topic and subjects, etc.) using the same reference point to reality; i.e., Se.

$$Se = \sqrt{\frac{S^2}{n}} = \frac{Sd}{\sqrt{n}} \qquad (1.7)$$

> We have to couple the mean with a measure of variability; either between the subjects of the group and their mean or between the latter and the mean of the population; i.e., either the Sd or the Se.

1.3.4.4　Extension to the Qualitative Variable

The reader can return to Schwartz and colleagues to verify that the variance of a proportion (p) equals [p(1 − p)]. The standard deviation is the square root of variance and the standard error of mean is the square root of variance divided by sample size, as usual "Eq. (1.8)" [4, 5].

$$Sd = \sqrt{p(1-p)} Se = \sqrt{\frac{p(1-p)}{n}} \qquad (1.8)$$

Those calculations assume that the qualitative variable is normally distributed in the population of interest. In short, statisticians have found that a qualitative variable follows approximately a normal distribution whenever both np and n(1 − p) are at least five [4]. For example, a researcher has found that complications occurred in as much as 10% of 100 patients undergoing a certain procedure. The variance of complications [p(1 − p)] will be equal to 0.09 (0.1 × 0.9) or 9%. The Sd equals 30% (square root of 0.9 = 0.3) and the Se equals 3% (0.3 divided by square root of sample size = 0.03). The calculation can be easily verified: np = 100 × 0.1 = 10 and n(1 − p) = 100 × 0.9 = 90; both being >5.

We have to note that calculations of proportions should be made in decimals (i.e., 10% = 0.1 in decimals) and then can be either ex-pressed in decimals or as a percentage.

1.3.4.5　Minimum, Maximum and Interquartile Range

One obvious measure of dispersion is the range between the lowest and highest values and is often expressed as the two extremes. As example, in a series of 13 (n) observations: 1, 2, 3, 4, 5, 6, 7, 8, 9, 10, 11, 19, and 20; the range is: 1–20. We can divide data into *quantiles*, which are values that divide the distribution into given proportions of observations above and below. *The median* is the central value of a distribution, with half of the data are above, and half are below. *The quartile* divides the distribution into four equal parts called *quarters or fourths*; the median is the second quartile. In our example, the median or the second quartile is 7 [value at 0.5 × (n + 1)], the first quartile is 3.5 [0.25 × (n + 1)] and the third quartile is 10.5 [value at 0.75 × (n + 1)]. *The interquartile range is the difference between the 1st and 3rd quartiles* = 3.5 − 10.5 = 7. The interquartile range can be either expressed as the two extremes (3.5 − 10.5) or as the net difference (7). *A box and whisker plot* is a convenient fire figure summary of a distribution showing the median, 1st, and 3rd quartiles as well as the two extremes (Fig. 1.6). The box shows the distance between the 1st and 3rd quartiles: the interquartile range. A horizontal line marks the median in the middle of the box. The whiskers represent the extremes. In addition, the plot will show *outliers*: any value that is away from the edge of the box (the quartile) by more than 1.5 times the length of the box (i.e., interquartile range).

1.4　The Normal Distribution

The data summary to use depends mainly on data distribution. Most biological variables obey the characteristic "*normal distribution*," which is a misnomer; otherwise, it would suggest that variables following other distributions, such as

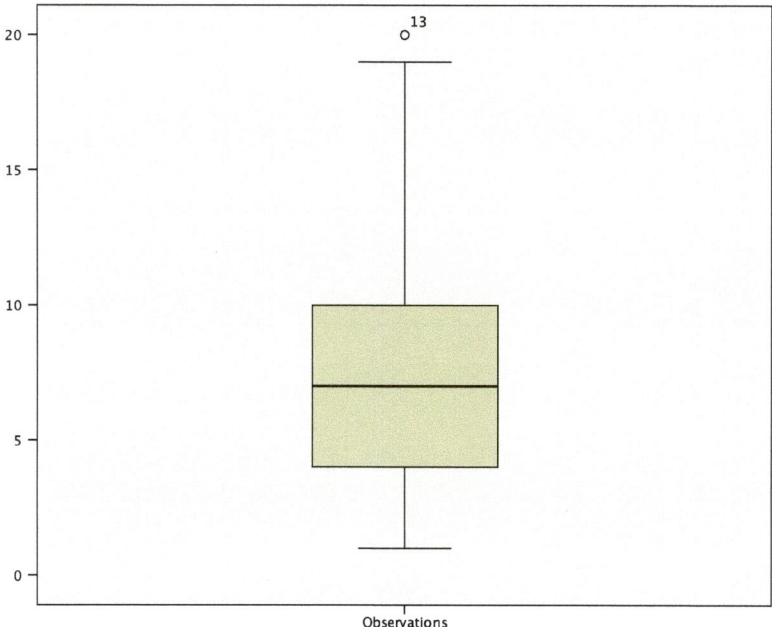

Fig. 1.6 Box and Whisker plot of a series of 13 observations: 1, 2, 3, 4, 5, 6, 7, 8, 9, 10, 11, 19, and 20

Student, Poisson, or else are "not normal." Normality is just a given name for being the most common. As will be shown in a moment, the mean, Sd, and Se of a normally distributed variable have special characteristics. Hence, they are the usually preferred measures for data expression in such a case. Otherwise, we typically express data as median and range for the absence of those characteristics.

A classic study on the birthweight distribution in 200 newborns has shown that infants' weight follows a normal distribution [4]. We repeated the study in a local maternity hospital and included 102 cases (Table 1.2). In order to compare both studies, we followed the classic analysis by arranging the babies in 13 classes, each in the 200 g range [4]. Table 1.2 shows the number of babies in each class in absolute (frequency) and relative values (relative frequency). Figures 1.1 and 1.2 are the corresponding histograms. *A histogram* is a diagram in which we scale classes (or intervals) on the x-axis as columns. The heights of those columns are either their frequency, cumulative frequency, or percentages and are presented on the y axis. In case

the variable is normally distributed, drawing a line across the heads of columns results in an *inverted bell-shaped or Gaussian–Laplace curve* (Fig. 1.7).

In our study, the mean birth weight, variance, Sd, and Se were equal to 3198 g, 289,919 g^2, 538 g, and 53 g, respectively. Data have characteristic distribution: the mean birth weight ($\bar{x}$ = approximated to 3200 g) is in the middle of values and includes the highest proportion. The frequency of values decreases bilaterally and symmetrically as we go further away from the mean. As an example, the frequency of babies weighing 3400–3600 g (14.7%) is less than those weighing 3200–3400 (18.6%) and so on. The frequency of the weight value ($\bar{x}$ + x) is nearly equal to that observed for the weight value ($\bar{x}$ − x). As an example, five babies (4.9%) are 700 g larger than the mean (3900; i.e., in the interval 3800–4000), compared to four babies (3.9%) who are smaller by the same amount (2500; i.e., in the interval 2400–2600). Replacing (x) by the Sd (approximated to 540 g), it was noticed that the birth weight of 72 out of 102 babies (70.6%) varied by 1 Sd (540 g) around the mean

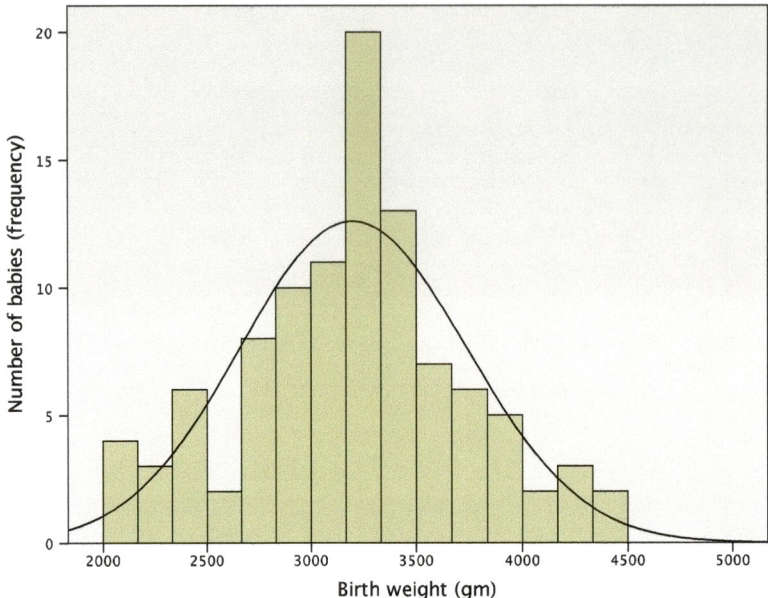

Fig. 1.7 Inverted bell-shaped (Gaussian–Laplace) curve of data presented in Table 1.2

(3200 g): 2660–3740 g. Similarly, the birth weight of 95 babies (93%) varied by two Sd on either side of the mean: 2120 and 4280 g. We can include all birth weights in an interval made by about three Sd on either side of the mean: 1580–4820 g. In general, the interval formed by one standard deviation on either side of the mean is expected to include about two-thirds of the values. A larger interval formed by two standard deviations is supposed to include about 95% of values. All or 99% of values are expected to lie within three standard deviations, on either side of the mean. The larger the sample, the more those expectations are correct. *A variable showing such characteristics is said to have a "normal distribution" or to follow the normal law.*

1.4.1 The Standardized Normal Distribution and the Z Score

Statisticians have taken repeated large samples of normally distributed data like ours, generalized these observations, and created the standard normal distribution curve to describe any normally distributed population (Fig. 1.8). *The frequency of normally distributed data is dependent upon how many standard deviations a data value is away from the mean (i.e., is smaller or larger than the mean).* Hence, the standard deviation of the population or sigma will be the standard measurement unit ($\sigma = 1$). Any data value that happens to be equal to the mean itself will have a sigma value of 0, and hence, the mean will be the zero units on the scale ($\mu = 0$). The interval formed by ($\mu - 1\sigma$) and ($\mu + 1\sigma$) is enclosing 68.2% of observations, 34.1% on either side of the mean (μ). Similarly, 95.4% of values are expected to be enclosed between ($\mu - 2\sigma$) and ($\mu + 2\sigma$) and 99.7% of values are expected to be enclosed between ($\mu - 3\sigma$) and ($\mu + 3\sigma$). We can calculate probabilities for fractions of (σ) as well and hence, 95% of observations are expected to be exactly between ($\mu - 1.96\sigma$) and ($\mu + 1.96\sigma$) and 99% of observations between ($\mu - 2.6\sigma$) and ($\mu + 2.6\sigma$) [4].

Applying the rule to our example shown in Table 1.1.2, 95% of babies have an expected birth weight between 3200 ± 1.96 (540); i.e., 2142–4259 g. By deduction, only 5% of babies are expected to be born outside this interval. View the bilateral symmetrical character of normal distribution; there is about 2.5% probability

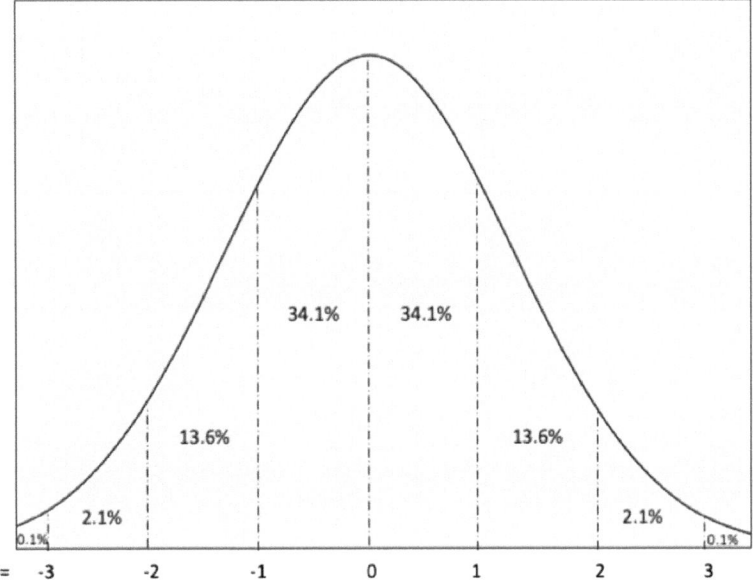

Fig. 1.8 The standard normal distribution curve showing the proportions of values per Z score units

for a baby to be smaller than 2142 g and another 2.5% probability of being larger than 4259 g. The mean and standard deviation of a study are the best estimates of the corresponding values in the population. In consequence, we can assign a probability for any normally distributed biological value (x) by just knowing how many standard deviations is (x) away from the mean ($\bar{x}$), which is called the standardized value or Z score of (x) "Eq. (1.9)".

$$Z = \frac{(x_i - \bar{x})}{Sd} \qquad (1.9)$$

Transforming any normally distributed data value (x) into its Z score permits us to assign a probability for (x), simply because we know the probability of Z. As an example, if the mean and Sd of a person's height are: 170 and 5 cm, the Z score of being as tall as 180 cm or taller is (+2). As we know the probability of having a Z score of that is (+2) or larger (more positive), we can estimate the same 2.5% probability for being 180 cm tall or taller; i.e., 2.5%. The probability of being a short as 160 cm or shorter is (−2) and, it is the mirror image of the previous one. A Z score can be negative or positive, depending on whether the value is smaller or larger than the mean. In the standard normal distribution, 50% of the z values are positive, and the other mirror image 50% will be negative. Hence, it was sufficient for statisticians to present the probabilities associated with the absolute values of Z: *the z table*. Statistical tables are freely available on the internet [6]. Details of consulting statistical tables is given in Sect. 2.2.

In short, the Z table gives the cumulative probability for z to acquire any smaller value than the one calculated for (x); i.e., the proportion of the area under the curve to the left of (z) to the total curve area. Hence, this probability is always smaller than one. Consequently, the chance to have a z value that is precisely equal to or larger than (x) is calculated by subtracting 1 from the probability given by the table (Fig. 1.9). For example, the probability of a z value between 0 and 1.96 is 0.975 (intersection of line 1.96 and column 0.06), and hence the chance to have a Z score of 1.96 or larger = 1–0.975 = 2.5%. The inverse probability of having any Z value between (−1.96) and 0 is just a mirror image of the latter. As a result, the likelihood of having a Z value outside the interval (−1.96 to 196) = (2.5 + 2.5%) = 5%.

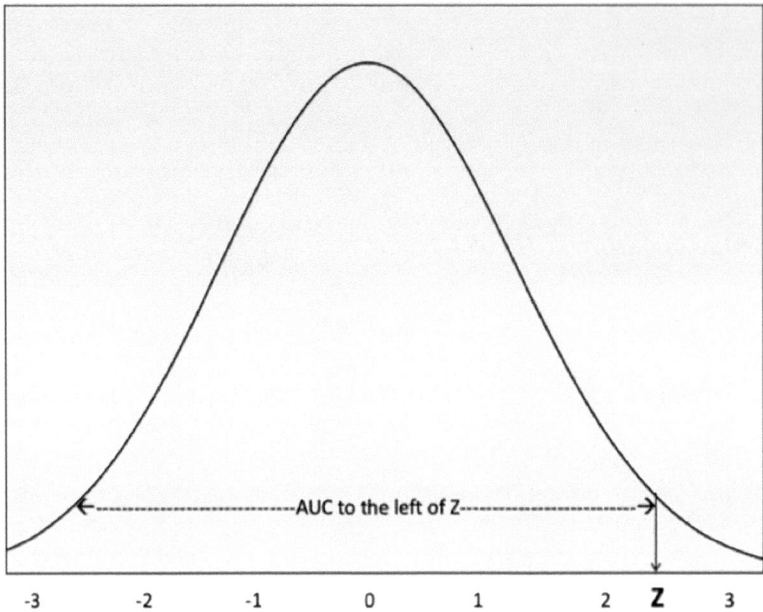

Fig. 1.9 The cumulative standardized normal distribution: gives the probability of a normal random variable (x) to have a standardized value that is smaller than Z. The probability for (x) to have a standardized value that is equal or larger than Z is calculated by subtracting 1 from the value given by the table

Fig. 1.10 The standardized normal distribution: gives the probability of a normal random variable (x) to have an absolute Z value that is smaller than the one given by the table. The probability of an equal or larger Z is calculated by subtracting 0.5 from that given by the table

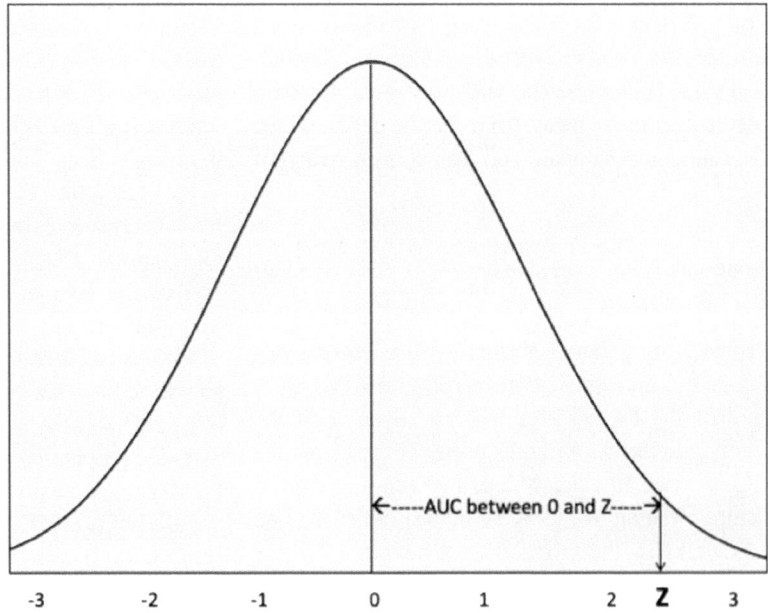

Returning to our birth weight example (Table 1.2), 95% of babies are expected to weigh between 2142 and 4259 g, with a 2.5% probability of having a baby heavier than 4259 g and another 2.5% probability of having a baby smaller than 2142 g. We can calculate the probability of having a baby with any given birth weight (e.g., 4100 g) by calculating his Z score; i.e., how many Sd is his birth weight away from the mean = (4100 − 3200)/540 = 1.67. The latter is checked out at the intersection of line 1.6 with column 0.07. The Z table indicates that the probability for any data value to acquire a Z score < 1.67 is 0.9525 (95.25%). Consequently, the probability of having a child weighing 4100 g or larger equals 4.75% (1–0.9525). The probability for his mirror image fellow whose Z score is (−1.67) for being 900 g smaller than the mean is equally 4.75% too. By deduction, the probability of having a baby who is 900 g larger or smaller than the mean birth weight is the sum of both probabilities (9.5%).

In conclusion, any normally distribution variable can be perfectly defined by only knowing the mean and the standard deviation. Knowing both, and for a given value (x), one can find the equivalent point on the standard normal distribution curve by calculating its z value. In the z-table, statisticians have calculated the areas under the curve to the left of (smaller than) all possible values of z. *The probability of having a z value that is at least equal or larger* than the one calculated is easily acquired by subtracting (1) from the probability given by the table.

We have to note that not all Z tables present the cumulative probability of Z values as we have shown. An alternative way is a "standardized normal distribution table" presenting the probability of having either a positive or a negative z value; i.e., *the probability of having a z value that is either larger from the mean (positive z) or smaller than the mean (negative z).* Consequently, the probability for a particular data value to be only larger than the mean (x > mean) and hence giving a positive z, is calculated by subtracting 0.5 form the probability inscribed in the table (Fig. 1.10). As example, the probability given by the table for a Z value of

1.67 is 0.4525 and hence the probability to have a Z value $\geq$ 1.67 = 0.5–0.4525 = 4.75%. Its mirror image probability (x < mean) and hence, giving a negative z, is the same (4.75%), simply because the table provides an absolute z. By deduction, the probability of having a baby who is 900 g larger or smaller than the mean birth weight (to lay outside the interval formed by $\bar{x} \pm x$) is the cum of both probabilities (9.5%). In conclusion, using any of those two forms of a Z table gives exactly the same result but we have to be careful during the calculation.

The invention of the Z score is as important as the invention of money because it permitted the transaction of any data value with unknown probability to a standardized value whose probability is perfectly known.

1.4.2 The Confidence Interval (CI)

Let us see how we can benefit from these observations. We know that two-thirds of observations are present in the interval formed by the (mean $\pm$ 1 Sd), 95% in the interval created by the (mean $\pm$ 1.96 Sd), and 99% are present in the interval formed by the (mean $\pm$ 2.6 Sd) and so on [4]. In fact, at each fraction of Sd, we are confident that we will find a certain percentage of observation, which is why we call those intervals: the intervals of confidence (CI). Taking the most commonly used CI at 95%, and like any other interval, it has an evident *descriptive value* for the study: the birth weight of 95% of babies varied between 2142 and 4259 g. It gives all needed information and from which one can deduct the mean (the number in the middle: 3200 g), and the Sd is equal to nearly half of the difference between the mean and any of its limits: 540 g).

Turning the table around, we are 95% confident (sure) that the birth weight of any future baby from the same population will be included within its lower and upper limits, which is *the predictive value* of CI. The more we include patients in our study, the smaller the Sd is, the tighter (narrower), and hence, the more valuable the CI will be [4]. Looking at the other side of the coin, babies from different populations will have different means, Sd and CI, of course. Consequently, the *comparative value* of CI becomes a handy tool in testing hypotheses and concluding upon the presence/absence of a statistically significant difference between different population groups [4].

1.4.2.1 The Confidence Interval of Subjects

As we can never be 100% sure of our results or decisions, the 95% CI is the usually adopted cutoff point for diagnosis and decision-making. The mean ± 1.96 Sd forms the 95% CI of a subject. As shown before, the Sd is the measurement of the variability of a subject (a person), indicating the average variability between the subjects of the sample and their mean value; i.e., it measures the in-between subject's variability. The "range" of normal values figured in laboratory sheets (leucocytic counts, serum hemoglobin, glucose levels in blood, serum creatinine, etc.) and radiological documents (cardiothoracic ratio, left atrial size, gall bladder size, etc.) are no more than "the upper and lower limits of the 95% intervals of confidence of normal persons". A particular patient is most probably diabetic when his fasting blood sugar lies outside the 95% CI calculated for normal persons. We are 95% sure of our decision, and hence, there is still a tiny 5% probability that he does not have diabetes, which is why we have to do a confirmatory test (post-prandial blood sugar) to ensure our diagnosis.

Similarly, we are 95% sure that a patient whose serum creatinine lies outside the "normal range" of laboratory values has a slim probability of being normal. His state should be confirmed by creatinine clearance to exclude a possible normal but extreme value of serum creatinine. *On the level of an individual patient, we are usually making decisions based upon whether a particular patient data value lies within or outside the 95% CI, as we will show in discussing the P-value in a moment (see Sect. 1.5).*

The so-called "normal ranges" of laboratory and radiological values are no more than the upper and lower limits of the 95% confidence intervals calculated for the "normal population". A subject has a 95% chance to be diseased whenever the result of his analysis exceeds this range.

1.4.2.2 The Confidence Interval of Mean

Returning to the birth weight example (Table 1.2). The results of our study were compared to those acquired in a larger study including 200 new born babies [4]. In the latter, the birth weight varied between 2100 and 5100 g, with a mean birth weight of 3309 (± 494). The results of any two studies can be different or comparable but can never be the same. Repeating the study for the third or the fourth time, even in the same hospital, during the same period, and by the same investigators, will never give the same mean value. The legitimate question would be: which value represents the true mean? In other words, what is the mean birth weight of this population (u)? Although nobody can give a definitive answer, we can calculate a range that includes (u).

In each sample (each study), the units are the birth weights of the individual babies, and those units are normally distributed around their mean value. Playing the same tune, the means of different samples are the units in the population. Those units are expected to be normally distributed around the population's true mean. For a given sample (study), the measure of variability by which the study units are distributed around their mean value is the Sd (1.3.4.2). On the other hand, the unit of the variability of the means of the different samples (studies) around the population's true mean is the Se (1.3.4.3). *As there is a 95% chance for an individual birth weight to lie within 1.96 Sd of its mean value, the population's mean is expected to lie within 1.96 Se of the mean of a given sample.* The smaller the Se of the mean of an individual sample, the more its mean approaches and is representative of the true mean of the population.

We typically report the confidence interval of the mean as follows: "The mean birth weight of our studied group of babies was 3200 g (95% CI, 3096 and 3304 g)". The confidence interval can be interpreted as follows: we are 95% confident that the mean birth weight of the population lies between 3096 and 3304 g, provided that our study is large and the cases are chosen at random. If we repeat the study, there is a 95% chance that the mean birth weight of the future study will acquire any value between 3096 and 3304 g, which is the predictive value of the confidence interval. Put it another way, our sample is compatible with any other sample drawn randomly from the same population and has a mean birth weight between 3096 and 3304 g, which is the comparative value of the confidence interval.

Figure 1.11 shows the 95% intervals of confidence of the subject and the mean. As the Se is smaller than the Sd for being equal to the latter divided by the square root of sample size, "*the CI of mean*" *is always smaller than that of the*

subject. Also, the more we include cases, the narrower our CI will be and the more we are supposed to approach the "true values." *The CI of mean has the same three practical descriptive, comparative, and predictive values* of the confidence interval of subjects: However, comparing 2 studies is technically different. The 95% CI of each study represents its personal space; hence 2 studies are significantly different from one another (i.e., coming from 2 different populations) whenever they respect their reciprocal spaces; i.e., their respective 95% CI of means are separated from one another. On the other hand, studies with overlapping intervals have a limited 29% chance of being significantly different (see Sect. 7.4.6.4). As example, a second study whose 95% CI excludes both the lower (3096 g) and the upper limits (3304 g) of our classic study (e.g., 2900–3095 g or 3305–3400 g) is significantly different from our reference study. A third study which includes either one or both limits (e.g. 2900–3096 or 3300–3400 g) is most probably comparable to our study. Another difference is that means of several samples are normally

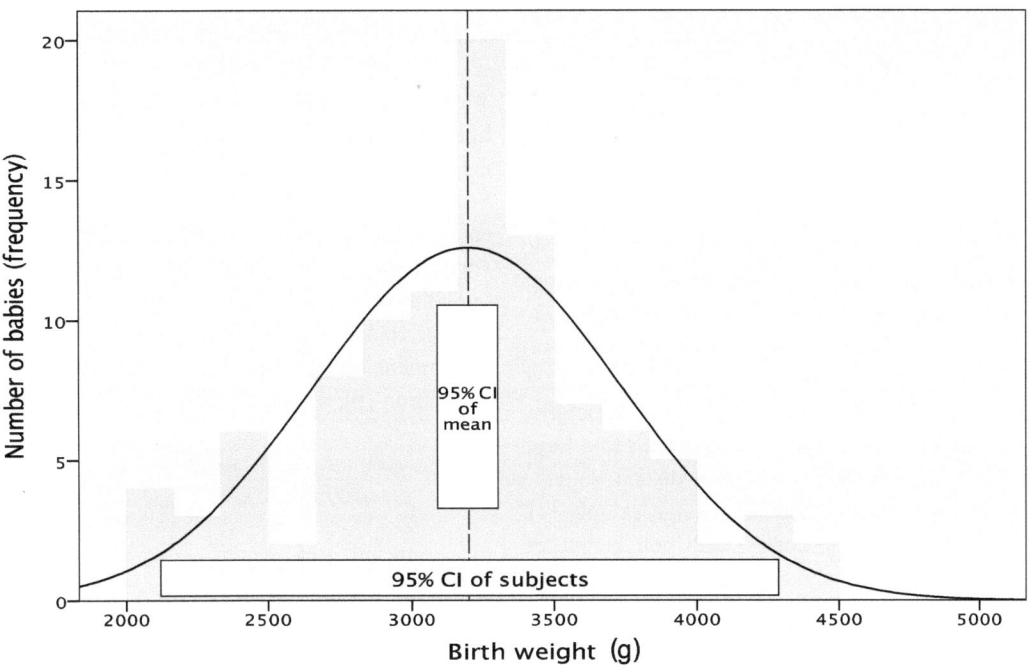

Fig. 1.11 The 95% interval of confidence (CI) of subjects (mean ± 1.96 Sd) is always larger than the 95% CI of mean (mean ± 1.96 Se). Calculated for data presented in Table 1.2

distributed themselves. Consequently, the CI of the mean does not necessitate the normal distribution of the studied variable in the population of interest.

> We are 95% confident that the mean of the population lies within the interval of confidence of the mean of our study. By deduction, a study that shares the same CI of mean is expected to issue from the same population. Put another way, the 95% confidence interval of the mean of a particular study represents the set of the still unknown (possible) data that are comparable with our study.

1.4.2.3 The Confidence Interval of the Small Study

The calculations of the different confidence intervals assume "the normal distribution" of the studied variable, which is practically accepted whenever the number of values (n) is at least 30. However, many clinical studies involve small samples and using the Z value (1.96) to calculate the CI becomes a source of bias and not a way for precision. William Sealy Gosset (1876–1937), widely known as "Student," has postulated that small samples selected from a known normally distributed variable follow a near normal distribution, called the Student or Student-Fisher distribution, later on. Small samples are less likely to represent the population, and this bias increases as the sample get smaller. The resultant is that *the CI estimated from the small sample is less precise, i.e., broader than that calculated with a large sample.* Because of the wide variability expected in a small sample, compared to a large sample, the calculated Sd is more distant from the mean compared to those of a large sample [4]. The Z values of the normal distribution that are standard as long as the sample size is >30 patients per group have to be replaced by larger Student "t" values dependent upon sample size. The smaller the sample, the larger the "t" and hence, the less precise the estimated CI is. Putting it

another way: in order to assume the same probability (e.g., 95%), a larger t-value (>1.96) will always be needed, compared to the corresponding Z value (1.96). *Consequently, the CI formed by the t-value will always be wider and hence less precise than that formed by the corresponding Z value for the sake of being less biased.* In order to get "t," we have to consult Student's table [6], which we will explain in detail in the appropriate chapter (see Sect. 2.2.3).

Returning to the example of the 102 newly born babies presented in Table 1.2 and suppose that we have observed the birth weights of 10 babies only and calculated the same mean birth weight (3200) and Se (53) g. Checking Student's table for 9 degrees of freedom (sample size-1), t = 2.26 and the 95% CI = m ± t Se = 3200 ± 2.26 × 53 = 3080–3320 g; which is wider and hence, lees precise than that calculated with z value: 3096–3304 g. It is always advisable to use the t-values in case we doubt normality, as Student's distribution and tests are more robust than Z values; i.e., still valid if "normality" is not perfectly respected. For large samples, both: t and z values merge (see Sect. 2.2.3).

1.4.2.4 The Confidence Interval of a Proportion

We have previously shown that the variance of a binomial qualitative variable of proportions: p and (p − 1) is equal to p(1 − p) (see Sect. 1.3.4.4). Afterward, the equations for calculating the confidence intervals of a qualitative variable [4, 5] are nearly the same as for a quantitative variable. The observation of a percentage (p_0) in a sample of (n) cases permits the assignment for the unknown percentage of the population (p), a 95% CI "Eq. (1.10)":

$$p_0 \pm 1.96\sqrt{\frac{p_0(1 - p_0)}{n}} \qquad (1.10)$$

For a 99% CI, 1.96 is replaced by 2.6, of course. Similarly, we can only apply the formula in case of large numbers; however, the rule of 30 is insufficient here, and the applied rule is that both: np and n(1 − p) are >5 and for both limits of the CI (see the example for details). Moreover, the formula is approximate, and some tables give the exact CI, especially when (n) is small [4]. Let us have the example of examining the prevalence of obesity among middle-class teenagers (boys and girls) attending private schools. A random sample of 100 students revealed an obesity percentage as high as 25%. Hence, $p_0 = 0.25$ and by simple deduction $1 - p_0 = 0.75$. The 95% CI is calculated as in "Eq. (1.11)"

$$= 0.25 \pm 1.96 \sqrt{\frac{(0.25 \times 0.75)}{100}} = 0.17 - 0.33$$

$$(1.11)$$

We will conclude that the percentage of obesity in our sample was 25% (95% CI: from 17 to 33%). Next, we have to check on the conditions of application for the lower limit of $p = 0.17$, $(1 - p) = 83$, $np = 17$, and $n(1 - p) = 83$. For the upper limit of $p = 0.33$, $(1 - p) = 0.67$, $np = 33$ and $n(1 - p) = 67$; and all conditions are verified. Checking the more accurate tables for $n = 100$ and $p = 25\%$, the 95% CI lies between 17 and 35% [4]; which shows the acceptable results given by the formula as long as the conditions necessary for its applications are well verified. The calculations can be easily made online [7–9].

The continuity correction

It is worth noting that the calculation of the CI of a binomial distribution approximates the normal distribution. A binomial variable of sample size (n) and proportion (p), is supposed to follow an approximately normal distribution with a mean of (np) and a variance of $[np(1 - p)]$. The approximation assumes that the sample is large, as indicated by both (np) and $[n(1 - p)]$ being ≥ 5 and (p) is close to 0.5 [4]. By default, any approximation invites imprecision, and hence, a mathematical correction was made to improve those approximations: the continuity correction. The Wald 95% CI calculated in "Eq. (1.11)" can be corrected by a factor $(1/2n)$ that is added to the upper limit $(0.33 + 0.005 = 0.335)$ and subtracted from the lower limit of the interval $(0.17 - 0.005 = 0.165)$. For a lay physician, the continuity correction was suggested by statisticians to compensate for the fact that they have approximated a discrete binomial variable to a continuous variable, aiming to improve the approximations they made. Although the continuity correction version of the CI is wider, it is more accurate, especially in the case of a small sample size.

1.4.2.5 The Confidence Interval of a Unilateral Versus a Bilateral Study Design

Figure 1.12 shows the 95% CI of a subject, as described above: 95% of the normally distributed variable observations are present in an interval formed by about 1.96 Sd, on either side of the mean. The birth weight of 95% of babies is expected to vary between 2142 and 4259 g (mean $\pm$ 1.96 Sd). Let us put it this way: we are 95% confident that the birth weight of any future baby from the same population will vary between 2142 and 4259 g. View the bilateral symmetry of the distribution; the probability of having a baby (<2141 g) is 2.5% and of having a larger baby (>4259 g) is 2.5% too. The Z table shows that this 2.5% probability (0.95) is at the intersection of line 1.9 and column 0.06. Hence, the corresponding critical Z value associated with either a larger or smaller birth weight is 1.96. In other words, the probability of a positive Z value > 1.96 (large baby weighting >4259 g) is 2.5%, and it is equal to the probability of a negative Z value < −1.96 (small baby weighting <2142 g). Such study design is described as being bilateral. It is made to answer the study question: what is the probability of having a baby who is *different* from those from the same population: whether by being smaller or larger than the 95% majority? As we will show later, this *bilateral study design* is used to compare two treatments, aiming to answer the study question: which is the better treatment: A or B?

On the other hand, whenever we compare a treatment to a placebo or a standard care regimen, the study question is not which is better but whether the treatment is effective or not? The other possibility that a placebo is better is never tested, of course. The design adopted to show that only one of the two comparators (treatment)

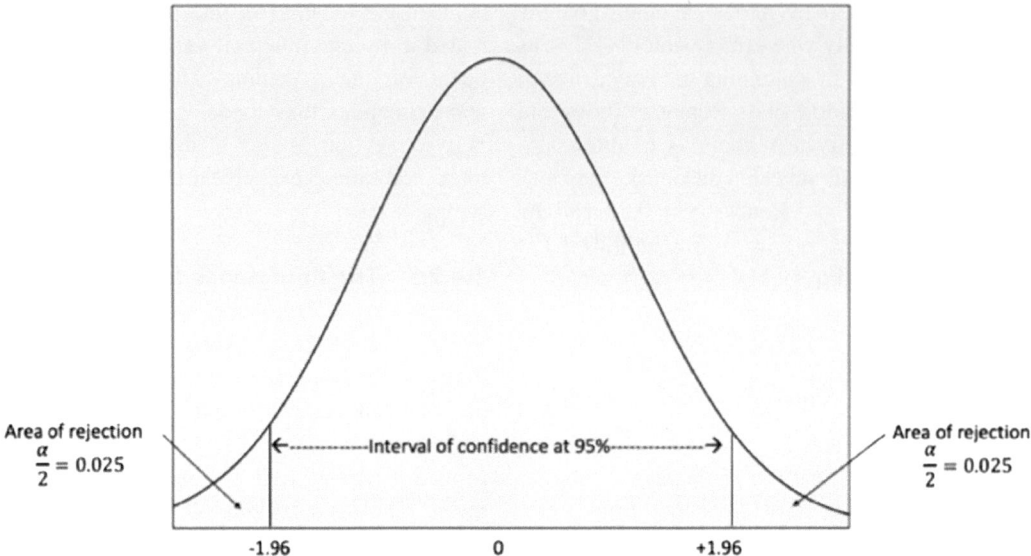

Fig. 1.12 Bilateral study design: the primary risk of error is equally split between the 2 examined possibilities, 2.5% on either side of the centralized 95% interval of confidence

is better than the other (placebo) but not the reverse is *a unilateral study design*. Applying the same concept to our survey on the birth weight of newly born babies, we may be only interested to know whether any future baby from the same population will be larger than the majority or not? We are not interested to know whether the baby is smaller than this 95% majority? We know that the birth weight of 2.5% of babies will be >4259 g, and by deduction, we are 97.5% confident that the birth weight of any baby from the same population will be smaller than 4259 g; which is *the upper limit of the 97.5% CI* of being >4259 g. However, the routine is to use the 95% CI and not the 97.5% CI. The 95% CI is the one that excludes 5% (and not 2.5%) of the observations in question; i.e., the one that will exclude 5% of the babies expected to be smaller than 4259 g. The Z table shows that the 5% probability (0.95) is at the intersection of line 1.6 and column 0.05. Hence, the critical Z value of the upper limit of the unilateral 95% CI of a unilateral design is 1.65 and *is equivalent to the bilateral 90% confidence interval*. The same applies when calculating the CI of means but with Se and not the Sd, of course.

Finally, compare Figs. 1.12 and 1.13, which show the 95% CI of subjects for bilateral and unilateral study designs, respectively. The critical Z value (the value that excludes 5% of the observations in question) associated with the former is larger (1.96) than that associated with the latter (1.65). The 95% CI of the bilateral design is centered around the mean and encloses 1.96 Sd on either side. On the other hand, the 95% confidence interval of the unilateral design extends to only 1.65 Sd on one side to the mean, and in fact, it corresponds to the 90% CI of a bilateral design. Kindly refer to Sect. 1.4.2.8 for using the unilateral 95% CI in the non-inferiority and the double unilateral 95% CI in the equivalence studies.

1.4.2.6 The Confidence Interval of the Difference Between Two Means

In the case of two groups, we were interested to know the difference between the birth weights of baby boys (mean birth weight = ma = 3186 g, number of babies = na = 50, and variance S^2a = 262,144) and baby girls (mean birth weight = mb 3210 g, number of babies = nb = 52 and variance

Fig. 1.13 Unilateral study design: the whole primary risk of error (5%) is confined to the only studied side, shifting the 95% CI to the other side

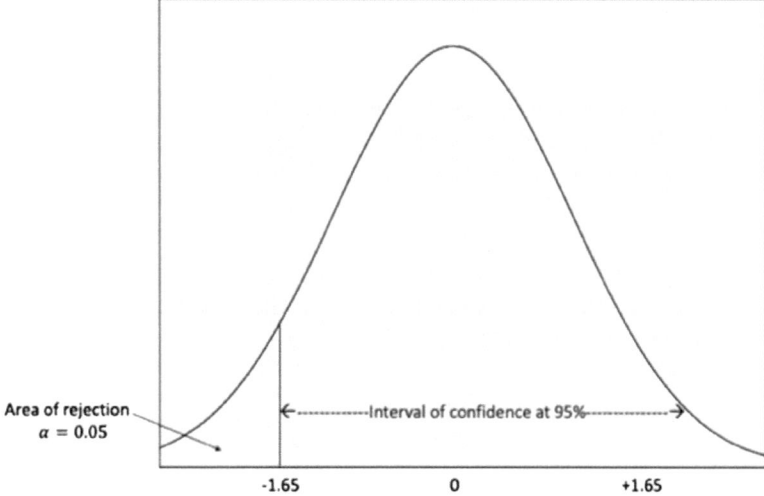

Area of rejection
$\alpha = 0.05$

←----------Interval of confidence at 95%----------→

-1.65   0   +1.65

$S^2b = 321{,}489$). We are interested in assigning a 95% CI to the calculated difference using the Z value (1.96) where both na and nb > 30. Otherwise, we have to use the t value for the corresponding df = (na + nb) − 2 "Eq. (1.12)"; (see Sect. 2.4.1). Note that the CI of the difference is the one used in meta-analysis (see Sect. 6.1). Interpretation: the mean difference in birth weight is 23 g, in favor of newly born females. However, the IC at 95% bypasses the null (no difference = 0 g), which means that this difference is not statistically significant and, sometimes, it can happen to be in favor of females. In other times, it can be in favor of males "Eq. (1.13)".

$$m_d \pm 1.96 \sqrt{\frac{S_a^2}{n_a} + \frac{S_b^2}{n_b}} \qquad m_d \pm (t) \sqrt{\frac{S_a^2}{n_a} + \frac{S_b^2}{n_b}}$$

$$\tag{1.12}$$

$$3186 - 3210 \pm 1.96 \sqrt{\frac{262144}{50} + \frac{321489}{52}} = -236 \text{ to } +189$$

$$\tag{1.13}$$

1.4.2.7 The Confidence Interval of the Difference Between 2 Proportions

We conducted a study to compare two antibiotics in the treatment of urinary tract infections. Two hundred patients were equally randomized between 2 groups. The primary outcome was the patient cure, as indicated by free urine culture and sensitivity analysis, three weeks after the onset of the treatment. The observed cure rates were 45% with treatment A (P_a), and 75% with treatment B (P_b), and the question was whether their difference ($p_d = 0.75 - 0.45 = 0.3$) is significant? As in the case of means, the variance of the difference between two proportions is the sum of both variances. The 95% CI of the difference between the two proportions (p_d) is all on one side of null. Hence, if we repeat the study, the difference is expected to favor treatment B 95% of the time "Eq. (1.14)".

$$p_d \pm Z \sqrt{\frac{p_a(1 - p_a)}{n_a} + \frac{p_b(1 - p_b)}{n_b}}$$
$$= 0.30 \pm 1.96 \sqrt{0.0087} = 30 \pm 18.3\%$$
$$= 11.7 - 48.3\%$$

$$\tag{1.14}$$

1.4.2.8 The Confidence Intervals of Non-Inferiority and Equivalence Studies

The Routine Superiority and Efficacy Studies

Most randomized clinical trials (RCTs) used to be *superiority clinical trials (SCT)* or *efficacy clinical trials (ECT)*. An SCT aims to determine whether one intervention is superior to another, while an ECT aims to shows that a (new) treatment is effective; compared to a control group receiving a placebo or a standard care treatment, the probability of the placebo or the standard care treatment being superior to new treatment is not tested. In Sect. 1.4.2.5, we have shown the calculation of the 95% CI for the bilateral SCT and the unilateral ECT. We have established the details of those calculations in the case where the outcome variable was quantitative (see Sect. 1.4.2.6) or qualitative (see Sect. 1.4.2.7). Figure 1.14 shows the interpretation of the calculated CIs for both ECT and SCT. The results of an SCT are statistically significant whenever the whole bilateral 95% CI of the difference is on one side of the null, whether in favor of standard or new treatment. In the case of ECT, the whole unilateral 95% CI of the difference has to favor the new treatment, without touching the null: i.e., excluding the probability that there is no difference between new treatment and placebo. Failure to demonstrate a statistically significant difference in those "*negative studies*" is easily visualized by a CI not excluding zero (the null) and, it should never be interpreted as both treatments are equal. The reasons are many: one is the fact that "equality" does not exist in life, even for identical twins, and hence, trying to find it or to prove it is just a waste of time. In second, many negative studies (absence of a statistically significant difference) may give positive results (finding a

statistically significant difference) by increasing sample size. Hence, *many of those negative studies are just due to a lack of study power.* We need unique study designs to reveal "a positive finding," proving that a difference is significantly so slight that it can be overlooked or neglected. Those are the "unilateral" non-inferiority (NIF) and the "double unilateral" equivalence (Eq) studies. The term double unilateral will be explained by the end of this section.

> In a superiority study, a confidence interval of the difference between two treatments that includes or bypasses the null is non-conclusive. If we repeat the study, sometimes the difference will favor the first treatment, and other times, it will favor the second treatment. Such a negative study should never be interpreted that both treatments are equal but just comparable. The correct way to conclude upon "equality" is to design a non-inferiority or an equivalence study.

The Non-inferiority Study

Whenever preliminary data indicates that the new treatment may fall just a few steps behind the classic one, investigators will be satisfied by a study showing that the new treatment is no worse than the classic one. *The question will be defining*

Fig. 1.14 Interpretation of the 95% CI of the bilateral superiority study and the unilateral efficacy study. The CI is statistically significant when it excludes the null

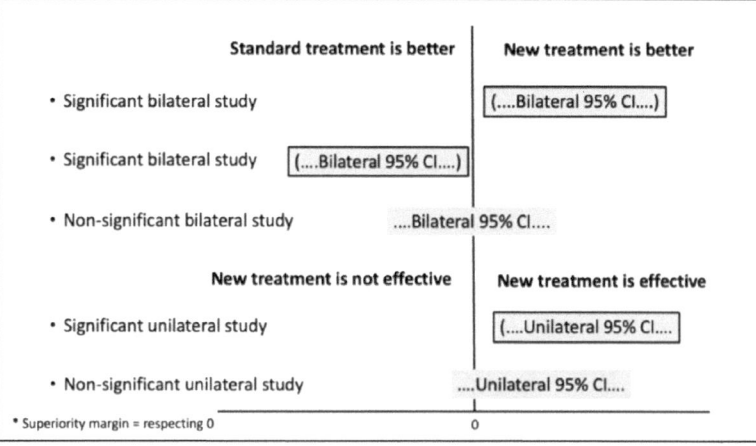

a *"non-inferiority margin (Δ)" that we can accept clinically and statistically.* The null hypothesis is that the new treatment is "more worse" than the classical treatment by an amount that is equal or more important than (Δ). The alternative hypothesis is that the new treatment is *"no more worse"* than the classic treatment (Δ). As an example, if the classic treatment gives a 95% success rate and the new one gives only 94%; the medical community can accept this slight 1% difference, especially if the new treatment is cheaper, associated with fewer side effects, can be safely used in conjunction with other treatments, etc. Once we prove that the difference is "no more worse" than (Δ)", the bargain is concluded, and the new treatment is considered to be *"not inferior to"* classic treatment, in exchange for the associated benefits. Statistically, (Δ) is usually chosen as a fraction of the lower limit of the 95% CI of the standard treatment when the latter was compared to placebo, whether in large randomized trials or from meta-analysis studies. In other words, *the new treatment should always behave better than the placebo vis-a-vis the classic treatment.* In studying mortality, the FDA suggests adopting 50% of the lower margin of this CI. Figure 1.15 shows the non-inferiority limits and the interpretation of the CI of the results accordingly. The new treatment is non-inferior as long as the

calculated difference acquires any value between Δ (highest limit of acceptable inferiority in favor of classic treatment) and passes by 0 (no difference between both classic and new treatments). Any extra positive value in favor of the new treatment is an acceptable bonus but not the reverse, of course. Put it this way, *the result has to fulfill two conditions: it should not bypass (Δ) otherwise, the new treatment is worse than the classic treatment and should include (0) otherwise, the new treatment is significantly worse than classic treatment.*

In addition, a difference bypassing both the null (0) and a (Δ) value in favor of the new treatment can be considered as a significant superiority. However, we should interpret it with caution. One reason is that the sample size of a "unilateral" study is smaller by about 20% of that calculated for a routine bilateral study aiming to show which is better the new or the classic treatment. The resultant is that the unilateral NIF study is usually underpowered to be interpreted as a bilateral superiority study. One more reason is that sample size calculation of the NIF trial is mainly dependent on the chosen value of (Δ), with small changes predominantly affecting study power [10]. Researchers can avoid this drawback by initially calculating the sample size for both aims: non-inferiority and superiority.

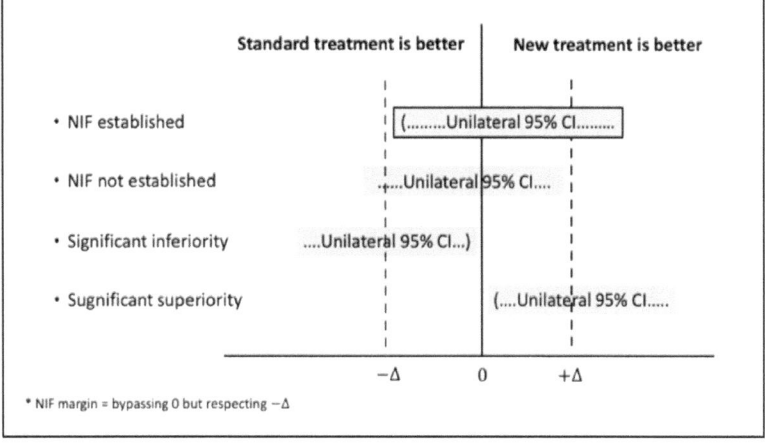

Fig. 1.15 Interpretation of the unilateral 95% CI of the non-inferiority (NIF) study The CI is statistically significant when it bypasses the null (0) and respects the lower limit of the NIF margin (Δ)

To conclude upon non-inferiority, the 95% confidence interval of the difference between the new and the classic treatment has to include zero (both treatments can equal) and, its lower limit has to respect the pre designed non-inferiority margin (new treatment is expected to always behave better than placebo when the latter was compared to the classic treatment).

The Equivalence Study

The aim of an equivalence study is not to prove that both treatments are strictly equivalent, simply because this can never be true. The term equivalence means that the efficacies of the two therapies are close enough so that one cannot be considered superior or inferior to the other. However, and like its unilateral NIF version, we have to define the clinically irrelevant (Δ) that we are willing to overlook. Equivalence is usually tested using a *two one-sided test (TOST) procedure*: one to prove that new treatment is "no more worse" than classic by more than (Δ) and the other to prove that classic is "no more worse" than new by more than (Δ). An approach that was found by many investigators to be more precise than routine bilateral study design [10]. Each of those unilateral tests adopts the usual primary risk of error (α) of 5%. Both treatments are equivalent if they exclude both possibilities;

i.e., 2α and hence, the CI of equivalence = $(1-2\alpha) \times 100\%$ and not the usual $(1 - \alpha) \times 100\%$; which is equal to a bilateral 90% CI. As shown in Fig. 1.16, the bilateral 90% CI is included between $(+\Delta$ and $-\Delta)$ and, in order to conclude upon equivalence, the difference between both treatments should be included in this interval and respecting both upper and lower margins. Figure 1.17 shows the interpretations of the superiority, non-inferiority and equivalence studies.

To conclude upon equivalence, the 90% bilateral confidence interval of the difference between the new and the traditional treatment has to include zero (both treatments can equal), together with respecting the pre-designed equivalence margin on either side.

1.4.2.9 The Confidence Interval of Variance

Whenever the variation of values –rather than the mean—is the most important, as in the case of laboratory measurements; an IC at 95% (or else) can be assigned to the calculated variance (S^2), provided that the distribution is normal "Eq. (1.15)" [4]. In small samples, t replaces z, as usual.

$$S^2 \pm 1.96 Se\sqrt{2} \qquad (1.15)$$

Fig. 1.16 Interpretation of the bilateral 90% CI of the equivalence study. The CI is statistically significant when it bypasses the null (0) and respects both NIF margins ($-\Delta$ and $+\Delta$)

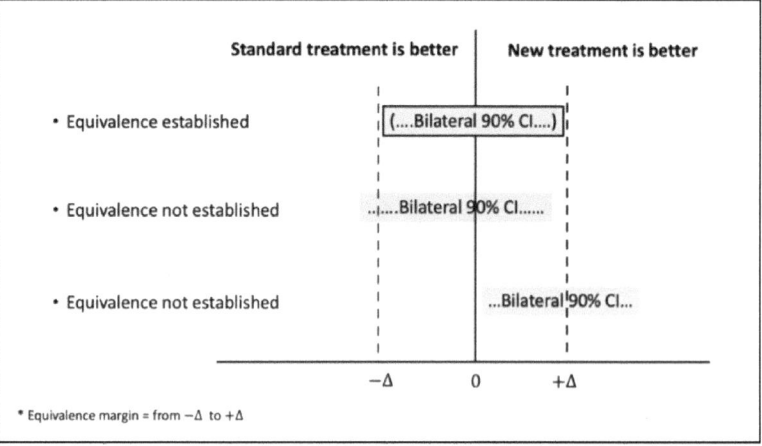

Fig. 1.17 The statistically significant bilateral 95% confidence interval (CI) of the superiority study, unilateral 95% CI of the non-inferiority (NIF) study and the bilateral 90% CI of the equivalence study

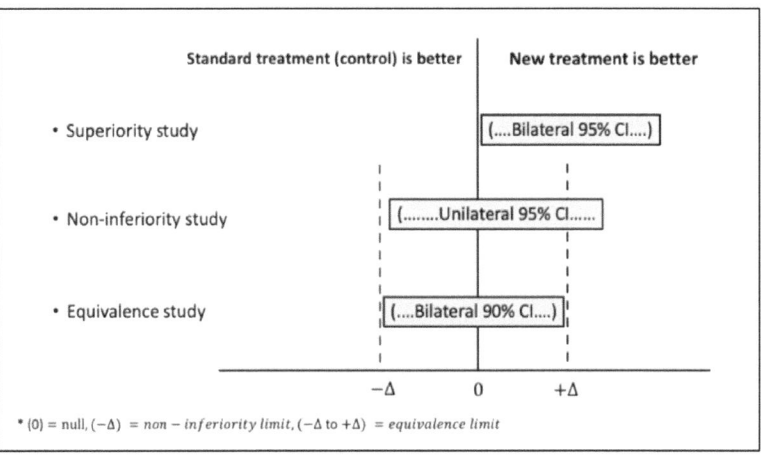

1.4.2.10 The Confidence Interval of an Event that Has Never Happened

The confidence intervals calculated for the small series of patients are wide compared to larger series and hence, they should not supply reliable evidence. Let us take the example when we apply a new procedure. The safety of the procedure should remain in question, even if the reported adverse events are nil. In fact, when the complication rate of a certain procedure is reported to be zero, the upper limit of the IC at 95% equals 3/n. This is Hanley's formula, where (n) is the number of procedures performed that should be at least 30 [11]. If for example only 10 procedures were performed without any complication, our result is still statistically compatible with a high complication rate of 30% (3/n = 3/10). It follows that the more we operate upon patients, the less is the expected maximum risk of adverse events. The calculations can equally be easily made online [7–9].

1.4.3 Verifying Normality

Normal distribution of a variable (sometimes called: normality) is not a universal rule, but rather a condition frequently met in biology. Normality does not mean "being normal" in the common sense of the term, otherwise, its absence would indicate an abnormality [4]. It usually refers to the normal distribution of the variable in population from which the sample was drawn rather than to the sample itself [1, 4]. A small sample taken from a normally distributed population may not be normal itself and, the larger the sample, the smaller is the variability and hence, the probability to show normality [1, 4, 12]. For example, serum albumin is normally distributed in the population. Consequently, we can assume normal serum albumin in any sample drawn from the same population, even if we cannot demonstrate it.

The normal distribution is practically expected to be verified if the number of values in the sample (i.e., studied patients) is >30 per group. In the case of a qualitative variable, we can expect a normal distribution in large samples, with both np and n $(1 - p)$ are >5; where p and $(1 - p)$ are the proportions of a 2-classes qualitative variable and n is the number of values [4]. As an example, if the proportion of males to females is 4:6, normality can be achieved if we include 13 males $(13 \times 0.4 = 5.2)$ and ten females $(10 \times 0.6 = 6)$, at the least. Normality can be checked out visually, by calculating skewness and kurtosis and by formal statistical testing.

1.4.3.1 Visual Check: The Histogram, Normal Q-Q Plot

Once data are collected, normality should be looked for because parametric statistical tests such as ANOVA, Student test, linear regression, etc. require that the dependent variable is approximately normally distributed for each category of the independent variable (see Sect. 2.1). For example, if we compare the duration of hospital stay in days (dependent variable) in patients benefiting from 2 different surgical techniques (independent variable) by the test of Student, the duration of hospital stay in days should have a near-normal distribution in both patients' groups. The simplest way is to plot a histogram of our data using excel or else and verify if the relative frequencies of observations are near a standard normal distribution. Returning to our example of baby boys and baby girls (Table 1.2), the 102 newly born babies were 50 males and 52 females, and hence, we should check out normality in both genders. Figures 1.18 and 1.19 show *the histograms* plotted for both genders and, apparently, both histograms satisfy normality. Note that we are not looking for strict normality but for near normality.

A good alternative would be a make a normal plot, which is a plot of the cumulative frequency distribution data against those expected in a standard normal distribution. In other words, we plot data against their equivalent Z values. If both

distributions match, the plot will give a more or less straight line, of course. Because we plot the quantiles of both distributions, this plot is also known as *the normal quantile or Q–Q plot.* Returning to our example of baby boys and baby girls (Table 1.2), data in both Q–Q plots performed for both genders coincide with the straight line, with few being on either side but still near the mainline (Figs. 1.20 and 1.21).

1.4.3.2 Calculation of Skewness and Kurtosis

Skewness

Unlike the normal distribution, a distribution is skewed when the distance between the central value and the extreme is much greater on one side than on the other. On the other hand, if the tail on the right (the part of the histogram next to the right extreme of the distribution) is longer than the one on the left, the distribution is said to be *skewed to the right or positively skewed.* Such distribution indicates that the frequency of values decreases in proportion to the value magnitude. An example, Fig. 1.22 shows the duration of ICU stay of 30 patients, where the majority of

Fig. 1.18 Histogram of birth weight in 50 newly born baby boys showing normal distribution

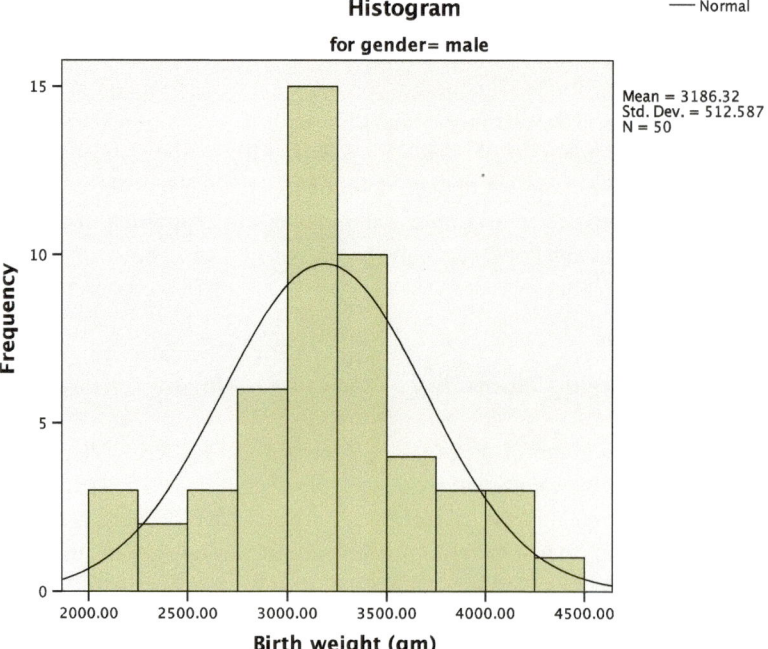

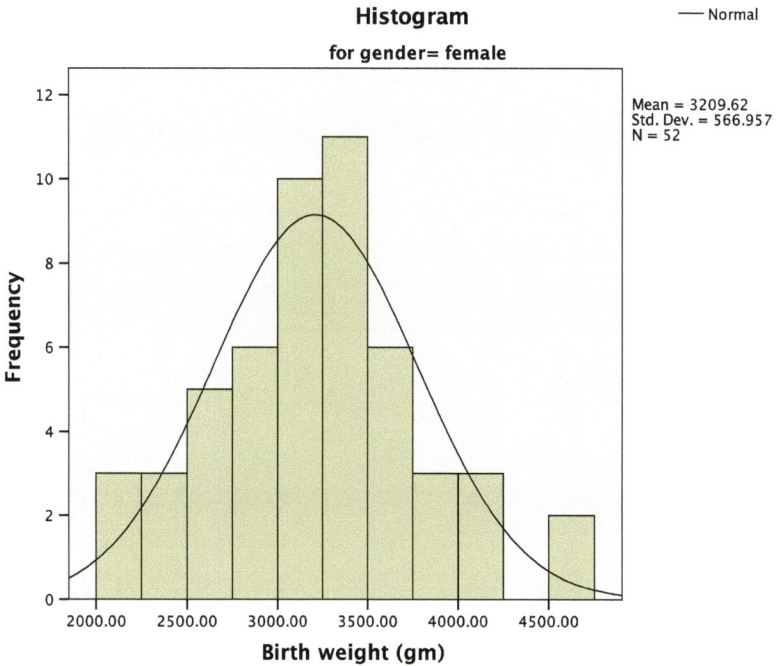

Fig. 1.19 Histogram of birth weight in 52 newly born baby girls showing normal distribution

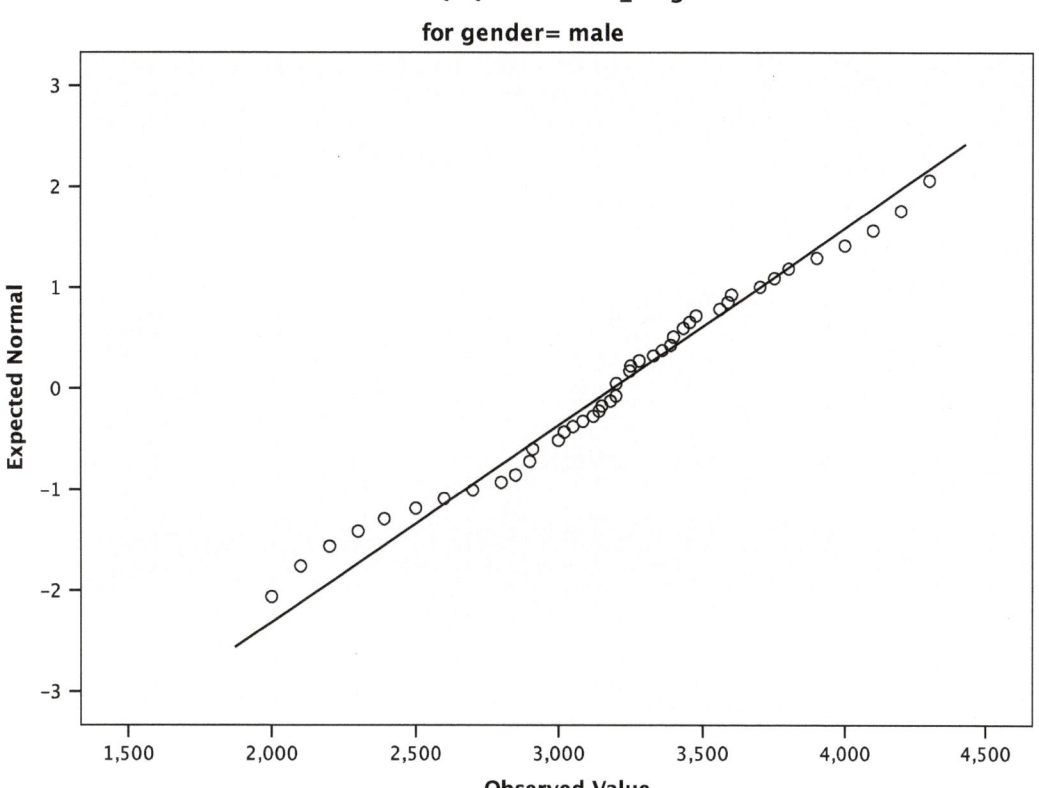

Fig. 1.20 Q–Q plot of birth weight in 50 newly born baby boys showing normal distribution

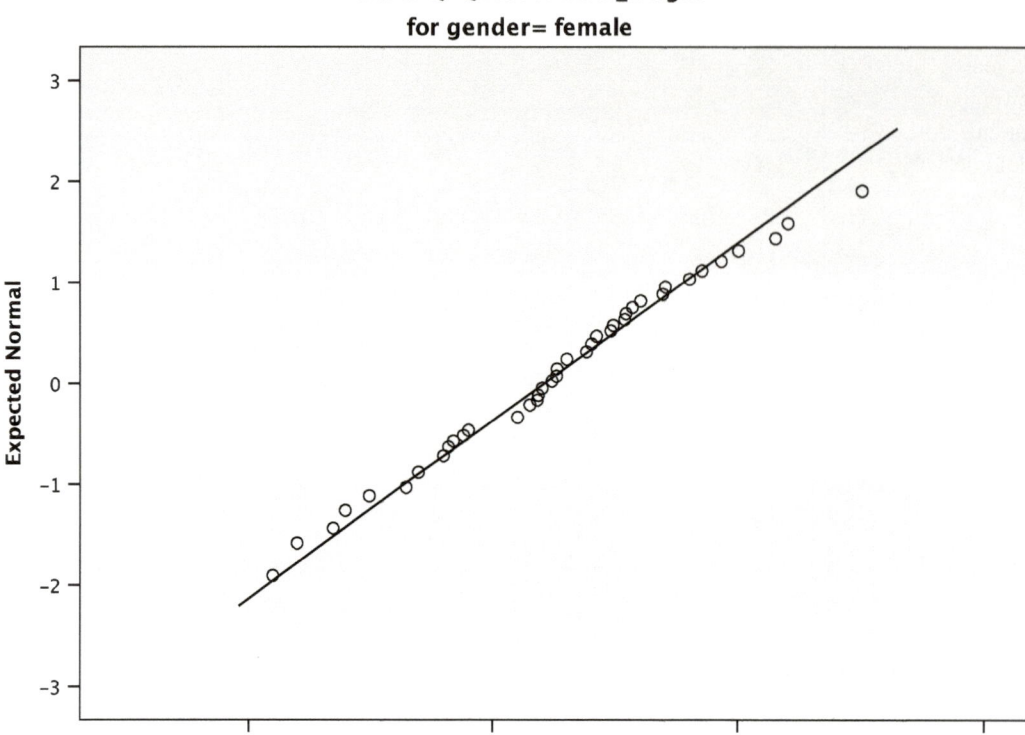

Fig. 1.21 Q–Q plot of birth weight in 52 newly born baby girls showing normal distribution

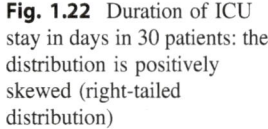

Fig. 1.22 Duration of ICU stay in days in 30 patients: the distribution is positively skewed (right-tailed distribution)

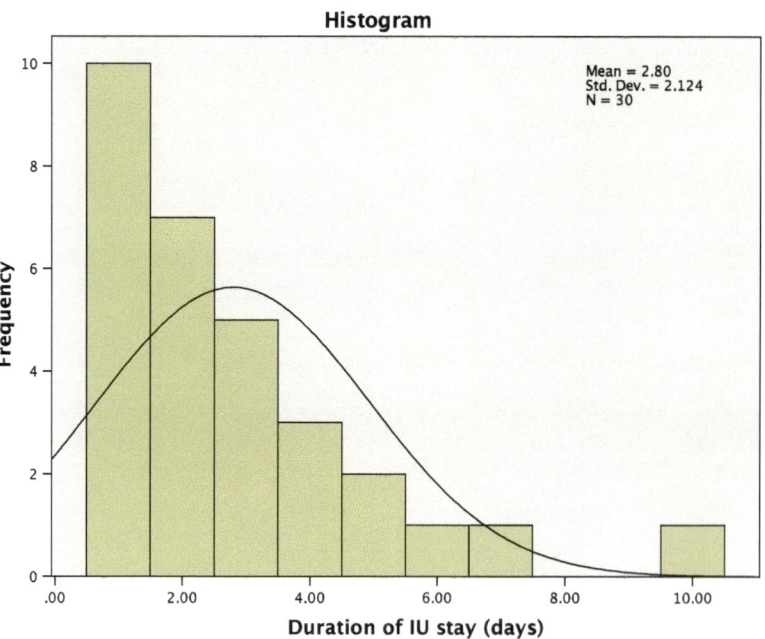

patients stayed for 1 or 2 days and the number of patients staying for more extended periods decreases in proportion to the length of stay: fewer patients stayed for three days and fewer patients for four days and so on. Most of the biological variables are either symmetrical (normal) or skewed to the right.

On the other hand, variables with data being less frequent with smaller values (*negatively skewed to the left*) are few. Data become more frequent as the magnitude of the value itself increases. We show an example: the duration of pregnancy in 30 live births (Fig. 1.23). Although babies can be born alive as early as 28 weeks, the percentage of live birth increases with the advancement of the gestational age. By 36–42 weeks, all babies are forced to be born, and hence the highest frequency will be among those born at the more considerable gestational age. *Statistically, skewness is the relative size of the two tails, and hence, a standard normal distribution has a theoretical value of 0.* Normally distributed samples usually present a certain

degree of skewness that should not significantly violate normality.

Kurtosis

Kurtosis is another measurement of symmetry indicating the combined sizes of the two tails. Many software like excel and SPSS calculate excess kurtosis after subtracting 3, kurtosis of a standard normal distribution. There are many guidelines for the evaluation of skewness and kurtosis. One popular guideline is to accept normality as long as the calculated z values is limited between +1.96 and −1.96. The z value is calculated by dividing the test statistics by the standard error, as usual. Table 1.3 show the calculated skewness and kurtosis reported by SPSS for the observed birth weight in 50 baby boys (Fig. 1.18) and 52 baby girls (Fig. 1.19), as well as for the duration of ICU stay in 30 patients (Fig. 1.22), and the duration of pregnancy recorded for mothers of 30 live-births (Fig. 1.23).

We can quickly note that all z values for skewness and kurtosis in both baby girls and

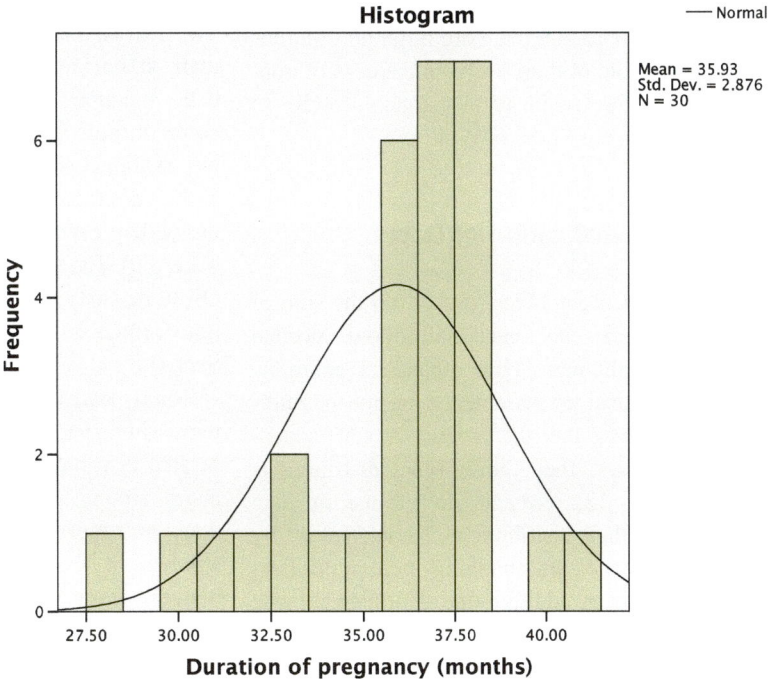

Fig. 1.23 Duration of pregnancy in mothers of 30 live births: the distribution is negatively skewed (left-tailed distribution)

Table 1.3 Part of SPSS output for skewness and kurtosis calculated for different samples

Example	Skewness	Se of skewness	kurtosis	Se of kurtosis
Birth weight of 50 baby boys[a]	−0.17	0.34	0.22	0.66
Birth weight of 52 baby girls[b]	0.14	0.33	−0.07	0.65
ICU stay in 30 patients[c]	1.72	0.43	3.47	0.83
Pregnancy duration in 30 patients[d]	−1.06	0.43	1.17	0.83

[a] = Fig. 1.18, [b] = Fig. 1.19, [c] = Fig. 1.20, [d] = Fig. 1.21

boys are within −1.96 and +1.96 (e.g., the z value of skewness of baby boys = −0.17/0.34 = −0.5), indicating the normal distribution of birth weight. On the other hand, z values of skewness and kurtosis of the positively skewed ICU stay and skewness of the negatively skewed gestational age are all larger than 1.96, indicating a significant difference from normality.

1.4.3.3 Tests of Normality

We can check normality by using the many available tests, such as the Kolmogorov–Smirnov test and the Shapiro–Wilk test. They check whether there is a statistically significant difference between observed data and a standard normal distribution, and hence, a statistically non-significant P-value > 0.05 indicates normality. We have to note that there are different opinions about the value of those tests. In the case of non-concordant results, many investigators prefer to depend upon the Shapiro–Wilk test.

1.4.4 Normalization of Data

Most biological variables result from the sum of many influences and, hence, will follow a normal distribution, human height being an example. Other biological measurements are not the additive result but rather the product of several factors, and hence, they follow other distributions than normal [12]. We can often transform data following other distributions to normality by linearization; i.e., by changing their multiplicative nature to an additive one. Normalization is often achieved by simply taking the logarithm, antilog, square root, reciprocal, or some other data function [12, 13]. Those simple transformations are readily available in many statistical

software such as Excel, SPSS, STATA, and R packages. However, there are cases where the need for a professional statistician is mandatory.

Mathematically, if we multiply two numbers, the log of the product is the sum of their logs, and the difference between two logs is the log of the ratio "Eq. (1.16)". In plain English, the product of 2 values (ab) is equal to their sum (a + b) on the logarithmic scale. It follows that a log transformation can make any multiplicative relationship additive. It can make a skewed distribution symmetrical "normal", and curves can become straight lines [12, 13].

$$\log ab = \log a + \log b$$
$$\log a - \log b = \log (a/b) \quad (1.16)$$

The next step is to analyze the transformed (normalized) data rather than the raw (un-transformed) data. A famous example is the odds ratio (OR), a common outcome used to express the results of observational studies and randomized clinical trials (see Sect. 1.8). Moreover, (OR) is the output of the widely used logistic regression analysis (see Sect. 3.5). The (OR) has to be transformed into log OR to be analyzed. The net results are then back-transformed into OR for final presentation (see Sect. 3.5.2).

Many statistical techniques, such as t-tests, regression, and analysis of variance, require normal distribution of data and equality of variances among the compared group. The latter does not mean strict equality but rather the absence of a statistically significant difference between those variances. *Fortunately, normalizing data often makes the variance uniform as well* [12]. The reader is invited to refer to chapter seven for more procedures of normalization (see Sect. 7.2.1.1).

Normality is a plus but not a necessity. It is a plus because it permits using many powerful and well-known parametric statistical tests. However, it is not always necessary because other tests (known as distribution-free or non-parametric) are not dependent on normality and may be sufficient for the analysis (see Sect. 2.1.2).

1.5   The P-value

We are returning to our example on the birth weight of 102 newborns (Table 1.2). The study showed that the mean birth weight was 3200 g, and the Sd was 540 g. Being normally distributed, 95% of babies from this population will be born with a birth weight that will vary by about 2 (precisely 1.96) Sd around the mean: between 2142 and 4259 g. Any baby whose birth weight falls outside this interval has a slim 5% chance to belong to this population. Once born, and if we decide that this baby is NOT from this population, we should couple this decision with the 5% probability of being wrong, which is nothing but the P-value of this decision. In other words, the P value is the probability that rejecting the null hypothesis was not correct because we could have the same result, while the null hypothesis is true: there is a 5% probability that the birth weight of a baby born from the same population is outside the 95% CI. IN other words, unlike a common misbelieve, the P value is calculated under the null hypothesis and not the alternative hypothesis.

1.5.1   The Primary Risk of Error (α)

Researchers know well that we can never be 100% accurate about our diagnosis, investigations, treatments, or any other decision related to biology. They have agreed that they can make a decision whenever the risk of being wrong is limited to 5% or less. The choice of this 5% cut-off point was just arbitrary for being a small round figure. Although a more negligible risk of error such as 1% may appear safer for our patients, it will deprive them of getting treatments with high margins of benefit between 96 and 98%, which will be unfair.

Nevertheless, this risk is *the primary risk of error, error of primary species or (α),* and a classic example of the terminology is a researcher comparing the effects of 2 treatments. If the study shows that patients receiving treatment (A) improved more than those receiving treatment B, the researcher will conclude that treatment A is better than treatment B. However, when treatment A was then used on other patients, it did not show any effectiveness, and the researcher asked himself: if treatment A is not effective, why did my patients improve in the first place? The answer is simple; if improvement was not due to treatment, it must have been related to the patients themselves, for being less ill, better risk than those receiving treatment B. The cause of the error was mend before (primary) giving treatment, and it should have been due to patients' (species) differences rather than treatment. This "sampling error" is almost inevitable, even in prospective randomized clinical trials.

The P-Value

Every researcher plans and conducts his study under this agreement: we should not accept a primary risk of error above 5%. The researcher collects the data and analyzes the results using the appropriate statistical tests. Each test will calculate the probability of acquiring the results under the null hypothesis, the P-value related to this particular study, and produced by this specific statistical test. If this P-value is at least equal to or smaller than the pre-settled primary risk of error (α), the researcher can conclude; otherwise, he cannot. As shown in Figs. 1.24 and 1.25, the P-value should never bypass the 5% ceiling of (α).

Fig. 1.24 The limit of
rejection (α) of a unilateral
study design

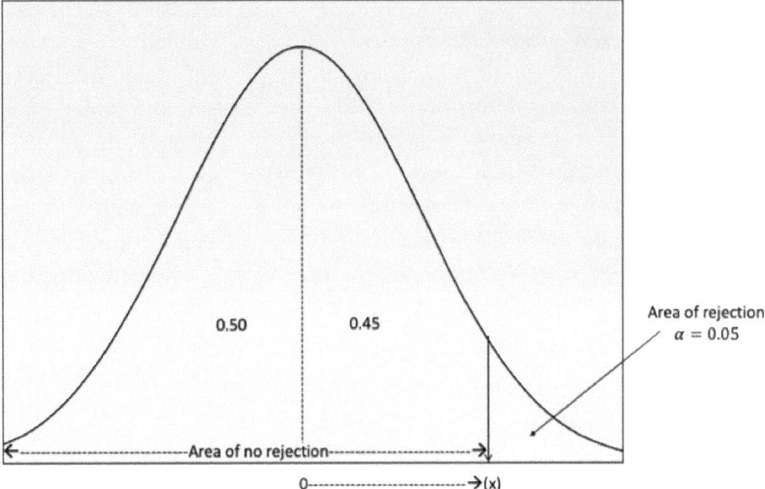

Fig. 1.25 Unilateral study
design: the relation between
the primary risk of error (α)
and P value: X1 and X2 are
two given data points

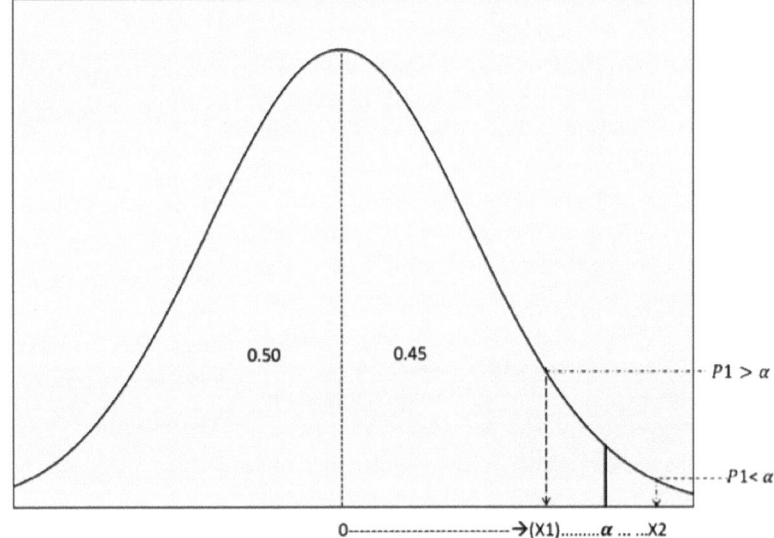

1.6 The Null and Alternative Hypothesis

Let us take the classic example of comparing two treatments A and B, in 2 separate (independent) groups of patients. In order to be fair, the study begins by suggesting that there is no (null) difference between both treatments (A = B), wishing that the experiment will disprove this hypothesis. We have shown before that equality does not exist in the strict sense of the term, and

hence, *the null hypothesis is just a virtual situation and a candidate for disproval but never for approval.* The null hypothesis is a benchmark against which we will test the study results. Once a study shows a considerable difference between treatments (A#B), we cannot support the null hypothesis. We have to admit that such a difference exists. However, as we can never be 100% sure of our decision, we must consider that finding the difference is still a hypothesis, even if this *alternative hypothesis* becomes much more probable than the previous one.

Let us think it over. In biology, variability is the rule, and there is no exception, as previously mentioned. A patient receiving a particular treatment twice will never respond the same both times. Consequently, there will always be a difference (variability) in the response of the "same" group of patients to the "same" treatment, even if small. Let us call this difference "*the within-group variability.*" On the other hand, if we give both groups "different" treatments, the variability of their response is expected to be larger, of course. Let us call the latter: "*the in-between group variability.*" The null hypothesis suggests that the within-group variability is equal to the in-between group variability, and hence treatment A is equally effective as treatment B. In other words, the in-between group variability is small, and hence, it can still be explained by (or considered due to) the expected within-group variability. The larger is the difference between both variabilities, the less we continue to support the null hypothesis. However, we will reach a point that the probability of the null hypothesis being true is as small as 5%. As per the universal agreement, we reject the null hypothesis and adopt the alternative hypothesis: treatments are significantly different (A#B), with *a small 5% risk that the null hypothesis is true (P-value).*

If the difference between both variabilities does not reach the limit of (α), we continue to "maintain the null hypothesis" and invite others to arrange for more studies to reject it. In such a case, our study will be termed a "*negative study*" because it failed to prove that the null hypothesis is not true. Remember that the null hypothesis is never true, simply because strict equality does not exist in life. In other words, the null hypothesis is meant to be rejected but never to be proved.

Figure 1.24 shows the limit of rejecting the null hypothesis. It is rejected whenever the probability of being true drops to as low as 5%, or more, of course. The larger is the difference (distance) between the data observed during the study (x) and the hypothesis of no difference (0),

the more (x) moves away from (0) till it reaches *the limit of rejection denoted by the triangular area on the extreme right-hand side of the curve.* At this point, the probability that (x) can still be equal to (0) drops to as low as 5%, and, per the universal agreement, we reject the null hypothesis. Note that the triangular rejection area represents 5% of the total surface area under the normal distribution curve.

Figure 1.25 shows the relation between the pre-designated primary risk of error (α) and the P-value calculated during an analysis of a particular research. The larger the observed difference, the more our data point (x) moves away from the point of no difference (0). The less probable that the within-group variability can still explain this difference. Although the difference between (0) and (X1) is large, yet the associated probability of the null hypothesis (P1) being true is still higher than the universal pre-designed limit of statistical significance (α). On the other hand, point (X2) is much larger than (X1) and has reached and even bypassed the area of rejection.

Consequently, we can now reject the null hypothesis and conclude that (X2) is significantly larger than (0). As we are never 100% sure of any decision, we have to couple our conclusion with the remaining small probability (<0.05) that the null hypothesis can still be valid. Note that the normal distribution curve is bilateral and symmetrical and that the null hypothesis assumes that there is no difference (0) between compared treatments. In consequence, the same logic will apply, either we were testing if the observed difference (X) is significantly larger (positive) or smaller (negative) than (0).

(α) is the "theoretical" primary risk of error that all studies should respect. The (P-value) is the probability of this error calculated in each study. The result of a particular study is statistically significant whenever its calculated (P) respects the limit of (α), which is conventionally 5%.

1.6.1 Statistical Significance and the Degree of Significance

A P value of 0.05 means that if the experiment is repeated 100 times, in 5 times of which we will reject the null hypothesis, while it is true. In other words, we should expect to reject the null hypothesis and declare a statistically significant, while it should not be, once in every 20 times the P-value is calculated [15]. Consequently, we should limit repeating testing our data to avoid such a bias. It inflates the risk of error and necessitates rigorous methodology and a penalty on the significance limit, as shown later in the post Hoc analysis section. Categorizing P values into borderline, significant, and highly significant has no theoretical background and should not be adopted. We have to report the P-value numerically; however, many investigators find no point in reporting values smaller than 0.001. A small P value of 0.01 means there is only a 1% chance of acquiring a difference at least equal to or larger than the one calculated, while the null hypothesis remains true. Such a small P value has already bypassed the 5% critical limit of statistical significance, but it does not mean that the results are truer but more credible. The truth always remains unknown. In addition, the P value is a function of the sample size. In other words, the larger the sample, the more the probability of getting a smaller P value and achieving the critical limit of statistical significance. Hence, there is no point in comparing the P values of different studies or within the same study [15]. Instead, we can compare effect sizes (see Sect. 4.1.1).

1.7 Testing Hypothesis

1.7.1 A Simple Parametric Test

In order to test the efficacy of a new antihypertensive treatment, 60 cases with mild to moderate hypertension were randomized to either receive the new treatment (treatment A) or Placebo (treatment B). The primary end-point was the

mean systolic blood pressure after three months: 127 ± 15 mm Hg and 132 ± 16 mm Hg for treatments A and B, respectively.

1.7.2 Unilateral Study Design

Every new treatment is primarily tested versus placebo or standard care in which patients do not receive a "real treatment." Such studies aim to prove whether the treatment is effective (and safe) or not? As we will show in a moment, the theoretical "possible" superiority of placebo is never reported, simply because it is never tested in the first place. Before defining the null (H_0) and the alternative hypotheses (H_1), let us think about the three possible results of any study comparing treatment (A) to placebo or standard care (B). There are three theoretical possibilities: (A = B), (A > B), or (A < B). As (A = B) is never true and is the hypothesis that we all want to overthrow, (A = B) is the essential part of the null hypothesis [H_0]. On the other hand, no researcher wants to prove that placebo is better than treatment; this possibility [A < B] then shifts from the alternative hypothesis (what we want to prove) to the null hypothesis (what we want to reject). Put it this way, the null hypothesis of a unilateral study is now composed of two components: treatment and placebo are equally effective (A = B) AND placebo is better than treatment (A < B) "Eq. (1.17)". On the other hand, the alternative hypothesis that we wish to prove is that treatment is better than placebo (A > B) "Eq. (1.18)".

$$H_0: \; (A = B) + (A < B) \qquad (1.17)$$

$$H_1: A > B \qquad (1.18)$$

We begin by examining the variable of interest. The systolic blood pressure is normally distributed, provided that the sample is large (>30 patients); which is our case. Consequently, we are in a position to use the standard normal probability (Z) table [6]. The question posed is the following: is the difference between both means so small that the mean value obtained by treatment (A) could be considered a variation of that obtained by (B) or, it is too large to support the null hypothesis? Remember that the mean of a normally distributed variable has a 95% chance to vary by 1.96 Se in case of a bilateral design and by 1.65 Se in case the design was unilateral (see Sect. 1.4.2.5). If the mean pressure of patients receiving treatment (A) falls outside the 95% CI of those receiving treatment (B), treatment (A) will have a slim 5% chance to be a "replica" of (B). As per the universal agreement, we will reject this small probability and conclude that (A) is significantly different from (B), with the usual 5% risk of error. Otherwise, we will consider that the blood pressure control associated with the new treatment is just an extreme variation of that obtained with placebo, and no conclusion can be drawn from this study.

Suppose that treatment B was a placebo or a standard care (salt restriction). Let us examine whether the mean blood pressure for patients following treatment A was >1.65 Se less than that achieved by those following treatment B; i.e., more effective. Remember that the Se is calculated by dividing the Sd by the square root of the sample size. As we have two standard errors for both A and B, the question is which one to use? We have to use the Se that best represents the population. The best representative is a rule of thumb, the Se of placebo or standard care, followed by that of the classic treatment, in this order. Statistically, the question is, how many standard errors are the two means apart? We proceed and calculate the difference between both means and then divide it by Se of treatment (B) to get the Z score "Eqs. (1.19) and (1.20)". The probabilities associated with those Z scores are perfectly known and are tabulated in the Z table [6], which permits us to assign those exact probabilities to the data values themselves, i.e., the difference between the two means in mm Hg.

$$Z = \frac{(\bar{x}_A - \bar{x}_B)}{Se} \qquad (1.19)$$

$$Z = \frac{(127 - 132)}{16/\sqrt{30}} = -1.71 \qquad (1.20)$$

Figure 1.26 shows our study data applied on the standard normal distribution curve. Note that in a unilateral study, the entire 5% risk of error is confined to the only possible conclusion permitted by a unilateral design; i.e., the new treatment is better than placebo or standard care. The whole (α) is being confined to one tail of the curve, which is why those studies are equally described as one-tailed. As shown, the difference between the sample mean (127) and the mean of the control (132) is translated as Z scores. The latter represents the population from which the sample is supposed to be drawn and hence, it has a Z value of (0). The larger is the mean of the sample, the more it will move to the left side of the population, acquiring a more negative score, as shown in the figure. Once the mean of the sample (in Z values) reaches the critical Z zone starting at 1.65 Se, the probability of being just a variation of the population becomes 5% or less and hence, we can reject the (H_0) and accept (H_1). Our calculated Z score (1.71) bypassed the critical level shown in the figure (1.65), and hence we can conclude that (A) gives significantly better blood pressure control than (B); $P < 0.05$ "Eq. (1.20)". Note that we simply ignored the whole right half of the curve, which can examine the possibility that treatment B gives a better control than A (Fig. 1.26). This possibility was deliberately put in the null hypothesis; hence, it cannot be found because it was not looked for in the first place. In conclusion, a unilateral study aims to show whether treatment is effective by being better than placebo or not, period?

The last step is to check on the degree of significance of 1.71. The cumulative probability given by the table at the intersection of row 1.7 and column 0.01 = 0.9564 is the probability of having any Z score between 0 and <1.71. The

Fig. 1.26 Unilateral study design comparing mean systolic blood pressure of patients receiving new antihypertensive treatment to those receiving placebo (control)

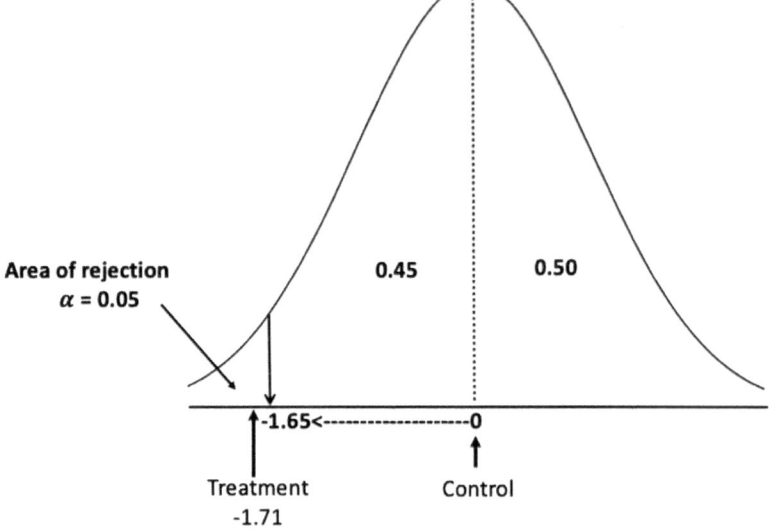

probability of having a Z value ≥ 1.71 is calculated by subtracting (1) from that given by the table: $1 - 0.9564 = 0.0436$. Finally, we can conclude that the new treatment is significantly more effective than the classic additive; P = 0.0436.

Symmetrically, Goldstone LA has tested the effect of a new infantile feeding additive versus standard care therapy [3]. Unlike our study, where treatment is expected to reduce blood pressure, the feeding additive is expected to increase weight, and hence, the calculated Z score will be positive, which will change nothing in the probability. The P value for a Z score of -1.71 is the same as that of a Z score of $+1.71$ due to the mirror image quality of the standard normal distribution curve. Like flipping a coin; the more effective the feeding additive, the more the sample mean moves to the right side of (0), acquiring a more positive Z score till reaching the critical point of Z = (+1.65). Similarly, the exact P-value will be calculated by subtracting (1) from the one given in the table [6].

> The unilateral study design (e.g., whether treatment is better than placebo or not?) permits to conclude upon a smaller difference, compared to the situation where the

study's design was bilateral; knowing that the other probability (placebo is better than treatment) was not tested.

1.7.3 Bilateral Study Design

Now let us suppose that B is not a placebo or a standard care treatment but another active treatment. In consequence, the researcher cannot neglect the probability that this treatment is better than the new one (A < B) and hence, he has to shift this possibility from the null hypothesis to the alternative hypothesis. Consequently, in a bilateral situation, the null hypothesis is formed of only one part: both treatments are equal (A = B) "Eq. (1.21)". The alternative hypothesis is formed of two parts: A > B or A < B "Eq. (1.22)".

$$H_0: A = B \qquad (1.21)$$

$$H_1: A > B \text{ or } A < B \qquad (1.22)$$

The bilateral design is interested in putting into evidence one of 2 probabilities: A > B or A < B; hence, the total 5% risk of error (α) is equally split

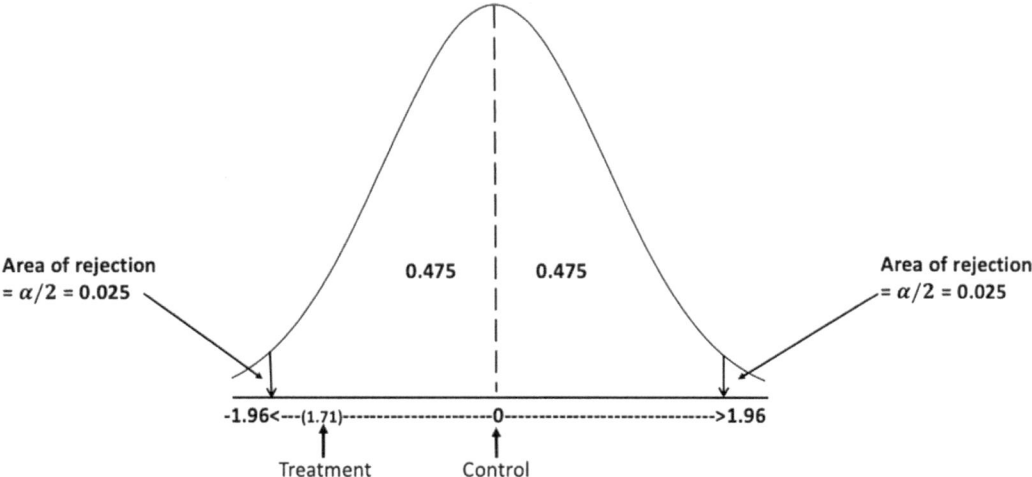

Fig. 1.27 Bilateral study design comparing mean systolic blood pressure of patients receiving new antihypertensive treatment to those receiving active comparator (control)

into two $\alpha/2$, each related to one of the 2 possible alternatives. As shown in Fig. 1.27, we have to have two mirror image critical zones of rejection corresponding to the two possible situations. Splitting the area of rejection into two small halves shifts the critical limits further away from (0), increasing the now two critical limits from 1.65 to 1.96 (-1.96 and $+1.96$). In other words, the new treatment has to be more effective to conclude upon statistical significance, compared to the situation if the same treatment was compared to a placebo. We will then proceed as usual by calculating the difference between the two means and standardizing the difference, using the appropriate Se of the classic treatment. Although we will get the same Z of (-1.71), the latter drops short of the higher critical Z score necessary to reject the null hypothesis in a bilateral study (-1.96). We will conclude that the new treatment did not show a significantly better control compared to the placebo ($P > 0.05$). The table gives the probability of acquiring a value that is either equal or larger than the one given by the table; hence, the probability to acquire a value that is either "equal or larger" OR "equal and smaller" than the one given by the table is simply double. In practice, the probability (area under the curve) associated with our Z value is calculated by subtracting (1) from the probability given by the

table and then multiplying it by 2; $P = 2$ $(1 - 0.9564) = 0.0872$. As the study is now bilateral, the P value ($P = 0.0872$) is larger than the critical limit of 0.05, and we cannot conclude the superiority of the new treatment, despite having the same data as in the previous section (see Sect. 1.7.2). Flipping the coin, if the new treatment gives a higher value than the comparator, the calculated Z score will be positive [3], which changes nothing in the P value [6].

1.7.4 The Secondary Risk of Error

We have previously shown that the primary risk of error (α) is the risk of rejecting the null hypothesis when the null hypothesis is true. Put it this way: it involves the conclusion upon a difference (or a relation) in the study that does not exist in reality. *The (α) error was committed before the beginning of the study (primarily)* by choosing a sample that was not representative of the aimed population or "species" and, in consequence, the conclusion itself will mismatch reality too. This sampling error is almost inevitable even in randomized studies. *The secondary risk of error, risk of secondary species, (β), or type II error* is exactly the other side of the coin. It is the failure to conclude upon a difference in the study despite its existence in reality. Returning to our example and suppose that a second researcher was testing the same anti-hypertensive treatments in a comparable group of patients. Being short of resources, he enrolled only 20 cases per group and observed the same results. As he recruited fewer patients, he had to expect a larger Se due to the smaller sample size; remember that Se = Sd/$\sqrt{n}$ = 16/$\sqrt{20}$ = 3.58. Consequently, the new Z value will be smaller: (127−132)/3.58 = 1.39; stopping short before reaching the 1.645 critical limit of significance.

We have to stop here too and analyze this result: the second researcher failed to demonstrate a difference that has been already demonstrated by the first one! Put it this way: he has failed to put into evidence a difference in the experiment, despite that it exists in reality; which is exactly "the secondary risk of error". The reason behind missing the evidence is obvious: he did not recruit enough patients to show it up. In other words, the study did not have enough power (sample size) to show the reality. This example reflects the high cost of the commonly committed error of not calculating (or underestimating) the number of patients necessary for his study.

The following scenario demonstrates the relationship between the two error types. In order to be "more sure" of results, one may suggest raising the limit of statistical significance (type I error) from the usual 5 to 1%. A 1% limit means that our risk of concluding upon a difference that does not really exist will be only once a hundred times. Although the idea looks attractive, this would also mean that researchers will pass by some significant (important) results between 1 and 5%, without concluding upon them, compared to the standard 5% limit. In other words, type II error increases concordantly, including all results with a P-value between >1 and 5%. On the other hand, lowering the limit of type I error to 10% decreases type II error as we will conclude upon more significantly different results [16, 17].

A 5% limit appeared to be the most reasonable and the universally accepted limit for the primary risk of error but what is the accepted limit of the secondary risk of error? There is no universal agreement on the limit of secondary risk of error but a consensus. It cannot be as large as 50% because it will not differ from tossing a coin. It cannot be as small as 5% because poor non-funded researchers, small pharmaceutical companies, and developing countries will not contribute to research due to the concordant increase in sample sizes and expenses, of course. A mid-way solution was adopted, and *the secondary risk of error is usually set at 10 or 20%*, with only a few researchers adopting a challenging negligible risk of 5%.

1.7.4.1 The Power of a Study

The power of a study is based upon its credibility, i.e., the ability to extend the results to the population. As the secondary risk of error (β) is missing this evidence, the power of the study equals 1 − (β). Setting the secondary risk of error at 0.2 (20%) means that the study has 80% power to detect the evidence, provided that the latter exists. Studies failing to demonstrate the evidence are sometimes called "negative studies" or "negative trials" because they just failed to show what exists in reality. We have to be cautious in interpreting these "negative" trials as being "the evidence of the ineffectiveness of the new treatments," which is wrong. What is more wrong is interpreting this failure that "both treatments are equal," which is wrong too. Studies aiming to show that one treatment is not inferior to the other (non-inferiority studies) or that both treatments are equally effective (equivalence studies) have a different design than the "routine" superiority studies.

The only conclusion we can get from negative studies is that we have failed to demonstrate a significant difference between both treatments [17]. Goodman and Berlin had an interesting comment upon the "extra" recommendation made by many researchers: "larger studies are needed to find the evidence". Setting the secondary risk of error to a certain limit before the study, e.g., 0.2; means that this study has an 80% probability of finding the evidence. In other words, it is designed to find the evidence 80 times out of every 100 possible results. The post-trial result is only one of those 100 possibilities. For example, if we designed a study to compare two hypnotics and the pre-trial minimal statistically significant difference of the duration of sleep was two hours, all the hundreds of differences >2 h are also significant. Hence, power is not only the probability of detecting "the single" 2 h difference but also all those hundreds of potentials statistically significant differences. Looking the other way around, the pre-trial probability of "all non-significant outcomes" taken together is 20%, and attempts to apply power to "the single non-significant outcome" of the study can be problematic. Once the study is terminated and the results are analyzed, power does not remain a meaningful concept. We share their point of view that *best way to express the low statistical power after the study is to calculate the confidence intervals*. The negative studies usually have small sample sizes, and hence, they will produce wide confidence intervals that best express their limited precision [16] (see Sect. 1.4.2.3).

Besides sample size, the power of a study depends upon *the magnitude of the difference* that we wish to demonstrate. The smaller the difference we are looking for, the more likely we will miss it and pass by significant results, and the more we need a powerful test $(1 - \beta)$ and vice versa [15]. More details about the relation between the magnitude of the difference and the study power will be given in Sect. 4.1.1. Power equally depends on *the type of comparison made: whether it is one or two-sided* [12–15]. A unilateral test is more powerful than a bilateral one because we conclude upon a smaller difference (e.g., a Z value of 1.65) than a bilateral design (a Z value of 1.96). A lousy practice uses a one-sided study as a device to make a conventionally non-significant difference significant. More details about factors affecting the power of a study will be discussed in Chap. 4.

1.8 Common Indices of Clinical Outcomes

Outcomes of observational studies, randomized clinical trials, systemic reviews and meta-analysis are usually summarized in meaningful indices; including odds ratio, likelihood ratio, relative risk, risk reduction or increase and number needed to treat or to harm.

1.8.1 The Risk and the Odds

The term "risk" is used to express the frequency (the probability) of a given event among a certain group of patients (population). It is calculated as the number of patients who developed the event to the total number of patients at risk. On the other hand, the odds are the proportion of patients who developed the event to those who did not [4]. As example, if only one case of mortality is recorded in every 4 patients treated, the risk of mortality is ¼ = 0.25 or 25%, while the odds are 1/3 = 0.33 or 33.3%. In this example, both the risk and the odds are indicators of a protective treatment effect however, the interpretation of the risk is straight forwards (treatment decreases mortality by 25%) and can point to causality while that of the odds is somehow ambiguous (the probability of remaining alive is 3 times that of being dead) and is more observational. Despite of this, the odds remain very useful, as will be shown later. Figure 1.28 shows the relation between the risk (probability) and the odds: outside 0, the risk will be always smaller than the respective odds, for having a larger denominator. Risk and odds are interchangeable by a simple equation "Eq. (1.23)"; in our small example, the risk of mortality can be calculated from the odds = 0.333/(1 + 0.333) = 0.248 = 25%.

$$Risk = \frac{odds}{(1 + odds)} \qquad Odds = \frac{risk}{(1 - risk)}$$

$$(1.23)$$

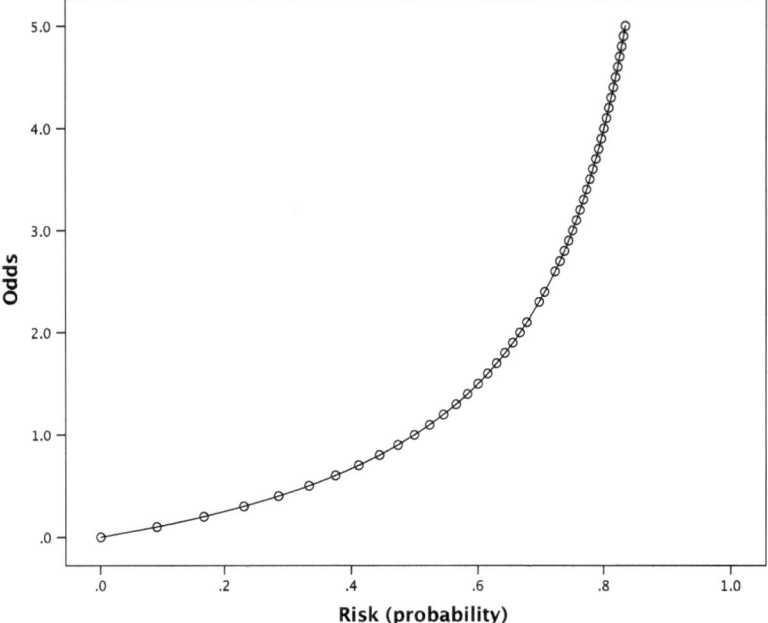

Fig. 1.28 The relation between the odds and the risk (probability), according to Eq. (1.23)

1.8.2 The Relative Risks and the Odds Ratio

Most clinical studies compare a treatment to a control group, with the latter being usually a placebo or a classic treatment. Table 1.4 shows the abbreviations used in this section to calculate the odds and the risk in both groups. N, (n_t) and (n_c) are the total number of patients, number of patients in the treatment group and number of patients in control group; (a) and (b) are number of patients who developed the event and those who did not, in the treatment group; (c) and

(d) are number of patients who developed the event and those who did not, in the control group.

The relative risk (RR) is the ratio between 2 risks: risk (probability) to develop the outcome in the treatment group and the risk (probability) in the control group "Eq. (1.24)". The odds ratio is between 2 odds: The odds in the treatment group and the odds in control "Eq. (1.25)". A (RR) of 1 means equal risks, and an OR of 1 means equal odds between the two groups. A ratio >1 means higher risk (or odds), and a ratio <1 means lower risk (or odds) in the treatment group compared to the control group. Returning to the interpretation

Table 1.4 Calculation of the risk and the odds in the treatment and the control groups

	Event (+)	No event (−)	Total
Treatment group	(a)	(b)	(a + b = n_t)
Control group	(c)	(d)	(c + d = n_c)
Total	(a + c)	(b + d)	N

(a), (b) and (a + b = n_t) = number of patients who developed the event, number of patients who did not develop the event and total number of patients; all being calculated in the treatment group. (c), (d) and (c + d = n_t) = number of patients who developed the event, number of patients who did not develop the event and total number of patients; all being calculated in the control groups. (a + c) = total number of patients who developed the event, (b + d) = total number of patients who did not develop the event, (N) = the grand total number of patients = (a + b = n_t) + (c + d = n_c) = (a + c) + (b + d) of the risk and the odds and completing the small example given above, the risk of mortality in the treatment group was 0.25 (1 mortality for every four patients treated), and the odds were 0.33. Suppose that there were two mortalities in every four patients in the control group; the respective risk and odds will be: 0.5 and 1. The RR and the OR will be equal to 0.5 (0.25/0.5) and 0.33 (0.33/1). Note that empty cells (a, b, c, d) can cause problems with computation of the relative risk, odds ratio, or their standard errors, which we can solve by adding (0.5) to all cells (a, b, c, d) [18].

$$\text{The relative risk} = RR = \frac{a/(a+b)}{c/(c+d)} = \frac{a/n_t}{c/n_c} = \frac{p_t}{P_c} \quad (1.24)$$

$$\text{The odds ratio} = OR = \frac{a/b}{c/d} = \frac{ad}{cb} \quad (1.25)$$

The straightforward interpretation of the RR (treatment decreases mortality by 50%) tempts the researchers to interpret the odds ratio similarly. In other words, instead of saying that "the proportion of mortalities/survivors in the treatment group is only one-third that recorded in the control group," they will be tempted to interpret the odds ratio as a risk ratio and say that "treatment reduces mortality by 33%". However, this "approximate" reduction is only 33%, compared to "a true" 50% reduction, as calculated by the "proper" estimate: relative risk. This approximation is only valid when the probability of the event is rare. We should avoid using the odds ratio as a relative risk when the event is common,

as in our example, and when there is a large discrepancy between the prevalence in both groups [19]. The more frequent is the outcome in the sample (>10%), the more the odds ratio overestimates the risk ratio when it is >1 and underestimates it when it is <1 and, the same applies to OR derived from logistic regression [20]. Zhang and Yu proposed a simple formula to calculate the RR from OR "Eq. (1.26)". Fortunately, the simple formula can be applied to calculate the lower and upper borders of the 95% confidence interval [20]. Applying the formula in our small example gives a RR of 0.5 "Eq. (1.27)".

$$RR = \frac{OR}{(1 - P_c) + (P_c \times OR)} \quad (1.26)$$

$$RR = \frac{0.33}{(1 - 0.5) + (0.5 \times 0.33)} = 0.5 \quad (1.27)$$

We advise the young researcher to calculate those indices by hand at least once. We believe that understanding "the formulation of the equation" is mandatory for a correct interpretation of the results. Afterwards, those indices can be easily calculated using an online calculator [7–9].

1.8.2.1   The Two Relative Risks

Table 1.5 shows the relationship results between having a history of rheumatic fever and the development of mitral valve stenosis. Looking at data prospectively: among the 60 patients with a positive history of rheumatic fever, 25 (42%) developed mitral stenosis. On the other hand, out

Table 1.5 Relation between the presence of a history of rheumatic fever and the development of mitral valve stenosis in 100 patients

		MS		Risk	RR	Odds	OR
		Yes	No				
RF	Yes	25 (a)	35 (b)	0.42		25/35	
	No	5 (c)	35 (d)	0.125	3.3	5/35	5
Risk		0.83	0.5				
RR		1.7					
Odds		25/5	35/35				
OR		5					

MS = mitral stenosis, RF = rheumatic fever, RR = relative risk, OR = odds ratio, (a) and (c) = number of patients who developed the event in the group at risk and in the control group, (b) and (d) = number of patients who did not develop the event in the group at risk and in the control group, respectively of the 40 patients who did not have this history, only five patients (12.5%) developed mitral stenosis. Authors can draw a straightforward conclusion: having a history of rheumatic fever triples the risk of developing mitral stenosis later on (RR = 0.42/0.14 = 3.3). *This straightforward relationship explains why the RR is the index of choice in clinical trials*, which main aim is to show the effect of a predictor (having a risk factor, following a particular type of treatment, etc.) on study outcome (developing a disease, attaining cure, etc.).

Looking the other way round: out of the 30 patients who have mitral stenosis, 25 cases (83%) had a history of rheumatic fever, compared to 35 cases out of the 70 patients (50%) who do not have mitral stenosis. Authors can deduct that the "presence" of mitral stenosis was associated by 66% increase (RR = 0.83/0.5 = 1.66 times) in the probability of having "a positive history" of rheumatic fever. We have 2 different relative risks here, depending upon which variable is the predictor and the outcome variable. The risk to develop mitral stenosis (outcome) if one has a rheumatic fever (predictor) is different from the risk of having a history of rheumatic fever (outcome) if the patient has already mitral stenosis (predictor). *The relative risk is a unilateral index that interprets the effect of the risk factor on the outcome; hence, switching the risk factor and the outcome gives a different relative risk.* In table 1.5, the risk of developing mitral stenosis in patients who had rheumatic fever = a/(a + b), while the risk of having a positive history of rheumatic fever in patients already presenting with mitral stenosis = a/(a + c); the numerator is the same but the denominator changes and hence, the risk changes too. The same calculation applies to patients in the control group, of course.

1.8.2.2 One Odds Ratio

Looking to data prospectively: the odds of having or not having mitral stenosis in the group at risk (patients with rheumatic fever) equals a/b (25/35), the respective odds in the control group equals c/d (5/35), and hence the OR = ad/cb = 5. Looking the other way round, the odds of having or not having a history of rheumatic fever in patients already having mitral stenosis = a/c = 25/5, the respective odds in the control group = b/d = 35/35, and the OR = ad/cb = 5. Unlike the relative risk, the odds ratio is always the same. *The OR expresses the tightness of the relation between two variables, irrespective of which is the predicting factor and which is the outcome variable?* The OR is a bilateral index and is more suitable for observational studies that are not usually concerned with causality.

The adjusted odds ratio in logistic regression

The multivariable analysis is commonly used to determine the independent contribution of multiple covariates or predictor variables (e.g., age, gender, weight, etc.) to an event or outcome (e.g., the development of hypertension). Multivariable models have multiple similarities but differ in the outcome variable (see Chap. 3). In binary logistic regression, the outcome is a dichotomous qualitative variable (e.g., the patient is cured or not, the treatment is effective or not, etc.), making the OR the perfect index to express the effect of the predictors on the outcome. The model calculates the effect of the predictor variable (e.g., age of patients) on the outcome (e.g., mortality), adjusted on the presence of other predictors in the model (e.g., type of treatment, gender, presence of other risk factors).

The adjusted OR ratio is interpreted as follows: "a unit change" in the predictor "changes the odds of the outcome" by an average amount equal to the calculated OR. For example, a binary logistic regression model showing that age (calculated in years) significantly affects mortality by an odds ratio of 2 is interpreted as follows: each year increase in age doubles the odds of mortality, holding other predictors constant (type of treatment, gender, other risk factors). If the OR of the female gender was 0.5: "being a female reduces the odds of mortality by half", holding other predictors constant. The model equally calculates the 95% confidence intervals of OR, and the reader is advised to refer to Sect. 1.8.7.2 for the accurate interpretation (see Sect. 1.8.1.2). We will discuss the logistic regression model and the use and interpretation of the resulting OR in Sect. 3.5.

Describing the relationship between two qualitative variables, we have two relative risks but a single odds ratio. The RR is a one-way index expressing the effect of one variable (the risk factor) on the other variable (outcome); switching the risk factor and the outcome yields a different RR. On the other hand, the OR is a standard two-way index expressing the tightness of the relation between the two variables, ignoring which is the predicting factor and which is the outcome variable?

1.8.3 The Hazard Ratio

1.8.3.1 The Hazard Ratio Versus the Relative Risk

Hazard ratio (HR) is the ratio between 2 hazards: the hazard of developing the event in the treatment group to the corresponding hazard in the control group "Eq. (1.28)". Hence, an HR of 1 means equal hazard between the two groups. An HR > 1 (or HR < 1) means higher hazard (or lower hazard) in the treatment group, compared to the control group, respectively. The HR is a commonly reported outcome in time to event analysis when we are primarily concerned—not with the total number of events—but rather on how long it takes for a particular event to occur. As the risk is technically different from the hazard, we should not interpret the calculated HR as the relative risk (RR). The risk is the probability of developing an event. It is calculated as the number of cases that developed the event to the total number of patients at risk. On the other hand, the hazard is the probability of developing the event, at a specific time (t), provided that the patient was still at risk and did not experience the event before that time. For example, if the outcome event is "cure" and a group of patients were followed up for five years, a RR of 2 means that twice as many patients in the treatment group are expected to be cured after five years as the control group. In other words, the RR is

cumulative. An HR of 2 means that any time during the five years, twice as many of patients in the treatment group are expected to be cured, compared to the control group; i.e., the HR is instantaneous.

$$
HR = \frac{H_T}{H_C}
$$
$$
= \frac{New\ cases_T/Patients\ remaining\ at\ risk_T}{New\ cases_C/Patients\ remaining\ at\ risk_C}
$$

(1.28)

Table 1.6 and Fig. 1.29 show the development of an event (cure) over a 5 years follow-up period in 200 patients, equally divided between treatment and control. By 5 years, a total of 53 patients in treatment group were cured, compared to only 25 patients in control group and hence, the RR = $(7 + 9 + 11 + 12 + 13)/(4 + 5 + 6 + 7 + 8) = 53/25 = 2.2$. Look at the five-time intervals from t1 to t5 and note the "changing" hazard ratios compared to the "one fixed" final relative risk.

1.8.3.2 The Hazard Function in Time to Event Analysis

We usually follow up our patients for multiple reasons, such as time to cure, recurrence of symptoms, or development of a particular complication. We use the hazard function to describe the probability for a patient to experience a specific event at a particular time (t), provided that he was free from that event till that time. In the case of mortality; it is a hazard for a person to die in the next few seconds, provided that he is still living just right now. As time is a continuous variable and the event is supposed to occur at random, the probability of the event happening strictly at the time (t) is extremely small. Theoretically, it is equal to zero. For example, what is the probability of someone dying exactly on August 23rd, the year 2022, at 13 h, 50 min, 33 s, and 0.000000… 1 fraction of a second? It is impossible to calculate the hazard that an event occurs precisely at a given time (t) = h(t) = 0. On the other hand, we can calculate *the probability for an event to occur in a specific interval of time*; e.g., from the beginning of the study and

Table 1.6 The hazard of cure in 200 patients equally randomized between treatment and placebo and followed up for 5 years period

Time intervals	Group	Patients at risk[a]	Cure	Hazard	Hazard ratio[b]
t1	Treatment	100	7	0.07	
	Control	100	4	0.04	1.75
t2	Treatment	93	9	0.09	
	Control	96	5	0.05	1.8
t3	Treatment	84	11	0.13	
	Control	91	6	0.07	1.9
t4	Treatment	73	12	0.16	
	Control	85	7	0.08	2
t5	Treatment	61	13	0.21	
	Control	78	8	0.1	2.1

t1 to t5 are five yearly time intervals, [a] = patients who were not cured and still living at the beginning of the (t) time interval, [b] = hazard in treatment group/hazard in control group

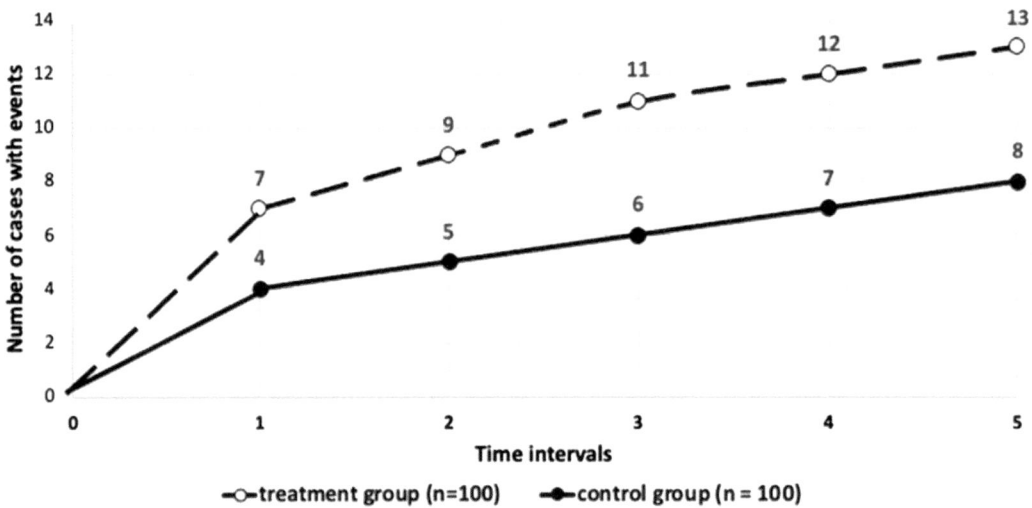

Fig. 1.29 The hazard of cure for patients presented in Table 1.5

up to time t = h(<t) or from time (t) up to a more significant time interval that we can call delta = h (t + dt).

The second question would be: *is the hazard stable, or does it change with time, and if it does change, what would be its direction and magnitude?* Hazard is dependent upon the variable of concern and the researcher has to study the distribution of this variable and choose the best fitting model. In this section, we will discuss the three most commonly used models, which mainly differ in the way by which hazard is

supposed to function. In *the exponential model*, the hazard is supposed to be constant; i.e., the hazard rate is the same for a given period (e.g., one month), regardless of whether this period is at the beginning of the study, in the middle or late in the study. In *the Cox proportional hazard model*, the hazard is supposed to be a function of time: it can sometimes increase and sometimes decrease with time, but it always keeps the same ratio between the treatment and the control groups. In other words, the hazard rates are changing, but the hazard ratio is constant. In *the*

Table 1.7 The baseline hazard in Cox regression in 200 patients equally randomized between treatment and control and followed up for three years

Time intervals	Group	Patients at risk[a]	Mortality	Censored cases	Mortality rate	Hazard ratio[a]
1st year	Treatment	100	3	0	0.03	
	Control	100	4	0	0.04	0.75
2nd year	Treatment	97	6	3	0.06	
	Control	96	8	1	0.08	0.74
3rd year	Treatment	88	9	1	0.10	
	Control	87	12	2	0.14	0.72

[a] = Hazard ratio calculated from raw data: mortalities/patients at risk

Weibull model, the hazard can decrease, can be constant, and can increase too. In conclusion, we can calculate the hazard during a certain period rather than at a specific time. There are several models for calculation depending upon the distribution of the variable of concern. It is up to the researcher to find the best fitting model for his study.

The hazard function in Cox proportional hazard model

Cox proportional hazard regression analysis is a combination between 2 techniques: survival analysis and regression analysis. The idea of the analysis is to divide the effect of time into a series of repeated observations over specific time intervals and to calculate the corresponding series of probabilities of new cases developing the event of interest; which will finally provide an overall reference: *the baseline hazard function* [$h_0(t)$]. Cox proportional hazard assumes that the basic hazard function is time dependent and is free to vary (to increase or to decrease), as time goes by. Meanwhile, the model assumes that the hazard ratio (hazard rate in the treatment group/hazard rate in the control group) is unrelated to time and hence, it remains constant at all times and at all hazard rates. Put it this way, the hazard of both groups can change with time but they have to maintain the same proportionality. Table 1.7 shows the calculated mortality rates and hazard ratios in 200 patients equally randomized between treatment and placebo and followed up for 3 years. In this example, the hazard of mortality increases overtime (nearly doubled by the second year and tripled by the third year) but the hazard ratios remain almost the same (0.72–0.75). As time to event do not follow a normal distribution, this part of Cox model is called the non-parametric component of Cox regression (Table 1.7).

The parametric part of the Cox model is "a routine" regression analysis. The model weights the effect of each predictor ($\times 1$, $\times 2$, $\times 3$, … $\times k$) on the outcome as the adjusted HR. *Because the HR is assumed to be constant throughout the study, any change is supposed to be due to the effect of the predictors.* The calculated HR ratio is interpreted as follows: "a unit change" in the predictor "changes the hazard of the outcome" by an average amount equal to the calculated HR. For example, a study has shown that age calculated in years and male gender were independent predictors of mortality, with respective hazard ratios of 1.1 and 1.5. The interpretation is as follows: there is an average 10% increase in the hazard of mortality, relative to each one-year increase in age or, the expected hazard is 1.1 times higher in a person who is one year older than another, holding other predictors constant. The expected mortality hazard is 1.5 times higher in men than women, holding all other predictors constant. The model equally calculates the 95% confidence intervals of HR, and the reader is advised to refer to Sect. 1.8.7.3 for the accurate interpretation of those intervals. Kindly refer to

Sect. 3.6 for the detailed calculations of the Cox model itself.

The hazard function in the exponential distribution

The famous French mathematician Poisson (1781–1840) described the probability distribution of a number of discrete events occurring in a fixed time interval, e.g., the number of attacks an asthmatic patient can experience during 24 h-period. Events are assumed to be independent: the occurrence of an event does not prevent, delay or invite another one, and hence, *the exponential distribution has no memory. Events are supposed to occur at a constant rate*: the probability of an event to happen in a specific time interval (e.g., during the day, the first year of follow-up, etc.) is the same for any interval with a similar length (during the night, during any other follow-up year, etc.). In the case those two conditions were fulfilled, Poisson found that the probability of occurrence of the event can extend from 0 to infinity and that it will be dependent upon the average number of times the event has occurred (λ). Examples in medical research include the probabilities of occurrence of attacks of asthma, the likelihood of a patient being cured of disease or gene mutation during a specific time (t), based upon our previous known average number of events (λ).

As Poisson describes how many times events occur during a fixed time, the exponential distribution describes the length of time between 2 successive events, and hence, it looks like the other side of the coin. It changes the question from how many events occur in a fixed time to how much time is needed until the next event? Taking the example of a study on 100 patients, where we have observed 50 events (recurrence of attacks of bronchial asthma) in one year. The average number of events recorded during one year = (λ) = 50/100 = 0.5 event (Poisson distribution of events). Flipping the coin, the average time between 2 successive events = (1/λ) = two years (exponential distribution of time). Put it this way: it took one year for a patient to have 0.5 events, and hence, we need two years to produce

a whole event. Note that Poisson distribution is discrete (we cannot have a "true" fraction of an event), while exponential distribution is continuous for fractions of time being true. A characteristic of both distributions is that their standard deviations are also equal to the means.

Based on this information, the question would be: what is the probability for a patient to experience an event within a specific time (<t), let's say two years. Remember that time is a continuous variable, and hence, the probability of having an event at any specific time (t) is zero. Consequently, we are looking for the cumulative probability: from the beginning of the study and up to 2 years (t). Provided that the variable in question fulfills the two assumptions required by a Poisson distribution, *the hazard of having the event (He) will be dependent upon the previously known average number of events* ($\lambda = 0.5$) *and the expected time frame in question* (t = 2 years) "Eq. (1.29)". By deduction, the probability of being alive or being free from the event at the time (St) is (1) minus the latter "Eq. (1.30)".

$$Exponential\ hazard = H_e(<t) = 1 - e^{-\lambda t}$$
$$(1.29)$$

$$Event\text{-}free\ cumulative\ probability\ (S_t)$$
$$= 1 - \left(1 - e^{-\lambda t}\right) \qquad (1.30)$$

Figure 1.30 shows the cumulative event-free hazard (St) for the 100 patients, calculated yearly for 10 years. The dotted horizontal lines represent (St) calculated for ≥ 1 year (61%), ≥ 2 years (37%), and ≥ 3 years (22%). We can directly calculate (St) by a hand calculator: upload (minus λt) and then click on the [e^x] key. The cumulative hazard at (<t) is then obtained by deducting (St) from (1). As an example, (St) at ≤ 2 years is calculated by uploading (-0.5×2) and then clicking on [e^x] key = 37%. By deduction, the exponential hazard (He) = 1 − St = 1 − 37% = 63%.

The interpretation of the results is that each patient has a 63% chance to experience an asthmatic attack during the next two years and, by deduction, an 37% probability of remaining free

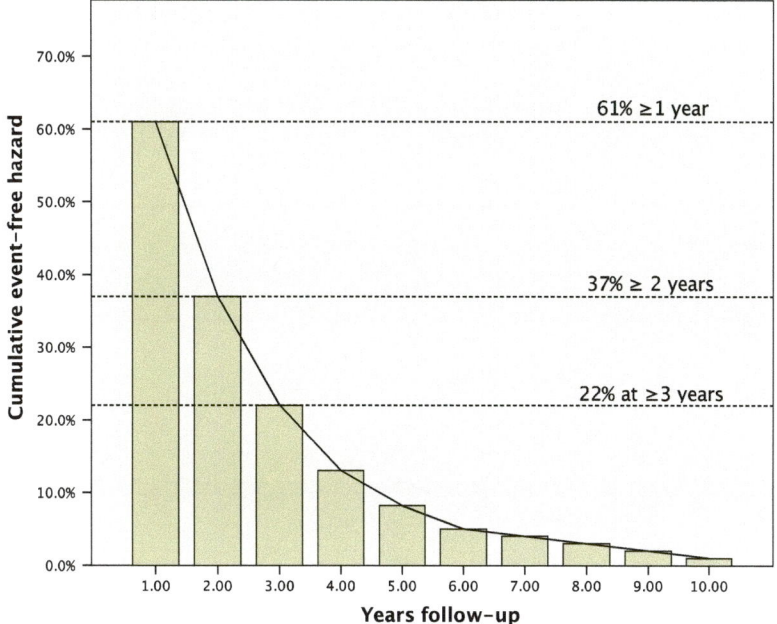

Fig. 1.30 Cumulative event-free rate (development of bronchial asthmatic attack) in 100 asthmatic patients followed up for ten years

from bronchial asthma. The mean time to event is = $(1/\lambda)$ = 1/0.5 = two patients/year; i.e., every patient's average duration needed to produce one event is two years. We can calculate the median time-to-event as $(\ln2/\lambda)$ = 0.693/0.5 = 1.39 patients/years. The interpretation is as follows: every patient has a 50% chance to produce one event every 1.4 years. Like in Cox regression analysis, the hazard function can be estimated by a regression model adjusting for multiple predictors in the study and calculating the effect of each predictor on the outcome; using the equations shown before. The main and essential difference will be that the basic hazard (b_0) does not change with time like in Cox regression, but it is supposed to be constant. In Fig. 1.30, it is quite clear that the cumulative event-free probability decreases with time, which means that the hazard increases, in contradiction to the basic assumption of the hazard being stable. As hazard = new events/number of patients at risk at the time (t), we remove the patients who developed the event

from the following calculation (t + 1), which gives this false impression of increased hazard.

The hazard function in Weibull distribution

The Weibull distribution is a continuous probability distribution named after the Swedish mathematician Waloddi Weibull (1887–1979), who initially proposed the distribution as a model for material breaking strength. Early after been manufactured, the "defective" products are diagnosed and are removed from the market. The remaining "good" products will then continue to function appropriately, experiencing constant random failures. In the end, instruments are affected by wear and tear due to "aging" and stop by failing in an accelerating fashion [21].

The model was extrapolated in many sciences, including economics and biology. In humans, the hazard of infant mortality is initially high, but it tends to decrease with time after all diseased babies have been eliminated by natural selection. The risk of mortality becomes constant and

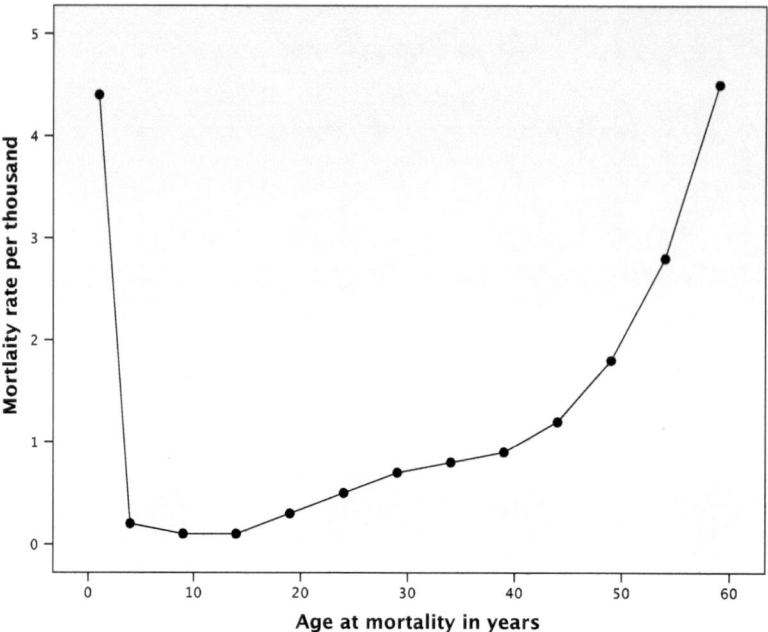

Fig. 1.31 The mortality rate in Canadian population (2019) till the age of 59 years. Dots represent mortality rates calculated for subjects who died before 1 year of age, from 1–4 years, then every 5 years till the age of 59 years

random during adulthood. However, it starts to increase with a progressive rate later with patients getting older [21]. Figure 1.31 shows the characteristic bathtub pattern in an extract taken from official mortality records for Canadian subjects who died before the age of 60 years [22]. The initial high infant mortality rate (0.44%) dropped sharply to 0.02% in subjects who died between one and four years. Following periods of stability during adulthood, mortality started to increase slowly then progressively till it regained its initial high rate (0.45%) in subjects who died between 55 and 59 years. However, looking at the global figure representing all subjects, the improvement in geriatric care extended life expectancy but with significant increase of mortality rates up to 18.8% in patients dying at the age of 90 years or older [22]; giving a more or less tongue-shaped pattern for the overall period of life (Fig. 1.32).

The main difference between Weibull distribution and the previous 2 models is *the basic hazard function that is supposed to be either stable, increasing with time or decreasing with time*. Looking to our bathtub or tongue shaped

pattern: there is a constant hazard of mortality, regardless of the patient's age, but there is a second hazard of mortality related to the phase or age period; being decreasing in children, stable during adulthood, and then increasing with aging. *The basic hazard of the Weibull model is the sum of 2 parts.* A constant hazard of random mortality that is not related to time (h_0), plus a second part related to time $\alpha(t)$; all being calculated in the log scale to normalize hazard, as usual "Eq. (1.31)".

Weibull basic hazard $= \log(h_0) + \log(\alpha) * \log(t)$

$$(1.31)$$

It is the value of (α) that dictates the direction and magnitude of baseline hazard. Remember the properties of the logarithmic scale, namely, log (1) is equal to zero, log (>1) gives a positive value, and log (<1) gives a negative value. In case ($\alpha = 1$), the part of the hazard related to time will be equal to zero [log(α) * log(t) = 0 * log (t) = 0], and the basic hazard is reduced to the constant part only (log h_0). In the case of ($\alpha > 1$), the part of the hazard related to time acquires a positive value that will be added to the constant

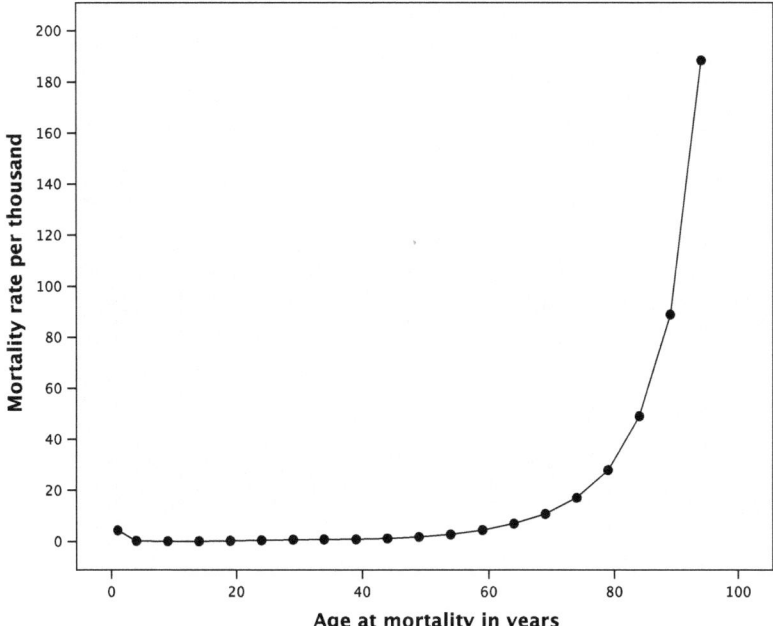

Fig. 1.32 The mortality rate in Canadian population (2019). Dots represent mortality rates calculated for subjects who died before 1 year of age, from 1 to 4 years, then every 5 years till the age of 89 years. The last rate represents subjects who died at the age of 90 years or after

part of the hazard and, the basic hazard will increase with time. In the case of $(\alpha < 1)$, the part of the hazard that is related to time acquires a negative value that will be subtracted from the constant part of the hazard and, the basic hazard will decrease with time.

> The relative risk (RR) is not the hazard ratio (HR). If the outcome is cure and follow-up is for 5 years; a RR of 2 means that after 5 years, twice as much of patients in the treatment group are expected to be cured, compared to the control group; i.e., the RR is cumulative, which is why it is the outcome of choice in randomized clinical trials. A HR of 2 means that any time during the 5 years, twice as much of patients in the treatment group are expected to be cured, compared to the control; the HR is instantaneous, which is why it is the outcome of choice in time-to-event analysis.

1.8.4 Relative Risk Increase (RRI) and Relative Risk Reduction (RRR)

Table 1.8 shows the results of 3 years follow up for the risk of sudden death, in a total of 800 patients with aortic valve stenosis (AS). Patients were divided into 4 equal groups according to the severity of the disease (moderate or severe) and to the method of treatment (medical treatment or aortic valve replacement). In both groups, surgery was associated with 5% mortality however, the rate of sudden death in patients treated medically was as high as 30% in cases presenting with severe AS, compared to only 15% in those presenting with moderate AS.

Although the outcome in each category was clear, we are more interested in the comparative results, that is, the outcome in one group relative to the outcome in the other. *The relative risk (RR) is the risk in the treatment group relative to (divided by) that in the control group.* In our example, the RR of surgery was 33% in patients

Table 1.8 Sudden death after three years in patients with either moderate or severe aortic stenosis

Aortic stenosis (n = 800)	Surgery	Medical treatment	RR	RRR (%)	ARR	NNT
Moderate (n = 400)	10/200 (0.05)	30/200 (0.15)	0.33	67	0.1	10
Severe (n = 400)	10/200 (0.05)	60/200 (0.3)	0.17	83	0.25	4

RR = relative risk, RRR = relative risk reduction, ARR = absolute risk reduction, NNT = number needed to treat

with moderate AS (0.05/0.15 = 0.33) and 17% in patients with severe aortic stenosis (0.05/0.3 = 0.17). In patients with moderate AS, the mortality risk due to surgery is one-third of that associated with medical treatment. The risk drops down to only one-sixth for patients with severe AS.

We can put it another way: surgery has reduced the risk of sudden death in patients with moderate AS by 67% (*relative risk reduction* = RRR = 1 − RR = 1 − 0.33 = 0.67) and in patients with severe AS by as much as 83% (RRR = 1 − RR = 1 − 0.17 = 0.83), compared to medical treatment. In general, if (P_c) is the probability of the event in the control group and (P_t) is the probability in the treatment group, the RR = P_t/P_c, with beneficial treatments giving relative risks below one. As RRR = (P_t/P_c) − 1, a RRR of zero indicates no benefit or harm associated with the active treatment, whereas a RRR of 1 could mean a "cure" [23]. It is worth saying that although both: RR and RRR are usually used in the context of preventing an adverse event, they can also be used to describe a favorable outcome that we intend to increase by treatment. In such a case, a beneficial treatment will give a RR > 1, and it becomes more logical to use the term "*relative risk increase*" (RRI) instead of the word "relative risk reduction" (RRR). In such a case, the relative risk increases (RRI) = 1 − RR.

1.8.5 Absolute Risk Increase (ARI) and Reduction (ARR)

Although the relative risk reduction (or increase) clarifies the comparison, it doesn't show precisely the weight of this 67% or that 83% change on the absolute scale. Simple subtraction shows

that the risk of sudden death has dropped by 10% in patients with moderate AS and by as much as 25% in patients with severe AS. A negative value indicates a beneficial treatment that reduces the risk on the absolute scale, while a positive value will indicate a harmful treatment. Unlike the RRR, the absolute risk reduction (ARR) may tell less about proportional effects. Yet, it says a great deal about whether an effect is likely to be clinically meaningful: beneficial or harmful and to what extent [23]. A negative ARR shows that surgery is always helpful for patients, regardless of the severity of the aortic lesion. On the absolute scale, surgery decreased the risk of sudden death in patients with severe AS 2.5 folds those presenting with moderate AS.

1.8.6 Number Needed to Treat Benefit (NNTB) and Number Needed to Harm (NNTH)

A closer look at the follow-up results of the 400 patients presenting with moderate AS (Table 1.8): we saved 20 lives by referring 200 patients to surgery instead of medical therapy. In other words, we can save ten lives out of every 100 patients referred to surgery and, by simple deduction, we can save one life each time we treat ten patients surgically, which is the number needed to treat (NNT). The NNT is the number of patients we have to treat to prevent one adverse event, which is mortality in our example. The NNT is simply the reciprocal of ARR = 1/0.1 = 10 patients. In the case of severe AS, the gain associated with surgery is much more impressive, and we can save one life by only treating four patients surgically = 1/0.25 = 4 patients. Although every life is precious, it remains small on the absolute scale, especially in the eyes of the decision-makers [23, 24]. View the inherent limitation of resources in all health care systems; it would be more reasonable to direct the resources to treat patients with severe AS before those presenting with moderate AS. As patients in both cases benefited from the treatment, the NNT just described is usually called: number needed to treat benefit (NNTB). In the case where treatment is associated with an increase in the risk of events, the absolute risk is increased (becomes positive). It is then called the absolute risk increase (ARI) and, its reciprocal value is better called the number needed to harm (NNTH). The NNTH is interpreted as follows: one more adverse event will be produced if the patients are given the treatment. Put it this way; those patients will be harmed instead of getting a benefit.

1.8.7 Calculation of the 95% Confidence Interval and Testing Statistical Significance

1.8.7.1 The 95% CI of the Relative Risk

As previously mentioned, the null of a ratio is 1, with values larger than 1 representing causative or positive effects and those smaller than one representing preventive or negative effects. In general, risk ratios (e.g., relative risk and odds ratio) have a skewed distribution but their logarithmic values are approximately normal. For example, the log of a risk ratio of 2 equals (0.69) and the log of its inverse value 1/2 equals (−0.69), the log of a risk ratio of 4 equals (1.39), and the log of its inverse value (1/4) equals (−1.39), etc. Normality permits the calculation of a standard error, the creation of a 95% confidence interval and testing statistical significance, all in the logarithmic scale. Afterwards, results are converted back to the arithmetic (original) scale for more comprehensive presentation. Although plotting the symmetrical logarithmic scale is also recommended, Rothman and colleagues suggested that the asymmetrical arithmetic scale is a better reflection of the quasi-important risk and ratio differences [25].

As shown in "Eq. (1.32)", we calculate the standard error (Se) of the normalized risk ratio (Log RR) as the square root of the sum of the reciprocals of a, c, (a + b) and (c + d), shown in Table 1.4 [26]. The standardized value of log (RR) is then routinely calculated by dividing log (RR) by its Se "Eq. (1.33)". The statistical significance of the standardized Log RR is then checked in the Z table, as usual. We can produce a 95% CI for Log RR by assigning 1.96 Se (Log RR), on either side "Eq. (1.34)". The resulting upper limit (UL) and lower limit (LL) of this interval are then anti logged (exponential) to get the corresponding upper and lower limits of the 95% CI of the relative risk itself, "Eq. (1.35)" [26, 27].

$$Se(\log RR) = \sqrt{\frac{1}{a} + \frac{1}{c} + \frac{1}{a+b} + \frac{1}{c+d}}$$
(1.32)

$$Z = \frac{(\log RR)}{Se(\log RR)}$$
(1.33)

$$95\% \ CI(\log RR) = (\log RR) \pm 1.96 \ Se(\log RR)$$
(1.34)

$$95\% \ CI(RR) = e^{LL \ 95\% \ CI(\log RR)} \ \text{to} \ e^{UL \ 95\% \ CI(\log RR)}$$
(1.35)

Taking the example of the RR of developing mitral stenosis in patients presenting with rheumatic fever, compared to those without rheumatic fever (Table 1.5). The relative risk is 3.33, Log RR = 1.2, the Se = 0.445, the 95% CI of Log RR = 2.07 to 0.328, the 95% CI of RR = 1.39 to 7.98, Z value = 2.7 and P = 0.007. The interpretation of the result is straightforward: the presence of rheumatic fever significantly increases the risk of developing mitral stenosis by 1.4 to 8 times that of the patients who did not have rheumatic fever. Let us check on the details of calculations by taking the example of the RR of sudden death after surgery in patients presenting with moderate AS, compared to those treated medically (Table 1.6). The RR = 0.3333, Log

RR = −1.099, Se Log RR = 0.38 "Eq. (1.36)". The 95% CI of Log RR = −1.85 to −0.35 "Eq. (1.37)", the z value = 2.89 and P = 0.0038 "Eq. (1.38)". The back transformation of the log values, produces a 95% CI of RR = 0.16–0.7 "Eq. (1.38)". The interpretation is that the risk of sudden death in patients presenting with moderate AS is between 16 and 70% of its preoperative value; i.e., surgery significantly decreases the risk (RRR) of sudden death in moderate AS by 30–84%.

$$Se(\log RR) = \sqrt{\frac{1}{10} + \frac{1}{30} + \frac{1}{200} + \frac{1}{200}} = 0.38$$
$$(1.36)$$

$$95\% \ CI(\log RR) = -1.099 \pm 1.96(0.38)$$
$$= -1.85 \ to - 0.35$$
$$(1.37)$$

$$Z = \frac{-1.099}{0.38} = 2.89; \quad P = 0.0038 \quad (1.38)$$

$$95\% \ CI(RR) = e^{(-1.84)} \ to \ e^{(-0.35)} = 0.16 \ to \ 0.7$$
$$(1.39)$$

Applying the same formula on patients presenting with severe AS, the RR equals 16.7%, the lower and upper limits of the 95% CI 9–32%; Z = 5.48 and P < 0.0001. The risk of sudden death after surgery in severe AS is only 9–32% of its preoperative value; i.e., surgery decreases the risk (RRR) by as much as 68–91%. Calculations can be easily made online [7–9]. Small differences in our example can be due to the approximations made during the hand calculations.

1.8.7.2 The 95% CI of the Odds Ratio

The odds ratio has a skewed distribution, too. Log OR is approximately normal, and its graphical presentation is usually plotted in the logarithmic scale. Playing the same tune, OR is normalized by a change in scale (Log OR), and its standard error (Se Log OR) is estimated as the square root of the sum of the reciprocals of the four frequencies showing in Table 1.4: a, b, c, and d "Eq. (1.40)" [28]. The statistical significance of the OR is checked by consulting the Z table for the P-value associated with the standardized value of Log OR, calculated as: (Log OR)/Se (Log OR) "Eq. (1.41)". The 95% CI of Log OR is produced by assigning 1.96 Se (Log OR), on either side of (Log OR) "Eq. (1.42)". The resulting upper limit (UL) and lower limit (LL) of this interval are then anti logged (exponential) to get the corresponding upper and lower limits of the 95% CI of the odds ratio itself "Eq. (1.43)" [28]. In the example given in Table 1.5, OR = 5. Log OR = 1.61 and the Se of Log OR = 0.545. We can produce a 95% confidence interval for the log odds ratio by assigning 1.96 standard errors on either side of the estimate (0.54–2.67). We can easily obtain the 95% CI of OR's upper and lower limits by simple antilog of the corresponding logarithmic limits (1.7–14.5).

$$Se(\log OR) = \sqrt{\frac{1}{a} + \frac{1}{b} + \frac{1}{c} + \frac{1}{d}} \quad (1.40)$$

$$Z = \frac{(\log OR)}{Se(\log OR)} \quad (1.41)$$

$$95\% \ CI(\log OR) = (\log OR)$$
$$\pm 1.96 \ Se(\log OR) \quad (1.42)$$

$$95\% \ CI(OR) = e^{LL \ 95\% \ CI(\log OR)} \ to \ e^{UL \ 95\% \ CI \ (\log OR)}$$
$$(1.43)$$

Applying the same equations on data presented in Table 1.5, the 95% CI for the odds ratio calculated for patients presenting with moderate AS (0.298) is 0.14–0.63, with a Z value of 3.18 and a P-value of 0.0015. The 95% CI for patients presenting with severe AS (0.123) is 0.06–0.25, with a Z value of 5.87 and a P-value < 0.0001. The interpretation is that there is a statistically significant tight negative relation (for OR < 1) between surgery and the occurrence of sudden death. In other words, surgery is associated with lower mortality compared to medical therapy. The association is more pronounced in those patients presenting with severe AS.

The Role of Prevalence

We invite the reader to compare the results of RR and OR calculated for patients presenting with moderate AS (RR = 16–70% versus

OR = 0.14–0.64 = 14–63%) as well as those calculated for patients presenting with severe AS (RR = 9–32% versus OR = 0.06–0.25 = 6–25%). The results of RR and OR are pretty comparable to one another because the prevalence of sudden death in the control group is only 5%. We have previously shown that for low prevalence up to 10%, the odds ratios can be interpreted as risk ratios. Consequently, we can conclude that surgery was associated with significantly smaller "risks" of sudden death (14–63% in patients with moderate AS and 6–25% in patients with severe AS), compared to those following medical treatment. Calculations can be easily made online using any available free online calculators [7–9]. Any detected small difference will be due to the approximations made during the hand calculations.

1.8.7.3 The 95% CI of the Hazard Ratio

We have to use a statistical package to estimate the Se and the 95% CI of HR calculated in Cox proportional hazard regression analysis. However, we can obtain an approximated confidence interval, assuming that the event rate is constant over time [29]. The hazard ratio can be estimated as the ratio between the median survival of the treatment (S_t) and the control groups (S_c) "Eq. (1.44)". The Se of log HR ratio can be estimated from the number of events in both treatment (E_t) and control groups (E_c) "Eq. (1.45)". We calculate the 95% CI of log HR "Eq. (1.46)" and invert its upper and lower limits to get the 95% CI of the HR "Eq. (1.47)".

$$HR = \frac{S_t}{S_c} \tag{1.44}$$

$$Se(\log HR) = \sqrt{\frac{1}{E_t} + \frac{1}{E_c}} \tag{1.45}$$

$$95\% \ CI(\log HR) = (\log HR) \\ \pm 1.96 \ Se(\log HR) \tag{1.46}$$

$$95\% \ CI(HR) = e^{LL \ 95\% \ CI(\log HR)} \ to \ e^{UL \ 95\% \ CI(\log HR)} \tag{1.47}$$

1.8.7.4 The 95% CI of the Absolute Risk Difference and the Number Needed to Treat

The absolute risk reduction (ARR) is the difference between two risks and hence, we can assign a 95% CI, like any other difference between two proportions "Eq. (1.48)". On the other hand, the NNT is like the "arithmetic mean" but is just one number, and hence, it cannot be used to create an interval of confidence. As the NNT is the reciprocal value of the ARR, the upper and lower limits of its 95% CI of the former will be the reciprocal values of those calculated for the latter [23]. Taking the example given in Table 1.5, we calculate the 95% CI of the absolute risk reduction (ARR). The latter is simply the difference between 2 risks (2 ratios): proportion of sudden death in the treatment group $(P_t = 0.05)$ and proportion of sudden death in the control group $(P_c = 0.15)$ and is equal to −0.1. The Se of the confidence interval of the difference (Se_d) equals the square root of the sum of both standard errors, as usual. We can produce a 95% CI by assigning 1.96 Se_d, on either side of the ARR "Eq. (1.49)". The same can be applied to patients presenting with severe AS, of course "Eq. (1.50)".

$$95\% \ CI(ARR) = ARR \pm 1.96 \ \sqrt{\frac{P_t(1-P_t)}{n_t} + \frac{P_c(1-P_c)}{n_c}} \tag{1.48}$$

$95\% \ CI(ARR) \ moderate \ AS$
$$= -0.1 \pm 1.96 \sqrt{\frac{0.05(0.95)}{200} + \frac{0.15(0.85)}{200}}$$
$$= -0.158 \ to \ -0.042 \tag{1.49}$$

$95\% \ CI(ARR) \ severe \ AS$
$$= -0.15 \pm 1.96 \sqrt{\frac{0.05(0.95)}{200} + \frac{0.3(0.7)}{200}}$$
$$= -0.18 \ to \ -0.32 \tag{1.50}$$

The upper and lower limits of the 95% CI of the NNT are just the reciprocal of those values. As we cannot have a fraction of a patient, we approximate calculations to the higher number, being 7–24 patients in moderate AS and only 4–6 patients in severe AS. Note that the ARR was negative, meaning that the risk is decreased by surgery; i.e., patients will benefit. In consequence, the calculated NNT are called numbers needed to treat benefit (NNTB).

Suppose that the study included only 80 patients in each disease category, equally divided between surgery and medical treatment, with the same proportions of success being achieved. In the 40 patients presenting with moderate AS, we had 1 case of sudden death in the 20 patients treated surgically (5%) and 3 cases of sudden death in the control (15%). Despite the same ARR of −10%, the 95% CI will widen because of the small sample size, overlapping the null (−0.283 to +0.083); i.e., the CI will include zero or the possibility of no difference between treatment and control (i.e., an ineffective treatment) "Eq. (1.51)". The 95% CI of the ARR can be presented as −0.283 to zero to +0.083. The reciprocal values will be (+3.55) to (∞) to (−11.99), which is approximated to the highest number: (+4) to (∞) to (−12). As we calculate the ARR by subtracting the risk of the treatment group from that of control, a "negative" value means a beneficial treatment effect. Its reciprocal value has to be "positive," indicating the number of patients we have to treat to prevent (1) adverse events. A positive number to treat is called number to treat benefit (NNT benefit = NTTB). On the other hand, a positive ARR means that the risk increases with treatment, i.e., a harmful treatment. Its reciprocal value will be negative, indicating the number of patients treated will result in an extra event (harm), which is why the latter is called the number needed to harm (NNT harm = NNTH) [27]. In this way, we can get rid of the disturbing negative sign by presenting NNT as NNTB and NNTH. Whenever treatment is associated with a bad (undesirable) outcome, as compared to the control group, it is better to use relative risk increase (RRI), absolute risk increase (ARI), and NNTH instead of RRR, ARR, and negative NNTB [27].

$95\% \ CI(ARR)$ moderate AS in a small sample

$$= -0.1 \pm 1.96 \sqrt{\frac{0.05(0.95)}{10} + \frac{0.15(0.85)}{10}}$$
$$= -0.283 \ \text{to} \ +0.083$$

(1.51)

According to Altman D, there are three difficulties with this confidence interval (+4) to (∞) to (−12). Firstly, one of the NNT is negative (−12). At the same time, logically, an NNT can only be positive. Secondly, if we can interpret an ARR of zero as the treatment is useless, how can we interpret its reciprocal value of an NNT that equals infinity? Finally, it may be difficult to imagine how the CI (−12 to 4) includes the calculated NNT of 10 [27].

We have just shown that a negative NNT is the reciprocal of a "positive" ARR, reflecting that the new treatment can induce harm by reducing the number of patients who can benefit by one, every time 12 patients receive the new treatment. Concerning the second difficulty, we have to go back to the origin of NNT, which is the ARR. In our example, the 95% CI of the latter ranges between an absolute risk increase of 28% (treatment has harmful effect) and an absolute risk reduction of 8.3% (treatment has a beneficial effect). Logically, the transition between being harmful and being beneficial, has to pass by having no effect. In other words, the upper and lower limits of the 95% CI passing from (+28%) and (−8.3) has to include zero. As the reciprocal value of zero is infinity, the 95% CI of the NNT (−12 to +4) includes infinity. The question is what does infinity mean? As an ARR of zero means that the treatment has no effect, its reciprocal value NNT (∞) means that the treatment makes no difference whatever is the number of patients treated (ARR = 0 and NNT = ∞).

Concerning the third difficulty, we have to interpret the scale of NNT Benefit or Harm while considering the ARR or ARI. The scale of the absolute risk difference (ARR or ARI) starts from −100% ARR (every patient will benefit from the treatment) and ends by 100% ARI (the treatment will harm every patient), passing in the middle by zero (treatment has no effect). The NNT is just the reciprocal of those values, and hence, the NNT has the following scale: on one extreme side, the unattainable value of an NNTB = 1 and on the other extreme end an NNTH = 1, passing by infinity. It is clear that, rather unusually, infinity is in the middle of the scale, not at the ends [24, 27]. In our example, going from an NNTB = 4 to (treating an infinite number of patients) will eventually include the best estimate (NNTB = 10). As (∞) is in the middle of the scale, progressing on the same scale will cross over to the other side (from NNTB to NNTH) and finally ends with an NNTH of 12. Reporting our results as 10 NNTB; 12 (NNTH) to ∞ to 4 (NNTB) solve both afro-mentioned problems by embracing the best estimate (NNTB 10) and avoiding the negative results.

NNT in Meta-Analysis

In a meta-analysis, NNT is calculated from a pooled ARR, which does not consider that studies may have included patients with different characteristics or prognoses. The source of bias is that different patients' groups have different basal risks: i.e., a different prevalence for each group: P_{c1}, P_{c2}, P_{c3}, etc. A more logical way is to multiply the reciprocal pooled ARR calculated for all trials by each basal risk to deduct a range of all possible numbers needed to treat for the different basal risks "Eq. (1.52)" [30, 31]. In the case of trials reporting odds ratio, we can also derive the NNT from the odds ratio (OR) and basal risk (P_c) "Eqs. (1.53) and (1.54)" [32].

$$NNT = \frac{1}{(RR \times P_c)} \quad (1.52)$$

$$NNT_{Benefit} = \frac{1 - P_c(1 - OR)}{P_c(1 - OR) \times (1 - P_c)} \quad (1.53)$$

$$NNT_{Harm} = \frac{P_c(OR - 1) + 1}{P_c(OR - 1) \times (1 - P_c)} \quad (1.54)$$

NNT in Time-to-Event Studies

The NNT is the number of patients who need to receive the treatment to prevent the occurrence of one adverse event, at a specific time (t) [30]. The longer is the follow-up duration, the more the difference between treatments is expected to increase, and hence, the smaller will be its reciprocal value (NNT). Assuming that the treatment effect is stable over time and that the events occur at a constant rate, the expected NNT for a given time (t_2) can be seen as a fraction of the one observed at the time (t_1) "Eq. (1.55)" [30]. For example, if the observed average duration of follow-up is five years and the calculated NNT is 100 patients, the NNT for ten years follow-up = 100 × 5/10 = 50 patients.

$$NNT(t_2) = NNT(t_1) \times \frac{t_1}{t_2} \quad (1.55)$$

To avoid making those two hard assumptions, Altman and Andersen suggested a direct calculation of the NNT at a particular time point (t) [33]. First, we calculate the absolute risk reduction (ARR) at the time (t) as the difference between survival in the treatment group (S_t) and survival in the control group (S_c) "Eq. (1.56)", provided that $S_t > S_c$. The NNT will be its reciprocal value as usual. As an example, if the survival probabilities of treatment and control groups are 60 and 40%, the NNT = 1/ (06 − 0.4) = 5 patients. The interpretation is as follows: giving the patients the treatment will lead to an extra survivor for every five patients treated. In many manuscripts, it is usually hard to find the Se of the ARR to create a 95% CI around the NNT. The manuscript may give the Se or the confidence interval of each survival probability. If not given, we can estimate the Se of each survival probability (Se_t and Se_c) as one-quarter of the width of its 95% confidence interval. We can then calculate the Se of (ARR) as the sum of the standard errors of both survival probabilities. "Eq. (1.57)". If neither were given, we could estimate the Se of ARR from the survival probabilities themselves (S_t and S_c) and the number of patients remaining at risk in both groups (n_t) and (n_c), at the time (t) "Eq. (1.58)". Using any of those means, we can finally produce the desired 95% CI by assigning 1.96 Se on either side of ARR "Eq. (1.59)". The upper and lower limits of the 95% CI of the NNT will be the reciprocal values, as usual "Eq. (1.60)". An illustrative example is given by Altman and Anderson, with $S_t = 62.2\%$, $S_c = 46.8\%$, $n_t = 59$ patients and $n_c = 43$ cases, giving an ARR from 0.013 to 0.295 and an approximate NNT of 7 (4–78) patients [33].

$$ARR = S_t - S_c \qquad (1.56)$$

$$Se(ARR) = \sqrt{(Se_t)^2 + (Se_c)^2} \qquad (1.57)$$

$$Se(ARR) = \sqrt{\frac{(S_t)^2(1 - S_t)}{n_t} + \frac{(S_c)^2(1 - S_c)}{n_c}} \qquad (1.58)$$

$$95\% \ CI(ARR) = ARR \pm 1.96 \ Se(ARR) \qquad (1.59)$$

$$95\% \ CI(NNT) = \frac{1}{UL \ 95\% \ CI(ARR)} \ \text{to} \ \frac{1}{LL \ 95\% \ CI(ARR)} \qquad (1.60)$$

In a time to event analysis, the HR is the ratio of 2 probabilities: experiencing the event in the treatment group to that of the control group at a certain time. In Cox regression, survival is not an output of the analysis, However, whenever authors supply the survival in control group (S_c), we can calculate survival in the treatment group (S_t) as $(S_c)^{HR}$. Consequently, we can calculate the ARR equals as the difference between both survival probabilities, and the NNT will be its reciprocal value, as usual, "Eq. (1.61)" [33]. It is evident that without knowing HR and S_c, we cannot estimate the NNT. The statistical software usually provides the upper and lower limits of the 95% CI of the HR, which can replace the average (HR) in "Eq. (1.61)", to calculate the 95% CI of the NNT "Eq. (1.62)". An illustrative example was given by Altman and Anderson, with $S_c = 0.33$, h = 0.72 (95% CI: 0.55–0.92) and an approximate NNT of 9 (5–33) patients [33].

$$NNT = \frac{1}{(S_c)^{HR} - (S_c)} \qquad (1.61)$$

$$NNT = \frac{1}{(S_c)^{UL \ of \ the \ 95\% \ CI \ of \ HR} - (S_c)} \ \text{to} \ \frac{1}{(S_c)^{LL \ of \ the \ 95\% \ CI \ of \ HR} - (S_c)} \qquad (1.62)$$

1.9 Diagnostic Accuracy

Theoretically, the diagnosis of a disease has to be made by a gold standard test, which could be microbiological, pathological, biochemical, radiological, genetic, final outcome, or set of criteria. Gold standard tests can rule in or rule out the disease; however, they are usually invasive, may be potentially harmful, not readily available, and maybe expensive and time-consuming. A diagnostic test is commonly used for deciding on as a proxy for the gold standard. Hence, it has to be relatively simple, readily available, cheap, harmless, etc., but it must be evaluated against the gold standard.

Diagnostic accuracy is the most fundamental characteristic of any diagnostic test measuring its ability to discriminate among alternative states of health, such as health and disease, two stages of a disease, etc. Measures of diagnostic accuracy are either *paired or single measures*. Paired measures include sensitivity and specificity, positive and negative predictive values and, positive and negative likelihood ratios. Examples of single measures are the size of the surface area under a ROC plot (AUC), Youden's index, and diagnostic odds ratio. Positive and negative predictive values help to interpret whether someone—in a *specific population*—has the disease because his test result was positive or he is disease-free because he had a negative test. On the other hand, other measures have the advantage of being *independent of the disease prevalence* in the population, such as sensitivity, specificity, and likelihood ratios. Sensitivity and specificity are used to indicate the presence or absence of the disease. Likelihood ratios can be used to express how likely a diseased patient of any population can give a positive (true positive) or a negative result to the test (false negative) compared to a disease-free patient.

1.9.1 The Discriminative Measures

Suppose that someone wants to protect his new car from being stolen by putting an alarm and, the first thing he will do is increase its sensitivity to the max, of course. The result is that the alarm will not only come off in case of a thief is trying to steal the car (a true positive alarm = TP) but also in the case of a kid just trying to touch it, or a speedy motor cycle comes too near to it (a false positive alarm = FP). Setting the sensitivity too high will get more FP results (we will be obliged to re-check the car too many times). While setting it too low, we will get many false-negative results. Note that the FN is the worst situation: the car is stolen, and the alarm did not get off). The best scenario is that the alarm does not get on because the car is safe (true negative = TN). Let us now translate this example into the medical field. The car is the subject who will be diseased if the car is stolen or healthy if the car is safe. The alarm is the test that can either give a positive result by the alarm getting on or a negative result by the alarm remaining silent. As the perfect alarm does not exist, the "ideal test" can perfectly discriminate between patients (who have the disease) and the healthy population (who do not have the disease). Figure 1.33 assumes the "wishful but impossible situation";

where the distribution of health and disease is perfectly distinct.

In reality, and as shown in Fig. 1.34, there will always be this intermediate zone where diseased subjects (D+) seem to be healthy while they are not (FN) and healthy subjects (D−) are giving false positive signs (FP). Consequently, whenever a diagnostic test is performed, the result could be either positive (R+) or negative (R−). In the case where the subject in concern is already diseased (D+), then a positive result of the test is a true positive (TP) while a negative result is a false negative (FN) one. On the other hand, if this person does not have the disease (D−), the positive result of the test is a false positive (FP), and the negative result is a true negative one (TN); (Table 1.9).

1.9.1.1 Sensitivity of the Test (Sn)

The sensitivity of a test is its ability not to miss a person who might have the dis-ease. In other words, it is the probability to give a positive result (R+) when the subject already has the disease (D +), i.e., sensitivity rules in the disease. As shown in Fig. 1.35, the diseased subject (D+) may either give a true positive result (TP) or a false negative result (FN). Consequently, *sensitivity can be defined as the proportion of true positive results from all test results in the diseased population*: $Sn = TP/(TP + FN)$; (Table 1.9).

The more sensitive the test, the less we expect FN results until the test reaches a maximum sensitivity of 1. Put it another way, Sn of a test is

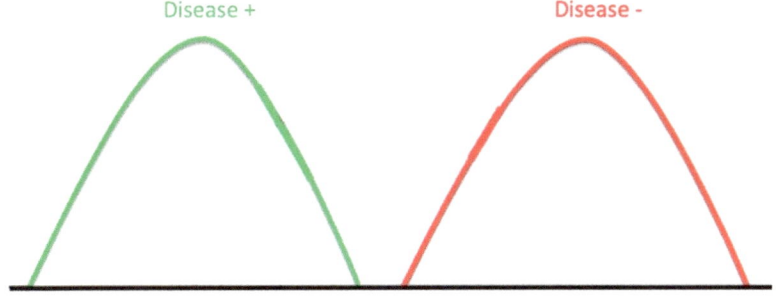

Fig. 1.33 A wishful distribution of health and disease

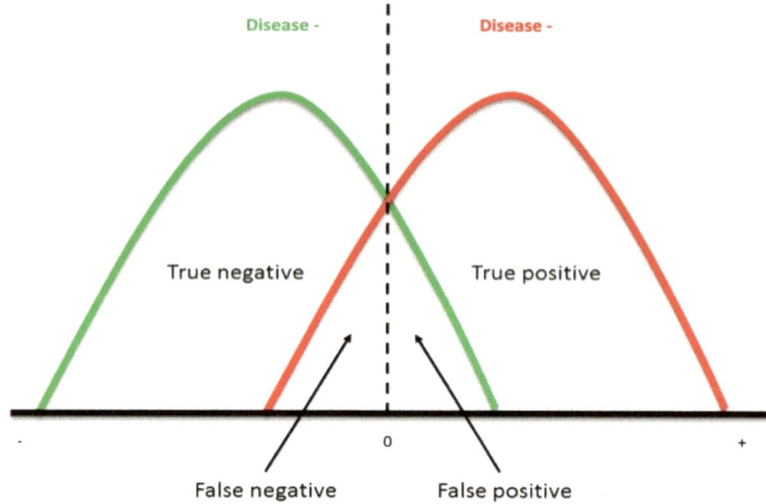

Fig. 1.34 A usual distribution of health and disease

Table 1.9 Sensitivity versus specificity

	Disease (D+)	Healthy (D−)
Positive test (R+)	TP	FP
Negative test (R−)	FN	TN
	TP/(TP + FN)	TN/(TN + FP)
	Sensitivity	Specificity

TP = true positive, FP = false positive, FN = false negative, TN = true negative

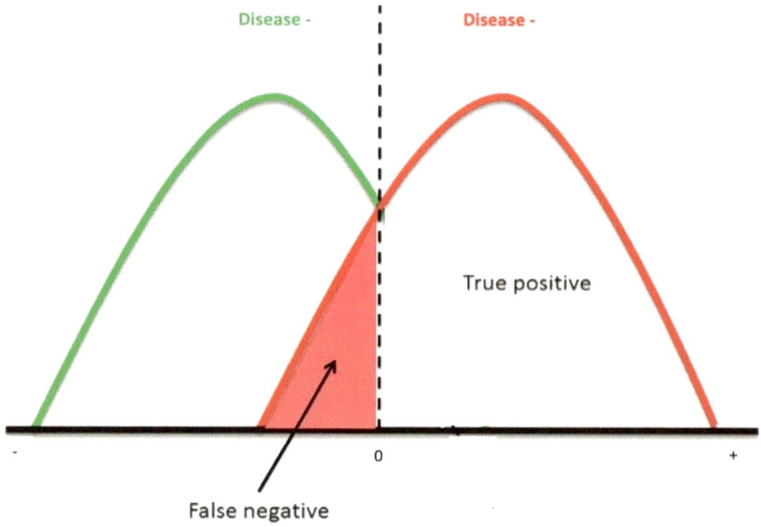

Fig. 1.35 The result of the diagnostic test in a diseased population

how many times the test is truly positive (TP) when the patient has the disease (TP + FN). As Sn describes the proportion of the test results in the diseased population, it is independent of its prevalence. On the other hand, researchers have to be careful that Sn can be largely dependent on the spectrum of the disease and the characteristic of subjects, such as being widely variable between early and late cases [34].

1.9.1.2 Specificity of the Test (Sp)

The specificity of a test is its ability to confirm the diagnosis by excluding normal subjects. In other words, it is the probability to have a negative result (R−) when the subject is not diseased (D−); i.e., a negative test rules out the diagnosis. As a healthy subject (D−) may either give a true negative (TN) or a false positive (FP) result (Fig. 1.36), *specificity can be defined as the proportion of true negatives that are correctly identified by the test*: $Sp = TN/(TN + FP)$; (Table 1.9).

The more specific the test is, the fewer FP results until the test reaches a maximum specificity that equals 1. Put it another way, the Sp of a test is how many times the test is truly negative

(TN) when the patient does not have the disease (TN + FP). As Sp describes the proportion of the results of the test in the healthy population, it is independent of the prevalence of the disease; i.e., Sp is unrelated to the distribution of health/ disease. On the other hand, researchers have to be careful that Sp can be largely dependent on the spectrum of the health and the characteristic of healthy subjects, such as being widely variable between young and old controls [34].

> The sensitivity of a test is how many times the test is truly positive when the patient has the disease. Specificity is how many times the test is truly negative when the patient does not have the disease. Sensitivity and specificity are properties of the test.

1.9.1.3 Calculation and Interpretation: Choosing the Appropriate Cut-Off Point

Unlike tests having only a single cut-off point such as presence or absence of a disease, tests

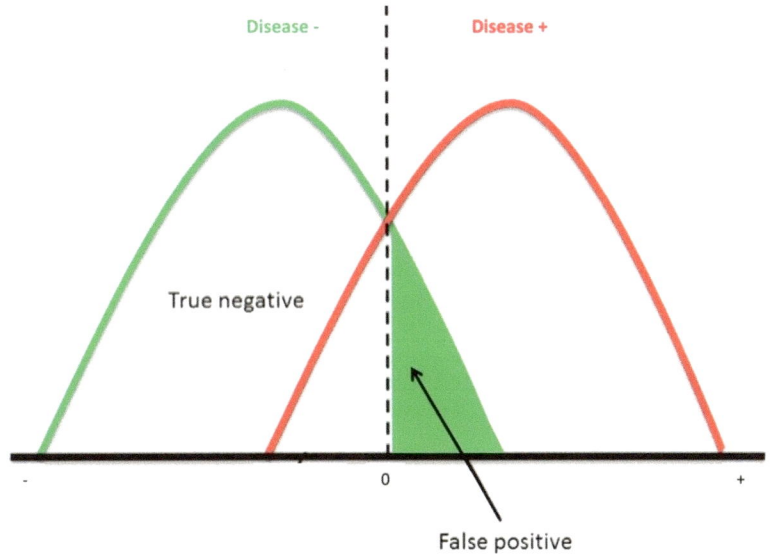

Fig. 1.36 The result of the diagnostic test in the healthy population

having results on a continuous scale require to carefully specify the test threshold, according to the prevalence and the severity of the disease. Missing a life-threatening disease (FN) is much more important than a FP diagnosis in a healthy patient. On the other hand, in a disease with high prevalence, costly FP tests may overweight a benign FN diagnosis. In all cases, one desirable characteristic of a good diagnostic test is that it has a sensitivity value close to 1. Hence, the test will be able to diagnose as many patients as it can. Likewise, the other side of the coin is the testability to exclude as many normal people as possible, which can be achieved as its specificity approaches 1. Unfortunately, achieving both aims simultaneously is usually not feasible. Increasing sensitivity will decrease specificity and vice versa due to the usual overlap between the distribution of both conditions: health and disease (Fig. 1.34). Figure 1.37 shows an attempt to maximize sensitivity by moving the test cut-off point from point (0) towards point (A) to rule in the disease in all patients (D+). Although none of the patients will escape

diagnosis (no FN), more controls will be falsely diagnosed as patients (FP results are increased). In concordance, the proportion of controls which will be correctly diagnosed will be reduced (TN results are decreased). The net result is that *increasing the test's sensitivity will reduce its specificity, depending on the overlap between the distributions of the two health conditions and how accurate the measurement scale will be.*

Figure 1.38 shows the reverse attempt to maximize the specificity of the test by shifting the cut-off point: from point (0) to point (B) to rule out the disease in all controls (D−). Although none of the controls will escape diagnosis (no FP results), more patients will be falsely diagnosed as healthy (FN results are increased). In concordance, the proportion of patients who will be correctly diagnosed will be reduced (TP are decreased). In either attempt, the amount of increase or decrease of proportions is dependent upon how much the distribution of the two conditions (health and disease) do overlap and on accurate is the used measurement. Although there are tests that have good

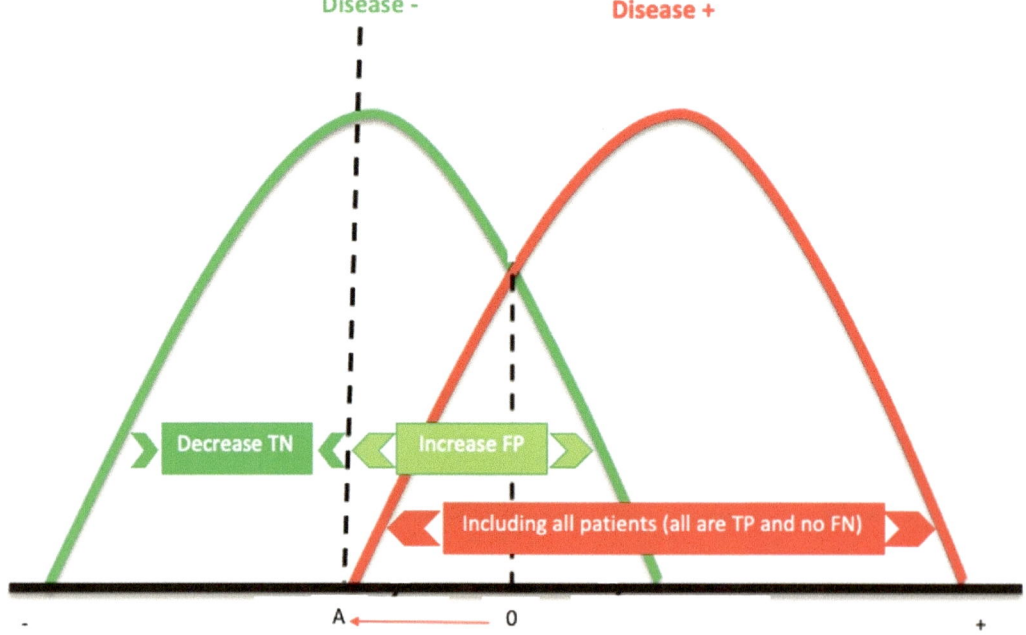

Fig. 1.37 Maximizing sensitivity by moving cut-off point from point 0 towards point A

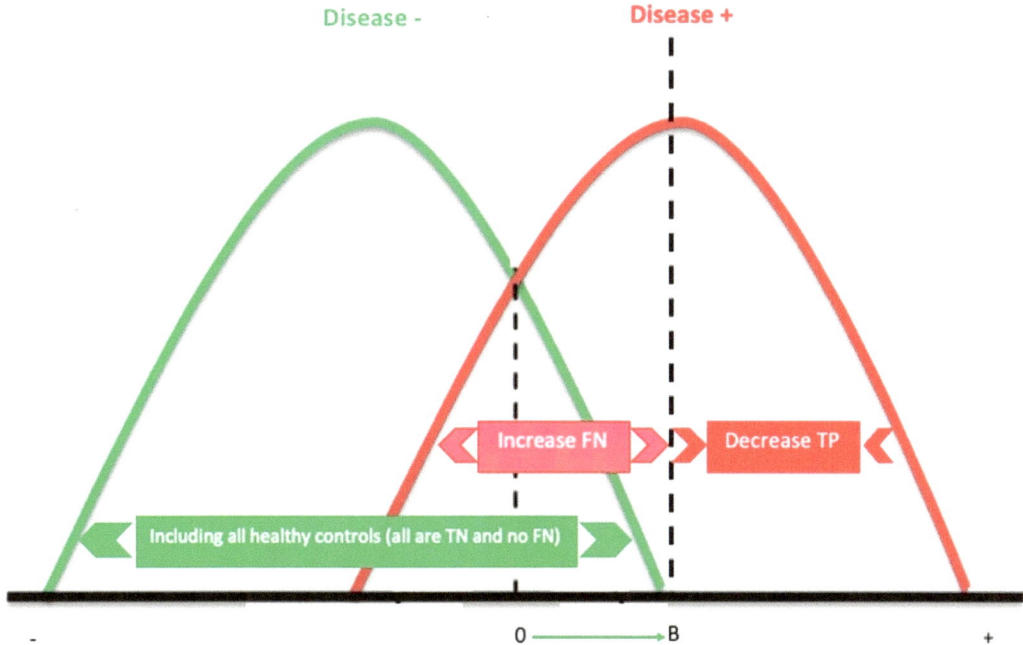

Fig. 1.38 Maximizing specificity by moving cut-off point from point 0 towards point B

Table 1.10 Fasting blood sugar levels in 30 diabetic patients and 30 normal controls

Diabetic patients	80, 90, 90, 90, 100, 100, 100, 100, 110, 110, 110, 110, 120, 120, 120, 120, 120, 120, 120, 130, 130, 130, 140, 140, 140, 150, 150, 160, 170, 180
Normal controls	40, 40, 50, 50, 50, 60, 60, 60, 60, 70, 70, 70, 70, 70, 70, 70, 70, 80, 80, 80, 80, 90, 90, 90, 100, 100, 110, 110, 120, 130

Values are fasting blood sugar levels (FBS) measured in mg/dL

sensitivity and specificity, in practice, many tests are designed to have maximum sensitivity to be used for screening patients. In contrast, others are designed to have maximum specificity to be used for confirmatory purposes.

Evaluation of a Single Sn and Sp Point

A study was carried out to define the appropriate limits of a "normal" fasting blood sugar (FBS) in a sample of 30 diabetic patients and 30 normal controls of comparable age, sex, and other risk factors (Table 1.10). The mean FBS for diabetic patients was significantly higher than that of normal subjects (121.7 ± 24 versus 76.3 ± 22.7 mg/dL; P < 0.001); however, both distributions do overlap. As shown in Fig. 1.39, the FBS of normal controls varies between 40

and 130 mg/dL, while that of diabetic patients varies between 80 and 180 mg/dL. The cut-off threshold of normality must be guided by the main indication of the newly proposed method, among other factors. If the test's main purpose is screening patients for the disease, one can choose the threshold of > 70 mg/dL. All diabetic patients had an FBS > 80 mg/dL, and this threshold will ensure a 100% sensitivity, and none of the patients will be missed. However, as many as 43% of normal subjects (13/30) will be considered as being diabetic, while they are not (false positive), (see Fig. 1.39).

On the other hand, a threshold of >130 mg/dL is appealing for a confirmatory test and will ensure excluding all disease-free patients or a 100% specificity; however, 26% of diabetic

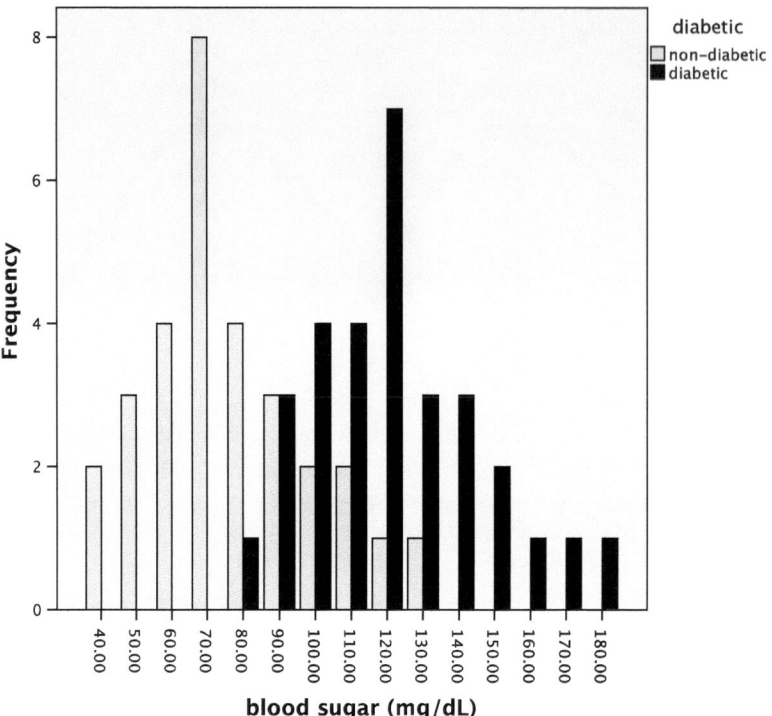

Fig. 1.39 The distribution of fasting blood sugar in diabetic patients and in normal controls. Data are presented in Table 1.10

patients (8/30) will be misdiagnosed as being free from the disease (false negative); Fig. 1.39. The consequences of the two choices are also visualized in Fig. 1.40, showing the cumulative distribution of fasting blood sugar measurements observed in both diabetic patients and controls. As changing the threshold will largely influence our diagnosis and further management, the researcher has to have a global view of the whole data spectrum before closing the test's best deal to achieve its main purpose.

Evaluation of the Whole Spectrum: ROC Plots

We have shown how one change in the cut-off limit can influence diagnosis and subsequent patient management. A wise attitude would be to examine all possible cut-off points and choose the most suitable one for the test's main purpose. Receiver (sometimes known as a relative) operating characteristic (ROC) plots provide such

whole spectrum analysis through graphing, not only one pair of data, but all spectrums of available sensitivity/specificity pairs, through continuously varying the decision threshold over the entire range of observed results. Besides choosing the best Se and Sp thresholds, ROC plots are used to evaluate the overall test performance and compare different tests, different groups of patients, or different observers within studies. View the multiple indications; we will discuss the ROC plot in detail in Sect. 1.9.1.4.

Interpretation of Sensitivity and Specificity

Sensitivity and specificity provide test accuracy in subjects belonging to either the diseased or the healthy population, which does not add much to a patient with an unknown situation. Put it this way, Sn and Sp may be the extra theoretical knowledge that satisfies a doctor but not the patient who is eager to know what is actually happening to him.

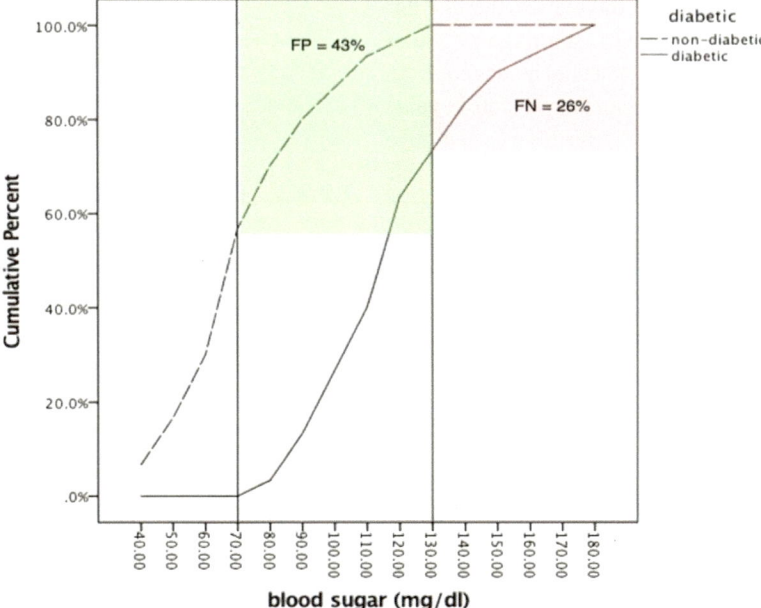

Fig. 1.40 The cumulative distribution of fasting blood sugar in diabetic patients and normal controls. FP = false positive results: with a cut-off point of 70 mg/dL, 43% (13/30) of non-diabetic subjects will be considered as being diabetics; FN = false negative: with a cut-off point of 130 mg/dL, 26% (8/30) of diabetics will be considered as being non-diabetic

1.9.1.4   What Should Be Reported

We can calculate a 95% confidence interval (95% CI) for both Sn and Sp using the large sample method, previously described for routine calculations of a CI of proportions, provided that the necessary conditions for calculation are fulfilled (see Sect. 1.4.2.4). In brief, the variance of a binomial qualitative variable of proportions p and $(1 - p)$ is equal to $p(1 - p)$. The observation of a percentage (p) in a sample of (n) cases permits the assignment of 95% CI that equals: $p \pm 1.96 \sqrt{(p(1 - p))}$ "Eq. (1.10)", provided that both: np and $n(1 - p) \geq 5$. In the case where those conditions cannot be verified, or when the proportion is near zero (0%) or one (100%); the CI calculated by the formula will be hyperinflated [35]. The exact confidence intervals should be looked for in special statistical tables [4] or otherwise calculated using a commercially available statistical computer package [7–9, 36]. The result is usually multiplied by 100 and expressed as a percentage. An Sn of 25% in 100 patients should be reported as follows: $p \pm 1.96$ $\sqrt{(p(1 - p))}$ = 17–33%. Checking on the conditions of using the formula: for the lower limit: p = 0.17, q = 83, np = 17, and nq = 83. For the upper limit: p = 0.33, q = 0.67, np = 33 and nq = 67; and all conditions are verified. The calculations can be easily made online through many links, which equally provides the 95% CI with continuity correction that should be presented if the previously mentioned conditions were not fulfilled [7–9, 36]. We will discuss reports of ROC plot in detail in Sect. 1.9.4.3.

1.9.2   The Predictive Values

A positive result can be TP or FP and a negative result can be TN or FN. Neither sensitivity nor specificity can answer the question: is this positive or negative result true or false? Doctors care about how sensitive and specific the tools they are using for diagnosis (i.e., the tests), but patients do not care much about this information. A patient will care about what those tests mean for him or their role in predicting whether: he has the disease if the test result is positive or he does not have the test if the test result is negative. In other words, he cares about the predictive value of his positive result (positive predictive value = PPV) and the predictive value of his negative result (negative predictive value = NPV). Neither Sn nor Sp will answer those questions.

1.9.2.1 Positive Predictive Value (PPV)

The positive predictive value (PPV) is the probability for the person to have the disease (D+) if the result of his test was positive (R+). A positive result may either be a TP or an FP one, and hence, a PPV is the proportion of patients with positive test results who are correctly diagnosed (PPV = TP/(TP + FP). Put it another way, PPV is how many times the patient will have the disease (TP) if the test is positive (TP + FP), as shown in Table 1.11.

1.9.2.2 Negative Predictive Value (NPV)

The negative predictive value (NPV) is the probability for a subject to be free from the disease (D−) if the result of his test was negative (R−). A negative result may either be a TN or an FN result, and hence, the NPV is the proportion of patients with negative test results who are correctly diagnosed (NPV = TN/(TN + FN)). Put it another way, NPV is how many times the patient will indeed be free from the disease (TN) if the test is negative (TN + FN).

> The positive predictive value is how many times the patient truly has the disease if the test is positive. The negative predictive

> value is how many times the patient is not having the disease if the test is negative.

1.9.2.3 Calculation and Interpretation: The Role of Prevalence

Prevalence is the proportion of new and pre-existing cases in a population who have a particular disease or attribute at a specified point or period. In the absence of sufficient information, whether in the literature or documented guidelines, prevalence can be interpreted as the probability that the subject has the disease before any test is carried out. Hence, it can be thought of as a prior probability of the disease. After doing the test, the positive and negative predictive values are the revised estimates of the same probability for those subjects. Hence, they could be defined as the posterior probabilities of the disease. Knowing Sn, Sp, and P, we can deduct both PPV "Eq. (1.63)" and NPV from a simple equation "Eq. (1.64)" or by using an online calculator [7–9, 36]. As for the construction of the 95% CI, we can apply the same rules given before to calculate those intervals in the case of Sn and Sp (see Sect. 1.9.1.3)

$$PPV = \frac{SeP}{SeP + (1 - Sp)(1 - P)} \quad (1.63)$$

$$NPV = \frac{Sp(1 - P)}{Sp(1 - P) + P(1 - Se)} \quad (1.64)$$

It is evident from the equation that both predictive values are largely dependent upon the prevalence of the disease. The higher the P, the more significant the expected PPV is, and the

Table 1.11 Positive versus negative predictive values

	Disease (D+)	Healthy (D−)		
Positive test (R+)	TP	FP	TP/(TP + FP)	PPV
Negative test (R−)	FN	TN	TN/(TN + FN)	NPV
	TP/(TP + FN)	TN/(TN + FP)		
	Sensitivity	Specificity		

TP = true positive, FP = false positive, FN = false negative, TN = true negative, PPV = positive predictive value, NPV = negative predictive value, R+ = positive test result, R− = negative test result, D+ = diseased subjects, D− = non-diseased subjects

Table 1.12 Role of Prevalence in predictive values: comparing two sphygmomanometers

			Mercury			
			Disease (D+)	Healthy (D−)		
Population 1 (P1 = 50%)						
	Digital	Positive test (R+)	80	5	94.1%	PPV
		Negative test (R−)	20	95	82.6%	NPV
		Sensitivity	80%	–		
		Specificity	–	95%		
Population 2 (P2 = 20%)						
	Digital	Positive test (R+)	80	20	80%	PPV
		Negative test (R−)	20	380	95%	NPV
		Sensitivity	80%	–		
		Specificity	–	95%		

Sn = sensitivity, Sp = specificity, PPV = positive predictive value, NPV = negative predictive value, P = prevalence of the disease, D+ = diseased subjects, D− = healthy subjects

smaller the expected NPV and vice versa. Table 1.12 gives an example of the change in PPV and NPV in response to carrying the same test in 2 different populations. A new test (digital sphygmomanometer) has 80% sensitivity and 95% specificity to diagnose hypertension, compared to the conventional mercury type. We apply the test in 2 different populations: a cardiac population where the prevalence of hypertension (P1) was as high as 50% and in a general population, where (P2) was as low as 20%. As shown, the positive post-test probability (i.e., the PPV) is higher in the population with a higher prevalence of the disease. The negative post-test probability (i.e., the NPV) is higher in the population with the lower prevalence. Consequently, PPV and NPV are valid only in the study population or similar population, but Sn and Sp are valid for everyone. Unless the study is genuinely representative, i.e., a well-randomized sample, one cannot extrapolate PPV and NPV to other patient groups with confidence [37].

Interpretation of Predictive Values

Interpretation of predictive values is straightforward for both doctors and patients. In addition, they provide the patient with the information that he needs to know. The probability of having the disease if his test was positive and of being disease-free in case of a negative test.

1.9.2.4 What Should Be Reported

Results have to be reported in percentages together with the 95% confidence intervals. We can calculate the latter by the large sample method, previously used to calculate the 95% CI of Se and Sp (see Sect. 1.9.2.4) and, initially described for routine calculations of a CI of proportions, provided that the necessary conditions for calculation are fulfilled (see Sect. 1.4.2.4). In brief, the variance of a binomial qualitative variable of proportions p and $(1 - p)$ is equal to $p(1 - p)$. The observation of a percentage (p) in a sample of (n) cases permits the assignment of 95% CI that equals: $p + 1.96 \sqrt{(p(1 - p))}$ "Eq. (1.10)", provided that both: np and $n(1 - p) > 5$. Using data presented in Table 1.12 and replacing (p) by PPV and by NPV gives an PPV (95% CI) of 94.1% (89.1–99.1%) and, an NPV of 82.6% (75.7–89.5%). Replacing (p) by Sn and Sp gives an Sn of 80% (72.2–87.8%) and an Sp of 95% (90.7–99.3%).

In the case where those conditions cannot be verified, or when the proportion is near zero (0%) or one (100%), the CI calculated by the formula will be hyper-inflated [35]. Consequently, we must look for the exact confidence intervals in unique statistical tables [4]. A more accessible alternative is to calculate using commercially available statistical software or simply online through many links [7–9, 36], providing the 95%

CI with continuity correction that we prefer to use if the previously mentioned conditions were not fulfilled.

1.9.3 The Likelihood Ratios

In general, *the likelihood ratio (LR) summarizes how many times more (or less) likely patients with the disease are to develop an event or have a particular test result than patients without the disease.* For example, suppose 10% of patients with rheumatic heart disease (RHD) have an elevated antistreptolysin O titer (ASOT) > 200, compared to only 1% of patients free from the disease. In that case, we can deduct that RHD patients are ten times more likely to have elevated ASOT than normal controls. In our case, the likelihood ratio (LR) is between the two probabilities: 10 and 1% or 0.1:0.01, and hence, LR = 10. This number (10) does not mean that cases with a positive ASOT are ten times more likely to have RHD; this is the PPV and not LR. This "10" means that if a patient has RHD, he is ten times more likely to give a positive ASOT test than someone who is RHD-free, which is the LR. *We constantly compare patients to controls and not the reverse,* regardless of whether we are describing how many times more or less likely the patients develop the event or give a particular result to the test. For example, suppose 5% of the usually young RHD patients have elevated blood sugar levels compared to 20% of normal controls. In that case, we conclude that RHD patients are four times less likely to have elevated fasting blood sugar than controls (LR = 0.25) and not those normal cases are four times more likely to have abnormally high fasting blood sugar than RHD patients. Remember that *the null of a ratio is one.* A likelihood ratio >1 indicates that the test result (or the event) is associated with the presence of the disease. In contrast, a likelihood ratio <1 indicates that the test result is associated with the absence of disease. The different likelihood ratios are from 1, the more substantial the evidence for the test's usefulness or the presence or absence of the disease [38]. *In the case of test results being either positive or negative*

(dichotomous), there will result in 2 likelihood ratios that are called: the positive LR and the negative LR.

1.9.3.1 The Positive Likelihood Ratio

In practice, physicians would prefer to order a particular diagnostic test only if the result enables them to rule in or rule out a particular disease. Ruling in the disease would follow if the probability of a true-positive outcome in a diseased individual (TP) is considerably more likely than a false-positive error in a disease-free subject (FP). The former probability is the test's sensitivity, and the latter is (1 − specificity) "Eq. (1.65)". Put it this way, if Sn is the probability to have a positive result among the diseased population (TP), 1 − Sp is the probability to have a positive result among the healthy (FP). The positive LR will be the ratio of these two positive probabilities and can be called: the likelihood ratio of a positive test result.

$$
\begin{aligned}
(1 - Sp) &= 1 - \frac{TN}{(TN + FP)} \\
&= \frac{(TN + FP)}{(TN + FP)} - \frac{TN}{(TN + FP)} = FP
\end{aligned}
$$

(1.65)

Graphically, the positive LR is the ratio between the two areas of TP and FP, shown in Fig. 1.41. The first is measured under the diseased population distribution curve (D+), with a base extending between the points 0 and D+ and, the second area is overlapping the first one but is measured under the disease-free population distribution curve (D−), with a base extending from point 0 to point D− on the basal measurement scale. As a rule of thumb, positive LR of 2, 5 and 10 increase (improve) our post-test probability by about 15%, 30% and 45%. A positive LR $\geq$ 10 has been considered to provide strong evidence to rule in diagnoses, in most circumstances [38].

1.9.3.2 The Negative Likelihood Ratio

The other side of the coin is a test that can help the physician to rule out the disease. It would follow when the probability of a negative test is more likely true (TN) than false (FN). Hence, the subject

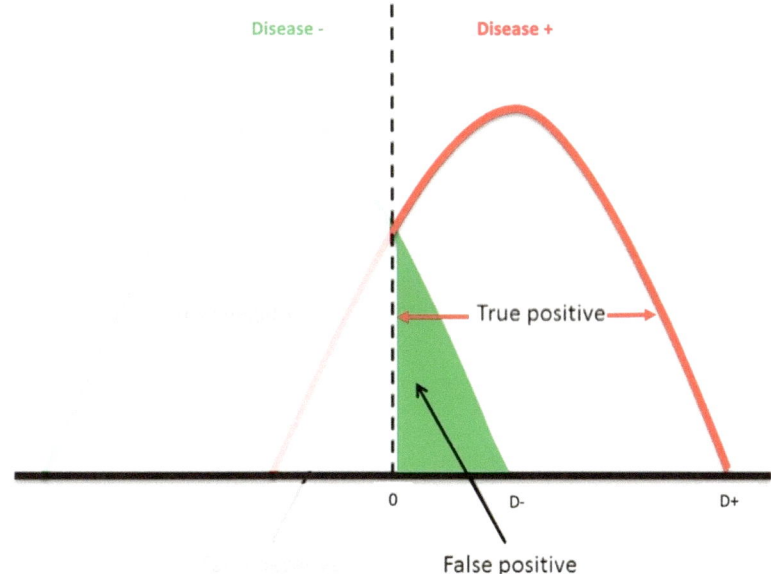

Fig. 1.41 The positive likelihood ratio: true positive/false positive

is likelier to be free from the disease than to have the disease. As Sn is the probability of having a positive result among the diseased population [TP/(TP + FN)], 1 − Sn is the probability to have a negative result among diseased: FN "Eq. (1.66)". Note that the negative LR is the proportion of those two probabilities: the probability of having a false negative result among diseased and probability of having a true negative result among healthy that is often called the likelihood ratio of a negative test result: (1 − Sn)/Sp.

$$1 - Sn = \frac{TP + FN}{TP + FN} - \frac{TP}{TP + FN} = FN \quad (1.66)$$

Graphically, the negative LR is the ratio between the two areas of TN and FN, shown in Fig. 1.42. The first is measured under the diseased-free population distribution curve (D−), with a base extending between the points 0 and D− and the second is overlapping the first one. However, it is measured under the diseased population distribution curve (D+), with a base extending from point 0 to point D+ on the basal measurement scale. The patients' results are always placed in the numerator, and hence, the negative LR is the

ratio between (FN = 1 − Se) in the patient and true negative in the healthy subject (Sp). Consequently, the values of likelihood ratios for negative test outcomes thus defined would typically be less <1 and ideally much smaller than one. As a rule of thumb, a negative LR of 0.5, 0.2, and 0.1 decrease our post-test probability by about −15, −30, and −45%; with a negative LR < 0.1 being considered to provide strong evidence to rule out diagnoses in most circumstances [38]. Note that the decrease mentioned above in post-test probability means that it improves our ability to rule out the disease and does not mean that it decreases our ability to do so.

1.9.3.3 Calculation and Interpretation: The Pre and Post-Test Odds

Returning to the example of the new sphygmomanometer that was shown to have a sensitivity of 80% and specificity of 95% to detect hypertension (see Sect. 1.9.2.3, Table 1.12) and the question posed was whether this instrument is useful or not? In general, any test's usefulness depends on the size of the difference between the

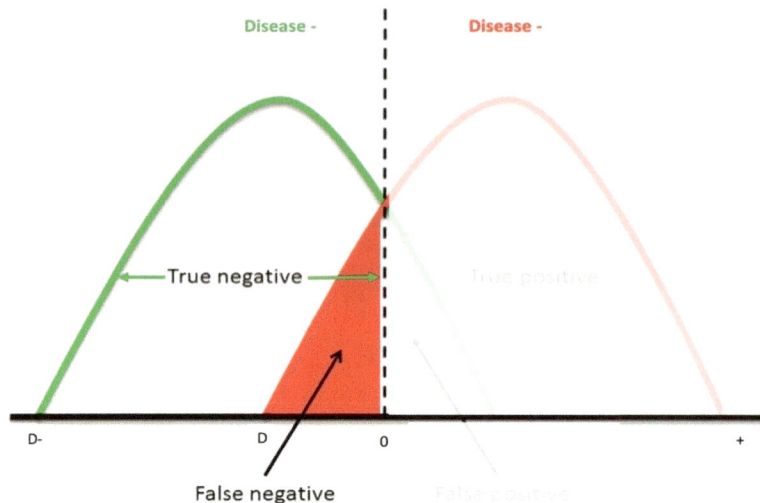

Fig. 1.42 The negative likelihood ratio: false negative/true negative

Table 1.13 Calculation of post-test probabilities

Pre-test odds	p/(1 − p)	0.2/(1–0.2) = 0.25
Positive LR	Sn/(1 − Sp)	0.8/(1–0.95) = 16
Negative LR	(1 − Sn)/Sp	(1–0.8)/0.95 = 0.21
Positive post-test odds	Pre-test odds × positive LR	0.25 × 16 = 4 (4:1)
Positive post-test probability	Odds/(1 + odds)	4/(1 + 4) = 80%
Negative post-test odds	Pre-test odds × negative LR	0.25 × 0.21 = 0.053
Negative post-test probability	Odds/(1 + odds)	0.053/(1 + 0.053) = 5%

P = probability, Sn = sensitivity Sp = specificity, LR = likelihood ratio

pre-test probability of making a correct diagnosis and the post-test probability. In our case, the question is about the value of the sphygmomanometer in diagnosing hypertension. We can search for the pre-test probability in the literature or valid guidelines. If unknown, we can use the prevalence in the general population, provided that there are no other risk factors associated with the disease in concern. The prevalence of HTN was around 20% in the general population and 50% in the cardiac population. We will take the example of the general population. We begin by calculating the pre-test odds from the pre-test probability, using the simple equation: odds = probability/(1 − probability). We calculate the positive and negative LR from Sn and Sp, as shown before. The positive and the

negative post-test odds are the products of the pre-test odds and the corresponding positive and negative LR. We calculate the positive and negative post-test probabilities by converting each post-test odds into probability, using the simple equation: probability = odds/(1 + odds) "Eq. (1.23)". Table 1.13 shows the steps and the results of our example.

Let us first define what does a positive test mean? It means that we will confirm hypertension by the new sphygmomanometer. Second, we have to interpret what does a positive LR of 10 means? A patient with the disease is ten times more likely to give a positive test compared to a disease-free patient, and not that any person (patient or control) who gives a positive test is ten times more likely to be a patient than to be

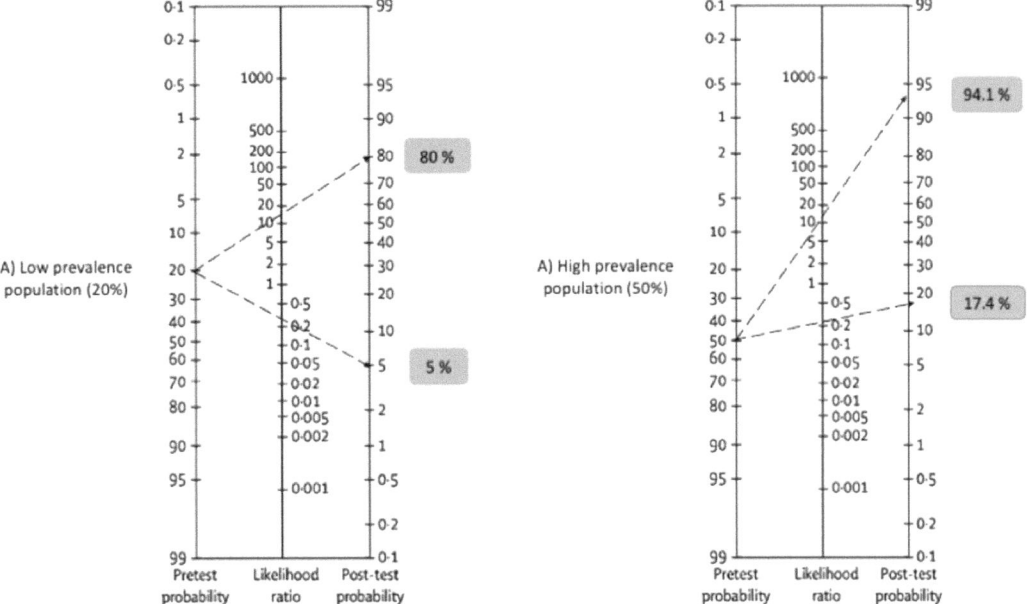

Fig. 1.43 Post-test probabilities calculated by Fagan's nomograph in; (**A**) low prevalence population of and, (**B**) high prevalence population of 50%. Positive likelihood ratio = 16 and negative likelihood ratio = 0.2. A line departing from the pre-test probability on the left of the nomograph, passing through the likelihood ratio in the middle, lands on the post-test probability on the right side of the nomograph

disease-free; this is the PPV. The same difference must be noted in predicting the negative LR, which should not be taken for the NPV. Finally, the LR permitted us to calculate the post-test probabilities from the corresponding pre-test values and show the test's usefulness: the sphygmomanometer has improved the physician's ability to correctly diagnose the disease from 20% (prevalence) to 80%. Put it this way, nearly 80% of subjects with a positive test will be sick.

On the other hand, if someone has a negative test, he has a limited 5% chance of being HTN than being normal or, 95% of subjects with a negative test are well. Those long calculations were only mending to show how does it work? Nearly five decades ago, Dr. Terrence G Fagan created a simple nomograph to interpret the post-test probabilities for a known pre-test probability (prevalence) and observed test results (likelihood ratios). A straight line drawn from a patient's pre-test probability will point to the disease's post-test probability through the likelihood ratios for the

test [39]. The nomograph can be automatically generated online [36]. Figure 1.43 shows the use of the nomograph to calculate the post-test probabilities for a patient drawn from the low prevalence population of 20% (Fig. 1.43A) and another patient drawn from the high prevalence population 50% (Fig. 1.43B); with a positive LR 16 and a negative LR of 0.21 (see Tables 1.12 and 1.13). In either case, a line passing from the pre-test probability on the left side of the nomogram, passing through the likelihood ratio in the middle of the figure, will land on the post-test probability on the right side. Complete results, with their 95% intervals of confidence, can be retrieved by numerous online calculators [7–9, 36].

The Likelihood Ratios Versus the Predictive Values

In brief, the PPV and NPV are the pos-test results calculated for a specified prevalence of the disease (P), while the positive and negative LR summarize the diagnostic ability of the test that we can use to predict the PPV and NPV for any given (P). In Sect. 1.9.3.4, we have evaluated the usefulness of the new sphygmomanometer, with 80% sensitivity and 95% specificity. We deducted the positive and negative likelihood ratios from those two probabilities: 16 and 0.21, respectively.

On the other hand, the post-test probabilities are dependent upon the pre-test values (prevalence). The positive post-test probability is equal to the PPV (80%), and the negative post-test probability equals $1 - NPV$ ($1-0.95 = 5\%$). Both negative post-test probability and NPV are the two faces of the same coin. The former describes the probability that someone who has the disease will give a positive test (5%), while the NPV is the probability for a person with a negative test to be free from the disease (95%).

In brief, the positive LR describes how likely a patient will give a positive test compared to a disease-free subject. In contrast, the PPV describes the probability of a subject who has a positive test being a patient or free from the disease. Similarly, the negative LR describes how likely a patient will give a negative test compared to a disease-free subject. In contrast, the NPV describes the probability of a subject who has a negative test being a patient or free from the disease. Although we did not show the details of the more diseased cardiac population, the positive post-test probability equals 94.1%, and the negative post-test probability is equal to $1 - NPV = 1-82.6 = 17.4\%$ (Fig. 1.43B). The interpretation is as follows: using the sphygmomanometer improves our ability to correctly diagnose a patient with hypertension from 50 to 94.1%. There is a limited 17.4% chance that a hypertensive patient will be diagnosed as disease-free, or 82.6% of cases giving a negative test are disease-free.

Another example may give more clarity on the difference between likelihood ratios and predictive values. Suppose that 90 out of every 100 patients presenting to a large tertiary cardiac center with chest pain due to myocardial ischemia have a positive CK-MB test (TP). The same test was positive for 15 out of 100 patients whose chest pain was due to other causes than myocardial ischemia (FP), and hence, the positive

LR = TP/FP = 0.9/0.15 = 6. This result does not necessarily mean that a patient presenting with chest pain in another hospital with a positive test result is six times as likely to have myocardial ischemia as not; this is the wrong interpretation of the positive LR. The latter means that if the patient already has myocardial ischemia, he is six times more likely to give a positive test than a patient without myocardial ischemia. LR does not predict the disease in a patient with a given test but the test results if the patient already has the disease. In a smaller hospital where the prevalence of such serious cases is only 10%, the pre-test odds = 0.1/(1–0.1) = 0.11. The post-test odds = 0.11 × 6 = 0.66 and hence, the post-test probability = 0.66/(1 + 0.66) = 0.397. In conclusion, given a patient with a positive test result, the post-test probability of acute myocardial infarction (40%) is less than half of that calculated for the tertiary center (90%).

> The positive LR describes how likely a patient will give a positive test compared to a disease-free subject. The negative LR describes how likely a patient will give a negative test compared to a disease-free subject. Interpretation is straightforward but the results are mainly directed to the physician helping him re-evaluate his decision for a particular patient.

1.9.3.4 What Should Be Reported

As the likelihood ratios are just the ratio of 2 proportions, we can calculate the 95% CI of LR as any other proportion, provided that the sample size is large with, say, 60 patients or more [38]. All calculations for the 95% confidence intervals have to be made in the logarithmic scale. Provided that n1 = number of patients and n2 = number of healthy subjects, we are calculating the 95% CI of positive LR, p_1 = Sn and p_2 = (1 − Sp). In case we are calculating the 95% CI of negative LR, p_1 = (1 − Sn) and p_2 = specificity. We begin by calculating the Se of log LR "Eq. (1.67)". We produce the 95% CI by assigning 1.96 logs Se on either side of log LR "Eq. (1.68)". We then produce the 95% CI of LR by the back transformation of the upper and lower limits of the logarithmic values "Eq. (1.69)". Applying the formulae on data presented in Table 1.13, the positive LR will equal 16 (95% CI: 10–25) and the negative LR equal 0.21 (95% CI: 0.14–0.31). Finally, we can consult the Z table to find the degree of significance of the standardized LR "Eq. (1.70)" or calculate the P-value ourselves by applying a formula given by Altman and Bland "Eq. (1.71)" [40]. Note that all confidence intervals are bilateral and all equations suppose that sample size is large.

$$Se(\log LR) = \sqrt{\frac{1 - p_1}{n_1 \times p_1} + \frac{1 - p_2}{n_2 \times p_2}} \quad (1.67)$$

$$95\% \ CI(\log LR) = \log LR \pm 1.96 \ Se \log LR \quad (1.68)$$

$$95\% \ CI(LR) = e^{LL \ 95\% \ CI(\log LR)} \ \text{to} \ e^{UL \ 95\% \ CI(\log LR)} \quad (1.69)$$

$$Z \ \text{for} \ LR = \frac{\log LR}{\log Se} \quad (1.70)$$

$$P \ \text{value} = \text{Exp}^{\left(-0.717 \times Z - 0.416 \times Z^2\right)} \quad (1.71)$$

1.9.4 Single Indicators of Test Performance

None of the previously mentioned paired indicators of diagnostic accuracies, such as Sn and Sp, PPV and NPV, positive LR, and negative LR, in itself represents the discriminatory test performance. As an example, a test can have a high sensitivity but low specificity. Hence, comparing competing tests can be misleading, significantly if one test does not outperform the other on both indicators. Overall accuracy measures were suggested to be more helpful in comparing different tests or the same test used in different groups drawn from the same population. Single indicators can either measure the performance of a diagnostic test at specific thresholds or, globally,

available thresholds. Examples of the former include the overall accuracy, diagnostic odds ratio (DOR) [41], and net benefit methods [42, 43]. Examples of the latter are the most widely used area under the receiver operating curve (AUC ROC) and the oldest method known after the name of its creator: the Youden index. Being created from Sn and Sp, those indices cannot appreciate the effect of the disease prevalence that dictates the number of false results, which can have significant clinical and budgetary effects. Net benefit methods were created to overcome this major disadvantage by looking at the benefits beyond instantaneous accuracy. Including the disease prevalence and impact of false positive and false negative results in the index itself overcomes the sequelae of misclassification [43].

1.9.4.1 Total Accuracy
One prominent approach was to combine sensitivity and specificity in one single number. In its simplest form, we can express the overall accuracy as the proportions of all correct results, i.e., the true positive and true negative results (TP + TN)/(TP + TN + FP + FN). Among the drawbacks of this simple approach is that it does not differentiate between Se and Sp, giving equal weight to a test with high Sn but low Sp and another test with low Sn but high Sp. Both tests do not have the same discriminative power, of course. The method equally ignores prevalence and hence, the sequelae of misclassification.

1.9.4.2 Diagnostic Odds Ratio (DOR)
Odds ratio (OR) is usually used to express the tightness of the association between 2 binary qualitative variables, such as the presence/absence of a risk factor or an event and the presence/absence of the disease. Consequently, it can be used to describe the strength of the relation between the result of a diagnostic test (positive or negative) and the health condition (disease or disease-free). Diagnostic odds ratio (DOR) is the ratio between 2 odds. The odds of having a positive or a negative test result, when the patient has the disease (TP/FN) and the odds of having a positive or negative test result, when the patient is

free from the disease (FP/TN) "Eq. (1.72)". Put it this way, DOR is the ratio of the odds of positivity in disease relative to the odds of positivity in the disease-free [41].

$$DOR = \frac{TP/FN}{FP/TN} \qquad (1.72)$$

Put it another way, Sn is the proportion of TP among the diseased, and hence, FN = 1 − Sn. Sp is the proportion of TN among disease-free patients playing the same tune, and hence, FP = 1 − Sp. Consequently, we can deduct DOR directly from Sn ad Sp, independently from the prevalence of the disease "Eq. (1.73)".

$$DOR = \frac{Sn/(1 - Sn)}{(1 - Sp)/Sp} \qquad (1.73)$$

Mathematically, (a/b)/(c/d) = (a/c)/(b/d); as example: (50/5)/(10/2) = (50/10)/(5/2) = 2. In consequence, Sn/(1 − Sn)/(1 − Sp)/Sp = Sn/(1 − Sp)/(1 − Sn)/Sp. As, Sn/(1 − Sp) is the positive LR and (1 − Sn)/Sp is the negative likelihood ratio, DOR can be directly calculated from the likelihood ratios "Eq. (1.74)":

$$DOR = \frac{positive\ LR}{negative\ LR} \qquad (1.74)$$

Being an odds ratio, DOR has a skewed distribution, can take any value and the null is (1), indicating that the test has no discriminative ability. The higher is the sensitivity or specificity, the larger would be the value of DOR and the more test can discriminate between patients and healthy subjects [41]. In order to assign a 95% CI around DOR, it has to be normalized by calculating log DOR and executing all calculations in the log scale. We can calculate the standard error of log DOR from the square root of the sum of the four inverse values (TP, FP, TN, and FN) "Eq. (1.75)". Log DOR follows an approximately normal distribution. We can proceed as usual and find the corresponding Z value by dividing log DOR by its standard error "Eq. (1.76)". The statistical significance of Z is

looked for in the Z table as usual. We calculate a 95% CI of log DOR "Eq. (1.77)," and then back transform its upper and lower limits to get the corresponding limits of the 95% CI of DOR "Eq. (1.78)".

$$Se(\log DOR) = \sqrt{\frac{1}{TP} + \frac{1}{FP} + \frac{1}{TN} + \frac{1}{FN}} \qquad (1.75)$$

$$Z = \frac{(\log DOR)}{Se(\log DOR)} \qquad (1.76)$$

$$95\%\ CI(\log DOR) = \log DOR \\ \pm 1.96\ Se \log DOR \qquad (1.77)$$

$$95\%\ CI(DOR) = e^{LL\ 95\%\ CI(\log DOR)} \text{ to } e^{UL\ 95\%\ CI(\log DOR)} \qquad (1.78)$$

The Example

Let us take the example of testing a new digital sphygmomanometer versus the classic mercury device. The new digital device has a known sensitivity and specificity of 80 and 95%, respectively and the example has been given before in the likelihood ratio (see Sect. 1.9.3, Table 1.12). As seen from the preceding equations, DOR can be calculated from either TP, TN, FP and FN values, sensitivity and specificity, or likelihood ratios "Eqs. (1.73), (1.74). and (1.75)". In our example, DOR is equal to 76 "Eq. (1.79)". The Se is calculated on the logarithmic scale "Eq. (1.80)" and the statistical significance of Log OR is tested by calculating the corresponding Z and P values "Eq. (1.81)". The 95% CI of OR is first calculated on the normalized logarithmic scale "Eq. (1.82)" and then its upper and lower limits (3.65–5) are back transformed to get the corresponding limits on the regular scale (39 and 148) "Eq. (1.83)". The interpretation of our results is that the odds of a positive test in a hypertensive patient is 76 (39–148) times the odds of a positive test in a disease-free patient; P < 0.001. The same calculations can be easily obtained online [8]

$$DOR = \frac{80/20}{20/380} = \frac{0.8/(1-0.8)}{(1-0.95)/0.95} = \frac{4}{0.053}$$
$$= 76$$

$$\text{(1.79)}$$

$$Se(\log DOR) = \sqrt{\frac{1}{80} + \frac{1}{20} + \frac{1}{380} + \frac{1}{20}} = 0.339$$

$$\text{(1.80)}$$

$$Z = \frac{(\log DOR)}{(Se \log DOR)} = \frac{4.33}{0.339} = 12.77;$$
$$P < 0.001 \quad \text{(1.81)}$$

$$95\% \ CI(\log 76) = 4.33 \pm 1.96(0.339)$$
$$= 3.65 \text{ to } 5 \quad \text{(1.82)}$$

$$95\% \ CI(DOR) = e^{3.65} \text{ to } e^5 = 39 \text{ to } 148$$

$$\text{(1.83)}$$

The diagnostic odds ratio is the ratio between two odds independently calculated in two populations. The odds of having a positive/negative test if the patient has the disease and the same odds if the patient is free from the disease. A value of 1 means that the test cannot discriminate between the two populations and that the test is useless for not telling whether the patient has or does not have the disease.

1.9.4.3   The Area Under the Receiver Operating Curve (AUC-ROC)

The analysis of the area under the curve (AUC) of a ROC plot began in observations made in Britain during World War II. Radar receiver operators were being assessed on their ability to differentiate between a genuinely positive signal (e.g., an enemy aircraft or submarine) or a false positive one (e.g., a group of birds or whales). This ability to differentiate between a true-positive test and a false-positive test soon found its place in the industry and later on in medicine.

The Idea Behind ROC Plots

The idea behind a ROC plot is simple. Sensitivity is the proportion of true positive results in the diseased population, while specificity (Sp) is the proportion of TN results in the disease-free population. As the test results in the disease-free population can be either TN or FP; Sp = TN/(TN + FP) and (1 − Sp) will be the proportion of FP results "Eq. (1.84)".

$$(1 - Sp) = 1 - \frac{TN}{(TN + FP)}$$
$$= \frac{(TN + FP)}{(TN + FP)} - \frac{TN}{(TN + FP)} = FP$$

$$\text{(1.84)}$$

As example, a test with an (Sp) of 0.8 means that 80% of the results are expected to be TN and 20% are FP. By simple deduction, (1 − Sp) = 1− 0.8 = 0.2 or 20%; which is the proportion of FP results in the disease-free population. Second, as Sn and Sp are known to be inversely proportional to one other, Sn and 1 − Sp will be directly proportional to each other (Fig. 1.44). Put it this way:

- Sn is the proportion of TP results among the diseased patients.
- 1 − Sp is the proportion of FP results among the disease-free subjects.
- Both are directly proportional to each other.

Now, by plotting the (Sn) on the y-axis and the (1 − Sp) on the x-axis, we can calculate for each paired data point the probability of being "a truly positive" result (Sn) and the probability of being "a false positive" result (1 − Sp). Repeating the same interpretation of all data points plots the whole spectrum of sensitivity and specificity. The area formed under this plot is called: the area under the curve (AUC). The size and the shape of the latter visualize the overall diagnostic performance of the test. In addition, the researcher can choose from all paired data points the cut-off values that best serve the purpose of designing the test. A high sensitivity cut-off value for a test used to screen the disease or a high specificity

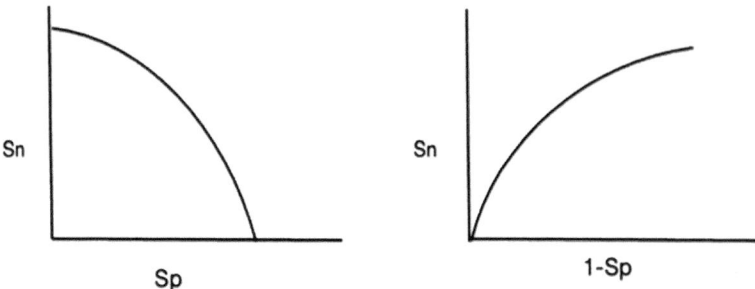

Fig. 1.44 The relation between sensitivity (Sn), specificity (Sp) and (1 − Sp)

(low 1 − Sp) threshold for a confirmatory test [15].

A Mini-Example

Although it is advised to include a minimum of 30 patients for a meaningful ROC plot, yet we will try to understand the mechanism by taking a "mini" sample of only five diabetic patients and five normal controls. The calculation of our "mini sample" is presented in Table 1.14. Column I show the five measures observed in the diabetic group: 50, 100, 110, 130, and 140 mg/dL, and column IV shows the five

measures observed in the control group: 60, 70, 80, 90, and 120 mg/dL. Column III shows the suggested cut-off points, which should embrace the whole range of values observed in the series (50–140 mg/dL), and hence, the suggested thresholds have to range from: <50 to >140 mg/dL. The 1st (49 mg/dL) has to lie just before the smallest observed value, and each of the following thresholds will lie at the mean of every two successive values. By definition, sensitivity is the number of TP cases/total number of diseased cases (D+). Hence, Sn is only calculated independently in the diseased group and shown

Table 1.14 Sensitivity and specificity thresholds in a mini-ROC plot

I	II	III	IV	V
FBS (D+)	Sensitivity	Cut-off points	FBS (D−)	1 − specificity
−	1	49[a]	−	1
50	0.8	55	−	1
−	0.8	65	60	0.8
−	0.8	75	70	0.6
−	0.8	85	80	0.4
−	0.8	95	90	0.2
100	0.6	105	−	0.2
110	0.4	115	−	0.2
−	0.4	125	120	0
130	0.2	135	−	0
140	0	145[b]	−	0

Values are fasting blood sugar (FBS) in mg/dL, Column I = FBS calculated for the 5 diabetic patients (D+), column II = sensitivity = proportion of positive cases among the diabetic group (the case is considered positive when its FBS ≥ respective value in column III), column III = cut-off points of FBS, column IV = FBS calculated for the 5 disease-free patients (D−), column V = 1 − specificity = proportion of positive cases among the disease-free group (the case is considered positive when its FBS ≥ respective value in column III), [a] and [b] = 1st and 11th cut-off values in column II in decimals. On the other hand, (1 − Specificity) is the number of FP cases/total number of disease-free cases (D−), and hence, (1 − Sp) is calculated independently in the disease-free group only and is shown in column IV in decimals too. Any FBS value is considered positive (either TP or FP) if it is equal to or larger than the suggested cut-off point shown in the same row of column III.

Starting by analyzing sensitivity: considering the 1st suggested threshold (49 mg/dL), all diabetic patients have an FBS > 49 mg/dL. Hence, this threshold will not miss a single diabetic patient from being diagnosed. In other words, this thresh-old will detect all 5 TP results. The Sn of the 1st threshold = TP/D+ = 5/5 = 1 or 100%. For the second line, with a threshold of 55 mg/dL, one diabetic patient has a smaller FBS value (50 mg/dL), and hence, he will escape diagnosis. This threshold will detect 4 TP results out of the five diabetic patients. The Sn of the 2nd threshold = TP/D+ = 4/5 = 0.8 or 80%; i.e., 20% of diabetic patients will be missed by this threshold. Nothing changed for the four successive threshold values of 65, 75, 85, and 95 mg/dL; till we reached the 7th threshold value of 105 mg/dL where one more diabetic patient had a smaller FBS value of 100 mg/dL and hence, he will be missed from being diagnosed. Only 3 TP cases will be detected among the 5 diabetic patients and hence, the Sn drops to =TP/D+ = 3/5 = 0.6 or 60%. In other words, 40% of diabetic cases will be missed if we choose the 105 mg/dL threshold. As shown in Table 1.14, the calculations go on in the same manner but have to stop as we reach the 11th and last threshold value of 145 mg/dL, where all diseased patients have smaller FBS levels reducing the Sn at this threshold to 0%.

We repeat the same procedure independently to calculate 1 − Sp in the disease-free subjects, along with the same cut-off values (thresholds). From the 1st cut-off point (49 mg/dL) to the 2nd cut-off point (55 mg/dL), all patients had FBS > 49 mg/dL and hence, they will be all considered as being FP and hence, 1 − Sp at those thresholds = FP/D− = 5/5 = 1 or 100%. At the 3rd cut-off point of 65 mg/dL, one patient

has a smaller value (60 mg/dL) and hence, 1 − Sp at this threshold = FP/D− = 4/5 = 0.8 or 80%. At the 4th cut-off point of 75 mg/dL, another case has a lower FBS level of 70 mg/dL and hence, 1 − Sp at this threshold = FP/D− = 3/5 = 0.6 or 60%. The calculation goes on but has to stop as we reach the 11th and last cut-off value of 125 mg/dL, where all diseased patients have smaller FBS levels reducing 1 − Sp to 0%. Specificity at those 11 thresholds is then calculated as 1 − (1 − Sp). The 11 cut-off points are presented in Fig. 1.45, which is the ROC plot of data presented in Table 1.14. Each one of those points represents a decision made, at a specific threshold. Kindly note that while those eleven decisions were based on paired data (sensitivity/1 − specificity), the two components of each pair were calculated independently from one another. Sensitivity was calculated in the diseased population, while (1 − specificity) was calculated in the healthy population. Hence, calculations are independent from the prevalence of the disease in the population of concern [44].

The Generation of the ROC Plot

Returning to our data points, the more significant is the probability that a particular data point is TP, the more it will acquire a higher position on the plot. On the other hand, the more significant is the probability that it is an FP result, the more it will move to the right side of the plot. In other words, the final position of each data point is a bargain between the two probabilities of being TP or FP? The more are the former probabilities for all data points (TP), the more the line (the curve) joining those points will be dragged up and to the left and, the more are the (FP) probabilities, the more the curve will be dragged down and to the right. Consequently, the proportion of the area under the curve to the total surface area increases with TP results, reflecting the discriminative ability of the test in making a correct diagnosis among diseased patients, i.e., in terms of sensitivity.

Now concerning specificity: a particular ROC plot that is dragged up and to the left and hence, increasing the area under the curve (AUC) means that the probability of FP results is low and, as

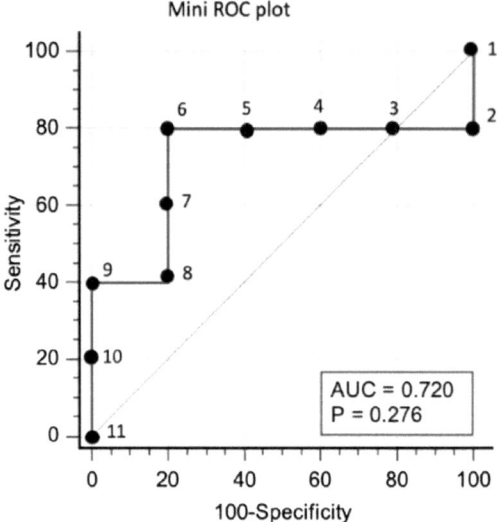

Fig. 1.45 Mini ROC plot of data presented in Table 1.14. The dots from the 1st to the 11th represent the 11 cut-off points figuring in Table 1.14, Sn = sensitivity, Sp = specificity, AUC—area under the curve (95% CI)

the latter is calculated in disease-free patients only, this means that the proportion of TN results increases among those patients. Put it this way, the more is the probability of making a correct diagnosis among disease-free patients (TN results), the more the ROC plot will move towards the opposite direction (upwards and to the left), and the larger will be the (AUC). Consequently, the AUC reflects the discriminative power of the diagnostic test in terms of both: sensitivity and specificity.

The Perfect and the Useless ROC Plot

If there is no overlap between the two distributions (e.g., health and disease), every positive result will be TP. Hence, all observed data points will lie directly on the y-axis, and the corresponding value on the x-axis will always be zero. Consequently, the area to the right of the line joining those data points (AUC) is equal to the total surface area = 1, or 100% (perfect) sensitivity, as shown in Fig. 1.46A. Put it this way, every positive test will be a TP result, and by deduction, every negative test will be a TN result; hence, an AUC that equals 1 means perfect specificity.

The other side of the coin is that both distributions are identical and perfectly overlapping. Every positive result will have equal chances of being either TP or FP. As shown in Fig. 1.46B, the distance between each data point and the x-axis is exactly equivalent to the distance between this point and the y-axis. The no-discrimination trend line is a 45° diagonal passing from the coordinates (0,0) to (1,1). The area under this curve is 50%, meaning that each data point has a 50:50 chance of being TP or FP and an utterly useless plot. In practice, most plots fall between these two extremes, and the closer the plot is to the upper left corner, the higher the test's overall accuracy [44].

Figure 1.47 shows The ROC plot of data presented in Table 1.10, as generated by IBM-SPSS statistical software. The probability for a data point to be TP (its value on the y-axis) is larger than the alternative probability to be FP (corresponding value on the x-axis), which is responsible for the shoulder made by the *useful ROC plot*. The probability of the TP data drags the curve more towards the upper left corner and increases the area under the curve (AUC). On the other hand, the probability of the FP data drags

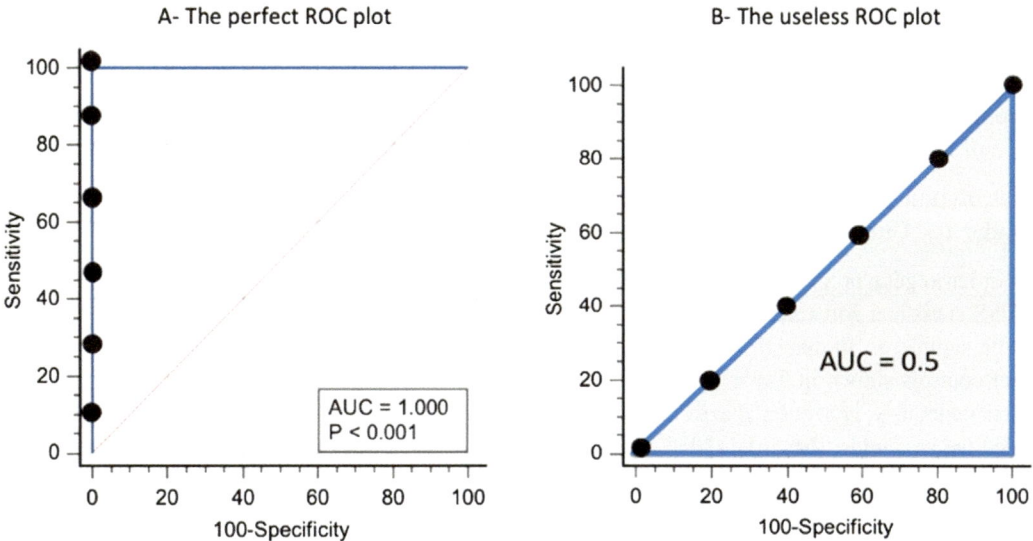

Fig. 1.46 The perfect and the useless ROC plot. A = the perfect plot, B = the useless plot, AUC = area under the curve

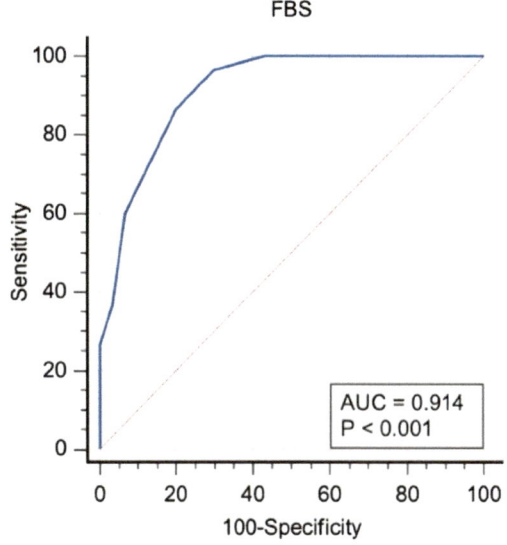

Fig. 1.47 The ROC plot of data presented in Table 1.10 generated by SPSS statistical software package, AUC = area under the curve (95% CI)

the curve towards the lower right corner, which tends to flatten this shoulder and decrease the area under the curve.

In conclusion, both the shoulder and the area under the curve reflect the usefulness of the ROC plot. As a rule of thumb, an AUC of 0.7–0.8 of the total surface areas indicates a good or useful discriminative power of the test, and AUC between 0.8 and 0.9 indicates an excellent test, and an AUC of 0.9 or higher indicates that the test has out-standing discriminative power [45]. As will be shown later, one of the oldest but still valid indices used to evaluate the overall discriminative power of a test is the Youden index, which is nothing but the distance between the shoulder and the no-discrimination 45° diagonal line of equality.

Calculation and Interpretation of the Area Under the Curve (AUC)

In order to get a proper ROC plot, we will use the SPSS statistical software package to analyze the large sample of 30 diabetic patients and 30 normal controls shown in Table 1.10. The software instantaneously generated the ROC plot, calculated the area under the curve (AUC = 0.914), its standard error (Se = 0.036), its 95% confidence interval of (0.843–0.98) and the P value < 0.001 (Fig. 1.47). The AUC can be interpreted as follows: if we randomly select a person from the diseased group and another person from the normal group, in 91.4 times out of 100, the first person will show a higher value of the test, compared to the latter. Put it another way, this area equals to a 91.4% probability that a random person with the disease has a higher value of the measurement than a random person without disease [37]. The test statistics is simple: comparing the no discrimination AUC of 0.5 (the null hypothesis) to our observed AUC of 0.914 (the alternative hypothesis) by calculating the standardized difference between both values; i.e., the Z value "Eq. (1.85)". Note that a Z value of ≥ 1.96 indicates a statistically significant discriminative power of the test (P < 0.05). Our Z value is much larger (11.5), indicating a highly significant discriminative power of the test (P < 0.001).

$$Z = \frac{(AUC - 0.5)}{Se} \qquad (1.85)$$

The Mini Versus the Conventional Plot

We have previously gone through the hand-made calculation for a mini-example which showed that a threshold of 95 mg/dL was associated with an 80% Sn and 80% Sp. Measuring the AUC and calculation of the its Sn and the 95% confidence interval is a tedious process, specially that they

are easily executed by many statistical software packages. Uploading the data of those 10 patients to SPSS, instantaneously generates the ROC plot and calculates the AUC as well as its 95% confidence interval: 0.72 (0.36–1), as shown in Fig. 1.45. Although this mini-ROC plot would have been considered as a useful ROC plot for having an AUC > 70%, yet neither this mini plot nor this interpretation can be accepted for publication anywhere, for the very small sample size and very wide interval of confidence.

Compared to the "conventional" example, the stairs appearance of the mini-example (Fig. 1.45) is replaced by diagonals due to the presence of ties (patients in the diseased and control groups who share the same FBS values) in the conventional example (Fig. 1.47) and obvious overlap of both distributions. Most importantly, the small sample of the mini example was responsible for the smaller discriminative power (AUC = 0.72), a much larger Se (0.185) and hence, a wider 95% interval of confidence (0.35–1) and a statistically non-significant P value; $Z = (0.72 - 0.5)/0.185 = 1.19$; P > 0.05.

Choosing the Appropriate Threshold

An overall ROC curve is most useful in the early stages of evaluating a new diagnostic test. Whether the test is primarily made to screen patients or confirm the diagnosis, a ROC plot offers the researcher the opportunity to form the whole spectrum the best threshold that fits the main test indication [46]. Let us continue working on the mini sample for the ease of viewing differences and effect of moving from one threshold to the other. Examining the 11 thresholds of our mini example shows that choosing the 6th threshold of 95 mg/dL or larger will provide 80% sensitivity and 80% specificity (1 − Sp = 0.2). In other words, by adopting this threshold, we will be able to correctly diagnose as much as 86.7% of diabetic patients and 80% of controls. Lowering our threshold will only decrease the test specificity from 80% down to 60, 40, and 20% and, the sensitivity will only be raised to 100% when we reach the threshold of 49 mg/dL. This threshold cannot be adopted because it is associated with 0% Sp, meaning that all disease-free cases will be misdiagnosed as having diabetes. The threshold of 95 mg/dL appears to be a good choice for a balanced test. Now returning to the large sample, it happens that the 95 mg/dL threshold also offers the best combined Sn (86.7%) and specificity (80%).

The Effect of Prevalence and Misclassifications

Every researcher should work to limit diagnosis errors, i.e., to decrease the proportion of FP and FN results. Although the calculation of both Sn and Sp are independent of prevalence (P), *the higher is (P), the more will be "the number" of healthy cases which give an (FP) result.* Concurrently, the less will be "the number" of diseased patients who give an (FN) result. The increased "numbers" of errors increases the financial and health burdens, and hence, when it comes to cost, prevalence has to be taken into consideration. The investigator has to look for those costs in previous records or studies. On the other hand, *false negative and false positive diagnoses, however, are rarely equally important.* Missing a life-threatening disease is much more serious than a false positive diagnosis in a healthy patient [43].

Zweig and Campbell suggested an equation to detect the best threshold on a ROC curve, while considering the costs of undesirable errors and prevalence [44]. First, all costs have to be expressed numerically and on the same scale. For example, if the health cost of an FN result is expected to be double that of an FP result, $FN_c = 2$ and $FP_c = 1$. The effect of prevalence and false results can be expressed as a line descending from above and to the left (maximum Sn point) downwards towards the ROC curve. The slope "m" of this line as it touches the ROC curve represents the threshold point that will yield the optimal mix of FP and FN results, given prevalence and the relative cost weights assigned to false results in the cost ratio [44]. As shown in "Eq. (1.86)" the costs of TN and TP results can be added to the original equation designed by the authors.

$$m = \frac{FP_c - TN_c}{FN_c - TP_c} \times \frac{1 - P}{P} \qquad (1.86)$$

As "m" has to be a positive number, costs of FP and TN as well as costs of FN and TP cannot be equal and, if the cost of TN > FP, the cost of TP has to be >FN and vice versa. An expected benefit from an FP or an FN result can be expressed as a negative cost. It is clear that if the cost of FP and FN results were equal, the cost of errors would be dependent on prevalence alone. The calculation of "m" can be made online by a statistical software package such as MedCalc statistical software. The software calculates for each threshold, not only the associated sensitivity (column II, Table 1.14) and the 1 − specificity (column V in Table 1.14) but equally the average cost of using the diagnostic test at this level, which does not include the overhead cost of using the test itself, of course [8].

The AUC of a ROC plot is the most commonly used indicator of test performance. The more significant is the AUC (>0.7), the more is the discriminative ability of the test. As the plotted paired data points (Sn/1 − Sp) are calculated independently in the diseased and the healthy populations, the AUC ignores prevalence and the clinical and financial costs of misclassifications (FP and FN results). Prevalence and costs of false results are better considered during the calculations, and they have to be reported, especially when comparing two ROC plots.

The partial AUC (AUCp)

A conventional ROC plot can be a disadvantage if thresholds that are clinically relevant are combined with those that are clinically nonsensical. The standard ROC AUC can be seen as an average across all possible thresholds. However, not all test thresholds are clinically important. As Sn is indirectly proportional to Sp, many high Sn thresholds (such as greater than 80%) are not clinically useful because their specificity can be too low and hence too many FP cases will be recruited with such threshold overwhelming diagnostic services [43].

Playing the same tune, the researchers will aim to reduce the amount of FP results in case of a hazardous test, where it will be unwise to subject too many patients for those hazards [43]. Figure 1.48 shows AUCp restricting comparisons between the Sn thresholds from 0 to 80%, giving a partial ROC AUC (AUCp) of 0.763. AUCp can be equally calculated for the interval between any two Se or Sp thresholds. Figure 1.49 shows AUCp (0.151) calculated for the interval of 80–100% specificity. As such, AUCp removes a lot of redundant thresholds from the evaluation, especially those cases below the diagonal line where 50% of patients are expected to be FP.

In Fig. 1.49, the partial area under the curve (AUCp) calculated for the limited Sp threshold between 80 and 100% equals 0.151, compared to a total area under the curve of (0.914) calculated for all specificity threshold calculated for the same patients (Fig. 1.47). The former can be interpreted as the average sensitivity for the prespecified specificity interval (80–100%), while the latter is interpreted as the average sensitivity over the overall specificity thresholds.

The Standardized AUCp

McClish has proposed to standardize the AUCp so as to be view from the same scale as the total AUC [47]. As shown in Fig. 1.49, the AUCp that is limited inferiorly by the horizontal dashed line extending between the two (1 − specificity) points 0 and 20, corresponding to 100–80% specificity. The AUCp above this line is divided by the tangential line of equivalence into two parts: an upper part above the line and a lower part below the line of equivalence. This lower part is the *minimum surface area* that AUCp can acquire (AUCp$_{min}$).

Now looking to the ROC curve, itself, the *maximum vertical position* that it can acquire is 100% and hence, the upper border of the dotted rectangle represents the upper limit of the maximum surface area that AUCp can acquire too (AUCp$_{max}$). The standardized AUCp (AUCps) will be the proportion between the "observed" AUCp and the "maximum expected" area under the curve (AUCp$_{max}$) after removal of the redundancy (AUCp$_{min}$) "Eq. (1.87)". The standardized

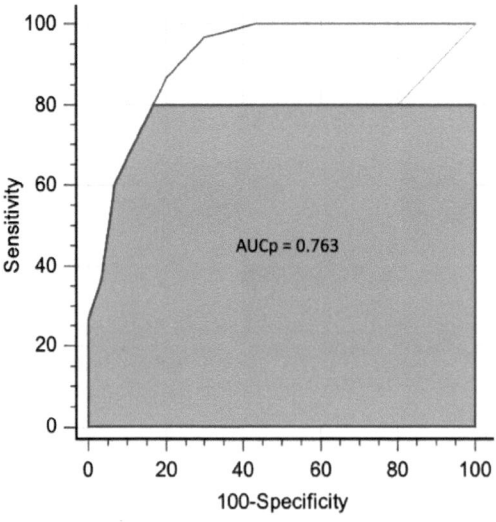

Fig. 1.48 The partial AUC of a ROC plot (AUCp) for sensitivity ≤ 80%

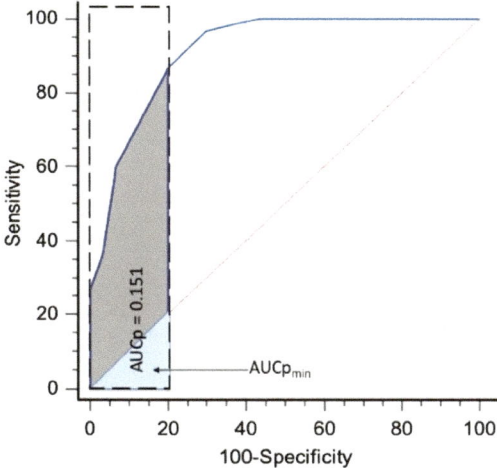

Fig. 1.49 The partial AUC of a ROC plot (AUCp) for sensitivity specificity between 80–100%. AUCp$_{min}$ is presented by the basal triangular light-shaded area below the tangential line of equivalence

AUCp has a maximum value of 1 and a minimum value of 0.5. Remember that 0.5 is a useless point and means nothing on the curve. The standardized AUCp for Figs. 1.48 and 1.49 were 0.943 and 0.863; respectively. They can be calculated by a commercial statistical software package such as MedCalc software [8]. As nothing is perfect, AUCp has the disadvantage of raising the arguments about which thresholds which would be clinically relevant and which are not, especially that changing a particular threshold on such a small scale can lead to a totally different clinical decision [43].

$$AUCps = 0.5\left(1 + \frac{AUCp - AUCp_{min}}{AUCp_{max} - AUCp_{min}}\right)$$
(1.87)

What Should be Reported

We have to report whether the total AUC or AUCp and standardized AUCp, with their 95% confidence intervals. Although we have to report the P value, yet the surface area is much more important that the calculated P value, which only points to a significant difference between the ROC curve and the equivalence line. We should report specificity and sensitivity and their 95% intervals of confidence, the prevalence of the disease and discuss the costs of misdiagnoses, whenever they were included in the calculations, with the selected references.

The AUC of standard ROC averages across all possible thresholds but not all thresholds are clinically relevant. Limiting comparison to those sensitive thresholds by a partial area under the curve (AUCp) was suggested to improve interpretation. However, researchers may argue about the relevance of the chosen sensible limits. In addition, the narrowed scale of an (AUCp) makes the test very sensible to changing cut-off thresholds and subsequent decisions. As the results of studies on (AUCp) were mended to exclude many FP results, it may be unwise to extrapolate those results on the whole population, where FP results can predominate.

1.9.4.4 Youden Index

Returning to our data points, the more significant is the probability that a particular data point is TP, the more it will acquire a higher position on the plot. On the other hand, the more significant

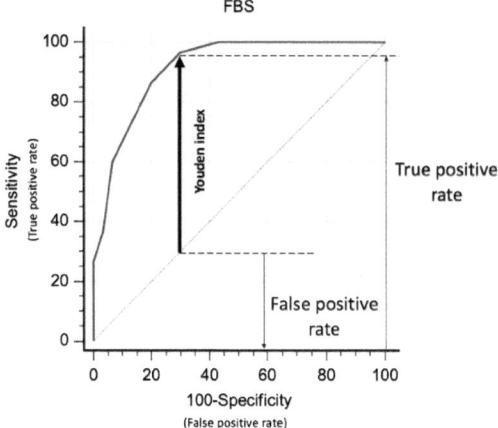

Fig. 1.50 Youden index

the probability that it is an FP result, the more it will move to the right side of the plot. In other words, the final position of each data point is a bargain between the two probabilities of being TP or FP? The more are the former probabilities for all data points (TP), the more the line (the curve) joining those points will be dragged up and to the left and, the more are the (FP) probabilities, the more the curve will be dragged down and to the right. Consequently, the distance between the shoulder of ROC and the first bisector of equality measures the rate of TP results, while its downward extension to the x-axis $(1 - Sp)$ measures the FP rate (Fig. 1.50). The former is the index suggested by Youden JW to describe the power of the test to discriminate between health and disease [48]. The reader is invited to calculate Youden index for the perfect and the useless ROC plots shown in Fig. 1.46. The shoulder of the perfect plot runs along the y-axis itself and hence it detected all TP results; i.e., it has a perfect sensitivity of 1 and the distance between the shoulder and the first bisector of equality (Youden index) = 1 (100% of the total vertical distance). The second question is what is the specificity of this perfect ROC plot? As shown, it has a $1 - Sp$ of (0) and hence it has perfect specificity of 1 (Fig. 1.46).

Consequently, another quick way to calculate Youden index is to subtract 1 from the sum of both Sn and Sp [49]. In our case, Youden

index $= (1 + 1) - 1 = 1$; which is the same value calculated graphically (Fig. 1.50). Now looking to the useless curve, its shoulder is on the first bisector line itself, and hence, its Youden index = 0. It is clear that Youden index can vary between 0 (a useless test) and 1 (a test with perfect discriminative power). One advantage of being calculated from Sn and Sp is to be immune to the changes in Prevalence. However, for the same reason of being calculated using the sum of both Se and Sn, Youden's index becomes insensitive to the differences between Sn and Sp [49]. In other words, two tests having the same index may have totally different discriminative Sn and Sp powers. Hence, although a higher index indicates a better discriminative ability of a test, Youden indices cannot be simply compared as numbers.

1.9.5 Choosing the Appropriate Diagnostic Test

A diagnostic test is commonly used for making a decision as a proxy for a gold standard. Some measures are used to assess the diagnostic test's discriminative property, such as Sn and Sp, area under the ROC plot, diagnostic odds ratio, and Youden index [49]. Sn and Sp are used to describe how having or not having the disease predicts the results of the test. In contrast, PPV and NPV describe the reverse: how a positive or a negative test result predicts that a patient has or does not have the disease. Unlike the Sn and the Sp, predictive values depend on the Prevalence; hence, they can only be generalized with extreme caution. The likelihood ratios provided a solution by predicting the post-test probability of having or not having the disease while adapting to prior probabilities, including the Prevalence. Consequently, unlike predictive values, likelihood ratios calculated for one study can be extrapolated to other studies and adapted to a specific group of patients [38]. We have shown an example in Sect. 1.9.3.3. We have used the solid positive (LR = 16) and meaningful negative LR of the test (LR = 0.21) discovered in one of the two populations to update the pre-test probabilities of the other. As mentioned, the equations are simple, and the instantaneous online calculations are freely available [7–9, 36].

The choice of a particular measure depends upon the primary indication of the diagnostic test. If we aim to screen a disease, we benefit from including all possibly diseased patients, even if some of the positive results later appear to be false. In other words, we should to minimize false-negative results (FN) so as not to miss any patient; in such a case, sensitivity [Sn] will be the crucial element. As Sn = TP/(TP + FN), it is evident that the smaller FN is, the more sensitive the test would be. The other side of the coin is the test's negative predictive value [NPV], which should also be demonstrated, i.e., its ability to exclude the presence of the disease if the result was negative (rendering false-negative results to a minimum too). Both Sn and NPV correlate positively: the higher the probability of identifying a single diseased patient, the more likely an individual who shows a negative result to the test does not have the disease.

On the other hand, if we aim to confirm the disease, we have to focus on the [Sp] of our method. In this setting, we have the interest to minimize false positive (FP) results. As Sp = TN/(TN + FP), the smaller FP, the higher Sp to approach (1 = 100%). Concordantly, the other side of the coin will be the [PPV] of the test, i.e., its ability to confirm the presence of the disease

when the subject shows a positive result. Both [Sp] and [PPV] correlate positively: the higher the probability of having the disease when the test is negative, the more the probability that an individual who shows a positive result to the test has the disease.

Choosing a particular test depends on the pre-test probability. If the latter is low, the primary aim will be to exclude the disease, and hence, we choose the most sensitive test, hoping that a negative result can rule out the disease. In case of a high pre-test probability, the primary aim will be to confirm the disease, and hence, we choose the most specific test, hoping that a positive result can rule in the disease. Alternatively, we choose the test with the highest positive LR in the former and the lowest negative LR in the latter.

1.9.6 Comparing Two Diagnostic Tests

A researcher comparing diagnostic tests in non-randomized group faces the major challenge of initial comparability between subjects. In contrast, he may expect the most accurate results when conducting a paired study or, at least, randomize his study groups [43].

1.9.6.1 Comparison of Paired Measures at a Specific Threshold

If we wish to compare a paired measure such as sensitivity or specificity, we must present each measure with its 95% CI. The appropriate statistical test will depend on the setting. If the diagnostic tests were studied on two independent groups of patients, the results would be compared by chi-square or Fisher's exact tests (see Sect. 2.3.1). If both diagnostic tests were performed on the same group of patients, then the paired data has to be compared by McNemar's test (see Sect. 2.3.2). The reader is requested to refer back to chapter two for the details of those tests, and, most importantly, he has to be careful in interpreting the absence of evidence. A statistically significant difference is interpreted that both measures are significantly different, while the absence of a significant difference should never be interpreted that both measures are the same but only comparable.

Sn and Sp are calculated independently in the diseased and in the healthy population and hence, they are independent of the disease prevalence (see Sect. 1.9.1). A change in prevalence changes the "number" of false positive and false negative results, which can have important clinical and financial costs. Sn and Sp ignore those costs, and hence, they are mainly helpful whenever the balance between false positive and false negative results is not of immediate importance. On the other hand, we can enhance their values by reporting alongside the actual number and costs of misdiagnosis.

1.9.6.2   Comparison of Summary Measures at Specific Thresholds

Several methods were suggested to develop a single measure of diagnostic performance at a specific clinically relevant threshold, such as diagnostic odds ratio (DOR). The test with the larger measure is considered to be more accurate. DOR is deducted from Sn and Sp and hence, it ignores the clinical and financial costs of false results and their importance in the decision-making process (see Sect. 1.9.4.2). Reporting DOR can also be enhanced by reporting alongside the actual number and costs of misdiagnosis, as in paired measures.

The Weighted Comparison Method (WC)

The newer net benefit methods aimed to cover the limitations of using Sn and Sp alone by extending the evaluation to the consequences of diagnosis, especially the financial cost of false results, and incorporating the prevalence. The weighted comparison (WC) is a good example [42, 43].

The difference between Sn and Sp of the two compared tests (Δ) is weighted by the relative cost of false results (FP and FN) and the Prevalence of the disease (P) "Eq. (1.88)" [42, 43]. As shown by Mallet and colleagues [43], the result interpretation is straightforward: a positive WC index means a benefit while a negative value translates into a net loss. Moreover, the statistical significance of the result can be evaluated by creating a 95% CI, as usual. The authors illustrated an informative example and provided references to other net benefit methods [43].

$$WC = \Delta Sn + \left(\frac{1-P}{P}\right) \times relative\ cost\left(\frac{FP}{TP}\right) \times \Delta Sp$$

$$(1.88)$$

1.9.6.3   Comparison of Single Measures Averaged Across Multiple Threshold

Unlike Sn and Sp, ROC plots are not dependent on the scale of the test results, and hence, they regain their importance once the researcher wishes to compare two or more test results on a common scale [50]. The AUC has the disadvantage of including the redundant information (the part of results below the diagonal line) in the comparison and not taking into consideration the cost of misclassifications. The AUC can be enhanced by introducing prevalence and the cost of false results in the calculations, as suggested by Zweig and Campbell [44]. Limiting the calculation to include the clinically relevant thresholds (AUCp) can be criticized by questioning the basis upon which those limits were chosen in the first place, the test becoming very sensitive to changing threshold due to the narrowed scale and the unsafe extrapolation of those "partial" results on the "whole" population. Knowing the AUC, we can compare two independent ROC curves for different tests, treatment groups or different test observers whether online or with a statistical software package [7–9].

1.9.7 The Standards for Reporting Diagnostic Accuracy (STARD)

STARD initiative was a crucial step toward improving the quality of reporting of those studies of diagnostic accuracy. The completeness and transparency of reports allow the readers to assess the potential for bias in the study (internal validity) and to evaluate its generalizability (external validity). The majority of scientific journals include the STARD statement in their instructions to authors in scientific journals. Editors encourage authors to use the STARD checklist whenever reporting their studies on diagnostic accuracy. STARD 2015 checklist, flow diagram, and updates can be checked out at the equator network website [51].

References

1. Altman DG, Bland JM. Statistics notes: the normal distribution. BMJ. 1995;310:298. https://doi.org/10.1136/bmj.310.6975.298.
2. Edelman A. Statistics-and-PCA. http://web.mit.edu/18.06/www/Spring17/Statistics-and-PCA.pdf (2018). Accessed 25 Oct 2021.
3. Goldstone LA. The standard deviation and other measures of variations. In: Goldstone LD, editor. Understanding medical statistics. London: William Heinemann Ltd; 1983. p. 25–35. https://doi.org/10.1002/sim.4780040216.
4. Schwartz D. Méthodes statistiques a l'usage des médecins et des biologistes. 3rd ed. Paris: Médecines-Sciences Flammarion; 1969.
5. Altman DG, Machin D, Bryant TN, Gardner MJ. Statistics with confidence: confidence intervals and statistical guidelines. 1st ed. London: BMJ books; 1989.
6. Dougherty C. Statistical tables. In: Introduction to econometrics, 2nd ed. Oxford: Oxford University Press; 2002. https://home.ubalt.edu/ntsbarsh/Business-stat/StatistialTables.pdf. Assessed 1 Oct 2021.
7. Lowry, R. VassarStats: website for statistical computation. http://vassarstats.net/ (1998). Assessed 23 Oct 2021.
8. MedCalc software Lt. SciStat.com online. https://www.scistat.com/sysreq.php (2021). Accessed 9 Oct 2021.
9. Sergeant, ESG. Epitools epidemiological calculators. Ausvet. https://epitools.ausvet.com.au (2018). Accessed 6 Aug 2021.
10. Walker E, Nowacki AS. Understanding equivalence and non-inferiority testing. J Gen Intern Med. 2011;26:192–6. https://doi.org/10.1007/s11606-010-1513-8.
11. Hanley JA, Lippman-Hand A. If nothing goes wrong, is everything alright? JAMA. 1983;259:1743–5 PMID: 6827763.
12. Bland JM, Altman DG. Statistics notes: transforming data. BMJ. 1996;312:770. https://doi.org/10.1136/bmj.312.7033.770.
13. Bland JM, Altman DG. Statistics notes: logarithms. BMJ. 1996;312:700. https://doi.org/10.1136/bmj.312.7032.700.
14. Goodman SN. Towards evidence-based medical statistics: 1. The P value fallacy. Ann Intern Med. 1999; 130:995–1004. https://doi.org/10.7326/0003-4819-130-12-199906150-00008.
15. Laplanche A, Com-Nougue C, Flamant R. Méthodes statistiques appliqués a la recherché Clinique, 1st ed. Paris: Médecines-Sciences Flammarion; 1987. http://bdsp-ehesp.inist.fr/vibad/index.php?action=getRecordDetail&idt=52329.
16. Sn G, Berlin JA. The use of predicted confidence intervals when planning experiments and the misuse of power when interpreting results. Ann Intern Med. 1994;121:200–6. https://doi.org/10.7326/0003-4819-121-3-199408010-00008.
17. Altman DG, Bland JM. Statistics notes. Absence of evidence is not evidence of absence. BMJ. 1995; 485:311. https://doi.org/10.1136/bmj.311.7003.485.
18. Pagano M, Gauvreau K. Principles of biostatistics, 2nd ed. Belmont, CA: Brooks/Cole; 2000. https://doi.org/10.1201/9780429489624.
19. Altman D, Deeks J. Odds ratios should be avoided when events are common. BMJ. 1998; 317:1318. https://doi.org/10.1136/2Fbmj.317.7168.1318.
20. Zhang J, Yu KF. What's the relative risk? A method of correcting the odds ratio in cohort studies of common outcomes. JAMA. 1998; 280:1690–91. https://jamanetwork.com/journals/jama/fullarticle/188182.
21. Cox DR, Oakes D. Analysis of survival data, 1st ed. Boca Raton: Chapman and Hall/CRC; 1984. https://doi.org/10.1201/9781315137438.
22. Statistics Canada. Table 13-10-0710-01 mortality rates, by age group. https://doi.org/10.25318/1310071001-eng (2020). Accessed 16 Oct 2021.
23. Sackett R, Cook D. The number needed to treat: a clinically useful measure of treatment effect. BMJ. 1995;310:452–4. https://doi.org/10.1136/bmj.310.6977.452.
24. McQuay R, Moore H. Using numerical results from systematic reviews in clinical practice. Ann Intern

Med. 1997;126:712–20. https://doi.org/10.7326/0003-4819-126-9-199705010-00007.

25. Rothman KJ, Wise LA, Hatch E. Should graphs of risk or rate ratios be plotted on a log scale? Am J Epidemiol. 2011;174:376–7. https://doi.org/10.1093/aje/kwr156.

26. Daly L. Confidence limits made easy: interval estimation using a substitution method. Am J Epidemiol. 1998;147:783–90. https://doi.org/10.1093/oxfordjournals.aje.a009523.

27. Altman D. Confidence intervals for the number needed to treat. BMJ. 317:1309–12. https://doi.org/10.1136/bmj.317.7168.1309.

28. Bland JM, Altman D. Statistics notes: the odds ratio. BMJ. 2000;320:1468. https://doi.org/10.1136/bmj.320.7247.1468.

29. Wiley online library: statistical formulae for calculating some 95% confidence intervals. https://doi.org/10.1002/9781444311723.oth2 (2021). Accessed 14 June 2021.

30. Sacket D, Haynes B, Guyatt G, Tugwel P. Clinical epidemiology: How to do clinical practice research. 3rd ed. USA: Lippincott Williams and Wilkins; 2006.

31. Smeeth I, Haines A, Ebrahim S. Numbers needed to treat derived from meta-analyses; sometimes informative, usually misleading. BMJ. 1999;318:1548–51. https://doi.org/10.1136/bmj.318.7197.1548.

32. Arsham H. Topics in statistical data analysis: revealing facts from data. http://home.ubalt.edu/ntsbarsh/stat-data/Topics.htm (2015). Accessed 25 Oct 2021.

33. Altman D, Anderson P. Calculating the number needed to treat for trials where the outcome is time to an event. BMJ. 1999;319:1492–5. https://doi.org/10.1136/bmj.319.7223.1492.

34. Reid M, MS L, AR F. Use of methodological standards in diagnostic test research: getting better but still not good. JAMA. 1995; 274:645–51. https://doi.org/10.1001/jama.1995.03530080061042.

35. Deeks JJ, Altman DG. Sensitivity and specificity and their confidence intervals cannot exceed 100%. BMJ. 1999;318:193. https://doi.org/10.1136/bmj.318.7177.193b.

36. Schwartz A. Diagnostic test calculator. http://araw.mede.uic.edu/cgi-bin/testcalc.pl (2002). Accessed 25 Oct 2021.

37. Altman DG, Bland JJ. Diagnostic tests 2: predictive values. BMJ. 1994;309:102. https://doi.org/10.1136/bmj.309.6947.102.

38. Jonathan JD, Altman DG. Diagnostic tests 4: likelihood ratios. BMJ. 2004;329:168–9. https://doi.org/10.1136/bmj.329.7458.168.

39. Fagan TJ. Letter: nomogram for Bayes theorem. N Engl J Med. 1975;293:257. https://doi.org/10.1056/nejm197507312930513.

40. Altman DG, Bland JM. How to obtain the P value from a confidence interval. BMJ. 2011;343: d2304. https://doi.org/10.1136/bmj.d2304.

41. Glas As, Lijmer JG, Prins MH, Bonsel GJ, Bossuyt PMM. The diagnostic odds ratio: a single indicator of test performance. J Clin Epidemiol. 2003; 56:1129–35. https://doi.org/10.1016/s0895-4356(03)00177-x.

42. Moons KG, Stijnen T, Michel BC, Buller HR, Van Es GA, Grobbee DE, et al. Application of treatment thresholds to diagnostic-test evaluation: an alternative to the comparison of areas under receiver operating characteristic curves. Med Decis Making. 1997;17:447–54. https://doi.org/10.1177/0272989x9701700410.

43. Mallet S, Halligan S, Thompson M, Collins G, Altman D. Interpreting diagnostic accuracy studies for patient care. BMJ. 2012;344:1–7. https://doi.org/10.1136/bmj.e3999.

44. Zweig M, Campbell A. Receiver-operating characteristic (ROC) plots: a fundamental evaluation tool in clinical medicine. Clin Chem. 1993;39:561–77 PMID: 8472349.

45. Hosmer D, Lemeshow S. Applied logistic regression, 2nd ed. New York: Wiley; 2000. https://doi.org/10.1002/0471722146.

46. Turner D. An intuitive approach to receiver operating characteristic curve analysis. J Nucl Med. 1978;19:213–20 PMID: 627904.

47. McClish DK. (1989) Analyzing a portion of the ROC Curve. Med Decis Making. 1989;9:190–5. https://doi.org/10.1177/0272989x8900900307.

48. Youden WJ. Index for rating diagnostic tests. Cancer. 1950;3:32–5. https://doi.org/10.1002/1097-0142(1950)3:1%3c32::AID-CNCR2820030106%3e3.0.CO;2-3.

49. Okeh UM, Okoro CN. Evaluating measures of indicators of diagnostic test performance: Fundamental meaning and formulars. J Biomet Biostat. 2012. https://doi.org/10.4172/2155-6180.1000132.

50. DeLong ER, DeLong DM, Clarke-Pearson DL. Comparing the areas under two or more correlated receiver operating characteristic curves: a nonparametric approach. Biometrics. 1998;44:837–45 PMID: 3203132.

51. The Equator network. STARD 2015: an updated list of essential items for reporting diagnostic accuracy studies. https://www.equator-network.org/reporting-guidelines/stard/ (2021). Accessed 6 Aug 2021.

Abstract

The aim of statistical analysis is not to have as many results as possible but mainly to be certain of the few credible ones that the researcher can defend and explain. The conditions of applying bivariate statistical tests are few and easily verified, and hence, the results are plausible, provided that the study design was appropriate. Reporting must be adequate, including sample size, the test statistics, the exact P-value, the 95% confidence interval and a proper measure of effect size.

The Use of Online Calculators and Statistical Software

Besides the well-known commercially available statistical software package such as IBM-SPSS and STATA, there are free statistical software and numerous links to perform analysis online [1–3]. Free software varies from the powerful R package [4] to much more user-friendly simple software like JASP statistical package [5]. We can agree on how difficult and dangerous it will be to chase a fly with a cruise missile. *Statistical packages are potent and sophisticated tools, and we advise the lay clinician to limit their use to the statistical tests that he understands and masters.* As an example, those packages cannot verify if two sets of data are coming from two independent patient groups or the same group of patients, such as the case of: "before and after studies" and hence, whether using a paired or unpaired test is at the researcher's own risk.

Many commonly statistical tests, such as the analysis of variance (ANOVA), necessitates normal data distribution. However, *the software will consistently execute the test, regardless of data is normally distributed or not.* Hence, accepting the software output becomes the sole responsibility of the researcher. *The software often verifies normality and gives "a clue" about the test conditions being violated.* However, the researcher lacking decent statistical knowledge may not appreciate the importance of those clues or may not even understand their meaning. It is up to the researcher to check upon normality first, using another test (e.g., Shapiro–Wilk test) that is equally provided by the software but is not programmed to be linked to those tests requiring normality, such as ANOVA.

On the other hand, *the software can generate a large number of results that may surpass our simple needs.* Unfortunately, the researchers cannot always resist the temptation to use those "foggy" or "unnecessary" results in their work. On the other hand, *if we confine the analysis to a professional statistician, we have to keep in mind that the research work is finally ours and not his.* Often, decisions have to be made during the analysis and, if those decisions were made by the statistician alone, the researcher has to know that he will be the only one who bears the consequences.

We hope that this chapter can allow researchers to "simply and fully" understand the idea behind each test and the mainframe of the used equations, enabling them to play their undeniable positive role during the analysis. *Most statistical tests and equations presented in this book do not need any formal mathematical or statistical background and will be explained thoroughly.* On the other hand, we know that sometimes the equations become too complicated to be executed manually, even for statisticians themselves. Statisticians usually describe those equations as being ugly. In those few cases, we will skip the details of calculation but will maintain the same focus on the conditions of applications, the interpretation of the results, and the practical use of outputs generated by the software.

Outside formal research, part of a biologist's main activity is building up his knowledge by participating in continuous medical education programs, reviewing his colleagues' work, or simply reading a published paper. *Without basic statistical knowledge, we cannot judge if a manuscript is suitable for publication or verify that a published paper is sound and valuable.* Decisions and conclusions are based on clinical relevance and statistical significance. Although we can reply on a separate report made by a professional statistician, this brings us to the previous point of discussion: we have to understand how and why all parts of the decision were taken, simply because it will be finally our decision, not anybody's else.

2.1 Choosing a Statistical Test

In broad terms, statistical analysis can be divided into two main types: bivariate and multivariable analysis. The former analyzes the relationship between two variables only, without considering the effect of any other or additional factors. The factors are supposed to not effect relationship in question for being absent, stationary, or evenly distributed between the compared groups. As a rule of thumb statistical tests assumes that patients are chosen at random, which maximizes the chance that studied and unstudied variables (factors) are more or less equally distributed between compared groups producing a balanced or no role. For example, comparing the effects of two diet regimens on weight loss by the bivariate test of Student assumes that patients were randomly chosen from those fulfilling specific inclusion and inclusion criteria. Hence, other influential variables such as age, gender, and physical activity are comparable between the two groups.

On the other hand, multivariable analysis investigates the effects of many *independent variables* (e.g., type of antihypertensive treatment, weight gain, age, sex, salt intake) on *a dependent variable* (e.g., diastolic blood pressure). The role of multivariable analysis (MVA) is to weigh the effect of each of the independent variables on the dependent variable (outcome). The former variables are "independent" because they exert their significant "own" effect on the outcome, independently from other variables. They are being called "*predictors*" because a given value (e.g., "x" amount of daily salt intake) can be used to predict outcome (how much the patient's blood pressure is expected to be "y"). They are also called *risk factors* for being associated with the risk of development of the outcome. They can also be called *confounder variables* because their presence confounds assessing a causal relationship between other variables and the outcome. Multivariable analysis will be the subject of a separate chapter in this book.

The choice of the appropriate bivariate statistical test depends upon many factors, including the type of variable, data distribution, number of measurements made, group independence, number of groups, and whether the factor time is taken into consideration. In general, data can be either quantitative or qualitative. As we are comparing just two variables, we can have one of three possible combinations: both variables are qualitative, both are quantitative, or one is qualitative while the other is quantitative.

2.1.1 Independence of Data: Paired Versus Unpaired Tests

A second factor is whether we are comparing the patient to himself or independent groups. Comparing a patient to himself significantly reduces variability. Consequently, a paired design comparing the effect of two treatments (two procedures, methods of investigation) on a single group of patients is much more powerful than a usual unpaired study comparing the effect of two treatments between two different groups of patients. Do we have to explain what we mean by *a more powerful test*? It means that it can put into evidence statistically significant results, with a smaller sample size and a smaller difference in magnitude between treatments, compared to the situation if the design was bilateral. The statistical tests used to analyze paired data are called paired tests (e.g., paired Student test), and those used to analyze independent data are called unpaired tests (e.g., unpaired Student test). *The equations used in both tests are designed to analyze different forms of variability, and hence, they are not the same.*

2.1.2 Data Distribution: Parametric Versus Distribution-Free Tests

A third factor is whether data is normally distributed or not? Many statistical tests necessitate the presence of this parameter (condition) and are hence called parametric tests. By deduction, tests not necessitating normality are called: nonparametric or distribution-free tests. It is worth noting that parametric tests are those directly based on the normal distribution and those based on distributions derived from normal, such as t and F distributions. Typically, these tests require that the analyzed variables are normally distributed in the population, a condition frequently met in biology. It is always advisable to check data for normality first (see Sect. 1.4.3) before the analysis. If data are significantly different from Normal, we can either tend to normalize data (see Sect. 1.4.4 and 7.2.4) or use a nonparametric test (see Sect. 2.5).

The use of parametric tests for the analysis requires two main conditions (parameters): The first is the normal distribution of the studied variable, and the second is the equality of variance among the compared groups, both of which should be verified before the application of those tests. Although we insist upon the reader to revise the section on Normal distribution for details yet, we will mention a few essential points in short: Most of the biological variables usually follow a normal or a "near normal" distribution. The means of values usually acquire a normal distribution when included values are at least 30 per group of patients. A change of the scale of a value (x), with a particular distribution other than Normal, into a log (x), (1/x) or else may achieve a normal distribution of the new scale and hence, permitting the use of parametric tests. Fortunately, the variances of normally distributed variables are usually equal among compared groups. Hence, normality usually verifies the second condition necessary for applying the parametric test. *Care should be taken not to "twist" variables to reach "normality,"* as we can always use the equally valid nonparametric tests. Most researchers will consider their use in case of a small sample size. Others are just comfortable with them in most situations for the additional benefit of being easy to use. Nevertheless, there is a complete armada of distribution-free tests, and we will only envisage some of the most widely used in the clinical literature.

Nonparametric tests involve ranking of observations rather than using the actual values. According to the central limit theorem, the sums of values, such as ranks, are normally distributed. Consequently, the statistical significance of the results obtained by mathematical equations based upon the summing of ranks can be checked out in normal distribution tables, such as the z-table or the student's table. It is worth noting that this is valid as long as the number of values (patients) does not drop below a minimum of 10 per group if we compare two independent groups and a minimum of 20 patients in case of one-group analysis. That is because this is an approximation, and otherwise, it is advised to check out the significance of our results directly in the unique tables of significance designed for nonparametric tests [7]. *A main disadvantage of the nonparametric tests is the inherent loss of information due to substituting the sensitive true data by crude ranks, which decreases the power of the test.* Compared to a parametric test, however, such loss of power is negligible and surpasses the application of a test without reliable verification [6]. Another drawback of ranking is the Ex-Aequo or ties, which is the case where several cases share the same values. Those cases can either be given "a mean rank," or we randomly choose which case will be given first and which will come later. Moreover, the types of analysis offered by non-parametric tests are.

2.2 Consulting Statistical Tables

2.2.1 The Test Statistics

Research is to analyze differences and not similarities. In its simplest form, the difference between two values (A and B) can be calculated by subtracting A from B, comparing the result to (0). Another simple alternative is to divide A by B, and compare the result to 1. The plan of any research starts by postulating the null hypothesis. Under the null hypothesis, there is no "true" difference between the two treatments, A and B. Hence, any observed difference maybe just due to chance. However, the more significant the difference we observe in our study, the less probable it is due to chance. In other words, the less probable the null hypothesis is true. The universal cut-off point was that if the observed difference is very large to the extent that the probability of being due to chance is as small as 5% or less, we will consider the difference true. Consequently, we reject the null hypothesis and accept the alternative hypothesis that this

difference is true, reflecting a real treatment effect. Put it this way, in order to make a decision; we have to be 95% confident that the observed difference is true and, by deduction, the risk of being wrong about its trueness has to be 5% or less, which is expressed as the P-value.

A statistical test is just the way to calculate those differences in the appropriate (standardized) form. *The standardized form is called the test statistics and is usually named after the name of the test itself.* Examples are the Z value, the Chi-square value calculated by a Chi-square test, the t-value calculated by a Student t-test, and the Fisher's F value calculated for ANOVA. The choice of a specific statistical test depends upon many factors, including study design, data distribution, number, and types of variables. Hence, the permutations and combinations of those factors are behind the numerous statistical tests available.

We have shown in Sect. 1.7.2 that the mean blood pressure achieved with the new treatment (127 mm Hg) was significantly lower than that of placebo (132 mm Hg). Under the null hypothesis, there should be no difference between both treatments, and any observed difference (d) can be only due to chance. We do not know the probability (the chance) of acquiring a raw difference in mm Hg (d). However, we know the probability of a standardized difference or the difference calculated in terms of Z value. *The test statistic (Z value) changes the difference from how many mm Hg the blood pressure is reduced to how many standard errors (Se) compared to the placebo?* We do so because we know exactly the probabilities associated with each fraction of standard error on the Normal distribution curve, which were tabulated in the Z table.

The calculation is simple: dividing *the raw difference* (d) by the appropriate standard error (Se) $= -5/2.92 = -1.71$; giving us how many (Se) does (d) deviate from the point of no difference (0). Consulting Z table shows that the probability of acquiring a test statistic of -1.71 under the null hypothesis is only 4%. Hence, we can reject the null hypothesis and adopt the alternative hypothesis that the new treatment is more effective than the treatment, with a small acceptable probability of error (P-value) of 4%.

Statisticians have calculated the probabilities of acquiring every possible value for a given test statistics under the null hypothesis, such as (χ^2) value, t-value, F value, and correlation coefficient r. The calculation was tedious but straightforward: first, any variable or value follows a certain distribution, such as the Normal distribution, t-distribution, Chi-square distribution, or F distribution. Second, the total area under any distribution curve represents the total probability space for this distribution, and hence, it sums to 1. Consequently, the probability of acquiring a particular test statistic is simply the fraction of the area related to this part to the total area under the curve. For example, Fig. 1.8 shows the standard Normal distribution curve where the probability of acquiring a Z score >2 = 2.1% and its mirror image score <2 = 2.1%. This 4.2% is no more than the proportions of the surface areas of those two extreme triangles to the total area under the Normal distribution curve. Statisticians have tabulated the probabilities corresponding with the minimum test statistics obtained under the null hypothesis to obtain those probabilities: the critical statistical values. The researcher can check on the statistical significance of his results by ensuring that his test statistic has at least reached the critical value inscribed in the tables. For example, the researcher has to ensure that the Z value of his study is at least (1.96) if the study was bilateral and at least (1.645) if the study was unilateral to assign to his results a P-value of 0.05 [8].

2.2.2 The Degrees of Freedom (Df)

Unlike the normal distribution, where the test statistic is only dependent upon the mean and standard deviation (see Sect. 1.4), other distributions such as Chi-square (see Sect. 2.3), Student's and Fisher's distributions (see Sect. 2.4) are dependent upon the degree of freedom (df), which entitles some explanation. In its most direct form, the (df) of a data set of size (n) is the

number of data that are free to vary = n − 1. We will estimate probabilities by taking a simple example of inviting three persons (n = 3) to have one out of three available chairs. The first person will enjoy the probability to choose one out of three chairs, the second will choose one out of the remaining two chairs, while the third person will have no choices to make and he is not free to choose. The last person is obliged to take the last chair. The number of persons who were free to choose or to vary (df) in this data set was only 2, which is equal to the sample size (n) minus one: n − 1 = 3 − 1 = 2. *In statistical tables we are concerned with calculating probabilities for our sample and hence, we have to exclude who are not free to vary; i.e., who have no probability to calculate.* Put it this way, we calculate probabilities only for those who are free to vary (df) and not for the whole sample (n).

2.2.2.1 The df of Student Distribution and Pearson's Correlation Coefficient

Concordantly, the df of any data set of size (n) of a particular distribution equals n − 1. The test of Student is used to compare the means of two groups of size n1 and n2. The df of Student's statistics (t value) is obtained by subtracting (1) from each data set: n1 + n2 − 2. The same applies to correlation coefficient (r), where the degree of freedom is equal to sample size minus two (df = n − 2), one for each measurement made. We have to note that in a paired design such as the paired Student's test, we are estimating a single parameter, which is the mean of the difference of paired data, and not the paired data themselves, and hence, the df = n − 1.

2.2.2.2 The df of the Analysis of Variance (ANOVA)

A more general definition of the df of a particular parameter is the number of free pieces of information used to calculate this parameter. One-way ANOVA is a test that compares the means of multiple groups (see Sect. 2.4.3). Suppose that we compare the mean duration of pain relief in k

(=3) groups of patients, each receiving a different treatment (A, B, and C). We have two different types of variability: variability between the three groups because each group received a different treatment ($V^2_{between-groups}$) and an expected minor variability within each group, despite the patients receiving the same treatment ($V^2_{within-groups}$). In other words, we have two parameters (two variabilities) to estimate, and hence, we have to estimate two degrees of freedom: (df$_{between-groups}$) and (df$_{within-groups}$).

The more significant is the variability between groups, the more we will believe that treatments are significantly different from one another, which is why the test statistic (Fisher's value: F) is the ratio between the two variances: ($V^2_{between-groups}$) and ($V^2_{within-groups}$). Concerning the *in-between groups' parameter*, knowing the total mean duration of pain relief in the three groups, it will be sufficient to know the mean durations of two groups to detect the mean duration in the third one. In consequence, the (df$_{between-groups}$) = K − 1. The basic rule applies on the second *within-groups parameter*: we deduct (1) from the sample size (n) of each (k) group and hence, the (df$_{within-groups}$) = N − k; where N is the total sample size, and K is the number of groups. The reader can refer to Sect. 2.4.3 for more details and a simple example (see Sect. 2.4.3).

2.2.2.3 The df of the Chi-Square Tests

The Chi-square test involves comparing the observed distribution of a single qualitative variable to a theoretical one or comparing the observed distribution of 2 qualitative variables. Each qualitative variable can be composed of two or more (k) classes such as gender (males, females), hypertension (mild, moderate, and severe hypertension). The question is whether the

patients belong to one class or another, and hence, *the units of comparison are the (K) classes and not the individual patients*. For example, if we examine a total number (N) of cases to see whether they are hypertensive or not? It is sufficient to detect the number of hypertensive cases (n) to deduct the number of normotensive patients = (N − n).

Consequently, the df of this two-class variable = number of classes minus one = 2 − 1 = 1. In general, the (df) of a single variable formed of k classes = k − 1. We usually test the distribution of a single K class qualitative variable to see whether it fits a theoretical one. An example is to test the ratio of baby boys to baby girls born in a particular maternity hospital to the theoretical universal 1:1 ratio. The test is called *the Chi-square test for goodness of fit* and the df of our example = k − 1 = 1. The Chi-square test of goodness of fit can also be used to see whether an observed distribution fits a theoretical binomial, Poisson, or Normal distribution. Take the example of using the test to verify that qualitative data are normally distributed or not? The sample is divided into k intervals and hence, df = K − 1 as usual. However, the mean and Sd of data are usually unknown, and in such a case, one extra degree of freedom is counted for each estimate made, and hence, df = k − 3.

On the other hand, the Chi-square test is more commonly used to check if the distribution or the K-classes of two qualitative variables are independent of one another? For example, testing whether being hypertensive or not is related to the patient's gender (Table 2.1)? The test is known as *the Chi-square test of independence*. As multiplications sum probabilities, the total df of the two variables is the multiplication of the df of the first variables (k − 1) by the df of the second variable (k − 1). For example, for the

Table 2.1 The distribution of hypertension between genders

	Males	Females	Marginal values
Hypertensive	40	10	50 (c)
Normotensive	60	90	150 (d)
Marginal values	100 (a)	100 (b)	200 (total)

Values are the number of patients in each category. (a), (b), (c) and (d) are the marginal values = total number of males, total number of females, total number of hypertensive cases and total number of normotensive cases; respectively simple 2×2 comparison shown above, the df of the test = $(2-1) \times (2-1) = 1$. The total numbers of each category (number of males and number of females, number of hypertensive patients, and number of normotensive cases) are known as the marginal numbers. *Knowing the marginal numbers of a two-by-two table, it will be sufficient to know the number of patients in only one of the four categories to deduct the other three, and hence, only one category is free to vary.* We are taking the example shown in Table 2.1. Suppose we know the marginal values (100 males, 100 females, 50 hypertensive cases, and 150 normotensive cases). In that case, it will be sufficient to know any of the four distributions (40, 60, 10, or 90) to deduct the other three. What is the df if we test the independence of a 3-class qualitative variable and a 4-class qualitative table? The df = $(3 - 1) \times (4 - 1) = 6$.

2.2.3 Consulting Individual Tables

Although the researcher can consult one of the many freely available sources of statistical tables to verify his results [8–10], all statistical software packages will automatically calculate the statistical significance of his results. Critical values can be equally checked online [1].

2.2.3.1 Consulting the Z Table
We have previously shown how to consult the Z table (see Sect. 1.7). In short, the table is usually consulted to calculate the probability to acquire a Z score that is at least equal or larger (in absolute value) than the critical value figured in the table. Note that the critical values are calculated under the null hypothesis. Hence, exceeding those values means that the chances of the null hypothesis being true are very slim. Once those chances are 5% or lower, we can reject the null hypothesis and accept the alternative hypothesis. The rows show the score units at one decimal fraction $(0.0, 0.1, 0.2, \ldots, 0.3.4)$ and the columns gives the complementary second decimal $(0.01, 001, 0.02 \ldots 0.0.09)$. For example, a bilateral study was organized to compare the duration of pain relief between two treatments. The standardized difference between mean durations

gave a Z score of +1.96, favoring the first treatment. The standardized difference between mean durations gave a Z score of +1.96, favoring the first treatment. The significance of Z is checked out at the intersection of the row (1.90) and the column (0.06). It shows a probability of 0.475 or 47.5%, which is the probability of having a positive Z score that is at least equal to or larger than +1.96, under the null hypothesis. Being a bilateral study, the other symmetrical probability of having a Z score of −1.96 (in favor of the second treatment) is also 47.5% (see Fig. 1.12) Consequently, the probability of having a Z score that is either larger or smaller than 1.96 is the sum of both probabilities $(0.4750 + 0.475$ or $0.475 \times 2) = 95\%$. The interpretation is as follows: there is a 95% chance of having a Z score of +1.96 in favor of the first treatment or a score of −1.96 in favor of the second treatment, which is what we are looking for in a bilateral study. By deduction, the probability of having a Z score that is either smaller or larger than 1.96 is 5%.

On the other hand, *a unilateral study aims to find if a particular treatment is better than a placebo but never the reverse.* The probability associated with the same Z score of +1.96 is calculated by adding 0.5 (50%) to the one figured in the table $(0.475 + 0.5 = 0.97.5$ or 97.5%) (see Fig. 1.13). We have to add this 50% probability that we did not look for in the first place (probability to have a negative Z score of −1.96) because no one is interested in showing that a placebo is better than treatment. This explains why the limit of statistical significance in a bilateral study is a Z score of 1.96, with a corresponding risk of error of $1 - (0.475 \times 2) = 1 - 0.95 = 5\%$; while the limit of statistical significance in a unilateral study is a Z score of 1.65, with the same corresponding risk of error of $1 - (0.45 + 0.5) = 1 - 0.95 = 5\%$.

2.2.3.2 Consulting the Chi-Square Table
The table gives the probability to acquire a Chi-square value that is at least equal or larger (in absolute value) than the critical value figuring in the table, calculated according to the df [8–10]. At 1 df, we have to have a Chi-square value of at least 3.84 to declare statistical significance with

the usual P = 0.05. On the other hand, a minimum Chi-square value of 11.07 is necessary to declare the same statistically significant result (P = 0.05), at 5 df. The critical values shown in our table are those of a bilateral test, with the primary risk of error (α) being split between both study tails: α/2 on each side. In the case of a unilateral design, the P-value is checked out under the column of 2α; for example, the usual 5% limit of statistical significance has to be checked out along the 0.1 column (0.05 × 2). In a unilateral study with 1 df, a Chi-square value of 2.71 will be sufficient to declare statistical significance, with the usual 5% significance limit.

2.2.3.3 Consulting the Student Tables

The table gives the probability of acquiring a Student (t) value that is at least equal to or larger (in absolute value) than the critical values figured in the table, calculated according to the df [8–10]. At 120 df, Student values coincide with those of the normal distribution. We know that those critical values depend on whether the study has a bilateral or a unilateral design (see Sect. 1.7.2 and 1.7.3). Some tables are bivalent, providing the critical values for both study designs, while other tables are designed for either bilateral or unilateral studies. Although the design is usually clearly noted, it still may be a source of confusion. The simplest solution is to consult a bivalent table, which shows the critical values for both study designs, and the researcher can pick up what he is looking for and disregard the other result. Another solution is to consult a table that conforms with our study design: a unilateral student table for a unilateral study design and a bilateral table for a bilateral design.

Going the hard way and consulting a bilateral table for the results of a unilateral study or vice versa, the researcher needs to know precisely what he is looking for. The probabilities (the P values) occupy the heads of the columns, and the critical values needed to acquire those probabilities are arranged in rows according to the degrees of freedom. In a unilateral study, the null hypothesis is rejected once the test value is at least equal to or larger than the critical value

necessary to reject the whole (α). In a bilateral study, we need a larger critical value, not to reject (α), but to reject the smaller (α/2). Consequently, a table designed for a unilateral study will place the critical values corresponding to the whole (α) under the P = 0.05 column, while a table designed for bilateral studies will place the larger critical values corresponding to (α/2) under the same column of 0.05. Put it this way, the critical values are the same in both tables but what is changing is the corresponding P values occupying the heads of the columns.

A table designed for unilateral studies will show the probabilities (P-values) to acquire the critical value necessary to exclude the whole (α). For example, at 60 df, we need a critical t-value of 1.671 to reject the null hypothesis, and hence (1.6.7.1) has to be logically placed under the P = 0.05 column. In contrast, a larger critical t-value, such as t = 2, has a smaller probability and is placed under the 0.025 column. Consequently, we can reject the null hypothesis when the t-value is at least equal to 1.671 (P = 0.05) while acquiring a larger t-value of 2 denotes a higher statistical significance (P = 0.025). In case we need to consult the same unilateral table for the results of a bilateral study, we have to remember that we need a larger t-value to reject the null hypothesis in a bilateral study. The t-value excludes the smaller (α/2) and not the whole (α).

Consequently, we have to look for P-value under the column of (α/2) and not under (α). The usual limit of statistical significance of 0.05 is looked for under the 0.025 column (0.05/2). All P-values are looked for under the P/2 columns, or, more practically, we can get the P-value of our bilateral study by multiplying the P-value shown in the table by two. Applying the rule to the example given above, if the study was bilateral, the P-values associated with 1.671 and 2 would be 0.1 (0.05 × 2 = non-significant) and 0.05 (0.025 × 2 = just significant). The procedure is reversed when we look for the critical values of a unilateral study in a table designed for bilateral studies. In short, the critical values are not verified under the expected P columns but in the 2P columns, and a more practical way is to divide the P-values figured at the column heads by 2.

2.2.3.4 Consulting Fisher Tables

Fisher's tables have unique characteristics: unlike other tables with only one df for each statistic (t, chi-square, Z value), the F statistic has two df, as shown in Sect. 2.2.2: $df_{between\text{-}groups}$ and $df_{within\text{-}groups}$. As the test statistics (F) is the ratio between the variance between groups ($V^2_{between\text{-}groups}$) and the variance within groups ($V^2_{within\text{-}groups}$), the df of the resulting F is the ratio between the respective degrees of freedom $df_{between\text{-}groups}/df_{within\text{-}groups}$. In other words, the numerator df (df_n) = $df_{between\text{-}groups}$ and the denominator df (df_d) = $df_{within\text{-}groups}$ and, the problem is that both degrees of freedom have to be placed in the table, leaving no room for the P values. Yes, because any table is formed of rows and columns. In other distributions, only one df was placed in the rows, and the P-value was placed in the columns. Now, we have two degrees of freedom, the first one (df_n) = $df_{between\text{-}groups}$ is placed along with the columns and the second one (df_d) = $df_{within\text{-}groups}$ is placed along the rows and no place will be left for the P-value. The simple solution was to create multiple Fisher's tables, each representing a specific P-value: one table for P-value of 5%, another table for P-value of 4%, the third table for a P-value of 3% and so on [8, 9]. Another solution was to subdivide the rows denoting the (df_d) into multiple rows, each indicating a specific P-value and the ones shown are those for P = 0.1, 0.05, 0.025, 0.01 and 0.001 [10]. As such, Fisher's table is quite crowded by including three information: the numerator df, the denominator df, and the P-value. We think that displaying F values for each cut-off P-value is a simpler and hence, a better presentation.

In all tables [8–10], the shown F values are the ratios between the two variances, with df_n/df_d and hence, the F ratio shown in the table has to be written as: F, df_n/df_d; which is not equal to F, df_d/df_n. For example, for the same P value of 0.001: the F, df_5/df_4 equals 51.71, while the F, df_4/df_5 equals 31.09. In other words, we have to be careful that the variable in question is the numerator of F ratio and not the reverse. In One-way ANOVA, F is calculated to prove that patient groups have significantly different means and hence, the in-between group variability ($V^2_{between\text{-}groups}$) with its corresponding ($df_{between\text{-}groups}$) is the numerator of the ratio and the ($V^2_{within\text{-}groups}$) with its corresponding ($df_{within\text{-}groups}$) is the denominator of F statistics. As example, in case of one-way ANOVA, F should be written as: (F, $df_{between\text{-}groups}/df_{within\text{-}groups}$). In the case where both variances have the same df, such as comparing 4 groups of patients (df between groups = k − 1 = 3) and having a total sample size of 6 patients (df within groups = N − K = 6 − 3 = 3), we will have the same F value of 141, regardless of which is used as numerator and which is used as denominator.

Consulting Fisher's Tables in a Unilateral Study Design

Fisher's distribution and tables are estimates of variances of random samples taken from Normal distributions, with approximately equal variances. The tables were essentially designed for the analysis of variance (ANOVA), where we are only interested if a variance is larger than the other or not. In consequence, F tables are readily applied as such to answer the ANOVA question. In practice, the tables can be used to compare two variances (A and B) to investigate whether: a variable is significantly larger than the other as in ANOVA (A > B) or a variable is significantly smaller than the other (A < B). The two questions are two unilateral designs in which the primary risk of error (α) is totally confined to a single available answer. We start by calculating the ratio between the two variances (F ratio). The latter is the test statistic, which statistical significance can be checked out in Fisher's tables; here, we have to be careful. As noted above, the critical values given by the F tables were constructed for a one-tailed test (α) to investigate whether the variance in the numerator is significantly larger than the denominator. Hence, we have to divide the larger variance by the smaller one (V^2_L/V^2_S).

We compare our F value with the one figured in the table, at the intersection of the column denoting the numerator df (df of the largest of the

2 variances = df_L) and the row denoting the denominator df (df of the smallest variance = df_S). Our F value must be identified by the degrees of freedom, written in this order: $F_{(dfL/dfS)}$ and not the reverse. For example, if the variance of a group of 7 patients equals 500 and the variance of a second group of 6 patients equals 100; F = 500/100 = 5. The latter is then compared to the critical F given by the table, at the intersection of the column denoting the numerator df_L (n − 1 = 7 − 1 = 6) with the row denoting the denominator df_S (n − 1 = 6 − 1 = 5). As our value is larger than that given by the table (4.95) at P = 0.05, we can conclude that the first variance is significantly larger than the second variance; P = 0.05.

On the other hand, if the study question is whether one variance is significantly smaller than the other, we calculate the reversed F ratio $(V_S^2/V_L^2) = 100/500 = 0.2$ and the numerator and denominator df have to be reversed too = (df_S/df_L) = column 5/row 6. As Fisher's tables were primarily constructed to give the ratio probability between a large and a smaller variance, F will always be > 1. The critical value of (V_S^2/V_L^2) is not found in the table. It has to be calculated by reciprocating (inverting) the one figuring at the table for the ratio (V_L^2/V_s^2), not at its original df, but at the reflected df (df_S/df_L). For the usual 5% limit of statistical significance, the critical Fisher's value found at the intersection of column 5 and row 6 equals 4.39, and it reciprocate = 1/4.39 = 0.228. As our value (0.2) is even smaller than the latter, we can conclude that the second variance is significantly smaller than the first variance.

Consulting Fisher's Tables in a Bilateral Study Design

In order to compare diagnostic methods or procedures, researchers are more interested in the variability of measurements rather than their mean values. Variability is usually tested bilaterally to know which is the better method: A or B? Another everyday use of bilateral testing is the routine check of homogeneity of variances before using a parametric test, such as the test of Student. In all those tests, the null hypothesis is that (A ≠ B), the alternative hypothesis is that (A > B or A < B) and the primary risk of error (α), is equally split between those two possibilities as (α/2). As previously noted, the F test is unilateral, with α being confined to only one of the two probabilities. In a bilateral design, the calculated F has to be compared to the critical value figured in the table at α/2. For example, and the usual 5% limit of statistical significance, the calculated F has to be compared to the critical F values presented in Fisher's table point 2.5%. An F value that is at least equal to or larger than the one figured in Fisher's table 2%, means that our value is significant at 1% only and so on.

A simple statistical test is designed to calculate the difference between the effects of 2 treatments in a standardized form. Those standardized differences are dependent upon the distribution of the variable in concern and the degrees of freedom. The result of the comparison is called the test statistic and is usually named after the test itself. Examples are the (t) value calculated by Student's t-test and the chi-square value calculated by a chi-square test. On the other hand, statisticians have calculated and tabulated the probabilities to acquire those test statistics under the null hypothesis, i.e., in the case where there is no difference between the two treatments (A=B).

Consequently, if our test statistic is equal or larger than the one figured in the tables, at the universal critical probability limit of 5%, the probability of test statistics being due to chance (A=B) is 5% or less. As per rule, we reject this small probability, and we conclude that there is a true difference between the two treatments (A≠B).

2.3 Inferences on Two Qualitative Variables

The Chi-square Tests

Numerous statistical tests are available to determine whether there is a significant relationship between qualitative variables, with Pearson's Chi-square tests being the most commonly used. Pearson Chi-square can be used to test whether the observed distribution of a single variable fits well a theoretical one such as Normal, Poisson, or binomial distribution: the Chi-square goodness of fit (see Sect. 2.3.1.1). A simple example is to compare the "observed" frequencies of baby boys and baby girls born in a maternity hospital to an "expected" worldwide ratio of 1:1. However, the Pearson Chi-square test is more commonly used to check whether the distributions (K classes) of two qualitative variables are independent of one another: Pearson Chi-square test of independence (see Sect. 2.3.1.2). A simple example is to examine whether there is a relation (dependence) between gender (male or female) and a particular disease such as hypertension (hypertensive or not). Although we have limited the given examples to the case of 2-class qualitative variables, both tests are readily applicable on multiple-class (k-classes) and ordinal variables such as mild/moderate/severe hypertension, man/woman/child. It was noted that Chi-square tests tend to inflate the calculated χ^2 value in small studies, and statistical significance can be declared while it should not. Yates [11] has suggested a modification to reduce this inflation (see Sect. 2.3.1.3). Cochran–Armitage made an interesting modification to test is a modification made to test whether there is a linear trend in the proportions of the binomial variable across the categories of an ordinal variable (see Sect. 2.3.1.4).

On the other hand, as all Chi-square tests assume data independence, a modification had to be made by McNemar to suit the paired design (see Sect. 2.3.2.1). As the test can only be applied in the case of two binomial variables, several modifications were made to suit the different combinations. The Bowker test is a modified McNemar if one of the two variables has >2 classes (see Sect. 2.3.2.2). The Cochran Q test is another modification, which can be applied to multiple qualitative variables, provided binomial (see Sect. 2.3.2.3).

2.3.1 The Unpaired Tests

2.3.1.1 Pearson's Chi Square Test Goodness of Fit

The Example

Table 2.2 shows the observed frequencies of boys (60) and girls (40) in 100 babies born in a maternity hospital. Under the null hypothesis of equal gender distribution among newly born babies, we expected to have 50 boys and 50 girls, and the question is whether the null hypothesis is true? The more significant is the difference between what we have observed (O) and what we expected (E), the less we will maintain our confidence in the null hypothesis being true. As the difference enlarges, the probability that the null hypothesis is true goes down till it reaches the 5% limit. At this point, we reject the null hypothesis and adopt the alternative hypothesis that the difference between the observed and the theoretical distribution is true, with the universally accepted 5% risk of being wrong about it.

Table 2.2 Chi-Square test goodness of fit: gender distribution among 100 newly born babies

	Observed	Expected	$(O - E)$	$(O - E)^2$	$(O - E)^2/E$
Baby boys	60	50	10	100	2
Baby girls	40	50	−10	100	2
χ^2 value					4

Values represent frequencies, O = observed frequency, E = expected frequency

The Equation

As in all statistical tests, we are looking for differences and not for similarities, which do not exist. The total deviation (difference) from the null hypothesis is the sum of the differences between all observed and expected frequencies in boys and girls. As previously described in Sect. 1.3.4, simple "raw" differences must be squared and standardized before being summed. Squaring prevents the positive and negative differences from annulling each other during summation. On the other hand, a raw difference does not mean much, and it has to be appropriately weighted through standardization. Let us take the example of the exam results of two students: the first student was expecting to have 80 marks (E), but he got only 60 (O) and hence, (O − E) = (60 − 80) = 20. The second student expected to get 40 and got only 20 and (O − E) = (20 − 40) = 20. As such, the simple row differences (O − E) gave the "wrong information" that both students experienced the same "amount of loss,"; which is untrue. Standardizing those differences by weighting each loss by the student's expectation (E) shows that the first student has lost 25% (20/80) of what he was expecting, while the second student has lost as much as 50% (20/40). In conclusion, dividing the squared differences by the expected values ($\frac{(O_i - E_i)^2}{E_i}$) before summing them gives proper weight to the loss (deviation) from the null hypothesis. Consequently, the test statistics or the Chi-square value (χ^2) will be the sum (Σ) of all squared and standardized differences "Eq. 2.1". The null hypothesis is that the observed values are equal to the ones expected and, the alternative hypothesis is that they are not.

$$\chi^2 = \sum \frac{(O_i - E_i)^2}{E_i} \qquad (2.1)$$

Table 2.2 shows the observed (O) and expected (E) frequencies for baby boys and baby girls, their squared (O − E)² and standardized squared differences (O − E)²/E, with a total Chi-square value of 4. The more significant is the value, the smaller is the probability of the null hypothesis

being true. The statistical tables show the sum of those squared standardized values [8–10] and hence, they cannot be negative. The result is that the Chi-square curve becomes positively skewed with a right-hand tail. Put it this way; the larger is the Chi-square value, the more it moves away from the extreme left-hand side point of no difference (0) towards the right-hand tail to meet the extreme small triangle of rejection. When the surface area of the latter gets as small as 5% of the total curve area, we reject the null hypothesis of no difference (or no association) and adopt the alternative hypothesis.

Now we have to know where to look in the table itself? The columns denote the probabilities, and hence, we will look first at the 5% column, denoting the universal limit of statistical significance. If our value exceeds that figured in this column, we shift to the smaller probability of 4% and so on. The second question is in which row, and the answer is simple: we look in the row corresponding to our degree of freedom? The df of our test = number of K classes −1 = 2 − 1 = 1(see Sect. 2.2.3.2). *In order to be statistically significant, our value should be at least equal or larger than that figure in the table, at the corresponding df.* Our value (4) is larger than that figuring in the table (3.84), and hence we can conclude that the proportion of baby boys to baby girls in our sample is significantly different from the theoretical 1:1 proportion; P < 0.05. Note that the tables [8–10] are just extracted from more detailed tables. Hence, they cannot always provide us with the exact P-value. It is advisable to report the exact P-value, readily obtained with a statistical software package. In our case, IBM-SPSS statistical software shows an exact P-value of 0.046.

The Interpretation

A statistically significant test means that the observed distribution does not fit the theoretical one. A non-significant P-value > 0.05 means that the observed distribution is not significantly different from the theoretical one. In our example, the proportion of baby boys to baby girls is significantly different from the universal 1:1 proportion (P = 0.046).

What Should be Reported

In addition to reporting the descriptive statistics (numbers and %), type of theoretical distribution (normal, binomial, Poisson, or else), and the P-value, it would be beneficial to report effect size, such as Cohen h or Odds ratio (see Sect. 4.3.1).

Conditions of Application

The sample should be a random sample of normal distribution. As shown in Sect. 14.2.4, normality can be assumed whenever the number of expected values is ≥ 5. In this setting, Cochran has suggested that Pearson's Chi-square test results can be accepted as long as 80% of the cells have expected values ≥ 5 and none is below 1 [12]. Otherwise, researchers can either correct the inflated results by applying the penalty proposed by Yates (see Sect. 2.3.1.3) or better use Fisher's exact test (see Sect. 2.3.1.5). Both tests, however, are only applicable in the case of 2 × 2 contingency tables, and hence, in the case where data have > 2-classes, researchers have to drop/regroup classes of data (see Sect. 2.2.1.2). In our example, we had two cells only (2 expected values: one for baby boys and one for baby girls), with each being equal to 50 and largely surpassing Cochran recommendation.

2.3.1.2 Pearson's Chi Square Test of Independence

The Example

A study was conducted to investigate whether there is a relation between being a doctor or a nurse and a particular disease (being hypertensive or normotensive). The study question is whether being in a specific class of one qualitative variable is dependent on being on a particular class of the other variable? Pearson Chi-square is the test of choice to investigate whether both distributions were independent or not. A statistically significant test will mean that both occupation and disease are dependent on one another.

The Equation

Table 2.1 shows the distribution of hypertension among 100 nurses and 100 doctors. As shown,

40% of doctors were hypertensive, compared to only 10% of nurses, and whether this discrepancy in observed frequencies violates the null hypothesis? We have an equal number of doctors and nurses. We expected equal frequencies of hypertensive and normotensive patients in both groups, which was not the case. The more significant is the difference between observed and expected values, the less is the probability that the null hypothesis is true. As shown, there were more hypertensive doctors than nurses and, it seems that being hypertensive or not is dependent upon one's profession.

The Chi-square value is calculated as usual: the sum of all squared standardized differences between observed and expected values. The statistical significance of the calculated Chi-square value is compared to the critical value inscribed in the Chi-square table at 1 df; $(k - 1) \times (k - 1) = (2 - 1) \times (2 - 1) = 1$ (see Sect. 2.2.2 and 2.2.3). The table shows that a value of 3.84 is sufficient to declare statistical significance at (1) df. As shown in "Eq. 2.2", our value is much larger (24), exceeding the critical value of P = 0.01 (6.63) and even that of P = 0.001 (10.83). However, researchers do not usually report smaller values and are just satisfied to report a P value of < 0.001.

$$\chi^2 = \sum \frac{(O_i - E_i)^2}{E_i} = \frac{(40 - 25)^2}{25} + \frac{(10 - 25)^2}{25} + \frac{(60 - 75)^2}{75} + \frac{(90 - 75)^2}{75} = 24$$

(2.2)

We have presented the most straightforward example: testing the independence of two qualitative binomial variables, with an equal number of patients in each group (100 doctors and 100 nurses). However, the Chi-square test is also applied on >2-class qualitative variables and unequal numbers or unbalanced design. Table 2.3 shows a study organized to compare the effectiveness of 3 treatment regimens in preventing thromboembolic complications among 80 patients with mechanical cardiac valves. Twenty-five patients were kept on oral anticoagulants (regimen A), 30 patients on

Table 2.3 Chi-square test of independence: the distribution of prosthetic cardiac valve complications among patients receiving 3 anticoagulation regimens

	PVT	PE	TIA	None	Total
Regimen A	4 (6.3)	6 (6.3)	5 (6.3)	10 (6.3)	25
Regimen B	15 (7.5)	10 (7.5)	3 (7.5)	2 (7.5)	30
Regimen C	1 (6.3)	4 (6.3)	12 (6.3)	8 (6.3)	25
Total	20	20	20	20	80

Observed values are presented as numbers, expected values are presented as numbers between brackets. PVT = prosthetic valve thrombosis, PE = peripheral embolism, TIA = transient ischemic attacks, None = no complications recorded. Regimens A, B and C are patients receiving oral anticoagulants, antiplatelets and combined oral anticoagulants and antiplatelet therapy, respectively

antiplatelets (regimen B), and 25 patients received a combined regimen of oral anticoagulants and antiplatelets (regimen C). Reported events were 20 cases of valve thrombosis (VT), 18 peripheral embolization events (PE), 17 transient ischemic attacks (TIA), while 25 patients were event-free. The study question was whether there is an association between following a particular regimen and the development of complications, including the patient being free of complications as one of the 4-classes of the complication variable? In other words, the df of this test will be equal to 6 [(4 classes of complications $-$ 1) $\times$ (3 regimens $-$ 1)].

Table 2.3 shows the repartition of the number of observed events and, in between brackets, the expected numbers of events in the case where both variables were truly independent. The expected value of each cell is calculated by multiplying the total of the relevant raw (total number of patients following a particular regimen) by the total of the relevant column (total number of patients developing a particular complication), divided by the grand total (number of all patients). As example, the number of expected values for the development of VT in patients following regimen (a) = 20 $\times$ 25/80 = 6.25. The number of patients free from complications among those following regimen (b) = 25 $\times$ 30/80 = 9.4. All calculations can be easily verified as the sum of the expected values in each row or column equals the corresponding sum of observed values. The larger is the difference between observed (O) and expected values (E),

the smaller is the probability that the null hypothesis is true and that both distributions are independent. Once this probability drops to 5% or less, we can reject the null hypothesis and adopt the alternative hypothesis that both distributions are dependent. The total Chi-square value of our example (22.8) largely surpasses that shown in the table at the intersection of df = 6 and P = 0.05 (12.59). Our Chi-square value is even larger than that figuring in the table for a P-value of 0.001 (22.46).

The Interpretation

The interpretation of a 2 $\times$ 2 Chi-square test is straightforward: doctors are significantly more hypertensive than nurses, but the interpretation of a > 2 class qualitative variable is more delicate. The test indicates a statistically significant association between the followed regimen and the four complications (P = 0.001), which does not explicitly mean that a particular regimen is significantly associated with a particular complication. Put it this way, the test rejected the complications being independent of the regimens but it did not indicate precisely which complication is specifically related to one of the regimens. In conclusion, this Chi-square test did not answer the study question entirely. We have to do further analysis (post hoc analysis) to link a specific regimen to specific complications.

Post Hoc Analysis

In order to prove such an association, we have to repeat the analysis with 2 $\times$ 2 tables. Concerning

Table 2.4 Chi-square test of independence: the occurrence of complications in patients following antiplatelets regimen B and combined therapy C. Data extracted from Table 2.3

	Complications	None	Total
Regimen B	28 (24.5)	2 (5.5)	30
Regimen C	17 (20.5)	8 (4.5)	25
Total	45	10	55

Observed values are presented as numbers, expected values are presented as numbers between brackets. Complications = patients presenting with prosthetic valve thrombosis, peripheral embolism or transient ischemic attacks, None = no complications recorded. Regimens B and C are patients receiving oral anticoagulants or antiplatelets, respectively

the variable regimen, we may be interested in comparing regimen C (the worst regimen) to either regimen A or B, and leaving regimen C aside. Suppose this second comparison gives a statistically significant result. In that case, it will only tell us that one of the two regimens (e.g., B) shows significantly less "overall complications" than the other. It cannot tell us which specific complication (PVT, PE or TIA) is significantly more in either regimen. In order to answer this question, we had to repeat the analysis, comparing two complications at a time. Another way to transform the variable complication into a binomial variable is to regroup complications into yes or no (Table 2.4). Put it this way; the Chi-square test can indicate exact independence between 2 binomial variables. Otherwise, it will indicate the "presence" or absence of independence between two K classes of qualitative variables without specifying the exact location (class) of independence.

Most importantly, we must be aware that each time we make a "fresh" comparison with the same data, we repeatedly test our results against chance. In our example, our data has been tested once with K-class variables (Table 2.3) and, we are proposing to reuse the same data once or even several times more. Each time we reuse our data, we get an extra chance to reach statistical significance. *Giving himself an extra second chance to win anything increases the probability of winning without truly deserving it, which is unfair. It is like throwing a dice several times without losing money until we do win!* We have

to have some penalty on this action. As the primary risk of error (α) is the probability to conclude upon a significant difference due to chance, re-testing our data inflates this probability. A simple remedy to raise the ceiling of making such a "false or undeserved" conclusion (P-value) was suggested by Bonferroni [13]; where the calculated P-value is not compared to ($\alpha = 0.05$) but to α divided by the number (n) of tests made. For example, if we are doing 2 Chi-square tests by comparing the same data twice (n = 2), we have to reach a P value of 0.025 ($\alpha/n = 0.05/2 = 0.025$) to declare a statistically significant result at the level of P = 0.05. When performing three tests, one has to achieve a P value of 0.0166 (0.05/3) to report a statistically significant result of 0.05. Take it as some penalty that we have to accept for the extra chances we were given to prove our point of view.

Table 2.4 shows the Chi-square test performed after removing the results of regimen (A) and regrouping complications into yes or no. As shown, regimen (B) was associated with more complications (93.3%), compared to only (68%) in patients following regimen (C). The calculated (X^2) value (5.88) is below the universal limit of 5% at 1df (3.84), corresponding to a P-value of 0.0153 "Eq. 2.3". However, as suggested by Bonferroni, multiple comparisons (n) inflate the risk of error, raising the limit of significance from the usual 0.05 to 0.05/n. A simple remedy is to multiply the calculated P-value by the number of comparisons made. In this study, we should report a P value of 0.0153 x 2 = 0.031.

$$\chi^2 = \sum \frac{(O_i - E_i)^2}{E_i}$$
$$= \frac{(28 - 24.5)^2}{24.5} + \frac{(2 - 5.5)^2}{5.5}$$
$$+ \frac{(17 - 20.5)^2}{20.5} + \frac{(8 - 4.5)^2}{4.5} = 5.88$$

(2.3)

What Should be Reported

In addition to descriptive statistics (numbers, %), (χ^2), and P values, we should report the post Hoc analysis and any P-value adjustment. It is highly recommended to report the effect size (ES). Unlike sample size, ES describes the true effect treatment in the population, regardless of the chosen risks of error, and is very useful to calculate sample size for future studies (see Sect. 4.1.1). ES can be calculated from binomial data itself as Odds ratio, relative risk, or sample size and (χ^2) value as Phi (φ) in case of 2-class variables or as Cramer's V in k-class qualitative variables (see Sect. 4.3.1). In the example shown in Table 2.1, $\chi^2 = 24, K = 2$, total sample size = 200 and Cramer's V = 0.346. In the example shown in Table 2.3, $\chi^2 = 22.8$, K = 3 (the smallest number of classes in both variables), total sample size = 80 and Cramer's V = 0.377. The reader is requested to refer to Sect. 4.3 for more details.

Conditions of Application

The sample should be random, have a normal distribution and, groups have to be independent. As shown in Sect. 1.4.2, normality can be assumed whenever the number of expected values $\geq$ 5. In this setting, Cochran has suggested that Pearson's Chi-square test results can be accepted as long as 80% of cells have expected values $\geq$ 5 and none is below 1 [12]. Otherwise, researchers can either correct the inflated results by applying the penalty proposed by Yates (see Sect. 2.3.1.3) or better use Fisher's exact test (see Sect. 2.3.1.5). However, both tests are only applicable in the case of 2 × 2 contingency tables. Hence, they can be applied to data given in Table 2.2 but not in the example given

in Table 2.3, unless we drop or regroup data as shown in Table 2.4.

2.3.1.3 The Corrected Chi-Square Test (Yates)

The Chi-square test is based on the condition that the qualitative variables of concern are normally distributed, with the number of expected frequencies (E) being 5 or larger. In the case of smaller (E), the numerator increases (O − E), the denominator (E) decreases, and the calculated Chi-square value (χ^2) tends to be larger than what it should be [12]. Yates suggested reducing the inflated (χ^2) by subtracting a small absolute value (0.5) from the difference calculated in each cell before being squared $(O - E - 0.5)^2$. The correction can be made in both Pearson's Chi-square and McNemar's Chi-square tests (Sect. 3.2.5) but can be only applied to a 2 × 2 contingency table. Some statisticians extended its use to a larger expected frequency of 10 per cell. Others considered the test as being too tight and do not recommend its application at all. View to the discrepancy of indications, statistical software packages such as IBM-SPSS, automatically include the corrected Chi-square test whenever the analysis concerns a 2 × 2 contingency table.

The Example

A new regimen of prophylactic antibiotics was suggested for patients benefiting from coronary bypass grafting. A double-blind, bilateral randomized trial was constructed to compare this new regimen (A) to the classical prophylactic regimen (B). Forty patients were randomized into two equal groups, each following one of the two regimens during the first three postoperative days. The success criterion was the absence of fever and a normal leucocytic count on the seventh postoperative day. The study results are shown in Table 2.5, together with the calculated expected values between brackets. A "regular" Chi-Square test calculated by hand will give a Chi-square value of 4.3, which is higher than the 3.84 value required to declare statistically significant results at 1 df "Eq. 2.4". However, it will be unwise to declare a statistically significant

Table 2.5 Corrected Chi-square test (Yates): the comparison of success rates between two prophylactic antibiotic regimens

	Success	Failure	Total
Regimen A	19 (16.5)	1 (3.5)	20
Regimen B	14 (16.5)	6 (3.5)	20
Total	33	7	40

Observed values are presented as numbers, expected values are presented as numbers between brackets

superiority of regimen A because a primary condition necessary for applying a regular Chi-square test was not fulfilled: two out of the four expected values (50%) were less than 5 (=3.5).

$$\chi^2 = \sum \frac{(O_i - E_i)^2}{E_i}$$
$$= \frac{(19 - 16.5)^2}{16.5} + \frac{(1 - 3.5)^2}{3.5} + \frac{(14 - 16.5)^2}{16.5}$$
$$+ \frac{(6 - 3.5)^2}{3.5} = 4.3$$

$$(2.4)$$

The Equation

Yates's correction was made to reduce the inflated Chi-square value (χ^2) due to small expected frequencies by systematically subtracting a small value (0.5) from the difference calculated in each cell before being squared "Eq. 2.5". In our example, the application of the correct test gives a much smaller corrected Chi-square value χ_C^2 of 2.7 and a statistically non-significant result "Eq. 2.6".

$$\chi_C^2 = \sum \frac{(O_i - E_i - \mathbf{0.5})^2}{E_i} \quad (2.5)$$

$$\chi_C^2 = \frac{(16 - 19.1 - \mathbf{0.5})^2}{19.1} + \frac{(9 - 5.9 - \mathbf{0.5})^2}{5.9}$$
$$+ \frac{(26 - 22.9 - \mathbf{0.5})^2}{22.9} + \frac{(4 - 7.1 - \mathbf{0.5})^2}{7.1} = 2.7$$

$$(2.6)$$

The Interpretation

The test is interpreted as a regular Chi-square test for independence. As the test is only applicable with 2-class qualitative variables, the df is always 1, and the significance of the test statistics (χ_C^2)

will be checked out in the first row of the Chi-square table; where a result > 3.841 is considered to be statistically significant, at the usual 0.05 level. Our result was statistically non-significant for having a value of only 2.7 "Eq. 2.4".

What Should be Reported

Besides the descriptive statistics (numbers, %) and P-value, it is advisable to report effect size as Cohen h, Odds ratio, or relative risk (see Sect. 4.3.1). In our example, with a total of 40 patients (N) and a χ_C^2 value of 2.7; $(\varphi) = \sqrt{(2.67/40)} = 0.26$. Cramer's V will give the same value.

Conditions of Application

The sample should be random, have a normal distribution and, groups have to be independent. Yates's correction is only applicable in 2 × 2 contingency tables and provided that each of the expected values is at least 2. Due to the absence of a universal agreement on when to apply Yates' continuity correction and Fisher's exact test, many commercially available statistical software packages such as SPSS automatically calculate both tests for every 2 × 2 contingency table. As shown, the test can be easily calculated by hand; however, unless there is the clear-cut statistical significance (or non-significance), it will be more coherent to use Fisher's exact test (see Sect. 2.3.1.5).

2.3.1.4 Chi Square for Trend (Cochran–Armitage Test)

In the case we are testing the relation between an ordinal variable (x) and a categorical variable (y), the researcher may be interested to know whether there is a linear trend in the proportions of the binomial variable (y) across the categories of the ordinal variable. An example will be investigating the association between cerebrovascular stroke (yes/no) across four levels of hypertension effects. A regular Chi-square test will just tell us whether the proportions of complications across the four levels of hypertension are significantly different from one another or not. However, as such, the test is not sensitive to investigate whether the proportion of complication constantly increases with the increasing order of hypertension and whether this relation is linear and statistically significant in itself? The question can be equally answered by simple regression analysis, with coding complication as a dependent variable (0, 1) and coding the hypertension levels as a predictor (1, 2, 3, and 4). As shown later, linear regression analysis will give nearly the same result that we are about to obtain here by Cochran–Armitage test, with F $(1,38) = 6.59$ and P = 0.014 (see Sect. 2.6.3).

The Example

Table 2.6 shows the results of a study carried out in 40 hypertensive patients. We recorded whether each patient had a cerebrovascular stroke (CVS) and the hypertension level, whether controlled, mild, moderate, or severe. Whether there is a significant association between the occurrence of complications and the levels of hypertension can be quickly answered by a chi-square test of independence? However, the test does not consider whether the increasing order of hypertension is significantly associated with an increasing percentage of complications. The proportion of CVS is constantly increasing following the increased level of hypertension. Sweeping the results of mild (8 patients with no

complications and 2 patients with complications) and severe hypertension (3 patients with no complications and 7 patients with complications) will never change the Chi-square results. However, it will disrupt the apparent positive correlation between an increasing level of hypertension and the sureness of more complications (20% in mild cases and 70% in severe cases). The Cochran–Armitage or the Chi-square test for trend was designed to answer this second question by considering the effect order in the calculations.

The Equation

Table 2.6 shows the proportion of cerebrovascular events in patients presenting with controlled, mild, moderate, and severe hypertension. If the level of hypertension does not affect the proportion of complications, the latter would be the same, regardless of the level of hypertension. Consequently, fitting a line through data points makes a perfectly horizontal line, which is the null hypothesis. The test aims to prove that the slope of the line is significantly different from the horizon, which is why we can obtain the same result by regression analysis, using the complication as a dependent variable and level of hypertension as a predictor (see Sect. 3.5). The test is based on a modification of the chi-square formula to disguise the nature of the method. We begin by assigning scores to describe the ordinal levels of the variable of interest. We have assigned the scored 1, 2, 3, and 4 to describe the increased risk associated with increasing order of the disease. Table 2.7. shows the detailed procedure: we begin by weighting the number of

Table 2.6 Chi-square test for trend: the effect of the level of hypertension on the occurrence of cerebrovascular complications

	Controlled HTN	Mild HTN	Moderate HTN	Severe HTN	Total
CVS (yes)	2 (20%)	3 (30%)	5 (50%)	7 (70%)	17 (42.5%)
CVS (no)	8	7	5	3	23
Total	10	10	10	10	40

HTN = hypertension, CVS = cerebrovascular stroke. Values represent number of patients who developed (yes) or did not develop (no) CVS. Numbers in paratheses are the proportions of patients who developed CVS in each HTN category and in total

Table 2.7 Chi-square test for trend: calculation of data presented in Table 2.6

Hypertension	Controlled	Mild	Moderate	Severe	Total	Mean
Score (x_i)	1	2	3	4	–	2.5
Event (r_i)	2	3	5	7	R = 17	P = R/N = 0.425
Sample size (n_i)	10	10	10	10	N = 40	
$r_i x_i$	2	6	15	28	51	
$n_i x_i$	10	20	30	40	100	
$n_i x_i^2$	10	40	90	160	300	

x_i = score assigned to the 4 levels of hypertension, r_i = number of observed events per patient level, R = sum of r_i in all levels, n_i = number of patients per level of hypertension, N = total number of patients, P = proportion of events in all patients

observed events (r_i) by the assigned score that denotes the severity of the event (x_i) and, we calculate the observed weighted events ($r_i x_i$) for each of the four levels of hypertension.

The sum of observed weighted scores (Total $r_i x_i$ = 51) should not be significantly different from the sum of the expected weighted events (Rx = 42.5), calculated as the total number of events (R = 17) multiplied by the mean score of all patients (x = 2.5) "Eq. 2.7". The Chi-square value is given as usual; the results of the standardized squared difference between observed and expected weighted events = 5.91; P = 0.015 "Eq. 2.8". The reader can refer to Agresti for more details on the equation [14].

$$\chi^2_{trend} = \frac{\left(\sum r_i x_i - R\bar{x}\right)^2}{p(1-p)\left(\sum n_i x_i^2 - N\bar{x}^2\right)} \quad (2.7)$$

$$\chi^2_{trend} = \frac{(51 - 17 \times 2.5)^2}{0.425\,(0.575)\,(300 - 40 \times 2.5^2)} = 5.91 \quad (2.8)$$

The Interpretation

Although the Chi-square value for trend (5.91) was smaller than that obtained by a regular Chi-square (6.036), it is a much more powerful test for following a chi-square distribution of only 1 degree of freedom, compared to 3 df for the standard test. The difference between both chi-square values: $\chi^2 - \chi^2_{trend} = 6.036 - 5.91 = 0.136$; representing the amount of variation that is not due to trend. In other words, we can

conclude that most of the detected variation in complications (97.8%) is due to the positive trend of increasing complications with increased severity of hypertension.

Mantel–Haenszel test for trend (Linear by linear association test)

The same result can be obtained comparing the assigned scores by a Mann and Whitney test, giving a z value of 2.4 and P = 0.016 (see Sect. 2.5.1.1). The Mantel–Haenszel test for trend, also known as the linear-by-linear Association (LLA) test for trends, is automatically given by IBM-SPSS when performing a Chi-square test, provided that one of the variables is dichotomous. The Chi-square value of the LLA test is calculated as $r^2 \times N$, where r is Pearson's correlation coefficient between the two variables and N is the total sample size = $(0.38)^2 \times 40 = 5.77$. The Chi-square value of the Cochran–Armitage test can be deducted by multiplying that of the LLA test by the quantity N/(N − 1) and the very near P-value can then be rechecked in the Chi-square table at 1 df [14].

What Should be Reported

Chi-square for trend, P value and correlation coefficient r as effect size.

Conditions of Application

The sample should be random, and groups must be independent, with one dichotomous and another k-class qualitative variable. We assign scores to express a constantly increasing or decreasing value. Although the values of those scores are arbitrary, it is usual to choose them equally spaced on either side of zero. Thus, for our four levels, the scores can be −3, −1, +1, and +3; however, the statistic is quite robust to other values for the scores, provided that they are steadily increasing or steadily decreasing. Note that the relative spacing of the scores will affect the strength of linear association.

Chi-square statistics χ^2 is a test that measures how a model compares the actual observed data. Data must be random, mutually exclusive, drawn from independent variables and a large sample, as indicated by 80% of expected values being >5. We can use the test to verify whether an observed distribution is different from a theoretical one (χ^2 test for goodness of fit) and, more commonly, to test whether the distributions of two qualitative variables are independent of one another (χ^2 test for independence). We can extend the test to verify whether there is a linear trend in the proportions of the binomial variable (e.g., the occurrence of a particular event) across the categories of an ordinal variable (χ^2 test for independence). In the case of a K (>2) class qualitative variable, the test has the disadvantage of not telling us which class in one variable is dependent on a particular class of the other variable. A repeated two-by-two analysis can answer this question provided to correct the P-value inflated by multiple testing. An index of effect size, such as Odds ratio, relative risk, Phi, or Cramer's V has to be reported.

2.3.1.5 Fisher's Exact Test

Fisher's exact test is used to analyze the statistical significance of the association of two independent binomial variables. It has the advantage of being applicable in small expected frequencies of 1 or 2 and that the results are more concordant with Pearson's Chi-square test, compared to a corrected Chi-square.

The Example

Table 2.8 shows the frequencies of cerebrovascular stroke (CVS) with mono versus dual antiplatelet therapy in a small group of high risk patients with ischemic heart disease The observed frequencies of stroke was (1) case in 30 patients on dual therapy (3.3%) and 4 cases in ten patients on monotherapy. Hence, the difference in success of preventing stroke was as high as 36.7% in favor of dual therapy. The question will be: what is the probability of acquiring a difference in a success rate that is at least equal or larger than the one observed, under the null hypothesis? Suppose this probability of having such difference in favor of either treatment is as small as 5% or less. In that case, we reject the null hypothesis of no difference and accept the alternative hypothesis that the success rate obtained with one treatment is significantly better than the other. Technically, two of the expected values are below 3 (2.5), so we cannot use neither Chi-square test (see Sect. 2.3.1.1) nor the corrected Chi-square test of Yates (see Sect. 2.3.1.3).

The Equation

As shown in Table 2.8, the marginal values in the first and second row are the total observed frequencies of success (5) and failure (35), respectively. The marginal values in the two middle columns are the total number of patients on dual (30) and monotherapy (10), respectively. The Total marginal value (40) inscribed at the intersection of the last row and the last column represents the sum of all marginal values = N. Remember that the total number of observations is equal to the total number of expected values, under the null hypothesis; i.e., in case of independence between the two variables.

Table 2.9 is a general 2 × 2 contingency table, i.e., cross-tabulation of the frequencies of any two binomial variables. The table represents the distribution of frequencies of two qualitative variables: x and y, each being formed of two

Table 2.8 Fisher's exact test: observed cerebrovascular stroke with mono versus dual antiplatelet therapy in high-risk patients

Cerebrovascular stroke	Dual antiplatelet therapy	Mono antiplatelet therapy	Marginal values
Yes	1 (2.5)	4 (2.5)	5[a]
No	29 (17.5)	6 (17.5)	35[b]
Marginal values	30[c]	10[d]	40 (N)[e]

Values are the observed frequencies, expected values are placed between brackets, (a) = cases with stroke, (b) cases without stroke, (c) number of patients on dual therapy, (d) number of patients on monotherapy, (e) = total number of patients (N), Marginal values a + b = c + d = N

Table 2.9 Fisher's exact test: a general contingency two-by-two table

	Variable x (1)	Variable x (0)	Total
Variable y (1)	a	b	R1
Variable y (0)	c	d	R2
Total	S1	S2	N

a, b, c and d represent the observed frequencies (1) or (0) of two variables (x) and (y). R1, R2, S1, S2 and N represent the marginal values which are the sums of those frequencies. R1 = a + b, R2 = c + d, S1 = a + c, S2 = b + d and N = R1 + R2 = S1 + S2

classes only (0, 1). The letters a, b, c, and d represent the observed frequencies, and the letters: R1, R2, S1, S2, and N represent the marginal values which are the sums of those frequencies. R1 = a + b, R2 = c + d, S1 = a + c, S2 = b + d and N = R1 + R2 = S1 + S2.

Now examine both Tables 2.8 and 2.9, the sum of rows (R1 + R2; 5 + 35) = the sum of columns (S1 + S2 = 30 + 10) = N (40). R1, R2, S1, S2, and N are called the marginal values. The idea of Fisher's exact test is to calculate all possible sets of data that keep the same marginal values of the observed set of data, i.e., to keep R1 = 5, R2 = 35, S1 = 30, S2 = 10, and of course, N = 40. The study question will be which therapy (or procedure) will achieve a difference that is at least equal or larger than the one which has been observed in the study?

Table 2.10 shows those possible sets of data, and the practical way to do so is to consider the smallest marginal value (total success rate = R1 in our example) and calculate all possible distribution of an R1 = 5 between the two treatments. It is evident that there are six possible distributions or frequencies; i.e., the number of possible distributions is equal to the smallest marginal value + 1, which equals 6 (R1 + 1 = 5 + 1) in our example. Then we fill in the empty spaces by the other distributions, which keep the same marginal values observed in our initial set of data; i.e., which keeps S1 = 30, S2 = 10 and N = 40, of course. Now we can

Table 2.10 Fisher's exact test: expected sets of frequencies keeping marginal values of data presented in Table 2.8

CVS	D1	M1		D2	M2		D3	M3		D4	M4		D5	M5		D6	M6	
Yes	0	5	R1	1	4	R1	2	3	R1	3	2	R1	4	1	R1	5	0	R1
No	30	5	R2	29	6	R2	28	7	R2	27	8	R2	26	9	R2	25	10	R2
	S1	S2	N	S1	S2	N	S1	S2	N	S1	S2	N	S1	S2	N	S1	S2	N

CVS = cerebrovascular stroke, R1 = total number of cases with CVS, R2 = total number of cases without CVS, S1 = number of patients on dual therapy, S2 = number of patients on monotherapy, N = total number of patients = R1 + R2 = S1 + S2. Values are all possible 6 combinations (from 1 to 6) that can be observed with dual (D) and mono therapy (M) while keeping the same marginal values (R1, R2, S1, S2 and N) observed in Table 2.8

answer the question: which of these possible six distributions give a difference in success rate in favor of dual therapy that is at least equal or larger than the one observed (>3)? As shown in Table 2.10, Set 1 gives a larger difference (5 − 0 = 5), and Set 2 gives an equal difference (4 − 1 = 3), compared to that given in Table 2.8 (4 − 1 = 3). The other 4 sets give a smaller or a negative difference (3 − 2 = 1; Set 3), (2 − 3 = −1; Set4), (1 − 4 = −3; Set 5) and (0 − 5 = −5; Set 6) [7].

This will lead us to the second question: what is the probability of those two sets to the total probability of the six sets, which is equal to 1 or 100%, of course? Remember that this probability (P) is the probability that dual therapy provides more protection than monotherapy; i.e., it is one side of the coin, and the other side of the coin is the probability that monotherapy provides better protection than dual therapy. This second probability is equal to the calculated P, and although the following equation will not directly give it, it should be taken into consideration during hypothesis testing. In other words, we will calculate P, but we will consider statistical significance only if double this quantity (i.e., 2P) is smaller than 0.05. Statisticians have demonstrated that P can be calculated by the "Eq. 2.9" [7].

$$P = \frac{R_1! + R_2! + S_1! + S_2!}{a! + b! + c! + d! + N!} \quad (2.9)$$

where R1, R2, S1, S2, and N are the observed marginal values, a, b, c, and d are the calculated frequencies of the data sets showing a difference that is at least equal or larger than the one observed. The probability is calculated for each set, and then P is obtained by the summation of those probabilities. The exclamation mark denotes "factorial" and means successive multiplication by cardinal numbers in descending series; for example, the quantity $4! = 4 \times 3 \times 2 \times 1 = 24$ and by convention, the quantity $0! = 1$. The probability of having a result that is at least equal to or larger than that observed in Table 2.8 is calculated by "Eq. 2.10" [7].

$$P = \frac{35! + 5! + 30! + 10!}{0! + 5! + 30! + 5! + 40!}$$
$$+ \frac{35! + 5! + 30! + 10!}{1! + 4! + 29! + 6! + 40!} \quad (2.10)$$
$$= 0.00495$$

As P = 0.00495, 2P = 0.0099, which is a quite small probability, and hence, the difference in success rates is statistically significant; P = 0.0099. The latter is usually approximated to P = 0.01. Although the calculation of the P-value looks complex, the factorial functions are available at many hand-held calculators for the interested reader. The test is difficult to calculate by hand but became a routine output of nearly all commercially available statistical software packages. Fisher's exact test practically replaced the corrected Chi-square for testing the statistical significance of 2 × 2 contingency tables.

The Interpretation

The test calculates the probability of a random association (independence) between the two classes of the qualitative variables in question. A small P-value of 5% or less permits the conclusion that both distributions are dependent on one another.

What Should be Reported

Besides the descriptive statistics (numbers, %) and P-value, it is advisable to report effect size such as Cohen h, Odds ratio, or relative risk (see Sect. 4.3.1).

Conditions of Applications

The sample should be random, and groups have to be independent. The test is only valid for 2 × 2 contingency tables; however, unlike the corrected Chi-square test, it can be applied in case of small expected values of 1 or 2. The test can even be applied if we have an empty cell. The minimum is to have 1 valid observation per row and one valid observation per column. The results given by Fisher's exact test are more concordant with those given by the Pearson's

Chi-square compared to the corrected Chi-square test. It is always advisable to use Fisher's exact test in the case where the results of the corrected Chi-square test are borderline. Finally, the difficulty of calculating the test by hand was removed by the development and availability of hand calculators and statistical software packages, which paved the way to replace the corrected Chi-square test.

2.3.2 The Paired Tests

2.3.2.1 McNemar Test (The Paired Chi-Square)

McNemar's test is applied to verify the independence of the distribution of two binomial variables or two responses of one binomial variable, whether in the same group of patients or two matched groups. The test can be used to examine whether the patient is being relieved or not is significantly related to one of two analgesic drugs. It can compare the pre to post-test results or the judgment of two raters, provided that the outcome is binary and the study is carried out in the same group or two matched groups of patients or other study material.

The Example

A study was conducted to compare the analgesic effects of 2 drugs (A and B) in a single group of 100 patients with chronic pain that was judged to be not amenable for a cure. Each patient received both drugs successively in a randomly assigned order. Each drug was used for one week, and the judgment criterion was patient satisfaction for the pain becoming tolerable by the end of the week (yes, no). Provided that there was no order effect (effect due to the order by which drugs are given), the pairs of answers recorded from each patient were as follows: 5 patients preferred drug A and not drug B, 15 patients preferred drug B and not drug A, 45 patients were satisfied from both drugs A and B and, 35 patients declare being unsatisfied from both drugs A and B.

The concordant pairs bring nothing to the main question: which of the two gives patients satisfaction and which does not? Consequently, a regular Chi-square test that will consider both concordant and non-concordant pairs will not give the desired answer to the question. As we compare the patient to himself, we should only concentrate on the non-concordant answers (a) = 5 and (b) 15 patients and drop the concordant answers from the analysis. McNemar has modified the regular Pearson's Chi-square to analyze the non-concordant pairs solely [15].

The Equation

Under the null hypothesis, both drugs should give the same satisfaction, and the 20 non-concordant answers (a and b) should be equally distributed between both groups. In our example, the expected number of satisfied patients should be 10 cases per group. The test should then compare the observed satisfaction numbers to the expected numbers by an ordinary Chi-square equation. Mathematically, the regular Chi-square equation applied to non-concordat pairs can be simplified into the squared difference between observed frequencies divided by the sum of expected frequencies of non-concordant answers (a) and (b) "Eq. 2.11".

$$\chi^2 = \sum \frac{(O_i - E_i)^2}{E_i}$$
$$= \frac{\left(a - \frac{a+b}{2}\right)^2}{\frac{a+b}{2}} + \frac{\left(b - \frac{a+b}{2}\right)^2}{\frac{a+b}{2}} = \frac{(a-b)^2}{(a+b)}$$

$$(2.11)$$

The Interpretation

The test statistics (χ^2) should be compared to the critical value shown in the Chi-square table, at 1 df = 3.841. Our calculated value ($\chi^2 = 5$) is higher, and hence, we can conclude that the patients significantly better appreciated the analgesic effect of drug B than that of drug A (P < 0.05).

What Should be Reported

Besides the P-value, we should report the number (%) of non-concordant pairs in total 20 (20%) and in each group: 5% in Group A and 15% in Group B. Effect size (ES) can be presented as Odds ratio = 0.15/0.05 = 3. Although the latter is calculated from non-concordant pairs only, the proportion of concordant pairs should also be known to calculate the total sample size (see Sect. 4.5.3).

Conditions of Application

The sample should be a random sample of paired dependent 2-class qualitative data. Any case missing one of the paired information is excluded from the analysis. The number of expected values should be at least 5. In the case of smaller values between 2 and 5, Yates's correction can be applied to reduce the inflated test statistics (χ^2), as shown before.

2.3.2.2 McNemar-Bowker Test

Bowker test is a generalized extension of McNemar's test, permitting the verification of the independence of an ordinal (K > two classes) and a binomial variable, whether in the same group of patients or two matched groups. Like McNemar's test, the Bowker test can be used to compare the effects of two treatments, the judgment of two raters, or the pre to post results; offering the additional advantage of dealing with an ordinal outcome variable or judgment criterion (e.g., improved, stable, deteriorating).

The Example

A study was organized to test the effectiveness of an analgesic in a single group of 150 patients. Patients' symptoms were recorded before and after treatment as being mild, moderate, or severe. The ordinal data are the patients' symptoms (mild, moderate, and severe), and the dependent binomial variable was the same

patient before and after treatment. The study question is not how many patients had a particular symptom (e.g., severe symptoms) before the treatment and how many had the same symptoms afterward, otherwise a regular Chi-square test would answer the question? The study question is whether the symptoms of an individual patient were changed by the treatment or not, considering the level of change? Put it this way, is the patient getting better or worse by changing from one level to the other and, what is the statistical significance of this change? Consequently, the 91 patients whose symptoms did not change will not be included in the analysis, as in McNemar's test. Those cases are shown between brackets along the diagonal of Table 2.11.

The Equation

Note that the McNemar test was testing the change on just one level of the binomial variable. In the previous example, patients were either improved on treatment A (a) or treatment B (b), and the test statistic was to compare (a) to (b). Bowker test is just an extension that will compare the change, not on the level of a binomial variable, but the K levels of an ordinal variable. Hence extending the comparison from just between (a) and (b) to between a1 and b1, a2 and b2, a3 and b3...ai and bi.

Under the null hypothesis, there should be no difference between those who improved by one level of symptoms (a1, a2, a3, ... ai) and those who got worse by the same level (b1, b2, b3, ... bi). For example, the number of patients whose symptoms improved from moderate to mild has to be equal to the number of patients whose

Table 2.11 McNemar-Bowker test: change of the patients' symptoms with treatment

		After treatment			
		Mild[a]	Moderate[a]	Severe[a]	Total
Before treatment	Mild[b]	(21)	15	7	43
	Moderate[b]	9	(30)	17	56
	Severe[b]	0	11	(40)	51
	Total	30	56	64	150

Values represent the number of patients in each class before (a) and after (b) receiving the treatment. Numbers presented along the diagonal between brackets (21), (30) and (40) = number of patients whose symptoms remained the same despite of the treatment symptoms worsened from mild to moderate. Put it this way, if the number of classes of the ordinal variable is k, the tests statistics (B) looks like the sum of the standardized differences of (K) variables 'Eq. 2.12". The test statistic deals only with the complete information provided by the cases which experienced a change. Cases with missing information and those providing constant response along the K classes of the ordinal variable (e.g., cases between brackets in Table 2.11) are not included in the equation "Eq. 2.13" [16].

$$\chi^2 = \frac{\sum (a_i - b_i)^2}{\sum (a_i + b_i)} \quad (2.12)$$

$$B = \frac{(15-9)^2 + (7-0)^2 + (17-11)^2}{(15+9) + (7+0) + (17+11)} = 9.8 \quad (2.13)$$

The Interpretation

The statistical significance of the test statistics (B) is checked out in the Chi-square table at k(k − 1)/2 degrees of freedom. Our χ^2 value (9.8) is much larger than the critical value shown in the table, at 3 df (3 × 2/2 = 3). Hence, we can conclude that treatment was significantly effective in improving the patients' symptoms. Bowker's test is a test of symmetry, and the result tells us that the distribution of the ordinal variable between the two categories of the ordinal variable is not symmetrical. It cannot tell us the exact position of this dissymmetry: is it between the mild and the moderate categories, the moderate and the severe categories, or the mild and the severe categories? Only repeated McNemar tests of those classes can answer this question, applying the Bonferroni correction as indicated (see Sect. 2.2.1.2).

What Should be Reported

Besides the descriptive statistics, χ^2 and P-values, we should report the effect size (ES). Campbell and colleagues suggested the cumulative OR as ES for unpaired data [17]. A more appropriate EF would be the OR calculated for paired 2 by 2 subgroups (see Sect. 4.5.3).

Conditions of Application

The sample should be a random sample of paired study design, with one binomial qualitative and one K class ordinal outcome variable. Any case missing one of the paired information is excluded from the analysis. The number of expected values should be at least 5. In the case of smaller values between 2 and 5, Yates's correction can be applied to reduce the inflated test statistics (χ^2), as shown before (see Sect. 2.3.1.3).

2.3.2.3 Cochran Q Test

Cochran Q test verifies the symmetry of the distribution of a binomial variable, whether measured several times (≥ 3) in a single group of patients or once in (≥ 3) matched groups or experimental conditions. An example of the former is the repeated assessment of one treatment's dichotomous effect (satisfied/not satisfied) on >3 different occasions (e.g., each week for ≥ 3 successive weeks). An example of the latter is single assessment of the dichotomous effect of ≥ 3 treatments, whether being given on intervals to the same patient group or, each being given to one out of 3 matched groups of patients. In all cases, the outcome variable has to be dichotomous.

The Example

A study was conducted to analyze the effect of an antidepressant in a randomly selected group of 10 patients. Patients were assessed by answering a single question, whether they felt relieved from depression or not? The assessment took place on four occasions: after brief counseling and before the treatment, and then every week for three successive weeks. Feeling depressed was coded (0), and being relieved from depression was coded as (1). The results are shown in Table 2.12. Compared to all patients feeling depressed before treatment, 60% were relieved after one week, 70% after two weeks, and finally 90% of patients were relieved by the end of the study at three weeks. Remember that the question was not about the difference between "crude" proportions of patients being relieved versus those who remained depressed in the paired situation. The

Table 2.12 Cochran Q test: repeated measurements of depression

Patients	Pretreatment	1 Week	2 Weeks	3 Weeks
I	0	0	1	1
II	0	0	0	0
II	0	0	1	1
IV	0	1	1	1
V	0	0	1	1
VI	0	1	1	1
VII	0	1	0	1
VIII	0	1	1	1
IX	0	1	1	1
X	0	1	1	1
% Success	0%	60%	70%	90%

I to X represent the 10 patients, numbers represent the coded outcome: 0 = feeling depressed, 1 = feeling relieved from depression

question is about the difference being observed within the same patient. Hence, patients whose response remains the same (patient II in our example) bring no answer to the question, and they are excluded from the analysis. As with other paired tests, patients missing a single piece of information have to be excluded too.

The Equation

The test is a modified Chi-square test comparing proportions among dependent groups; like McNemar and Bowker tests, it removes patients with the same outcome across measurements and those with a missing outcome from the analysis. Compared to McNemar's test, the Cochran Q assesses the "within-subject variability" across the repeated measurements (or measurements of different experimental designs) and not only two measurements. Under the null hypothesis of all measures being the same, the observed differences are expected to be small due to random variation (i.e., due to chance). The alternative hypothesis is that they are not. A significant test tells us that at least two of the measurements are different, but it does not tell us specifically which two measures?

If the four measurements in our example were those of four different types of treatments, the null hypothesis would be that treatments are equally effective. The alternative hypothesis

would be that at least two treatments are significantly different from each other. Although the equation involves simple additions and multiplications, the calculations are lengthy and rarely performed by hand. Suppose that k is the number of treatments (= four groups in our example), xj is the column total for the Jth treatment (the four percentages of success in our example), b = number of blocks (ten patients in our example), xi is the row total for the Ith block (the four observations made for each patient in our example), N is the grand total (40 observations in our example), the test statistics Q is calculated by "Eq. 2.14" [18].

$$Q = k(1-k) \frac{\sum_{j=1}^{k} \left(x_j - \frac{N}{k}\right)^2}{\sum_{i=1}^{b} x_i(k - x_i)} \qquad (2.14)$$

The Interpretation

Feeding the data to a statistical software package such as IBM-SPSS gives a Cochran Q value of 18.87. The calculated Q can be approximated to a Chi-square value at a degree of freedom equal to the number of measurement categories minus one (k − 1). At three df, the critical Chi-square value is 7.81, and our Q value (18.87) is much larger, permitting us to conclude that there is a statistically significant difference between the four measurements of an; P < 0.001.

Post hoc analysis

As far as the Q test can go, it is to conclude that the four measurements are significantly different. The test was not designed to tell us where this difference came from, which is the same problem that we usually encounter with a regular Chi-square test, at >1 df. On the other hand, it is only after ensuring a statistically significant test that we can further answer the question: which two proportions are significantly different from one another and which are not? This post hoc analysis can be achieved by multiple McNemar tests comparing every two proportions two by two. One point of caution is to compensate for the expected P value inflation due to repeatedly testing the same data against the hazard. The simple method suggested by Bonferroni has been explained before (see Sect. 2.2.1.2). In short, the critical value to declare a statistically significant difference at the usual 0.05 level will be the one that is present under the P-value column of 0.05/number of comparisons made. In our case, six two-by-two comparisons will be made, and a P-value of 0.0083 or less will be necessary to declare a statistically significant difference at the usual 5% limit. Table 2.13 shows the results of the six two-by-two comparisons made by McNemar's tests. The shown P values should not be taken for granted and the only statistically significant difference ($P \leq 0.0083$) will be the one comparing the pretest to the observation made after 3 weeks show ($P = 0.004$).

What Should be Reported

Besides the descriptive statistics, we report P value, results of post hoc analysis and effect size (see Sect. 4.5.3).

Conditions of Application

Subjects (N) are randomly selected from the population. The k groups represent the number of times measurement was repeated or the number of experimental conditions being compared, such as different types of treatments, different methods of diagnosis. As in the McNemar test, we exclude from the analysis subjects with similar answers in all (k) measurements and those with any missing measurements for groups that have to be equal.

The sample has to be large, as indicated by $n > 4$ and $nk > 24$; (n) the number of cases remaining in the analysis after excluding cases with the same or missing results. K is the number of repeated measurements or compared experimental designs. In our study, both conditions were satisfied for n and (nk) equal 9 and 36, respectively. In the case of small samples, a more complicated exact calculation will be needed [18].

We have discussed three tests using the Chi-square equation to verify the independence of distribution of two qualitative variables, whether in the same group of patients or matched patients' groups or other study material. McNemar's test is designed for the case of two binomial variables. Bowker's test is an extension of McNemar made to adapt for a K class (>2) categorical outcome. On the other hand, the Cochran Q test was designed to test whether a binomial outcome is symmetrically distributed across repeated

Table 2.13 Post-hoc analysis of data presented in Table 2.12: repeated McNemar's tests

	Pretest versus 1st week	Pretest versus 2nd week	Pretest versus 3rd week	1st week versus 2nd week	1st week versus 3rd week	2nd week versus 3rd week
Sample size	10	10	10	10	10	10
P value	0.32	0.008	0.004	0.625	0.25	1

measurements or several measurements made in matched experimental designs.

As paired tests evaluate accuracy or symmetry, cases with the same response or a single missing observation are removed from the analysis. The tests have the inherent disadvantage of the multiple-class Chi-square test. A statistically significant result indicates that at least two classes are different and post-hoc analysis will be necessary to evaluate all classes two-by-two. The inflated P value must be corrected by applying some penalty, such as Bonferroni correction.

2.4   Inferences on Means and Variances of Normal Distribution: The Parametric Tests

We have previously shown that most biological variables obey the characteristic normal distribution, which has been the subject of extensive analysis. Normality refers to the normal distribution of the variable in the population of concern. Hence, the more we increase our sample size, the more we expect it to follow the normal distribution (see Sect. 1.4 and 2.1.2). Fortunately, the variances of normally distributed variables are usually equal, permitting the analysis of those variables by a group of statistical tests necessitating both parameters normality and equality of variances: the parametric tests.

2.4.1   The Comparison of Two Means

Among the numerous statistical tests applied in the medical literature, the Student test is the most popular for being straightforward, readily applicable even with few patients. Lastly, the conditions necessary for its application can be easily verified. For respecting his work regulations in the Guinness beer factory, William Sealy Gosset (1876–1937) published his research work under the nickname: "Student" [19]. The main part of his research was focused on the behavior of small samples drawn from a normal population. He noted that the smaller is the sample, the more it deviates from normality. Hence, in front of "the one" normal distribution that fits all, we have "multiple" near-normal distributions, each fitting for a particular sample size, which were later on named after his nickname.

The Normal versus the Student Distribution

We have previously discussed how values are distributed in the "normal" population. Statisticians have modeled it graphically as the standard normal distribution curve (see Fig. 1.8). In short, values tend to group in the middle around their mean. A decreasing frequency characteristically disperses them as we go further away from the mean. The more is a particular value different from the mean (larger or smaller), the less is its proportion in the "normal population". The "Z score" was the scale on which those values move near or away from the mean. The Z score indicates how many standard deviations is a particular value away from its mean or how many standard errors the sample mean is away from the population's grand mean. Ideally, about 95% of values are included between two 1.96 standard deviations around their mean value. We have a 95% chance to find the population (true) mean in the interval formed by the mean of the sample and 1.96 standard errors. Consequently, any value having a Z score outside this range (>1.96<) has a limited 5% of being part of this population. Researchers have decided that a 5% probability is too small, and it can be neglected. Hence, the Z score of 1.96 was chosen as the limit of statistical significance in the normal population. These calculations were based on the assumption that the sample size is always large.

On the other hand, a rule of thumb is that the more we include values, the more those values will tend to group around the mean (in the middle) and, by deduction, the less will be the values in the periphery of the "normal distribution." The reverse is expected when the sample is getting smaller: the proportion of values in the middle will decrease, and those in the peripheries will increase. Hence, variability increases. Graphically, the result is also a bell-shaped curve but with a smaller height (flattened top) for a smaller number of values being in the middle and, with a broader spread (larger SD) for a more significant number of values being in the periphery; compared to a standard normal distribution curve (Fig. 2.1).

Put it this way, the "normal" curve flattens, more values are pushed away from the mean towards the periphery, and, in consequence, the limit of significance is pushed away from its original position in the population (1.96 Se from the mean) to a more distal position > 1.96 Se. The more the sample size decreases, the critical limit is pushed further away from the mean. The same applies to a unilateral study, whose original limit of statistical significance of 1.65 is equally pushed further away from the mean, in concordance with the decreasing sample size.

In conclusion, the variability of the mean of a large sample drawn from a normal population is measured by the Z score, which is the number of Se between the sample mean and the mean of the population. The z value is stable, provided that the sample is sufficiently large to show the characteristics of being normally distributed. The Z distribution is not dependent upon the sample size, and hence, there is "one" Z distribution that fits any normally distributed variable. On the other hand, the variability of the mean of a small sample drawn from "the same" normal population cannot fulfill those characteristics and is not stable but varies with sample size. The larger is the sample, the more it approaches the normal distribution and vice versa. In consequence, "the one" Z distribution that fits any normally distributed variable is replaced by "multiple" t distributions, each calculated for a specific sample size. By definition, any random t-variable is larger (further away from the mean) than a random Z variable drawn from the same population. Numerically, the "stable" limit of the statistical significance of a normal distribution that is equal to a Z value of 1.96 in a bilateral study (1.65 in a unilateral study) is replaced by a "variable" t-value that gets larger as the sample is getting smaller.

Finally, both distributions depend upon the mean and the standard deviation. The mean represents "the signal" of the measure. The standard deviation represents "the noise" due to the variability around this mean. The mean alone does not tell us much, and it has to be standardized by being divided by the proper Se. In the same way, we try to get ride-off the noise to appreciate the signal better. The more noise we have, the less is the value of the signal and vice versa. The standardized value is how many Sd a particular (x) value is away from its mean or how many Se a mean is away (different) from the population mean calculated in Z scores in the normal distribution and the t-scores in Student distributions.

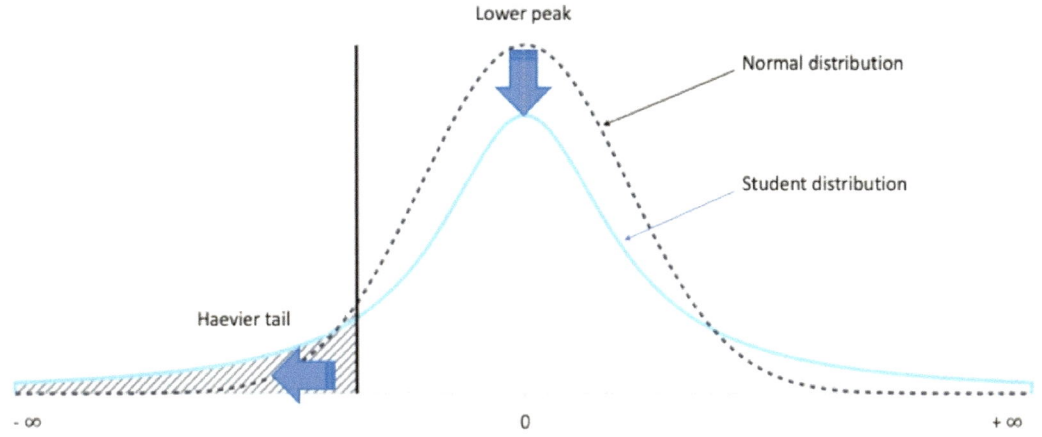

Fig. 2.1 The normal versus Student distribution

Consulting Student's Table

We can verify the statistical significance of the test statistic (t-value) in one out of the many freely available Student tables [8–10]. The reader is advised to refer to Sect. 2.2.3.3 to calculate the degrees of freedom in the Student table. it is equally important to refer to Sects. 1.7.2 and 1.7.3 for memory refreshment about the main difference between a unilateral and a bilateral study design. In a unilateral study, the entire primary risk of error (α) is confined to the only "available" conclusion (e.g., treatment is better than placebo). The other "possible" conclusion (e.g., placebo is better) is not looked for. A bilateral study comparing two treatments A and B, (α) is equally split between two possibilities: A > B ($\alpha/2$) or B > A ($\alpha/2$). The net result is that (α) of every study is maintained at the 5% level, whether the study is unilateral (α) or bilateral (2 times $\alpha/2$). Put it this way; a unilateral study examines whether our test statistic (t-value or else) is at least equal or larger than (α)? If the study is bilateral, we examine whether the test statistic is either equal or larger than ($\alpha/2$) or equal or smaller than ($\alpha/2$).

Another point is that some tables figure the probability of being equal or larger than (α) [Stat Perdu 2015]. Other tables figure the probability of being at least equal or larger than ($\alpha/2$), the same as the probability of being equal or smaller than ($\alpha/2$). Many tables figure both probabilities [8.9]. Calculations are the same but what is reported is different (α or $\alpha/2$) and, we have to be vigilant. In practice, if our study is unilateral (e.g., comparing treatment to placebo) and we are consulting a one-tail table reporting the probability of (α), the critical t-value will figure under the 0.05 column. The critical value is looked for under the ($\alpha/2$) or the 0.025 column if we are consulting the same tables for a bilateral study. In the tables figuring both (α) and ($\alpha/2$) values [8, 9], we have to know what we are looking for? At 10 df, the table shows that the critical limit of a bilateral study comparing treatment A to treatment B is 2.228. The researchers can conclude

that the comparison is statistically significant (P = 0.05), as there is a limited 5% chance to find such standardized difference (t = 2.228), in favor of either treatment A ($\alpha/2 = 2.5\%$) or treatment B ($\alpha/2 = 2.5\%$). On the other hand, if the study was unilateral, the same test statistic of 2.228 corresponds to a lower P-value of 2.5%. The researchers can conclude that the comparison is statistically significant (P = 0.025), as there is a limited 2.5% chance to find such standardized difference (t = 2.228), in favor of the treatment ($\alpha = 5\%$). The other possibility that a placebo is better than treatment was not tested. In this unilateral study, the critical limit necessary to conclude upon a P-value of 0.05 is 1.812, at the expense of not testing the possibility that a placebo is better than the treatment.

The Interval of Confidence of Mean in Student's Distribution

The confidence interval is a property of the normal distribution, from which the Student's distribution is derived. However, the Z value of the normal distribution has to be replaced in the equation by the larger t-value "Eq. 2.15". The latter has to be looked for in the Student's tables at the intersection of the degree of freedom (e.g., 10 df) and the desired level of confidence that we want to assign to our interval (e.g., the 0.05 column for the usual bilateral 95% confidence level). For example, if the mean body weight of 11 patients (n) is 80 kg and the standard deviation (Sd) is 5 kg, the standard error (Se) equals Sd/√n = 1.51 and the 95% IC = m ± (t) Se = 80 ± (2.228) 1.51 = 80 ± 3.36 kg = 76.6–83.4 kg. The interpretation is as follows: there is a 95% chance that the body weight will vary be between 76.6 and 83.4 kg. If we want to assign a unilateral confidence interval as in non-inferiority studies, the unilateral 95% CI is equal to the bilateral 90% CI (see Sect. 1.4.2.8). In our case, the unilateral 95% CI is calculated by replacing 2.228 with 1.812. The interpretation of the unilateral 95% CI is not always straightforward, and it is better interpreted bilaterally: there is a 90% chance that the bodyweight will vary between 77.3 and 82.7 kg.

$$95\% \; CI \; of \; mean \; (\bar{x}) = \bar{x} \pm (t) \; Se \qquad (2.15)$$

2.4.1.1 The One-Sample Student Test

The one-sample test of Student is used to compare an observed mean to a theoretical one.

The Example

A researcher was interested to know whether the systolic blood pressure (SBP) of a small group of 20 young female patients was significantly different from that of the population. In other words, the study had a bilateral design that aims to show a difference in favor of either party: sample or population. Recorded SBP values varied between 80- and 130-mm Hg, with a mean value of 96.8 mm Hg and an Sd of 13.9 mm Hg. Previous studies have shown that the mean SBP of the population was 120 mmHg, and the question was whether the mean SBP of the sample was significantly different from (higher or lower than) that of the population? The null hypothesis is that both the sample and the population have the same SBP.

The Equation

Following the usual path of testing hypothesis, we begin by assuming a certain distribution to our variable of interest. Systolic blood pressure is a continuous variable known to be normally distributed in the population. With such a small sample, it will most probably follow the near-normal distribution described by Student. The next step is to see whether the "observed" mean $(\bar{x})$ is significantly different from the mean of the population (μ) but, as usual, the raw difference between means $(\bar{x} - \mu = 96.8 - 120 = -23.2 \text{ mm Hg})$ has to be standardized by dividing it by the proper Se. As statisticians have already calculated and tabulated the probabilities associated with each t-value, we only have to calculate the t value of our results "Eq. 2.16". The proper Se of the Student's equation is the population Se, which is usually unknown but can be estimated from the sample

itself by dividing its Sd by the square root of sample size. Se = Sd/√n = 13.9/√20 = 3.1.

$$t = \frac{(\bar{x} - \mu)}{Se} \qquad (2.16)$$

The Interpretation

The calculated t-value (−7.45) is smaller (more negative) than the critical t (−2.093) inscribed in the Student table, at the intersection of the row denoting 19 df (n − 1) and the column denoting the usual critical limit of statistical significance of P = 0.05 [8]. Although we can conclude that the mean SBP is significantly smaller than the mean SBP of the population (P < 0.05), yet we have to calculate the degree of significance or the exact P-value (0.001). Note that if the study was unilateral; i.e., we were just interested in proving that sample blood pressure is lower than that of the population and not the reverse, the critical limit of statistical significance will be 1.729.

What Should be Reported

We have to report the descriptive statistics: mean, Sd, and 95% CI of observed systolic blood pressure. The Se and the df can be easily deduced from the Sd and sample size, and hence, reporting both information is redundant. Concerning the inferential statistics, we have to report the t and the P values.

We advise reporting two additional essential pieces of information: the 95% CI of the difference "Eq. 2.17" and the effect size. Effect size (Cohen ds) can be either calculated from the (t) value and sample size or both means and Sd and is equal to −1.66 (see Sect. 4.2.1.1). View the expected inflation of ES due to our small sample size; ES is better expressed as Hedges g = −0.96 (see Sect. 4.2.1.2). The second important information is the 95% CI of the difference, which provides the set of the unknown but true information compatible with our results. Although both the mean of the difference ($\overline{x_d}$ = mean of the sample—mean of the population = 96.8 − 120 = 23.2 mm Hg) and the Se (Sd/square root of sample size= 13.9/4.47 = 3.11) can be calculated from the descriptive data, yet the t-value used in calculating the 95% CI of the difference is not the t-value of the test result (−7.45). The t-value used to calculate the bilateral 95% CI of the difference is the bilateral 5% critical limit of significance that figures in the Student table, at the intersection of the corresponding (n − 1 = 19) df and the 0.05 probability column; i.e., 2.093 [8]. Unless reported, the reader will be obliged to check it out by himself in the Student table, which is not an easy task for a lay reader. Note that if the study was unilateral, the 95% CI would be created with the corresponding critical limit of the significance of 1.729 and not the 2.093 limits of the bilateral design.

$$
\begin{aligned}
95\% \; CI \; of \; the \; difference &= \overline{x_d} \pm t \; Se \\
&= -23.2 \pm 2.093 \times 3.1 \\
&= -29.7 \; to \; -16.7 \; mm \; Hg
\end{aligned} \tag{2.17}
$$

Conditions of Application

The sample has to be chosen at random, and the analyzed variable has to be continuous and normally distributed in the population of interest. As a rule of thumb, a minimum of 20 cases is needed to comfortably apply the test.

2.4.1.2 The Unpaired Student Test

The unpaired Student test is used to compare the means of a continuous normally distributed variable in two independent groups of patients.

The Example

A small study was conducted to compare the effect of two oral hypoglycemic drugs in type two diabetic groups of patients. Sixty-four cases were randomly selected to either receive oral hypoglycemic A or B. Following one week of regular intake, the mean (Sd) of fasting blood sugar (FBS) were: 94.8 ± 11.5 mg/dL for patients receiving treatment A and 60.6 ± 7 mg/dl for those receiving treatment B. The study question was whether the observed difference is true and reflects different hypoglycemic effects of both treatments. Is it just due to chance, and both treatments have comparable effects? The null hypothesis is no difference between treatments

(H_0: A = B), and the alternative hypothesis is that both treatments are different (H_1: A ≠ B). The more significant is the observed difference between means, the less is the probability that the null hypothesis is true. The null hypothesis is finally rejected when the probability of being true drops to 5% and, we accept the alternative hypothesis of the difference being true.

The Equation

The test is simple and follows the usual path of the testing hypothesis. We begin by assuming a certain distribution to our variable of interest. Fasting blood sugar is normally distributed in the population, and with such a small sample, it will follow the near-normal distribution of Student. The next step is to look for the difference between both means (mean a − mean b) and standardize this by dividing it by the proper Se, as usual, "Eq. 2.18". Although the mean is "the signal" of efficacy, the Se is "the noise" due to variability around this mean. Standardization brings "all differences" that can be calculated in variable scales such as gm/dl, cm, years, etc..; to "a common standardized scale (t-value)", which has a perfectly-known probability distribution as figured in Student's table. The probability of this (t-value) can then be assigned to the initially calculated difference.

$$
t = \frac{(\overline{x}_a - \overline{x}_b)}{Se} \tag{2.18}
$$

In case the two variances were homogenous

Here we have to define: which is the proper Se of the equation? The answer is straightforward because we all know that the proper Se is that of the populations of concern. However, the latter is hardly known, and, we almost always have to estimate it from the sample. If we assume that both groups issue from the same population, their variances have to be homogenous. Consequently, it will be logical that those "homogenous" variances are pooled together into a common variance (Variance pooled) "Eq. 2.19", from which we deduct the proper Se for Student's equation "Eq. 2.20". Homogeneity is said to be assumed as long as both groups are of nearly equal size and with a minimum number of 30 patients per group. However, this is not always the case, as we will show in our example. Hence, it is advisable to test variance homogeneity by a frank statistical test before proceeding to compare the two means by the test of Student. A statistically non-significant Levene's test means that the assumption of homogeneity can be maintained. In such a case, the statistical significance of (t) is checked out in Student's table at (na + nb − 2) df. Our calculated t-value "Eq. 2.21" is much higher (14.45) than that figured in the table, at 62 df. Feeding our data to a commercial statistical software package returns a P-value of < 0.001. The results of the analysis based upon the assumption of variance homogeneity are shown in the first line of Table 2.14.

$$S^2_{pooled} = \frac{(n_a - 1)S^2_a + (n_b - 1)S^2_b}{n_a + n_b - 2}$$
$$= \frac{(31 - 1)11.5^2 + (33 - 1)7^2}{31 + 33 - 2} = 89.3$$

$$(2.19)$$

$$Se_{pooled} = \sqrt{\frac{Se^2_{pooled}}{n_a} + \frac{Se^2_{pooled}}{n_b}}$$
$$= \sqrt{\frac{89..3}{31} + \frac{89..3}{33}} = 2.37 \quad (2.20)$$

$$t = \frac{(\bar{x}_a - \bar{x}_b)}{Se_{pooled}} = \frac{(94.8 - 60.6)}{2.37} = 14.45 \quad (2.21)$$

In case the two variances were significantly different

A statistically significant Levene's test simply means that both variances are significantly different from one another, and hence, pooling two significantly different entities (variances) into a single one (pooled variance), as we just did, does not make much sense. In fact, in our example, Levene's test produced a high F ratio of 16.7 and hence, pointed to a statistically high significant difference between both variances with a P value < 0.001. Interestingly, and despite of showing a significant heterogeneity between both variances, IBM-SPSS produced the two results

(Table 2.14). Results assuming variance homogeneity are shown in the upper line and those assuming non-homogeneity are shown in the lower line of Table 2.14. We have to be careful that many software executes all possible analyses and leave the researcher to choose the most appropriate one.

Nevertheless, view the heterogeneity of the two variances, the proper "common" variance cannot be the pooled variance but the (larger) variance of the difference (Variance$_{diff}$), calculated by summing the variances of both groups. The proper standard error will be the square root of it (Se$_{diff}$) "Eq. 2.22". As shown in Table 2.14, the larger (Se$_{diff}$) will produce a wider 95% CI and a smaller t-value, of course. Most importantly, the latter is not checked at the usual df (na + nb − 2 = 62) but at a smaller df (49.1, in our example), calculated by a more complicated formula "Eq. 2.23" [7] and making it more difficult to achieve statistical significance. Put it this way, the test of student is most powerful when sample sizes are equal, with homogeneity of variances.

$$Se_{difference} = \sqrt{\frac{Se^2_a}{n_a} + \frac{Se^2_b}{n_b}} = \sqrt{\frac{11.5^2}{31} + \frac{7^2}{33}}$$
$$= 2.4$$

$$(2.22)$$

$$df = \frac{\left(s^2_a/n_a + S^2_b/n_b\right)^2}{\left(S^2_a/n_a\right)^2/(n_a - 1) + \left(s^2_b/n_b\right)^2/_{(n_b-1)}}$$

$$(2.23)$$

The Interpretation

Although homogeneity of variances could not be assumed, the test could still be used after using (Se$_{diff}$) instead of the (Se$_{pooled}$) and adapting the degrees of freedom. In conclusion, there was a statistically significant difference between the hypoglycemic effects of both treatment; P < 0.001.

What Should be Reported

We should report the descriptive statistics: mean, Sd, sample size, and 95% CI of the mean in both

Table 2.14 The unpaired Student's test: extract of IBM-SPSS output comparing the fasting blood sugar in two groups of patients receiving different oral hypoglycemic

	t-value	df	P-value	Mean of the difference[a]	Se of the difference[a]	95% CI of the difference[a]
Equal variances assumed	14.45	62	<0.001	34.23	2.37	29.5–38.9
Equal variances not assumed	14.243	49.1	<0.001	34.23	2.40	29.4–39

[a] = fasting blood sugar in mg/dL

groups. View the absence of variance homogeneity; we have to ignore the analysis results shown in the first line of Table 2.14 and report the values figured in the second line. The t-value (14.243), df (49.1), P-value (<0.001), and 95% CI of the difference (29.4–39). In case Levene's test was non-significant, we would report the same values from the first line of the Table, of course. It is highly recommended to report the effect size (ES). Unlike sample size, ES describes the true effect treatment in the population, regardless of the chosen risks of error, and is very useful to calculate sample size for future studies (see Sect. 4.2.1). We can calculate Cohen's d from the t-value and total sample size; however, the inherent large variability of small groups like ours tends to inflate ES, and Hedges was suggested to be a better estimate. In our example, Cohen's ds equals 3.56 "Eq. 2.24", and the smaller but more correct Hedges g equals 3.5 "Eq. 2.25".

$$Cohen\ ds = t\sqrt{\frac{1}{n_a} + \frac{1}{n_b}} = 14.234 \times 0.25$$
$$= 3.56$$

$$(2.24)$$

$$Hedges\ g = Cohen\ ds\left(1 - \frac{3}{4(n_a + n_b) - 9}\right)$$
$$= 3.5$$

$$(2.25)$$

Conditions of Application

Both samples have to be independent and chosen at random. The variable of concern (FBS in our example) must be continuous and normally distributed in the population. Both groups have to have homogeneous variances, which can be assumed as long as they are of nearly equal sizes, with each including ≥ 30 patients. As a rule of thumb, a minimum of 20 patients is required per group to "comfortably" use the Student test. It is advisable to test homogeneity of variances by Levene's test. Suppose the test shows a statistically significant deviation from homogeneity. In that case, the difference between both means has to be standardized by the "larger" (Se_{diff}) instead of the (Se_{pooled}), which decreases the calculated t-value. The statistical significance of the latter has to be checked, not at the df of ($na + nb - 2$), but at the lower df "Eq. 2.23."

2.4.1.3 The Paired Student Test

Comparing data acquired from the same person or two well-matched persons reduces the in-between group variability and increases study power. We can acquire data from the same person before and after treatment, such as measuring fasting blood sugar in a diabetic patient before and after insulin has been given. Another design is the same person receiving the two treatments on two occasions. An example is to measure fasting blood sugar in a diabetic patient while receiving treatment A and then measure it another time when he shifts to treatment B. A matched design is to give the two treatments, each to a separate group of patients; provided that the two groups have been well-matched regarding demographics and known disease-related risk factors, both groups can be considered identical, as being one group. The paired test of Student is the most commonly used test to compare the means of 2 paired groups, whether dependent or matched.

The Example

Twenty hypertensive patients were randomized to either receive treatment A first, then treatment B, or the reverse. Each patient receives one treatment for one week before measuring the diastolic blood pressure (DBP). As shown from previous studies, a washout period of 5 days of no therapy was sufficient to ensure no residual effect of the first on the second treatment. Mean diastolic blood pressure (±Sd) was 97 ± 6.6 mm Hg and 83.3 ± 5.7 mm Hg with patients' receiving treatment A and B, respectively. Unlike the bilateral design, where the study question was: which is better: treatment A or treatment B; the question of the paired design is whether there is a difference between A and B or not? In other words, the null hypothesis is that both treatments are equal (H0: A–B = 0), and the alternative hypothesis is that they are not (H1: A–B ≠ 0). Hypothesis testing follows the usual path; the larger is the observed (standardized) difference, the less we are confident that the null hypothesis is true. Once our confidence (probability of the null hypothesis being true) drops down to the universally accepted critical 5% limit, we reject the null hypothesis and adopt the alternative hypothesis that the difference between treatment effects is true and not due to chance.

The Equation

We start by the assumption that the variable in concern follows a Student distribution. Note that, unlike the unpaired design, we do not start by comparing both variances by Levene's test. The patient is compared to himself and not to another (different) group of patients. Moreover, the same person receiving both treatments is much less variable than the response of two patients, each receiving one of the two treatments. We directly proceed to the test of Student. However, we have to be careful, we will not compare the two means observed with each treatment (mean A versus mean B), but we will calculate the difference between the effects of treatment A (x_{ai}) and treatment B (x_{bi}) for each patient: ($x_{ai} - x_{bi}$) (x_{Di}). We sum those calculated differences to get the mean of the differences ($\bar{x}_{Di}$) and Se of the

differences (Se_{Di}). If the treatment is ineffective, the mean of the difference will equal zero ($\bar{x}_{Di} = 0$); which is the null hypothesis. The alternative hypothesis is that it is not ($\bar{x}_{Di} \neq 0$). The equation dictates itself: we compare the mean of the difference to zero, standardized by the only available Se, the Se of the difference. The zero is removed from the equation, of course "Eq. 2.26". The significance of the t is then checked out in the Student table at 19 (n − 1) df.

$$t = \frac{(\bar{x}_{Di} - 0)}{Se_{Di}} = \frac{\bar{x}_{Di}}{Se_{Di}} \qquad (2.26)$$

The paired versus the unpaired test of Student

The paired test is also known as a one-tailed test for confining the entire 5% primary risk of error (α) to one tail (one side) of the distribution. It is the only site where we expect to find what we were looking for: is there is a difference or an effective treatment (see Fig. 1.13)? Table 2.15 shows an extract of the results of DBP measurements in 5 out of the 20 patients. The 4th column shows the observed differences calculated for each of the five patients (10, 10-, 10-, 5-, and 15-mm Hg), which are not equal to zero. The mean of the differences is calculated as the sum of all differences divided by their number (10 + 10 + 10 + 5 + 16)/5 = 10 mm Hg. We calculate the variance as usual: we subtract each of the five differences from the mean difference and square each result before summing them all. We calculate the variance as the mean of those squared differences. The Sd of the difference is the square root of the variance and, the Se is the Sd divided by the square root of sample size, as routine (see Sect. 1.3.4). Although we can deduct the mean of the difference from the means of both groups yet we cannot deduct the Sd of the difference (1.58 mm Hg) and, in consequence the 95% CI of the difference, from the mean (±Sd) DBP of treatment A (98 ± 7.6 mm Hg) and treatment B (88 ± 8.4 mm Hg). The mean of the difference is the information used in the paired equation and should be reported by the researcher, together with its 95% CI: 5.6 ± 14.4 mm Hg (Table 2.15).

In the unpaired design, (α) is equally split between the two tails (two sides) of the curve to

Table 2.15 Calculation of the paired Student's test

	Treatment A	Treatment B	Difference (A–B)
Patient I	110	100	10
Patient II	100	90	10
Patient III	90	80	10
Patient IV	95	90	5
Patient V	95	80	15
Mean	98	88	10
Sd	7.6	8.4	3.5
Se	3.4	3.7	1.58
95% CI*	–	–	5.6–14.4
t-value	–	–	10/1.58 = 6.3

Values are diastolic blood pressure measurement (mm Hg). * = confidence interval of the difference, calculated for the paired design

give the probability of a "wrong" answer of one of the two raised questions: is A better than B or B better than A (see Fig. 1.12)? In the case our actual study was bilateral, the comparison would have been between the mean DBP of treatment A (98 ± 7.6 mm Hg) and mean DBP of treatment B (88 ± 8.4 mm Hg) (Table 2.15). Unlike the paired design, we have to begin by testing homogeneity of variances by Levene's test. Feeding the data of this small subgroup of five patients to IBM-SPSS statistical software produces a statistically non-significant Levene's test (F = 0.086; P = 0.776). Hence, we can use the data output shown in the first line of Table 2.16. If the test showed significant heterogeneity, we should use the data presented in the second line instead. Compared to the unilateral design, the mean of the difference does not change; of course, it is 10 mm Hg. What changes significantly is the variability. The variability of a bilateral study is much more considerable than that of a unilateral study. The pooled Se is much higher (5 mm Hg), and hence, the confidence interval is much wider, and the t value is smaller = 10/5 = 2, compared to the unilateral t-test. Moreover, check the statistical significance of the t-value at eight df (na + nb − 2), compared to only four df (n − 1) for the unilateral design. The net result, if the study was bilateral, we had to conclude that both treatments were comparable to one another.

The Interpretation

Our test statistic (t = 6.3) is larger than the critical value figured in Student's table at 19 (n − 1) df for a unilateral study (t = 1.729). Our result is even larger than the one figure for a P-value of 0.001. We can conclude that there is a statistically significant difference between the effects of both treatments. Treatment B significantly lower the DBP than treatment A; P < 0.001.

Table 2.16 Calculation of the unpaired Student's test. Data extracted from Table 2.15

	t-value	df	P-value	Mean of the difference[a]	Se of the difference[a]	95% CI of the difference[a]
Equal variances assumed	1.98	8	0.083	10	5	−1.6 to 21.6
Equal variances not assumed	1.98	7.9	0.83	10	5	−1.7 to 21.7

[a] = diastolic blood pressure in mm Hg

What Should be Reported

We have to report the descriptive statistics: mean, Sd, and 95% CI of diastolic blood pressure observed in both groups. View the small sample size; we have to repeat that those confidence intervals are calculated as mean ± (t) Se. The latter is not the (t) value calculated by Student's test but the critical (t) value, figured in Student's table at 19 df (= 1.729).

We have to report the inferential statistics, including the mean of the difference (10 mm Hg), it's Se (1.56 mm Hg), and the 95% CI of the difference (5.6–14.4 mm Hg). We have to report the t value (6.3) as well as the P-value (<0.001). In addition, most statistical software automatically calculates the correlation coefficient r between the two measurements and its P-value. We have to report our r value (r = 0.082: P = 0.73) for being useful in estimating ES and future sample size calculation based upon the actual study. Cohen has suggested expressing ES (Cohen dz) by standardizing the mean of the difference by the standard deviation of the difference that can become more precise by including coefficient r. Cohen dz can also be calculated by dividing our t-value by the square root of sample size or simply derived from Cohen ds (see Sect. 4.5.1). In our study, Cohen $dz = 6.3/\sqrt{20} = 3.14$. Kindly refer to Sect. 4.5 for the details on effect size.

Conditions of Application

They are the same as for all other parametric tests dealing with quantitative variables: the sample has to be chosen at random, and the analyzed variable has to be normally distributed in the population of concern. The test is said to be robust. The larger is the sample, the more those conditions of application can be verified. As a rule of thumb, it is advised that the sample size has to be at least 20.

The Student test is the most commonly used to compare the means of a normally distributed continuous variable, whether between two independent groups, two dependent groups, or one group, to a theoretical distribution. The test is robust and can be comfortably applied in groups as small as 20 cases, following a near-normal distribution and showing heterogeneity between variances. The unpaired Student is most potent when sample sizes are equal and homogeneity is being verified. Otherwise, the penalty is to use the large Se of the difference instead of the pooled Se and to decrease the degrees of freedom.

2.4.2 The Comparison of Two Variances

Normal distribution and equality of variances are pre requisites of parametric tests. Equality is not in the strict sense of the term but rather the absence of a statistically significant difference between the variances, providing sufficient evidence that groups do not issue from different populations. Comparing two variances has many other applications. For example, suppose we want to test the accuracy of FBS measured with a bed-side strip, compared to regular laboratory procedures. In that case, the comparison of means cannot answer the study question. What is most important in such a study would be that the variability of measures "variances" given by our tested strips rather than their "means" would not be significantly different from those given by laboratory analysis, which denotes their accuracy. The use of the Student's test or else to compare means has no place in such a study. The test that should be applied is the comparison of both variances, hoping not to find a significant difference in the variability between strips and lab. Whenever we compare methods of investigation or diagnostic procedures in 2 groups of patients, we have to compare variances rather than means.

The Example

We will recall the same example used to compare the effects of 2 oral hypoglycemics in 2 independent groups of patients (see Sect. 2.4.1.2). The study question was whether the observed difference between mean fasting blood sugar (FBS) measurements in both groups is true and reflects different hypoglycemic effects or is it just due to chance? As patients were selected at random and FBS is known to be normally distributed in the population, the researchers have to ensure homogeneity of variances to complete the conditions necessary for the application of a "classic" unpaired Student test.

The Equation

The homogeneity between two groups can be assumed whenever the ratio between the larger and the smaller standard errors (Se) is less than two or when the ratio between the larger and the smaller variance (Fisher's value) is smaller than that figuring in Fisher's table point 2.5% at the corresponding df. On the other hand, homogeneity of two or multiple variances can be examined by formal hypothesis testing using Brown-Forsythe, Levene's test, or else.

Testing variance homogeneity by the ratio between the two standard errors

Two variances can be homogenous whenever the ratio between the larger Se (Se_L) and the smaller Se (Se_S) is less than 2. Applying this to our example given in Sect. 2.4.1.2, $Se_L/Se_S = 2.07/1.22 = 1.69$. We already knew that Levene's test showed significant heterogeneity, and hence, this ratio is not sensitive. Put it this way; if the ratio between both standard errors is >2, both variances are heterogeneous; however, the reverse is not always true, giving a false negative result.

Testing variance homogeneity by the ratio between the two variances

Two variances are significantly different when their Fisher's ratio (ratio between the larger variance (V_L^2) and the smaller variance V_S^2) is smaller than Fisher's value figured in Fisher's table point 2.5%, at the intersection of the larger variance df to the smaller variance df : (df_L/df_S). The reader may need to go back to Sect. 2.2.3.4 to verify we look for statistical significance in Fisher's table at point 2.5% and not 5%. Although the variance per se (V^2) is not a common output of many statistical software packages, it can be easily calculated by squaring the omnipresent Sd. The Sd of group A and group B patients are 11.5 and 7 mg/dL, and the respective sample sizes were 31 and 33 patients (see Sect. 2.4.1.2). Fisher's ratio $F_{31,33} = 132.25/49 = 2.699$. Both variances are heterogenous because our F ratio is larger than the critical value of 2.041, calculated for a numerator df of 31 and a denominator df of 33. [1, 8].

Testing variance homogeneity by formal hypothesis testing

The equations of Levene's test, Bartlett's test, and Brown-Forsythe test are ugly [20], and hence, they are among the few commonly used equations that we decided not to present here. Nevertheless, Levene's test is the most applicable and is built up in most statistical software packages, such as IBM-SPSS and STATA. In our example, Levene's test gave an F ratio of 16.7 and a statistically significant heterogeneity; P < 0.001.

The Interpretation

Homogeneity could not be verified for the presence of a statistically significant difference between both variances.

What Should be Reported

The F ratio and the P-value of Levene's test.

Conditions of Application

The sample was chosen at random and the variable in question (FBS in our example) is normally distributed in the population.

2.4.3 The Comparison of Multiple Means

Although multiple means are sometimes primarily compared two-by-two by a series of

Student tests, repeated comparisons inflate type I error and, unless corrected, it becomes a significant source of bias. One-way ANOVA avoids this situation by comparing multiple means in one step. In addition to the normal distribution, a regular one-way ANOVA requires homogeneity of variance among compared groups [21]. In case of significant differences between variances, we can still compare means by the robust Welch's F test [22] or the Brown and Forsythe test [23]. Commercial statistical software such as IBM-SPSS usually offers the option of producing both tests along with ANOVA.

On the other hand, a statistically significant ANOVA tells us that at least two of the multiple groups are significantly different from each other, but it does not tell us which two groups? In other words, the null hypothesis is that all means are equal, and the alternative hypothesis is that at least one pair of means is not. Unless a priori comparison of contrasts was pre planned before the analysis, a post hoc analysis is then required to compare the groups two by two if required.

2.4.3.1 One-Way Analysis of Variance (One-Way ANOVA)

Variability is not a single block, and the role of ANOVA is to partition variability into its originating components and to test the statistical significance of each one of them, as well as any possible interaction. For example, the duration of hospital stay after surgery is not the result of a single factor but the product of many factors such as type of surgery, surgeon experience, hospital facilities, and several patient-related risk factors. ANOVA first quantifies the amount of variation related to the hospital stay, then weights, and finally tests the statistical significance of the effect of each of those risk factors on the duration of stay. In this section focusing on bivariate analysis, we will only deal with one-Way ANOVA analyzing the effect of one variable (e.g., type of surgery) on the outcome (duration of hospital stay). The analysis of the effect of 2 factors (e.g., type of surgery and surgeon experience) is called 2-way ANOVA. The analysis of

three factors is called 3-way ANOVA, and up to full factorial ANOVA, which tests the effect of all possible factors and their interaction on the outcome, will be dealt with in a future section (see Sect. 3.2).

ANOVA: How Does it Work?

Although ANOVA is mainly used to compare multiple means, we will only compare two means to simplify calculations. The computations can then be extended to compare means among any number of groups. We have previously shown that variance (S^2) is the measurement of variability and is computed as the sum of squared deviations (SS) of the individual values from their mean, divided by the degrees of freedom, which is estimated from sample size (see Sect. 1.3.4.1). Thus, given a specific sample size, S^2 is a function of "SS". Put it this way; the SS represents the total variation in a sample, and S^2 is the mean variation. We will begin by discussing variation in terms of SS, and then we will recall df to calculate the variance. Consider the data set in Table 2.17 showing the duration of hospital stay in 9 patients, equally randomized between laparoscopic (Group a), minimal invasive cholecystectomy (Group b), and conventional cholecystectomy (Group c). What should be done is to compare the 3 groups by a single test, which is one-way ANOVA. In case of a significant ANOVA, the three groups can be compared two-by-two by post-hoc analysis, taking into consideration the inflation of the P value due to the repeated comparisons (see Sect. 2.4.3.4). In order to demonstrate how ANOVA works, we will not follow this correct approach but we will compare group a to group b then group a to group c.

1. *Comparison of Group a to Group b*

Ignoring group membership, the overall mean duration of hospital stay for the six patients in group a and b is four days, which varies between patients, of course. Let us calculate the total variability observed in this comparison,

Table 2.17 How does ANOVA works?

Observations	I	II	III	Mean stay	SS
1-Group a versus b					
Group a (n = 3)	1	2	3	2	2
Group b (n = 3)	5	6	7	6	2
Total mean	–	–	–	4	–
SS$_{within}$	–	–	–	–	4
SS$_{total}$	–	–	–	–	28
2-Group a versus c					
Group a (n = 3)	1	2	3	2	2
Group c (n = 3)	9	10	11	10	2
Total mean	–	–	–	6	–
SS$_{within}$	–	–	–	–	4
SS$_{total}$	–	–	–	–	100

Values are durations of hospital stay in days, n = number of observations, I, II and III = identification of observed cases in each group, Group a = patients benefiting from laparoscopic surgery, Group b = patients benefiting from minimal invasive surgery, Group c = patients benefiting from conventional surgery, SS = sum of squared deviations, calculated in days-square

regardless of the group membership. In terms of SS, this total variability SS$_{total}$ equals 28 "Eq. 2.27".

$$SS_{total} = (2 - 4)^2 + (3 - 4)^2 + (1 - 4)^2$$
$$+ (6 - 4)^2 + (7 - 4)^2 + (5 - 4)^2 = 28$$
$$(2.27)$$

Considering group membership, we calculate the variability within each group, always in terms of SS. The variability within the first group (SS$_{within\ a}$) equals (2) "Eq. 2.28" and, the variability within the second group (SS$_{within\ b}$) equals (2) too "Eq. 2.29", which is just due to chance. However, it shows us an important point: although the mean hospital stay of the two groups is quite different (2 and 6 days; respectively), the within-group variabilities can be the same. The within-group variabilities represent variability recorded among patients receiving the same treatment modality and calculated independently from the other group. Their sum (2 + 2 = 4) is the within-groups variability for both: (a) and (b) treatment groups "Eq. 2.30". In other words, it represents the overall part of variability that we cannot explain: why do patients receiving the same treatment react differently?

$$SS_{within\ a} = (1 - 2)^2 + (2 - 2)^2 + (3 - 2)^2 = 2$$
$$(2.28)$$

$$SS_{within\ b} = (5 - 6)^2 + (6 - 6)^2 + (7 - 6)^2 = 2$$
$$(2.29)$$

$$SS_{within-groups} = 2 + 2 = 4 \qquad (2.30)$$

As we do not know precisely why patients receiving the same treatment have different responses, the SS$_{within-groups}$ are also called the SS$_{error}$ for being possibly due to a measurement error. It can also be called the SS$_{residual}$ for being the part of variability that we still need to explain by further analysis; i.e., we may need to know why this happens? Returning to our example, variability within both groups SS$_{within-groups}$ explains a small part of the total variability SS$_{total}$: 4/28 = 14%. In order to explain the remaining 86%, let us compare "Group a" to a third group of patients undergoing conventional cholecystectomy: "Group c" (Table 2.17).

2. Comparison of Group a to Group c

We have intentionally fixed the three values of Group c patients (9, 10, and 10 days), to keep the same within group variability of (2), for the three groups of patients "Eqs. 2.31" and "2.32". In other words, whether we are comparing: Group a versus Group b or Group a versus Group c; the within-groups variability will be the same: $SS_{within-groups} = 4$ "Eq. 2.33".

$$SS_{within\ a} = (1-2)^2 + (2-2)^2 + (3-2)^2 = 2$$
$$(2.31)$$

$$SS_{within\ c} = (9-10)^2 + (10-10)^2 + (11-10)^2 = 2$$
$$(2.32)$$

$$SS_{within-groups} = 2 + 2 = 4 \qquad (2.33)$$

Comparing the two situations: Group a versus Group b and, Group a versus Group c. The total SS in the second comparison ($SS_{total\ ac}$) is much increased up to 100 and hence, the within-group variability (2 + 2 = 4) which explained 14% of the total variability in the first comparison, now explains a much smaller amount of total variability (4%). In consequence, the remaining part of the total variability has increased from 86% "Eq. 2.34" to 96% "Eq. 2.35"; which can only be explained by the only change: increasing the difference between compared means from 4 days (mean a − mean b = 2–6 = −4) to 8 days (mean a − mean c = 2 − 10 = −8). Subtracting the within-group from the total variability reflects the difference between both means, and hence, it deserves to be called: the between-groups variability. It is also called the effect variability for reflecting the difference between the effects of compared treatments.

$$SS_{total\ ab} - SS_{within-groups\ ab} = SS_{between-groups\ ab}$$
$$= 28 - 4 = 24$$
$$(2.34)$$

$$SS_{total\ ac} - SS_{within-groups\ ac} = SS_{between-groups\ ac}$$
$$= 100 - 4 = 96$$
$$(2.35)$$

Now calculate the proper variance, also called mean square (MS), by dividing each SS by the appropriate df. We have analyzed the total variability into variability between the two groups due to differences between treatments effects and variability within groups that we cannot explain. In order to calculate the respective variances (variance between groups and variance within groups), we have to calculate their degrees of freedom. The df of groups is equal to the number of groups minus one and, as we have only two groups, our between-groups df = 1. The df within each group = sample size minus one. Hence, the df within both groups a and b = (3 − 1) + (3 − 1) = 4. Now we proceed and calculate the variances:

$$Variance_{between-groups\ ab} = 24/1 = 24 \quad (2.36)$$

$$Variance_{within-groups\ ab} = 4/4 = 1 \qquad (2.37)$$

$$Variance_{between-groups\ ac} = 96/1 = 96 \quad (2.38)$$

$$Variance_{within-groups\ ab} = 4/4 = 1 \qquad (2.39)$$

Concerning the comparison of group a and group b, it becomes evident that the variance explained by the difference between means is 24 times that explained by the difference in patients' response to the same treatment "Eqs. 2.36 and 2.37". The patient response will not vary if the treatments have no effect, so variability is the effect. Put it this way, the effect of different treatments is 24 times that observed in patients receiving the same treatment. For comparison of group a to group c, the effect we can explain by the difference between treatments is 96 times the residual effect that we cannot explain "Eqs. 2.38" and "2.39". The statistical significance of those effects will be explained in the coming formal example.

Although ANOVA is mainly used to compare multiple means, we have used it to compare two means only for the simplicity of calculations. The computations can be readily extended to compare means among any number of groups. Suppose we are comparing three groups, each formed of 30 patients. The total SS will be computed for all 90 patients as shown before, regardless of a group membership. The total df = 90 − 1 = 89. The within-group SS will be the sum of SS calculated for each of the three groups and the within-group df = 9 + 9 + 9 = 27. The between-group SS will be computed by subtracting the within-group SS from the total SS, and the between-group df = number of groups −1 = 2. Another point is that our sample included only three patients per group, and ANOVA should never be used to compare the means of such extremely small groups. This was deliberately made to ease calculations, and it should not be used as a formal illustrative example for AONVA.

The Example

A study was conducted to compare the fasting blood sugar (FBS) of patients with liver cirrhosis, with or without hepatocellular carcinoma (HCC). The researchers randomly selected 78 patients with liver cirrhosis, among whom 44 cases had HCC as well. Patients were compared to a group of 44 matching normal controls. The study question was whether the mean FBS measured in gm/dL was significantly different among the three groups. The null hypothesis (H_0) states that the means are equal, and the alternative hypothesis (H_1) is that at least two means are significantly different. The FBS ranged from 68 to 125 mg/dl, with an overall mean FBS of 97.5 ± 16.9 mg/dL. Mean (Sd) of FBS were 108.7 ± 13.4, 95.35 ± 16.1, and 88 ± 14.2 mg/dL for patients presenting with liver cirrhosis with HCC, without HCC and controls, respectively.

The Equation

We begin by assuming a specific distribution to our variable of interest. FBS is normally distributed among the population, and normality can be tested by several methods, including graphical presentation and formal statistical tests such as the Shapiro–Wilk test (see Sect. 1.4.3). In the absence of normality, we may think about data transformation, which can be easily achieved by transforming data into their logarithmic, reciprocal or squared values (see Sect. 1.4.4). However, transformation can be more demanding and need the help of a professional statistician. Otherwise, we can shift to a non-parametric alternative such as Kruskal and Wallis test.

The second step is to verify the equality of variances among the three groups by Levene's test; which has to be statistically non-significant,

in order to use the regular ANOVA. The third step is to perform the analysis of variance after assuming homogeneity of variance. As shown in our simple example outlined in Table 2.17, one-way ANOVA calculates the three sum of squares (total, within-groups, and between-groups SS) and their corresponding df to compute two sources of variability (2 variances): effect variance (between-groups) and residual variance (within-groups). The ratio between the former and the latter indicates how much of the total variability is explained by effect variance; i.e., by group membership.

1. *Calculation of the Sums of Squares*

In order to avoid long calculations, statisticians have derived quick formulae to compute SS, especially in the case of large samples. For a specific quantitative value (x) compared among groups (g); if Σx = sum of (x) values, Σx^2 = sum of squared (x) values, Ti = sum of individual (x) values in each group, TG = sum of (x) values in all groups, ni = number of patients in each group, N = total number of patients and g = number of groups; the total "Eq. 2.40", within-groups "Eq. 2.41", and between-groups SS "Eq. 2.42" can be calculated by the following formulae:

$$SS_{total} = \sum x^2 - TG^2/N \qquad (2.40)$$

$$SS_{within-groups} = \sum x^2 - \sum \left(\frac{Ti^2}{n_i}\right) \qquad (2.41)$$

$$SS_{between-groups} = \sum \left(\frac{Ti^2}{n_i}\right) - TG^2/N \qquad (2.42)$$

The reader can check on the validity of those equations by himself, using the simple data shown in Table 2.17. For example, the total SS $= (2^2 + 3^2 + 1^2 + 6^2 + 7^2 + 5^2) - (2 + 3 + 1 + 6 + 7 + 5)^2/6) = 28$.

2. *Calculation of the Degrees of Freedom*

Kindly refer to Sect. 2.2.2 to verify the basics of calculating the degrees of freedom. In short, the total df of a study is equal to the total sample size minus one = (N − 1). The within-groups df = the sum of degrees of freedom for each group, calculated by subtracting the number of groups from the total sample size (N − g). Finally, the between-groups df = number of groups minus one = (g − 1) (see Sect. 2.2.2).

3. *Calculation of Variances and their F Ratio*

As usual, both within-groups and between-groups variances are calculated by dividing each SS by its corresponding df. The between-groups variance is the amount of variability explained by patients' groups, and the within-groups variance is the amount of variability that remains unexplained. The F statistics is the ratio between the former and the latter: the larger is the effect variance, the more "factor groups" explains a considerable part of the total variability "Eq. 2.43".

$$F\ ratio = \frac{SS_{between-groups}/df_{between-groups}}{SS_{within-groups}/df_{within-groups}}$$
$$= \frac{Effect\ variance}{Residual\ variance}$$
$$(2.43)$$

Table 2.18 shows the partitions of the sum of squares in our example. The total SS is portioned into: between groups SS (9629.2; df = 2) and within groups SS (25,003; df = 119). Fisher's value ($F_{2,119}$) is the ratio between the in-between groups' variance and the residual variance = 22.9. The F ratio should be equal to or larger than the critical value (F = 3.072) figured in F point 5%, at the intersection of the numerator df (column number 2) and the denominator df (row number 119). Otherwise, we cannot conclude upon a statistically significant difference between at least two out of the three

compared groups at the universal level of 5%. Our value was much larger and the software produced a P-value < 0.001.

The Interpretation

Unless Levene's test reinforces homogeneity of variances by showing statistically non-significant results, it is not advisable to use ANOVA. It is better to choose Welch's F ANOVA that does not require variance equality. The test is also preferred when sample sizes are significantly different from each other (see Sect. 2.4.3.2). In our example, Levene's test showed that heterogeneity could be assumed (P = 0.226).

Many statistical tests represent explained to unexplained variability ratios, and ANOVA is an excellent example of this. The test is based on the comparison of the variance due to the between-groups variability (called Mean Square Effect, or MS effect) to the within-group variability (called Mean Square Error, or MS Error). Under the null hypothesis, their F ratio should be (1), and the alternative hypothesis is that it is not. In our example, F = 4813.6/210 = 22.914; hence, the amount of variation explained by the disease is nearly 23 times the unexplained amount. The final step is to find the statistical significance of the calculated Fisher's ratio. Our F value is larger than the critical value figured by the (3.072), and the software produces a P value < 0.001. Note that we can check the critical value online, and the only data we need to upload is the numerator df (2) and denominator df (119) and choosing 5% level of significance [1].

What Should be Reported

We have to report the descriptive statistics: overall and individual mean, Sd, and 95% CI of FBS. We have to report the exact P-value of

Table 2.18 One-way ANOVA comparing fasting blood sugar levels among patients with cirrhosis with and without hepatocellular carcinoma and normal controls

Source of variation	Sum of squares	df	Variance	F ratio	P-value
Between groups	9629.18	2	4814.59	22.91	<0.001
Within groups	25,003.3	119	210.1		
Total	34,632.49	121			

ANOVA (<0.001) and effect size as Eta squared η^2, Omega squared ω^2, or Cohen's F. As an example, Eta squared $\eta^2 = SS_{effect}/SS_{total}$ = 9629.182/34632 = 0.278 (see Sect. 4.6.1). Finally, we have to report the results of an "a priori" as well as "a posteriori" contrasts when performed (see Sect. 2.4.3.3).

Conditions of Application

Groups have to be independent and chosen at random. The quantitative variable of concern has to be normally distributed with equal variances among the compared groups. In the case of small sample size and variance inequality, the Welch F test is the most recommended by statisticians than ANOVA. In case of a very small sample size of less than 6 per group, such as in animal studies, Brown-Forsythe test [22] was chosen to be a better fit.

2.4.3.2 Welch's F ANOVA

In the cases where the assumption of variance homogeneity is violated, and in studies involving groups of unequal size, studies have shown that ANOVA inflates type I error. Welch's ANOVA has null and alternative hypotheses like a regular one-way ANOVA and calculates the F ratio between the group and residual variances. However, the test has the advantage of adjusting the calculated F ratio and uses more degrees of freedom to compensate for any violated assumptions of variance homogeneity. The test is equally applicable in all sets of situations and was even found to be more s than a regular ANOVA [22].

The Example

We will use the same example used for the regular ANOVA. As a reminder, the researchers randomly selected 78 patients with liver cirrhosis, among whom 44 cases had HCC. Patients were compared to a group of 44 matching normal controls. The FBS ranged from 68 to 125 mg/dl, with an overall mean FBS of 97.5 ± 16.9 mg/dL. Mean (Sd) of FBS were 108.7 ± 13.4, 95.35 ± 16.1, and 88 ± 14.2 mg/dL for patients presenting with liver cirrhosis with HCC, without HCC and controls, respectively.

The Equation

1. *We Replace the Raw Means with the More Appropriate Weighted Means*

Unlike the regular ANOVA, Welch's ANOVA is not based upon the equality of variances. Hence, the first step is to weigh each mean ($\bar{x}_K$) by its size (n) and the inverse of its variance ($1/S^2$). The weighting quantity is calculated independently for each mean value from its sample size (n) and its variance = n/S^2 "Eq. 2.44". Put it this way, the larger is the mean, and the smaller is its variability, the more it is representative to the population and hence, the more weight it should have. Consequently, the overall grand mean ($X_{Welch\ grand}$) will be equal to the sum of weighted means divided by the sum of all weights "Eq. 2.45". For our example, the weighted mean of FBS in patients with cirrhosis and HCC = $108.7 \times 44/(13.4)^2 = 26.46$ g/dL. The weighted means of patients with cirrhosis without HCC and controls = 12.5 and 19.2 g/dL. The weighted grand mean = sum of weighted means/sum of weights = (26.5 + 12.5 + 19.2)/(0.245 + 0.13 + 0.218) = 58.19/0.59 = 98.6 g/dL.

$$W_K \bar{x}_K = \frac{n\,\bar{x}_K}{S^2} \qquad (2.44)$$

$$X_{Welch\ grand} = \frac{\sum W_K \bar{x}_K}{\sum W_K} \qquad (2.45)$$

2. *We Calculate the Weighted SS and Effect Variance (MS)*

We calculate the SS and MS (variance) of weighted means at the usual degree of freedom; i.e., number of classes −1 = K − 1. Note that what we did here was just to replace the individual and grand means of a regular ANOVA by their Welch alternatives. For our example $SS_{Welch} = 0.245(98.6 - 26.5)^2 + 0.13(98.6 - 12.5)^2 + 0.22(98.6 - 19.7)^2 = 1273 + 964 + 1370 = 3608$ and an MS_{Welch} (variance) $= 3608/(3 - 1) = 1804$ "Eq. 2.46".

$$MS_{Welch} = \frac{SS_{welch\,M}}{df} = \frac{\sum W_K\left(x_K - X_{Welch\,grand}\right)}{K-1}$$

$$(2.46)$$

3. *We Correct the Model df to Compensate for Variance Inequality and Calculate the Residual Variance and F_{welch}*

What may look entirely unfamiliar is the calculation of the residual variance and its degree of freedom. We cannot continue with hand calculations, and we have to trust the computer software package. The calculation is based on the term (λ), which is also based on the weights (w_k), the number of patients per group (n_k) and the number of groups (k) "Eq. 2.47" [24, 25]. Finally, we calculate (F_w) and check out on its statistical significance in Fisher's at the same numerator as a regular ANOVA $df_{(k-1)}$ but at a much smaller denominator $df_{(1/\lambda)}$ "Eq. 2.48". The result of applying Welch ANOVA on our example, gives a much lower df of 74.5, a higher F_w ratio of 25.1 and a P-value of <0.001.

$$\lambda = \frac{3 \sum \dfrac{\left(1-\dfrac{w_K}{\sum w_K}\right)^2}{n_K - 1}}{K^2 - 1} \qquad (2.47)$$

$$F_W = \frac{MS_{Welch\,M}}{1 + 2\lambda(K-2)/3} \qquad (2.48)$$

The Interpretation

The Welch's F ratio was (25.08), its degrees of freedom (df1, df2: 2, 74.563), and its statistical significance was <0.001. In conclusion, the three means were statistically significant from each other, and post Hoc tests are necessary to discover from where this difference comes from, as with a regular ANOVA (see Sect. 2.4.3.3).

What Should be Reported

As in a regular one-way ANOVA, we have to report the descriptive statistics, the exact P-value of Welch's test, effect size as well as the results of any preplanned a priori comparisons or Post Hoc tests.

Conditions of Application

Groups have to be independent and chosen at random. The quantitative variable of concern has to be normally distributed among the compared groups. The test works regardless of equality of variance or groups sizes [22, 24, 25] and, compared to regular one-way ANOVA, Welch's test is said to be the most s at all levels [22].

2.4.3.3 ANOVA Contrasts: A Priori and Post-Hoc Analysis

We have to be careful that both regular and Welch's ANOVA compare the means of the groups to the grand mean. Hence, a statistically significant result should never indicate that one specific group is significantly different from the others. In other words, those tests only alarm that there is a difference, and then other tests have to be performed to find where exactly this signal (difference) comes from? In general, there are two main types of tests for comparing individual means: "A priori contrasts" set up before running the study and "A posteriori contrast or Post Hoc tests" used after the study.

A Priori Contrasts

Before launching his study, the researcher can set a scheme (a contrast) for comparing the individual means of the different groups, with one group chosen as a reference; which may be the placebo, the reference treatment group, the group with the highest level of ordered categories, or else. In other words, comparisons are not limited to a repeated series of two-by-two tests (series of pairwise contrasts). However, they can be nested into more comprehensive plans (comparing one or more groups on one side to one or many groups on the other side).

Suppose that the study question is which disease type is associated with significantly higher FBS. Instead of comparing the three groups to one another by three tests of Student, the investigators pre-planned only two contrasts (two comparisons) that will give the same answer (Table 2.19). The first contrast compares both cirrhotic groups to controls (contrast 1), and the second contrast the cirrhotic group with HCC to the cirrhotic group without HCC (contrast 2), excluding controls. The software permits the creation of those contrasts by assigning codes (dummy numbers) to the compared variables. It is wise to keep the sum of the codes in each contrast equal to 0. For example, in the first contrast, we can assign code 1 to both diseased groups and code -2 to the control group. The sum of the three codes $(1 + 1 - 2)$ will be zero and, the software will compare the groups with a code of 1 (diseased groups) to the group with the other (-2) code (the control group). In the second contrast, we wish to compare the two diseased groups and exclude the control group. We can assign the code (0) to the latter, a message to the software to exclude those patients from the comparison. We code the two diseased groups as $(+1)$ and (-1), which will be compared with the software. Note that the sum of the second comparison $(0 + 1 - 1)$ is zero too.

Table 2.19 shows the comparison of the two contrasts by the test of Student, and, by default, the software will produce the comparison twice: with and without the assumption of variance equality (see Sect. 2.4.1.2). As we have just shown that equality was assumed (Levene's test; $F = 1.34$; $P = 0.266$), we will only consider the first two lines assuming equal variances. The first contrast showed that both disease states have a significantly higher FBS compared to controls $(t = 5.11, P < 0.001)$, while the second contrast showed that HCC patients have significantly higher FBS than those presenting with cirrhosis without HCC $(t= -4; P < 0.001)$. Note that the t-tests performed had the same df of ANOVA $(df = 119)$ and that the results did not include

any penalty on the repeated comparisons made. In concordance with the rule of thumb, the Se of the (large) main group is more representative of the population than any other (small) subgroups.

The reader must consider that clinical trials are not always as simple as our example, and more complex comparisons among groups are sometimes mandatory. Commercially available statistical software packages offer many types of contrast designs for comparing the mean value of each group to the overall mean (deviation contrast), one specified mean (simple contrast), the mean of subsequent level (repeated contrast), the mean of subsequent levels (Helmet contrast) and the mean of previous levels (difference or reversed Helmet contrast). They also offer the possibility to test whether there is a linear positive or negative trend across the subgroups of patients. For example, whether there is a positive linear increase in the time of wound healing measured in days across the subgroups of diabetic patients classified in increasing order of duration of the disease (<5 years, < 10 years, < 15 years < 20 years). The software will calculate the part of SS related to the linear term, the same way it calculated the part of SS.

A Posteriori Contrasts: Post Hoc Analysis

Unlike "A priori contrasts," where the investigator limits the preplan to the specific follow-up comparisons that can answer his study questions, "A posteriori contrasts" perform all possible comparisons between all ANOVA groups after the analysis. Table 2.20 shows the results of three commonly used post hoc analyses, as applied to our example.

Table 2.19 A priori contrasts of fasting blood sugar levels among patients with cirrhosis with and without hepatocellular carcinoma and normal controls

Equality of variances	Contrast	Value of contrast	Se	t-value	df	P-value
Assumed	1	28.03	5.48	5.11	119	<0.001
	2	−13.3	3.31	−4.03	119	<0.001
Not assumed	1	28.03	5.48	90.85	90.8	<0.001
	2	−13.3	3.43	63.77	63.7	<0.001

Contrast 1 = cirrhotic patients with or without hepatocellular carcinoma versus normal controls, contrast 2 = cirrhotic patients with versus those without hepatocellular carcinoma

Table 2.20 Post-hoc analysis of fasting blood sugar levels among patients with cirrhosis with and without hepatocellular carcinoma and normal controls

Method	Groups	Mean of the difference	Se of the difference	P	95% CI of the difference
LSD[a]	HCC versus non-HCC	13.3	3.31	<0.001	6.78 to 19.9
	HCC versus Control	20.68	3.09	<0.001	14.56 to 26.8
	Non-HCC versus control	7.35	3.31	0.028	0.8 to 13.9
Tukey HSD	HCC versus non-HCC	13.3	3.31	<0.001	5.47 to 21.2
	HCC versus Control	20.68	3.09	<0.001	13.35 to 28
	Non-HCC versus Control	7.35	3.31	0.072	−0.5 to 15.2
Bonferroni	HCC versus non-HCC	13.3	3.31	<0.001	5.29 to 21.4
	HCC versus Control	20.68	3.09	<0.001	13.18 to 28.19
	Non-HCC versus Control	7.35	3.31	0.085	−0.68 to 15.39

HCC = cirrhotic patients with hepatocellular carcinoma, non-HCC = cirrhotic patients without hepatocellular carcinoma, a = using harmonic mean sample size

The least significant difference (LSD)

The first post Hoc test was suggested by Fisher as a series of multiple t-tests [26]. The least significant difference (LSD) test calculates the difference between a pair of means required to declare that both means are statistically significantly different, at the usual 5% primary risk of error. The calculated "critical LSD value" is then compared across all possible pairs of (k) means of ANOVA, and hence, the number of comparisons made will be equal to $k(k - 1)/2$. In our example, with k = 3, the number of required comparisons = 3, which will inflate by nearly three times the real P-value. The test does not suggest any correction, and hence, the LSD test is termed as being liberal and is not routinely used.

Tukey's honestly significant difference (HSD) test

John Tukey (1915–200) views that making multiple two-by-two comparisons (multiple t-tests) inflates the P-value and is dishonest unless reported. The P-value should be controlled, and hence, it was the name of the test: "honestly significant difference". In comparing two means, the test uses the studentized range distribution rather than the Student's distribution. Both distributions are similar, comparing the standardized differences. However, the latter considers the number of compared means and adjusts the critical value (P-value) accordingly. The more means under consideration, the more comparisons are made and the larger the critical value is.

We have previously explained Student distribution (see Sect. 2.4.1). Now let us explain what does a Studentized distribution means in simple terms. Suppose we take multiple samples from a particular normal distribution, the range between the mean of the smallest sample (μ_S) and mean of the largest sample (μ_L) standardized by the Se of all samples will follow a certain distribution: the studentized range distribution (q). Note that we have standardized the difference using the Se of all samples and not that of the two differences. Tukey has calculated and tabulated those extreme standardized variations (variation between the largest and smallest means) under the null hypothesis: the critical q statistics (q_{crit}). In other words, (q_{crit}) is the largest difference attributed to chance, according to the number of groups and sample size, i.e., adjusted for multiple comparisons. The (q_{crit}) can be acquired either from Tukey's tables [27] or through an online calculator after uploading the number of groups (k) and the within-groups df (N − K) [1]. The next step was to calculate the critical HSD of a particular study, which is also dependent upon the variability of the study. The best estimation of the latter was a standard error derived from the within-group variance of the whole study ($MS_{within\text{-}groups}$) and group sample size (n_K). Note that those two information are related to the study that we are about to analyze, unlike the (q_{crit}) values that was basically calculated by Tukey. The critical HSD is the maximum expected difference that we can attribute to chance in this particular study, adjusted for the multiple comparisons.

The HSD test does not compare the means of the two groups but their "absolute difference" to the "critical HSD" "Eq. 2.49". If the former is larger than the latter, the difference between both means cannot be attributed to chance and we can conclude that both groups are significantly different, adjusting for the multiple comparisons made. There are critical HSD values calculated for different probability points other than the usual 5%, such as 2.5% and 1% [27]. In case we have no access to q tables or calculators, we can acquire q from the t value by the equation: $t_{crit} = \frac{q_{crit}}{\sqrt{2}}$.

$$HSD = q_{crit}\sqrt{\frac{MS_w}{n_k}} \qquad (2.49)$$

Although the test was designed to fit groups of equal size, yet it can be adapted to unequal groups by using the harmonic mean instead of (n) "Eq. 2.49". The harmonic mean is known to better fit fractions, and it is calculated by dividing the total number of observations by the sum of their reciprocals. As example, the arithmetic mean of the three observations: 2, 4 and 5 = (2 + 4 + 5)/3 = 3.66, while their harmonic mean = 3/(1/2 + 1/4 + 1/4) = 3.16. Applying the test in our example with unequal group sizes, the harmonic mean = 3/(1/34 + 1/44 + 1/44)

= 40.1 mg/dl. Using the online calculator, with k = 3 and N−K = 119, the critical q = 3.36 [1]. With a within-group variance of 210.1 (Table 2.18) and a harmonic mean of 40.1, the critical HSD = 7.69. The difference between the mean FBS of cirrhotic patients without HCC and controls (95.35 − 88 = 7.353) did not reach the calculated HSD (7.69), and hence, those two groups are not significantly different from one another (P > 0.05). On the other hand, the difference between the means of the other groups (HCC versus controls and HCC versus cirrhotic without HCC) were all larger than the calculated HSD, and hence, these groups are significantly different from one another (P < 0.05), (Table 2.20).

Games-Howell test

Tukey HSD was based upon variance equality and Games-Howell test is a modification used in case the groups have unequal variances. The test is based on Tukey's studentized ranged distribution but uses the degrees of freedom to compensate for the violated equality assumption. Remember that the same procedure was used by Welch ANOVA to compensate for variance inequality (see Sect. 2.4.3.2). In practice, instead of checking on the value of (q_{crit}) at the usual N − K df, we use the smaller df calculated for the unpaired Student's test, with unequal variances "Eq. 2.23" (see Sect. 2.4.1.2). As variances are no more assumed to be equal, it was quite logical to use a different variance to compare each pair, instead of using a common variance for all. In the equation, we replace the common Se ($\sqrt{MS_w/n_k}$) with a different Se, calculated for each (a and b) pairs of means of different sample sizes (na and nb) "Eq. 2.50".

$$GH = q_{crit}\sqrt{\frac{1}{2} \times \left(\frac{S_a^2}{n_a} + \frac{S_b^2}{n_b}\right)} \qquad (2.50)$$

Dunnett's test

Dunnett's test can be seen as a variant of HSD that compares the means from several experimental groups to a control group mean. Hence, reducing the number of comparisons and pro- ducing a narrower confidence interval, at the expense of testing many to only one group and not testing the experimental groups against one another. The test calculates the minimal differ- ence ($D_{Dunnett}$) required to declare a statistically significant difference between any groups and the control by Student's t-statistics, controlling for the number of comparisons made. The basic elements of the equation are nearly the same. The Se error is calculated from MS_W and the sample size per group (n_K). The $t_{Dunnett}$ critical values were equally calculated according to type I error, number of groups (k) and $df_{within\text{-}groups}$. In order to serve experimental conditions, the $t_{Dunnett}$ critical values were tabulated for both one-sided (the most positive or negative t-value) and two-sided comparisons (the largest absolute t-value) [28]. The net result is that the Dunnett equation "Eq. 2.51" is similar to HSD equation "Eq. 2.49", with (q_{crit}) being replaced by (t_{crit} $\sqrt{2}$). The absolute difference between the experi- mental and control groups has to be at least equal or larger than $D_{Dunnett}$ value to declare a statis- tically significant difference between the experi- mental group and the control. Applying the equation in to example, with k = 3 and N − K = 119, the critical $t_{Dunnett}$ at 5% = 2.238 [28]. With a within-group variance of 210.1 (Table 2.18) and a harmonic mean of 40.1, the critical $D_{Dunnett}$ = 7.25. The absolute difference between control and HCC and non-HCC cirrho- sis was 20.68 and 7.35; indicating a statistically significant difference between cirrhosis with HCC and control and a non-significant difference between cirrhotic non-HCC and control group. Checking on Dunnett tables, the critical $t_{Dunnett}$ at 1% was 2.845 [28]; giving a critical $D_{Dunnett}$ of 9.21. Hence, we can conclude that the mean FBS of patients with cirrhotic HCC was significantly lower than control; P < 0.01.

$$D_{Dunnett} = t_{Dunnett}\sqrt{\frac{2MS_w}{n_k}} \qquad (2.51)$$

Bonferroni test

Bonferroni is another commonly used test that requires equality of variance but corrects the P-value inflation more simply [29]. Under the null hypothesis, the probability of having a non-significance result is 0.95 (1 − α), and having a significant result—which is untrue—is 0.05 or 5%. Remember that probabilities are summed by multiplication. If we test 2 independent null hypotheses, the probability that neither of them will be non-significant = 0.95 × 0.95 = 0.90 and, if we test 20 such hypotheses, the proba- bility that none of them will be significant drops down to: 0.9520 = 0.36 or 36%. Hence, and in general, if we have (k), independent compar- isons, the probability that we will get no signif- icant difference equals $(1 − α)^K$. Refreshing our basic mathematical information "Eq. 2.52":

$$(1 − α)^K = 1^K + α^K − (k \times 1 \times α) \approx 1 − α^K \qquad (2.52)$$

Regardless of the number of comparisons made (k), 1^k will always be equal (1) and, postulating that (α) is too small that we can neglect $α^k$, the quantity $(1 − α)^k$ will approximately be equal to (1 − kα). We deducted here that the primary risk of error (α) has to be replaced by the quantity (kα) to maintain the same primary risk of error of 0.05. Put it another way, in case of multiple comparisons (k), and in order to maintain the usual primary risk of error of 0.05; (kα) = 0.05 and hence, (α) = 0.05/k. Consequently, if we compare two treatments within five groups of patients in a clinical trial, the treatment will be significantly different at only 5% if there is a P value less than 0.01 (0.05/5) within any of the subsets compared. Put it more simply, the cal- culated P-value from any (k) number of signifi- cance tests will be penalized by being multiplied by the number of compared groups. We have to note that Bonferroni does suffer from loss of power due to several reasons, including that type II error rates are high for each test. In other words, it overcorrects the type I errors.

Table 2.20 shows "A posteriori comparisons" of the means of our example, using three post hoc tests. As shown, the most liberal LSD test showed a statistically significant difference between each pair of the three groups for not putting any penalty on re procession of data. On the other hand, both Bonferroni and Tukey's tests corrected for P-value inflation. Hence, both failed to show a significant difference between 2 closely related means: mean fasting blood sugar of cirrhotic patients without HCC and mean controls ($P > 0.05$). Let us check on the different P values those three tests gave for the same t (mean of the difference/Se = $-7.353/3.31$ = 2.221) and the same df (df of ANOVA =119). The calculated t is larger than that required to declare statistical significance, at the usual 5% α limit (=1.96). Hence, the comparison was statistically significant with the liberal LSD test that puts no penalty on the inflated P-value. On the other hand, the Bonferroni test corrects α to = 0.05/3 = 0.0166, which necessitates a minimum t value of 2.4 to declare statistical significance. Using another approach, the difference between the means of those two groups (= -7.353) did not reach the minimum difference required to declare statistical significance by Tukey's honestly significant difference (HSD) test (HSD = 7.69).

The experiment wise or family-wise error correction

The family-wise error rate (FWE or FWER) can be defined as the probability of having at least one false conclusion (one Type I error) in a series of hypothesis tests. Synonyms include experiment-wise error, cumulative Type I error, or alpha inflation. If α = Type I error of one comparison (usually 0.05), FWER for a number of comparisons (c) is calculated by the following equation "Eq. 2.53", which shows that the error rate can jump up to 26%, when six comparisons are made. In the case of 15 comparisons, a false positive result is almost guaranteed >99.5%.

$$FWER < 1 - (1 - \alpha)^c \qquad (2.53)$$

FWER need to be controlled, and two main procedures that are usually used are either performed as a single step or as sequential steps. An example of a single-step procedure is the Bonferroni correction. We have already discussed this: we divide alpha by the number of comparisons made and apply the new alpha to each test for finding P values. As mentioned before, the correction has been criticized for being of low power, with a high probability of Type II error. Sequential control is similar to Bonferroni but makes adaptive adjustments to each p-value, which increases the test power. Several sequential methods exist; the easiest is probably Holm's Sequential Bonferroni Method (HB) [30].

Holm's Sequential Bonferroni Method (HB)

The idea behind the test is to distribute the "overall common" penalty posed by Bonferroni in proportion to the degree of significance achieved with each comparison made. P values associated with the number of comparisons made (n_c) are ranked from the smallest (highest significance) to the largest, and the smallest P will take the biggest share of penalty, followed by the larger P taking a smaller share and so on "Eq. 2.54".

$$HB = \frac{target \propto (usually\ 0.05)}{n_C - rank\ of\ pairs\ (by\ degree\ of\ significance + 1)}$$
$$(2.54)$$

In order to apply the equation to our example, we will arrange the "uncorrected" P values resulting from multiple comparisons with the LSD test in ascending order. The first, second, and third ranks will then correspond to HCC versus controls, HCC versus cirrhotic without HCC, and finally, cirrhotic patients without HCC versus controls, respectively. HB1 = 0.05/(3 − 1 + 1) = 0.0166 and hence, we reject the null hypothesis for the actual P-value being smaller ($P < 0.001$) than HB1. HB2 = 0.05/(3 − 2 + 1) = 0.025 and here too we reject the null hypothesis for the actual P-value being smaller ($P < 0.001$) than HB2. On the other hand, HB3 = 0.05/(3 − 3 + 1) = 0.05, so we cannot reject the null hypothesis for the actual P-value being larger than HB3. The testing stops when we reach the first non-rejected hypothesis. All subsequent hypotheses will be non-significant (i.e., not rejected).

Which post hoc test to choose?

Post Hoc tests are too many to be fully outlined, and the young investigator usually questions which one is the most suitable test for his study? We are not able to give a straightforward answer but we can outline a few recommendations. In the case where equality of variances is assumed, we recommend using Tukey's honestly significant difference (HSD) or Bonferroni test to compare all means together. As the latter inflates type II error, Tukey's HSD is preferred when a large number of comparisons have to be made. Other alternatives include Duncan multiple range and Student–Newman–Keuls (S–N–K) tests; both make pair-wise comparisons using a step-wise order. The means are ordered from highest to lowest and extreme differences are tested first. In case of unequal group sizes, alternatives include Tukey's test with harmonic mean, Gabriel test, and Hochberg's GT2 test, with the latter being the most suitable test in extreme deviation. In case of inequality of variances, the researcher can choose among Tamhane's T2, Dunnett's T3, Dunnett C, and Games-Howell tests.

> In multiple group comparison, the first question would be which type of ANOVA is suitable for a particular study? After ensuring normality, subgroups have to be tested for variance equality. Regular ANOVA necessitates equal variances and equal sample sizes among groups. Brown-Forsythe ANOVA was designed for experimental studies. The robust Welch ANOVA is preferred by many statisticians and can be applied in all cases. The second question would be if we can compare groups two-by-two? Further comparisons are not permitted unless ANOVA shows a statistically significant difference among groups. Comparisons can be pre-planned during the preparation of the study or just performed after getting the

results. Nesting an "A priori contrast" during the preparation of the study permits the comparison of individual groups to one another after the study while avoiding the inflation of the type I error, which is a good option. Otherwise, post-hoc-analysis can be performed after the data collection, with measures to control the bias of type I error. The third question would be: what type of post-hoc test is the most suitable for a particular study? We will follow the same logic of choosing the type of ANOVA. In the case of variance equality, we can use Tukey's HSD or Bonferroni tests, adjusting unequal samples using harmonic means, if necessary. We can use the Games-Howell test to compare means with unequal variances and different sample sizes.

2.4.3.4 One-Way Repeated Measures ANOVA (RMANOVA)

Repeated measures ANOVA (RMANOVA) is the equivalent of one-way ANOVA for dependent groups, aiming to analyze the within-subject variability across the repeated sampling. RMANOVA can also be thought of as an extension of the paired t-test to compare multiple dependent groups. This section will discuss the bivariate version of RMANOVA with only one dependent continuous and one independent categorical variable. The dependent variable is repeatedly measured three or more times in the same condition or measured once under different conditions. An example of the first design is repeatedly measuring blood pressure in one group of patients, such as before treatment, after one week of treatment, and two weeks after treatment. The aim is to study the effect of time on the patients' response to detect the best time to get maximum efficacy or avoid certain complications. An example of the second design is to measure blood pressure in one group of patients only once after receiving each of 3 or more different treatments.

An alternative is to give the three treatments to three groups, matched for age, sex, and other disease-related risk factors. Put it this way, the investigator will compare changes in the mean score measured over time under the same level or condition (e.g., treatment) or measured once but under different levels or conditions (e.g., different treatments).

The Example

We have to admit that the following example is too small to be analyzed by an RM-ANOVA. However, it allows an easy calculation by hand, which removes our "inherent" fear from statistics and repulsion of mathematical calculations. Nevertheless, we will verify other conditions of using RM-ANOVA, such as normality and variance equality.

A study was conducted to compare warfarin doses given for the anticoagulation of patients with deep venous thrombosis (DVT). Warfarin dose is usually adjusted to reach a target therapeutic INR level between 2 and 3 days. Table 2.21 shows reported warfarin doses adjusted to three repeated INR measurements in a small group of ten patients. RM-ANOVA is used to test whether there is a statistically significant difference between the three measurements. The null hypothesis (H_0) will be that the three means are equal, and the alternative hypothesis (H_1) is that they are not, in that at least one mean is different from the others. If we reject the null hypothesis, RM-ANOVA is just an omnibus test that cannot tell us exactly where the difference between repeated measurements lies. A post hoc test will be necessary to compare the groups two by two, using the same rules shown in Sect. 2.4.3.3.

The Equation

We have previously shown that variability is not one block. ANOVA aims to analyze the study's total variability by partitioning it into its originating components. In short, the total variability in independent groups one-way ANOVA (SS_{total}) was partitioned into: variability between groups ($SS_{between-groups}$) that can be explained by the difference between the effects of compared group (e.g., treatments) and, variability within groups

($SS_{within-groups}$) that expresses the variability in outcome observed among the patients of the same group (e.g., receiving the same treatment). Note that the model explains only the between-groups variability and all the remaining within-group variability is not explained and hence, ($SS_{within-groups}$) expresses the total error term of the model (SS_{error}). The relevant variances ($MS_{between-groups}$ and MS_{error}) are just the mean values of the sum of squares and are calculated by dividing each SS by its df. Fisher's value is the ratio between the 2 variances: between-groups variance (e.g., variance explained by treatment groups) and the remaining unexplained error variance. In independent groups ANOVA, the whole $MS_{within-groups}$ was not explained. Put it this way, in independent groups ANOVA, the (MS_{error}) = ($MS_{within-groups}$).

One-way RMANOVA follows the same general rules but is much more powerful in explaining variability. The (SS_{total}) is partitioned into the two main components: variability "between measurement groups" and variability "within groups". As all measurements are carried out in the same group of patients, ($SS_{between-groups}$) can be noted either as: ($SS_{conditions}$) referring to the repeated measurements being one measurement per condition (e.g., one measurement per type of treatment) or as (SS_{time}) referring to the repeated measurements being observed over time but always under the same condition (e.g., multiple measurements for the same treatment). Although ($SS_{conditions}$) or (SS_{time}) express a different way by which the repeated measurements are observed, yet both represent the variability between measurement groups ($SS_{repeated\ measurements}$) and are analyzed similarly. At this point, both independent and repeated measurement models look mathematically the same, in the way of calculating the in-between group as well as the within-group variability.

RM-ANOVA takes a further step and reduces the unexplained variability (SS_{error}) by explaining (i.e., calculating) part of the within-group variability ($SS_{within-groups}$). As shown in Table 2.21, warfarin dose has been measured three times for each subject: first dose, a second dose, and a third dose. The mean of the three

Table 2.21 Repeated measures ANOVA: repeated dosing of warfarin in ten patients presenting with deep vein thrombosis (DVT)

Subjects	First dose	Second dose	Third dose	Subject's mean dose
I	5	5	8	6
II	2	7	7	5.3
III	3	4	7	4.6
IV	5	7	7	6.3
V	3	5	6	4.6
VI	5	6	6	5.7
VII	4	5	8	5.7
VIII	5	5	9	6.3
IX	4	6	8	6
X	3	3	2	2.6
Dose means	3.9	5.3	6.8	–

Grand mean 5.3

Values are warfarin doses in mg, calculated for the 10 subjects from I to X. Grand mean = sum of all values divided by the total 30 measurements

measurements varied differently for the ten subjects: being 6 mg for the first patient, 5.3 mg for the second, … and 2.6 mg for the 10th patient. This variability of the response of different subjects to different measurements ($SS_{subjects}$) can be calculated as the sum of squared differences between each of those mean subject doses and the grand mean dose of all patients shown in the last row (5.3 mg). The $SS_{subjects}$ now explained part of the unexplained within-group variability and can be deducted from it. The net result is that the unexplained variability (SS_{error}) of independent group ANOVA that was totally formed by the "whole within group variability" ($SS_{within-groups}$) becomes smaller in RMANOVA for being now formed by ($SS_{within-groups} - SS_{subjects}$) "Eq. 2.55". Concordantly, the denominator of the F ratio calculated for RM-ANOVA is smaller than that calculated for independent groups ANOVA, which usually increases the calculated F value and, in consequence, the power of the test to detect a statistically significant difference "Eq. 2.56".

Put this way, a regular one-way ANOVA partitions the total variability into variability between groups (explained by the difference between means) and variability within groups that remains unexplained (error). One-way RMANOVA further explains part of the latter by calculating and removing the variability between subjects themselves, leaving a smaller within-group variability (error). As such, a more significant part of the model is explained by one-way RMANOVA, making it a much more robust test than its regular variant.

$$MS_{error} = MS_{within\ groups} - MS_{subjects} \quad (2.55)$$

$$F_{RMANOVA} = \frac{MS_{repeated\ measures}}{MS_{error}} \quad (2.56)$$

1. Calculation of the Sum of Squares

Although $SS_{repeated\ measures}$ can be precisely calculated as the $SS_{between-groups}$ of independent groups ANOVA, yet we will show another variant of the equation that gives the same result; where n = number of subjects, x is the grand mean of all measurements and xi is the mean of each of the three measurements observed in the patients (see

Table 2.21) $SS_{repeated\ measures} = 10[(3.9 - 5.3)^2 + (5.3 - 5.3)^2 + (6.8 - 5.3)^2] = 42.1$ "Eq. 2.57".

$$SS_{repeated\ measures} = \sum n_i(\bar{x}_i - \bar{x})^2 \quad (2.57)$$

Equally, the $SS_{within-groups}$ is calculated as its homologous in independent groups ANOVA: the sum of squared differences between: each individual measurement (x_i) observed in one group and the mean value of that group $\bar{x}$. The $SS_{within-groups}$ is the sum of all those squared differences, calculated for the K groups "Eq. 2.58" and "Eq. 2.59".

$$SS_{within-groups} = \sum_1 (x_i - \bar{x}_1)^2 + \sum_2 (x_i - \bar{x}_2)^2 + \cdots + \sum_k (x_i - \bar{x}_k)^2$$

$$(2.58)$$

$SS_{within-groups} = (5 - 3.9)^2 + (2 - 3.9)^2 + (3 - 3.9)^2 + (5 - 3.9)^2$
$+ (3 - 3.9)^2 + (5 - 3.9)^2 + (4 - 3.9)^2 + (5 - 3.9)^2 + (4 - 3.9)^2$
$+ (3 - 3.9)^2 + (5 - 5.3)^2 + (7 - 5.3)^2 + (4 - 5.3)^2 + (7 - 5.3)^2$
$+ (5 - 5.3)^2 + (6 - 5.3)^2 + (5 - 5.3)^2 + (5 - 5.3)^2 + (6 - 5.3)^2$
$+ (3 - 5.3)^2 + (8 - 6.8)^2 + (7 - 6.8)^2 + (7 - 6.8)^2 + (7 - 6.8)^2$
$+ (6 - 6.8)^2 + (6 - 6.8)^2 + (8 - 6.8)^2 + (9 - 6.8)^2 + (8 - 6.8)^2$
$+ (2 - 6.8)^2 = 58.6$

$$(2.59)$$

Under the null hypothesis, the mean of the repeated measurements taken for any subject ($\bar{x}_i$) should not be different from the grand (average) mean calculated for all subjects ($\bar{x}$). Consequently, $SS_{subjects}$ is calculated as the squared difference between the mean value of measurements taken for the same subject at different (k) timing or under different (k) conditions and the grand mean "Eq. 2.60" and "2.61".

$$SS_{subjects} = k. \sum (\bar{x}_i - \bar{x})^2 \quad (2.60)$$

$SS_{subjects} = 3[(6 - 5.3)^2 + (5.3 - 5.3)^2 + (4.6 - 5.3)^2 + (6.3 - 5.3)^2 + (4.6 - 5.3)^2$
$+ (5.7 - 5.3)^2 + (5.7 - 5.3)^2 + (6.3 - 5.3)^2 + (6 - 5.3)^2 + (2.6 - 5.3)^2] = 33.3$

$$(2.61)$$

Unlike the case of independent group ANOVA where the within-group variability remained unexplained and constituted the error term of the model (SS_{error}), RM-ANOVA was able to explain part of this variability by being able to

calculate the outcome variation per patient: ($SS_{subjects}$). Removing the latter from $SS_{within-groups}$, reduces the unexplained variability (SS_{error}) to a much smaller variability = 58.6–33.3 = 25.3 "Eq. 2.62".

$$SS_{error} = SS_{within-groups} - SS_{subjects}$$
$$= 58.6 - 33.3 = 25.3 \quad (2.62)$$

2. Calculation of the Degrees of Freedom

The degree of freedom (df) of the three repeated measurements is calculated as the number of (k) measurements minus one, and hence, it equals 2 in our example. On the other hand, the error df is calculated as the total number of patients (n) minus 1, multiplied by the df of repeated measurements (k − 1), and hence it equals 18 in our example. Put it another way; we have three measurements made in ten patients. We know the marginal (total) value of each measurement, e.g., the total starting warfarin dose was 39 mg. Hence, we need to know the doses for 9 patients to detect the dose of the 10th case, i.e., df = n − 1 = 9 per measurement (see Table 2.21). On the other hand, we know the total dose received by each patient, e.g., the total dose received by the 1st patient is 18 mg. Hence, we need to know two doses per patient to deduct the third one, i.e., df = k − 1 per patient. By deduction, the error df = (n − 1) × k − 1 = 9 × 2 = 18 df.

3. Calculation of Mean Squares and F Ratio

Applying the routine equation, we can calculate the two variances, each is equal to its SS, divided by its df "Eqs. 2.63" and "2.64". We compute the F ratio, as usual "Eq. 2.65"

$$MS_{repeated\ measures} = \frac{SS_{repeated\ measures}}{df_{repeated\ measures}} = \frac{42.1}{2}$$
$$= 21$$

$$(2.63)$$

$$MS_{error} = \frac{SS_{error}}{df_{error}} = \frac{25.3}{18} = 1.4 \quad (2.64)$$

$$F_{(2,18)} = \frac{MS_{repeated\ measures}}{MS_{error}} = \frac{21}{1.4}$$
$$= 14.98; P < 0.001 \qquad (2.65)$$

The Interpretation

The study showed a statistically significant difference between the three repeated measurements; P < 0.001. The major advantage of running a repeated measures ANOVA over an independent ANOVA is that the test is generally much more powerful. We want to show how much RM-ANOVA is more powerful than ANOVA. As $MS_{repeated\ measurements}$ is exactly equal to $MS_{between-groups}$ and F ratio is calculated in either case by dividing this MS by the respective MS_{error}, let us run our analysis as a regular independent group ANOVA and calculate SS_{error}, df_{error} and MS_{error}.

In independent group ANOVA, SS_{error} is equal to the whole $MS_{within-groups}$ = 58.6. With a df = 27, the MS = 2.17. It is obvious that RMANOVA has decreased the amount of unexplained variance by as much as 57%: from 58.6 "Eq. 2.59" to 25.27 "Eq. 2.62". Despite the lower df in RMANOVA (18), compared to ANOVA (27); the resulting MS_{error} of the former (1.4; "Eq. 2.64") is still smaller by about 48% of the latter (2.17); which is because $SS_{subjects}$ have explained a large part of variability. The net result is that the F ratio calculated by RMANOVA (14.98) was 1.5 times what would have been calculated by regular ANOVA (9.69).

What Should be Reported

As in a regular one-way ANOVA, we have to report the descriptive statistics: mean and Sd of the first, second and third doses were: 3.9 + 1.1, 5.3 + 1.25, and 6.8 + 1.93 mg, respectively. Inferential statistics reporting includes the F-statistic and P-value: F (2, 18) = 14.98; P < 0.001. Remember that a statistically significant RM-ANOVA cannot tell us where the difference came from. A priori two-by-two comparisons or post-hoc analyses are necessary to answer this question. Table 2.22 shows three pre-planned paired t-tests to compare the results two-by-two, indicating a significant change in dose at each level of measurement. Note that if Bonferroni equation was applied to correct for a post-hoc analysis, the critical limit of P will be 0.0125 and hence, the adjusted P-values of the three comparisons shown in Table 2.22 (0.016, 0.001 and 0.022) will be 0.049, 0.002 and 0.066; respectively.

In order to increase their chances of being cited, authors are encouraged to report Effect size and Spearman's correlation coefficient r, both of which are important for sample size calculation for future studies (See Sect. 2.4). Effect size can be reported as partial eta-squared, calculated as $SS_{repeated\ measurements} / (SS_{repeated\ measurements} + SS_{error})$ = 0.625. Table. 2.22 shows the results of correlation coefficient.

Conditions of Application

Samples have to be chosen at random. The within subject factor has to be a k-class qualitative variable and the outcome has to be a continuous variable. Observations must be independent in the sense that making any observations is not influenced by another observation. Data must be checked out for outliers and for (approximate) normality across all within-subject levels (the repeated measures). One specific assumption of RMANOVA is sphericity, which is the equality of repeated measures across all within-subject levels. Mauchly's test is automatically generated by many statistical software packages and is commonly used to examine whether there is a significant difference between data and sphericity. Hence, a statistically non-significant test means that sphericity was respected. For our example, the statistically non-significant Mauchly's test assumed sphericity; P = 0.849. In case sphericity was not assumed, several methods are proposed to adjust the degrees of freedom to calculate within-subject effects, such as Greenhouse–Geisser and Huynth–Feldt. Those methods are discussed in more details in the section of the ANOVA family (see Sect. 3.2.5.1).

The Use of Statistical Software

Before the analysis, we can verify the assumptions related to the study design. Namely, the sample is chosen randomly, observations are independent, the outcome is a continuous variable, and the within-subject predictor variable is a k-class categorical variable. The analysis begins by uploading data as arranged in Table 2.21. Data are arranged as three variables (columns), each representing a series of measurements made at one class of the within-subject predictor variable.

1. *The Execution of the Analysis*

Provided that we are using IBM-SPSS, we start by clicking on the "analyze" button, then "general linear model," then "repeated measures" to open the repeated measures NOVA first panel. We begin by "naming" our within-subject (dose) and the "number of levels" (=3), and we "add" it to the panel. We click on "define," which will take us to a second new panel. We shift our now three levels to the "within-subject variables" in the same order. We click on "plots" and shift dose to the panel "horizontal axis," and then we click to "add" the plot and click "Continue". We click on the "save" button to request the creation and save on the "studentized residuals", which discover outliers and click on "continue". We click to open the "options" and shift the within-subject predictor (dose) predictors to the "display

means" and request to "compare main effects" by "Bonferroni test". Finally, we choose to "display descriptive statistics" and "effect size" and close this final panel. As such, we are all set and we click on the "ok" button to start getting our results.

2. *Verification of the Remaining Assumptions*

Note that the software was requested to calculate and save six studentized values for each case (patient). We test normality by clicking on the "analyze" button, then on "descriptive statistics" then "crosstabs". We shift the within-subject three levels to the "dependent list", click on "plots" then request "normality plots and tests". We verify that the outcome scores are normally distributed across the three levels, as shown by non-statistically significant Shapiro Wilk tests. In our example, the studentized residual for the third dosage deviated from normality ($P = 0.21$). We accept it and continue the analysis.

We check on the absence of outliers by verifying that none of the cases had a studentized value larger than +3sd or −3Sd. In our example, the largest studentized value was (−2.62), calculated for the 3rd dose of patient number ten and hence, we can conclude that we have no outliers. Concerning homogeneity of variances across the repeated measures (sphericity), IBM-SPSS automatically produces Mauchly's test. In our example, the test was statistically non-significant (Chi-square = 0.33; $P = 0.849$) and

Table 2.22 Repeated measures ANOVA for data presented in Table 2.21: results of correlation and post-hoc student tests

Pairs	N	r	P value[a]	Mean of the difference	Sd of the difference	95% CI of the difference	t-value	df	P value[b]
1st does to 2nd dose	10	0.186	0.61	−1.4	1.5	−2.48 to −0.32	−2.94	9	0.016
1st dose to 3rd dose	10	0.408	0.24	−2.9	1.79	−4.18 to −1.62	−5.12	9	0.001
2nd dose to 3rd dose	10	0.487	0.15	−1.5	1.71	−2.73 to −0.27	−2.76	9	0.022

Values are the results of correlation and paired Student test to compare the paired results two-by-two. N = number of patients, r = Spearman's correlation coefficient, t = unpaired Student test statistic, a = P value for correlation, b = P value for paired Student test hence, we can use the produced F values without any adjustment for the degree of freedom. Kindly refer to Sect. 3.2.5.1 for more details on managing deviation from sphericity (see Sect. 3.2.5.1).

3. *Calculation of the Within-Subject Effect and Post-Hoc Analysis*

The software will give the same results that were calculated manually. However, we have to know that we cannot calculate Mauchly's test manually and that software result are more reliable and accurate than manual calculation, provided that we can understand and interpret the results correctly. In addition, the software calculated the effect size of the within-subject predictor as partial Eta square (0.744 in our example).

2.5 Inference on Medians and Other Distributions Than Normal: Non-parametric Tests

All the tests discussed in Sect. 2.4 necessitated the fulfillment of certain conditions (parameters) to be applied, mainly normality and variance equality. Distribution-free or "non-parametric tests" can be used whenever those two conditions are not verified. Many researchers will choose a non-parametric test in a small sample size for the difficulty of verifying normality. Others may be comfortable with them in most situations for the relatively few assumptions to be made. There is a complete armada of non-parametric tests, and we will only envisage some of the most widely used in the medical literature.

According to the central limit theorem, the sums of values, such as ranks, are "normally" distributed. The non-parametric tests 'normalize' values by replacing proper data with ranks. The following step will compare the sums or means of those (normal) ranks and finally verify the statistical significance of the results in the usual tables of a normal distribution or unique tables designed for a small sample size. Due to this ranking transformation, the non-parametric tests

acquire the advantage of being less sensitive to (not being affected by) extreme data or outliers compared to parametric tests. On the other hand, the inevitable loss of information associated with the substitution of valid data by ranks decreases the power of the tests to detect the evidence. In statistical terms, the non-parametric tests are more likely to commit a type II error than a parametric approach. For example, suppose we have the results of two classrooms A and B. In class A, the scores obtained by the students were 100, 90, and 80. Hence, those three students will acquire the ranks: 1st, 2nd, and third. The scores obtained by the students of classroom B were: 50, 40, and 30. Hence, they will be ranked as "1st, 2nd, and 3rd too". A non-parametric test will forget about the scores and will deal only with ranks. For the test, the 1st patient in class A has an equal rank as the first patient in class B, regardless of whether the former score was double the latter. Both classes A and B have the same mean rank of (2), regardless that the score of class A is double that of the latter.

However, such loss of power remains negligible, compared to the bias of applying a parametric test without reliable verification of the conditions necessary for its use. Another drawback of ranking is known as "the Ex-Aequo" or "ties," where several cases share the same value (same rank). Those cases can be assigned "a common mean rank," or the researcher can randomly choose which case will be given the first rank and which will come later.

2.5.1 The Comparison of Two-Groups

2.5.1.1 Mann & Whitney (U) Test

The Example

A researcher wished to compare the effect of two analgesics ("x" and "y") in two independent groups of patients suffering from chronic pain. Twenty patients (n = 20) were randomly assigned to either receive one of the two treatments. Recorded durations of pain relief among the ten patients (n_1 = 10) who received treatment "x" was: 23, 15, 28, 26, 13, 8, 21, 25, 24, and 29 h. The respective durations recorded among group 2 patients ($n_2 = 10$) receiving treatment "y" were: *18, 22, 33, 34, 19, 12, 27, 32, 31* and *30* h. The question was, which is the more effective analgesic? Viewing the small sample size in each group and the inability to verify normality, the researcher decided to use a non-parametric test.

The Equation

Regardless of the patient's group, all observed values will be classified in a single list by increasing order, and then, each value will be replaced by the group symbol "x" or "y". For the sake of a better visualization, durations of pain relief observed in patients receiving analgesic "y" were put between parentheses.

$$8, (12), 13, 15, (18), (19), 21, (22), 23,$$
$$24, 25, 26, (27), 28, 29, (30), (31), (32),$$
$$(33), (34).$$

$$x, y, x, x, y, y, x, y, x, x, x, x, y, x, x, y, y, y, y, y.$$

- The test starts by choosing one of the two groups—let's say "x"- to be replaced in the list by the number of smaller "y_s". The result will be as follows:

$$y \cdot 1 \cdot 1 \cdot y \cdot y \cdot 3 \cdot y \cdot 4 \cdot 4 \cdot 4 \cdot 4 \cdot y \cdot 5 \cdot 5 \cdot y$$
$$\cdot y \cdot y \cdot y \cdot y.$$

- We sum the ranks of the "ys" that are smaller than "x" and, we will call it the U_{yx} index:

$$U_{yx} = 0 + 1 + 1 + 3 + 4 + 4 + 4 + 4 + 5 + 6$$
$$= 31.$$

- Similarly, we can choose to replace each "y" with the number of smaller "x_s" and calculate the sum of ranks of those smaller "xs" and call it U_{xy} index:

$$U_{xy} = 1 + 3 + 3 + 3 + 8 + 10 + 10 + 10$$
$$+ 10 + 10 = 69.$$

What we just did is that we have calculated the sum of ranks of "ys" that are smaller than "x" and the sum of ranks of "xs" that are smaller than "y." If "x" and "y" were equal, they have to have equal ranks and, U_{xy} and U_{yx} have to be equal. We did so because we know the mathematical rule that the sum of both indices equals the product of their numbers.

- Knowing that both groups have an equal sample size of 10, let us check on this: $U_{yx} + U_{xy} = 31 + 69 = n_1 \times n_2 = 10 \times 10 = 100$.

Under the null hypothesis, (U_0) equals $(U_{yx} + U_{xy})/2 = (n_1 \times n_2)/2$. The alternative hypothesis is that U_{yx} or U_{xy} is larger than (U_0). The difference between the sum of observed ranks $(U_{yx}$ or $U_{xy})$ and (U_0) has to be standardized by the appropriate standard deviation (Sd_U), and the statistical significance of the standardized difference is checked out in the Z table "Eqs. 2.66" and "2.67". To conclude upon statistical significance, our value has to be at least equal or larger than the usual critical limit of 1.96 for a bilateral study or 1.65 for a unilateral study. What will follow is that if one of the groups has a significantly higher rank than the other, it would be reasonable to conclude that the observed values themselves are significantly larger than in the other group.

$$Z = \frac{U_{xy} - U_0}{Sd_u} = \frac{U_{xy} - (n_1 \times n_2)/2}{\sqrt{n_1 \times n_2(n+1)/12}} \quad (2.66)$$

$$Z = \frac{31 - (10 \times 10)/2}{\sqrt{10 \times 10(20+1)/12}} = 1.44 \quad (2.67)$$

It is clear that all calculations are based on the sample sizes and have nothing to do with the true data themselves. In case of small sample size of less than 10 patients per group, it is not advised to use the approximated formula shown above "Eq. 2.66". The statistical significance of the calculated (U_{yx}) is checked in the appropriate U table; where (U_{yx}) is the smallest of both indices [31, 32]. Unlike the rule of thumb of many statistical tables, our value (31) should be at least equal or smaller than the one figured in the table (23) to conclude upon a statistically significant difference at the usual 5% limit.

The Interpretation

In our example, the calculated Z (1.44) is smaller than the limit of statistical significance of a bilateral study (1.96). Hence, it appears that we have failed to put into evidence a significant difference between the analgesic effects of both drugs. Non-parametric tests are usually interpreted as comparing medians of non-normally distributed data, which is an incomplete statement. Remember that the median is the value lying in the middle of a frequency distribution, such as there is an equal probability of falling above or below it. We will work on the illustrative example given by Campbell and Swinscow [33] concerning data for two groups of patients, A and B, each with 100 cases. The outcome was the number of times (x) a patient misses his medication during a limited follow-up period. Results in group A were: 98 patients did not miss any dose (x = 0), one patient missed one dose (x = 1), and another patient missed two doses (x = 2). The median or the value that splits group A patients into two equal halves is (0): 50% of patients did not miss any dose (x < 0), and the other 50% missed one or two doses (x > 0). Results in group B were: 51 patients did not miss any dose (x = 0), one patient missed one dose (x = 1), and 48 patients missed two doses (x = 2). The median or the value that splits group B patients into two equal halves is (0) too: 50% of patients did not miss any dose (x < 0), and the other 50% missed one or two doses (x > 0). In conclusion, both groups have the same median, and hence, according to the interpretation that a non-parametric test just compares medians, one should expect a non-significant result of such a test. However, Mann and Whitney test will show a statistically significant difference between both groups. Uploading data on SPSS showed that mean ranks of the two groups were 76.77 and 124.24, the Z value equals 7.669 and P < 0.001. Unlike the parametric t-test, which directly calculates the standardized difference between the two means (see

Sect. 2.4.1.2), the non-parametric version is based on ranking all individual values of the group, with the median being only one of those values. The wider is the distribution of the values of one group (group B in our example), the larger is the mean of smaller ranks compared to the other group. The same results will be obtained if the study was analyzed by another non-parametric test, such as the Wilcoxon rank test (see Sect. 2.5.1.2). In fact, it is only when both groups are assumed to have the "same" distribution then the non-parametric test can be considered as being comparing the medians and, a statistically significant difference can be attributed to a significant difference between medians [33].

Moreover, it can also be assumed that a shift in the central location of similar distributions will move, not only medians but also means by the same amount. Thus, the non-parametric test can also be assumed as a test for the difference in means. In our example, and despite the two identical medians, the statistically significant difference is due to the fact that both distributions are different from each other, and hence, we have to appreciate that the non-parametric tests compare spread and not only medians [34]. Our report has to include the description and the analysis of the spread, alongside the median, so the reader can appreciate from where the significant difference is coming. The reader is invited to refer to the simple and illustrative examples given by Anna Hart [35].

What Should be Reported

We have to report descriptive statistics, namely, median and spread, P value, and effect size. Spread can be reported as minimum and maximum, interquartile range or percentiles. Concerning median, we have to report the upper and lower limits of the 95% CI of the median of each variable and the difference between the two medians.

The confidence interval of the median

Although the 95% CI of the median can be easily checked online [36], we will present an illustrative example. The recorded durations of pain relief associated with the use of the analgesic (x) in the ten patients were: 29, (28), 26, 25, 24, 23, 21, 15, (13), 8. Note that a decreasing order of magnitude arranges durations. The median duration equals (23 + 24)/2 = 23.5. We will substitute values by their ranks to fulfill the normality assumption. The 95% CI of the median rank depends on sample size (n = 10) and is computed by the formula given below "Eq. 2.68". Note that calculated upper (1.99) and lower limits (8.1) have to be approximated to the nearest next positive integer, i.e., 2 and 9 "Eq. 2.69". The lowest 2nd rank points to the highest value (28), and the highest 9th rank points to the lowest value (13). In conclusion, the median (95% CI) is equal to: 23.5 (13, 28).

$$95\% \ CI \ of \ median = \frac{n}{2} \pm 1.96 \frac{\sqrt{n}}{2} \qquad (2.68)$$

$$95\% \ CI \ of \ median = \frac{10}{2} \pm 1.96 \frac{\sqrt{10}}{2} = 5 \pm 3.1$$
$$= 1.88 \ to \ 8.1 \approx 2, 9$$
$$(2.69)$$

The confidence interval of the difference between 2 medians

The 95% CI of the difference between the two medians is more complicated, and, unfortunately, it is directly given by only a few statistical software, such as Minitab. We return to the previous example and compare the durations of analgesia recorded in the "x" group to those observed in group "y." The durations of analgesia recorded in the latter were: 12, 18, 19, 22, 27, 30, 31, 32, 33 and 34 h, as shown before. The median duration is (27 + 30)/2 = 28.5 and hence the difference between the two medians = 28.5–23.5 = 5. We want to calculate the 95% CI around 5, not to present only one expected difference, but a whole set of 95% of difference compatible with 5. We need software to calculate those 100 probable differences between media in terms of rank. In our example, the software ranked all values and calculated 100 possible ranked differences between both groups. The

median rank = (number of differences − 1)/ 2 = (100 + 1)/2 = the 50.5th rank.

The next step is to convert the chosen upper and lower limits of the 95% CI of those ranks to durations in hours. Here comes the value of the index (K) proposed by Campbell and Gardener, it just points to the upper and lower limits of the 95% CI [37]. The index K was calculated and tabulated by Campbell and Gardener and can be checked online or calculated by the following equations for unpaired (sample size = n_1 and n_2) "Eq. 2.70" and paired studies (sample size = n) "Eq. 2.71". Applying the equation to our example produces a K value of 24 "Eq. 2.72", which can be interpreted that the limits of the 95% CI are: the smallest 24th ranked value and the largest 24th ranked value.

$$K_{unpaired} = \frac{n_1 n_2}{2} \pm \left(1.96 \sqrt{\frac{n_1 n_2 (n_1 + n_2 + 1)}{12}} \right)$$
$$(2.70)$$

$$K_{paired} = \frac{n(n+1)}{4}$$
$$\pm \left(1.96 \sqrt{\frac{n(n+1)(2n+1)}{24}} \right) \quad (2.71)$$

$$K_{unpaired} = \frac{10 \times 10}{2}$$
$$- \left(1.96 \sqrt{\frac{10 \times 10(10 + 10 + 1)}{12}} \right)$$
$$= 24$$
$$(2.72)$$

Now we convert all those ranks back into durations of analgesia in hours. The value corresponding to the median rank (50.5th) will be the median value of (5) hours. The corresponding lower and upper limits of the 95% CI of the difference of medians themselves will be (−2) and (10). The conclusion will be that the median of the difference between the two treatments (95% CI) = 5 (−2, 10) hours. Put it this way; we could not put significance the superiority of either drug, although the median duration was in favor of treatment "y" by 5 h, yet the result is unstable and is expected to be sometimes in favor of one treatment, while in other times in favor of the other.

Effect size

Grisson and Kim have suggested that P_{ab} and Pearson's correlation coefficient r are suitable estimates of the effect size of non-parametric data [38] (see Sect. 4). In short, P_{ab} is the probability that an individual picked up at random from the group (a) has a higher score than an individual from the group (b). It is calculated from the (U) statistics and sample sizes of both groups (n_a and n_b). In our example, $P_{ab} = U/n_1n_2 = 31/100 = 0.31$, and hence, there is a 31% chance that a score randomly chosen from patients receiving analgesic (y) will be greater than a score randomly chosen from those receiving analgesic (x). For the r conversion formula, $r = z/\sqrt{n} = 1.436/4.472 = 0.321$, which can be interpreted according to Cohen's rule of thumb or better compared with previously reported effect size in the literature.

Conditions of Application

Samples have to be chosen at random. The variable of concern has to be continuous, ordinal, or ordered categorical. The tests assume the independence of data and the symmetrical distribution of ranks, which can be checked by eye-balling on a graph. If the latter assumption is strongly violated, it is either to change the variable scale or to use the less powerful sign test that does not require this assumption. The normal approximation made by the equations shown above is only valid for a minimum of 10 per group. Otherwise, it is advised to check out the significance of our results directly in the special tables of significance designed for non-parametric tests [32].

2.5.1.2 Wilcoxon Rank (W) Test

The Example

We will analyze the same example used in Sect. 2.5.1.1. In brief, a researcher wished to compare the effect of 2 analgesics ("x" and "y") in 2 independent groups of patients suffering

from chronic pain. Twenty patients (n = 20) were randomly and equally assigned to receive one of the two treatments. Recorded durations of pain relief among the 10 patients ($n_1 = 10$) who received treatment "x" was: 23, 15, 28, 26, 13, 8, 21, 25, 24, and 29 h. The respective durations recorded among group 2 patients ($n_2 = 10$) receiving treatment "y" were: *18, 22, 33, 34, 19, 12, 27, 32, 31* and *30* h. The question was, which is the more effective analgesic? Viewing the small sample size in each group and the inability to verify normality, the researcher decided to use a non-parametric test.

The Equation

- As in U-test, each value in the list is replaced by its symbol. We choose one of the symbols —let us say "x"—and we replace it with its rank in the list:

$$1, y, 3, 4, y, y, 7, y, 9, 10, 11, 12, y, 14, 15, y,$$
$$y, y, y, y$$

- We calculate the W_x index; which equals to the sum of ranks of x:

$$W_x = 1 + 3 + 4 + 7 + 9 + 10 + 11 + 12 + 14 + 15$$
$$= 86.$$

- Similarly, the W_y index equals 124

$$W_y = 2 + 5 + 6 + 8 + 13 + 16 + 17 + 18 + 19 + 20$$
$$= 124.$$

- Note that the sum of both indices ($W_x + W_y$) is equal to the sum of the positive integers in both groups:

$$W_x + W_y = n(n+1)/2 = 20(20+1)/2$$
$$= 210.$$

Under the null hypothesis of no difference between the rankings of values of both groups, the calculated W_x for the (n_1) patients in group 1 should not be significantly different from the expected value W_{x0}, which is equal to n1 (n + 1)/2 = 10 (20 + 1)/2 = 105, in our example. In our example, concordantly, the calculated

Wy should not be significantly different from the expected value W_{y0}, which is equal to n2 $(n + 1)/2 = 105$. Note that the sum of observed values, the sum of expected values as well as the sum of the first positive integers are all equal: $(W_x + W_y) = (W_{x0} + W_{y0}) = n (n + 1)/2$. In our example, this value equals: $86 + 124 = 105 + 105 = 20$ $(20 + 1)/2 = 210$.   Before checking the Z table, the difference between W_x and W_y has to be standardized by (Sd_U) "Eq. 2.73". The test will yield the same result as before (1.44) and both tests are strictly identical.

$$Z = \frac{W_x - n_1(n+1)/2}{\sqrt{n_1 \times n_2(n+1)/12}} \qquad (2.73)$$

The Interpretation, What Should be Reported and Conditions of Application

They are exactly the same as for Mann and Whitney test (see Sect. 2.5.1.1).

2.5.1.3 Wilcoxon Signed Rank Test (Paired T)

The test is the non-parametric alternative of paired Student t-test, using "ranked" medians rather than means. Hence, it can be used to compare the median of a sample to a hypothetical median or the ranked medians of paired data, whether acquired from the same group or 2 matched groups. The test can be equally used to compare medians calculated for ordinal variables such as Likert's items (e.g., a 7-point time from strongly agree to disagree strongly). The test can equally be used to compare ordered categorical data, for example, by assigning the ranks of 1, 2, 3, and 4 to ascending ordered categories such as patients having controlled, mild, moderate, and severe hypertension.

The Example

A study was conducted to compare the duration of analgesia of two analgesics A and B. The material of the study was ten cases chosen at random from a population of patients suffering from chronic pain. Patients were randomized to receive treatment A for one week followed by treatment B for another week or the reverse.

A suitable wash-out period was looked for in the literature and was allowed between the intake of both treatments. As shown in Table 2.23, the differences were ranked in absolute ascending order, regardless of the sign. The sign itself was recorded in a separate column.

The Equation

The study question is whether there is a difference between the two analgesics. Hence, zero differences will not answer the question and have to be eliminated from the analysis (patient number VII and patient number X). Equally, cases with a single observation have to be eliminated. We calculate the differences and rank their absolute values in ascending order: column A–B in Table 2.23. We note the sign in a separate column: column Sign in the same table. Now we can calculate the sum of positive ranks $(P = 7 + 2 + 4 + 8 + 5 + 6 = 32)$, the sum of negative ranks $(N = 3 + 1 = 4)$, and the sum of all ranks $(T = P + N = 32 + 4 = 36)$: last row in Table 2.23.

Under the null hypothesis of no difference between both treatments, the sum of P ranks has to be equal to N ranks = 18 (36/2). We have previously shown in the Wilcoxon test that the sum of all ranks $(N + P)$ is equal to the sum of the first positive integers: $(N + P) = n (n + 1)/2$ (see Sect. 2.5.1.2). By deduction, $(N + P)/2 = n (n + 1)/4$. Note that (n) will be the number of ranked patients and not the original total number of patients as we did exclude those two cases who showed no favor regarding either treatment. Let us verify the equation: in our example, we expect to have equal number of P and N ranks = n (n + 1)/4 = 8 (8 − 1)/4 = 18.

If the null hypothesis is true, there should be no difference between our observed positive (or negative) ranks and expected ranks. The larger is the difference; the smaller is the probability of a true null hypothesis. As usual, we standardize the difference by the appropriate Sd "Eq. 2.74". The statistical significance of the standardized difference is checked out in the Z table to see whether our observed value reaches the universal critical limit of 1.96 for a bilateral study "Eq. 2.75". In the case the study was unilateral as comparing a treatment to a placebo, the critical limit would be 1.65, as usual. As our study was bilateral, the results of the equation suggest that there is a statistically significant difference between both treatments.

$$Z = \frac{P - n(n+1)/4}{\sqrt{n(n+1)(2n+1)/24}} \qquad (2.74)$$

$$Z = \frac{32 - 8(8+1)/4}{\sqrt{8(8+1)(2 \times 8 + 1)/24}} = \frac{14}{7.14} = 1.96 \qquad (2.75)$$

The Interpretation

The equation given above is a normal approximation of the test, and it is not advisable to use it in case of a small sample size like ours. Note that we are speaking about the number of ranked cases and not the total number of patients. In case of a small total ranked sample size of less than 20, like ours, the statistical significance of the results should be directly checked out in the specialized Wilcoxon T table [31, 32]. Unlike the rule of thumb of many statistical tables, our value should be at least equal or smaller than the one figured in the table to conclude upon a statistically significant difference at the usual 5% limit. For our example, the smaller sum of ranks (whether N or P) should be at least equal or smaller than the value inscribed at the Wilcoxon T-rank table, at the line corresponding to the total number of ranked patients (n). For n = 8, the smaller calculated sum must be equal to or smaller than 3 for a two-tailed study. As our study was bilateral and our T value was larger than the one figured in the table at n = 8 in contrast to the results given by the approximative formula, we have to conclude that we have failed to show a statistically significant difference between both treatment effects. In the case our study was unilateral, our smaller rank (N) equals (4) and, it is smaller than the one figured in the table (5), and, in such case, we can conclude upon the efficacy of our treatment.

What Should be Reported

We must report descriptive statistics, namely, medians (95% CI) and spread (minimum and maximum, interquartile range or percentiles), P-value, and effect size. We can report effect size as PS_{dep}, equal to the number of positive ranks (n+) to the total number of ranks (N) = 6/8 = 0.75. In

Table 2.23 Wilcoxon sign rank test: comparison of the durations of pain relief with two analgesics (A and B) in a single group of 10 patients with chronic pain

Patient ID	A	B	(A − B)	Rank	Sign
I	10	2	8	6	P
II	17	4	7	8	P
III	9	7	2	2	P
IV	14	3	11	7	P
V	8	1	7	5	P
VI	14	15	−1	1	N
VII[a]	6	6	0		
VIII	13	7	6	4	P
IX	16	21	−5	3	N
X[a]	14	14	0		
Sum of ranks				36[b]	4N[c]/32P[d]

A and B = durations of pain relief in hours due to treatments A and B, A–B = difference between the two durations of pain relief in each patient, Rank = ascending ranks of the differences (A–B) in absolute value, Sign = sign of the difference (A–B), P = positive rank (in favor of treatment A), N = negative rank (in favor of treatment B), a = patients not ranked for not showing any difference in favor of either treatment, b = total sum of all ranks, c = sum of negative ranks (3 + 1 = 4), d = sum of positive ranks (7 + 2 + 4 + 8 + 5 + 6 = 32) our example, we can interpret PS_{dep} as a 75% chance that analgesic B would be superior to analgesic A (see Sect. 4.6).

Conditions of Application

Patients have to be chosen at random. The paired information is acquired, either from the same patient or matched pairs. A minimum number of 20 cases is required to use the approximative equation. Otherwise, it is advised to check out the significance of our results directly in the special tables of significance designed for non-parametric tests [31, 32].

2.5.2 The Comparison of Several Groups

2.5.2.1 Kruskal & Wallis (H) Test

Kruskal–Wallis test is the non-parametric alternative of one-way ANOVA. It is usually indicated when the number of cases per group is smaller than 30, even if other conditions of ANOVA are verified, namely normal distribution and equality of variance. Another common indication is when the variable of concern is following other distribution than normal, such as when we are comparing scores or ranks given to ordered categorical data. Like ANOVA, the H test assumes that groups have an equal sample size and equal variance and shares the same disadvantage of testing the overall difference between groups, without showing where a statistically significant difference came from?

The Example

NYHA is a functional classification established by the New York Heart Association to classify cardiac patients by increasing the severity of the disease. Hence, a patient in class I NYHA is in better shape than someone in Class IV. A study was conducted to compare the cardiac output (CO) in 20 patients (n = 20), classified into four groups according to the New York Heart Association (NYHA) functional classes. The study question was whether the four groups have significantly different cardiac outputs, as measured

in Liters/minute? The number of patients was only five in each group (ni = 5), and hence, the analysis of variance could not be applied. As groups have equal sizes, the researchers decided to use the non-parametric version: the H test of Kruskal and Wallis. The results of CO measurements (in liters/minute) were the following:

Class I patients: 4.9, 4.6, 4.5, 4.2 and 3.8,

Class II patients: 5.0, 4.1, 4.8, 4.7 and 3.8,

Class III patients: 4.0, 4.4, 3.9, 2.8 and 3.1,

Class IV patients: 2.7, 2.6, 3.0, 3.2, and 3.3.

The Equation

- As with previous tests, values are classified in one single row by increasing order and then substituted by their symbols:

    2.6, 2.7, 2.8, 3.0, 3.1, 3.2, 3.3, 3.8, 3.8, 3.9,
    4.0, 4.1, 4.2, 4.4, 4.5, 4.6, 4.7, 4.8, 4.9, 5.0.
    IV, IV, III, IV, III, IV, IV, II, I, III, III, II, I,
    III, I, I, II, II, I, II.

- We calculate the mean rank of each class = sum of ranks/number of patients = W_i/n_i.

- Finally, we calculate the Grand mean of all ranks = $W/n = (W1 + W2 + W3 + W4)/n$.

    For Class I patients: $W_1/n_1 = (9 + 13 + 15 + 16 + 19)/5 = 14.4$

    For Class II patients: $W_2/n_2 = (8 + 12 + 17 + 18 + 20)/5 = 15$.

    For Class III patients: $W_3/n_3 = (3 + 5 + 10 + 11 + 14)/5 = 8.6$

    For Class IV patients: $W_4/n_4 = (1 + 2 + 4 + 6 + 7)/5 = 4$

    $$W = (W1 + W2 + W3 + W4)/(n)$$
    $$= (14.4 + 15 + 8.6 + 4)/4 = 10.5.$$

Under the null hypothesis, the "observed" mean rank in each of the four classes ($\frac{W_i}{n_i}$) is "expected" to be equal to the overall mean rank ($\frac{W}{n}$). The test statistic (H) is a Chi-square equation calculating the standardized sum of squared differences between each mean rank and the total average rank "Eq. 2.76". The value of H was found to approximate the Chi-square value whenever the groups are of equal size, with a minimum of 5 patients per group. Consequently, the statistical significance of (H) can be checked out in the Chi-square table, at a df that is equal to the number of classes minus one: df = k − 1. Otherwise, the exact significance of H has to be directly checked in Kruskal and Wallis tables [31, 39]

For our example, the critical value figured in the Chi-square table for 3 df is much smaller (7.185) than ours (11.6) "Eq. 2.77" and hence, we can conclude that our test showed a statistically significant difference between compared groups. Uploading our data to an online calculator or statistical software package gives the same H value (11.6) and an exact P-value of 0.0088.

$$H = \frac{\sum n_i \left(\frac{W_i}{n_i} - \frac{W}{n} \right)^2}{n(n+1)/12} \qquad (2.76)$$

$$H = \frac{5(14.4 - 10.5)^2 + 5(15 - 10.5)^2 + 5(8.6 - 10.5)^2 + 5(4 - 10.5)^2}{20(20+1)/12} = 11.6 \qquad (2.77)$$

The Interpretation

There is a statistically significant difference between the CO in at least two groups, but the test does not tell us which groups. Only a series of two-by-two comparisons using the Mann and Whitney test, with measures to control the inflated primary risk of error, can answer this question. The simplest is to apply Bonferroni correction and raise the P-value ceiling to P/n, where n is the number of repeated comparisons (see Sect. 2.4.3.3). For example, if we wish to compare the four groups by a series of two-by-two comparisons, n = 6. Hence, we have to reach a pretty small P-value of 0.00833 (0.05/6) to conclude a statistically significant difference at

the usual 5% level. Note that we are not obliged to make all six comparisons. For example, we can limit our comparisons to three contrasts: class I and class II patients together versus class III versus class IV, provided it is clinically relevant. As such, our critical limit of declaring statistical significance will be more reachable (0.05/3 = 0.0125) than if all six comparisons were made.

What Should be Reported

We have to report descriptive and inferential statistics: median (95% CI), spread (minimum and maximum, interquartile range or percentiles), and P-value. We have to report the inferential statistics of post-hoc analysis when performed. In such a case, the effect size can be reported as P_{ab} and interpreted as previously shown with Mann and Whitney test (see Sect. 2.5.1.1).

Conditions of Application

Patients have to be chosen at random, and groups have to be independent. Groups have to have an equal sample size, with a minimum of five patients per group. Otherwise, we need to check on the statistical significance of H in special tables [31, 39].

2.5.2.2 Friedman Test (Paired)

Friedman test is the non-parametric alternative of one-way repeated measures ANOVA. Hence, it is used to detect the differences between (k) repeated measurements of a quantitative variable in one group of patients (n). The test can also be used to detect the differences between (k) experimental designs such as several treatments, different methods of investigations, whether carried out in the same patient or in matched groups of patients. The test is mainly indicated whenever the quantitative outcome variable does not follow a normal distribution or has been recorded in a small group of patients. However, in concordance of repeated measures ANOVA, Friedman's test assumes that the repeated measurements are performed at equal intervals and are independent within each group.

The Example

The efficacy of an antihypertensive drug is tested over time by being repeatedly measured in 15 individuals on three different occasions: before treatment, one month, and three months after treatment (K = 3). Cases were chosen at random from a population of patients with chronic hypertension. Measurements were independently made and recorded.

The Equation

Like many non-parametric tests, the test of Friedman uses the ranks rather than the raw values to calculate the statistics. Suppose that columns represent the (k) groups of repeated measurements and rows represent the (n) measurements made for each patient; the test involves ranking each row together, then considering the values of ranks by columns. As shown in Table 2.24, the measurements made for each patient on the three different (k) occasions are ranked in decreasing order. For

example, those measurements made for patient I (100-, 95-, and 75-mm Hg) are ranked (3, 2, and 1; in this order). If two measurements have the same value, as in the first and second measurements made for patient IV, they can be given a mean rank, i.e. (3 + 2)/2 = 2.5.

The second step is to calculate a mean rank for the three occasions; i.e., values that were ranked by rows (patient) are now evaluated by columns (groups). The null hypothesis is that the mean ranks (2.67, 2.17, and 1.17) are not significantly different across occasions (groups). The calculated "Fr" or Friedman's Q statistics can be approximated to a Chi-square value at $k - 1$ degrees of freedom, provided that the number of patients (n) is at least 15 "Eq. 2.78". Otherwise, the significance of the value of Friedman Q can be checked out in special Q tables [31]. Our "F_r" value is larger than the critical Chi-square value at 2 df (5.99) and is even smaller than that calculated for a P value of 0.001 "Eq. 2.79".

Table 2.24 Friedman's test: repeated measurement of diastolic blood pressure on three occasions

Patient Number (n)	A	B	C	Rank A	Rank B	Rank C
I	100	95	75	3	2	1
II	95	75	80	3	1	2
III	90	100	80	2	3	1
IV	95	95	70	2.5	2.5	1
V	100	85	90	3	1	2
VI	90	100	75	2	3	1
VII	90	80	80	3	1.5	1.5
VIII	105	95	90	3	2	1
IX	95	80	75	3	2	1
X	90	100	80	2	3	1
XI	90	100	75	2	3	1
XII	100	100	70	2.5	2.5	1
XIII	110	105	80	3	2	1
XIV	95	90	85	3	2	1
XV	100	95	90	3	2	1
Sum				40	32.5	17.5
Mean				2.67	2.17	1.17

(n) = subject number, (A), (B) and (C) are the three measurement occasions of diastolic blood pressure in mmHg. Rank (A), (B) and (C) are their respective ranks, independently calculated for each patient. Sum and mean are the sum and mean of ranks independently calculated for each occasion

$$F_r = \frac{12}{nK(K+1)} \sum R_K^2 - 3n(K+1) \quad (2.78)$$

$$\begin{aligned} F_r &= \frac{12}{15 \times 3(3+1)} \left(40^2 + 32.5^2 + 11^2\right) - 3 \\ &\quad \times 15(3-1) \\ &= 17.5 \end{aligned}$$

$$(2.79)$$

The Interpretation

There is a statistically significant difference between the three groups of measurements (P < 0.001). A Post hoc analysis, using a series of Wilcoxon rank tests, is then necessary to test those groups two by two, correcting the inflated P-value by Bonferroni equation. The respective Z values (and P values) for the comparison of pre-treatment (A), one month (B), and three months (C) after antihypertensive therapy; i.e., A vs. B, B vs. C, and A vs. C were: 1.1 (0.27), 2.8 (0.004) and 3.44 (0.001). Applying the Bonferroni equation gives the corrected P values: 0.81, 0.012, and 0.003. Hence, C measurement is significantly different from A and B measurements, while A and B measurements are quite comparable. We can conclude that, overall, the treatment appears to be effective. However, it seems that we will have to wait for three months to expect a significant treatment effect (P = 0.012). After another three months, the treatment is even significantly better than before treatment (P = 0.003).

What Should be Reported

We have to report descriptive and inferential statistics of main statistics: median (95% CI), spread (minimum and maximum, interquartile range or percentiles), and P-value. We have to report the descriptive as well as inferential statistics of post-hoc analysis when performed. In such a case, the effect size can be reported as PSdep and interpreted as previously shown with Wilcoxon sign Rank test (see Sect. 2.5.1.3).

Conditions of Application

Patients have to be chosen at random. Paired information is acquired from the same patient or matched pairs. Measurements have to be independent, and the sample size should be large, with at least four groups or measurement occasions (k > 4) and a minimum sample size of 15 patients per group (n > 15) is at least 15. Otherwise, it is advised to check out the significance of our results directly in special tables [31].

There is a complete armada of non-parametric tests (NPT) that many researchers do not efficiently use. They allow statistical inference without making previous assumptions that the sample was taken from a particular distribution. The required sample size is usually smaller than the minimum required by a parametric version and can even be executed with few patients per group. The NPT come at the rescue in small studies and whenever we are not sure about the distribution of the variable in concern.

In practice, there is a non-parametric version for the commonly used tests such as independent-samples Student test (Mann-Whitney test), paired Student (Wilcoxon-Sign rank test), one-way ANOVA (Kruskal and Wallis test), and repeated measures ANOVA (Friedman's test). They are safer (less commonly making type I error) but less powerful than their parametric versions (more commonly making type II error). Put it this way, NPT are more likely to miss the evidence but less likely to conclude upon something untrue.

2.6 Inference on the Relation of Two Quantitative Variables

Correlation and regression are two statistical techniques that can be used to analyze the relation between two quantitative variables. The use of either technique is mainly dependent upon the study question. Suppose the study is about the strength of the association between the two variables. In that case, correlation can quantify the magnitude and direction of such association, provided that the relationship is linear and is entirely symmetrical and bidirectional: the effect of (x) on (y) is the same as the effect of (y) on (x). Correlation, per se, cannot point to causality.

On the other hand, if the study question is about how much a variable (y) changes for a given (x) value, a regression can analyze the "effect" of (x) on (y). However, and unlike correlation, the regression equation is not symmetrical and cannot be used to deduct the effect of (y) on (x). A second and a completely different regression equation must be constructed to predict (x) for a given (y) value. Both equations "can" point to causality: the first can show how much (x) is responsible for the changes in (y), while the second can be used to analyze how much (y) influences (x); which are not the same as will be shown in Sect. 2.6.2.

Choosing between correlation and regression is sometimes unclear. Statistically, it is safer to describe the effect of each variable on the other by a separate regression equation unless both variables are interdependent by their nature and distribution. Hence, the single correlation equation can describe their relationship. However, we must note that not every regression can be "safely" interpreted as being a "reliable" indicator of a cause-effect relationship. Causality is dependent on all other elements of the study, and regression is just a tool that can put it into evidence.

2.6.1 Correlation

In one of the earliest attempts to quantify the "correlation" between 2 variables, Sir Francis Galton (1822–1911) noted that: "the adult son tends to have his father's stature, with a degree that differs from case to case." Since then, Karl Pearson (1857–1936) and other statisticians have worked on studying correlation in different situations and according to many factors. Those factors include the nature of the variable (quantitative or qualitative), its distribution (Normal or else), considering the effect of other variables, and much

more. The result is that we have many correlation coefficients. This section will analyze two commonly used correlation coefficients analyzing the relation between 2 quantitative variables, whether those following a Normal (correlation coefficient r) or another distribution (Spearman rank correlation coefficient).

2.6.1.1 Pearson Correlation Coefficient "r"

We will consider the typical case where correlation describes the association between two quantitative variables (x and y), e.g., birth weight and gestational age, duration of surgery, and amount of blood loss. Provided that such relation does not change direction during the period of the study, correlation can be described as being positive whenever the increase in the value of one variable is associated with a proportional increase in the value of the other variable. An example is a proportionate increase in the pulse rate secondary to the increase in the body temperature. On the other hand, a negative correlation describes the relation between 2 variables, where the increase in the value of one of the variables is associated with a decrease in the value of the second variable, e.g., the number of cigarettes smoked per day and life expectancy in years.

Graphically, each pair of related data (each "x" and its corresponding "y") could be represented by one point, and the "cloud" formed by the aggregation of those points may suggest the type (linear or other relationship) as well as the sign (positive, negative) of correlation. A linear correlation could be visualized by taking a ruler and fitting a straight line by eye, subjectively, to the data points on the graph, passing through as many points as possible and minimizing the distances from others. Figure 2.2 shows a positive (Fig. 2.2A) and a negative linear correlation (Fig. 2.2B). In the absence of correlation, the series of points will be scattered over the graph paper, with an overall vague or pointless distribution (Fig. 2.2D). This chapter will not discuss non-linear, such as quadratic, exponential, and polynomial, where we cannot fit a straight in the center of the cloud of data points (Fig. 2.2C). We

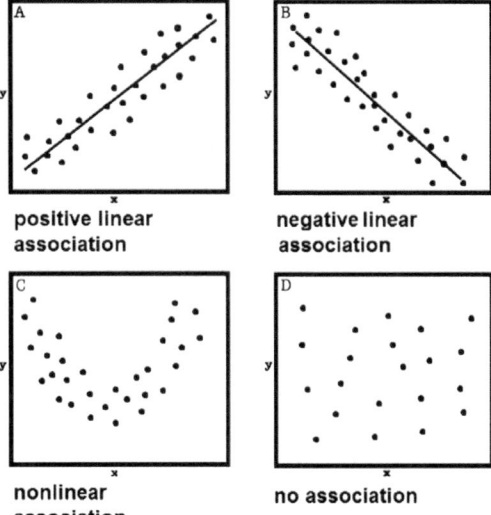

Fig. 2.2 The association between two quantitative variables (x and y). Each point on the graph represents the paired x and y data

insist that the reader plot his data first and ensure a linear relationship; otherwise, the information provided in this chapter should not be applied (Fig. 2.2).

The Trend Line

The trend line has as leverage the central point (m_{xy}), which coordinates are the means of the (x) and (y) variables (Fig. 2.3). In the case where the change in one variable is always associated with the "same" change in the other variable, the line will equally pass by all data points, which is practically impossible. In fact, there will be always some fluctuations of data and the line will join as much points as possible but there will be always variable distances between the line and many of those points. In practice, we have to be satisfied by the "best fitting line" (regression line, trend line, line of least squares, or moving average), which brings those distances (deviations) to a minimum. Following the general rule in statistics of squaring all differences before summing them, the best fitting line is the one that can reduce to a minimum the sum of squared deviations (differences) of all points from their mean value, on the (y) scale. Figure 2.3 shows a graphic presentation of the differences between

each "observed y value" and its corresponding point on the regression line (y′) and "the best fitting line" is expected reduce to a minimum those (y y′) lines. Pearson's correlation coefficient "r" is a measure on how well those points fit the line, the closer are those points to the line, the more is the magnitude of r.

The Example

A study was conducted to analyze the relationship between the duration of surgery (x) and the amount of blood loss in deciliters (y) in ten poly traumatized patients (Table 2.25). The study question was whether there was a significantly positive correlation between both variables? The first thing to do is to visualize data by forming a simple scatter plot, which suggests a positive correlation between both variables: the longer is the duration of surgery, the more the patient will bleed and vice versa (Fig. 2.4). The question now will be about the magnitude and the statistical significance of the relation. Consequently, our researchers decided to proceed and quantify the relation by the correlation coefficient r and to analyze its statistical significance, provided that the conditions of application are fulfilled.

The Equation

Before proceeding, we advise the reader to have a look at Table 2.25 where we have easily calculated three variabilities: Sx (the standard deviation of the x variable = 2.49), Sy (the standard deviation of the y variable = 2.26), and the Covariance of (x, y = 5). The correlation coefficient r is directly computed from those three numbers, and we can stop here and directly calculate r [40]. However, we decided to present the sequence of equations to give the interested reader the chance to understand the idea behind the calculations and the meaning of each number.

The first thing to do is make a scatter plot to visualize the relation between data points. Provided that there is a linear relationship between both variables, the statistical software fits the trend line passing by the central point (m_{xy}). In a perfect 100% correlation, the line will pass by all data points, which is only hypothetical. There will always be differences (deviation, variation) between many data points and the trend line. The correlation coefficient (r) was created to quantify those variations, and an (r) value of 1 means that there is 100% correlation, and an (r) value of zero means that there is no correlation at all between both variables. In other words, the value of (r) is indirectly proportional to variability. The larger is (r), the smaller is the variability between data points and the "perfect" correlation line.

A correlation may be either positive or negative, (r) can acquire any value between −1 and +1. Let us now proceed and calculate this variability.

1. *Calculation of the covariance (x, y)*

The general rule of expressing individual variability of an (x) variable is to calculate the variance, which is the average of the sum of squared deviations (SS) of those values from their mean "Eqs. 1.3" and "1.5" (see Sect. 1.3.4.1). In our example, we have to consider that each data point is not formed by one variable (x or y), but it represents a pair of data (an x value and its corresponding y). Hence, it is better-called covariance. Most importantly, the variability of each paired data point (x_i, y_i) has to be calculated considering both means (mx as well as my), and hence, it is neither a squared ($x_i − m_x$) nor a squared ($y_i − m_y$) but the product of the two = ($x_i − m_x$) ($y_i − m_y$). Note that the latter will be a squared value too. As usual, the covariance (x, y) will be the sum of those products divided by the degree of freedom (n − 1) "Eq. 2.80".

Table 2.25 shows covariance calculation, starting by calculating mean x (=5) and mean y (=6). This is followed by the calculation of ($x_i − m_x$) and $y_i − m_y$) to compute the product ($x_i − m_x$) ($y_i − m_y$) for each case. The covariance (x, y) equals the sum of those products (=45), divided by n − 1 (=9) = 5. Now we understand what

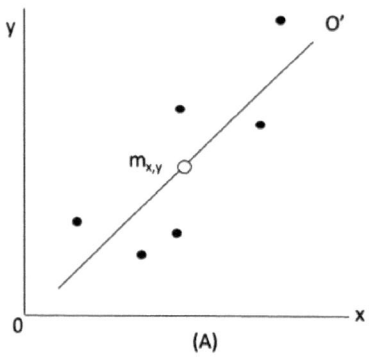
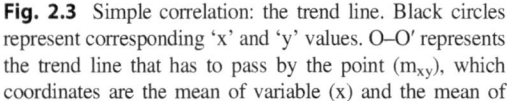
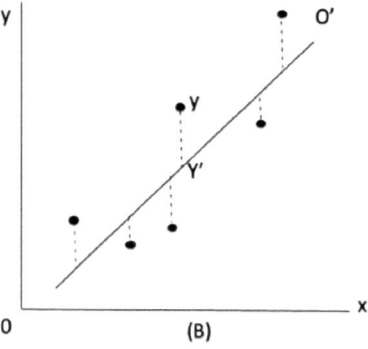

Fig. 2.3 Simple correlation: the trend line. Black circles represent corresponding 'x' and 'y' values. O–O′ represents the trend line that has to pass by the point (m_{xy}), which coordinates are the mean of variable (x) and the mean of variable (y). The line renders to a minimum the sum of squared deviations [$\sum (y − y')^2$] of those black circles calculated parallel to the vertical 'oy' scale; $\sum$ = sum, y = individual values of y, y′ = mean value of y

Table 2.25 Correlation between the duration of surgery and the total amount of blood loss in ten poly traumatized patients

1	2	3	4	5	6	7	8	9
Number	x	y	(x − mx)	(y − my)	(x − mx) (y − my)	(x − mx)^2	(y − my)^2	y_{fit}
I	2	3	−3	−3	9	9	9	3.59
II	5	7	0	1	0	0	1	6
III	3	5	v2	−1	2	4	1	4.39
IV	2	4	−3	−2	6	9	4	3.59
V	6	5	1	−1	−1	1	1	6.8
VI	8	9	3	3	9	9	9	8.41
VII	3	4	−2	−2	4	4	4	4.39
VIII	9	10	4	4	16	16	16	9.21
IX	5	7	0	1	0	0	1	6
X	7	6	2	0	0	4	0	7.61
Sum	50	60	0	0	45	56	46	60
Mean	mx = 5	my = 6						my_{fit} = 6
V^2					5	6.22	5.11	
Sd						2.49	2.26	

Numbers in Latin represent individual patients, x = duration of surgery in hours, y = amount of blood loss in deciliters, mx and my = mean values of x and y; respectively. Column 6 = sum of squares of covariance (x, y) = (x − mx) (y − my), columns 7 and 8 = sum of squares of x and y, Column 9 = the predicted values of y (y_{fit}). V^2 = variance, Sd = standard deviation

covariance is? It is the variation of the paired data points in relation to the means of both variables.

$$Covariance\ (x, y) = \sum (x - m_x) \frac{(y - m_y)}{(n - 1)}$$

$$(2.80)$$

2. Calculation of the correlation coefficient r:

Although the covariance calculated the differences (variability) between data points and trend line, it cannot express correlation. The covariance calculated the "raw" differences, which is dependent upon the measurement scale, and hence, as such, the covariance cannot be used to compare measurements of different scales. As for any raw measurement, the covariance has to be standardized by dividing by the proper standard deviation. Remember that we have two variables. The acceptable standard deviation of their

covariance is the product of the standard deviations of both variables S_x and S_y, as calculated in Table 2.25 "Eq. 2.81". Figure 2.4 shows an example of the standardized variability of a single (x_1, y_1) point: it is the product of the standardized differences, calculated for its 2 components = $[(x_1 - m_x)/S_x]/[(y_1 - m_y)/S_y]$. In consequence, the coefficient of correlation (r) of a sample = 0.89

$$r = \frac{Covar(x, y)}{S_x S_y}$$

$$(2.81)$$

3. Verification of Calculations

Uploading our data to SPSS or an online calculator produces means and Sd of both x (5, 2.49) and y variables (6, 2.26), the sum of squares of duration of surgery (56) and amount of blood loss (45), covariance (5), coefficient r (0.887) and P-value (0.001).

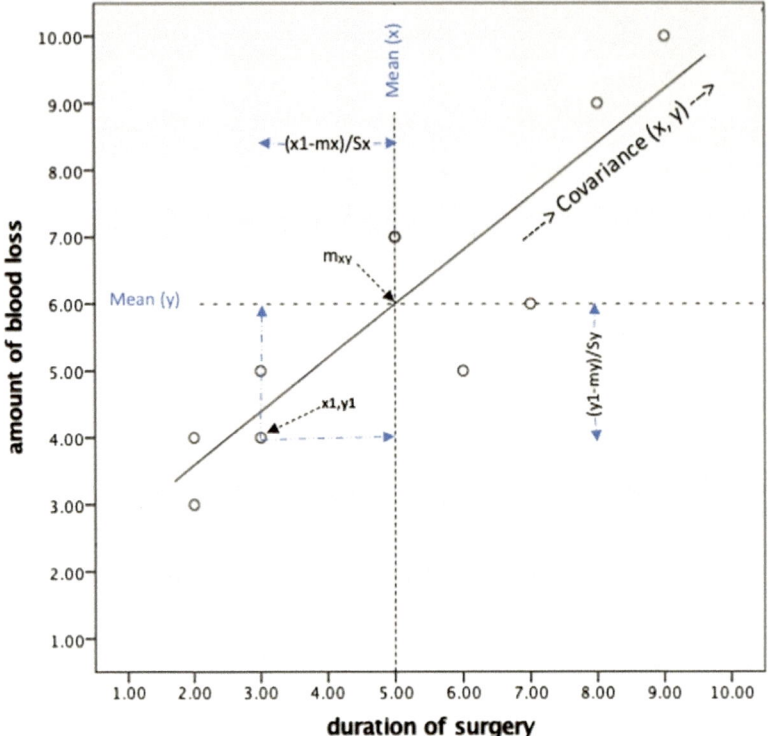

Fig. 2.4 Correlation between the duration of surgery and the amount of blood loss in ten polytraumatized patients (see Table 2.25). Open circles represent paired (x,y) data. Dotted horizontal and vertical lines denote mean x (duration of surgery) and mean y (amount of blood loss in deciliters), respectively. Point m_{xy} = point of leverage of the covariance, with the coordinates: mean x, mean y (5, 6). Point x1y1 = point that varies from mean x by (x1 − mean x)/Sx and from mean y by (y1 − mean y)/Sy. Sx = standard deviation of (x), Sy = standard deviation of (y)

The Interpretation:

A correlation coefficient of 1 means that knowing (x) perfectly explains (y), and an r value of zero indicates no correlation. Theoretically, r varies between −1 (perfect negative correlation) and +1 (perfect positive correlation); however, it is something in-between in practice. On the other hand, a rule of thumb is that if the absolute value of (r) is at least equal for larger than 2/√n, then the relationship does exist. Arbitrary, absolute value of: <0.2, <0.4, <0.6 and <0.8, and <1 can be considered as being weak, moderate, strong and very strong correlation.

The statistical significance of r can be checked out by calculating a Student t-value based upon (r) and the number of paired data (n) "Eq. 2.82". The t-value is compared to that figured in

Student's table, at df = n − 2 = 8. Our result (5.4) is even larger than that in the Student's table (5.041) for a P-value of 0.001. Our conclusion will be a statistically significant high positive correlation between the amount of blood loss and the duration of surgery (r = 0.89; P < 0.001).

$$t = \frac{r\sqrt{(n-2)}}{\sqrt{1-r^2}} \qquad (2.82)$$

What Should be Reported

We have to report the descriptive statistics: mean and Sd of each variable. Inferential statistics include r, R square, the P-value, and effect size. R square, or simply the square of (r), represents the part of the variation of outcome (y) that can be explained by (is dependent on) the independent variable (x). In our example, R square = 0.792. It can also be expressed in percentage and, in such a case, it is called: the coefficient of determination. It can be interpreted as follows: 79.2% of the variation in blood loss is accounted for by the duration of surgery. The remaining unexplained part may be due to other factors or random causes. Finally, the effect size can be reported using Fisher's transformation (see Sect. 4.9.1). In our example, effect size C = 1.42.

The 95% CI of (r)

There are two main methods to calculate a 95% CI for Pearson's correlation coefficient r. We will begin by presenting the first method based upon the "Fisher's z to r transformation" and, it is the one preferred by most researchers. For samples of correlation coefficient, the calculated correlation is not normally distributed, even if the x and y data values were normal [41]. In consequence, Fisher proposed transforming r into its normalized logarithmic value (z_r) "Eq. 2.83", calculate the standard error of (z_r) and its the 95% confidence interval and, finally, antilog its upper and lower limits to get the upper and lower limits of (r) "Eq. 2.84". In our example, r equals 0.89 and its normalized logarithmic value (z_r) equals 1.42 "Eq. 2.83". The 95% CI of z_r is calculated as usual from the Z score (1.96) and the Se, which is estimated as $1/\sqrt{n-3}$. In our example, the 95% CI of $z_r = z_r \pm Z\,(Se) = 1.42 \pm 1.96\,(0.38) = 2.16$ to 0.68. The upper and lower limits are then back transformed to the original correlation scale by the "Eq. 2.84"; replacing r' one time by 2.16 and the other time by 0.68. The upper and lower limits of the 95% CI of the correlation coefficient are 0.97 and 0.56. The method is not appropriate when (x) and (y) significantly deviate from normality, even if sample size is large. there is a significant deviation from normality of both x and y variables

$$z_r = \frac{1}{2}\log\frac{1+r}{1-r} = \frac{1}{2}\log\frac{1+0.89}{1-0.89} = 1.42$$

(2.83)

$$r = \frac{e^{2z_r} - 1}{e^{2z_r} + 1} = \frac{e^{2\times2.16} - 1}{e^{2\times2.16} + 1} = 0.97;\ \frac{e^{2\times0.68} - 1}{e^{2\times0.68} + 1} = 0.56$$

(2.84)

Unlike the first method which is based upon normalizing r, the second method is based upon normalizing the unexplained part of variability. As the squared value of the correlation coefficient r (r^2) measures the part of variability of (y) that can be explained by (x); ($1 - r^2$) represents the unexplained part. In our example, (r^2) was 0.79 and, as the maximum value of (r^2) is 1; ($1 - r^2$) = 0.21. Put it another way, the maximum expected value of (r^2) = 1 = (r^2) + (1 − r^2) = 0.792 + 0.208. If our data are normally distributed, we can expect that (r^2) which increased by a maximum value of +(1 − r^2) can decrease by the same amount of −(1 − r^2). In other words, (1 − r^2) can be assumed as being the quantity by which our correlation coefficient (r) varies (increases/decreases); i.e., (1 − r^2) is the variance of (r). At that point, the Se can be routinely calculated from "Eq. 2.85". View the small sample size, we cannot use the z value (1.96) in the calculation but the critical t-value (2.3) figured n Student table, at 8 (n − 2) df. The 95% CI can be directly estimated as: r ± t (Se) = 0.89 ± 2.3 (0.16) = 0.52 to 1.26. We can easily note that the 95% CI of our example is completely misleading, giving a proportion >1. Although this second approach gives a symmetrical 95% CI of r, yet it is not advised in case of r near to zero or 1 and in small sample size, like ours.

$$\text{Se } r = \frac{r^2\sqrt{(1-r^2)}}{n-2} = \frac{0.79\sqrt{(1-0.79)}}{10-2} = 0.16$$

(2.85)

Conditions of Application

Samples should be drawn at random, observations should be independent, and both variables have to be normally distributed. Normality can be simply checked visually by plotting a histogram or more formally by a Shapiro–Wilk test (see Sect. 1.4.3). Other assumptions include linearity and homoscedasticity. Linearity assumes a straight-line relationship between each of the two variables, provided that it does not change in sign or magnitude during the studied intervals. Homoscedasticity or homogeneity of variance assumes that data is equally distributed about the regression line. Kindly refer to Sect. 2.6.2. for details on checking on linearity and homoscedasticity (see Sect. 2.6.2).

The correlation coefficient necessitates that at least one of the two tied distributions (distribution of "y" for a given value of "x" or the distribution of "x" for a given value of "y") is normal and of a constant variance; conditions that are usually realized in biology. The tied distribution of a variable (y) is the distribution of (y) for a given value of the other variable (x). In other words, it describes the variations of the (y) values as tied to a specific value of (x) and hence, was given the name of the tied distribution. In our example, the distribution of the amount of blood loss (y) of all cases with "one" defined duration of surgery (x) has to be normal and of constant variance. It differs from the well-known total distribution, which describes the variation of all (y) values, regardless of (x) and, which is called the total variance.

However, the test is robust and can be applied even if the necessary conditions of its use are not perfectly verified, provided that the number of studied patients is large (n > 30). In the case of a statistically significant "r", the latter can be pushed far beyond being just an indication of the association of two variables to become a measure of the strength of such association. In such a case, other (extra) application conditions need to be verified; both -and not only one-tied distributions have to be normal, and with a constant variance, both total distributions have to be normal and, both regressions have to be linear.

2.6.1.2 The Coefficient of Correlation of Ranks (Spearman's Rank Test)

Spearman's rank test is the non-parametric version of the correlation coefficient (r) that is

indicated whenever the number of patients is small (n < 30) or the conditions of application of (r) are hard to verify.

The Example

The example is the same used in Sect. 2.6.1.1. Data are presented in Table 2.26. View the small number of patients; the authors have decided to test the association between the duration of surgery and the amount of blood loss by the non-parametric test of Spearman.

The Equation

As with all non-parametric tests, data will not be used as such and will be replaced by their ranks (see Sect. 2.5). Each of the 2 variables of concern is reclassified separately by increasing order. For each patient, we calculate the difference between his two ranks (di): his rank in the duration of surgery and his rank in the amount of blood loss. In order to sum the differences calculated for each patient, we have to square them first (di2), as usual, to calculate the sum of squared difference ($\sum$di2). Calculations are shown in Table 2.26.

If both variables correlate perfectly with one another, there should be no difference between the ranks of a patient; hence, every (di) should be equal to zero. As an example, a patient who is ranked as number 3 in the duration of surgery should be ranked as number 3 in the amount of blood loss, and hence, the difference between this patient's two ranks should be equal to zero (3 − 3 = 0). In other words, all calculated (di)s will be zero as well as any value deducted from them, such as the squared differences (di^2), the sum of squares ($\sum di^2$) and the standardized sum of squares ($6\sum di^2$)/n(n − 1).

On the other hand, under the null hypothesis of no association between the two variables, all (di) will be >0 and ($6\sum di^2$)/n(n − 1) will reach a maximum value of 1. The alternative hypothesis of perfect correlation is that all (di) will be equal to zero, and in consequence, ($6\sum di^2$)/n(n − 1) will be equal to zero too. In practice, correlation is between zero and 1; hence, it can be quantified by subtracting this quantity from 1 "Eq. 2.86". In our example, this quantity equals 0.16 and hence, r = 1 − 0.16 = 0.84.

$$r_s = 1 - \frac{6 \sum d_i^2}{n(n^2 - 1)} \quad (2.86)$$

Management of ties

As shown in Table 2.26, a known ranking problem is the presence of ties (Ex-Aequo) or cases sharing common values. The duration of surgery in both: patient number I and number IV are 2 h and that of both: patient number III and number VII is 3 h and that of both: patient number II and number IX is 5 h. Also, Patients number IV and VII, number III and V, and numbers II and IX share the same amounts of blood loss: 4, 5, and 7 L, respectively. In order to rank those patients, we have given each of the two patients sharing the same value a mean rank. As an example, patients I and IV who should occupy the ranks of 1 and 2 in the duration of surgery are both given the common rank of 1.5 [(1 + 2)/2 = 3/2 = 1.5], patients III and VII who should occupy the ranks 3 and 4 are both given the common rank 3.5 [(3 + 4)/2 = 7/2 = 3.5].

The Interpretation

A Spearman's correlation coefficient of 1 means that knowing (x) perfectly explains (y) and an (r_s) value of zero indicates that there is no correlation

at all. Theoretically, (r_s) varies between −1 (perfect negative correlation) and +1 (perfect positive correlation). In our example, there was a powerful correlation between the duration of surgery and the amount of blood loss. Note that (r_s) was smaller than Pearson's correlation (r), which can be explained by the loss of information due to the ranking process. We have to repeat that this relatively small power of the non-parametric test largely surpasses the bias of applying a parametric test whenever to should not be.

There are special statistical tables that directly give the critical values of (r_s) for rejection of the null hypothesis [31] however; it was found that (r_s) will follow a Student's distribution whenever the number of cases is at least 10. Hence, and as previously done in the case of coefficient of correlation (r), we can calculate a t-value for $(r_s) = 4.38$ "see Eq. 2.82". The statistical significance of t can be checked out at Student's table at df = n − 2; where (n) is the number of pairs. Checking Students' table, at 8 df (n − 2 = 10 − 2 = 8), shows that our result (4.38) is statistically significant with a P-value >0.01%. Compared to Pearson's correlation coefficient, the calculated r and t-values are smaller, and hence, the P-value is larger due to the loss of information associated with ranking.

Table 2.26 Spearman's rank test: correlation between duration of surgery and total amount of blood loss in ten poly traumatized patients

Patients number	X	Y	Rank of X	Rank of Y	Difference of ranks (di)	di^2
I	2	3	1.5	1	0.5	0.25
II	5	7	5.5	7.5	−2	4
III	3	5	3.5	3.5	0	0
IV	2	4	1.5	2.5	−1	1
V	6	5	7	3.5	3.5	12.25
VI	8	9	9	9	0	0
VII	3	4	3.5	2.5	1	1
VIII	9	10	10	10	0	0
IX	5	7	5.5	7.5	−2	4
X	7	6	8	6	2	4
$\sum$di^2						26.5

Numbers in Latin represent individual patients, X = duration of surgery in hours; Y = amount of blood loss in deciliter's, $\sum$ = sum, di = difference in ranks

What Should be Reported

We have to report descriptive statistics, namely, median and spread, (rs), P-value, and effect size.

Conditions of Applications

Samples should be drawn at random. Both (x) and (y) should be independent continuous or ordinal variables. A minimum sample size of 10 cases without too many ties is preferable. Normality and homoscedasticity are not required.

2.6.2 Regression

Unlike correlation which studies the "mutual" relation between the 2 variables, the question in simple regression is whether one of the 2 variables is dependent on the other. If a person's body weight depends on his height, is the number of bacterial colonies in a blood film dependent upon the dose of a given antibiotic (x)? The term regression is a historical anomaly that was first used in the nineteenth century to describe how the height of children of tall or short parents tends to "regress" towards the mean (average) height. Regression simply means that the average value of one variable (called the dependent or outcome variable; e.g., "y") is a "function" of the other variables (called independent or control variables; e.g., "x"), that is, it changes with "x."

2.6.2.1 Simple Regression

Simple regression can describe the situation where the relationship is linear and with only one independent variable. A linear relation means that a given change in (x) produces a corresponding change in (y), and hence, when paired data are plotted, the cloud of points forms what looks like a straight line. As an example, a 10% increase (or decrease) in (x) will produce the same 10% increase (or decrease) in (y). The reader is invited to refer to the section on multiple regression, where the outcome variable is a function of multiple independent variables (see Sect. 3.4).

The Example

Let us take the same example used in correlation: duration of surgery in hours and amount of blood loss in deciliters (Table 2.25). We have already shown that there is a statistically significant positive correlation between both variables. In regression, the study question is not just the association between the two variables but to find whether the amount of blood loss is dependent on the duration of surgery, to quantify this dependence and up to predict the "average" amount of blood loss, based upon a specific duration of surgery. Provided that the application conditions are fulfilled, the researchers decided to use simple regression, with the duration of surgery as the independent predictor (x) and the amount of blood loss as the dependent outcome (y). Once more, this is a quite small example mainly used to permit hand calculation but is far from being an accurate model fulfilling the conditions necessary for applying the test.

The Equation

A primary helpful step is to create a simple scatter plot to visualize the relation's shape between variables and suggest the best curve to fit in the data: linear, logarithmic, quadratic, exponential, or other. A linear relation is common in biology and, in its simplest form, can be thought to be a straight line. The following equations are based upon the assumption of linearity, among other assumptions that will be detailed in the section on conditions of applications.

Let us start by supposing that the amount of blood loss is not related to the duration of surgery and that regardless of the latter, the patient is expected to lose the same amount of blood. As the "mean" is the best-predicted value of a normally distributed variable, we should expect that patients with variable durations of surgery will lose the same "mean" amount of blood, which is "6 dl" (Table 2.25). In consequence, under the null hypothesis of no effect of (x) on (y), variability becomes limited to the variability of

Fig. 2.5 Simple regression of the amount of blood loss (y) on the duration of surgery (x) in ten polytraumatized patients. Data presented in Table 2.25. P_0 = the slope that measures the effect of independent variable (x) on outcome (y)

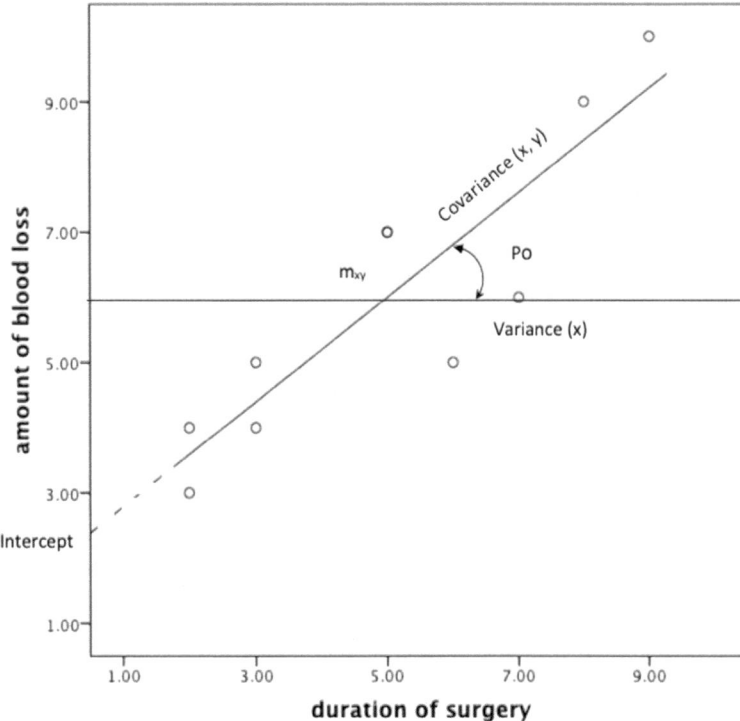

(x) alone, as (y) does not vary, being six dL every time. In other words, the "total" variability recorded in the study will be the "variance of the duration of surgery" alone (S^2x), simply because (y) does not change. Joining the paired data points representing a changing (x) with a constant (y) will form a straight line parallel to the x-axis; which is the null hypothesis: (x) changes but has no effect on (y) (Fig. 2.5).

On the other hand, the alternative hypothesis is that the amount of blood loss increases in proportion to the duration of surgery. Consequently, the data points will not follow the same horizontal line but will tend to swipe up and to the right progressively, and hence, joining the series of data points will make a slope; that is angled on the horizon (Po) (Fig. 2.5). Put it another way, the variation of paired data that was limited to the variance of x (S^2x), also becomes dependent on the mutual variability of the 2 variables (covariance x, y) and, the difference between the 2 situations (the horizontal line and the slope) measures the strength of the effect of

(x) on (y). The more is the effect of (x) on (y), the more the slope deviates from the horizon.

The calculations include calculation of the regression equation, the slope of regression, intercept, standardized coefficient beta, residuals and model fit, and calculation of R-square and coefficient of determination.

1. *The Regression Equation*

As we showed earlier, the line that best fits the series of the scattered data point is the one that can render to a minimum the sum of squared differences between those data points and the line itself (Fig. 2.3). In order to fulfill this requirement, the regression line has to pass by the point (m_{yx}), which coordinates are the means of the variables (y and x). This point is also called the centroid and acts as leverage to the line. Imagine that the line is anchored to the centroid, and then it keeps swinging up and down to settle when it reaches its best-fitting position finally. Figure 2.5 shows the regression line of our example. The line terminates at the smallest observed surgery duration of 2 h. Hence, it raises some questions, including what is the expected amount of blood loss in case of surgery requiring a shorter time and, is there any basic amount of blood loss that we have to expect, regardless of the duration of the surgery? Although the smallest paired data we had was 2 h and 3 deciliters, yet we can extend the regression line (dashed part) towards the y-axis to get the answers to both questions. The line will intercept (meet) the y-axis at a point that represents the basic amount of blood that should be expected, regardless of the duration of surgery. The intercept can be considered the value of (y) when (x) equals zero.

Taking another example of running a hospital and we want to calculate the cost (y) with the number of consultations made (x). First, a basic running cost (salaries, electricity, rent of equipment, etc.) should be paid, even if we had no patients at all, which is the intercept of the equation. To the latter, we have to add an average cost per patient. This average is (Po), and logically, it has to be multiplied by the number of consultations made (x). Now the equation became simple: the cost of running this clinic equals the basic running cost (intercept) to which we have to add an average cost that is dependent on (multiplied by) the number of patients. In our first example, there is a basic amount of blood loss that we have to expect, regardless of the duration of surgery. We then add to this "basic" amount (intercept) the "average" amount that is expected to be lost per hour due to the effect of duration of surgery on the amount of blood loss (Po), multiplied by the "number" of hours (x) "Eq. 2.87".

$$y = intercept + Po(x) \qquad (2.87)$$

2. Calculation of the Slope (Po)

As shown in Fig. 2.25, (Po) is the difference between 2 models: the first being the model where (x) has no effect on (y), and hence, the total variability of this model is the variance of x (S^2x) that will eventually follow a horizontal line parallel to its own axis; telling us that while (x) is changing, (y) remains the same. The second model is the one where (y) is influenced by (x), and hence, their (covariance x, y) becomes part of the total variability. The larger is the effect of (x) on (y), the more is the covariance deviates from the horizon and the larger the (Po) slope will be. We have previously shown that variances are not compared by subtraction but as proportions. Consequently, (Po) is calculated as: (covariance x, y)/(S^2x) "Eq. 2.88". After deduction of the df $(n - 1)$ from both numerator and denominator, (Po) becomes the proportion between the respective sum of squares that were already calculated in Table 2.25 = 5/6.22 = 0.804, in our example. Revise "Eq. 2.81" and note that (Po) is the product of the correlation coefficient r and the proportion of variation between both variables, in terms of standard deviation.

$$Po = \frac{Covariance(x, y)}{Variance(x)} = \frac{\sum (x - m_x)(y - m_y)}{\sum (x - m_x)^2}$$
$$= r\frac{S_y}{S_x}$$
$$(2.88)$$

3. Calculation of the Intercept

Knowing (Po = 0.804) and replacing both (x and y) values by their respective means (=5 and 6) shown in Table 2.25, the intercept (=1.98) is easily calculated from the regression equation "Eq. 2.87".

4. Calculation of the Standardized Coefficient Beta

The slope (Po) quantifies the effect of the independent variable on the outcome and is commonly called the "unstandardized b coefficient," and the name warrants some explanations. We have previously shown a measurement (x) can be standardized by a simple equation: (x − mean x)/ Sd; which gives how many standard deviations is

(x) away from its mean (see Sect. 1.3.4). All measurements are brought to this common scale, and hence, they can be compared on a common background. (Po) is called the raw data (duration of surgery in hours and amount of blood loss in deciliters). Hence, it is called the "unstandardized beta coefficient." It quantifies the effect of the predictor on the outcome and is used to test whether this effect is statistically significant or not, but it cannot be compared to the effect of other predictors on the outcome because they are usually calculated in different scales. The beta coefficient was standardized so that we could compare the effects of different predictors on the outcome.

Let us compare the meaning of both coefficients: an unstandardized b coefficient of 1.25 means that we should expect a mean of 1.25 units increase in (y), with each 1 unit increase in (x). In our example, we should expect an increase of 1.25 deciliters in the amount of blood loss, with each one hour increase in the duration of surgery. A standardized beta coefficient value of 1.25 indicates that a change of one standard deviation in the independent variable (x) results in 1.25 standard deviations increase in outcome (y), regardless of the units of measurements. Fortunately, the standardized b coefficient does not necessitate repeating the calculations with the standardized paired data and it can be easily deduced by multiplying the unstandardized coefficient by the ratio of the standard deviations of the independent variable and dependent variable "Eq. 2.89". In our example, with Sx and Sy = 2.49 and 2.26, the standardized beta coefficient = 0.887.

This brings us to the second point; the standardized beta coefficient gave exactly the same result as the correlation coefficient (r), calculated when the study question was about the correlation between the two variables (see Sect. 2.6.1); which is not a coincidence. Remember that both coefficients are standardized measurements of the difference between observed data and data expected by either models that is the same, whether the model is correlation or regression. Both coefficients will be equal as long as there is only one predictor and one outcome. The

standardized coefficient is commonly termed as "coefficient beta", the unstandardized coefficient as "B coefficient"; which is usually numbered as b_1, b_2, b_3, etc.; to allow for the inclusion of multiple predictors in case of multiple regression.

$$Coefficient\ Beta = b\left(\frac{S_x}{S_y}\right) \qquad (2.89)$$

Playing the same tune, the intercept is also called beta zero (b_0), for representing the value of outcome in the case where (x) equals zero. The intercept is sometimes also referred to as the constant. The regression equation is more commonly written after substituting the intercept by (b_0) and (Po) by ($b1$) "Eq. 2.90". The regression equation, ($b1$) is the unstandardized b coefficient, calculated in hours and not the standardized coefficient beta.

$$\hat{y} = b_0 + b_1(x) \qquad (2.90)$$

5. Calculation of the Residuals and Model Fit

The value of the regression equation is to predict an outcome as close as possible to the observed one. The more the predicted value is close to the one observed, the more the model "fits" our data, which is why the expected outcome is sometimes called (y_{fit}). Both observed and predicted values are presented in columns number 3 and number 9 in Tables 2.25 and 2.27 As an example and, according to the regression equation, with $b_1 = 0.804$ and $b_0 = 1.98$; the expected amount of blood loss after 2 h of surgery (x = 2) is 3.59 dl. In Table 2.25, patients I and IV had the same duration of surgery of two hours. However, the observed amounts of blood loss were different: three dL for patient number I and four dL for patient number IV. The expected blood loss calculated for both patients was 3.59 dL. The differences between observed and expected outcome values (three dL and four dL), calculated for the same predictor (two hours), are the model residuals or error due to the model equation (y_{resid}); the smaller it is, the more the model is said to fit our data.

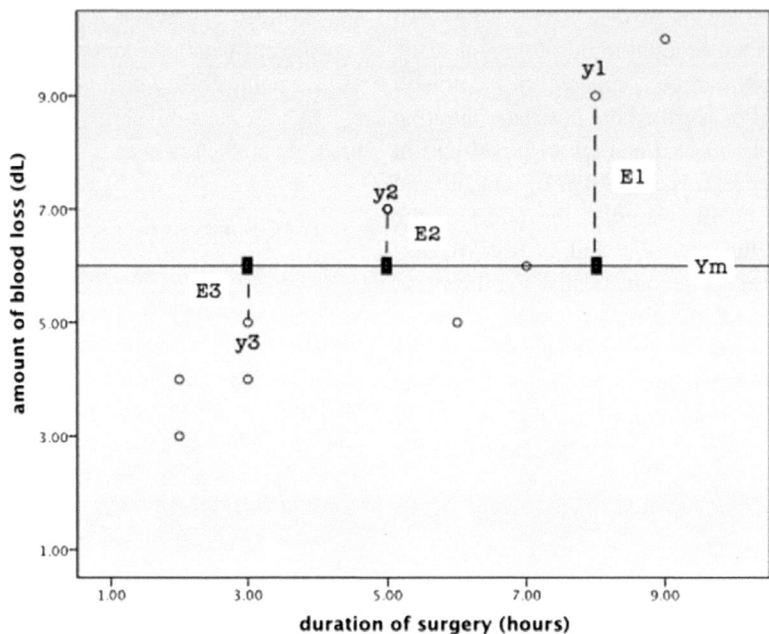

Fig. 2.6 Model error under the null hypothesis. Open circles = observed amount of blood loss (y1, y2, y3, etc.), solid squares = expected amount of blood loss under the null hypothesis (mean y = my), E1, E2, E3, etc. = error under the null hypothesis = observed − expected values = (y1 − my), y2·my), (y3 − my)

Table 2.27 Calculation of predicted (y_{fit}) and error sum of squares (SSE) of data presented in Table 2.25

1	3	5	8	9	10	11
Patients number	y	$(y - my)$	$(y - my)^2$	y_{fit}	$y_{resid} = (y - y_{fit})$	$(y_{resid})^2$
I	3	−3	9	3.59	−0.59	0.35
II	7	1	1	6		1
III	5	−1	1	4.39	0.61	0.37
IV	4	−2	4	3.59	0.41	0.17
V	5	−1	1	6.8	−1.8	3.24
VI	9	3	9	8.41	0.59	0.348
VII	4	−2	4	4.39	−0.39	0.15
VIII	10	4	16	9.21	0.79	0.62
IX	7	1	1	6	1	1
X	6	0	0	7.61	−1.61	2.59
Sum	60	0	46	60		9.8
Mean	my = 6			$my_{fit} = 6$	$my_{resid} = 0$	
V^2			5.11			
Sd			2.26	2	1.04	

The head of columns represent serial column numbers: the numbers 1, 3, 5, 8 and 9 are copies taken from Table 2.25, to which we added the column numbers 10 and 11 representing the difference and squared differences between observed (y) and expected outcome (y_{fit}), calculated for each patient ($y - y_{fit} = y_{resid}$). Other abbreviations are those used in Table 2.25: numbers in Latin represent individual patients, X = duration of surgery in hours, y = amount of blood loss in deciliters, mx and my = mean values of x and y; respectively. Column 6 = sum of squares of (x, y), columns 7 and 8 = sum of squares of x and y, Column 9 = the predicted values of y (y_{fit}). V^2 = variance of (x), variance of (y) or covariance (x, y). Sd = standard deviation

The analysis is carried out as usual by comparing the two models: the (null) model, which assumes that (x) has no effect on (y) and, the (alternative) model, which assumes that (y) is a function of (x). Under the null hypothesis, with (x) is being changing, the outcome variable is always acquiring the same mean value (y_m); the difference is wide: between "multiple observed outcomes" $(y_1, y_2, y_3,$ etc.) and "one constant expected" mean outcome (y_m), as shown in Fig. 2.6.

Under the alternative hypothesis, however, the difference is reduced; for the expected outcomes now lie at a much smaller distance of observed outcomes; being along the regression line, which passes through the center of the cloud formed by observed outcomes themselves: $(y - y_{fit})$ (Fig. 2.7). The gain acquired by regression is equal to the difference between those two models. Put it another way: the total variability $(y - y_m)$ is split into two parts: a part that is reduced by—explained by—regression $(y_{fit} - y_m)$ and the remaining residual part $(y - y_{fit})$ that still needs to be explained (Fig. 2.8) "Eq. 2.91".

$$(y - y_m) = (y - y_{fit}) + (y_{fit} - y_m) \qquad (2.91)$$

6. *Calculation of R-Square and Coefficient of Determination*

In statistical terms, the total variability (total sum of squares = $SS_{total} = (y - y_m)$ is reduced to a much smaller variability (error sum of squares = $SS_{error} = (y - y_{fit})$, and the difference is the gain achieved by regression (sum of squares gained by regression = $SS_{regression} = y_{fit} - y_m$) "Eq. 2.92". Both "Eqs. 2.91" and "2.92" are two sides of a coin.

$$SStotal = SS_{regression} + SS_{error} \qquad (2.92)$$

In the regression equation, the intercept (b_0) represents SS_{error}, b_1 represents $SS_{regression}$, and the ratio between $SS_{regression}$ and SS_{total} expresses the amount of variation explained by the model or the coefficient of determination. Being a proportion out of a total, R^2 is always between 0 and 1. In case there is no effect of "x" on "y", the

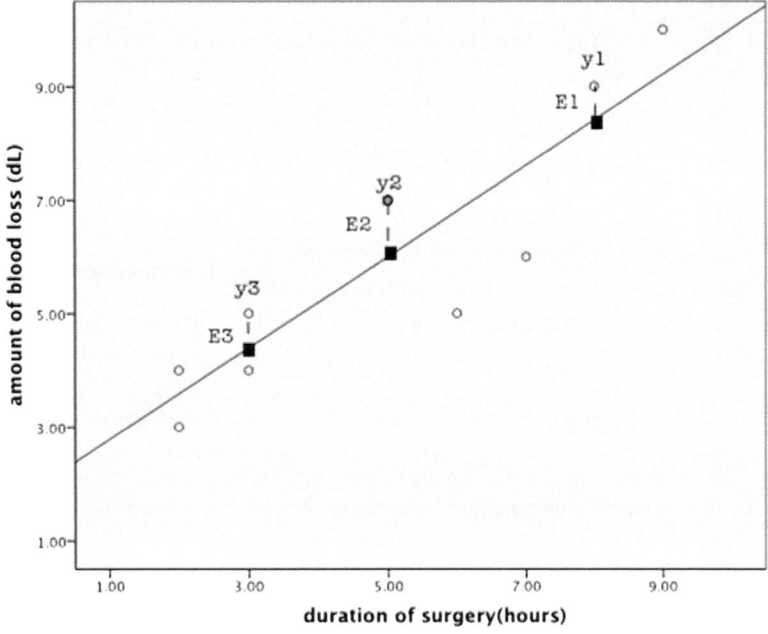

Fig. 2.7 Model error under the alternative hypothesis. Open circles = observed amount of blood loss (y1, y2, y3, etc.), solid squares = expected amount of blood loss under the alternative hypothesis (mean y = my), E1, E2, E3, etc. = error under the null hypothesis = observed − expected values = (y1 − my), y2·my), (y3 − my)

Fig. 2.8 Gain in error due to regression. Open circles = observed amount of blood loss (Y), solid square = expected amount of blood loss under the alternative hypothesis (Yfit), solid circle = expected amount of blood loss under the null hypothesis (Ym = mean Y). Error = error under the alternative hypothesis (Y − Yfit), Gain = gain in error due to regression (Yfit − Ym)

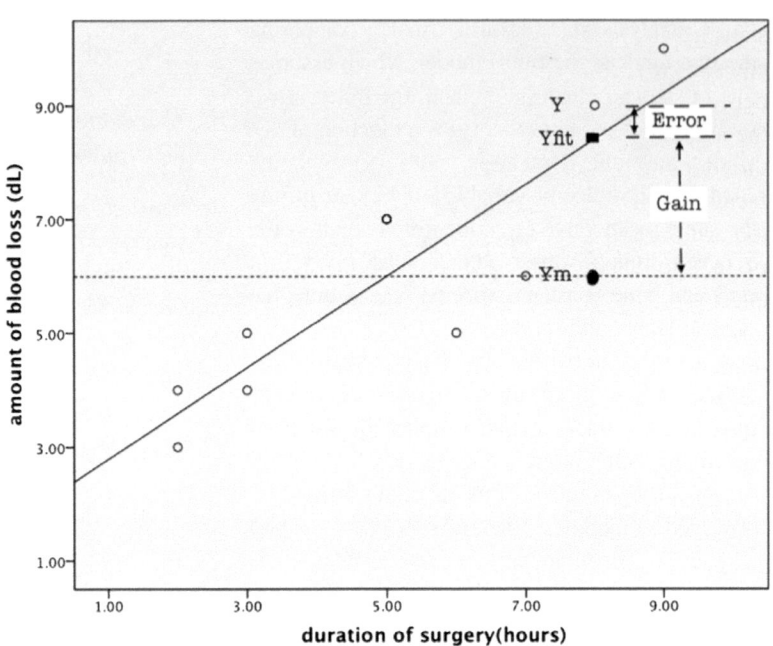

Table 2.28 Simple regression: model fit

Model	Sum of squares	df	Mean square	F ratio	P value
Regression[a]	36.16	1	36.16	29.4	0.001[b]
Residual	9.8	8	1.23		
Total	46	9			

a = outcome: amount of blood loss in dL, b = predictors: duration of surgery in hours, constant

regression line itself will be horizontal; SS error will be equal to SS total and, according to "Eq. 2.93", R^2 will be equal to (0). In case the data points are perfectly placed on the regression line, there will be no residuals and SS error itself will be equal to (0). Applying "Eq. 2.93", R^2 will be equal to 1.

$$R^2 = \frac{SS_{regression}}{SS_{total}} = \frac{SS_{total} - SS_{error}}{SS_{total}} \qquad (2.93)$$

In our example, the predictor (duration of surgery) explains 78.6% of the variability of the dependent variable (amount of blood loss), with 21.4% of the latter remaining unexplained. As there is only one predictor whose correlation with the dependent variable was estimated by an

(r) value of 0.887, raising (r) to the same squared scale (R^2) gives the coefficient of determination in decimals (0.786).

The Interpretation

The interpretation includes the model fit, interpretation of model coefficients (b_1 and b_0), and the regression equation. Finally, we will consider the situation when we switch the predictor and the outcome.

1. *The Model Fit*

One important point is to know how much of the variation of the dependent variable (amount of blood loss) can be attributed to the effect of the independent variable (duration of surgery). In statistical terms, how much does the regression equation explain the variability observed in the dependent variable? It will be illogic to think that the amount of blood loss varied only because of the duration of surgery. Other (independent) factors have to exist and have to have an effect too and, the question is how to separate the effect of the studied "duration of surgery" from the effect of those "unknown or unmeasured factors." Here comes the role of ANOVA in partitioning the total overall variation recorded in the amount of blood loss into the part due to the effect of duration of surgery and a remaining part due to other unknown or unmeasured factors.

Mathematically, the variances measuring those variations are the total variance, regression variance, and residual variance, respectively. In terms of the sum of squares, ANOVA partitions the total sum of squares (SST) into the sum of squares due to regression (SSR) that expresses the effect of predictor (x) on the outcome (y) and a remaining error sum of squares (SSE) that is represented by the intercept. The latter is also called the residual sum of squares to represent the part of variability that remained unexplained by regression. As shown in Tables 2.7 and 2.8, SST equals 46, SSE = 9.8, and by deduction, SSR = 36.2, which are the same results that were calculated by hand. As in a regular ANOVA, variances are compared in proportion. The statistical significance of SSR is tested by calculating Fisher's value, which is the proportion between the variances (Mean squares) of regression and the residual variance "Eq. 2.43" (see Sect. 2.4.3.1). The F value must be at least equal or more significant than the one presented in Fisher's table point 5% at (df1/df2 = 1/8), equal to 5.32 [10]. Our value (29.4) is much larger and is statistically significant, with a P-value of 0.001.

2. The Model Coefficients

The Predictor (b_1 Coefficient)

The statistical significance of the predictor is tested by comparing the two models. The model under the null hypothesis, (x) has no effect on (y). Hence, the linear relation between both variables will be a horizontal line parallel to the

(x) axis and making a zero angle with the horizon. The second is the alternative model, where (y) is a function of (x), and hence, the trend line will make a slope on the horizon (Fig. 2.5). The difference between the angle made by this slope and the zero angle of the first model ($P_O - 0$) can be tested by a regular test of Student "Eq. 2.94". The proper standard error of the difference is the square root of the variance of (P_O) that is deducted from the variances of both variables "Eq. 2.95". In our example, variance $P_O = 0.023$ and our t-value = 5.4. The t-value is larger than the critical value (2.306) figured in Student's table at the intersection of the line denoting the number of paired data minus 2 (df = 8) and the column denoting the limit of statistical significance (P = 0.05); P-value < 0.001.

$$t = \frac{P_0 - 0}{\sqrt{variance\ P_0}} \tag{2.94}$$

$$Variance\ P_O = \frac{\left(\frac{Sy}{Sx}\right)^2 - Po^2}{(n-2)} \tag{2.95}$$

The first two lines in Table 2.29 show the model coefficients. As the b1 coefficient is just an expected mean effect, we have to calculate a 95% CI around it. View the small sample size, the latter is not calculated using the critical Z value (1.96) but the corresponding t-value shown above (2.306) = b1 ± (t) Se. The upper and lower boundaries of the 95% CI will be equal to 0.46 to 1.145. The interpretation is straightforward: each hour increase in operative time increases the amount of blood loss by an average amount of 0.8 dL (95% CI = 0.46–1.15 dL). We are 95% confident in this result, with a small probability of chance (P < 0.001).

The Constant (b_0 Coefficient)

The same rules apply, the statistical significance of the difference between the interception of the y axis by the slope (b_0) and zero ($b_0 - 0 = 1.98 - 0$) is tested by a regular Student's test and the resulting t-value (t = **b_0**/Se = 1.98/0.82 = 2.418) was larger than the same critical value presented in Student's table (2.306). We can conclude that

Table 2.29 Simple regression. Effect of switching predictor and outcome on model coefficients

Model		B coefficient	Se	95% CI	t-value	P value	Coefficient B (standardized)
1	Duration of surgery	0.804	0.148	0.46–1.15	5.42	0.001	0.887
	Constant	1.98	0.82	0.09–3.87	2.42	0.042	–
2	Amount of blood loss	0.978	0.18	0.56–1.39	5.42	0.001	0.887
	Constant	−0.87	1.15	−3.52 to 1.78	– 0.76	0.47	–

1 = first scenario: the effect of the duration of surgery (predictor) on the amount of blood loss (outcome), 2 = second scenario: the effect of the amount of blood loss (predictor) on the duration of surgery (outcome)

a significant part of the variability is still unexplained by regression and other variables have to be introduced in the model to explain this remaining part; (P = 0.042). Table 2.29 equally gives the upper and lower limits of the 95% CI of (b_0) along the 2nd line.

3. *The Regression Equation*

There is a statistically significant positive effect of the duration of surgery on the amount of blood loss (P < 0.001). This statistically significant result allows us to pose essential questions concerning our sample and the population of concern: how much can we rely on the precision of the slope; i.e., is the slope of the sample close to its "true" value in the population? We can assign to our regression slope an IC that has a 95% chance to include the "true" value by the ordinary equation: Po ± t Se = 0.46 to 1.145. There is a 95% chance each hour increase in the operative time will increase blood loss between 0.5 and 1.1deciltres. If the number of paired data is large (n > 30), the t-value in the equation can be replaced by a z-value of (1.96). The smaller is the value of Se, as compared to that of the slope, the more precise the slope would be.

Assuming that the association is linear, it supposes that the dependent variable increases or decreases by a fixed amount for each unit increase or decrease in the predictor. Consequently, a further application is to try to predict the amount of blood loss (y) from a given duration of surgery (x). As an example, what would be the amount of blood we have to prepare

for a patient whose expected duration of surgery is 4 h? Expected mean blood loss (95% CI) in dl. = 1.982 ± 0.804 × duration of surgery in hours = 1.982 ± 0.804 × 4 = 5.2 (2 − 8.5) dL. Bearing in mind that the regression equation gives an expected average, we have to take into consideration the expected variability around the average, especially if the study that we rely upon has a small sample size or a large Se. Acknowledging the lower and upper limits of the 95% CI of both intercept and slope, the surgeon has to request the preparation of the "expected average volume" of 5.2 dl., but he has to note that the needed amount may be as low as 2 dL and as high as 8.5 dl.

The equation can only be applied to "comparable": patient population, type of surgery, operating surgeons, hospital facilities, etc. We have to be cautious and respect the studied limits of the predictor: between 2 and 9 h. Outside this range, the paired data may get more dispersed than before, significantly changing the slope's direction and intercept position, giving a different regression equation. Imagine that surgeons get tired with prolonged durations (x) and become less careful doing hemostasis, resulting in more blood loss (y); compared to the situation where they were operating within more reasonable time limits.

4. *Switching Predictor and Outcome*

Suppose that the researchers would like to answer a different question: what was the duration of surgery (x) that necessitated a specific amount of blood (y)? As there is only one predictor and one dependent variable, the correlation between the two variables (r) and its squared value (R^2 or RSS/TSS) denote how much predictor explains outcome is the same. Similarly, the standardized coefficient Beta measuring how much predictor affects outcome in "the common" units of standard deviation (0.887) is also the same. However, the unstandardized coefficient b and its 95% CI expressing the effect in the predictor's units are different (0.978; 0.562–1.394) as well as the "new" regression slope that intercepts the "new" (y) axis at a "new" position (−0.87) are different, of course (see Table 2.29).

It worth noting that in simple regression with a single predictor and a single outcome, the b_1 coefficient of the predictor can be obtained from (r) by the equation: $b_1 = r$ ($sd_{predictor}/sd_{outcome}$); where $sd_{predictor}$ and $sd_{outcome}$ are the Sd of predictor and outcome respectively "Eq. 2.96". In the first example, where the duration of surgery was the predictor, $b_1 = 0.89$ (2.26/2.49) = 0.8. In the second model where blood loss is the predictor, $b_1 = 0.89$ (2.49/2.26) = 0.98. The standard deviations used here were previously calculated in Table 2.25.

$$b_1 = r \frac{S_{predictor}}{S_{outcome}} \qquad (2.96)$$

What Should be Reported

We have to report the descriptive statistics: mean and Sd of each variable (Table 2.25). Inferential statistics include r, R-square, the model fit and its P-value (Table 2.28), the regression equation and the statistical significance of the predictor (Table 2.29). We may point to normality, independence and linearity being tested, especially in small sample size. Finally, effect size can be reported as R^2 (0.786), the b coefficient (0.804), the standardized coefficient Beta (0.887). The following equation calculates the standard deviation of regression and, in our example, it equals 1.067 "Eq. 2.97".

$$S_{regression} = \sqrt{(S_y)^2 - (P_0)^2 (S_x)^2} \qquad (2.97)$$

Conditions of Application

Regression is demanding. Many assumptions have to be verified before the analysis. Moreover, other assumptions are only verified during the analysis, such as analysis of residuals. Samples should be drawn at random, and a minimum of 20 observations must be recorded for each independent predictor included in the model. Observations should be independent. Both variables must be normally distributed; otherwise, residuals must have a normal distribution with few outliers, if any. Independent and predictor should be strongly correlated, with a minimum r value of 0.3. Other assumptions include linearity and homoscedasticity. Linearity assumes a straight-line relationship between each of the two variables, provided that it does not change in sign or in magnitude during the studied intervals. Homoscedasticity or homogeneity of variance assumes that data is equally distributed about the regression line. Verification of assumptions is facilitated by statistical software packages such as IBM-SPSS. Regression is robust, and the larger our sample size, the more the application conditions are expected to be fulfilled.

We have shown that the regression equation can be used to predict the outcome (y_{fit}) and the residuals (y_{resid}), which are the differences between observed and predicted outcomes (y − y_{fit}). We have also shown that to compare outcomes; they have to be standardized by being divided by the proper Sd. Hence, besides the predicted and residual values, we can also calculate the standardized predicted (Z_{pred}) and standardized residual (Z_{resid}) outcome values. Remember that a standardized value is how many standard deviations is a value away from its mean = (value − mean value)/Sd. Note that the mean and Sd of predicted blood amount are: 6 and 2 dl, as calculated in column 9 of Table 2.27. Similarly, the mean and Sd of residual blood loss are 0 and 1.04, as shown in column 10 of the same table. Let us verify the calculation of the first case as an example. The unstandardized predicted (y_{fit}) = $b_0 + b_1 x = 1.982 + 0.804 \times 2$

= 3.59. The unstandardized residual $(y_{resid}) =$ $(y - y_{fit}) = 3 - 3.59 = -0.59$. The $Z_{pred} = (y_{fit} -y_m)/Sd = (3.59 - 6)/2 = -1.2$. The $Z_{resid} =$ $(y_{resid} -0)/Sd = -0.59/1.04 = -0.57$.

We have executed those calculations for explanatory purposes and to know the real meaning. Afterward, we do not need to make them by hand as they are generated by most statistical software packages upon request.

1. Checking on Normality

The normality of data can be visualized on a histogram. A statistically non-significant Shapiro–Wilk test is a good indicator of normally distributed data (see Sect. 1.4.3). In our example, both variables were found to be normally distributed. Strict normality is not a must, and the normality of residuals is sufficient for many statisticians.

2. Checking on Linearity

Concerning linearity, the first and simplest thing to do is to look at the scatter plot, inspect the relationship between (x) and (y) and fit a regression line; this will give a rapid (rough) idea about the possibility of a linear relationship. A more formal test plots the standardized residuals (on the

y-axis) versus standardized predicted values (on the x-axis) to show whether the residuals increase in size as predicted values increase, which is a good indicator of linearity (Fig. 2.9).

3. Analysis of Residuals

We can test the independence and homoscedasticity (equality of variances) of residuals in the same way by plotting the standardized residuals on the (y-axis) and the standardized predicted values on the x-axis. As shown in Fig. 2.9, the data distribution looks like a rectangle, and most points are between −3 and + 3 on either axis. In our example, IBM-SPSS calculated a quite acceptable small range of standardized residuals between −1.6 and 0.9.

Normality of residuals can be visualized by a normal P–P plot of standardized regression residuals, with expected cumulative probability on the y-axis and observed cumulative probability on the x-axis. (Fig. 2.10) The more data points follow the line, the more the distribution of the observed unstandardized residuals is normal. Our small sample size is responsible for the remarkable deviation of points from the line. Similarly, the normality of unstandardized residuals can be visualized by plotting

Fig. 2.9 Checking on independence and homoscedasticity of residuals

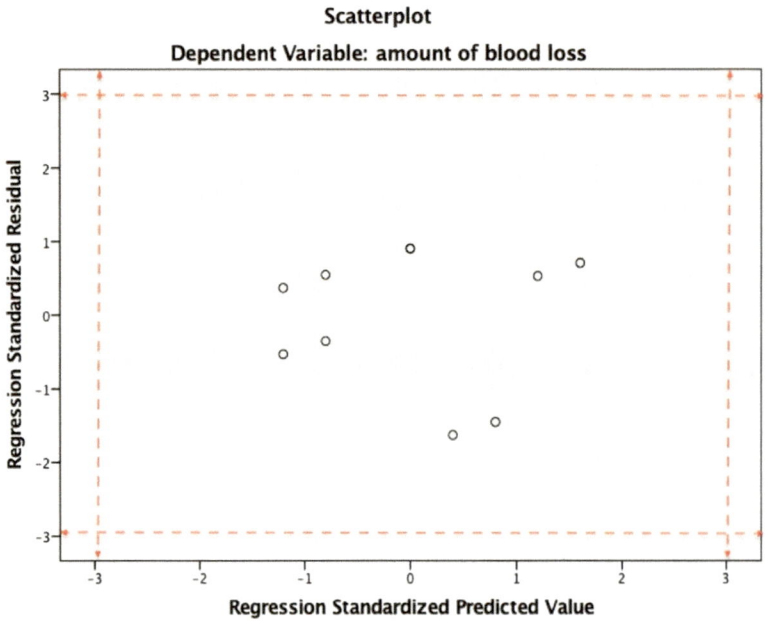

Fig. 2.10 Checking on normality of residuals

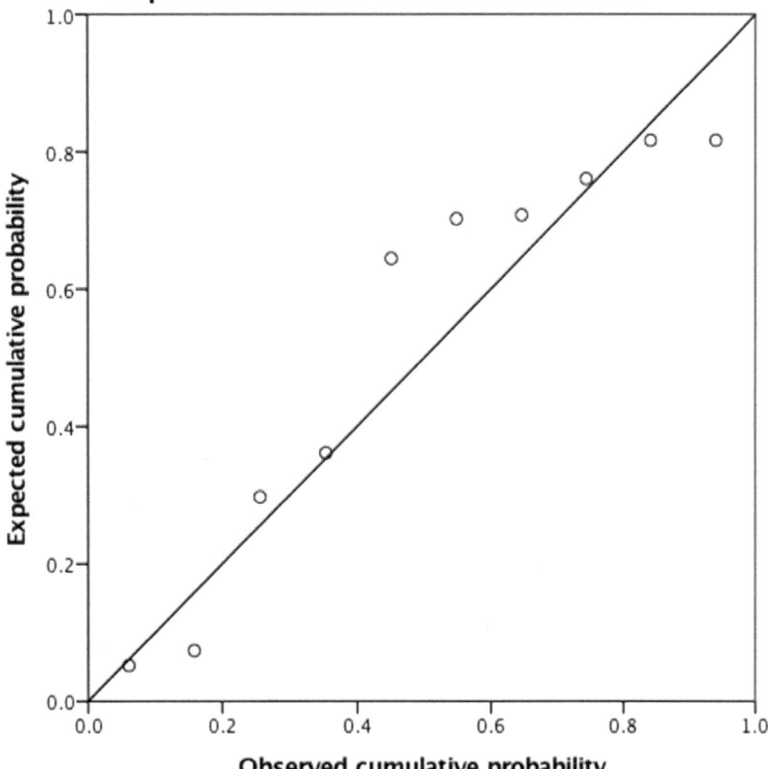

unstandardized residuals on the (y-axis) and the unstandardized predicted values on the x-axis, but it is not needed as it will give the same results obtained by the standardized residuals.

Finally, the normality of either standardized or unstandardized residuals can be formally tested by the Shapiro–Wilk test, as we already tested our observed data. A statistically non-significant Shapiro–Wilk test is a good indicator of data being normally distributed.

4. Checking on Outliers

We have shown the leverage point of a trend line in the mean point of both variables ($m_{x,y}$) (see Fig. 2.3). An outlier is a point with either extremely high or extremely low value. The more it is away from the mean, the more it influences this leverage, negatively affecting the regression model. The higher the leverage effect of the outlier, the higher the residuals in the model. An influential outlier has to be identified and is better removed from the analysis. The presence of too many outliers >10% questions our model itself.

Cook's distance is a method used to find those influential outliers among predictor variables. An outlier is said to be influential if the variability (Sd) is significantly changed when removed. The method removes the outlier and re-calculates regression. There is no general agreement on the critical limit of Cook's distance for the value to be removed. Suggested critical Cook's distances include 1, three times the mean value, larger than 4/sample size. In our example, the largest Cook's distance was 0.016, and hence, none of the paired values was removed.

5. Correlation Between Predictor and Outcome

Predictor strongly correlated with outcome, with an (r) value of 0.79, which is much larger than the minimum required r > 0.3

In the context of bivariate statistical analysis, the relation between two quantitative variables can either be answered as a question of correlation or regression. Pearson's correlation coefficient (r) describes the magnitude and direction of a linear relationship for normally distributed variables. Spearman's rank coefficient is the non-parametric alternative for other distributions than normal. Both tests should not be extrapolated as measures of agreement or indicators of causality.

Regression describes the dependence of one outcome variable on another predictor or explanatory variable but not the reverse. ANOVA partitions the total outcome variability into the part explained by the predictor and a remaining residual part and tests the statistical significance of each partition. The ratio explained to total variability expresses the effect of the predictor on the outcome. It is called the coefficient of variation, and it equals R square. Provided a proper study design and a large sample size, the regression equation permits interpretation of causality in the actual study and prediction of outcome in future studies.

2.7 Inference on Survival Curves

2.7.1 Introduction: Assumptions and Definitions

Time to event studies focus on the time that elapsed between the beginning of the study (e.g., the day of surgery) and the event's occurrence (e.g., hospital discharge). It has a different meaning from the occurrence of the event itself. A patient discharged two days after surgery is different from another patient who was discharged two weeks later. Something happened in those two weeks that need to be investigated. If the event of concern is mortality, survival analysis will study the probability of being free from mortality at a specific time. For example, the probability that a patient will be still alive 20 years after coronary bypass surgery (CABG). We are usually accustomed to using "survival analysis" not only as an indicator of "survival" over time but as an example of the time till the occurrence of "the event." It can be an adverse event, such as being free from stroke, tumor recurrence, or need for rehospitalization, or a good event, such as successful in vitro fertilization. In this section, all that we mend to apply to "survival" is readily applicable to any other event, as long as it remains easier to talk about "survival" rather than be free from another particular event at a certain period [42].

In time to event analysis, patients are categorized as those who experienced the event and censored cases. The latter are those patients who did not experience the event during the follow-up period, cases lost to follow-up, and patients who were cut off from the study by an accident or another competitive event, like death from another disease. As we will show in the next section, the power of the time-to-event study is its ability to estimate the survival probability from the information collected in all cases, whether they developed the event or have been censored [42] (see Sect. 2.7.2).

Another point is that patients are recruited in the study overtime and never in the same day, of course. As patients cannot be followed-up indefinitely but till the end of the study, which is a fixed date; not all patients will be followed for the same duration and hence, not all of them will be at the same risk of experiencing the event. It is mainly because of those 2 points (patient censoring and variable follow-up periods) that we cannot use ordinary statistical tests such as Chi-square or Student's tests to compare groups of patients because those tests cannot take censored data into account and hence, special tests were put to take those points into consideration during the analysis [42].

Assumptions

We have to make three main assumptions to carry on the analysis [42]. Because of the patients being censored, we have to assume that censored patients will have the same prognosis as those still followed in the study, and hence, we should always thoroughly investigate if censoring was not related to the event of concern. For example, to investigate whether the patient is lost to follow-up simply because he was getting well and did not feel that he should seek medical advice anymore. A patient may be censored for being a victim of a car accident (competitive event) or, he experienced the event of concern and died?

The second assumption is that the event really happened and is not just being discovered at the specified time. Follow-up has to be as meticulous and as complete as possible. Mixing true "event dates" with "false supposed" dates gives the wrong answer to the main question: did the event occur, and when did this happen?

Because patients are followed up for variable periods, another assumption is that all those patients have to have the same prognosis, regardless of follow-up duration and when they were recruited for the study. Here comes the importance of ensuring the stability of studied events and prognostic factors over time. Put it this way: patients with short follow-up periods have the same prognosis as patients with longer follow-up durations.

Definitions

The analysis of a time-related event is best calculated by forming a table & is best presented in the form of a curve, e.g., survival curves. Three methods will be discussed in this section, together with their corresponding indications and advantages. As an example, we will give the analysis of survival expectancy, which, as we have mentioned, could be replaced by any other event related to time without any change in the method of analysis or the graphic presentation. Before discussing the methods of life table analysis, specific terms should be defined:

- The Date of origin (O) is the chosen date for the beginning of the study, e.g., date of randomization, date of clinical diagnosis, date of the operation, date of hospital discharge, etc. Each patient has his "own date of origin" that notes when he participated in the study.
- The last date (L) at which we have contacted the patient.
- The patent's state (S) at the last date should also be noted: either having the event or is being censored (did not have the event, lost to follow-up, experienced a competitive event).
- The participation time (P) is the time of participation of every patient in the study, i.e., the time that elapsed between the date of origin (O) & the last date (L).
- The end date of study (E) is the pre-planned specified end date of the study. Events occurring after the end date are neglected, which means that if a patient dies (experiences the event) after the end date of the study, he will be considered as being alive (free from the event).

In practice, all we need to know to make the analysis is to know for each patient: his participation time (P) and his state (S) at last date. Put it in another way: we need to have two information for every patient: how long did he participate in the study and, did he experience the event or he has been censored? Depending on the expected rate of the event, the investigator usually divides the total period of his study (T) into the accrual period (A) and the follow-up period (F). The accrual period in which we only recruit legible patients. It starts by the first patient being recruited and ends by including all required participants, and hence, no patients should be recruited afterward. The follow-period (F) to monitor and record the events in those patients.

2.7.2 Kaplan Meier Method

Patients have unequal participation times. Unless he experiences the event, a patient can be censored in a way or another. Whether by being lost to follow-up, experiencing a competitive event, or safely reaching the end of the study. We will use mortality as an example of the event. The Kaplan–Meier method [43] divides the total time of the study (T) into successive intervals; each includes all patients living at the beginning of the interval and ends just before the occurrence of one or multiple mortalities at a specific time (t). Consequently, the first interval starts with the beginning of the follow-up period and ends just before the first mortality at a specific time (t_1). Note that no patient dies in the first interval because it ends just before the occurrence of the first death and hence, the probability of survival (being free from the event) of the first interval is always 100%.

The second interval follows the first one, and hence it starts just before the occurrence of first mortality and ends just before the occurrence of the second mortality. The third interval starts before the occurrence of the second mortality and ends just before the third mortality, and so on. Finally, the last interval begins just before the last event and ends with the longest participation time (P).

We have to note a few important details: First, mortality or any other biological event usually occurs at random, and hence, Kaplan Meier intervals are unequally spaced by default. Second, we have to note that a Kaplan Meier interval begins before the occurrence of mortality and not with it, and hence, a patient who dies during this interval was still living at its beginning. Third, an interval can also begin and end just before the occurrence of multiple mortalities recorded simultaneously. Consequently, the number of intervals equals the number of times we had one mortality or simultaneous multiple mortalities. We have to add the first interval that does not include any mortality by default. The following example will clarify those details.

The Example

A small group of 5 patients was operated upon for a malignant tumor of the pleura (mesothelioma). All patients benefited from extra pleural pneumonectomy without an operative mortality. The researchers were interested in studying intermediate-term survival after tumor resection. The day of surgery was set as the date of origin (O), and follow-up was planned to continue till the end of June 2020 (E). Table 2.30 shows the date of origin (O) of each patient, the date when the patient was last seen (L), his state at that date as well as at the end of study (S), patient participation time (P = O − L), and total time (T = O − E). Patients were arranged in ascending order of their participation times. For example, patient (I) was the first to be operated upon on 5/2018, he was alive when last seen one month later at 6/2018 but was lost of follow-up, and hence, he will be considered censored. Patient II was operated upon on 4/2019 and died from the disease four months later, on 8/2019. Note that if this patient has died from a car accident or other competitive event, he will be considered censored and not mortality. Patients III and V were operated upon on 10/2019 and 12/2018 and were still living till the end date on 6/2020. Hence, both patients were considered censored. Their respective follow-up periods: were 8 and

Table 2.30 Survival data of five patients undergoing surgery for mesothelioma

Patient number	Date of origin (O)[a]	Last date (L)	State at last date (S)	State at end date (S)	Participation time (P)[b]	Total time (T)[b]
I	5/2018	6/2018	Living	Lost	1	31
II	4/2019	8/2019	Dead	Dead	4	8
III	10/2019	6/2020	Living	Living	8	14
IV	9/2018	9/2019	Dead	Dead	12	27
V	12/2018	6/2020	Living	Living	18	18

a = date of surgery, b = time in months

18 months. Finally, patient IV was operated in 9/2018 and died from the disease eight months later on in 9/2019. Similarly, if this patient has died from a competitive event, he should have been considered a censored case and not mortality.

The Kaplan–Meier method assumes that all patients have the same prognosis, regardless of their follow-up durations and particular recruitment dates. Hence, the date of origin (O) and date of last visit (L) are only used to calculate the patient's participation time (P = O − L). Under the same assumptions, the quality of information collected from short participation periods is the same as that reported from extended periods. In practice, data presented in Table 2.30 are reduced to the following three pieces of information: the total number of patients at the beginning of the study (5), their respective participation times (1, 4, 8, 12, and 18 months) and state (2 mortalities and 3 censored cases). The specific reasons for being censored have to be included in our report. However, all censored cases are managed the same during the calculations.

As previously shown, the number of Kaplan Meier intervals is equal to the number of times we had an event (or multiple events occurring at the same time), in addition to the first interval. As we had two mortalities occurring at two different timings (patient number II at four months and patient number IV at 12 months), our analysis will include three intervals. If those two events had coincided (e.g., both mortalities were recorded at four months) or if one of the two patients was lost due to a competitive event, we would have a total of 2 intervals only. If both mortalities were due to competitive events, we would have a single interval and a 100% survival; i.e., all patients were free from mortality due to the disease and not due to any other cause, of course.

Figure 2.11 shows the diagrammatic presentation of our data. We had three intervals; each is included between two vertical dotted red lines. The number of patients being alive (event-free) at the beginning of each interval is shown between brackets. By definition, the first interval starts with the inclusion of all (5) patients and ends just before the occurrence of the first death, and hence, the first interval of any Kaplan Meier analysis will always end with zero mortality and 100% survival. Put it another way, the number of patients who were at risk of developing the event

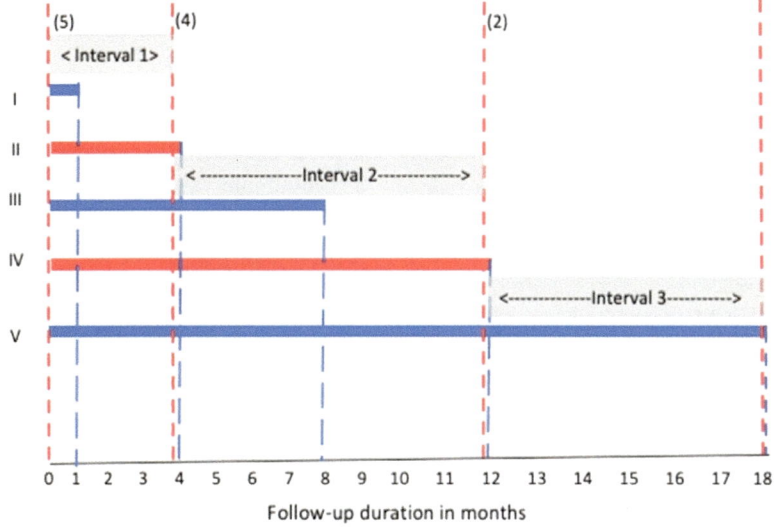

Fig. 2.11 Kaplan–Meier intervals. Data is reported in Table 2.30. There were three intervals, each included between two vertical red lines. Numbers between brackets are the number of patients alive at the beginning of each interval. Vertical blue lines point to the participation times of the five patients. Red horizontal bars are the participation times of the two mortalities (patients II and IV). Blue horizontal bars are the participation times of the three censored cases (patients I, III, and V)

during the first interval (n) is the total number of patients included in the study, i.e., five patients. As the first interval ends just before the occurrence of the first event, the number of patients who develop the event during the first interval (e) is zero. Hence, all patients survive the first interval, by definition.

We will define each of the following two intervals and calculate the same information: number of patients at risk of developing the event (n) and number of patients who did experience the event (e). The former is the number of alive patients at the begging of the interval, of course. Patients whose participation times ended before the beginning of the second interval by being either dead or censored are not considered as being at risk of mortality. In consequence, patient I, whose participation time ended after one month of surgery, will not be considered at risk of mortality in the second interval, which begins "just before" the occurrence of the first mortality at four months and hence, n = 4. Out of the latter, only one patient died at four months, and hence, e = 1. The third interval begins "just before" the occurrence of the second mortality at 12 months, and, as it is the last interval, it ends with the most extended follow-up period at 18 months. The number of patients at risk equals those who were at risk in the previous interval (4) minus who died (patient II who died at four months) or were censored (patient number II whose participation time ended at eight months) before the beginning of the third interval. Consequently, only two patients remained at risk of mortality during the third interval (n = 2) and, out of the latter, only one patient died at 12 months (e = 1).

In the Kaplan Meier method, an interval neither begins with the occurrence of an event nor ends with the occurrence of the next one, which is a common erroneous belief. As shown in Fig. 2.11, the vertical red line denoting the beginning of the second interval is just before (precedes) the vertical blue line indicating the occurrence of the first mortality at four months. Similarly, the vertical red line denoting the beginning of the third interval is just before (precedes) the vertical blue line indicating the

occurrence of the second mortality at 12 months. By definition, the first interval begins with the beginning of follow-up at the time (0), and the last interval ends with the most extended follow-up period at 18 months. In consequence, the first interval can be presented as [0, 4[to show that the first interval includes all patients since the beginning of follow-up at the time (0) and ends just before the occurrence of the first mortality, at four months; i.e., the first mortality is not included in the first interval.

Similarly, the second interval can be presented as [4, 12[and the third as [12, 18[. The former means that the second interval will include all patients whose participation times are at least four months and excludes events that occurred strictly at 12 months. The latter means that the third interval will include all patients whose participation times are at least 12 months and exclude events that occurred strictly at 18 months.

The Equation

Suppose that n_i is the number of patients living at the beginning of a given interval. (n_1) = the number of living patients at the first interval, which begins by the time (0) and ends just before the occurrence of the first mortality at four months. (n_2) = the number of living patients at the beginning of the second interval and n_3 = number of living patients at the beginning of the third interval, etc. Suppose that (e_i) is the number of patients experiencing the event during a specific interval. As no events occur during the first interval, e_1 = is always equal to zero; e_2 = number of events in the second interval, e_3 = number of events in the third interval etc. The probability of being free from the event (alive) during a specific interval is called the survival probability (SP). It is equal to the proportion of patients who remained alive during the interval $(n_i - e_i)$ to the total number of patients (n_i) exposed at risk of the event (alive) at the beginning of the interval = $(n_i - e_i)/n_i$ "Eq. 2.98". Note that because the first interval ends by definition just before the occurrence of the first event, its survival probability is always equal to 1 (100%): $SP_1 = (n_1 - 0)/n_1 = n_1/$

$n_1 = 1$. We proceed by calculating the survival probability of each of the following intervals: SP_2, SP_3, etc. In conclusion, each SP represents the probability of a patient remaining alive during an interval, provided that he was alive at its beginning.

$$SP_i = \frac{n_i - e_i}{n_i} \qquad (2.98)$$

Survival analysis is mended to calculate the survival probability of all patients, whether living at the beginning of each interval (SP) or censored during follow-up. We have to calculate a cumulative probability (CP) for all patients: whether they are still living or have been censored. The following example better explains the meaning of the cumulative probability (CP). Suppose that ten persons applied for a job opportunity ($n = 10$) and they have to pass two interviews to get it. Failure in the interview will be the adverse event that they want to avoid (e), of course. Five were eliminated out of the ten candidates who presented to the first interview ($n_1 = 10$) ($e_1 = 5$). Consequently, the probability to present to the second interview $SP_1 = (n_1 - e_1)/n_1 = (10 - 5)/10 = 50\%$. The remaining five candidates who are still at risk of elimination presented to the second interview ($n_2 = 5$), four were eliminated ($e_2 = 4$), and one got the job. In other words, $SP_2 = 4/5 = 20\%$. The question is, what was the probability of getting the job in the first place? It is 10%: one out of the ten candidates will get the job. How was this 10% calculated? It was the product of the two survival probabilities: $SP_1 \times SP_2 = 0.5 \times 0.2 = 0.1\,(10\%)$. As previously mentioned, probabilities are cumulated by multiplication and not by addition and the cumulative probability (CP) that we are looking for is calculated by multiplying the probability to survive failure in the first interview (SP_1) by the probability to survive failure in the second interview (SP_2) $= 50\% \times 20\% = 10\%$ "Eq. 2.99". In other words, every candidate had a 10% chance of getting the job, which is the correct interpretation of cumulative probability.

$$CP = \frac{n_0 - e_0}{n_0} \times \frac{n_1 - e_1}{n_1} \times \frac{n_2 - e_2}{n_2}$$
$$\times \ldots \ldots \frac{n_i - e_i}{n_i} \qquad (2.99)$$

On the other hand, we can never guarantee that the interviewer will give the job to one out of each ten candidates. Sometimes all ten candidates may fail, and at other times, the interviewer may even recommend hiring two equally distinguished candidates if the company needs to expand. In biology, variability is the rule, and there is no exception. Hence, we have to calculate the variance of CP "Eq. 2.100" and assign a 95% CI to every biological value "Eq. 2.101".

$$var\ CP = CP^2 \times \sum \left[\frac{e_i}{SP_i}\right] \qquad (2.100)$$

$$95\%\ CI\ of\ CP = CP \pm 1.96\ \sqrt{var\ CP} \qquad (2.101)$$

- Interval $[0, 4[$

The interval $[0, 4[$ begins by the date of origin and ends just before the occurrence of the first death at four months. By definition, the first interval ends just before the first event; hence, both SP and CP will always be equal to 1. $SP_1 = (n_1 - e_1)/n_1 = (5 - 0)/5 = 1$. $CP_1 = SP_1 = 1$.

- Interval $[4, 12[$

The second interval begins just before the first death at four months (e_2) and ends just before the second death at 12 months. One has to note that patient number I, who was lost to follow up after one month, did not reach the begging of this interval, and hence, he was not among those considered at risk (alive) at the beginning of the interval. On the contrary, patient number II, although he died "at" four months, yet was living (at risk) at the beginning of the interval (just before four months). Consequently, the only patient who was not at risk at the beginning of the second interval was the one who was censored at one month, and hence, $n_2 = 4$. $SP_2 = (n_2 - e_2)/n_2 = (4 - 1)/4 = 0.75$. $CP_2 = CP_1 \times SP_2 = 1 \times 0.75 = 0.75$.

- Interval [12, 18[

The third interval begins just before the second death at 12 months and ends with the longest participation time at 18 months. Two patients only have reached this interval $n_3 = 2$. Three patients did not reach the third interval: the first patient who was lost to follow-up after one month, the patient who died on the four months, and the patient whose participation time ended (was censored) at eight months. All calculations are shown in Table 2.31. Moreover, at 18 months, the survival rate of the five patients is 37.5 + 56%, and the upper and lower limits of the confidence interval at 95% are +93.5 and −18.5 months, respectively. We have to note that the "unrealistic" 95% CI (wide interval and including negative probability) is due to the small sample size that was deliberately chosen to allow the reader to do the calculations by hand.

Graphic Presentation

As shown in Fig. 2.12, the survival curve is composed of successive horizontal lines (steps) that are better relayed by vertical rather than oblique lines to distinguish the Kaplan Meier graph from an actuarial survival curve. Interestingly, all patients are presented on the curve (open circles for dead patients and closed circles for living ones) at the time corresponding to their death, disappearance, or last contact. In the case of a large number of patients, the curve becomes overcrowded and loses this advantage. By adding the number of patients living at the beginning of each interval and the cumulative survival (Sd), the curve becomes complete, and the reader will not need to return to the text for further information.

The Interpretation

Unfortunately, a typical false interpretation of cumulative survival is that 37.5% of patients will be alive (free from the event) at 18 months, which is not valid. The cumulative survival means that every patient who participated in this study has a 37.5% to be alive at 18 months. The question of whether a particular patient will be

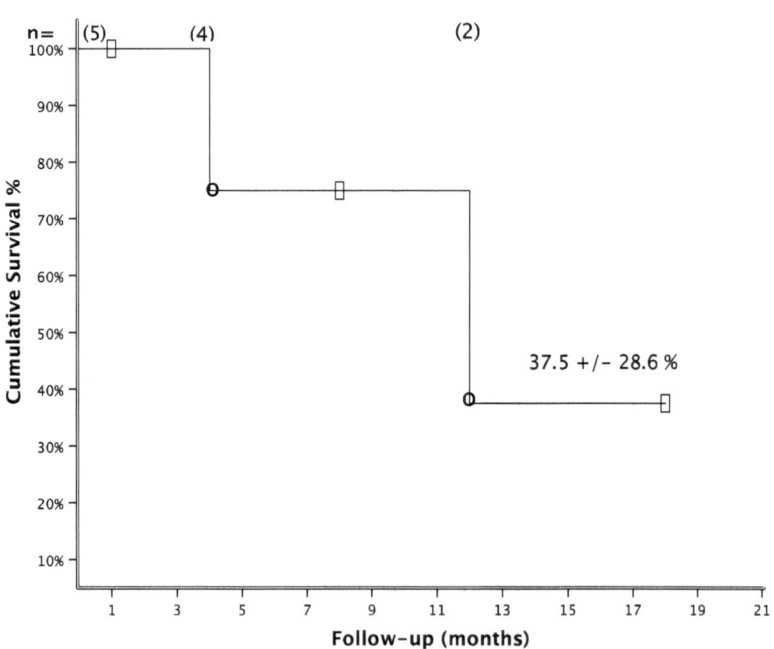

Fig. 2.12 Kaplan Meier curve for data reported in Table 2.30. n = numbers of patients living at the beginning of each interval. Rectangles represent censored cases; open circles represent mortalities. Cumulative survival is presented as mean ± standard error %

Table 2.31 Kaplan Meier analysis of data reported in Table 2.30

Interval	n	e	SP	CP	Var CP	95% CI
[0, 4[	5	0	$(5-0)/5$ $=1$	$5/5$ $=1$	–	–
[4, 12[	4	1	$(4-1)/4$ $=0.75$	0.75×1 $=0.75$	$0.75^2(1/12)$ $=0.047$	$0.75 \pm 1.96\sqrt{0.047}$ $=0.75 \pm 0.42.$
[12, 18[	2	1	$(2-1)/2$ $=0.5$	0.7×0.75 $=0.375$	$0.375^2(1/12+1/2)$ $=0.082$	$0.375 \pm 1.96\sqrt{0,086}$ $=0.375 \pm 0.56.$

n = number of patients alive at the beginning of each interval, e = umber of events (mortality), Sp = survival probability, CP = cumulative probability, Var CP = variance CP

censored remains alive or dead at 18 months is just a question of his luck, as long as he had his full opportunity, like everybody else. Once more, the small sample size does not permit us to interpret the CI. Suppose the sample was large and the Sd was 2.5%, the interpretation will be as follows: each patient entering the study has a 35–40% chance to be alive at 18 months.

Besides the descriptive part of the analysis, comparable patients from the same population will have the same survival probability, which is the predictive value of the analysis. Patients from different populations will show a different survival probability, which is the comparative part of the analysis.

What Should be Reported

We should report cumulative survival ($37.5 \pm 28.6\%$ at 18 months), mean and median survival with their respective 95% CI. View the non-parametric distribution of survival, most of the studies focus on reporting the median, which is when 50% of cases have experienced the event, leaving the other 50% free from the event. The median can be easily visualized on the curve by drawing a horizontal line that departs from the 50% cumulative event-free rate on the y-axis to hit the curve and then descends vertically to hit the median duration on the x-axis; which corresponds to 12 months in our example (Fig. 2.12). In our example, median survival = 12 ± 6.11 months. Kindly refer to Sect. 2.5.1.1 for calculation of a 95% CI around the median (see Sect. 2.5.1.1).

The mean survival can be reported as the mean duration of follow-up periods for all patients, whether those experiencing the event or censored, equal to $(1+4+8+12+18)$ $/5 = 8.6$ months. However, the mean survival reported in SPSS (12.25 ± 2.86 months) is estimated as the area under the survival curve: from the first interval (t_0), the maximum follow-up period (t_{max}), calculated according to Klein and Moeschberger [44]. Different software may use other calculation methods for mean, but the median is always the same.

Conditions of Application

We have previously discussed in our introduction, the assumptions necessary for the analysis. In short, the survival probability is the same for censored and uncensored subjects; the likelihood of the occurrence of the event is the same for the participants enrolled early and late; the probability of censoring is the same for different groups; finally, the event is assumed to occur at the defined time.

2.7.3 Actuarial Method

Unlike the Kaplan Meier method, time is divided into equal intervals, e.g., three months, six months, one year, or else. Every patient is placed in the interval corresponding to the length of his participation time.

For each interval, we must define the number of cases living at the beginning of the interval (l_i) and the number of cases whose participation times terminate before the end of the interval but without experiencing the event: i.e., censored patients (c_i). On the one hand, the way by which the actuarial method deals with censored cases is different from Kaplan Meier's analysis. The actuarial method considers censored cases to have a 50:50 chance to develop the event. In consequence, the number of patients at risk of the event during a specific interval (n_i) will be calculated as: the sum of all living patients (l_i) plus 50% of censored patients (c_i); (n_i) = (l_i) + ($c_i/2$). All censored patients (c_i) and those experiencing the event (e_i) during the interval will be excluded from the following interval, of course.

On the other hand, both methods disregard any event that occurs exactly at the end of a specific interval and amend it to the following interval. Any interval is symbolized by being included between 2 successive open brackets. For example, the interval between 3 and 6 months is symbolized as [3, 6[to show that the interval starts at three months and ends just before six months.

The Example

The difference in calculation between both methods can be clear if we use the same example shown in Sect. 2.7.2. The researcher usually chooses a "reasonable" constant length for his intervals, in concordance with the nature of the

disease and the total follow-up duration. We will take a 3-months interval, and hence, the first interval starts with the date of origin and ends just before three months, the second interval starts at three months and ends just before six months, and so on. Three patients were censored during the study; each will be counted as (1/2 case) that will be added to the number of living patients at the beginning of the corresponding interval. On the other hand, we had two events: one at four months and one precisely at 12 months. The first will be counted in the second interval [2, 6[. As per rule, the second event that occurred strictly at the end of the fourth interval has to be counted in the following fifth interval [12, 15[(Table 2.32).

The Equation

Although the actuarial method calculates SP and CP for each interval, it differs from the Kaplan Meier in a few calculation details. The way by which it partitions the intervals and deals with censored cases have been shown above. The equation used to calculate Var CP is also different "Eq. 2.102" however, the results of calculated cumulative probabilities by either method are pretty comparable, as shown in Tables 2.31 and 2.32.

Table 2.32 Actuarial analysis of data presented in Table 2.30

Intervals	l_i	c_i	n_i	e_i	SP	CP	Var CP
[0, 3[	5	1	$5 - 0.5 = 4.5$	0	1	1	–
[3, 6[	4	1	4	1	0.75	0.75	$0.75^2[0 + (1 - 0.75)/(4 \times 0.75)]$ $= 0.75^2[0 + 0.083] = 0.047$
[6, 9[	3	1	$3 - 0.5 = 3.5$	0	1	0.75	$0.75^2[0 + 0.083 + 0] = 0.047$
[9, 12[	2	0	2	0	1	0.75	$0.75^2[0 + 0.083 + 0 + 0] = 0.047$
[12, 15[	2	0	2	1	0.5	0.375	$0.375^2[0 + 0.083 + 0 + 0 + (1 - 0.5)/(2 \times 0.5)]$ $= 0.082$
[15, 18[	1	0	1	0	1	0.375	$0.375^2[0 + 0.083 + 0 + 0 + 0.5 + 0] = 0.082$
[18, 21[	1	1	$1 - 0.5 = 0.5$	0	1	0.375	$0.375^2[0 + 0.083 + 0 + 0 + 0.5 + 0 + 0]$ $= 0.082$

Data are derived from those presented in Table 2.30. Intervals = calculated in months follow-up after surgery, l_i = number of patients living at the beginning of the interval, c_i = number of patients censored during the interval, n_i = number of patients at risk at the beginning of the interval, e_i = number of patients experiencing the event during the interval, SP = survival probability (probability of being free from event (e)), CP = cumulative probability, Var CP = variance of CP

$$var\ CP_{actuarial} = CP^2 \times \sum \left[\frac{(1 - SP_i)}{n_i(SP_i)} \right]$$

$$(2.102)$$

Graphic Presentation

As shown in Fig. 2.13, each point represents an estimate of a cumulative probability (CP) at a particular time: the probability to "remain" alive (free from the event) during a time interval, provided that the patient was alive (at risk to develop the event) at the begging of that time. The number of living patients at the beginning of each interval is marked beside each point. Each point is connected to the preceding and the following by a straight line, forming the actuarial survival (event-free) curve. In addition, each patient is presented on the curve corresponding to his state being changed, i.e., the time when he developed the event or when he was censored. Each of the two states is represented by a different symbol, of course. As usual, the curve has to have a title, legends, and a 95% CI of CP.

The reader has to note that our example included only five patients for explanatory purposes and to permit an instructive hand calculation. Usually, an actuarial analysis has to deal with many patients, and tracing of the curve usually stops whenever the number of cases exposed to the risk of the event drops below 10.

The Interpretation

The interpretation is the same as for the Kaplan Meier analysis. The only exception is the fixed timing of intervals, compared to the timing related to an event's development in the Kaplan Meier method.

What Should be Reported

The same as in the Kaplan Meier method (see Sect. 2.7.2).

Conditions of Application

The same as in the Kaplan Meier method (see Sect. 2.7.2).

2.7.4   Comparison of Survival Curves

Theoretically, any biological event will happen one day or another and, the more patients are followed up, the more we encounter events (e.g.,

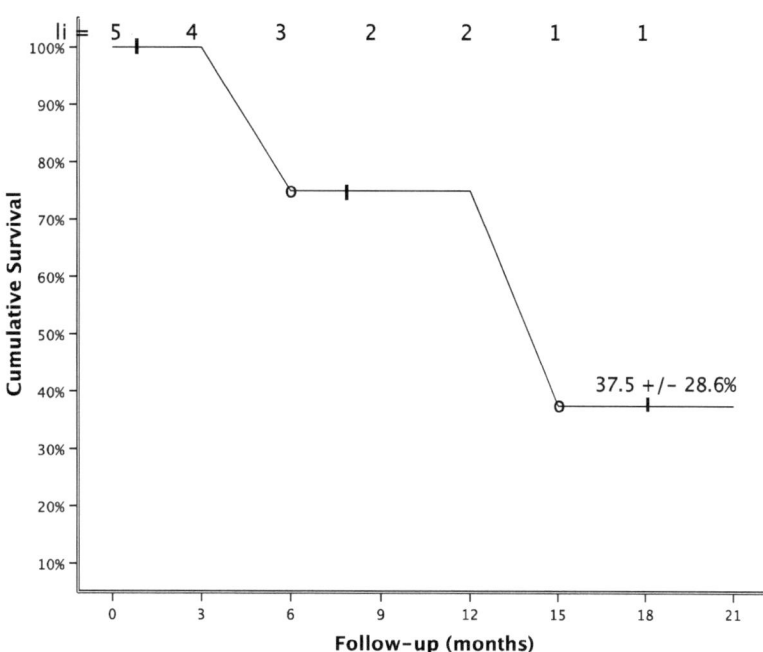

Fig. 2.13 Actuarial survival curve for data reported in Table 2.30. Open circles represent mortalities and "I" represent censored cases, li = number of patients living at the beginning of the interval

mortalities). Put it this way, survival data are positively (right) skewed and have to be analyzed by a non-parametric test. However, those tests that we described in Sect. 3.4. do not consider censored data, and hence, statisticians had to design special tests to analyze time to event studies.

2.7.4.1 The Log-Rank Test (Mantel–Haenszel or Cox–Mantel Test)

The most commonly known test is a Mantel–Haenszel, or log-rank test, proposed firstly by Mantel in 1966 [45] and then by Cox in 1972 [46]. As a result, some researchers refer to the procedure as to the Cox–Mantel test. In addition to the three assumptions of time to event analysis, the test assumes the proportionality of hazard among the compared groups (see Sect. 1.8.3) and is most powerful when the comparison is limited to two groups [47].

The Example

In order to permit hand calculation, we will propose a small study conducted to compare survival after resection of virulent pleural malignant tumor: mesothelioma. Sixteen patients were equally randomized to benefit from either surgery followed by adjuvants therapy (Group A) or surgery alone (Group B). The study endpoint was overall survival. Follow-up varied between 2 and 12 months, and it was complete. Only one patient in group A died at nine months, but all group B patients died at different timings. As shown in Table 2.33, patients are classified according to their participation times. The only second information needed for the analysis is whether the patient developed the event or has been censored.

The Equation

The equation is based upon comparing the number of "observed" events to those "expected" if the compared groups have similar events rates, i.e., under the null hypothesis. In other words, the aim will be to test the statistical significance of the relation between two qualitative variables: a 2-class qualitative variable (having the event or not) and another 2-class qualitative variable (group A or Group B). We invite the reader to refer to Sect. 2.3.1.2 to realize that Chi-square is the test of choice to evaluate the statistical significance of such association (see Sect. 2.3.1.2). However, the test has to consider that data is not collected only once at the end of the study. Observations are recorded and expectations are calculated, at each time interval when an event is observed. In other words, calculations are ranked by the intervals; which is behind the name of the test. Finally, a Chi-square test will compare the sum of all observations to the sum of all expectations in both groups.

We begin by classifying all patients in a single list, in increasing order of their participation times (Table 2.34). Note that we identified each patient by his group (Group A or Group B) and his state when last seen: either having the event (e) or is censored (c). Patients sharing the same participation time were placed in a single line, regardless of being censored or did develop the event. Namely, three patients in group B and two patients in group A shared the same follow-up duration of 9 months and, two patients in Group B and one patient in Group A shared the same follow-up duration of 11 months.

Let us revise how Kaplan Meier analyzes survival data. The first interval starts with the beginning of the study and ends just before the first event. Hence, by definition, there will be no

Table 2.33 Comparison of overall survival after resection of pleural mesothelioma

Treatment Group								
Group A	(2)	(4)	(7)	(8)	(9)	9	(11)	(12)
Group B	3	5	7	9	9	9	11	11

Values are follow-up durations in months, in an increasing order, values between brackets are those of censored cases, Group A = patients benefiting from surgery and adjuvant therapy, Group B = patients benefiting from surgery alone

Table 2.34 The Logrank test: comparison of overall survival after resection of pleural mesothelioma

Follow-up[a]	C_A	C_B	O_A	O_B	O_T	N_A	N_B	N_T	E_A	E_B
2	1	–	–	–	–	8	8	16	–	–
3			0	1	1	7	8	15	0.47	0.53
4	1									
5			0	1	1	6	7	13	0.46	0.54
7			0	1	1	6	6	12	0.50	0.50
7	1									
8	1									
9	1		1	3	4	4	5	9	1.78	2.22
11	1		0	2	2	2	2	4	1	1
12	1									
Total			1	8					4.21	4.79

a = duration of follow-up in months, C_A and C_B = number of censored patients in Group A and B. O_A, O_B and O_T = number of observed events in Group A, B, and total. N_A, N_B, and N_T = number of patients exposed at risk in Group A, Group B, and total. E_A and E_B = number of expected events in Group A and Group B. Expected events are only calculated when new events are produced: at 3, 5, 7, 9, and 11 months

observed or expected events during any first interval. On the other hand, each of the subsequent intervals will start just before an event (or multiple events occurring at the same time) and have to end just before the occurrence of the next event (events) at a different time. At each interval, we have to define the patients at risk of developing the event during the interval (t). They are those patients who did not develop the event before time (t) but are still living at that time. For example, a patient censored at nine months remains at risk during this month and till the occurrence of a new event.

As the number of patients at risk and the number of observed events differ from one interval to another, we must calculate the number of expected events for each time interval. Under the null hypothesis, patients are expected to have the same event-free rates. Hence, they are expected to have the same number of events at all-time intervals and regardless of being related to one group or another but in proportion to their sizes. For example, if one group is double the size of the other, we should expect twice as many events in the former compared to the latter. At each time interval (t), the number of expected events in each group (E_g) is calculated from the

total number of observed events (e) in proportion to the relative size of the patients at risk in this group. Provided that the number of patients at risk in one group is (N_g) and the total number of patients at risk is (N_t); the following equation calculates the number of events expected in this group "Eq. 2.103":

$$E_g = (e)\frac{N_g}{N_t} \qquad (2.103)$$

The first data line in Table 2.34 shows that one patient in Group A was censored (C_A) at two months. A censored case is a patient still at risk during the actual interval but is removed from the following one. Consequently, the number of patients at risk in Group B remained eight patients, despite the censored case. The second data line shows a single event observed at three months in a Group B $(O_{B1} = 1)$ patient, none in group B $(O_{A1} = 0)$, and no censored cases in either group. As Group A has already lost to follow-up one patient at two months, the number of patients at risk becomes seven in Group B patients but remains eight in Group A, with a total of 13 patients at risk in both groups. Under the null hypothesis, this single event is expected to be equally distributed between groups, in concordance with the relative group sizes. Applying Eq. 2.103, we expect to have 0.47 events in group A ($E_{A1} = 0.47$) and 0.53 events in group B ($E_{B1} = 0.53$). At four months, another patient is censored from group A, reducing the number of patients at risk in the following interval to six patients only.

At five months, we have six patients at risk in group A (two patients were censored at two and four months) and seven patients at risk in group B (one patient developed the event at three months). The total number of patients at risk is 13 cases. Another patient in group B developed the event during this interval ($O_{B2} = 1$) and none in group A ($O_{A2} = 0$). Under the null hypothesis, this event is expected to be distributed between both groups according to their relative sizes i.e., 6/13 = 0.46 events in group A ($E_{A2} = 0.46$) and 7/13 = 0.54 events in group B ($E_{B2} = 0.54$).

At seven months, six patients remained at risk in group A (two patients were censored at two and four months), but the number of patients at risk in group B is reduced to six patients (two patients already developed the event at three and five months). The total number of patients at risk is 12, six in each group, and hence any developing event is expected to be equally split between both groups ($E_{A3} = E_{B3} = 0.5$ events. However, we observed one event in group B ($O_{B3} = 1$) and none in group A ($O_{A3} = 0$).

At nine months, only four patients were at risk in group A. The other four cases were censored at two, four, seven and eight months (see column CA in Table 2.34). Three patients in group B already developed the event 3, 5, and 7 months after surgery, the number of patients at risk in group B is reduced to only five cases (see column OB in Table 2.34). Any future event is expected to be distributed in this 4:5 ratio between group A and B patients. While the observed numbers of events were ($O_{A4} = 1$) and ($O_{B4} = 3$), the expected number of events has to be ($E_{A4} = 4 \times 4/9 = 1.78$ events and, $E_{B4}\ 4 \times 5/9 = 2.22$. Note that the case in group A that was censored at nine months is at risk during this interval. It will be removed in the following interval.

At eleven months, Group A has lost six patients by censoring, and 1 case developed the event. Group B has lost the same number of cases. However, all developed the event. In other words, two patients remain at risk in each group, and hence any future event is expected to be equally distributed between both groups: $E_{A5} = E_{B5} = 0.5$ event. However, we observed two events in group B ($O_{B5} = 2$) and none in group A ($O_{A5} = 0$).

The last row of Table 2.34 shows the total number of observed and expected events in both groups: ($O_A = 1$), ($O_B = 8$), ($E_A = 4.21$), and ($E_B = 4.79$). Note that the total number of observed events (8 + 1) is equal to the total number of expected events (4.21 + 4.79). The study question is whether this balance (observed = expected) is maintained in each group or is it so unbalanced, suggesting that both groups are different from each other? Under the null hypothesis, there should be no difference between observed and expected events calculated for each group at each time interval. Any slight random difference can be attributed to chance. The alternative hypothesis is that the difference is significant and systematic, and hence, it may be attributed to the given regimen. As the difference enlarges, we become less confident in the null hypothesis till we reach a point where the probability of the null hypothesis being true is only 5% or lower. At this point, we reject the null hypothesis, and we adopt the alternative hypothesis that the difference is true and can be related to the type of regimen.

It is now the time to have a gentle reminder on how the Chi-square test works. We cannot sum crude differences simply because negative differences can annulate some positive ones, and hence, we have to square differences before summing them. Second, the test weights differences by their expected values to produce the final general Chi-square equation: $(O - E)^2/E$ (see Sect. 2.3.1.1). The log-rank test is a modified Chi-square test that calculates the weighted difference between the sum of observed (O_g) and the sum of expected values (E_g), in each group of patients (g) and, the Chi-square value is the sum

Fig. 2.14 The Logrank test. Comparison of the survival after resection of lung mesothelioma with (Group A) or without adjuvant therapy (Group B). Data presented in Table 2.33

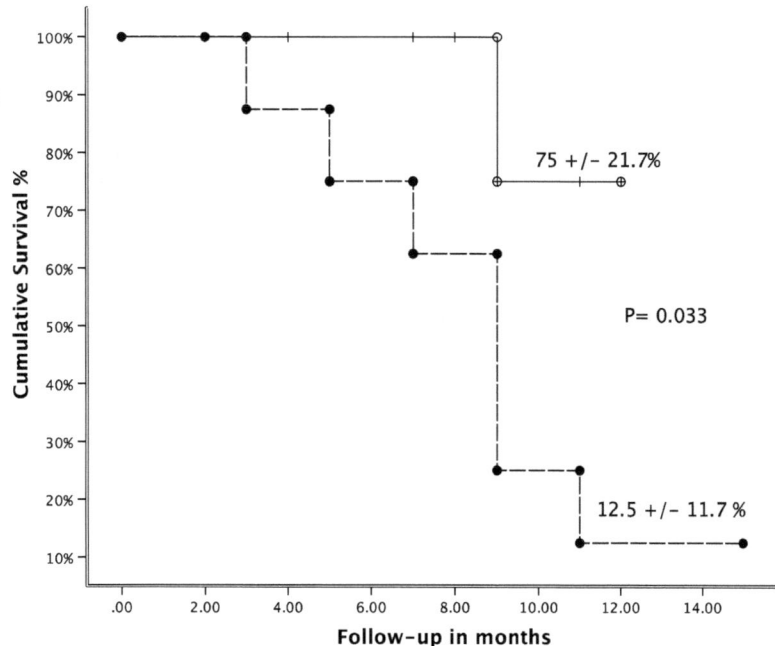

The Interpretation

Consulting the Chi-square table shows that, at one df (number of groups minus one: $g - 1 = 2 - 1 = 1$), a Chi-square statistic of 4.59 has a minimal probability of 3.3% due to chance [10]. Hence, we reject the null hypothesis and adopt the alternative hypothesis. If the study was randomized of sufficient sample size, adequately designed and conducted, and provided that the conditions of application of the test were fulfilled (see Sect. 2.7.4.1: conditions of applications); we can conclude that regimen A offers significantly

of values obtained in all groups "Eq. 2.104". Applying the equation to our example produces a large Chi-square value of $4.59 : (1 - 4.21)^2 / 4.21 + (8 - 4.79)^2 / 4.79$ "Eq. 2.105"

$$\chi^2_{log-rank} = \sum \frac{(O_g - E_g)^2}{E_g} \quad (2.104)$$

$$\chi^2 = \left[\frac{(O_A - E_A)^2}{E_A} + \frac{(O_B - E_B)^2}{E_B} + \cdots \frac{(O_i - E_i)^2}{E_i} \right] \quad (2.105)$$

better overall survival after resection of pleural mesothelioma; P = 0.033.

What Should be Reported

We have to report the cumulative survival rates of both groups, with the standard errors and 95% CI, mean and median survival with standard errors, and the Chi-square and P values of the Logrank test (Fig. 2.14). Statistical software usually automatically generates all this information. Although the test gives the statistical significance of the difference between survival curves, it does not report any effect size. Hence, it is advisable to report one, such as the relative risk of developing the event [48, 49]. The relative risk of mortality for a given group can be calculated as the observed proportion to the expected number of events. The relative risk between both groups can be calculated as the proportion between both relative risks [48]. In our example, the relative risk of mortality in group A patients = OA/EA = 1/4. 21 = 0.24 and the relative risk of mortality in group B patients = OB/EB = 8/4.79 = 1.67. The relative risk of mortality between both groups = 0.14.

Put it his way, the relative risk of mortality of the new treatment is only 14% of the relative risk of the classic treatment. Put it another way; the new regimen reduces the relative risk of mortality by 86%.

Conditions of Application

The test is based on the same three assumptions as of the Kaplan Meier survival curves. However, the test has three more assumptions. The left censoring has to be minimal; the hazard of the event has to be proportional, and the censored cases have to be equally distributed among groups [48, 49]. Left censoring occurs when the starting point of the study is not precisely identified. As an example, including patients early after being diagnosed, while others are included late. The "recorded" survival time of the latter will be shorter than the "true but unrecorded" time.

The Log-rank assumes that the hazard of the event is proportional among groups at all times during follow-up. This assumption can be visualized by the survival curves being parallel throughout the study, guarding a more or less constant distance. As shown in Fig. 2.14, both curves have a common point of departure at the beginning, and then they start to diverge from one another, which is quite normal because the survival of all first intervals is 100%. Moreover, the curves may converge and even touch each other at one or several points. Sometimes, they may even slightly cross one another then rapidly return to their original parallel course. All those patterns and limited variabilities are expected and accepted. On the other hand, we should not accept a frank crossing and the change of direction of the difference between both groups; e.g., being in favor of group A during the first part of follow-up then turning in favor of group B at another part [48].

On the other hand, our mini-example violated the assumption that censored cases are equally distributed between groups. None of the patients receiving the classic treatment was censored, compared to seven out of the eight patients who received the new treatment. Consequently, the statistical significance of our results is questionable and Tarone Ware test appears to be a suitable alternative (see Sect. 2.7.4.4).

2.7.4.2 The Adjusted (Stratified) Log-Rank Test

The Stratified log-rank test can be used to control for a factor, such as gender, categories of age or weight, the presence of a disease or other risk factor [50]. Strata can be either binary, or discrete qualitative variables, such as age groups.

The Example

We will forward the comparison of 2 or more survival rates, or any other time-related event, with adjustment on a 2-class qualitative variable. Suppose that we are analyzing survival rates in 2 treatment groups A and B, and we want to adjust on a 2-class qualitative variable (class 1 and class 2) known to affect survival.

The Equation

Instead of forming a single list in which we classify all patients by increasing participation time, we form two separate lists, one for each of the two classes of adjustment variable (e.g., class 1 and class 2). All calculations are those of a "regular" Log-rank test but are made separately for each of the two lists. Hence, for class 1 patients, we note the observed events in group A and group B, calculate the corresponding expected events, as well as the sums of observed (OA1 and OB1) and expected events (EA1 and EB1). The same is repeated with class 2 patients, and we end by calculating the sums of observed (OA2 and OB2) and expected events (EA2 and EB2). The total observed events with treatment A (OA = OA1 + OA2) and treatment B (OB = OB1 + OB2). The total expected events with both treatments are (EA = EA1 + EA2) and (EB = EB1 + EB2).

Put it this way, in a regular Log-rank test; calculations of expected events are made per interval; i.e., calculations are ranked by the intervals. In the adjusted log-rank test, adjustments are made inside each interval, i.e., calculations are double ranked by the adjustment variable, then by the interval. In the case of a "g" class adjustment variable, "g" lists are made instead of only two lists. The differences between total observed and total expected events are tested as demonstrated. Then we proceed as in the case of a regular Log-rank test by calculating the Chi-square value, the sum of all standardized differences calculated for (g) groups.

The Interpretation

Under the null hypothesis, the sum of observed values has to be equal to the sum of expected values in each group and should not differ from one group to another. The larger is the calculated Chi-square value, the less probable the null hypothesis is to be true. In order to reject the latter and conclude that survival curves are significantly different, the test value should be at least equal to or larger than the critical value present in the Chi-square table, at the intersection of the column of $P = 0.05$ and the line corresponding to $(g - 1)$ degrees of freedom.

However, the drawn conclusion is not the same. Suppose that our adjustment variable was the presence of diabetes mellitus, and treatment A showed significant superiority over treatment B. We can conclude that taking into consideration the factor diabetes; treatment A was superior to treatment B. In other words, treatment A was superior to treatment B, in both diabetics and non-diabetics, i.e. regardless of the patient was diabetic or not.

What Should be Reported

As in a regular Log-rank test Note that the adjusted test gives the statistical significance of the difference between survival curves but does not report any effect size. It is advisable to report one such as the adjusted relative risk of developing the event in both groups (OA/EA and OB/EB as well as in comparison of one group to the other [(OB/EB)/(OA/EA)].

Conditions of Application

Besides the usual conditions of applying a regular Log-rank test, another two assumptions have to be satisfied. The stratification variable should not be a confounder (i.e., should not be in the causal pathway between independent variable and time to event). Events are supposed to be equally distributed between strata.

2.7.4.3 The Generalized Wilcoxon (Gehan, Breslow) Test

The generalized Wilcoxon procedure does not require the assumption of the proportional hazards to be met [51]. As a result, some scientists use it as the alternative to the Mantel–Haenszel statistic. Studies indicated that the test might also yield more reliable results for the data with a constant hazard ratio. However, like the Log-rank test, the test becomes unreliable when the survival curves frankly cross [52].

The test is a modified log-rank to fit the situations where we believe that certain parts of the survival curves being compared are of greater interest than others. Hence, instead of assigning equal weight to each event at whatever time it occurs, like in a regular Log-rank test, more weight has to be assigned to those interesting parts. For instance, when surgery is compared to medical treatment, more events are expected with surgery during the early follow-up period. In contrast, events associated with medical treatment tend to occur at a later time. If a new treatment is known to be helpful to avoid early mortality, then it would be useful to compare the first part of the survival curves without paying too much attention to the subsequent time intervals. Since the weighting element in the Gehan test is the number of patients at risk in each group, the test gives more weight to the early failures, where the number of patients at risk is the highest.

The weighting element in the Gehan test is the number of patients at risk in each group and for each time point (Rt). Placing (Rt) in the original log-rank equation's denominator increases the test statistics, giving more weight to early intervals than late ones. Otherwise, the equation is similar to a log-rank test, where Ogt and Egt are the sums of observed and expected events, calculated for each category (g) and per time interval (t) "Eq. 2.106". The test is executed by many statistical software packages, such as SPSS.

$$\chi^2_{Gehan} = \sum \frac{\left(O_{gt} - E_{gt}\right)^2}{R_t^2 E_{gt}} \qquad (2.106)$$

2.7.4.4 Tarone Ware Test

When the survival curves cross, both the Mantel–Haenszel, and the Gehan test do not work well. The Tarone-Ware test can be used instead. The test emphasizes that failures happen in the middle but unlike the Log-rank test, it neither requires proportionality assumption nor equal censoring and works well for more than two groups [53]. Unlike the Gehan test, where the weighting element is the number of patients at risk in each group, Tarone Ware uses the square root of the number of individuals at risk. Hence, the weight given is greater than Log-rank but smaller than Gehan test [52]. We have used the Log-rank test to compare survival after resection of pleural mesothelioma with (Group A) and without adjuvant therapy (Group B) (Table 2.33). Although we have used the Log-rank test for comparison, the application conditions were not completely satisfied due to marked unequilibrated censoring and small sample size (Table 2.34). In this setting, the Tarone Ware test is a better alternative for not requiring equal censoring and working well with small groups [52]. Although the test produces a smaller Chi-square value (4.412) and a larger but still significant P-value (0.036), those results are much more credible than those produced by a non-verified Log-rank test. The test is executed by many statistical software packages, such as SPSS.

2.7.4.5 Harrington and Fleming Test Family

Preventive treatments may require some exposure before the appearance of the treatment effect. Consequently, events are expected to occur late in preventive clinical trials. Hazards are almost the same during the early period of the study, and the survival curves take a considerable time to diverge. In this setting, the Log-rank test that assumes proportionality of hazard throughout the study will not be the ideal test for the analysis, which may be the reason behind many

of those studies yielding non-significant results for being analyzed by the log-rank test [54].

Choosing a specific weight at a particular follow-up period is thus a crucial issue in practice. The Harrington and Fleming (F–H) test is the most flexible test for choosing weights "Eq. 2.107" [55]. Put it this way, the Gehan test weighs events by the number of patients at risk, giving more weight to early events. Tarone-Ware test weighs events by the square root of this number, giving more weight to events occurring in the middle. F–H is a family of tests that can assign different weights to events occurring at different periods. F–H weighs events by the Kaplan–Meier estimator of survival function itself: survival probability × cumulative probability = St (1 − St) (see Sect. 2.7.2), raised to the power a specific binomial parameter (p, q) that can be equal to zero or acquire any positive value (p, q > 0).

$$W^{pq} = St^p \times 1 - St^p \qquad (2.107)$$

By assigning different values to (p) and (q), more weight can be given to early events, events occurring in the middle, or late events. When p and q are equal, the test ensures equal distribution of weights on the whole study, and the F–H test becomes equivalent to the Log-rank test. If treatment is thought to impact earlier periods, then q is chosen to be (0) with increasing values of p to ensure more weight is given to earlier events. When p equals 0, increasing values of q ensure that more weight is placed on late events [52]. The test is mostly used in the latter situation, W^{0q} but raises two significant difficulties. First, the weight is now dependent on (q) that must be set before collecting the data. For example, by assigning 0 to (p), a zero weight is given to the early part of the study, where the number of subjects being at risk is the highest, and more weight is given to later periods where most of the events occur. In this case, assigning the quantities 1, 2, 3, or else to (q) gives significantly different weights to late events. Moreover, the weight given to (q) will largely influence sample size calculation too. A specific quantity will be dependent upon the literature review or the investigator's judgment. Recent simulation studies have shown that assigning 3 to q may be a general choice to test late effects [54].

In biology, variability is the rule, with no exceptions. The time to change a biological variable with the production of a new event is the interest of many clinical studies. The probability of a random event occurring at a specific time is practically nil, and calculations are usually made for an interval of time (see Sect. 1.8.3.2). The interval usually begins with the patient is being given a particular medication or is benefiting from a specific procedure. Then, it ends with either an adverse event (e.g., mortality or morbidity) or a good event (e.g., with the patient being cured). Kaplan Meier and Actuarial analysis are the most commonly used methods of predicting the cumulative probability of a particular patient free from an event up to a specific time. Both methods assume the proportionality of hazard and the independence of censoring from the events, each being recorded in its exact timing. They differ in dealing with censored data and partitioning of intervals but produce comparable overall results and survival (event-free) curves.

Because of the non-parametric distribution of random events and patients being censored, special statistical tests had to be designed to analyze censored data. The classic Log-rank test is the most commonly used for being simple. However, it requires numerous assumptions: mainly proportionality of hazard, equality of censoring, large samples, and a small number of groups. Modifications have been made to accommodate different situations. The Generalized Wilcoxon test gives more weight to events during early follow-up, while the Harrington and Fleming test is a good choice for events suspected at the end of the study. Tarone-Ware is robust, not requiring proportional hazard nor equal

censoring. It can work with small and multiple groups, and it is the test of choice when curves do frankly cross. Unfortunately, survival curves can neither estimate an effect size nor include predictors in the model, which can be complemented by the semi-parametric model of Cox regression analysis (see Sect. 3.6).

2.8 Choosing the Appropriate Bivariate Statistical Test

2.8.1 Introduction

Choosing the appropriate bivariate statistical test is dependent upon many factors including the study main hypothesis, study design and data [33].

2.8.1.1 Independence of Data

Data are said to be dependent (related) when they are collected from the same patient or matched groups of patients. The example is to compare the effects of two treatments A and B, given to the same patient, with a suitable washout period in between. As each paired information (effect of treatment A and effect of treatment B) is observed in the same patient, both are dependent on (related to) one another. Data collected from matched groups of patients or case–control studies are treated similarly [33].

In the case we assign the 2 treatments to 2 different groups of patients, the effect of treatment (A) given to the first group will be totally unrelated to that of treatment B given to the second group and hence, data collected from those unrelated groups are independent from one other. The variability of the response of the "same" patient receiving 2 treatments is expected to be smaller than that observed when those treatments are given to 2 "different" patients. We have previously shown how the unpaired statistical equations and tests used to compare independent data have to be modified to paired

Table 2.35 Choosing the appropriate bivariate statistical test (independent groups)

		Output variable		
Input variable	Qualitative	Qualitative	Quantitative (normal)	Quantitative (other distribution than normal
		Chi-square test[a, b] Spearman's rank[c]	Student test[d], One-way or Welch ANOVA[e]	Mann and Whitney[d], Kruskall Wallis[e]
	Quantitative (normal)	Logistic regression[f]	Pearson's correlation, linear regression[g]	Spearman's rank
	Quantitative (other distribution than normal)	Logistic regression[f], Spearman's rank[h]	Spearman's rank	Spearman's rank

a = use Fisher's exact test if both variables are binomial, b = use Chi-square test for trend if one of the variables is ordinal, c = in case of ordinal input and output, d = in case of a binomial input, e = in case of a categorical or ordinal input, f = in case of a dichotomized binomial output, g = in case we assume causality, h = in case of a categorical or ordinal output

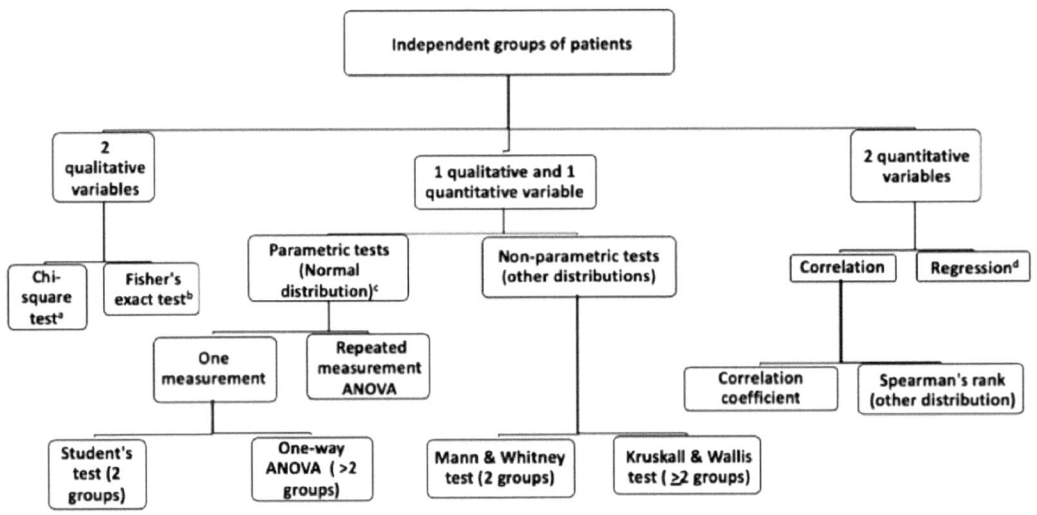

Fig. 2.15 Unpaired bivariate statistical tests. a = expected values ≥ 5 in $\geq 80\%$ of cells, b = two binomial qualitative variables, c = normal distribution and equality of variance, d = if causality is assumed

equations and tests, in order to assimilate change in variability due to data dependence. As analysis has to follow design, unrelated or unpaired data have to be analyzed by unpaired statistical tests (Table 2.35) and (Fig. 2.15) and related or matched data have to be analyzed by paired or matched statistical tests (Fig. 2.16).

2.8.1.2 Variable Type and Distribution

The type of a bivariate statistical test is then dependent upon the type, distribution and the role played by each variable, number of patient groups, number of measurements made and, whether factor time is taken into consideration. In broad terms, a variable can be either qualitative or quantitative. A qualitative variable can either be binomial (e.g., male or female), can have more than 2 categories (e.g., doctor, nurse and technician) or is said to be ordinal for having ordered categories (e.g., mild, moderate and severe). On the other hand, a quantitative variable may be formed of "continuous" unlimited

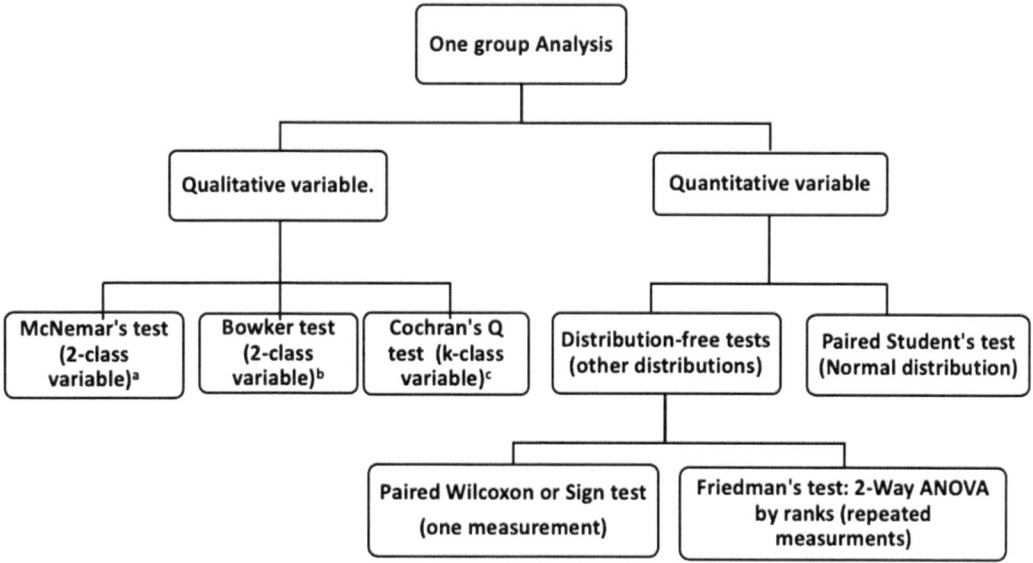

Fig. 2.16 Paired bivariate statistical tests. a = binomial qualitative variable, b = K-class qualitative variable, c = repeated binomial qualitative variable

values and their fractions and, follows a normal or other distribution. Alternatively, a quantitative variable can be just "discrete" formed of a countable limited number of values. Examples of a continuous quantitative variable are: age, fasting blood sugar and follow-up duration. Examples of discrete quantitative variables are data scores such as performance rated as 1, 2, 3, 4 and 5, or temperature rounded to the nearest degree. All qualitative variables have limited number of categories by default and hence, they are all discrete. One can benefit and enrich his analysis by changing an ordinal qualitative variable into a discrete quantitative variable, which can be further analyzed by statistical tests designed for the latter, such as Mann–Whitney, Kruskal–Wallis or Spearman's rank test (Table 2.35).

2.8.1.3 Variable Role

The researcher has to decide which of the two variables provides the data (input variable) that are supposed to produce the outcome (output variable). Table 2.35 shows bivariate statistical tests commonly used to analyze possible combinations of variables types, distributions, and roles [33]. Logistic regression analysis is the procedure of choice to test the significance of the

effects of multiple quantitative and qualitative predictors on a binary outcome. However, it can be used to analyze the effect of a single continuous or discrete quantitative variable on a binomial outcome (see Sect. 3.5).

2.8.2 The Unpaired Statistical Tests

2.8.2.1 The Association of Two Qualitative Variables

The observed distribution of a (k-class) qualitative variable can be compared to a theoretical one by the Chi-square goodness of fit test (see Sect. 2.3.1.1). On the other hand, the significance of the association between two (k-class) qualitative variables is usually tested by the Pearson's Chi-square test of independence, provided that the conditions of applications of the test are fulfilled (see Sect. 2.3.1.2). Otherwise, Fisher's exact test becomes the test of choice for not necessitating the fulfillment of any parameter except that both variables have to be binomial (see Sect. 2.3.1.5). In the case where one of the two qualitative variables is ordinal, and the other is binomial, either the Cochran–Armitage Chi-square test (see Sect. 2.3.1.4) or the Mann and Whitney test (see

Sect. 2.5.1.1) can verify the significance of the effect order (see Table 2.35) (see Fig. 2.15).

2.8.2.2 The Association of Two Quantitative Variables

On the other hand, the relation between 2 quantitative variables (e.g., body weight in kg and diastolic blood pressure in mm Hg) can be tested in one of two ways, either correlation or regression (Fig. 2.15). The former analyzes the tightness of the mutual relation between those two variables, as expressed by the correlation coefficient (r) (see Sect. 2.6.1.1). Spearman's rank correlation coefficient is the non-parametric alternative in case of a small sample size or variables following other distributions than normal (see Sect. 2.6.1.2). If causality is assumed, we can regress the predictor or explanatory variable on the outcome variable. Regression permits the quantification and testing of the significance of the effect of the former on the latter. For example, the more a person gains weight, the more his diastolic blood pressure increases by a specific mean value. Moreover, the regression equation permits the prediction outcome (diastolic blood pressure in mm Hg) for a given independent variable (body weight in kg) (see Sect. 2.6.2.1). Unlike correlation, the non-parametric version of regression analysis is beyond the scope of this chapter.

2.8.2.3 The Distribution of a Quantitative Outcome Across a Two- or Multiple-Class Qualitative Variable

The algorithm of choosing the appropriate test to compare quantitative data among patients' groups (see Table 2.35 and Fig. 2.15) starts by verifying the distribution of data in the study population. In the case of normal distribution and equality of variance, the unpaired test of Student (see Sect. 2.4.1.2) and either regular or Welch ANOVA (see Sects. 2.4.3.1 and 2.4.3.2) are the tests of choice for two and multiple groups, provided that the measurement is only made once. In the absence of normality and small studies, the

Mann and Whitney test (see Sect. 2.5.1.1) and the Kruskal and Wallis test (see Sect. 2.5.2.1) are the respective non-parametric alternatives. Although non-parametric tests are described as not necessitating any parameter for their application, the validity of the used equations becomes limited when the number of patients per group drops below ten. In such a case, the significance of the results should be checked out in specific tables.

2.8.3 The Paired Statistical Tests

Figure 2.16 shows an algorithm to choose the appropriate test for analyzing dependent data. McNemar (see Sect. 2.3.2.1) and Cochran Q tests (see Sect. 2.3.2.3) are the tests of choice to analyze binomial and K-class qualitative variables. The Bowker test is a modified McNemar if one of the two variables has more than two classes (see Sect. 2.3.2.2). The paired test of Student usually analyzes continuous paired parametric data (see Sect. 2.4.1.3), with the Wilcoxon Sign Rank test being its non-parametric alternative (see Sect. 2.5.1.3). In the case of repeated measurements made in a single or matched group of patients, Friedman's test (see Sect. 2.5.2.2) is often described as being "a weak" alternative of One-way repeated measures ANOVA (see Sect. 2.4.3.4).

2.8.4 The Comparison of Survival Curves

Choosing the test largely depends upon the available data [52].

- Log-rank: requires large sample size, assumption of proportional hazard, and equal censoring between groups. The test is most powerful in the case of comparing two large groups with suspected equal weights throughout the whole follow-up period.
- The generalized Wilcoxon sign (Gehan) test does not assume proportional hazard but requires equal censoring. The test gives more

weight to the early follow-up period, and it works well with small samples.

- Tarone-Ware: Like Gehan, the weighted element is the number of patients at risk; however, the given weight is smaller; being the square root of that number. Hence, it gives more weight to the intervals early and in the middle. Tarone-Ware is a robust test for not requiring proportional hazard nor equal censoring and can work with small and multiple groups. It is the test of choice when curves do frankly cross.

- Harrington and Fleming (F–H) tests are a good choice in case of prolonged follow-up and preventive studies, where events are suspected to occur late. The choice of (q) value has to be made before the study and can largely influence effect size and study power.

2.9 Adjusting Bivariate Analysis: Prognostic Studies

2.9.1 Introduction

A main aim of a clinical study is to link the predictor (e.g., a given type of treatment) to the study outcome (e.g., survival after treatment). A prognostic variable is a third variable that is linked to the study outcome, such as the histological type of cancer affecting the patient's survival. Prognostic factors are not always an integral part of the underlying pathology (internal) and many them are additional variables (external) that influence the study outcome too. A famous example is the association of low birth weight (outcome) with tobacco smoking (prognostic variable) during pregnancy (predictor). Prognostic variables can be the reason behind patients reacting differently to treatments and, unless those factors are properly identified before the study, they become a major source of bias and false interpretation of the results during the analysis. For confounding the direct link between predictor and outcome, those factors are also called confounding variables or confounders. In order to siege confounders, they have to be identified before the study by a full comprehensive literature review and then to be taken into consideration in the study design as well as during the statistical analysis.

For example, a prospective randomized study was conducted to compare the effects of 2 antihypertensive treatments. Review of the literature has shown that treatment effect can be significantly dependent upon the patient being diabetic or not. Not knowing or ignoring this information during randomization may lead to the creation of unbalanced study groups, with the play of hazard confining more diabetic patients to one group rather than to the other. The result that the effect of the treatment received by this group will be largely suppressed by the majority of patients being diabetic rather than being due to a modest treatment effect. As randomization per say can never guarantee a strictly equal distribution of risk factors between the study groups, this possible bias can be avoided by primarily creating 2 strata: diabetic and non-diabetic patients, prior to randomization. The second step is to separately randomize each stratum between the 2 treatment groups; permitting a balanced study design that evenly distribute the risk factor between the study groups.

Although a stratified analysis is easy to do, stratifying on multiple factors is hazardous. Suppose that besides diabetes, the researcher wishes to stratify on gender, smoking and three age groups (between 20–39 years, 40–59 years, and 60 years and above). The process will create 24 strata (2 × 2 × 3 = 24) or 24 "small" groups. Some of those small groups, will include very few patients, and none of which remain representative of the population As such, stratification itself becomes a major source of bias, and hence, it is always advisable to stratify on 1 or 2 main risk factors. More details on stratification will be given in the protocol section. The aim of this section is to show how to take into consideration the effect of a prognostic variable during a planned bivariate statistical analysis. In case of multivariable analysis, the effects of predictors on study outcomes are adjusted on prognostic variables by default and will be discussed in the relevant chapters.

The Source of Bias

A study was conducted to compare the effects of two antibiotic regimens in the prophylaxis of wound infection after major abdominal surgery. Two hundred patients were randomized into two equal groups to receive antibiotics A or B. The result of the study was negative: the success rates were 80% for regimen A compared to 70% with regimen B; hence, the investigator was unable to recommend either regimen (P = 0.1). On second thought, the researcher noticed that group A included more diabetic cases (60%) than group B (50%). Hence, he was tempted to independently verify the results in the persons with diabetes and the non-diabetic cases. Although non-diabetic cases showed the same overall negative comparison (66.6% with regimen A versus 70% with regimen B; P = 0.7), regimen A provided significantly higher success rates than regimen B (90% versus 70%; P = 0.02).

As such, the study is not allowed to recommend any regimen, even after showing that regimen A gives a significantly more protective effect in non-diabetic cases. The researcher follows the basic rule of thumb: we cannot compare subgroups (diabetic and non-diabetic) unless the main comparison shows a statistically significant treatment effect. Put it this way; the researcher has no point in comparing subgroups because he has not shown a treatment effect in the first place. The source of bias was that the researcher ignored the importance of the prognostic variable (diabetes) while planning the work, and he could not appreciate its value at the time of the analysis, as it should be.

The Approach

Patient groups have to be initially comparable before the beginning of the study so that differences observed at the end can be attributed to the difference between given treatments or procedures. Randomization is expected to achieve this initial comparability and can be reinforced by stratification. On the other hand, taking the prognostic variable into consideration during the analysis itself can evaluate two effects on study outcome: the independent effect of prognostic variable and the effect of interaction between prognostic variable and dependent variable. The proper approach is to create two comparable groups via randomization, which can be ensured by stratification on the prognostic factor. The second step is to exclude the presence of a reverse interaction; i.e., one stratum (e.g., diabetic cases) will respond positively to one treatment while the other (e.g., non-diabetic cases) will respond to the other treatment. It simply means that those are not just strata but two different populations, and hence, each population merits a separate study. After creating two comparable groups, which include the same proportion of risky and non-risky cases, the third step is to test the treatment effect while adjusting for (i.e., considering) the prognostic factor.

1. Stratification and Randomization

As briefly noted in the introduction section, stratification involves considering the role of the prognostic variable while planning of the analysis. In our study, patients have to be initially divided into two distinct strata: those with (diabetic cases) and those without the risk factor (non-diabetic cases). The procedure must be based on the same clinical and laboratory tests in all cases. The second step will be to randomize each stratum between the study groups, ensuring that each treatment group will contain the same proportions of patients with and without the risk factors. By the end of the study, the researcher can safely attribute the result achieved to the treatment effect and not to the different species (different proportions of risky and non-risky cases in each group). The protocol section will provide more details on randomization and stratification modalities.

2. Excluding a Reverse Interaction

Before proceeding to the test, we should ask ourselves an important question: does the prognostic variable affect the patients' response quantitatively or qualitatively? In our example, non-diabetic cases responded significantly better to regimen A than diabetic cases, which can be expected. What has to be excluded is a qualitative difference, where one group responds positively to one treatment, while the other group shows the inverse and responds significantly better to the second treatment. A quantitative interaction is expected and accepted but a qualitative interaction is not and should raise questions about our adjustment strategy. Its presence means that part of our studied group behaves as if it was extracted from a different population and hence, merits being studied alone. The Z test can be used to test a reverse interaction in case the adjustment variable is only limited to two classes, such as having or not having a certain risk factor (see Sect. 2.9.2.1). In case of multiple class adjustment variable, Berslow-Day and Tarone tests are common alternatives (see Sect. 2.9.2.2).

3. *Adjusting Two Proportions*

Continuing with our example and suppose that the authors successfully stratified diabetes and equally randomized 90 diabetic cases between the two treatment groups. Moreover, a Z test excluded reverse interaction. A poor analysis is to perform two statistical tests instead of one. A first analysis tests the treatment effect in all 200 cases and a second analysis to test the treatment effect independently in the 90 diabetic patients and in 110 non-diabetic controls. In this poor scenario, performing two statistical tests inflates the primary risk of error (see Sect. 2.3.1.2), and performing subgroup analysis on nearly half the sample increases the second risk of error. It is double jeopardy and a significant source of bias. A much more powerful scenario involves a single test that evaluates treatment effect, while adjusting for the prognostic variable by weighting its role on outcome; i.e., testing interaction of the prognostic variable (presence or absence of diabetes). In our case where the prognostic variable is qualitative, Cochran–Mantel–Haenszel test becomes the procedure of choice. Logistic regression is

another alternative usually performed in multi-variable analysis (see Sect. 3.5).

4. *Adjusting Two Means*

Unlike the case of a qualitative outcome, the analysis of variance (ANOVA) is used when the outcome is a normally distributed quantitative variable. ANOVA offers the researcher the opportunity to evaluate the effect of the predictor, the prognostic variable as well as any possible interaction between both variables on the outcome.

5. *Adjusting a Biserial Correlation*

Partial correlation investigates the association of two quantitative variables while considering (adjusting for) a third quantitative one that we believe it has an effect on the two variables of concern.

2.9.2 Excluding a Qualitative (Reverse) Interaction

2.9.2.1 The Z Test

Before proceeding to adjustment, the researcher has to exclude the presence of a statistically significant difference between the effects of the two classes of the prognostic variable on the outcome. In the presence of a significant difference, the idea of adjusting "contradictory effects" becomes absurd.

The Example

A study was planned to compare two arterial vasodilators in the treatment of intermittent claudication of the lower limbs. Knowing that the presence of diabetes mellitus affects the improvement of such patients, stratification was first performed on this risk factor. Patients of each stratum were then separately randomized between both treatment groups, and hence, instead of forming two lists of patients: one receiving treatment (a) and the other receiving treatment (b), four lists were performed: diabetics receiving treatment (a1), non-diabetics receiving treatment (a2),

Table 2.36 Comparison of the effect of 2 arterial vasodilators (a and b) in patients with intermittent claudication with adjustment on the presence or absence of diabetes mellitus: exclusion of qualitative interaction

Adjustment variable	Treatment (a) $n_a = 120$	Treatment (b) $n_b = 120$	Total n = 240
1. Diabetic patients:			
– Success	24 (60%)	18 (45%)	42
– Failure	16 (40%)	22 (55%)	38
Total	na1 = 40	nb1 = 40	n1 = 80
2. Non-diabetics patients:			
– Success	56 (70%)	40 (50%)	96
– Failure	24 (30%)	40 (50%)	64
Total	na2 = 80	nb2 = 80	n2 = 160

Values are presented as numbers and (%). n_a, n_b and n = number of patients on treatment a, number of patients on treatment b and total number of patients; respectively. na1, nb1, na2, nb2, n1 and n2 = number of diabetic patients on treatment a, number of diabetic patients on treatment b, number of non-diabetic patients on treatment a, number of non-diabetic patients on treatment b, total number of diabetic patients and total number of non-diabetic patients

diabetics receiving treatment (b1) and non-diabetics receiving treatment (b2). The outcome binomial variable was the success or failure to duplicate the claudication distance. The results are shown in Table 2.36, where we can easily notice that results of treatment (a) tended to be better than those achieved with treatment (b) and that non-diabetic patients were more improved than those who have diabetes. The question was whether those observations were statistically significant or not? To answer such a question, the investigators have chosen to use the Cochran–Mantel–Haenszel test, which allows to compare the effectiveness of both treatments and, at the same time, to consider (adjusting for) the risk factor (diabetes mellitus). However, we have to exclude a qualitative interaction between the effect of the treatment and the prognostic variable by a simple Z test. In other words, excluding that one group (e.g., diabetics) significantly improves using one treatment (e.g., treatment a). In contrast, the other group (e.g., non-diabetics) improves on the other treatment (e.g., treatment b).

The Equation

The Z test can be applied on a 2-class prognostic variable and hence, is ideal to evaluate the effect of the presence/absence of a risk factor. It is sufficient to show no significant difference between the success proportions between diabetic and non-diabetic patients to ensure the failure rates are comparable. We code the binomial prognostic variable as 1 for diabetic patients and 2 for non-diabetic controls. Pa_1 and Pa_2 are the proportions of success in patients with and without diabetes on treatment "a" and, Pb_1 and Pb_2 are the proportions of success in patients with and without diabetes on treatment "b". na_1 and na_2 are the numbers of diabetic and non-diabetic patients on treatment "a" and, nb_1 and nb_2 are the numbers of diabetic and non-diabetic patients on treatment b. The differences between the effects of both treatments in diabetic (d_1) and non-diabetic patients (d_2) are equal to ($Pa_1 - Pb_1$) and ($Pa_2 - Pb_2$), respectively.

As a routine, we have to standardize the difference by the appropriate standard deviation, i.e., the square root of variance. In our case, we have four proportions (Pa_1, Pa_2, Pb_1, and Pb_2), with four different sample sizes (na_1, na_2, nb_1, and nb_2). As the variance of a proportion (P) of sample size n equals $P(1 - P)/n$, our standard deviation will be the sum of the square roots of the four variances: $Pa_1(1 - Pa_1)/na_1$, $Pa_2(1 - Pa_2)/na_2$, $Pb_1(1 - Pb_1)/nb_1$, and $Pb_2(1 - Pb_2)/nb_2$.

Under the null hypothesis, there should be no difference between d_1 ($Pa_1 - Pb_1$) and d_2 ($Pa_2 - Pb_2$), and the alternative hypothesis is that the difference is true. We test the alternative hypothesis by comparing the calculated standardized difference (Z value) to the critical value figured in the Z table at the usual degree of significance of 5%; i.e., 1.65 for a unilateral study and 1.96 in the case where the study was bilateral "Eq. 2.108".

$$Z = \frac{d_1 - d_{12}}{\sqrt{\frac{Pa_1(1-Pa_1)}{na_1} + \frac{Pb_1(1-Pb_1)}{nb_1} + \frac{Pa_2(1-Pa_2)}{na_2} + \frac{Pb_2(1-Pb_2)}{nb_2}}}$$

$$(2.108)$$

The Interpretation

In our example, the calculated Z value is only 0.37 and is much smaller than the critical limit of 1.96. There is no evidence of a reverse interaction between diabetes mellitus and the outcome of therapy. Concordantly, we can proceed to adjust the outcome of therapy on the prognostic variable.

What Should be Reported

Besides the descriptive statistics (numbers, %), we have to report the Z and P values.

The Conditions of Application

The Z test can only be applied in case of a 2-class adjustment variable and with both: nP and n (1 − P) > 5; where n is the smallest number of patients per group and, P and (1 − P) are the proportions of the binomial qualitative variable (see Sect. 14.2.4). In our example, the conditions of the use of the test are verified. Our prognostic variable has two classes: the presence or absence of diabetes. The smallest number n = 40 and, the smallest proportion = 30% and hence, nP = 40 × 0.3 = 12.

2.9.2.2 Berslow-Day and Tarone's Tests

If we have more than two strata (K > 2), the Z-test cannot be used, and the Breslow-Day and Tarone tests are among the standard methods for testing the homogeneity of strata. Tarone test is a modification of Breslow-Day that gives more accurate results that are only apparent at three decimals.

The Example

As the test is applicable in the case of two strata, we will proceed by the same simple example shown above (see Sect. 2.9.2.1).

The Equation

We start by calculating the adjusted odds ratio as described by Mantel–Haenszel: ORMH. The adjusted OR is not the common OR calculated for all patients, regardless of the adjustment variable (diabetes mellitus). On the contrary, the adjusted OR is calculated while considering the adjustment variable [12, 56]. In our example, ORMH = 2.15 (see Sect. 2.9.3.2).

If the K strata of the adjustment variable (presence/absence of diabetes) are perfectly homogenous, the odds ratio of each stratum ORK must be equal to the adjusted ORMH. In our example, the ORK was 1.83 in diabetic patients and 2.33 in non-diabetic cases. Note that the OR is the ratio between two odds: the odds of having/not having the outcome of interest (success) among patients (a/c) and the odds of having/not having the outcome among controls (b/d). For example, the ORK in diabetic patients = (24/16)/(18/22) = 1.83 and, the ORK in controls = (56/24)/(40/40) = 2.33 (see Table 2.36).

The next step is to recalculate the expected proportions out of those observed during the study (a, b, c, and d), provided to satisfy the expected ORMH. In diabetic patients, we recalculate the observed proportions a_1, b_1, c_1, and d_1 that can give an OR of 2.15, instead of the observed ORK (1.83). Let us denote the recalculated expected proportions as A_1, B_1, C_1, and D_1. We calculate the expected proportions A_2, B_2, C_2, and D_2, out of those observed in controls (a_2, b_2, c_2 and d_2). The former are the proportions that can eventually give an OR of 2.15 instead of the observed ORK of 2.33. As such, we end by having two types of proportions in each stratum: observed proportions (a_i, b_i, c_i, and d_i) and expected proportions (A_i, B_i, C_i, and D_i). As usual, we compare the difference between observed and expected proportions, standardized by the proper variance. It is the variance of OR $(1/A_i + 1/B_i + 1/C_i + 1/D_i)$, but it is raised to the power of (−1) (see Sect. 1.8.7.2) "Eq. 2.109".

Let us see how those expected proportions are calculated out from the observed ones? Table 2.36 shows the observed proportions in diabetic patients: $a_1 = 24$, $b_1 = 18$, $c_1 = 16$ and

$d_1 = 22$. The observed OR is calculated from those four values as shown above: $(24/16)/(18/22) = 1.83$. If we want to change this OR from 1.83 to 2.15, it is sufficient to change only one of the four values (a, b, c, or d), the other three values will be automatically fixed. Remember what the degree of freedom is? In a two-by-two table with four values, the degree of freedom equals 1; i.e., only one value is free to vary. For example, we know that we had a total of 42 successes and 38 failures in the 80 diabetic patients and that the number of patients receiving each treatment is 40. If those marginal values are kept constant (42, 38, 80, 40, and 40), it will be sufficient to find the expected number of successes (A_1) to deduct B_1, C_1, and D_1. let us suppose that (A_1) was found to be 25 cases; the number of failures with treatment (a) must be 15 cases (40–25), the number of successes with treatment (b) must be 17 (42–25), and the number of failures with treatment (b) must be 23 (40–17) cases. We have presented the idea behind the computation of an expected proportion (A1). The details of those computations are demanding and beyond the scope of our book.

Nevertheless, only one proportion is free to vary in each stratum and hence, only one expected proportion is computed for each stratum. In our example, we have to compute only A_1 and A_2 for diabetic and non-diabetic patients. Now we can build up a modified Chi-square equation to test homogeneity of the distribution of the prognostic variable among the different strata: it is the sum of the standardized squared differences between observed (a_i) and expected numbers of successes (A_i), calculated per stratum. Taking the number of failures instead of the numbers of successes will give the same result, of course. Uploading our data to IBM-SPSS statistical software produces a small Chi-square of 0.185 and a P-value of 0.67.

$$\chi^2_{Berslow-Day} = \sum_{i=1}^{K\ strata} \frac{(a_i - A_i)^2}{\left(\frac{1}{A_i} + \frac{1}{B_i} + \frac{1}{C_i} + \frac{1}{D_i}\right)^{-1}}$$

(2.109)

The Interpretation

Fortunately, our Chi-square value is well below the critical limit of statistical significance figured in the Chi-square table at df (k − 1): 3.86. Hence, we can assume homogeneity and adjust the therapy outcome on the prognostic variable by the Mantel–Haenszel test.

What Should be Reported

Besides the descriptive statistics (numbers, %), we have to report the Chi-square and P-values.

Conditions of Application

The application conditions are the same as those of the Chi-square test of independence (see Sect. 2.3.1.2). In short, the sample size should be relatively large in each stratum, and at least 80% of the expected cell counts should be greater than 5.

2.9.3 Adjusting Two Proportions

2.9.3.1 Cochran–Mantel–Haenszel Test

The Cochran–Mantel–Haenszel is also known as the Mantel–Haenszel test. It assumes that there is no significant difference in the overall distribution of outcome as well as the individual distributions among the different classes of the prognostic variable [12, 56]. The role of the Mantel–Haenszel test in our example is to show whether there is a significant difference between the success rates observed in patients receiving treatment (a) and those receiving treatment (b), while taking into consideration (adjusting for) the effect of diabetes; all in a single step. Under the null hypothesis, we expect both treatments to have similar effects, and the alternative hypothesis is that the observed effects are not. A modified Chi-square equation tests the "adjusted" difference between what we were expecting and what we observed during the study. The larger the difference, the less is the probability for the null hypothesis being true. Once the difference is so large that this probability drops to only 5%, we reject the null hypothesis and adopt the alternative hypothesis.

The Example

We will use the same simple example shown above (see Sect. 2.9.2.1, Table 2.36). The exclusion of a significant qualitative (reverse) interaction by the Z, Berslow-Day, and Tarone tests gave us the green light to proceed and to the Cochran–Mantel–Haenszel test.

The Equation

Table 2.37 shows the observed number of successes, with the expected numbers between brackets. Remember that the expected numbers are calculated under the null hypothesis (hypothesis of no difference between the treatment effects). The reader is advised to refer to the chapter on the Chi-square test for more details (see Sect. 2.3.1.2). The expected number is generally calculated by multiplying the total number of observations by the group proportion. As shown, the expected number of successes in diabetic patients receiving treatment (a) equals the total number of successes in diabetic patients (42) multiplied by the proportion of the patients receiving treatment (a) among all diabetic patients $(40/80 = 21)$. Similarly, the expected successes in non-diabetic patients receiving treatment (a) $= 96(80/160) = 48$.

Provided that n_a = number of patients receiving treatment (a), n_b = number of patients receiving treatment (b), O = total number of observed successes, n = total number of patients; the variance of observed mortalities in patients receiving treatment a (Var Oa) is calculated by the equation "Eq. 2.110":

$$Var\ O_a = \frac{n_a\,n_b\,O\,(n-O)}{n^2(n-1)} \qquad (2.110)$$

Consequently, Var Oa_1 for observed successes in diabetic patients receiving treatment a $= 40 \times 40 \times 42\,(80 - 42)/80^2(80 - 1) = 5.1$ and Var Oa_2 of non-diabetic patients receiving the same treatment $= 80 \times 80 \times 96\,(160 - 96)/(160 \times 160 \times 159) = 9.6$. Under the null hypothesis, there should be no difference between the sum of observed successes in patients receiving treatment a $(\sum O_a = 24 + 56 = 80)$ and the sum of expected successes $(\sum E_a = 21 + 48 = 69)$. The difference between both sums is standardized by being divided by the sum of variances calculated for all classes $= \sum Var\ O_a = Var\ O_{a1} + Var\ O_{a2} = 5.1 + 9.6 = 14.7$. The standardized difference between the observed and expected values follows a Chi-Square distribution with 1 degree of freedom "Eq. 2.111". Applying the equation on our example produces a Chi-square value of $8.5\ (\chi^2 = (80 - 69)^2/14.7 = 8.5)$. All calculations can be generated either by a statistical software package such as IBM-SPSS or through an online calculator [25, 36].

Table 2.37 Cochran–Mantel–Haenszel test: Comparison of success of 2 arterial vasodilators in patients with intermittent claudication with adjustment on the presence or absence of diabetes mellitus

Adjustment variable	Treatment (a) n_a = 120	Treatment (b) n_b = 120	Total n = 240
Diabetic			
– Success	24 (21)	18 (21)	42
– Failure	16 (19)	22 (19)	38
Total	na1 = 40	nb1 = 40	n1 = 80
Non-diabetic			
– Success	56 (48)	40 (48)	96
– Failure	24 (32)	40 (32)	64
Total	na2 = 80	nb2 = 80	n2 = 160

Values are observed numbers and values between brackets are expected numbers. n_a, n_b and n = number of patients receiving treatment a, treatment b and total number of patients; respectively. na1, nb1, na2, nb2, n1 and n2 = number of diabetic patients receiving treatment a, number of diabetic patients receiving treatment b, number of non-diabetic patients receiving treatment a, number of non-diabetic patients receiving treatment b, total number of diabetic patients and total number of non-diabetic patients

$$\chi^2 = \sum \frac{\left(\sum O_a - \sum E_a\right)^2}{\sum Var\, O_a} \qquad (2.111)$$

The test can be simply extended to adjustment on K-class qualitative variable; e.g., 3-class variable. The difference between the sum of the observed events with treatment a $\left(\sum O = Oa1 + Oa2 + Oa3\right)$ and the sum of expected events $\left(\sum E = Ea1 + Ea2 + Ea3\right)$ is standardized (divided) by the sum of its variances $\left(\sum Var\, Oa = Var\, Oa1 + Var\, Oa2 + Var\, Oa3\right)$. The result follows an approximated Chi-square value, provided that the conditions of the test are fulfilled (see Sect. 2.3.1.2), and hence, their statistical significance is checked out in Chi-square table at K − 1 df.

The Interpretation

Checking on the Chi-Square table at 1 degree of freedom, our value (8.5) exceeds the critical (3.84) value necessary to reject the null hypothesis for a bilateral study. Consequently, we can conclude that treatment (a) is significantly more effective than treatment (b), adjusting for diabetes mellitus (P < 0.001). We must note that the same result would have been obtained if calculations were made for failures instead of successes or group (b) patients instead of patients in group (a).

What Should be Reported

Besides the descriptive statistics (numbers, %), we have to report effect size as the adjusted odds ratio or risk ratio with the 95% CI (see Sect. 2.9.2.4).

Conditions of Application

Being a modified Chi-square test, we have to assume all its assumptions (see Sect. 2.3.1.2). Patients (or any other study material) are chosen at random; observations are independent (one observation per case) and the number of expected values ≥ 5 in 80% of cells. Otherwise, we have to apply Yate's correction (see Sect. 2.3.1.3). In addition, we must avoid mixing observations taken by different methods and, we have to verify

that the prognostic variable does not have a qualitative (inverse) effect by Z test or else.

2.9.3.2 The Mantel–Haenszel Adjusted Odds Ratio and Risk Ratio

The value of one treatment, compared to another, can be expressed by the Mantel–Haenszel adjusted OR and its 95% CI. The OR is the ratio between 2 odds (2 proportions): the odds (proportion) of success/failure in diabetic patients (patients with the risk factor) and the odds (proportion) of success/failure in non-diabetics (controls). The reader is requested to refer to the chapter on the odds ratio (see Sect. 1.8.2.2) to know how to calculate its 95% CI and interpret the results statistical significance (see Sect. 1.8.7.2). Provided that (a) and (b) are the number of successes with treatment (a), and treatment (b) in diabetic patients and, (c) and (d) are the corresponding numbers of failure; the OR for diabetic patients = ad/bc = $(24 \times 22)/(18 \times 16) = 1.83$. The OR of non-diabetic patients = $(56 \times 40)/(40 \times 24) = 2.33$ and the combined OR = $(80 \times 62)/(40 \times 58) = 2.15$ "Eq. 2.112".

On the other hand, the Mantel–Haenszel OR is not the common OR that disregards the presence/absence of diabetes, but an OR adjusted to the relative size of diabetic and non-diabetic groups. As the OR does not follow a normal distribution, the 95% CI is primarily calculated as a log OR "Eq. 2.113". The exponential values of the lower and upper limits are 1.27 to 3.62, pointing to a statistically significant superiority of treatment (a).

$$OR_{MH} = \frac{\sum \left(\frac{ad}{n}\right)}{\sum \left(\frac{bc}{n}\right)} = \frac{\left(\frac{24 \times 22}{80} + \frac{56 \times 40}{160}\right)}{\frac{16 \times 18}{80} + \frac{24 \times 40}{160}} = 2.15$$
$$(2.112)$$

$$95\%\ CI\ OR_{MH} = OR^{1 \pm 1.96/\sqrt{Var\ OR}}$$
$$= 2.15^{1 \pm 1.96/\sqrt{8.2}} = 1.27\ to\ 3.62$$
$$(2.113)$$

The results are interpreted as follows: treatment (a) is associated with significantly more success, compared to treatment (b), adjusted for diabetes mellitus (Mantel–Haenszel OR = 2.15; 1.27 to 3.62: P = 0.04). The response was significant among non-diabetic patients (OR = 2.33; 1.22 to 4.26; P = 0.015) but did not reach statical significance in the diabetic subgroup, and hence, treatment (a) could not be recommended for diabetic patients. Note that the small difference between the combined and adjusted Odds ratio indicates that diabetes is not a significant confounder. All calculations can be generated either by a statistical software package such as IBM-SPSS or through an online calculator [25, 36].

The Adjusted Risk Ratio

The value of one treatment in relation to the other can be also expressed by the adjusted relative risk. The risk of success in diabetic patients $a/(a+b) = 24/(24+18) = 0.571$ and that of failure $= c/(c+d) = 16/(16+22) = 0.42$ and the relative risk = 1.36. The relative risk for non-diabetic patients = 0.583/0.375 = 1.55 and combined risk ratio $= 80/138 = 0.588/0.39 = 1.5$. As the risk ratio $[a/(a + b)]/[c/(c + d)]$ can be easier calculated as: $a(c + d)/c (a + b)$, the Cochran Mantel–Haenszel adjusted risk ratio equals 1.48; meaning that the expected success with treatment (a) is nearly one and half times what could be expected with treatment (b), adjusting for diabetes mellitus "Eq. 2.114".

$$RR_{MH} = \frac{\sum\left(\frac{a(c+d)}{n}\right)}{\sum\left(\frac{c(a+b)}{n}\right)} = \frac{\left(\frac{24\times38}{80} + \frac{56\times64}{160}\right)}{\frac{16\times42}{80} + \frac{24\times96}{160}} = 1.48$$

$$(2.114)$$

The Odds Ratio Adjusted by Logistic Regression

If the investigators plan to adjust on multiple prognostic variables, Mantel–Haenszel may become a source of bias in itself for fragmenting the sample size. Logistic regression is the model of choice in observational studies and is also used in clinical trials, provided that the outcome is a qualitative variable. By default, the model adjusts the outcome on the researcher's multiple qualitative and quantitative predictors. The outcomes are calculated in adjusted Log Odds ratios

that are usually extrapolated in the manuscripts to the more comprehensible form: the adjusted odds ratios. For more details, the reader can refer to chapter three (see Sect. 5.3).

2.9.4 Adjusting Two Means

2.9.4.1 Two-Way ANOVA

Before proceeding, we advise the reader to refer to the section on one-way ANOVA to get the basic information on the meaning of ANOVA and how it works (see Sect. 2.4.3.1)? ANOVA offers the researcher the opportunity to evaluate the effect of different predictor variables on the outcome variable. For example, groups of patients receiving different treatments are expected to respond differently, and hence, measuring this first part of variability (difference in response) reflects the treatment effect. On the other hand, difficult cases (e.g., diabetics) are expected to show a modest cure compared to other patients (e.g., non-diabetics). Hence, this second part of variability reflects the confounding effect of the risk factor (diabetes) on the outcome variable (cure). Likewise, the results of patients treated in a certain hospital can differ (can be worse/better) from those treated in another medical facility. Hence, this third part of variability (difference between cure rates in different hospitals) reflects the effect of factor hospitals.

Moreover, patients in one hospital may be better improved on a particular treatment, while those in another hospital improve on another treatment. Unfortunately, such interaction between two factors (treatment and hospital) reduces the power of ANOVA to evaluate the individual effect of each of them up to the point of discarding the results of ANOVA, in the case of a statistically significant interaction. In other words, the first thing to do in a two-way ANOVA or higher is to ensure the absence of a significant interaction; otherwise, the results of involved factors become questionable and have to be discarded.

ANOVA begins by measuring the overall variability observed in the outcome (dependent variable). The measured variability in all patients regardless of the type of treatment received or the place of recruitment, or any other patient or study-related risk factor. This variability is called "the total variance" due to the contributions of all factors together. Then, ANOVA partitions (analyzes) this total variability into its originating components, such as the variability due to the type of treatment received, the risk factors, and any possible interaction. The collection (the sum) of those variabilities is called "the model variance," i.e., the part of the total variability explained by the factors we have presented for the analysis. As no study is perfect, there will always be other factors that we did not include in our study (model), whether because they were unknown to us or simply because we did not collect the relevant data. Hence, our study cannot explain the part of variability due to those factors. Consequently, there will always be a difference between the total variance (variability due to known and unknown factors) and the model variance (variability explained by the factors we included in our study).

The difference is the part of variability that we could not explain by our study, which is known as "the residual or error variance." The amount of variation explained by the model and its individual components is weighted against the unexplained variation. The test statistics (Fisher's value) is nothing but the ratio between those variances and the residual variance. The larger is a particular F ratio; the more is the importance of this particular variance; e.g., overall model, effect treatment, factor hospital, the interaction between treatment and hospital, or any other factors. The statistical significance of each factor is found by matching its F ratio with the critical values figured in the Fisher's tables at the corresponding degrees of freedom.

The Example

Although the idea behind two-way ANOVA is simple, the calculations are lengthy, and the test is rarely performed by hand. We advise the researcher to attempt those calculations at least once to see and feel how the process is running. We will use a mini example that may not fulfill all the "hard" requirements of ANOVA but can be easily calculated by hand. Any deviations from those requirements will be criticized by the end. A multicenter trial compared two antihypertensive regimens (A and B) in treating adult patients presenting with essential chronic hypertension. The study included 24 patients from three participating hospitals (1, 2, and 3). The eight patients recruited in each hospital were equally randomized between the two treatments. As shown in Table 2.38, patients were grouped into six subgroups according to the hospital and the type of treatment received. The mean blood pressure values observed among the six subgroups represent the combinations of four measurements (m = 4) taken from patients receiving one of two treatments (c = 2) in three different hospitals (r = 3). The study has to answer three questions, whether there is a significant difference between the results of both treatments or various hospitals and if there is substantial interaction between factor treatment and factor hospital? A significant interaction means that one treatment is significantly better than the other in one hospital but significantly worse in another hospital, which jeopardizes the results of ANOVA concerning the significance of both factor treatment and factor hospital.

Table 2.38 Two-Way ANOVA: comparing the effects of two antihypertensive regimens among three hospitals

	Treatment A (n = 12)	Treatment B (n = 12)	Total
Hospital 1 (n = 8)	108	115.8	111.9
Hospital 2 (n = 8)	125.3	135.8	130.5
Hospital 3 (n = 8)	143	155.5	149.3
Total	125.4	135.7	130.5

Values represent mean systolic blood pressure in mm Hg, n = number of patients. Sum of all measured values = TG = 3133, sum of all squared values = 415313

The Equations

We start by analyzing variability as sum of squares (SS). Then, we calculate the corresponding degrees of freedom (df) to compute the variances as (SS/df). In the case of One-way ANOVA, we have included only one factor in the model: the type of treatment received. The total sum of squares (total SS) was portioned into a part explained by the treatment effect and a residual SS that remained unexplained. In other words, the model was formed by only one factor (factor treatment), and a large part of the total SS remained unexplained (residual variance). The two-way ANOVA opens a second venue to explain the latter by adding two more factors: hospital and possible interaction between treatment and hospital factors. The net result is that the model is getting larger for being formed of three factors instead of only one and, the residual variance is getting smaller. Remember that the significance of factor treatment and any other factor is tested in proportion to the size of the residual variance (F = variance treatment/residual variance). Consequently, the effect of factor treatment will become more significant because of the relative decrease of its dominator, making a two-way ANOVA a more robust test than its one-way version.

1. The Total Sum of Squares

The total sum of squares (SS_{total}) is the SS calculated for all outcome values, regardless of participating hospital or type of treatment received. It can be calculated routinely as the sum of squared deviations of all 24 measurements form their mean value. A more straightforward formula is to calculate (SS_{total}) from the sum of all 24 measurements (TG) and the sum of their squared values $(\sum x^2)$ "Eq. 2.115" and "2.116".

$$SS_{total} = \sum (x - \bar{x})^2 = \sum x^2 - \frac{TG^2}{N} \quad (2.115)$$

$$SS_{total} = 415313 - \frac{3133^2}{24} = 6325.9 \quad (2.116)$$

2. The Columns Sum of Squares (Factor Treatment)

We have chosen to place the factor treatment in columns (c = 2) and the factor hospital in rows (r = 3), and we could have chosen the reverse order. However, we must remember what we have chosen to avoid miscalculations (see Table 2.38). Under the null hypothesis, both treatments have the same effect, regardless of the hospital factor. In other words, there should be no difference between the mean value of measurements in each column (treatment) and the overall mean. Knowing that we have four measurements (m = 4) made in three hospitals (r = 3), the mean of each column (treatment) is denoted as $(\bar{x}_c)$ and the overall mean as $(\bar{x})$; the following formula calculates the (SS_c) "Eq. 2.117" and "2.118".

$$SS_c = mr \sum (\bar{x}_c - \bar{x})^2 \quad (2.117)$$

$$SS_c = 4 \times 3[(125.4 - 130.5)^2 + (135.7 - 130.5)^2]$$
$$= 630.4$$
$$(2.118)$$

3. The Rows Sum of Squares (Factor Hospital)

Under the null hypothesis, there should be no difference between the measurements made in any of the three hospitals, regardless of the treatment received. In other words, there should be no difference between the mean value of measurements in each row (hospital) and the overall mean. Knowing that we have four measurements (m = 4) made in each treatment group (c = 2), the mean of each row (hospital) is denoted as $(\bar{x}_r)$ and the overall mean as $(\bar{x})$; the following formula calculates the (SS_r) "Eq. 2.119" and "2.120".

$$SS_r = mc \sum (\bar{x}_r - \bar{x})^2 \qquad (2.119)$$

$$SS_r = 4 \times 2[(111.9 - 130.5)^2 + (130.5 - 130.5)^2$$
$$+ (149.3 - 130.5)^2] = 5587.6$$
$$\qquad (2.120)$$

4. The Interaction Sum of Squares (Columns × Rows: Treatment × Hospital)

As shown in Table 2.38, the six subgroups represent the combinations made by the two treatments, as received in the three hospitals. Any significant difference between the six measurements will indicate an interaction between both factors. Under the null hypothesis, there should be no interaction and hence, there should be no difference between the mean value observed in a particular subgroup (x_{irc}) and the mean values recorded in the same hospital (x_{ir}), in patients receiving the same treatment (x_{ic}) or the overall mean $(\bar{x})$. In other words, the difference between those four values has to be equal to zero and any observed difference reflects some interaction between both factors. For example, under the null hypothesis, there should be no difference between the mean value of the first subgroup (108) and the mean values recorded in his hospital (111.9), among patients receiving the same treatment (125.4) and the overall mean (130.5). Knowing that we have four measurements (m = 4) and denoting the means of the six subgroups, the three rows, the two columns, and the overall mean as $(\bar{x}_{irc})$, $(\bar{x}_{ir})$, $(\bar{x}_{ic})$ and $(\bar{x})$; the following formula calculates the sum of squares of interaction (SS_{irc}) "Eq. 2.121" and "2.122".

$$SS_{cr} = m \sum (\bar{x}_{irc} - \bar{x}_{ir} - \bar{x}_{ic} + \bar{x})^2 \qquad (2.121)$$

$$SS_{cr} = 4[(108 - 111.9 - 125.4 + 130.5)^2$$
$$+ (115.8 - 111.9 - 135.7 + 130.5)^2$$
$$+ (125.3 - 130.5 - 125.4 + 130.5)^2$$
$$+ (135.8 - 135.7 - 130.5 + 130.5)^2$$
$$+ (143 - 149.3 - 125.4 + 130.5)^2$$
$$+ (155.5 - 149.3 - 135.7 + 130.5)^2] = 22.7$$
$$\qquad (2.122)$$

5. The Model Sum of Squares

Unlike the one-way ANOVA where the model was only formed by one factor, the model is formed of three factors: factor treatment (SS_c), factor hospital (SS_r), and interaction (SS_{irc}) : $630.4 + 5587.6 + 22.7 = 6240.7$ "Eq. 2.123".

$$SS_{model} = SS_c + SS_r + SS_{icr} \qquad (2.123)$$

6. The Residual Sum of Squares

The residual SS is the amount of variation that was left unexplained by the model, and hence, it is simply calculated by subtracting the model SS from the total sum of squares: $6325.9 - 6240.7 = 85.2$ "Eq. 2.124".

$$SS_{residual} = SS_{total} - SS_{model} \qquad (2.124)$$

7. Calculation of the Degrees of Freedom

The degree of freedom of the total sum of squares equals the total sample size minus one = N − 1 = 23. As the interaction between several variables is their product, the df of interaction is the product of their degrees of freedom too. In our case, the df of interaction will be the df of factor treatment and hospital = 1 × 2 = 2. Put it another way, we have two columns and three rows, and hence, the df of their interaction will be equal to the number of columns minus one multiplied by the number of rows minus one = (2 − 1) × (3 − 1) = 2. The df of the model will be the Sum of the df of its three components: factor treatment, factor hospital, and interaction = 1 + 2 + 2 = 5. By deduction, the residual df will remain after deducting the model's df from the total df = 23 − 5 = 18. The reader can refer to Sect. 2.2.2 to refresh his memory about the degrees of freedom calculations.

8. *Calculation of the Variance (Mean Square)*

The variances are calculated by dividing each SS by its respective df. Hence, the model variance = 6240.7/5 = 1248.1, the variances of the columns (treatments), the rows (hospital) and interaction will be equal to: 630.4/1 = 630.4, 5587.6/2 = 2790.8 and, 22.7/2 = 11.4; respectively.

9. *Calculation of the F Ratios*

Each F ratio is calculated by dividing the respective variance by the residual variance (4.7). Hence, the F ratios of the model, treatment factor, hospital factor, and interaction are 263.5, 133.1, 589.9, and 2.4, respectively.

The Interpretation

The statistical significance of the model and each of its components is tested by comparing its F ratio with the critical F value figured in F tables point 5% [8]. Statistical significance is declared whenever any of the former is at least equal or larger than the latter and higher degrees of significance can be checked out at smaller points such as 1% or 0.1%. As previously noted, the values shown in the F tables are the critical values of the proportion of two variances: variance in the column/variance in the row and we have to be careful not to swap this order (see Sect. 2.2.3.4).

1. *The Significance of the Interaction*

Testing interaction is what we have to do first. In the presence of a statistically significant interaction, we cannot separate and test the statistical significance of the individual effect of each factor. The F ratio of interaction = variance of the interaction/residual variance, and hence, its df = df of interaction (2): df of the residual variance (18) and it should be expressed as $F_{2,18}$. The statistical significance is looked for in the F table point 5%, at the intersection of column number 2 and row number 18. Fortunately, the value figuring in the table equals (3.55) is much larger

than our calculated value (2.4). Hence, there is no significant interaction, and we can proceed to test the statistical significance of the factors included in the model.

2. *The Significance of the Model*

The F ratio of the model = variance of the model/residual variance, and hence, its df = df of the model (5)/df of the residual variance (18). The model F ratio should be expressed as: $F_{5,18}$. The statistical significance is looked for in the F table point 5%, at column number 5 and row number 18. The value figured in the table equals 2.77, and our value is much higher. Note that reversing the order by looking at the intersection of column 18 and row 5 gives a different critical F value (4.58). Nevertheless, our model explained a significant variation, and our P-value is less than 0.001.

3. *The Significance of the Factor Treatment (Column)*

The F ratio of the factor treatment = variance of the columns/residual variance, and hence, its df = df of the column (1)/df of the residual variance (18) should be expressed as $F_{1,18}$. The statistical significance is looked for in the F table point 5% at column number 1 and row number 18. The value figuring in the table (4.41) is much smaller than our calculated value (133.1), and our P-value is less than 0.001.

4. *The Significance of the Factor Hospital (Row)*

The F ratio of the factor hospital = variance of the rows/residual variance, and hence, its df = df of the rows (2)/df of the residual variance (18) should be expressed as $F_{2,18}$. The statistical significance is looked for in the F table point 5% at column number 2 and row number 18. The value figured in the table (3.55) is much smaller than our calculated value (589.9), and our P-value is less than 0.001.

5. *Interpretation of the Study*

These results allow us to conclude the following: taking into consideration the factor hospital, the mean blood pressure observed with treatment A (125.4 ± 15.1 mm Hg) was significantly smaller than the one achieved with treatment B (135.6 ± 16.9 mm Hg); P < 0.001. If the study was randomized and comparability was kept throughout the study, we can recommend using treatment A in treating comparable groups of patients presenting with essential hypertension. The study put into evidence the factor hospital, considering the treatment effect. The mean blood pressure recorded among the three hospitals 1, 2, and 3 were: 111.9 ± 4.5, 130.5 ± 6, and 149.3 ± 7 mm Hg; P < 0.001. The study could not prove a significant interaction between treatment and hospital factors.

6. *Post Hoc Tests*

Regarding the treatment effect, the results of ANOVA were net and clear: treatment A controls blood pressure more than treatment B, which is not the same regarding factor hospital. A statistically significant ANOVA between more than two groups tells us that the measurements acquired from at least one of the three groups (hospitals) is significantly different from the other two but could not tell us which of which? A post hoc analysis that compares the three subgroups two-by-two will provide this answer and correct the inflated P-value by the multiple two-by-two corrections (see Sect. 2.4.3.3). The means of the differences between measurements made in hospitals 1 and 2, hospitals 2 and 3 and, hospitals 1 and 3 were: 18.6 ± 2.9, 18.8 ± 2.9, and 37.4 ± 2.9 mm Hg; P < 0.001. We used the Bonferroni correction that standardizes the difference between every two means by the same residual variance (2.9) initially calculated when ANOVA compared the three means. This residual variance is more representative of the population than the pooled variance or the variance of the difference used by the test of Student. Moreover, it corrected the inflated P-value by raising the usual limit of significance (0.05) to

the power of the number of comparisons made; i.e., $0.05^3 = 0.0125$ (see Sect. 2.4.3.3).

7. *Effect Treatment: One-Way Versus Two-way ANOVA Models*

Suppose that all the researcher cares about is finding whether there is a statistically significant difference between both treatments, regardless of the factor hospital. A regular test of Student will be the procedure of choice; however, one-way ANOVA is also feasible and will give the same results. Hence, we will perform one-way ANOVA for the sake of comparison. The details of calculations were given before (see Sect. 2.4.3.1), so we will only provide the final result.

By applying one-way ANOVA, neither the total sum of squares (6325.9) nor the treatment SS will change (630.4), of course. What will change is what remains from the total SS after the part explained by the treatment has been removed, i.e., the residual SS. One-way ANOVA left over a large part of residual variance (5695.6), compared to what remained unexplained by the two-way technique (85.2); it was 66 times larger. Concordantly, the residual variance of one-way ANOVA (258.9) was 55 times the residual variance of two-Way ANOA (4.7). As the significance of any factor is tested in proportion to the residual variance, two-way ANOVA increased the chances of a significant treatment effect 55 times, compared to a one-way version. How was this done simply by giving a chance to factor "hospital" to explain a large part of the residual variance?

What Should be Reported

We have to report the descriptive statistics: means and Sd of all patients, the two main treatment groups, and the six subgroups. Inferential statistics have to be reported, including the exact P values of ANOVA, treatment effect, prognostic factor interaction, and post hoc analysis. It is favorable to report effect size, such as Eta squared η^2, Omega squared ω^2 or Cohen's F and, the reader is advised to refer back to 4.8 for more details.

Conditions of Application

Groups have to be independent and chosen at random. The quantitative variable of concern must be normally distributed with equality of variances among the compared groups. A statistically significant qualitative interaction between the two factors must be tested first; otherwise, the study groups must be considered as being issued from different populations and should not be compared.

2.9.5 Adjusting Two Quantitative Variables

2.9.5.1 Partial Correlation

Partial correlation investigates the association of 2 quantitative variables while considering a third one that we believe affects the variables of concern. In a previous example on correlation, we have tested the significance of the association between the duration of surgery (x) and the total amount of blood loss (y) in poly traumatized patients, without taking into consideration the probable effect of other factors, such as the nature of trauma, the delay in patient transfer, the patient's age, or the hospital facility. However, if we believe that the delay in hospital transfer (z) may also have a significant effect on (x) and (y), removing the effect (z) can give better information on the "true" association between the two variables of concern. Controlling for (removing the effect of) a third quantitative variable (z) while testing the correlation between the other two (x and y) is called partial correlation. Although we can extend the technique to consider more than one variable (>1 z), it is better in such a case to use multiple regression [57].

The Example

Table 2.39 shows the corresponding duration of surgery (x), amount of blood loss (y) and delay in hospital transfer (z) in 10 polytraumatized cases. In a previous section on simple correlation (see Sect. 2.6.1.1), we have found a statistically significant positive correlation between x and y (rxy = 0.887; P < 0.001). The researchers were

then able to get additional information, which is the time to hospital transfer (z). They now wish to correlate x and y, controlling for z; i.e., after removing any possible effect of delayed transfer on both variables. The researchers have considered partial correlation because all three elements were continuous variables. The first step would be to measure this possible influence by calculating another two correlation coefficients between the third variable and both: duration of surgery (rxz) and amount of blood loss (ryz). The second step will be to remove the effects of both (rxz) (ryz) from (rxy), so as to quantify and to test the statistical significance of the "pure" correlation between the duration of surgery and the amount of blood loss. Table 2.39 shows the detailed calculation of only one of the two suggested coefficients (rxz), as the calculation of the other coefficient (ryz) will follow the same steps.

The Equation

The reader is requested to refer back to the detailed calculations in the section on correlation coefficient (see Sect. 2.6.1.1). In brief, providing a linear relationship between paired data points (e.g., each x and its corresponding z), the correlation coefficient r measures how well they fit the trend line. Theoretically, r varies from 0, indicating non-fitting (no correlation), to +1 or −1, indicating a perfect negative or perfect positive correlation. We have already calculated rxy in the section on correlation, which showed a significantly positive correlation between the duration of surgery and the amount of blood loss. The question is whether a third quantitative variable (z) influences rxy?

To answer this question, we have to study how much the prognostic variable (z) influences x and y by calculating the corresponding correlation coefficients: rxz and ryz? We will present only one calculation (rxz), as an example. The next step is to remove the effect that (z) has on both (x) and (y); which permits the evaluation of the "pure" relation between (x) and (y), outside the influence of (z). Put it this way, to control the effect of a third variable (z) on the correlation between two variables (x and y), we calculate three correlation coefficients (rxy, rxz

Table 2.39 Partial correlation: correlation between the duration of surgery, the total amount of blood loss and the delay in hospital transfer in ten poly traumatized patients

1	2	3	4	5	6	7	8	9
Patients number	x	y	z	(x − mx)	(z − mz)	(x − mx) (z − mz)	(x − mx)^2	(z − mz)^2
I	2	3	1	−3	−1.1	3.3	9	1.21
II	5	7	3	0	0.9	0	0	0.81
III	3	5	2	−2	−0.1	0.2	4	0.01
IV	2	4	1	−3	−1.1	3.3	9	1.21
V	6	5	2	1	−0.1	−0.1	1	0.01
VI	8	9	3	3	0.9	2.7	9	0.81
VII	3	4	1	−2	−1.1	2.2	4	1.21
VIII	9	10	3	4	0.9	3.6	16	0.81
IX	5	7	3	0	0.9	0	0	0.81
X	7	6	2	2	−0.1	−0.2	4	0.01
Sum	50	60	21	0	0	15	56	6.9
Mean	mx = 5	my = 6	mz = 2.1					
V^2						1.67	6.22	0.77
Sd							2.49	0.88

Numbers in Latin represent individual patients, x = duration of surgery in hours, y = amount of blood loss in deciliters, z = delay in hospital transfer in hours, mx, my and mz = mean values of x, y and z. Column 7 = sum of squares of covariance (x, y), columns 8 and 9 = sum of squares of variables x and y. V^2 = variance or covariance, Sd = standard deviation

and ryz). Then we control (z) by removing its relation with x (rxz) and with y (ryz) from (rxy); permitting a more comprehensive evaluation of the correlation between x and y (rxy) [57].

1. Calculation of the Correlation Coefficients

We have already presented the detailed calculation of (rxy), presenting the calculations of another correlation coefficient (rxz). The first step is the calculation of the individual variances of x and z as SS/df. The respective SS are shown in columns 8 and 9 of Table 2.39. The df = sample size-1 = 9. Consequently, the respective variances of x and z = 6.22 and 0.77, and the respective standard deviations are Sx and Sz = 2.49 and 0.88.

The second step is the calculation of the covariance (x,z). The SS of the covariance is equal to the product of both sums of variability = (x-mx) (z-mz) and hence, the covariance (x,z) = SS/df "Eq. 2.80". In our example, the covariance = SS/df = 15/9 = 1.67.

As such, the covariance is just a raw statistic that has to be standardized by being divided by the proper standard deviation, and the best is the product of both standard deviations = (Sx) (Sz) "Eq. 2.81". The correlation coefficient r is hence the standardized value of the covariance. In our example, (Sx) (Sz) = 2.49 × 0.88 = 2.19. and hence, ryz = covariance (x,z)/(Sx) (Sz) = 0.76. The next step is to test its statistical significance in Student's table at n − 2 df, using the corresponding t value "Eq. 2.82". We can calculate a Se for r, as in "Eq. 2.85" (Se = 0.23), normalize r "Eq. 2.83" to assign a 95% CI (0.36–1.42), as shown in Sect. 2.6.1.1. Finally, we have to calculate the third correlation coefficient (ryz) correlating the amount of blood loss and the delay to hospital transfer. In our example, ryz = 0.989 and P = 0.001.

2. Calculation of the Partial Correlation Coefficient (rxy, z)

The three bivariate simple correlation coefficients (rxy, rxz and ryz) are also called "zero ordered correlation" for limiting the analysis to the two variables of concern and not controlling for the effect of any other variable. On the other hand, our example showed that the third variable (z) correlated positively and significantly with the duration of surgery (x) and the amount of blood loss (y). The more was the delay in hospital transfer; the longer was the operative time and the more the patient will lose blood. Hence, to have a more comprehensive analysis of the correlation between those two variables (x and y), we have to remove (control for) the effect of z. Statistically, the equation aims to subtract from (rxy) both: (rxz) and (ryz). Put it another way: instead of testing the significance of (rxy)—which was shown to be influenced by (z)—we will test the significance of (rxy) − (rxz).(ryz). As a routine, the latter quantity has to be standardized by the proper Se, and the question will always be: what is the variance from which we can deduct the Se. The variance of (r) is equal to $(1 - r^2)$; the variance of the effect of (z) on both (x) and (y) will be equal to the multiplication of both variances = $(1 - r^2xz) (1 - r^2yz)$. The coefficient of partial correlation (rxy, z) is the standardized correlation between (x) and (y) after removing the effect of (z), as in"Eq. 2.125". Its statistical significance can be checked out in the table of Student, at df = n − 3, as in "Eq. 2.126". In our example, (rxy, z) equals 0.71 and t-value = 2.68; P = 0.033.

$$r_{xy,z} = \frac{(r_{xy} - r_{xz}r_{yz})}{\sqrt{(1 - r_{xz}^2)(1 - r_{yz}^2)}} \qquad (2.125)$$

$$t = \frac{r\sqrt{(n-3)}}{\sqrt{1 - r^2}} \qquad (2.126)$$

We can use the same formula to calculate the partial correlation coefficient between any 2 of the three variables, after controlling for the effect of the third one. In other words, we can calculate (rxz, y) as well as (ryz, x) but we have to take care of re-ordering the bivariate coefficients in the equation. As an example, in calculating (rxz, y), the numerator becomes (rxz − rxy, rzy) and the denominator becomes the square root of $(1 - r^2xy) (1 - r^2zy)$.

The Interpretation

Note that in partial correlation, we start by doing zero-order correlation first, and hence, we have two null hypotheses: the first, is there an association between each of the two variables, and the second, does this association holds while controlling for the third, fourth or fifth variable? Zero ordered correlation has shown a statistically significant positive correlation between duration of surgery (x) and amount of blood loss (y). However, it also showed that time to hospital transfer (z) was positively and significantly correlated with both (x) and (y), and hence, removing the effect (z) provides a better assessment of the direct association between duration of surgery and amount of blood loss. The statistical significance of the partial correlation coefficient (rxy, z) is tested by calculating the corresponding t-value at a df of sample size minus the number of variables = n − 3.

Although there is still a statistically significant positive correlation between the duration of surgery and amount of blood loss, yet this correlation dropped from "a zero-order correlation" of (rxy = 0.887; P = 0.001) to "a partial correlation" of (rxy, z = 0.708; P = 0.033). The difference between (rxy,) and (rxy, z) reflects the importance of the time factor on both (x) and (y) or the importance of rapidly transferring the patient to the hospital. Let us quantify this importance and calculate the R square in both scenarios. Remember that R square represents the average variation in (y) due to (x). The respective R square values of zero ordered and partial correlation are 0.792 and 0.5. In other words, the duration of surgery which was thought to be responsible—on average—for 79% of the variations in the amount of blood loss, is most probably responsible for only 50% of the changes. The difference can be accounted for by the delay in transfer to the hospital after trauma.

What Should be Reported

We have to report the descriptive statistics: mean and Sd of each variable. Inferential statistics zero ordered correlation as well as partial correlation, R-square, the P-value, and the effect size; which can be reported using Fisher's transformation: $C = 0.5 \log (1 + r)/(1 - r)$ (see Sect. 2.6.1.1). However, unlike the scatter plot of zero ordered correlation that can be directly obtained from the data, the scatter plot of partial correlation needs some manipulation. We need to plot both (x) and (y) variables after removing the effect of (z). In statistical terms, we need to plot "the residuals" of both variables or, in plain English, what remains in the correlation of (x) and (y), after removing the effect of (Z).

We can use any commercially available software such as SPSS and calculate the unstandardized residuals of (x) and (y). The latter can be calculated by regressing the time to hospital transfer (as the independent variable) once from (x) and once from (y) and saving the unstandardized residuals. Figure 2.17 shows the scatter plot of unstandardized residuals of the duration of hospital stay and amount of blood loss.

Conditions of Application

Samples should be drawn at random, observations should be independent, and both variables have to be normally distributed. Other assumptions include linearity and homoscedasticity. Linearity assumes a straight-line relationship between each of the two variables, provided that it does not change in sign or in magnitude during the studied intervals. Homoscedasticity or homogeneity of variance assumes that data is equally distributed about the regression line. The test necessitates that at least one of the two tied distributions (distribution of "y" for a given value of "x" or the distribution of "x" for a given value of "y") is Normal and of a constant variance; conditions that are usually realized in biology. Moreover, the test is robust and can be applied even if the necessary conditions of its use are not perfectly verified, provided that the number of studied patients is large ($n > 30$). The chapter on correlation coefficient gives more details on homoscedasticity and tied distribution (see Sect. 2.6.1.1).

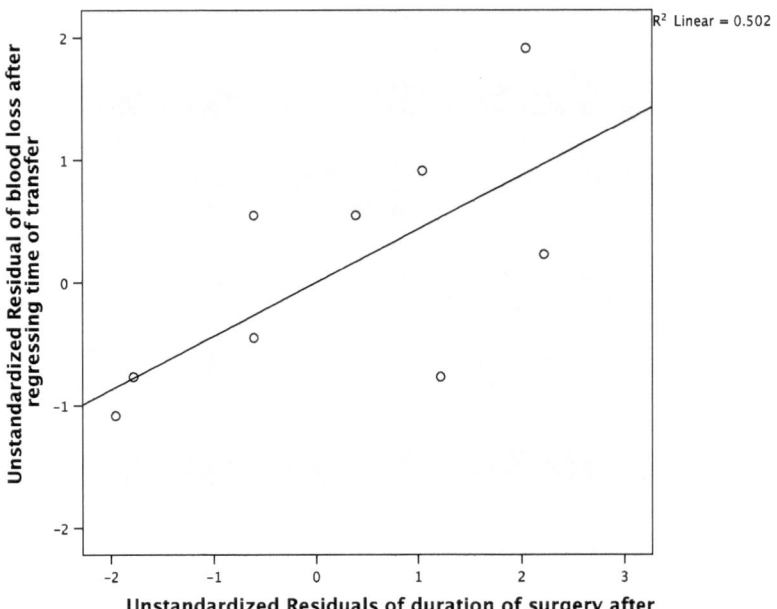

Fig. 2.17 Partial correlation between the duration of surgery and the amount of blood, controlling for the time to hospital transfer for data presented in Table 2.39

A primary aim of a clinical study is to link the predictor or explanatory variable to the study outcome. A prognostic factor is a third variable that increases the outcome variability, destabilizing this link, and hence, it should be controlled. Adjusting the outcome is not a single test or procedure but a strategy covering the study design, analysis methods, and interpretation of results.

Measures of adjustment include stratification of the randomized groups on the most important one or two prognostic factors. During the analysis, the researcher has to ensure the absence of a significant qualitative (reverse) interaction before adjusting a qualitative outcome by the Cochran–Mantel–Haenszel test. A two-way ANOVA can adjust a quantitative outcome. However, ANOVA cannot identify the independent roles of predictor and prognostic variable on outcome, unless it overrules a statistically significant interaction between them. Reporting should include both adjusted and unadjusted results to display the role of the prognostic variable. If they were multiple, a repeated adjustment could become a source of bias itself, and it should be replaced by multivariable analysis.

2.10 Measuring Agreement and Testing Reliability

Agreement between measurements refers to the degree of concordance between two or more sets of measurements. In addition to the type and distribution of the variable, measuring agreement depends on the operator, the used method or tool, and whether measurements are repeated or not? Measuring agreement aims to answer one or more of the following questions usually encountered in biology: whether the measurement by two different methods agrees so as one

method can replace the other? Is the measurement made by two different operators and using the same method reproducible, or is the measurement repeated by the same operator and using the same way precisely producing essentially the same result? The agreement is about answering three questions: is the measurement accurate and precise, is it reliable, and, finally, is it valid or not?

2.10.1 Introduction

Accuracy and Precision: Sampling and Systematic Errors

Before proceeding, we have to make a clear distinction between 2 terms: accuracy and precision. Accuracy means that the measurement is close to the true value (the target). For example, comparing the fasting blood sugar by a simple bedside test (test A) to the standard laboratory result gives 79 mg/dl versus 80 mg/dl, respectively. The result of test (A) is near to the standard, which represents the truth; hence, test (A) was thought to be accurate enough to replace the standard test. However, repeating test (A) 4 times and using the same blood sample gives very variable results: 75, 80, 80, 85 mg/dl (Table 2.40). Although the four measurements on average (80 mg/dl) are close to the truth, it is evident that this instrument lacks precision, which is how close the results are upon repeatability. Test (A) appears to be accurate but lacks precision, and the question would be: whether we can rely on (test A) to make a decision?

Another instrument (test B) gave less accurate results on the average: 69.5, 70, 70, and 70.5 mg/dl (mean 70 gm/dl) compared to the standard instrument (80 mg/dl), yet it was noticed that the results are very close to each other (Table 2.40). In other words, although test (B) is not accurate yet, it appears to be more precise than (A), and the question would be: whether we can rely on (test B) to make a decision? The difference between the results here and the truth is systematic that is present in all

Table 2.40 Accuracy versus precision

	1st	2nd	3rd	4th	Mean	Sd
Test A	75	80	80	85	80	4
Test B	69.5	70	70	70.5	70	0.4
Test C	79	79	81	81	80	1.1

Values represent 1st, 2nd, 3rd, 4th, the mean and standard deviation of fasting blood sugar readings in mg/dL, acquired from the same patient by three different test instruments: A, B, and C

readings, and is more or less constant (a systematic error). Hence, one can think to use the test and add a systematic correction to the results: e.g., adding 10, for example, the reading will be: 79.5, 80, 80, and 80.5 mg/dl. Note that a "similar constant" correction could not be applied to the results of test A that are due to chance: it is a random (sampling) error.

Accuracy means that the measurement is close to the true value/target, despite being precise (close to one another when repeated) or not. Precision means that the results are close to each other, despite being accurate (close to the target/truth) or not. Measurement has to be both: accurate and precise. As shown in Table 2.40, a third test (test C) gave accurate results on the average (79, 79, 81, and 81 mg/dl), which were precise as well (close to one another).

In conclusion, the agreement is concerned with both: accuracy and precision. Accuracy is how an "observed value" of a quantity agrees with the "true value" in the population. A measurement error is simply calculated as the difference between those two values. When the observed value is sometimes higher and sometimes lower than the true value but finally tends to balance out, this is called a random (sampling) error. An example was test A.

On the other hand, precision measures the extent to which repeated observations conform. The lack of precision is a systematic error where the observed values tend to be consistently high (or low) because of some known or unknown external factor, which must be eliminated to prevent bias. An example was test B. Put it this way, the variation of measurements is called measurement error. It can be of two kinds: A random error that is expected due to sampling

and a systematic error that has to be eliminated to prevent bias.

Reliability: Reproducibility and Repeatability

It is only after eliminating a systematic bias that we can proceed to test whether the new instrument (test, tool) is reliable. Reliability is the extent to which results are consistent or stable across time (repeated measurements), groups (different experimental conditions), etc..... Reproducibility aims to establish the between-methods or between-observers agreement. In other words, it aims to establish whether two persons using the same method of measurement obtain the same result or whether two techniques used to measure a particular variable, under identical circumstances, produce essentially the same result. Repeatability aims to establish a satisfactory within-observer agreement: will a 2nd measurement in the same subject by the same observer under identical conditions be the same? Fortunately, both reproducibility and repeatability can be assessed by the same test, as will be shown later. For the clinician, repeatability and reproducibility mean that the test is reliable.

Validity

In case the reliability being satisfactory, we can proceed to measure the usefulness of the new method to discriminate between two health conditions, between health and disease, etc. Measures of diagnostic accuracy were previously discussed in Sect. 1.9. In brief, there are paired measures assessing the condition independently in the 2 populations of concern (e.g., patients and controls, positive and negative test result) and, single measures that combine the assessments of the 2 populations in a single number. Paired measures include: sensitivity and specificity, positive and negative predictive values and, positive and negative likelihood ratios. Single measures include the size of the surface area under a ROC plot (AUC), Youden's index and diagnostic odds ratio. Some measures indicate the presence or absence of the disease, such as sensitivity, specificity and AUC of a ROC plot. Others are useful to interpret whether someone— in a specific population—has the disease because his "test" result was positive (positive predictive value) or he is disease-free because he had a negative test (negative predictive value). Likelihood ratios are independent from the prevalence of the disease in the population and hence, they can be used to express how much likely a diseased "patient" of any population can give a positive test result (true positive) or a negative test result (false negative), compared to a disease-free patient. For details on validity, the reader is advised to check on Sect. 1.9.

2.10.2 Plan of the Analysis

The plan begins by defining the study material, predictors and outcome; overruling a systematic bias by the appropriate statistical test and finally, measuring agreement itself, testing its statistical significance, interpreting and adequately reporting the findings.

2.10.2.1 Variable Definition

The plan of the analysis starts by defining the dependent variable (the outcome) that we want to measure and the independent variable (the predictor), which is supposed to explain the outcome. Note that we decided to use the terms "predictor and outcome variable" to prevent any confusion, especially that the terms: "dependent and independent variables" were initially used to describe that the former (e.g., the patient being cured) is dependent on the latter (e.g., type of treatment) and, by deduction, the type of treatment was termed as being independent. If the two compared treatments were given, not to 2 different groups of patients, but sequentially to

the same group, treatments are said to be dependent. It will be confusing to describe the type of treatment (predictor) as being independent of the outcome (cure) and, at the same time, as being dependent on being given to the same patient; which is why we have preferred to use the term "predictor variable" rather than the independent variable. We preferred to use the term outcome to describe the dependent variable to prevent raising the argument of dependent versus independent variables another time.

The Predictors

The predictor is responsible for the outcome. Classically, the predictor is a binomial qualitative variable. Common examples are testing agreement between 2 raters, two tests (usually a golden standard versus a new diagnostic test), or two experimental conditions (the use of conventional versus a new treatment in the same group of patients). The aim is to test whether the outcome is reproduced under those different conditions. The trimmer is "the variability between" subjects, tests, or diagnostic conditions; the more the test is considered reliable.

On the other hand, the same predictor can be compared to himself (itself) by repeating the measurement twice or several times, under the same condition and at fixed intervals. The smaller is "the variability within" the same subject, test, or experimental condition, the more the test is considered reliable. Less commonly, the predictor is a several-class categorical variable such as evaluating the agreement between three or more raters, tests, experimental conditions or, repeating the exact measurement under the same condition three times or more. Predictors have to be independent of each other: e.g., observers have to be blind from the decisions made by their colleagues, the performance of one test should not contaminate the other test, the effect of a specific drug should not overshadow the results of the second drug. Put it this way, the use of one predictor should not change "the basal condition" of the study material, which should be initially the same for every fresh predictor. Predictors have to be primarily chosen at random. However, they have to remain fixed and unique for the whole study material (all patients), except for Fleiss kappa. The latter assumes that predictors (usually two raters or sets of raters) are chosen at random, each time a new study material (a patient) is presented for evaluation (Kindly refer to Sect. 2.9.4.3. for details).

The Outcome

The outcome can be either qualitative or quantitative. The qualitative outcome is usually binomial, such as testing whether the patient has the disease or does not have the disease, e.g., being diabetic or not, depressed or relieved. The outcome can also be categorical or ordinal, such as the patient's symptoms have been relieved, were improved, or remained the same. The quantitative outcome can either be normally distributed or following other distribution than normal. An example of the former is a patient losing weight in kgs or getting his blood pressure improved in mmHg. Example of the latter is a change of a particular score, such as the pain visual analog score or Glasco Coma scale. Remember that score units represent discrete categories, and hence, they are not continuous and follow other distributions than normal.

The Study Material

The study material is usually the patients in medical practice, tissue samples, body fluids, electrocardiographic or radiological studies, or other patient-related documents. The material must be equally chosen at random and then fixed to be examined by both predictors or repeatedly over fixed time intervals by the same predictor. In the case of multiple predictors, a new material (e.g., a new patient, new blood sample) is chosen at random from a large population. It is examined once by the multiple predictors who are equally chosen at random from their respective populations. The material just examined is excluded from the next random selection so that no material is being selected twice for examination by the second set of predictors. The random selection process of both study material and predictors is repeated until all material has been examined.

2.10.2.2 Overruling a Systematic Bias

The researcher usually starts by eliminating the presence of a systematic error between the new method and the golden standard; otherwise, it will be pointless to proceed and test the agreement. As previously noted, the same test used to assess reproducibility is used to assess repeatability. Put it this way, the test used to eliminate a systematic bias in comparing a golden standard to a new diagnostic test is the same test used if either test is repeated twice. As shown in Table 2.41, the test used depends on the type of variable and its distribution and the number of predictors (raters or tested equipment). Although those tests were designed to prove a statistically significant difference between comparators yet, we hope that those tests fail to do so in the agreement context. It will not be meaningful to test agreement between two measures that were shown to be significantly different from one another by one of those tests. On the other hand, failure should never be translated that both tests are equal or in agreement, simply because the null hypothesis can never be true [29]. Eliminating systematic bias is just a preliminary step that turns the green light on to go one step further and test agreement by the appropriate measure. Eliminating systematic bias reinforces the proper tools of the agreement but should never be considered to replace those tools.

Tests used to eliminate systematic bias have been previously discussed in chapter two, and the researcher is invited to refer back to it for more details about the indications, the idea behind the equation, the interpretation, what should be reported, and the conditions of application. In brief, the McNemar test is used to eliminate a systematic bias in case two predictors judge on a binomial outcome or a single predictor evaluating a binomial outcome twice (see Sect. 2.3.2.1). Bowker test is a modification of the McNemar test. It eliminates systematic bias between two predictors judging on a categorical outcome or the same predictor judging twice on the same categorical variable (see Sect. 2.3.2.2). The paired test of Student (see Sect. 2.4.1.3) and the Wilcoxon sign rank test (see Sect. 2.5.1.2) are the respective

Table 2.41 Measuring agreement: plan of the analysis

(1) Outcome	(2) Predictor	(3) Eliminating systematic bias	Measures of agreement
Binomial	2 raters, 2 tests or 2 experimental conditions	McNemar test	Cohen Kappa
Categorical or ordinal	2 raters, 2 tests or 2 experimental conditions	McNemar Bowker test	Weighted Kappa
Binomial, categorical or ordinal	≥ 3 raters, 3 tests or 3 experimental conditions	Cochran Q test[a]	Fleiss or Randolph Kappa[b]
Quantitative, Normal	2 raters, tests or experimental conditions	Paired Student test	Bland Altman plots Lin's CC MDC/BSRC ICC
	≥ 3 raters, test or experimental conditions	RMANOVA	ICC
Quantitative, other distributions	2 raters, tests or experimental conditions	Wilcoxon sign rank test	KCC
	≥ 3 raters, tests or experimental conditions	Friedman's test	KCC

CC = correlation coefficient, MDC = minimal detectable change, BSIC = British standard institution coefficient, ICC = intraclass correlation coefficient, KCC = Kendall concordance coefficient
[a] = is only applied in case of a binomial outcome
[b] = does not take into effect weighting of categories or effect order

alternatives in case of a normally distributed continuous outcome and in case the quantitative outcome is following other distribution than normal. Finally, Cochran Q test, One-way repeated measures ANOVA (see Sect. 2.4.3.4) and Friedman's test (see Sect. 2.5.2.2) can eliminate a systematic bias if the outcome was a binomial variable, a normally distributed continuous variable, or a quantitative variable following other distributions than normal; respectively.

2.10.2.3 Measuring Agreement

Table 2.41 shows the most commonly used measures of agreement, depending upon the combinations of the type and distribution of outcome variable and the number of predictors. Classically, testing agreement was designed for two predictors, and modifications were made to include multiple predictors.

Cohen's Kappa and derivatives are the most commonly used measures to test agreement on a qualitative outcome. Cohen's Kappa was originally designed to test agreement between mutually exclusive nominal or categorical variables. It was later modified to consider the relative weights of different variable categories or orders, giving birth to the more "refined" weighted Kappa. The inclusion of more than two predictors necessitated another modification, with the emergence of Fleiss' Kappa and Randolph's Kappa, even at the expense of losing the property of weighting variable categories. Those are just the most commonly used measures that include a long list of other measures and indices of agreement [58].

In case the outcome is a continuous, normally distributed variable, Altman and Bland have shown that Pearson's correlation coefficient, even though precise, lacks accuracy and cannot be used to measure agreement. They proposed their famous plots, which display and measure the extent and limits of agreement. The agreement can then be expressed in a single measure (number) and, in this section, we will present two indices: Lin's correlation coefficient, and the intraclass correlation coefficient (ICCC). Lin's correlation coefficient gives the same results as ICCC, with the latter having the advantage of including multiple predictors. Hence, ICCC can test agreement between repeated measures carried over fixed time intervals. Finally, in the case of outcome variables following other distribution than normal, Kendall's W is the commonly used measure of agreement that can accommodate multiple predictors.

2.10.3 The Qualitative Outcome

2.10.3.1 Cohen' Kappa

Cohen's Kappa measures agreement between two predictors on a binomial or categorical outcome or one predictor evaluating the same material twice. Playing the same tune, it can measure agreement between 2 groups of individuals collectively giving a joint decision or a non-human agency such as a computer program giving one answer based on specific criteria [2]. Note that this is different from the situation where we wish to test agreement between multiple predictors, each giving his independent evaluation. We cannot use Cohen's Kappa as described in such a case.

As agreement per se can be just due to chance, Cohen's Kappa was designed to measure the proportion of agreement over and above the agreement expected by chance. It expresses agreement on a numerical scale ranging between −1 and +1. A positive Kappa indicates that agreement is better than chance, up to a (+1) Kappa, which means a perfect agreement (100%). A negative Kappa is rare and indicates a less-than-chance agreement [59].

The Example

A study was conducted to compare the results acquired with "the relatively new" multislice computerized axial tomography (MSCT) with the more invasive "gold standard" coronary angiography (CA). The material was 80 patients suspected of in-stent restenosis after percutaneous coronary intervention (PCI) (Table 2.9.3). Each pair of measurements was made in the same patient, acquired within a reasonable time (1 week), provided that the patient was stable between both measurements. The study question was whether the new technique agrees with the classic one sufficiently enough to be thought of

as a reliable replacement or not? McNemar's test produced a smaller Chi-square value (1.6) than the critical value indicated in the Chi-square table, at 1 df (3.84). The test failed to demonstrate a systematic (constant) error between the two measurements (P = 0.34), and we will proceed to measure agreement. PS. The reader can refer to Sect. 2.2.1.5 for the detailed calculations of this example.

The Equation

The new technique has diagnosed 73.3% (59/80) of cases as having a patent stent (73.7%) and the remaining 26.3% (21/80) as having ISR. Put it this way, every case benefiting from MSCT has a 73.7% chance of having a patent stent and a 26.3% chance of being diagnosed as having ISR, regardless of the "true diagnosis" made by the gold standard CA. We will begin with the 55 patients the gold standard has shown to have a patent stent. If the diagnosis made by MSCT was only due to chance, the number of cases that will be diagnosed as having a patent stent has to be equal to 73.7% of the 55 cases = $55 \times 73.7\%$ = 40.6 patients and not 52 cases, as observed. Each theoretical value (e.g., patent stent) can be calculated by multiplying the marginal values observed by both tests (59 and 55) and dividing the result by the total number of paired values (80) = $55 \times 59/80$ = 40.6.

Similarly, the number of cases that have a patient stent by CA but are expected to be diagnosed as having ISR by MSCT has to be equal to 26.3% of the 55 cases = $55 \times 26.3\%$ = 14.4 cases ($21 \times 55/80$ = 6.6 cases) and not 3 cases as observed. The same calculations can be repeated to get the expected values for the 18 cases diagnosed by both tools as having ISR ($21 \times 25/80$ = 6.6 cases) as well as the 7 cases shown by CA as having ISR but diagnosed by MSCT as having a patient stent ($59 \times 25/80$ = 18.4 cases). Table 2.42 shows theoretical values between brackets. Those expected numbers represent any agreement that may be due to chance. Hence, the differences between observed and expected numbers reflect the amount of agreement above what can be due to chance.

Table 2.42 Cohen Kappa: Measuring agreement between multislice CT (MSCT) and coronary angiography (CA) in patients with in-stent restenosis (ISR)

	CA (ISR)	CA (patent stent)	Total
MSCT (ISR)	18 (6.6)	3 (14.4)	21
MSCT (patent stent)	7 (18.4)	52 (40.6)	59
Total	25	55	80

Values are the observed number of cases, numbers between brackets are the theoretical numbers reflecting the amount of agreement that can be due to chance. MSCT = multislice computerized axial tomography, CA = coronary angiography, ISR = in-stent restenosis

Unlike the McNemar test, we have to look to the other side of the coin and concentrate on agreements, keeping the non-concordant results aside. Both procedures agreed on the diagnosis in 70 cases: na = 52 + 18 = 70. The observed percentage of agreement is the proportion of this number out of the total number of patients (n = 80): Pa = na/n = 70/80 = 0.875. The next step is to calculate the number of agreements that is expected due to chance: nc = 40.6 + 6.6 = 47.2 cases and, the percentage of agreement due to chance: = Pc = 47.2/80 = 0.59. As a perfect agreement (100%) is equal to 1 in decimals, Cohen Kappa is calculated as the proportion of agreement (Pa) to the perfect agreement (1), corrected for the part due to chance (Pc); i.e., both being corrected by taking (Pc) out "Eq. 2.127". In our example, Cohen's Kappa = 0.695. The Se of kappa (0.09) can be calculated by the Cohen formula given below "Eq. 2.128" [59] or by a more correct and complex formula suggested by Fleiss and colleagues [61]; both values can be easily calculated online [2].

$$k = \frac{(P_a - P_c)}{(1 - P_c)} = \frac{(n_a - n_c)}{(n - n_c)} \qquad (2.127)$$

$$Se_k = \sqrt{\frac{P_a(1 - P_a)}{n(1 - P_e)^2}} \qquad (2.128)$$

As Kappa (K) follows an approximately normal distribution, we can calculate a z value as: K/Se = 0.695/0.09 = 7.7, construct a 95% confidence interval (mean Kappa ± 1.96 Se = 0.52–0.87) and deduct a more approximate P value from Z table: P < 0.001. All calculations can be simply made online using one of the many freely available calculators [2, 62]. According to Cohen: Kappa values of: <0.00, 0 to <0.2, 0.2 to <0.4, 0.4 to <0.6, 0.6 to <0.8 and 0.8–1; indicate poor, slight, fair, moderate, substantial, and almost perfect agreement [59]. The interpretation of the result is as follows: there is a statistically significant substantial agreement between both tests: Kappa (95% CI) = 0.695 (0.52–0.87): P < 0.001.

The Kappa Paradoxes

It was noticed that the value of Kappa tends to decrease with significantly higher or lower prevalence of the disease and tends to increase the more raters disagree; which has been described as the two Kappa paradoxes [63]. The role of prevalence is greater when Kappa is large, while bias has been shown to be greater when Kappa is small [64]. Table 2.43 shows the results of testing agreement between the gold standard CA and the new diagnostic tool MSCT. The total number of agreements (na) is the sum of the number of positive agreements (na1 = 18) and the number of negative agreements (na2 = 52) and is equal to 70 cases. The total number of disagreements (nd) is the sum of the number of positive disagreements (nd1 = 7) and the number of negative agreements (nd2 = 3) and is equal to 10 cases. Note that positive or negative agreement is used here because the case was considered as being positive or negative by the gold standard. According to the gold standard, the total number of patients with the disease = na1 + nd1 = 25 cases and, the total number of disease-free cases = na2 + nd2 = 55 cases. According to MSCT, the total number of patients with the disease (ISR) = na1 + nd2 = 21

Table 2.43 Role of prevalence and bias between raters in Kappa. Data presented in Table 2.42

	CA (ISR)	CA (patent stent)	total
MSCT (ISR)	18 (na1)	3 (nd2)	21 (na1 + nd2)
MSCT (patent stent)	7 (nd1)	52 (na2)	59 (nd1 + na2)
total	25 (na1 + nd1)	55 (na2 + nd2)	80 (n)

MSCT = multislice CT, CA = coronary angiography, ISR = in-stent restenosis, na1 = number of positive agreements, na2 = number of negative agreements, nd1 = number of positive disagreements (as judged by CA), nd2 = number of negative disagreements (as judged by CA), na1 + na2 = na = total number of agreements, nd1 + nd2 = nd = total number of disagreements, n = total number of pairs

cases and the total number of disease-free cases = nd1 + na2 = 59 cases. We will begin by discussing the role of prevalence.

The Prevalence Index

Sensitivity (Sn) is the number of TP cases (na1) among the patients with the disease and is independent of the prevalence; i.e., if the prevalence of the disease increases, the number of positive cases (na1) increases too, in order to maintain the same Sn. On the other hand, specificity (Sp) is the number of TN cases (na2) among the healthy (52/55 = 0.945) and is also independent of prevalence; i.e., if the prevalence of the disease decreases, the number of negative cases (na2) has to increase too, in order to maintain the same Sp. A significant change (an increase or a decrease) in prevalence widens the gap between those two numbers (na1 − na2), which can be expressed as a proportion from the total number of cases: the prevalence index "Eq. 2.129". The latter is reported in absolute value = (18 − 52)/80 = 0.425, in our example. The higher is this index, whether due to a considerably high or low prevalence, the more are the "chances" of agreement. As Kappa is the proportion of agreement over what is due to chance, the smaller Kappa will be [65]; a phenomenon that has been described as one of the two paradoxes Kappa [63].

$$Prevalence\ index = \frac{(na1 - na2)}{n} \quad (2.129)$$

The Bias Index

The other phenomenon of the Kappa paradox is the bias index [63]. As previously mentioned, the

number of expected positive cases due to chance (nc1) is the product of the marginal values divided by the total number of pairs. The total number of positive cases diagnosed by CA (25 cases) and the total number of positive cases diagnosed by MSCT (21 cases) are divided by the total number of pairs (80 patients). As shown in Table 2.43, the total number of positive cases diagnosed by CA (25 cases) can be rewritten as 18 + nd1, and the total number of positive cases diagnosed by MSCT (21 cases) can be rewritten as 18 + nd2. The same applies to the number of expected negative cases due to chance, and the total number of expected cases due to chance (nc) will be the sum of nc1 and nc2, of course. As Kappa is the amount of agreement over what is due to chance, the larger (nc), the smaller Kappa will be. Now let us keep up with nc1 because what implies on nc1 will imply on nc2, and finally on nc.

In our example, the clinicians disagreed on 10 cases, in the proportion 7:3 (nd1: nd2) and hence, nc1 = 6.6(25 × 21/80). Now suppose that there was more disagreement between both clinicians, let us say 9:1, recalculation shows that nc1 decreases to 6.4 (27 × 19/80) and, consequently, Kappa will finally increase. It seems logical; the larger is the disagreement, the less are the chances that they will eventually agree, and hence, the larger Kappa will be. Looking the other way round and suppose that they agree more so that the disagreement proportion becomes 6:4; recalculation shows that nc1 increases to 6.6 (24 × 22/80), and Kappa is expected to decrease. The highest nc1 value is obtained when there is no disagreement between clinicians (nd1 and nd2 = 0) or when nd1

= nd2 = 5; in both cases, nc1 will attain the smallest value: 4.05. It is clear that the wider is the difference between nd1 and nd2, the less we expect an agreement due to chance, and hence, the larger Kappa will be "Eq. 2.130". In consequence, it is advised to report the bias index: $(nd1 - nd2)/n = (7 - 3)\,80 = 0.05$.

$$Bias\ index = \frac{(nd1 - nd2)}{n} \qquad (2.130)$$

In conclusion, the higher (or lower) is the Prevalence of the disease, "the more are the chances" to meet positive (or negative) cases, and hence, Kappa tends to decrease. The more raters disagree, "the less are the chances" that they agree, and hence, Kappa tends to increase. Remember that Kappa is the proportion of agreement beyond chance and is inversely proportional to it. Put it this way, Prevalence increases the chances of agreement and reduces Kappa and, bias decreases those chances and increases Kappa. The value of adjusting Kappa on Prevalence by calculating a prevalence-adjusted bias-adjusted kappa (PABAK), using the mean values of (na1 and na2) and (nd1 and nd2), is debatable but may be supplied alongside the original Kappa value [66].

Kappa Max. (K_{max})

Dunn recommends reporting K_{max}, which is the maximum value that Kappa can achieve within the constraint of the data set [67]. In our example, the total positive cases identified by CA and MSCT were 25 and 21. The total negative cases identified by CA and MSCT were 55 and 59. Those are the marginal values that indicate the limits of our material. Regardless of agreement,

MSCT can diagnose 21 out of the 25 positive cases diagnosed by CA and 55 out of the 59 negative cases diagnosed by CA (93.2%); this is the maximum MSCT can achieve.

Provided that MSCT was able to agree with CA in every one of those cases, the maximum number of agreements between both methods will be 21 positive cases and 55 negative cases, and the number of disagreements will change accordingly, of course. Those maximal values are presented in paratheses along the diagonal cells in Table 2.44. Note that they are the smallest marginal values in each category. Kappa max (K_{max}) can be calculated using Kappa equation "Eq. 2.127", after replacing (na = 70 in our example) by the sum of those maximal values (n_{am} = 76 in our example) "Eq. 2.131". The maximum value that Kappa can reach within the given limits of our study will be = (76–47.2)/(80–47.2) = 0.878. The difference between Kappa and Kappa max reflects the imbalance in the marginal tools on the magnitude of Kappa, which is due to pre-existing conditions before the test, such as difference in scales, specificity of the used tools, the experience of raters, or else.

$$k_{max} = \frac{(n_{am} - n_c)}{(n - n_c)} \qquad (2.131)$$

2.10.3.2 Weighted Kappa
As such, Cohen Kappa considers disagreement (yes/no) between 2 raters but not the degree (the extent) of disagreement that we may need to address in the case of a categorical variable. In fact, the presence of multiple categories, not just two, invites the researcher to examine whether the "internal" difference between those categories

Table 2.44 Calculation of Kappa Max (K_{max}). Data presented in Table 2.42

	CA (ISR)	CA (patent stent)	Total
MSCT (ISR)	**18 (21)**	3 (0)	21
MSCT (patent stent)	7 (4)	**52 (55)**	59
Total	25	55	80 (n)

Values represent the actual observations, values between parentheses represent the smallest marginal value in each category for agreements and, the remaining values for disagreements, MSCT = multislice CT, CA = coronary angiography, ISR = in-stent restenosis, n = total number of pairs may influence the degree of agreement between predictors. Hence, Cohen Kappa has to be modified to take this into account. The agreement can be weighted by the classes or the categories of the qualitative variable. The weighted kappa indicated the agreement better and is very similar to ICC used for numerical data.

The Example

A randomized study was conducted to measure how much clinicians can agree on the evaluation of the patients' symptoms. Two clinicians were requested to classify the symptoms of 50 patients with depression as being either: mild, moderate or severe symptoms (Table 2.45). Before proceeding to the testing agreement, the researchers have to show first that there is no statistically significant disagreement between the clinical evaluation of both researchers. As the outcome is an ordinal variable (mild, moderate, and severe symptoms), the McNemar-Bowker test can be used to test whether there is a significant difference between the classification made by both researchers.

The Equations

1. Calculation of Unweighted Kappa

For instructive purposes, we will measure agreement by both the conventional (unweighted) and the weighted Kappa to show how much the latter is more sensitive than the former. We will begin by supposing that all categories have the same magnitude, and hence, we calculate the unweighted Kappa by ignoring the non-concordant results. We concentrate on the concordant results shown along the diagonal of Table 2.45, i.e., 10, 16, and 18.

As Kappa measures the degree of agreement over what is due to chance, we have to calculate the numbers expected by chance. The expected number of agreements for the patients' symptoms diagnosed as being "mild" is calculated by multiplying the total number of cases diagnosed as mild by the first rater (15) by the total number of cases diagnosed as "mild" by the second rater (16), divided by the total number of patients in the study (50) = $15 \times 16/50 = 4.8$. Playing the same tune, the expected number of agreements due to chance for the "moderate" diagnosis = $24 \times 23/50 = 11$ and the "severe" diagnosis = $11 \times 11/50 = 2.4$.

The next step is to calculate the total number of concordant cases (na = $10 + 16 + 8 = 34$ cases) and the percentage of observed agreement, which is the proportion of this number to the total sample size (Pa = $34/50 = 0.68$). We do the same for the total number of expected cases (nc = $4.8 + 11 + 2.4 = 18$ cases) and the percentage of expected agreement (Pe = $18.2/50 = 0.364$). As a perfect agreement (100%) is equal to 1 in decimals, Cohen Kappa is calculated as the proportion of agreement (Pa) to the perfect agreement (1), corrected for the part due to chance (Pc); i.e., both the observed (Pa) and the perfect agreements (1) are corrected by taking (Pc) out "Eq. 2.127". The Se of Kappa equals 0.11 "Eq. 2.128". According to Cohen's suggestion [59], there is a statistically significant moderate agreement between the two raters: Kappa (95% CI) = 0.496 (0.365–0.753); P < 0.001. As previously mentioned, all calculations can be simply made online using one of the many freely available online calculators [2, 62].

Table 2.45 Unweighted kappa: 2 clinicians judging on a 3-class categorical variable

		Clinician 1			
		Mild	Moderate	Severe	Total
Clinician 2	Mild	10 (4.8)	4	1	15
	Moderate	6	16 (11)	2	24
	Severe	0	3	8 (2.4)	11
	Total	16	23	11	50

Values are the observed number of cases, numbers between brackets are the theoretical numbers reflecting the amount of agreement that can be due to chance

2. *Calculation of Weighted Kappa*

It is more logical to consider an inherent disagreement (difference) between the ordered categories of the outcome. A common way to give an ordered weight is to put a linear penalty by assigning 1, 2, 3, ….x weights to values as far as they go further away from the complete agreement's diagonal (0) value. A more severe quadratic penalty is equally provided by statistical software and online calculators [2, 62]. Before applying, a simple linear penalty to our example, we must know that weighted Kappa is calculated differently from the regular unweighted version.

First, while the latter calculates the proportion of agreement, weighted Kappa calculates the proportion of disagreement! As a perfect (100%) agreement equals 1 in decimals, Kappa can be finally expressed as 1 minus this proportion of disagreement. Second, a considerable disagreement by two levels, such as one clinician diagnosing the symptoms as mild while the other clinician considers those symptoms severe, should be given more weight compared to both clinicians disputing on a difference of one level only. Weighting the levels of disagreement differently by multiplying cases of a complete agreement by zero, disagreement on just one level by 1, a disagreement on two levels by 2, …, in an increasing linear order appears to be a fair way to weigh those values. Third, unlike the unweighted Kappa, we need to calculate the expected values due to chance for all observations and not for the diagonal values only, as shown in Table 2.46. Fourth, expected values are calculated as before: product of the marginal

values/total sample size. Fifth, observed and expected values in the diagonal cells (no disagreement) will be multiplied by zero (to be discarded), those with only one class difference will be multiplied by 1, and values in the bold cells with a difference of two classes will be multiplied by 2. Finally, we calculate the sums of all weighted observed values (Wo = 17) "Eqs. 2.132" and "2.133". We calculate the sum of all weighted expected values (We = 38.6) "Eq. 2.134" and Kappa will be equal to 1 minus the standardized observed proportion = $1 - Wo/We = 1 - (17/38.6) = 0.559$ "Eq. 2.135". The Se of Kappa = 0.099 and the 95% CI = 0.36–0.75; $P < 0.001$. Quadratic weighting will give a higher Kappa value of 0.636, Se = 0.129, and 95% CI = 0.38–0.89. As previously mentioned, all calculations can be made online [2, 62].

$$\sum W_o = (W_o \times 0) + (W_1 \times 1) + (W_2 \times 2) + \cdots \\ \cdot (W_i \times i)$$

(2.132)

$$\sum W_o = (10 \times 0) + (4 \times 1) + (1 \times 2) + (6 \times 1) \\ + (16 \times 0) + (2 \times 1) + (0 \times 2) \\ + (3 \times 1) + (8 \times 0) = 17$$

(2.133)

$$\sum W_e = (4.8 \times 0) + (6.9 \times 1) + (3.3 \times 2) \\ + (7.7 \times 1) + (11 \times 0) + (5.3 \times 1) \\ + (3.5 \times 2) + (5.2 \times 1) \\ + (2.4 \times 0) = 38.6$$

(2.134)

Table 2.46 Weighted kappa: 2 clinicians judging on a 3-class categorical variable

		Clinician 1			
		Mild	Moderate	Severe	Total
Clinician 2	Mild	10 (4.8)	4 (6.9)	**1 (3.3)**	15
	Moderate	6 (7.7)	16 (11)	2 (5.3)	24
	Severe	**0 (3.5)**	3 (5.1)	8 (2.4)	11
	Total	16	23	11	50

Values are the observed number of cases. Values between brackets are the expected numbers of the agreement due to chance. All values in the bold cells (3.3 and 3.5), values outside the diagonals, and values along the diagonals will be weighted by being multiplied by 2, 1, and 0, respectively

$$k_w = 1 - \frac{\sum W_o}{\sum W_e} \qquad (2.135)$$

Weighting increases the kappa value by considering the expected weight of each category on the degree of agreement. This salutary effect of weighting is becoming more pronounced, with increasing outcome category. It was noticed that the value of unweighted Kappa was reduced with increasing outcome categories [68]; i.e., the more the qualitative variable is subdivided into categories, the more predictors will disagree and, finally, Kappa is reduced. However, the increased sensitivity of Kappa with weighting was found to have a salutary effect on Kappa value, especially with quadratic weighting where Kappa was even found to increase in the proportion of categorization, especially between 2 and 5 categories [69].

2.10.3.3 Fleiss and Randolph Kappa for Multiple Categories

Cohen Kappa measures the degree of agreement between two raters who evaluate the same study material on a scale of mutually exclusive outcome categories. Several extensions of Cohen Kappa and different independent models have been proposed to evaluate more than two raters [58]. We will limit our discussion to the two most commonly used measures of agreement between multiple predictors: Fleiss Kappa and Randolph Kappa.

Fleiss Kappa

Fleiss is a modification of Cohen's Kappa that accommodates multiple predictors providing a binomial outcome. It is helpful in clinical studies aiming to test agreement between physicians' nominal diagnoses and in meta-analysis to determine how well different studies agree [70]. The introduction of the variable "multiple predictors" into the Kappa model necessitated the removal of the variable "weighting of outcome categories"; hence, the calculated Kappa is unweighted. However, this is partially compensated by the ability of Fleiss Kappa to calculate an overall Kappa value for the outcome variable

and an individual Kappa for each level of the categorical variables separately versus the other categories combined.

Randolph free-marginal Kappa

One of the assumptions of Fleiss kappa is that predictors have to assign a fixed number of cases to each outcome category, resulting in fixed marginal values, which is why those studies are sometimes called: "fixed-marginal studies." In "free-marginal studies", predictors are free to assign cases to categories with no limits on how many cases must go into each category, resulting in fluctuations of marginal values. We have previously shown that marginal values are used to calculate the expected values due to chance and, finally, the part of the agreement due to chance (Pc) (see Sect. 2.10.3.1). Consequently, (Pc) of free-marginal studies has to be calculated differently from that of fixed marginal studies, which is why Randolph modified Fleiss Kappa to accommodate better free-marginal studies [70]. As the fluctuations in marginal values are mainly due to prevalence and bias between predictors (see Sect. 2.10.3.1), we can assume that Randolph Kappa is calculated independently from both factors.

The Example

A study was conducted in a large tertiary center to examine the degree of agreement between cardiologists in referring patients with ischemic heart disease for either medical therapy, percutaneous angioplasty, or surgery (3 mutually exclusive categories). Ten patients (N = 10) were randomly chosen from all inpatients and, each patient was examined by three cardiologists (n = 3) who were randomly chosen, on each occasion, from all attending cardiologists. The principal researcher had to ensure that no patient was examined twice, but it can happen that the set of 3 cardiologists, who are randomly chosen each time to examine one patient, includes a cardiologist who has been chosen to examine another patient before. This play of chance is expected and accepted; however, the larger is the pool of cardiologists from which we randomly choose the set of three cardiologists, the smaller will be this chance. The assumptions behind multi-rater Kappa depend upon the fact that both the pool of study material (patients) and the pool of predictors (cardiologists) have to be large. The results of the study are shown in Table 2.47. The first column shows the ten patients. The values shown in the three middle columns are the number of cardiologists who agreed on a specific decision for the given patient at the row's top (the beginning). As the three cardiologists examine each patient, the sum of the three values in the middle of each row is always equal to 3. As an example, concerning the first patient (I), two cardiologists agreed that he is a good candidate for medical treatment. In contrast, one cardiologist suggested that the patient is a good candidate for surgery. The fifth and last column shows the proportion of agreement for each patient (Pi), while the last row shows the proportion of agreement for each outcome category (PJ).

We will use the same example to execute both fixed-marginal Fleiss and free-marginal Randolph Kappa to show the points of similarities and differences and, most importantly, their effect on the calculated Kappa value and, later on, on reporting and interpretation.

The Equation

1. *Calculation of the Proportion of Observed Agreement (Pa)*

We begin by calculating the proportion of observed agreement per patient (Pi): how many raters agree on each outcome category, relative to the number of all possible agreements. P_i of each patient is the sum of the squared values in the row, subtracted from the total number of cardiologists ($n = 3$) and divided by $n \times n - 1$. Pi for the first patient (I) "Eq. 2.136":

$$P_i = \frac{(2^2 + 0^2 + 1^2) - 3}{3(3-1)} = 0.333 \qquad (2.136)$$

In the case all cardiologists agree on the same decision, (P_i) will be 1 (100%); indicating a perfect agreement, which was the case in patients V, VI, VII, and X "Eq. 2.137":

Table 2.47 Fleiss Kappa: Measuring agreement between three cardiologists on the best way to manage ten patients with ischemic heart disease: medical therapy, percutaneous angioplasty or surgery

Patients (N = 10)	Outcome categories			
	Medical treatment	Percutaneous angioplasty	Surgery	Pi
I	2	0	1	0.333
II	0	2	1	0.333
III	2	1	0	0.333
IV	3	0	0	1
V	0	3	0	1
VI	0	3	0	1
VII	0	3	0	1
VIII	0	0	3	1
IX	1	2	0	0.333
X	0	3	0	1
Sum/N*n	8/30	17/30	5/30	
Pj	$(0.266)^2$	$(0.566)^2$	$(0.166)^2$	

Values are the number of cardiologists who agreed on a particular decision for the patient presented in each row, N = total number of patients, n = number of categories, P_i = proportion of observed pairs of agreement, relative to the number of all possible pairs, P_J = squared proportion of each outcome category (decision)

Table 2.48 Fleiss Kappa: SPSS input for data presented in Table 2.47

Patients (N = 10)	Predictors		
	First cardiologist	Second cardiologist	Third cardiologist
I	1	1	3
II	2	2	3
III	1	1	2
IV	1	1	1
V	2	2	2
VI	2	2	2
VII	2	2	2
VIII	3	3	3
IX	1	2	2
X	2	2	2

1 = medical treatment, 2 = percutaneous angioplasty, 3 = surgery

$$P_I = \frac{(0^2 + 3^2 + 0^2) - 3}{3(3-1)} = 1 \qquad (2.137)$$

In the case all cardiologists disagreed, with each one adopting a different decision (not shown in Table 2.47); (Pi) will be equal to zero, indicating no agreement whatsoever "Eq. 2.138":

$$P_I = \frac{(1^2 + 1^2 + 1^2) - 3}{3(3-1)} = 0 \qquad (2.138)$$

The proportion of observed agreements per patient is simply the average of the proportions calculated for the ten patients "Eq. 2.139":

$$
\begin{aligned}
P_a &= \sum P_i/n \\
&= (0.333 + 0.333 + 0.333 + 1 + 1 + 1 + 1 \\
&\quad + 1 + 0.333 + 1)/10 \\
&= 0.73
\end{aligned}
$$

$$(2.139)$$

2. *Calculation of the Proportion of Agreement Due to Chance (Pc)*

The second step is to calculate the proportion of agreement that is due to chance, regardless of an individual patient and here, comes the main difference between Fleiss kappa and Randolph Kappa.

Fleiss Kappa

Fleiss Kappa assumes that marginal values (Pj) are "more or less" fixed, and hence, it calculates the part of the agreement that is due to chance from these marginal values. (Pj) of each category is the squared value of the sum of the column divided by all possible combinations. The latter is the product of the number of outcomes and the number of patients = n × N = 3 × 10 = 30. The proportion of agreement that is expected due to chance for medical therapy "Eq. 2.140":

$$
\begin{aligned}
P_J &= \left(\frac{2+0+2+3+0+0+0+0+1+0}{(3 \times 10)}\right)^2 \\
&= (0.266^2) = 0.07
\end{aligned}
$$

$$(2.140)$$

The respective (Pj) for patients who will be referred to PTCA and to surgery are 0.32 and 0.27. The proportion of agreement due to chance (Pc) in Fleiss Kappa is the sum of (Pj) calculated for the three outcome categories "Eq. 2.141":

$$P_c = \sum P_J = (0.07 + 0.32 + 0.27) = 0.42 \qquad (2.141)$$

Randolph Kappa

We have previously shown the effect of prevalence (P) and bias on a binomial outcome, such as the presence or absence of a certain disease (see Sect. 2.10.3.1). Logically, their proportion (presence/absence) will also depend on the (P) and bias between the two raters. The same logic can be applied to our example here: suppose that the study population has a low prevalence, more cases will be assigned to medical treatment, compared to those referred to surgery and, the reverse is expected in case of a population with a high prevalence of ischemic heart disease. On the other hand, if one rater was a cardiologist in a hospital with no intervention facility and the second rater was an interventional cardiologist, the first will tend to assign the patients to medical treatment and the latter to intervention. "Tending" here means without clear evidence but guided by his feeling, i.e., just by chance. Hence, both prevalence and bias significantly affect the part of the decision due to chance (Pc) and lower kappa value, in the case of free-marginal study (Pj). Randolph and colleagues designed the free-marginal Kappa to be independent of the effect of prevalence and bias by setting Pc equal to the reciprocal value of the number of categories 1/k, where k is the number of outcome categories. As an example, our outcome variable has three categories, and hence, under the null hypothesis, any two raters would be expected to agree on 1/3 of the cases [58, 70]. In case of a four-class outcome, the two raters will be expected to agree on ¼ of the cases and so on.

3. Calculation of Kappa

As usual, Kappa is the proportion of observed agreement (Pa) that is over and above the part of agreement due to chance (Pc). Kappa is calculated by the routine equation "Eq. 2.127" and the only difference will be the value of (Pc); being 0.42 in Fleiss Kappa and 0.33 in the free-marginal Randolph Kappa.

Uploading our data as shown in Table 2.47 to an online calculator gives both Fleiss (0.054; 0.2–0.88) and Randolph Kappa values (0.6; 0.28–0.92) and their 95% confidence intervals [62]. It is clear that Randolph free-marginal Kappa levels kappa value to the degree of agreement. Uploading our example to SPSS version 24 or higher has the advantages of providing the exact P-value of Fleiss Kappa, individual kappa value for each category, its 95% CI, and P values for comparing each category to the other categories combined. The reader must note that data are not uploaded as shown in Table 2.10.47; i.e., the number of cardiologists who agreed on a specific diagnosis but instead as dummy indicator of outcome categories, per evaluating cardiologist (Table 2.48). Table 2.49 shows an extract of SPSS output for our example. There is an overall statistically significant moderate agreement Kappa between the three cardiologists: Kappa 0.54 (0.28–0.81); P < 0.001. Cardiologists showed a significantly larger moderate agreement on which patient is referred to PTCA than to medical treatment and surgery combined: Kappa 0.59 (0.23–0.95); P = 0.001. They agreed less on which patient to

Table 2.49 Extract of SPSS output of overall Fleiss Kappa and Kappa for individual categories of data presented in Table 2.48

Category	Kappa	Se	Z	P value	95% CI
Overall	0.54	0.135	3.987	<0.001	0.28–0.81
Medical treatment	0.49	0.183	2.68	0.007	0.13–0.85
PTCA	0.59	0.183	3.25	0.001	0.23–0.95
Surgery	0.52	0.183	2.85	0.004	0.16–088

PTCA = percutaneous coronary angioplasty, CI = confidence interval refer to surgery: Kappa 0.52 (0.16–0.88); P = 0.004 or, to continue medical therapy: Kappa 0.49 (0.13–0.85); P = 0.007; compared to the other two categories combined.

2.10.3.4 Interpretation, Reporting and Conditions of Application of Kappa

The Interpretation

Cohen's have suggested that Kappa values of: <0.00, 0 to <0.2, 0.2 to <0.4, 0.4 to <0.6, 0.6 to <0.8 and 0.8–1; indicate poor, slight, fair, moderate, substantial, and almost perfect agreement. However, we have to note that in order to interpret the value of Kappa correctly, we have to enclose the values of other factors that can influence its magnitude, including; the weighting of Kappa, the number of outcome categories, the prevalence of the disease, and the extent of disagreement [66].

What Should be Reported

We have to report: the number of outcome categories, Kappa value and the derivative used (weighted, unweighted, Fleiss or Randolph Kappa), the 95% confidence interval, and P-value. In the case of weighting, we have to report the weighting method (linear, quadratic, or else). In Fleiss kappa, we have to report kappa values, 95% confidence interval, and P values of individual categories. It is advisable to report alongside indices that were shown to influence calculation or interpretation, such as the prevalence index, the bias index, prevalence adjusted PABAK, and Kappa Max [66].

Conditions of Application

The conditions of application concern the trio of the relation: outcome, observations, and predictors. The outcome has to be a qualitative variable with mutually exclusive categories. The observations should be paired (e.g., each patient is examined by both clinicians); hence, incomplete observations must be discarded. The predictors have to be fixed and unique: the same clinicians assess all patients, the same raters judge on all observations. The exception is the multiple rater

kappas modified to allow randomly chosen raters for each observation. In such a case, Randolph Kappa is more preferred than Fleiss Kappa in case of the disease's significantly high or low prevalence or significant bias between predictors. Finally, both: study material and predictors have to be independent; e.g., each patient has to serve for a single paired examination (no patient should be observed twice by the same observer), and each observer should ignore the decision made by his colleague, of course.

2.10.4 Quantitative Outcome

Before we test agreement, we have to exclude the presence of a systematic bias between the quantitative measures in question. A statistically non-significant paired t-test can exclude bias in normally distributed data but does not indicate agreement. Remember that we cannot prove the null hypothesis. Wilcoxon-sign rank test is the non-parametric alternative for data following other distributions than normal. In the case of normality, the agreement can then be visualized by a Bland Altman plot (see Fig. 2.18) or by showing the paired data point falling on the 45-degree diagonal line passing through the origin of a scatter plot (see Fig. 2.20). Agreement can be quantified by Lin's concordance correlation coefficient or intraclass correlation coefficient (ICCC) for multiple groups. Kendall W is the non-parametric alternative for data following other distributions than normal.

2.10.4.1 The Bland Altman's Plots

In biology, variability is the rule and there is no exception, and hence, the role of the researcher is to assess differences rather than look for similarities. Consequently, we can assume that two measuring methods agree as long as the difference between their results does not change the clinical interpretation. For example, suppose digital and mercury blood pressure manometers give readings that differ by not more than 1–5 mm Hg. In that case, one can replace the other. However, the agreement cannot be assumed if the difference is several times larger than

Fig. 2.18 Bland Altman plot of data presented in Table 2.50

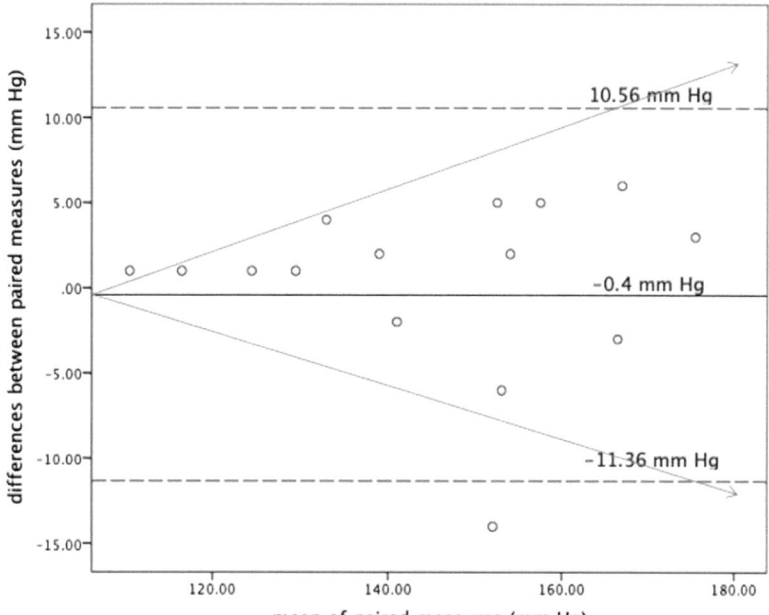

clinically accepted. Measurements can be far apart without causing difficulties is a question of judgment. [71].

The Example

Table 2.50 shows the results of measuring systolic blood pressure in 15 patients by two mercury sphygmomanometers A and B and the researchers aimed to test whether there is sufficient agreement between both instruments so that they can use them interchangeably.

The Equations

The first step is to test data for normality. Shapiro–Wilk test failed to show a statistically significant difference between any of the two series of measurements and normality $(P > 0.05)$; (Sect. 1.4.3.). The second step is to exclude the presence of a systematic bias between both instruments by the paired test of Student, whether by hand or by using an online calculator or a statistical software package (Sect. 2.3.1.6). The absence of a statistically significant difference between blood pressure measurements $(144.6 + 19.37$ versus $145 + 19.3$ mm Hg; $P = 0.776)$, gives the green light to measure the

extent of agreement between both instruments by a Bland–Altman plot.

We calculate the difference (d) and the mean value of each pair of measurement acquired from the same person by both instruments. The difference is supposed to reflect how close are the two measurements from one another; the smaller is the difference, the closer is the two measurements. On the other hand, the mean is the closest value that we can get to reality and, hence, it can be used as a benchmark to analyze how those differences vary in reality. Put it this way, do both measurements maintain a constant level of agreement across the variations of reality?

1. *Analyzing the Extent and Distribution of Agreement*

Provided that both measurements are normally distributed, 95% of their differences (d) are expected to lie within two standard deviations of their mean value (m_d); which is a characteristic of normality. Table 2.50 shows the mean of the difference $(m_d = -0.4$ mm Hg) and the standard deviation $(Sd_d = 5.11$ mm Hg). The upper and lower limits of the 95% confidence interval of the

Table 2.50 Paired measurements of systolic blood pressure in 15 patients using two mercury sphygmomanometers A and B and a digital manometer C

Patients	Mercury A	Mercury B	Difference of paired readings (A − B)	Mean of paired readings (A + B)/2	Digital C
I	110.00	111.00	1.00	110.50	82.00
II	116.00	117.00	1.00	116.50	88.00
III	124.00	125.00	1.00	124.50	95.00
IV	129.00	130.00	1.00	129.50	102.00
V	131.00	135.00	4.00	133.00	102.00
VI	138.00	140.00	2.00	139.00	110.00
VII	142.00	140.00	−2.00	141.00	115.00
VIII	150.00	155.00	5.00	152.50	130.00
IV	153.00	155.00	2.00	154.00	135.00
X	155.00	160.00	5.00	157.50	140.00
XI	156.00	150.00	−6.00	153.00	145.00
XII	159.00	145.00	−14.00	152.00	133.00
XIII	164.00	170.00	6.00	167.00	145.00
XIV	168.00	165.00	−3.00	166.50	150.00
XV	174.00	177.00	3.00	175.50	140.00
Mean ± Sd	144.6 ± 19.37	145 ± 19.3	−0.4 ± 5.11	144.8 ± 19.6	120.8 ± 22.8

Values are paired measurements of systolic blood pressure in mm Hg, Sd = standard deviation

difference are calculated as: $m_d + (t)\ Sd_d = -0.4 \pm (2.145)\ 5.11 = (10.56)$ and (-11.36) mm Hg. Note that due to our small sample size, we could not use "the usual critical limit: 1.96", and we have to refer to Student's table to find the critical value corresponding to our 14 df. As shown in Table 2.50 and Fig. 2.18, 14/15 (93.3%) of the differences lie within those limits, which is an expected and accepted small deviation due to the small sample size. As both measurements are normally distributed, 95% of their differences (d) are expected to lie within two standard deviations of their mean value (md); which is a characteristic of normality. Bland and Altman have presented an estimate by which the upper and lower limits of the 95% confidence interval themselves vary in the population. They vary by a standard error that is equal to $\sqrt{3(Sd_d)^2/n}$ [71]. In our example, the $Se = \sqrt{3(5.11)^2/15} = 2.28$.

2. *Analyzing the Pattern of Agreement*

The second point is that the researcher would like to know whether this agreement is related to the magnitude of the measurement? Put it this way, whether both measurements do agree on all levels or only a particular magnitude of measurement, such as high or low values. A Bland Altman plot addresses both issues by plotting the differences between paired values on the y-axis and the mean of pairs on the x-axis. It visualizes both: the extent as well as the pattern of agreement. Regarding the extent, 93.3% of measurements lie between the upper (10.56 mm Hg) and lower limits of the 95% CI and (−11.36 mm Hg). The arrows in Fig. 2.18 delineate the special pattern of distribution; the differences diverge from the mean of the differences, with the increased magnitude of the difference (the means of paired values). In other words, the extent of the difference between both measurements

Fig. 2.19 Bland Altman plot of log data presented in Table 2.50

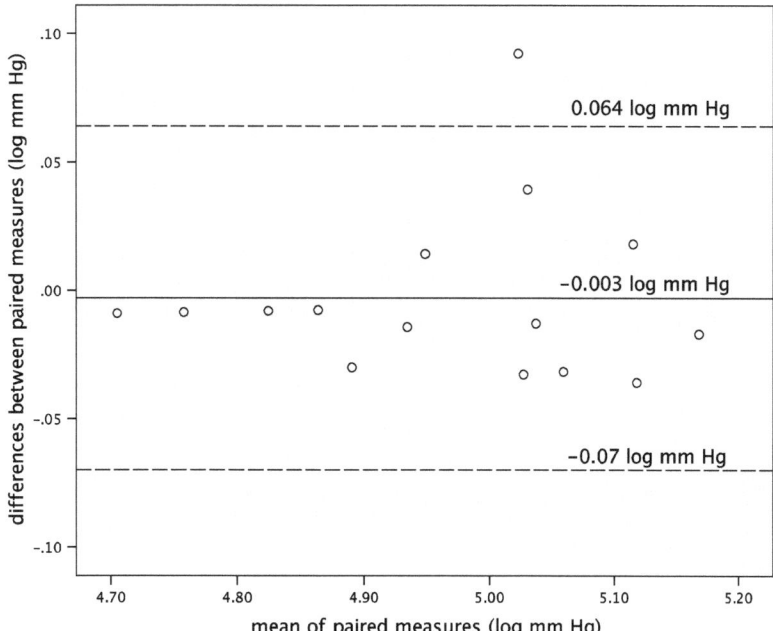

increases (indicating smaller agreement) with the increase in the magnitude of the measurement (with higher blood pressures).

The significance of this pattern can be tested statistically by regressing the mean of paired differences (independent variable) on the difference between paired measurements by simple regression. The presence of a statistically significant effect of the magnitude on the agreement will question the consistency of our results, especially in patients with severe hypertension. It will equally question any calculated numerical index of agreement, such as Lin's concordance correlation coefficient or ICC, since those single indices of agreement suppose a more or less a consistent agreement that does not change significantly with change in magnitude of measurement. Fortunately, uploading our data to SPSS statistical software shows a statistically non-significant effect of the magnitude of measurement on the agreement, with a beta coefficient of (−0.004), a (b$_0$) of 0.929 and a P-value of 0.96 (see Sect. 2.6.2.1).

3. *Improvement of Data by Log Transformation*

Bland and Altman have shown that when the differences vary with the mean, as in our example, a logarithmic transformation may improve the measurements [71]. We transform the measurements into their logarithmic values (Fig. 1.19) and we calculate the mean log difference (−0.003), the log Sd (0.0034) and the 95% upper and lower limits of agreement: 0.064 and −0.07. The antilogs of these limits are 1.07 and 0.93. The antilog of the difference between two values on a log scale is a dimensionless ratio [71]. Hence, Bland and Altman's limits tell us that the manometer B in 95% of cases will vary by 7% around manometer A (Fig. 2.19).

The Interpretation

The reading with manometer B may be higher up to 10.56 mm Hg or 11.36 mm Hg lower than with manometer A. If this variation is clinically accepted, manometer B can substitute manometer A. An easier interpretation would be with the logarithmic transformation. Readings of manometer B vary by 7% around manometer A, in 95% of cases. Only when the researcher accepts those differences can manometer B replace manometer A.

What Should be Reported

We should report the mean difference, the upper and lower limits of the 95% confidence intervals, and their antilog values if a logarithmic transformation was performed. The interpretation of those values has to be reported in conclusion as well.

In our example, the mean of the difference (m_d) equals (−0.4), the Se_d is equal to (5.11/$\sqrt{15}$ = 1.24) and hence the 95% CI of m_d = $m_d \pm$ (t) Se_d = (−0.4) ± (2.145) 1.24 = (−3.06) to (2.26) mm Hg. The small sample size lies behind this very wide 95% confidence interval. Besides being statistically non-significant, an interval of confidence that includes zero like ours, is confusing and devaluates any study (Sect. 1.4.2). The equation calculates the expected limits of the 95% CI in the population: *imit* $\pm$ $(t)\sqrt{3(Sd_d)^2/n}$ [71]. In our example, the upper limit is expected to vary between 5.7- and 15-mm Hg (10.56 ± 2.145 × 2.28) and, the lower limit is expected to vary between −6.5- and −16.3-mm Hg (−11.36 ± 2.145 × 2.28). A larger study would have given a more precise result, of course.

Conditions of Application

Observations should be taken at random, and measures should be independent in the sense that the operator of one instrument should not be aware of the result gained by the other instrument. Both measurements have to be normally distributed, and a statistically significant systematic error has to be eliminated by the paired test of Student. Conditions of using the latter should be equally satisfied (Sect. 2.3.1.6).

2.10.4.2 Lin's Concordance Correlation Coefficient (CCC)

More than three decades have passed since Bland and Altman have clearly shown that Pearson's

correlation coefficient (r) measures the strength of the relation between two variables but not their agreement [71]. The test of significance of (r) is whether data of both variables fall on a straight line may indicate precision but is irrelevant to the question posed in agreement, which is whether both measures are accurate as well as precise so as one can replace the other? The statistically significant correlation demonstrated in many agreement studies is because the magnitude of (r) is dependent upon the true quantity in the sample and, as those studies are usually concerned with the demonstration of agreement on a wide range of values, a statistically significant (r) is almost guaranteed [71]. In other words, data can "produce" correlation but still they "have" poor agreement.

Table 2.50 shows the results of measuring systolic blood pressure in 15 patients. Two mercury sphygmomanometers (A and B) and a digital sphygmomanometer C took each measurement. The digital manometer recorded lower measurements than the other two instruments. The difference was vast and systematic, and the paired test of Student showed a statistically significant difference between the digital measurements and both manometers A and B, with respective means of the differences as high as 23.8 ± 6.4 mm Hg (P < 0.001) and 24.2 ± 8.5 mm Hg (P < 0.001). On the other hand, Pearson's correlation coefficient (r) showed a statistically significant high positive correlation between manometers A and C (r = 0.967; P < 0.001) as well as between manometers B and C (r = 0.932; P < 0.001).

There is no contradiction between the results of both tests. Because, in order to conclude upon agreement, any measurement has to satisfy both components of agreement: accuracy and precision. The statistically significant Pearson's correlation coefficient showed that measurements did satisfy only one of the two components, i.e., precision. The statistically significant Student's test showed that both measures disagree; i.e., failed to satisfy both components together. Put it this way, both measures succeeded in satisfying precision but failed to satisfy accuracy.

As previously mentioned, Pearson's correlation coefficient is a measure of "precision" or how well the data are about the line of best fit. The latter is different from the line of agreement, which is the 45-degree line passing by the origin. Lin's correlation modifies Pearson's correlation by assessing the distance between those two lines [72]. Figure 2.20 shows the reference line and the best fitting line for paired data acquired by the mercury sphygmomanometer A and the digital manometer C (Table 2.50). Both lines are well distant from each other. Correlation coefficient r tested whether the 15 pairs of data (represented by open circles in the figure) are fitting a straight line (the dotted line (r = 0.967; P < 0.001) and nothing more.

It is clear from Fig. 2.20 that any point on the best fitting (dotted) line has a lower landing point on the y scale than on the x-axis. The digital manometer gives a smaller reading than the mercury sphygmomanometer for any given patient. On the other hand, the line indicating

perfect agreement is the one where each point representing paired data will have precisely similar landing points on both: the x and y axes, indicating that both instruments give exactly similar readings. The bias is the distance between those two lines. Hence, Lin's correlation coefficient (rc) was designed to express the percentage of agreement by subtracting this distance (bias) from 1, which indicates a perfect or 100% agreement. Consequently, (rc) varies between + 1 and −1, and a (0) value means complete disagreement.

The Example

We have previously shown that there was a considerable agreement between the two mercury manometers, with a clinically acceptable difference of 7% (see Sect. 2.10.4.1 and Table 2.50). A second step would be to quantify this agreement in a single number that can be easily reported, universally interpreted, and compared between studies. Lin's concordance coefficient

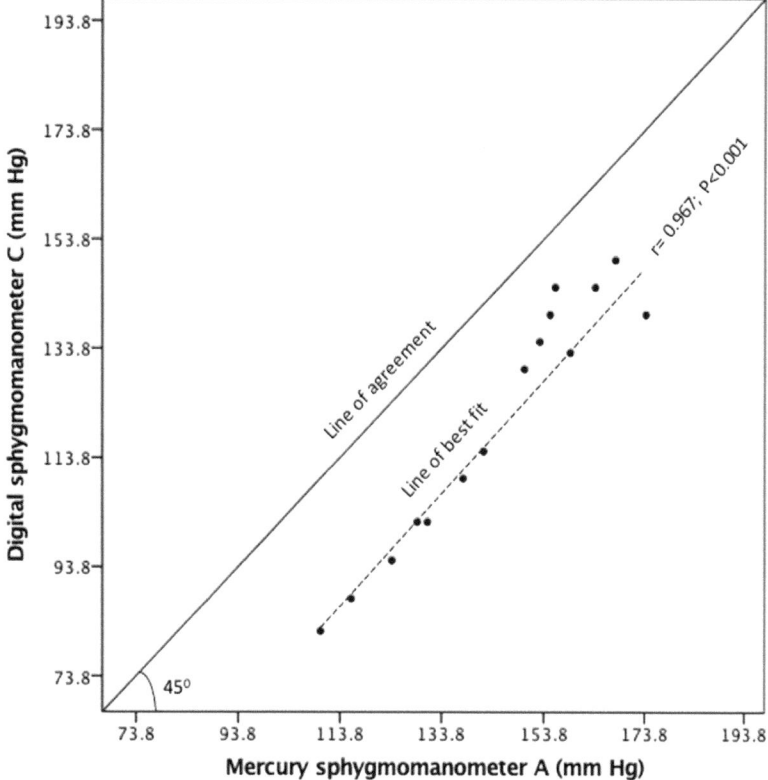

Fig. 2.20 Line of best fit versus line of agreement for paired data acquired with mercury sphygmomanometer A and digital manometer C presented in Table 2.50

satisfies some of those requirements and is also valid in small studies as ten paired [72, 73].

The Equation

The degree of concordance between two measures (x and y) can be expressed as the expected value of their squared differences $(x - y)^2$, where $\bar{x}$ and $\bar{y}$ are the respective mean values, Sx and Sy are the r standard deviations, Sx^2 and Sy^2 are the respective variances and r is Pearson's correlation coefficient "Eq. 2.142" [72, 73].

$$(\bar{x} - \bar{y})^2 + S_x^2 + S_y^2 - 2rs_x s_y \qquad (2.142)$$

In the case of total disagreement, with the paired values are totally independent of one another, r = 0 and, hence the degree of concordance, in terms of squared differences, will be only equal to: $(\bar{x} - \bar{y})^2 + S_x^2 + S_y^2$.

In order to calculate an index of agreement between 1 and minus 1, Lin's concordance correlation coefficient (rc) is 1 (indicating perfect agreement) minus the ratio between the degree of concordance in the sample and the degree of concordance assuming total independence "Eq. 2.143". This ratio expresses the distance between the best fitting and the agreement lines.

$$r_c = 1 - \frac{(\bar{x} - \bar{y})^2 + S_x^2 + S_y^2 - 2rs_x s_y}{(\bar{x} - \bar{y})^2 + S_x^2 + S_y^2}$$
$$= \frac{2rs_x s_y}{(\bar{x} - \bar{y})^2 + S_x^2 + S_y^2} \qquad (2.143)$$

The 95% CI of Lin's CCC (rc)

For samples of any correlation coefficient, whether Pearson's correlation coefficient (r) or Lin's concordance correlation coefficient (rc), the calculated coefficient is not normally distributed, even if the x and y data values were normal. We have to apply Fisher's transformation to any given (r'c), calculate the standard error of log (r'c), the 95% confidence interval of Log (r'c) and finally, antilog its upper and lower limits to get the upper and lower limits of Lin's CCC (rc) itself. We have previously shown those

calculations for Pearson's correlation coefficient (r) in Sect. 2.6.1.1. In our example, Lin's CCC (rc) = 0.965. Applying "Eq. 2.83" produces a normalized log value (rc') = 2.012 "Eq. 2.144". Unlike Pearson's correlation r, the calculation of the Se for (rc') is not as straightforward, even if it is calculated out of known quantities: Pearson's r, Lin's (rc) and $u = (\bar{x} - \bar{y})/\sqrt{S_x S_y}$ "Eq. 2.145" [25]. Fortunately, (rc') and Se (rc') can be generated by an Adds-in to Microsoft excel [25] or a macro for SPSS [74]. The software gives a Se (rc') of 0.277. The 95% CI of (rc') is shown in "Eq. 2.146". Applying "Eq. 2.147" back transforms the normalized log values into the original correlation scale. The 95% CI of Lin's CCC equals 0.89–0.99. In other words, we are 95% confident that Lin's CCC ranges between 0.89 and 0.99 in the population of concern.

$$rc' = \frac{1}{2}\log\frac{1 + rc}{1 - rc} = \frac{1}{2}\log\frac{1 + 0.965}{1 - 0.965} = 2.012 \qquad (2.144)$$

$$Se(r_c') = \sqrt{\frac{1}{n-2}\left[\frac{(1-r^2)r_c^2}{(1-r_c^2)r^2} + \frac{2(1-r_c)r_c^3 u^2}{(1-r_c^2)^2 r} - \frac{r_c^4 u^4}{2(1-r_c^2)^2 r^2}\right]} \qquad (2.145)$$

$$95\% \; CI \; r_c' = r_c' \pm 1.96\left(Se \; r_c'\right)$$
$$= 2 \pm 1.96\left(0.277\right) = 1.47 - 2.55 \qquad (2.146)$$

$$r = \frac{e^{2rC'} - 1}{e^{2rC'} + 1} = \frac{e^{2 \times 2.55} - 1}{e^{2 \times 2.55} + 1} = 0.99;$$
$$r = \frac{e^{2 \times 1.47} - 1}{e^{2 \times 1.47} + 1} = 0.89 \qquad (2.147)$$

Figure 2.21 shows Lin's concordance coefficient calculated for paired data acquired with mercury sphygmomanometers A and B, with the data points being aligned and grouped around the line of agreement. In other words, both elements of the agreement were satisfied. Kindly compare with Fig. 2.22 showing the paired data acquired with mercury sphygmomanometer A and digital manometer. Although data points are well aligned, yet they are far from the line of agreement, with rc being as low as 0.569 (0.34–0.73); P > 0.05.

Fig. 2.21 Lin's concordance correlation coefficient of paired data presented in Table 2.50: mercury sphygmomanometers A and B

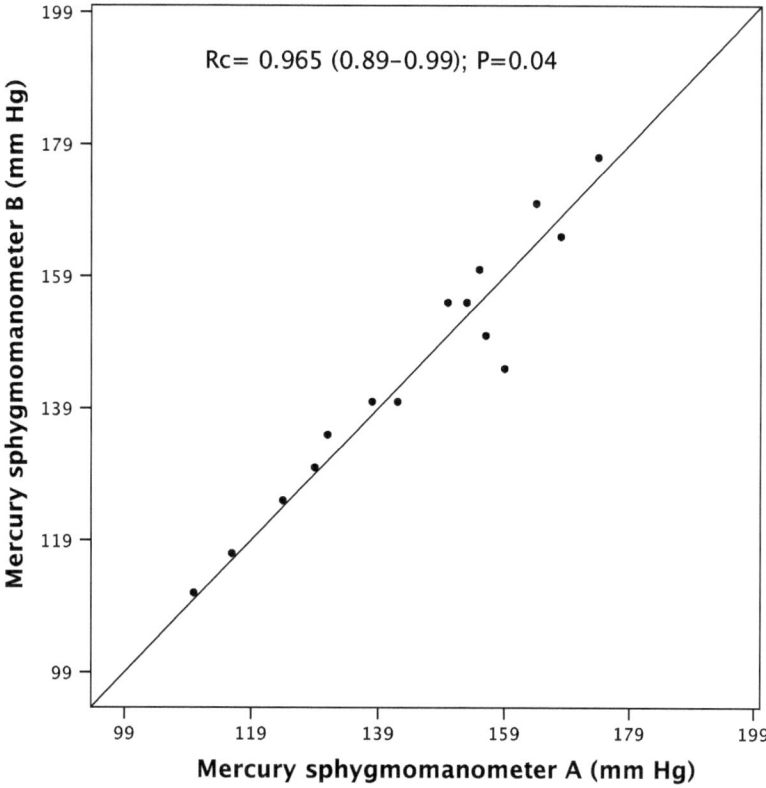

Fig. 2.22 Lin's concordance correlation coefficient of paired data presented in Table 2.9.11. Mercury sphygmomanometers A versus digital C

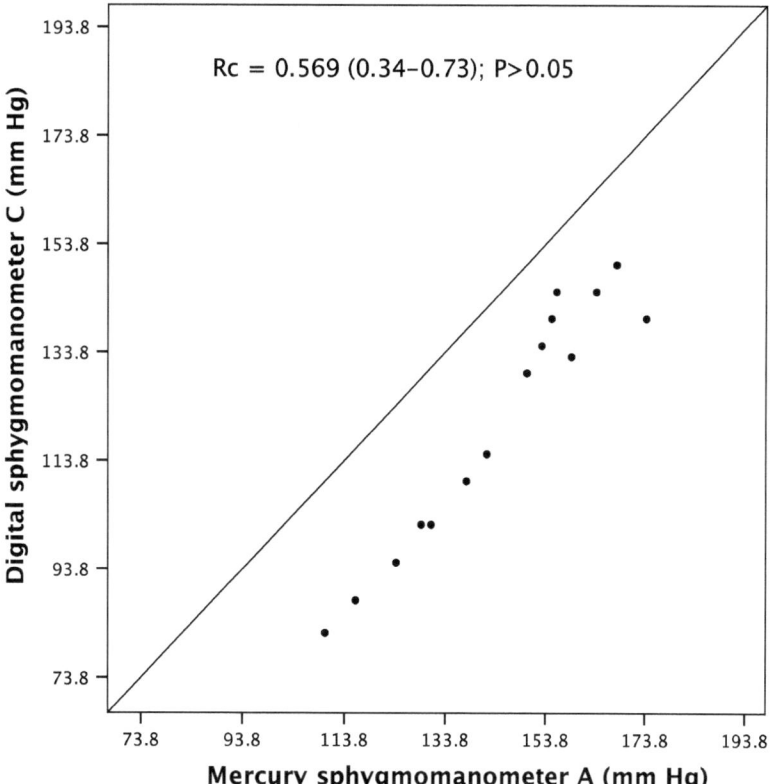

The Interpretation

There is a universal agreement that an (rc) value of zero indicates complete disagreement, and a value of 1 indicates perfect agreement. However, there are many controversies in between. Altman suggests applying the" usual" limits for 0.2 being poor and 0.8 being excellent [38]. McBride recommends much more stringent requirements: less than 0.9 is poor, 0.90–0.95 moderate, 0.95–0.99 substantial, and greater than 0.99 is excellent [25]. The reader is simply advised to report his own value and to compare it with those reported by others in the same field of research.

What Should be Reported

We have to report the descriptive statistics, including each measurement's mean values and standard deviation. The inferential statistics have to be reported, including the paired test results of Student, mean of the difference, and standard deviation of the difference. Measures of agreement: Bland and Altman plot with its upper and lower limits of agreement, Lins' concordance correlation coefficient, 95% confidence interval, and P-value.

Conditions of Application

Observations should be taken at random, and measures should be independent in the sense that the operator of one instrument should not be aware of the result gained by the other instrument —normal distribution of measurements and elimination of a statistically significant systematic error by the paired test of Student. Conditions of using the latter should be equally satisfied (see Sect. 2.4.1.3).

2.10.4.3   Intra Class Correlation Coefficient (ICC)

Intraclass correlation coefficient (ICC) can measure reproducibility and repeatability in paired numerical data acquired from 2 or more predictors. We will follow our definition that the predictor can be a rater, a condition, a test, an instrument evaluating a subject or other patient-related or study material. ICC can test inter-rater

reliability by measuring agreement between 2 or more predictors evaluating the same material. It can also be used to test intra-rater reliability or how much a single predictor agrees on measuring two or more sets of material. Finally, ICC can be used to assess what is called test–retest reliability by measuring the amount of agreement between the repeated measurements performed by the same predictor on the same material [75].

The Example

We have previously shown a considerable agreement between the readings of two mercury manometers (Table 2.50). Bland and Altman's limits of agreement showed a clinically acceptable 7% difference between both instruments' readings (see Sect. 2.10.4.1). Lin's CCC produced a statistically significant high concordance correlation coefficient of 0.965 (0.89–0.99); P < 0.001. On the other hand, there was a poor agreement when sphygmomanometer A was compared with a digital manometer C, with a small (rc) of 0.569 (0.34–0.73); P > 0.05. We will repeat the analysis by measuring the agreement between the two mercury sphygmomanometers by ICC to show that it will give the same results as Lin's CCC. Second, we will show the advantage of ICC that allows the comparison of the three instruments (multiple groups) in one step. Finally, we will demonstrate the difference between ICC when calculated for absolute agreement between measurements and, if calculated, just to express the consistency of measurements.

The Equation

When first proposed by Fisher, ICC assumed that diagnostic tests follow a one-way repeated measures ANOVA [76]. The total variability in the model (σ^2_{total}) is partitioned into the repeated measures of the same subject by different raters or tests (σ^2_{within}) and, the variability between the different subjects ($\sigma^2_{between}$). ICC will be the ratio between the latter and the total variability "Eq. 2.148". ICC will vary between 0 (no agreement) and 1 (perfect agreement), being a proportion out of a total.

Table 2.51 Intraclass correlation coefficient (ICC) models

Variation	I-Model	Comment
One-way random	Random effect comes from either raters or subjects	Not practical
Two-way random	Both subjects and raters are chosen at random	Aim is to validate a clinical model for general use
Two-way mixed	Subjects chosen at random for fixed raters	Best model for intra-rater or reliability or test-pretest
	II-Type	
Single rater	To answer a specific question: how accurate would a single rater be?	
K raters	Based on means of multiple raters (the usual posed question)	
	III- Definition	
Absolute	The same score is given for the same subject by all raters	Best model for intra-rater reliability or test-pretest
Consistency	Scores are correlated in an additive manner	

$$ICC = \frac{\sigma^2_{between}}{\sigma^2_{between} + \sigma^2_{within}} \qquad (2.148)$$

As with Cohen Kappa, the model further developed with time to answer more questions such as a two-way ANOVA model, equally accounting for the effect of the predictors (raters, tests, instruments, conditions) replications or repetitions and possible interaction. Variations also included whether study material and predictors are fixed or chosen at random and whether the analysis shows consistency between measurements or absolute agreement [77]. Shrout and Fleiss defined six forms of ICC based on the combinations of the model and Type [78]. McGraw and Wong raised this number to ten by adding two definitions to choose in between for the two-way models (Table 2.51) [79].

• The model

The "Model" included three varieties: one-way random, two-way random, and two-way mixed models. One-way random is rarely used for being unpractical. It may be feasible in a multicenter study, where different raters examine different patient subgroups [75]. Two-way random means

that both material and predictors are chosen at random, and hence, it is usually performed in large centers, aiming to extrapolate the results on the population. The two-way mixed model is when the raters are fixed, and the patients are chosen at random and; it is frequently used, but the results cannot be generalized, and hence, it is less commonly used to compare inter-rater reliability. According to Shrout and Fleiss classification, the model is the first number assigned to the ICC coefficient. The one way-random, two-way random and two-way mixed models are assigned the numbers: ICC (1), ICC (2), and ICC (3) [78].

• The type

The "Type" depends upon whether the unit of the analysis will be the result of a single measurement made by one predictor or it would be the mean value of multiple (K) measurements or raters [78]. The former will be assigned the number 1 and the latter will be assigned the letter K; both figuring after the model. As example, a one-way random model with a single rater or measure is expressed as: $ICC_{(1,1)}$ and a two-way random model with multiple raters or measures should be expressed as: $ICC_{(2, K)}$. The resulting six classes are ICC (1, 1), (1, K), (2, 1), (2, k), (3, 1) and ICC (3, k).

- The definitions

"Definitions" depend on whether we are just concerned that different results are consistent or in absolute agreement, in two-way models. The result is the increase of the categories of ICC from six to ten by subdividing each of the four two-way models (random or mixed), whether being designed for single or multiple measures, to measure either consistency between measures or absolute agreement. Measuring consistency gives the same results as correlation coefficient "r"; i.e., results are precise but not accurate. Absolute agreement measures both precision and accuracy, making it a choice model for inter-rater reliability or test-pretest [79]. Note that the uncommonly used one-way random variants ($ICC_{1, 1}$ and $ICC_{1, k}$), where the subjects are not rated by the same raters cannot be used to measure consistency and hence, it was left unchanged as being initially classified by Shrout and Fleiss [78].

- Choosing a specific ICC

The choice of a specific ICC is dependent on those three factors: Model, Type, and Definitions. In practice, two points have to be settled first. First, a one-way random model is rarely used, except few examples like the one just given by Koo and Lie [75]. Second, the type of measurement unit, whether based on a single measurement made by one predictor or the average of multiple measurements or predictors, is independent of the model and definition.

In the case of a study aiming to analyze the intra-rater reliability or a test-pretest, a two-way mixed model aiming to show absolute agreement between the fixed raters (or test-pretest) is the design of choice. Taking the average of multiple rates (type) permits the generalization of the model's results on the population [78].

In the case we intend to measure inter-rater reliability, the researcher has the choice between a two-way mixed or a two-way random that permits the generalization of the results on the population. Taking the average of multiple measurements will serve the same aim at the expense of organizing a large study that involves many raters and more material to measure. Unlike intra-rater reliability and test pretest, the researcher can then choose between showing an overall correlation between the different results or seeking an absolute agreement between measurements.

The ten relevant statistical formulae were nicely detailed by Koo and Li [75] and hence, there is no point of repeating them here. However, we will present the details of the calculation of two formulas to solve our examples. The first is a two-way mixed effect model, where 15 cases were randomly assigned to be measured once by one of two fixed mercury sphygmomanometers. The number of cases will be denoted as "n" and the number of instruments will be denoted as "k". The study aimed to show absolute agreement between the two measurements and not just consistency. The second example will be to measure consistency between the measurements made by the three instruments.

1. *Exclusion of a Statistically Significant Difference Between Instruments*

We will perform a two-way ANOVA either by hand (see Sect. 2.9.4.1) or using a statistical software package such as SPSS. We need a two-way ANOVA to analyze two sources of variability: the variability between both sphygmomanometers (in-between group) and the variability of measures within measures (within-group). Meanwhile, we are interested to exclude a statistically significant difference between the two instruments, which is shown in Table 2.52; F (1, 14) = 0.92, P = 0.76.

2. *Measuring Agreement: Two-way Mixed Model, Single Measure, Testing Absolute Agreement Between Two Instruments*

Table 2.52 ANOVA comparing the measurement of blood pressure acquired by two mercury sphygmomanometers in 15 patients. Data presented in Table 2.50

Source of variation	Sum of squares	df	Variance (MS)	F ratio	P value
Between columns[a]	1.2	1	1.2	0.92	0.76
Between rows[b]	10,282.8	14	734.5		
Residual	182.8	14	13		
Total	10,466.8	29	360.9		

MS = mean square (variance); a = predictors, instruments, tests or raters; b = study material or subjects

As there was no statistically significant difference between both instruments, we can proceed to test how much they agree? In this setting, the ICC measures the proportion of variation between subjects MS_R to the total variation ($MS_R + MS_C$), after removal of the part of variability that is due to chance (MS_{error}), the following equations calculate it "Eq. 2.149". Although the calculation of ICC by hand is simple "Eq. 2.150", there are many privileges for using statistical software, such as the correctness of computations and, most importantly, the production of the 95% CI of ICC and its statistical significance. In our example, it equals 0.91–0.98, $F_{14,14} = 56.2$ and P value <0.001. The software equally calculates the ICC for the case where the uploaded measurements were not single measurements but the means of multiple measurements: 0.983 (0.95–0.994); P < 0.001. However, as usual, we insist on attempting hand calculation at least once to understand the meaning behind the numbers.

$$ICC = \frac{MS_R - MS_E}{MS_R + (k-1)MS_E + \frac{K}{n}(MS_C - MS_E)}$$

(2.149)

$$ICC = \frac{734.5 - 13}{734.5 + (2-1)13 + \frac{2}{15}(1.2 - 13)}$$
$$= 0.967$$

(2.150)

The Interpretation

In our study, 91–98% of the total variability is present between subjects themselves, unrelated to the tested instruments. There is no universal agreement on the interpretation of ICC. Koo and

Li suggested that an ICC value <0.5, 0.5–0.75, 0.75–0.9, and >0.90 indicates poor, moderate, good, and excellent reliability [75]. According to the rule of thumb, our result indicates excellent reliability between both sphygmomanometers; P < 0.001.

Bland and Altman have criticized the use of ICC in assessing agreement for ignoring ordering and treating the compared methods as if they were randomly sampled from a population of methods, which is different from the actual practice of choosing specific methods [80]. Suppose that our example was about clinicians scoring patients' symptoms. Wouldn't the order by which patients are assigned to a particular clinician influence his judgment? For example, the clinician's judgment upon receiving successive severe cases then mild cases may differ from the same clinician examining alternating mild and severe cases. Effect order can influence judgment and, it is not examined here. On the other hand, how would we extrapolate the results acquired by two specific - not random-predictors on the whole population?

Moreover, as ICC measures the proportion of variability between subjects out of the total variability, it tends to increase with the increased number of subjects and the increased variability between the measures themselves [81]. Being so dependent on data is a source of bias in comparing the ICC results of different studies, even from the same population.

What Should be Reported

Reporting ICC should include the Model, Type, Definition, and reason behind each selection. Software information and ICC estimates for single and average measures, their 95% confidence intervals, and P values [75].

Conditions of Application

Normal data distribution and random study material, predictors or both. The value of ICC is proportional to the variability among patients, sample size, and the number of raters. As a rule of thumb, the recommended smallest sample is 30, and least number of raters is three [75]. Hence, our mini example, mainly designed to ease hand calculation, violated both rules.

A Second Example

Our second example will be to analyze the blood pressure measurements acquired by the three sphygmomanometers at one step, which Lin's CCC cannot achieve. We will use the ICC to measure whether the three measures are consistent and whether there is an absolute agreement between the three instruments.

1. *Exclusion of a Statistically Significant Difference Between Instruments*

We will proceed as usual by excluding the presence of a statistical significance between the three means followed by measuring agreement. Unfortunately, ANOVA shows a statistically significant difference between the three means of values, with an F ratio of 123.7 and a P-value < 0.001 (see Table 2.53). Consequently, we should obstinate from testing agreement. However, we will proceed and calculate the ICC for the purpose of training.

2. *Measuring Agreement: Two-Way Mixed Model, Single Measure, Testing Absolute Agreement Between Three Sphygmomanometers.*

The ICC (95% CI) equals 0.65 (0.056–0.89), indicating poor agreement between the three instruments "Eq. 2.151".

$$\text{ICC} = \frac{1222.4 - 23.3}{1222.4 + (3-1)23.3 + \frac{3}{15}(2880.6 - 23.3)} = 0.652$$

$$(2.151)$$

3. *Measuring agreement: Two-Way Mixed Model, Single Measure, Testing Consistency Between Three Sphygmomanometers*

At this point we will examine the consistency and not the absolute agreement between the three instruments. It will not change the results of ANOVA, of course, but ICC will change. ANOVA examines the difference between the three means, and hence, it examines how those means are close to the overall "grand" mean value representing the truth. In other words, it examined the accuracy of measurements. A statistically significant ANOVA tells us that at least one of the three measurements lacks accuracy (Table 2.53).

On the other hand, the question posed by ICC has now changed from testing absolute agreement to measuring consistency between the three measures. The calculation of ICC in this case,

Table 2.53 ANOVA comparing the measurement of blood pressure acquired by two mercury sphygmomanometers and a digital manometer in 15 patients. Data presented in Table 2.50

Source of variation	Sum of squares	df	Variance (MS)	F ratio	P value
Between columns[a]	5761.2	2	2880.6	123.7	<0.001
Between rows[b]	17,113.9	14	1222.4		
Residual	652	28	23.3		
Total	23,527.2	44	534.7		

MS = mean square (variance), a = predictors, instruments, tests, or raters, b = study material, or subjects will exclude the variability between the three measures presented along the three columns (MS_c) from the total variability of the study (denominator of the equation). Hence, we have to expect a higher ICC $_{(3,1)}$ value "Eq. 2.152". Put it this way, the question changed from the proportion of patients' variability, considering that the three instruments will give different measures for the same patient; to just disregarding the latter information. Put it another way, the question changed from how precise, and consistent the measurements are to only how precise? The calculated ICC $_{(3,1)}$ value of 0.945 (0.87–0979) indicates good consistency (precision) between the three measurements.

$$ICC_{(3,1)} = \frac{MS_R - MS_E}{MS_R + (k-1)MS_E}$$
$$= \frac{1222.4 - 23.3}{1222.4 + (3-1)23.3} \quad (2.152)$$
$$= 0.945$$

In conclusion, the three instruments show good consistency between measures ICC $_{(3,1)}$ (0.945; 0.87–0979) but poor agreement (0.65; 0.056–0.89). A high ICC testing does not always mean agreement, and we should never judge it unless it is fully reported.

2.10.4.4 Kendall Coefficient of Concordance (W)

Kendall's coefficient of concordance (W) is a measure of the agreement among multiple predictors (m) measuring several quantitative or semiquantitative variables (n) following other distribution than normal [82]. For example, if five raters (m = 5) were invited to rank ten different manuscripts (n = 10) and the question was which

is the best manuscript, Friedman's test would be the procedure of choice. The null hypothesis is that the ten manuscripts are taken form the same population and, the alternative hypothesis is that they are not (see Sect. 2.5.2.2). In other words, the question is about the manuscripts. Kendal W test answers the opposite question: to what extent do the five raters agree on their ranking? The question here is about the judges. Both Kendal W and Friedman's test, use the same data, apply the same Chi-square equation and produce the same statistics but answering a different question.

The perfect agreement versus the total disagreement

We will begin with a small example to explain the difference between a perfect agreement and a total disagreement. Three raters (rater 1, rater 2, and rater 3) were invited to rate three manuscripts (n1, n2, and n3). As shown in Table 2.54, the three raters disagreed totally, and hence, the sums of the rates given to each manuscript SUM_D were all equal (6, 6, and 6). This is the perfect disagreement that leads to zero variability between the SUM of ranks. The same three manuscripts were given to another set of raters (rater 4, rater 5, and rater 6) who perfectly agreed on their rankings and, as shown, the sums of the ranks (SUM_A) were in total disagreement (1, 6, and 9). Put it this way, the more raters agree; the more variable the SUM will be. Hence, measuring variability between SUMs reflects agreement; i.e., the larger is the variability, the more agreement is. In practice, the observed variability (SUM_O) will be something in between SUM_D and SUM_A, and Kendall W will be the ratio between the observed variability (SUM_O) and the maximal possible variability of perfect agreement

Table 2.54 Perfect agreement versus total disagreement: a working example

	Rater1	Rater 2	Rater 3	SUM_D	Rater 4	Rater 5	Rater 6	SUM_A
n1	1	2	3	6	1	1	1	1
n2	2	3	1	6	2	2	2	6
n3	3	1	2	6	3	3	3	9

Values are the ranks of three manuscripts (n1, n2 and n3) as judged by six raters, SUM_D = sum of ranks per n manuscript for raters 1, 2 and rater 3. SUM_A = sum of ranks per manuscript for raters 4, 5 and rater 6

(SUM$_A$), provided that both are calculated in the standardized form, as usual.

The Example

Five raters, m1, m2, m3, m4, and m5 (m = 5), were invited to rank ten manuscripts (n = 10), and the question is to what extent the five raters agree on their ranking. Kendall W can express their level of agreement in a single number. Table 2.55 shows the ranks given by the five raters arranged in columns, and the ranked manuscripts are displayed in rows. The column (SUM) shows the sum of the ranks of the five raters for each manuscript (SUM). Column D shows the difference between each SUM and the average rank of all manuscripts (27.5), and column D^2 shows the squared values for each D.

Note that if the values were continuous data, they must be transformed into ranks first before the analysis. Table 2.24 is an example of transforming numbers into ranks, where data were ranked per patient (study material) to perform Friedman's test (see Sect. 2.5.2.2). As mentioned, Kendall W is the other side of the coin, and hence, data must be ranked per predictor (per rater), as shown in our example (Table 2.55).

The Equation

We start by calculating the variability between manuscripts (material) in the usual way, as the sum of squared differences between each SUM of ranks and the mean rank (27.5) = (D^2). The more agreement is, the larger the variability over the SUMs and their squared values (D^2). The concordance coefficient W is the proportion between D^2 and the maximal possible variation of a perfect agreement "Eq. 2.153". The more the agreement, the larger the variability between SUMS, and hence, the higher Kendall W coefficient will be and vice versa. Being a proportion out of a total, Kendall W can vary between 0 (total disagreement) and 1 (perfect agreement). In our example, W = 76%, indicating good agreement "Eq. 2.154"

$$W = \frac{12 \times \sum D^2}{m^2(n^3 - n)} \tag{2.153}$$

$$W = \frac{12 \times 1566.5}{5^2(10^3 - 10)} = 0.76 \tag{2.154}$$

The equation presented above is valid as long as there are no many ties. In presence of multiple

Table 2.55 Kendall W test. The results of five raters ranking ten manuscripts

	m1	m2	m3	m4	m5	SUM	D	D^2
n1	9	8	6	7	10	40	12.5	156.25
n2	5	6	5	1	2	19	−8.5	72.25
n3	4	3	1	4	3	15	−12.5	156.25
n4	2	1	4	3	1	11	−16.5	272.25
n5	1	2	3	2	4	12	−15.5	240.25
n6	6	5	10	8	7	36	8.5	72.25
n7	7	10	8	9	8	42	14.5	210.25
n8	10	7	9	6	5	37	9.5	90.25
n9	8	9	7	10	9	43	15.5	240.25
n10	3	4	2	5	6	20	−7.5	56.25
Total						275		1566.5
Average						27.5		

Values are the ranks of the ten manuscripts (n1 to n10), as judged by five raters (m1 to m5), SUM = sum of ranks per n manuscript, D = difference between each SUM and the average rank (27.5), D^2 = squared differences ties, the equation has to be corrected by subtracting the quantity mT from the denominator. m is the total number of predictors as shown before. T equals the sum of $(t^3 - t)$ calculated per (n) row, with t being the number of the group of ties in the n row. For example, if a row has three ties (three numbers sharing the same rank), then its t value = $(3^3 - 3 = 24)$, if another row has 2 groups of ties, each formed of two ties, its t value = $(2^3 - 2 = 6) + (2^3 - 2 = 6) = 12$. If the remaining rows have no ties, their t values = 0. The total T value of the study = 24 + 12 = 36 and, provided that m equals 5, we have to subtract mT or $5 \times 36 = 180$ from the denominator of the equation "Eq. 2.155"

$$W = \frac{12 \times \sum D^2}{m^2(n^3 - n) - mT} \qquad (2.155)$$

The Interpretation

A χ^2 equation commonly tests the statistical significance of W "Eq. 2.156". In our example, the calculated χ^2 value (34.1) is much larger than the one figured in the Chi-square table at nine df $(n - 1)$; P < 0.001. Another alternative is recommended, especially for small sample size, is to compute the F statistics and checking its statistical significance in Fisher's table at the df $_{(1,2)}$ of: $n - 1 - (2/m)$, $n - 1 - (2/m)(m - 1)$ [82, 83] "Eq. 2.157". In our example, we can conclude that there is a significantly good agreement on the ten manuscripts.

$$\chi^2 = m(n - 1)W \qquad (2.156)$$

$$F = \frac{W(m - 1)}{(1 - W)} \qquad (2.157)$$

What Should be Reported

We have to report the median and range of the quantitative variable, the value of W, the test of significance, whether being Chi-square or F test and the resulting P value.

Kendall's W can be used to calculate another overall measure of concordance: Spearman's correlation coefficient of ranks (r_s) [83], which is equal to 0.7 in our example "Eq. 2.158".

$$r_S = \frac{(mw - 1)}{(m - 1)} \qquad (2.158)$$

Conditions of Application

Kendall W provides a common ranking of a set of materials and the test is unilateral. Hence, the test should not be used to analyze variables having equally significant positive and negative correlations [83]. In the case of a small sample size with $n \leq 7$ and $m \leq 20$, F statistics better tests the statistical significance of W than the Chi-square test [83].

A common question encountered in biology is whether two measures can agree when repeated by the same operator, by another operator or by using a different tool? Before proceeding to measuring agreement, we have to exclude a statistically significant difference between the two measures. and then proceeding to measuring agreement itself.

Afterward, a qualitative agreement is usually measured by Cohen Kappa or its derivatives. Two normally distributed quantitative measures are supposed to agree if the Bland and Altman plots show that 95% of their differences exclude a clinically significant difference across the range of test results. Another alternative to visualize agreement is to show paired data falling on the 45-degree diagonal line of agreement passing through the origin of a scatter plot. Finally, we have to express quantitative agreement by a single number: Lin's concordance correlation coefficient (CCC) in case of 2 measures and by intraclass correlation coefficient (ICCC) for two measures or more, with Kendall W concordance coefficient being the nonparametric alternative.

References

1. Statistics calculators. In: Social science statistics 2018. https://www.socscistatistics.com/tests/. Accessed 27 Oct 2021.
2. Lowry, R. VassarStats: Website for statistical computation. 1998. http://vassarstats.net/. Assessed 23 Oct 2021.
3. MedCalc software Lt. SciStat.com online; https://www.scistat.com (2021). Accessed 9 Oct 2021.
4. R Core Team. R: A language and environment for statistical computing. R Foundation for Statistical Computing, Vienna, Austria. URL http://www.R-project.org/ (2021). Accessed 27 Oct 2021.
5. JASP Team. JASP (0.15). Amsterdam. Netherlands https://jasp-stats.org (2021). Accessed 27 Oct 2021.
6. Goldstone LA. The standard deviation and other measures of variations. In: Goldstone LD, editor. Understanding medical statistics. London: William Heinemann Ltd; 1983. p. 25–35. https://doi.org/10.1002/sim.4780040216.
7. Schwartz D. Methodes statistiques a l'usage des medecins et des biologistes. 3rd ed. Paris: Flammarion Medecines Sciences; 1988. http://bdsp-ehesp.inist.fr/vibad/index.php?action=getRecordDetail&idt=194892.
8. Dougherty C. Statistical tables. In: Introduction to econometrics. 2nd ed. Oxford: Oxford University Press; 2002. https://home.ubalt.edu/ntsbarsh/Business-stat/StatistialTables.pdf. Accessed 1st Oct 2021.
9. Statistical tables. In: Hawkes learning. 2011. http://www.hawkeslearning.com/documents/statdatasets/stat_tables.pdf. Accessed 27 Oct 2021.
10. Statistical tables. Fundamental statistical inference distribution In: stat. purdue.edu. 2015. https://www.stat.purdue.edu/~jtroisi/STAT350Spring2015/tables/index.htm; Accessed 2 November 2021.
11. Yates F. Contingency tables involving small numbers and the $\chi 2$ test. J Roy Stat Soc. 1934;1:217–23. https://doi.org/10.2307/2983604.
12. Cochran WG. Some methods for strengthening the common χ^2 tests. Biometrics. 1954;10:417–51. https://doi.org/10.2307/3001616.
13. Armstrong RA. When to use Bonferroni correction. Ophthalmic Physiol Opt. 2014;34:502–8. https://doi.org/10.1111/opo.12131.
14. Agresti A. Categorical data analysis. 2nd ed. New York: John Wiley and Sons; 2002. https://doi.org/10.1002/0471249688.
15. McNemar Q. Note on the sampling error of the difference between correlated proportions or percentages. Psychometrika. 1947;12:153–7. https://doi.org/10.1007/BF02295996.
16. Bowker AH. A test for symmetry in contingency tables. J Am Stat Assoc. 1948;43:572–4. https://doi.org/10.1080/01621459.1948.10483284.
17. Campbell MJ, Julious SA, Altman DG. Estimating sample sizes for binary, ordered categorical, and continuous outcomes in two group comparisons. BMJ. 1995;311:1145–8. https://doi.org/10.1136/bmj.311.7013.1145.
18. Sheskin DJ. Handbook of parametric and nonparametric statistical procedures. 5th ed. Boca Raton: Chapman & Hall/CRC; 2011. https://doi.org/10.1201/9780429186196.
19. Student. The probable error of a mean. Biometrika. 1908;6:1–25. https://doi.org/10.2307/2331554.
20. Brown MB, Forsythe AB. Robust tests for the equality of variances. J Am Stat Assoc. 1974;69:364–7. https://doi.org/10.2307/2285659.
21. Altman DG, Bland JM. Statistics notes: comparing several groups using analysis of variance. BMJ. 1996;312:1472–3. https://doi.org/10.1136/bmj.312.7044.1472.
22. Tomarken AJ, Serlin RC. Comparison of ANOVA alternatives under variance heterogeneity and specific non-centrality structures. Psychol Bull. 2021;1986 (99):90–9. https://doi.org/10.1037/0033-2909.99.1.90.Accessed8Nov.
23. Brown MB, Forsythe AB. The small sample behavior of some statistics which test the equality of several means. Technometrics. 1974;16:129–32. https://doi.org/10.1080/00401706.1974.10489158.
24. Field A. Discovering Statistics Using SPSS. 3rd ed. London, UK: Sage publications Ltd.; 2009. https://doi.org/10.1002/bjs.7040.
25. Zaiontz C. Real statistics using excel. 2021. https://www.real-statistics.com. Accessed 10 Nov 2021.
26. Least Significant Difference Test. In: The Concise Encyclopedia of Statistics. New York, NY. Springer, 2008. https://doi.org/10.1007/978-0-387-32833-1_226. Accessed 8 Nov 2021.
27. Harter HL. Critical Values for Duncan's New Multiple Range Test. Biometrics, 1960;16:671–85. http://www.jstor.org/stable/2527770?origin=JSTOR-pdf.
28. Dunnett CW. New tables for multiple comparisons with a control. Biometrics. 1964;20:482–91. https://doi.org/10.2307/2528490.Accessed9Nov2021.
29. Bland JM, Altman DG. Statistics notes: Multiple significance tests: the Bonferroni method. BMJ. 1995;310:170. https://doi.org/10.1136/bmj.310.6973.170.
30. Holm S. A simple sequential rejective multiple test procedure. Scandinavian Journal of Statistics. 1979;6:65–70. http://www.jstor.org/stable/4615733.
31. Lee PM. Statistical Tables. Department of mathematics. The University of York. 2005. https://www.york.ac.uk/depts/maths/tables/. Accessed 13 Nov 2021.
32. Dugard P. Appendix 1. Statistical tables. In: Online library Wiley. Wiley and Sons. Inc. https://onlinelibrary.wiley.com, https://doi.org/10.1002/9780470776124.app1. Accessed 12 Nov 2021.
33. Swinscow TDV. Statistics at square one. 9th ed. London: BMJ Publ. Group; 1997. https://doi.org/10.1002/(SICI)1097-0258(19971130)16:22%3C2629::AID-SIM698%3E3.0.CO;2-Z

34. Altman DG. Practical statistics for medical research. 1st ed. London: Chapman and Hall; 1991.

35. Hart A. Mann-Whitney test is not just a test of medians: differences in spread can be important. BMJ. 2001;323:391–3. https://doi.org/10.1136/bmj.323.7309.391.

36. Sergeant, ESG. Epitools Epidemiological Calculators. Ausvet. https://epitools.ausvet.com.au. (2018). Accessed 6 Aug 2021.

37. Campbell MJ, Gardner MJ. Calculating confidence intervals for some non-parametric analyses. BMJ. 1988;296: 1369–71. https://doi.org/10.1136/bmj.296.6634.1454.

38. Grissom RJ, Kim JJ. Effect size for research: univariate and multivariate applications. New York, NY, Routledge. 2012. https://doi.org/10.4324/9780203803233.

39. Critical values for the Kruskal-Wallis test. DataAnalytics.org.uk. Understanding data. 2019 https://www.dataanalytics.org.uk/critical-values-for-the-kruskal-wallis-test/#approx; Accessed Nov 2021.

40. Goldstone LA. Correlation and regression analysis. Understanding medical statistics. 1st ed. London: William Heinemann Medical Books; 1983. P. 86–121. https://doi.org/10.1002/sim.4780040216.

41. Fisher RA. On the probable error of a coefficient of correlation deduced from a small sample. Metron. 1921;1:3–32. https://hdl.handle.net/2440/15169.

42. Altman DG, Bland JM. London. Statistics notes: Time to event (survival) data. BMJ. 1998;317: 468–9. https://doi.org/10.1136/bmj.317.7156.468

43. Kaplan EL, Meier P. Nonparametric estimation from incomplete observations. J Am Stat Assoc. 1958;53:457–81. https://doi.org/10.2307/2281868.

44. Klein JP, Moeschberger ML. Survival Analysis Techniques for censored and truncated data. 2003. 2nd ed. New York: Springer Publishers.

45. Mantel N. Evaluations of survival data and two new rank order statistics arising in its consideration. Cancer Chemother Rep. 1966;50:163–70 PMID: 5910392.

46. Cox DR. Regression models and life-tables (with Discussion). J R Stat Society Ser B. 1972;34:187–220. https://www.jstor.org/stable/2985181.

47. Peto R, Peto J. Asymptotically efficient rank invariant test procedures (with discussion). J R Stat Soc Ser A. 1972;135:185–206. https://doi.org/10.2307/2344317.

48. Laplanche A, Com-Nougue C, Flamant R. Methodes statistiques appliquées a la recherche Clinique. Paris: Flammarion-Medecine-Sciences; 1987. http://bdsp-ehesp.inist.fr/vibad/index.php?action=getRecordDetail&idt=52329.

49. Bland JM, Altman DG. Statistics notes. The Logrank test. BMJ 2004;328:1073. https://doi.org/10.1136/bmj.328.7447.1073.

50. Yang S, Prentice R. Improved Logrank-type tests for survival data using adaptive weights. Biometrics. 2010;66(1):30–38. https://onlinelibrary.wiley.com.

https://doi.org/10.1111/j.1541-0420.2009.01243.x. Accessed 19 Nov 2021.

51. Gehan EA. A generalized Wilcoxon test for comparing arbitrarily single-censored samples. Biometrika. 1965;52:203–23. https://academic.oup.com/biomet/article/52/1-2/203/359447. Assessed on 24 Nov 2021.

52. Karadeniz PG, Ercan L. Examining tests for comparing survival curves with right censored data. Stat. in Trans. New series 2017;18:311–28. https://doi.org/10.21307/stattrans-2016-072.

53. Tarone RE, Ware J. On distribution-free tests for equality of survival distributions. Biometrika. 1977;64:156–60. https://doi.org/10.1093/biomet/64.1.156.

54. Garès V, Andrieua S, Dupuy JF, Savy N. On the Fleming-Harrington test for late effects in prevention randomized controlled trials. J Stat Theory and Pract. 2017;11:418–35. https://doi.org/10.1080/15598608.2017.1295889.

55. Fleming TR, Harrington DP. Counting processes and survival analysis. 2nd ed. New Jersey: John Wiley & Sons; 1991. https://doi.org/10.1002/sim.4780111314.

56. Mantel N, Haenszel W. Statistical aspects of the analysis of data from retrospective studies of disease. J Natl Cancer Inst. 1959;22:719–48. https://doi.org/10.1093/jnci/22.4.719.

57. Schwartz D. Methodes statistiques a l'usage des médecins et des biologistes. 3rd ed. Paris: Flammarion Medecines Sciences; 1988. http://bdsp-ehesp.inist.fr/vibad/index.php?action=getRecordDetail&idt=194892.

58. Warrens M. Inequalities between multi-rater kappas. Adv Data Anal Classif. 2010;4:271–86. https://doi.org/10.1007/s11634-010-0073-4.

59. Cohen J. A Coefficient of Agreement for Nominal Scales. Educ Psychol Meas. 1960;20:37–46. https://doi.org/10.1177/001316446002000104.

60. Agresti A. Categorical data analysis. 3rd ed. Hoboken, NJ: Wiley; 2013. https://mregresion.files.wordpress.com/2012/08/agresti-introduction-to-categorical-data.pdf.

61. Fleiss J, Cohen J, Everitt B. Large sample standard errors of kappa and weighted kappa. Psychol Bull. 1969;72:323–7. https://doi.org/10.1037/H0028106.

62. Randolph J. Online Kappa calculator (computer software). 2008. http://justusrandolph.net/kappa/. Accessed 14 Aug 2021.

63. Feinstein A, Cicchetti D. High agreement but low kappa, I: the problems of two paradoxes. J Clin Epidemiol. 1990;43:543–9. https://doi.org/10.1016/0895-4356(90)90158-l.

64. Byrt T, Bishop J, Carlin J. Bias, prevalence and kappa. J Clin Epidemiol. 1993;46:423–9. https://doi.org/10.1016/0895-4356(93)90018-v.

65. Brennan P, Silman A. Statistical methods for assessing observer variability in clinical measures. BMJ. 1992;304:1491–4. https://doi.org/10.1136/bmj.304.6840.1491.

66. Sim J, Wright CC. The Kappa statistic in reliability studies: use, interpretation, and sample size requirements. Phys Ther. 2005;85:257–68. https://doi.org/10.1093/ptj/85.3.257.

67. Fleiss JL. Design and analysis of reliability studies: the statistical evaluation of measurement errors. New York: Oxford University Press; 1989. https://doi.org/10.1002/sim.4780100120.

68. Maclure M, Willett WC. Misinterpretation and misuse of Kappa statistic. Am J Epidemiol. 1987;126:161–9. https://doi.org/10.1093/aje/126.2.161.

69. Brenner H, Kliebsch U. Dependence of weighted Kappa coefficients on the number of categories. Epidemiol. 1996;7:199–202. https://doi.org/10.1097/00001648-199603000-00016.

70. Randolph J. Free-marginal multirater kappa: An alternative to Fleiss´ fixed-marginal multirater kappa. Joensuu Finland, the Joensuu University Learning and Instruction Symposium. 2005. https://files.eric.ed.gov/fulltext/ED490661.pdf. Accessed 21 Dec 2021.

71. Bland JM, Altman DG. Statistical methods for assessing agreement between two methods of clinical measurement. Lancet. 1986;327:307–10. https://doi.org/10.1016/S0140-6736(86)90837-8.

72. Lin L. A concordance correlation coefficient to evaluate reproducibility. Biometrics. 1989;45:255–68. https://doi.org/10.2307/2532051.

73. Lin L, Hedayat AS, Sinha B, Yang M. Statistical methods in assessing agreement. J Am Stat Assoc. 2002; 97:257–70. https://dor.org/, https://doi.org/10.1198/016214502753479392.

74. Nass SA, Hossain I, Sanyang C, Baldeh B, Pereira DIA. SPSS macro for Lin's concordance correlation coefficient. [Internet]. PLOS ONE; 2020. https://doi.org/10.1371/journal.pone.0239931.s002. Accessed 21 Dec 2021.

75. Koo TK, Li MY. A guideline of selecting and reporting intraclass correlation coefficients for reliability research. J Chiropr Med. 2016;5:155–63. https://doi.org/10.1016/j.jcm.2016.02.012.

76. Fisher RA. Statistical methods for research workers. Edinburgh: Oliver and Boyd; 1954. https://doi.org/10.1002/qj.49708235130.

77. Morgan CJ, Aban I. Methods for evaluating agreement between diagnostic tests. J Nucl Cardiol. 2016;23:511–3. https://doi.org/10.1007/s12350-015-0175-7.

78. Shrout PE, Fleiss JL. Intraclass correlations: uses in assessing rater reliability. Psychol Bull. 1978;86:420–8. https://doi.org/10.1037/0033-2909.86.2.420.

79. McGraw KO, Wong SP. Forming inferences about some intraclass correlation coefficients. Psychol Methods. 1996;1:30–46. https://doi.org/10.1037/1082-989X.1.1.30.

80. Bland JM, Altman DG. A note on the use of the intraclass correlation coefficient in the evaluation of agreement between two methods of measurement. Comput Biol Med. 1990;20:337–40. https://doi.org/10.1016/0010-4825(90)90013-F.

81. Bruton A, Conway JH, Holgate ST. Reliability: what is it, and how is it measured? Physiotherapy. 2000;86:94–9. https://doi.org/10.1016/S0031-9406(05)61211-4.

82. Kendall MG, Babington SB. The problem of m rankings. Ann Math Stat. 1939;10:275–87. https://doi.org/10.1214/aoms/1177732186.

83. Legendre P. Species associations: The Kendall coefficient of concordance revisited. JABES. 2005;10:226–45. https://doi.org/10.1198/108571105X46642.

Abstract

A multivariable analysis is a statistical tool for determining how independent predictor variables can explain or predict an event or outcome, whether as a set or independently. In general, the multivariable analysis combines regression and ANOVA; hence, it has to satisfy the many assumptions behind both techniques. The model of multivariable analysis is mainly dependent on the outcome variable. This chapter will discuss the three main types: the multiple linear regression to analyze a continuous outcome, the logistic regression in case of a binary outcome, and the Cox proportional hazard in the presence of censored data.

Keywords

ANOVA · ANCOVA · Mixed models · Logistic regression · Linear regression · Cox proportional hazard

3.1 Introduction

The terms multivariable and multivariable analysis are often used interchangeably. Statistically speaking, multivariate analysis refers to statistical models with two or more dependent outcome variables. On the other hand, multivariable analysis (MVA) refers to models with multiple independent variables and only one outcome variable [1], which is the main topic of this section. However, we will give one example of multivariate analysis as a demonstration (see Sect. 3.2.4).

We have previously shown that bivariate statistical analysis allows the researcher to measure and test the statistical significance of the tightness of the relation between two variables, such as the number of cigarettes smoked per day and the person's life expectancy in years. The bivariate analysis takes only a few easily verified assumptions, giving the researcher confidence in the results. However, relating smoking to life expectancy neglects the role of other associated variables of utmost importance, such as the patient's age, his gender, body weight, daily physical activity, family history, etc.... The analysis assumes that all those variables are either not present, stationary, or equally distributed among the compared groups, which is not valid, even in controlled randomized studies. Studying the role of a third variable, such as the patient's age, on life expectancy may clarify the effect of age on survival. Still, it cannot relate, at the same time, the patient's age to the number of cigarettes smoked per day. It may be the younger a person's starts smoking, the shorter is his life expectancy and not smoking per say, at any age. Even if we can adjust for age, we cannot adjust for multiple factors. In other words, the bivariate analysis cannot study the combined effect of age, smoking and physical activity on the life expectancy nor the unique effect of every one of those factors after removing (controlling for) the effects of others. Those are among the many roles played by the multivariate analysis [2].

We have previously demonstrated how stratification and adjustment analysis can also assess the effect of a risk factor on an outcome while holding other variables constant (see Sect. 2.9). However, stratification works well when there are only two or three confounders. When there are many potential confounders (adjustment variables), stratifying for all of them will create hundreds of groups literally with small sizes and unstable estimates of risk. We need to construct a statistical model that can relate the multiple predictors to the outcome and, at the same time, quantify the effect of each predictor independently from the others "Eq. 3.1". We have already discussed "simple regression," where the outcome variable (G) was a function (b) of only one predictor variable (x) (see Sect. 2.6.2). Multiple regression is just an extension of the simple regression discussed before. The effects of the multiple predictors $[(x_1), (x_2), (x_3)]$ on outcome are independently quantified as $[(b_1), (b_2), (b_3)]$. The mean value of the outcome (G) will be equal to the intercept $[b_0]$ plus the sum of all $[b_i(x_i)]$ "Eq. 3.1". Remember that the intercept is the mean value of the outcome (G) in case of the absence of all predictors, and hence, all their corresponding beta values will be all equal to zero (b_0). The reader is advised to return to Sect. 2.6.2 to get more details.

$$G = b_0 + b_1(x_1) + b_2(x_2) + b_3(x_3)... + b_i(x_i)$$
(3.1)

As such, multiple regression quantifies the effect of each predictor on the outcome and tests its statistical significance. However, it cannot test the statistical significance of the combined effect of all predictors, i.e., the effect of regression itself. Moreover, it cannot test the possibility of interaction between predictors. The presence of a statistically significant interaction between predictors may question the results of their individual effects (see Sect. 2.9.4.1). Only ANOVA

can answer those two questions, and hence, multiple regression is the mating product of both techniques: regression and ANOVA. Before proceeding to the next section, the reader is advised to revise the meaning and how to calculate the variance (see Sect. 1.3.4) and one-way ANOVA (see Sect. 2.4.3.1).

3.2 The ANOVA Family

The analysis of variance (ANOVA) is basically used to uncover the main as well as the interaction effects of categorical independent variables (also called "factors" or grouping variables) on one or more numeric outcome variables (also called dependent variables). A "main effect" is the direct effect of an independent variable on the outcome. An "interaction effect" is the joint effect of two or more independent variables. We have previously discussed simple forms of ANOVA, including one-way ANOVA, to analyze the main effect of one independent variable (see Sect. 2.4.3.1). One-way repeated measures ANOVA aiming to analyze the within-subject variability among repeated sampling (see Sect. 2.4.3.4) and two-way ANOVA to analyze the main and interaction effects of 2 independent variables on the outcome (see Sect. 2.9.4). In this section, we will over-review the main features of the technique. We will show how to use a higher-way ANOVA to analyze the main and interaction effects of multiple independent variables on outcome. In addition, we will outline the commonly used unique variants of ANOVA, (ANCOVA), (RMANOVA), and (MANOVA). Analysis of covariance (ANCOVA) studies the effect of including a concomitant numeric independent variable, usually called a "covariance". Repeated measures ANOVA (RMANOVA) is the case where the measures of outcome variable are no more independent but are rather repeated on the same subject. Multivariate ANOVA (MANOVA) is the case where the outcome is not a single but multiple numeric variables.

We have to admit that going higher than two-way ANOVA renders calculations difficult, exhausting, and a source of sizeable manual error. Hence, the use of a computer statistical software package becomes a must. On the other hand, those statistical packages have to be used with extreme caution, especially in the situations mentioned above. Before rushing to an "appealing, sophisticated test", the clinician has to understand his data's nature and use the package to verify or rectify this nature. For example, a simple histogram can give an important clue about the Normality of our data. The package can then supply additional evidence by applying a Normality test or can "normalize" our data by a suitable transformation. The question is which test to use and how to interpret it correctly; this is something that one has to know before using the sophisticated statistical software package.

We have to be careful in verifying the many assumptions made by those tests and choosing among the many options and variants offered by those packages. If we do not already understand the meaning and consequences of choosing an option, how can we evaluate the results? A sizeable delicious meal may end by a nightmare if the person does not choose the type and quantity of food that he can digest. In fact, after executing one of those tests, a clinician can be amazed by the quantity and the apparent "high quality" results. Be careful of the hidden bias due to unverified assumptions, lousy choice of options, and erroneous interpretation of results; only one of them is sufficient for turning a study into an absolute nightmare.

General Assumptions Behind ANOVA

Besides randomization, a primary necessity for any statistical test, ANOVA assumes that the outcome is a continuous, normally distributed variable. The independent variable(s) splits the outcome into multiple groups of nearly equal sizes and similar variability. The outcome distribution is assumed to remain normal within each group. Suppose that the outcome is the duration of pain relief, and we have one independent variable, which is studying a treatment's effect: aspirin versus paracetamol. ANOVA analyses how the distribution of outcome variability (duration of pain relief) is different between the two groups (aspirin versus

paracetamol) and within each group as well. The treatment effect can explain the between-group variability (difference in pain relief between those receiving aspirin and those receiving paracetamol). On the other hand, it remains obscure why patients receiving the same treatment (e.g., patients in the aspirin group) reacted somehow differently from one other. The latter represents the residual or the unexplained part of variability.

The key statistic in ANOVA is the F ratio (F-statistics), which is the ratio between the variability explained by the independent variable and the unexplained residual variability. The higher F, the more important the effect of the independent variable on the outcome and the smaller the probability that it can be due to chance. As usual, a statistically significant effect is declared whenever this probability drops to 5% or smaller.

Now let us understand how ANOVA compares means. The null hypothesis is that the independent variable (treatment in our example) does not affect the outcome. Hence, the mean durations of pain relief are equal in the two groups. The alternative hypothesis is that the independent variable has an effect; hence, not all group means are equal. In other words, if we have two groups only, such as in our example, a significant ANOVA tells us that the mean of one group is significantly larger than the other. However, if we have three groups or more, ANOVA just tells us that not all groups are equal. Consequently, ANOVA is an omnibus test, which points to the difference among the group but does not compare the groups two-by-two. A post-hoc analysis can answer this question [3, 4] (see Sect. 2.4.3.3).

3.2.1 Testing the Main Effects

3.2.1.1 One-Way ANOVA

Although we can always compute a Student test to compare two groups, ANOVA is a much more flexible and powerful technique to apply to more complex research issues. Let us take a simple example where a study was designed to compare the durations of pain relief achieved with either

Table 3.1 One-Way ANOVA: comparison of the duration of pain relief in hours in two-independent groups of patients receiving different analgesics A and B

Observations	Group A	Group B
Observation 1	2	6
Observation 2	3	7
Observation 3	1	5
Observation 4	4	8
Observation 5	5	9
Observation 6	3	7
Mean	*(3)*	*(7)*
Within-group sum of squares	*(10)*	*(10)*
Total mean = 5		
Total Sum of squares = 68		

Values are durations of pain relief in hours, values in parentheses are mean values and sum of squares per patient group

analgesic A or analgesic B that were randomly allocated to 12 patients divided into two equal groups. As shown in Table 3.1, the mean duration of pain relief is 3 h in group A and 7 h in group B patients, and the within-group sum of squares (SS) are 10 in each group, with a combined "within-group SS" of 20. On the other hand, the mean duration of pain among the 12 patients is 5 h, and "the total SS" is 68, regardless of the patients' group. Table 3.2 shows the one-way analysis of variance produced by a commercially available statistical software package. In terms of SS, a major part of the total variance (68) is explained by the group membership (48), and the part remaining unexplained is (20). The statistical significance of the main effect is tested by calculating the ratio between two variances: the variance of the main effect and the residual variance. The variance of the main effect = main effect SS/main effect df = 48/1=48. The residual variance = within-group variance/within-group df = 20/10 = 2. The F ratio = 48/2 = 24 and, its statistical significance is checked out in the F tables at F (1,10) df (see Sect. 2.4.3.1); $P < 0.001$. In conclusion, group membership was statistically significant, in the

sense that the mean duration of analgesia offered by analgesic B is significantly longer than that offered by analgesic A ($P < 0.001$).

3.2.1.2 Two-Way ANOVA

Now suppose that we introduce another grouping factor, gender, for example, and let's say that gender is equally distributed in both groups; i.e., we have three males and three females in each group (Table 3.3). Before performing any computations, it is clear that the total variance is partitioned into at least three sources:

- Variability due to group membership.
- Variability due to gender.
- A residual (within-group variability) is neither explained by the type of analgesia nor gender.
- There is an additional source of variation—interaction—that we will discuss shortly (see Sect. 3.2.2).

As shown in Table 3.3, we now have four small subgroups; each is formed of three patients: three males in Group A, three males in Group B, three females in Group A, and three females in Group B. The SS within each of them equals (2),

Table 3.2 One-way ANOVA table: analysis of data presented in Table 3.1

	Sum of squares	df	Mean square	F	P value
Between groups	48.00	1	48.00	24.00	<0.001
Within groups	20.00	10	2.00		
Total	68.00	11			

df = degree of freedom

Table 3.3 Two-Way ANOVA: comparison of the duration of pain relief in hours per type of analgesic and per gender

		Group A	Group B
Observation 1	Male	2	6
Observation 2	Male	3	7
Observation 3	Male	1	5
Mean		*(2)*	*(6)*
Sum of squares		*(2)*	*(2)*
Observation 4	Female	4	8
Observation 5	Female	5	9
Observation 6	Female	3	7
Mean		*(4)*	*(8)*
Sum of squares		*(2)*	*(2)*

Values are durations of pain relief in hours, values in parentheses are mean values and sum of squares per gender and per patient group

and the combined "within groups SS" equals 8 (2 + 2 + 2 + 2). Compared to Table 3.1, the within-group SS of the study has decreased from a total of 20 to only 8. We can deduce that the within-group (residual) SS becomes smaller when including gender. The difference is because the means for males (2 and 6) were systematically lower than those for females (4 and 8), and this difference in means adds variability (increases calculated SS) if we ignore this factor.

Table 3.4 shows the results of data analysis by two-way ANOVA. Out of the total SS of 68, a significant part (60) is now explained by both predictors collectively: group membership and gender, i.e., by the regression model itself. The statistical significance of the latter is tested by calculating the F ratio: the ratio between the model variance and the residual unexplained variance = 30/0.889 = 33.75. The statistical significance of the latter is checked out in Fisher's table at F (2,9) df (see Sect. 2.4.3.1). In conclusion, the model (type of analgesia + gender) explained a significant part of the duration of analgesia; P = 0.001.

Introducing the second factor in the model (gender) had decreased the residual variance more than before when only group membership was considered. In other words, controlling for error (residual) variance increases the test's sensitivity (power), offering the researcher the luxury that fewer patients are needed to demonstrate a statistically significant effect. Up to this point, ANOVA tested the statistical significance of the main effect of one (type of analgesic) or more predictors (analgesic + gender) on the outcome variable (duration of pain relief) and quantified the residual variation (residual variance) that remained unexplained. The more the added factor's effect, the more it decreases the residual variance and, the larger is the latter, the more we need to include factors in our model.

3.2.2 Testing Interaction Effects of Qualitative Variables

We may want to examine the consistency of an observed relation across two or more subgroups

Table 3.4 Two-way ANOVA table: analysis of data presented in Table 3.3

Model[a]	Sum of squares	df	Mean square	F	P value
Regression[b]	60.00	2	30.00	33.75	<0.001
Residual	8.00	9	0.889		
Total	68.00	11			

a = predictors: constant, gender, group. b = dependent variable: duration of pain relief, df = degree of freedom of the individuals studied in several studies. We have presented the example of a multicenter trial that was conducted to compare the effect of two antihypertensive treatments in two independent groups of patients (see Sect. 2.9.4.1). Twenty-four patients were recruited from three hospitals (eight patients per hospital), and patients were equally randomized between the two treatment groups, A and B. The results are shown in Table 2.38.

The researcher aimed to find a treatment effect, a hospital effect, and possible interaction. In other words, the researcher had three questions to answer, and the problem will be if he receives the wrong advice that separate statistical tests can obtain those answers. For example, he can use a Student test to compare the two treatment groups and a one-way ANOVA to compare the results among the three hospitals. Unfortunately, comparing the results of the two treatments by a t-test will not achieve a statistically significant difference between the two treatments. As shown in Table 2.38, the mean blood pressure of the 12 patients receiving treatment A was 125.4 ± 15.1 mm Hg, and the mean blood pressure of the other 12 patients receiving treatment B was 135.7 ± 16.9 mm Hg; $t = 1.56$ and $P = 0.133$. Comparing the three hospitals by one-way ANOVA will produce a statistically significant result (111.8 ± 4.5 mm Hg versus 130.5 ± 6 mm Hg versus 149.3 ± 7 mm Hg; $P < 0.001$). However, the comparison would be of no value since the two treatments were not different from one another in the first place. In conclusion, if the researcher had applied those two separate tests, he would have never reached a conclusion achieved by two-way ANOVA: the compared treatments were significantly different, considering the factor hospital (see Sect. 2.9.4.1

). *Two-way ANOVA can link the two factors (type of treatment and recruiting hospital) and the outcome variable (blood pressure measurement), but multiple t-tests cannot.*

In our example, two-way ANOVA equally tested a statistically significant interaction between the two independent variables? We already know that there is a difference between the effects of the two treatments (factor treatment) and that there is a difference between the results acquired from the three hospitals (factor hospital). However, those two factors have to be independent of one another. Put it this way; the effect treatment has to be the same, regardless of the treating hospital. Testing interaction is to find whether those two main effects are genuinely independent or interact with one another? *In other words, whether the results of a particular treatment are dependent on the patient's managing hospital?* In our example, we had six patient subgroups, each representing a subgroup of patients receiving one of two treatments in one out of the three hospitals. Any significant difference between those six measurements will indicate the presence of a significant interaction between the two factors. However, there was no statistically significant interaction between the two factors; $P = 0.119$ (see Sect. 2.9.4.1)

We will propose a second scenario; we will remove the results of the hospital (2) and analyze the study as if it was carried out in hospitals 1 and 3 only (Table 3.5). As shown in Table 3.6, the new study revealed statistically significant treatment and hospital factors. However, unlike the first scenario, the second study showed a statistically significant interaction between treatment and hospital factors; $P = 0.044$. The reader is kindly advised to refer to Table 3.6 to understand what changed. The mean results acquired

Table 3.5 Two-way ANOVA: comparison of the effects of two antihypertensive regimens in two hospitals

	Treatment A (n = 8)	Treatment B (n = 8)	Total
Hospital 1 (n = 8)	108	115.8	111.9
Hospital 3 (n = 8)	143	155.5	149.3
Total	125.4	135.7	130.5

Values represent mean systolic blood pressure in mm Hg, n = number of patients. Sum of all measured values = TG = 2089, sum of all squared values = 278,819

Table 3.6 Two-way ANOVA: analysis of data presented in Tables 2.38 and Table 3.5

	SS	df	MS	F	P value
(A) First scenario[a]					
1—Model	6240.7	5	1248	263.5	<0.001
2—Treatment	630.4	1	630.4	133	<0.001
3—Hospitals	5587.8	2	2793.8	589.9	<0.001
4—Interaction	*22.7*	*2*	*11.4*	*2.4*	*0.119*
5—Error	85.2	18	4.7		
6—Total	6325.9	23			
(B) Second scenario[b]					
1—Model	6020	3	2006.7	448	<0.001
2—Treatment	410	1	410	91.5	<0.001
3—Hospitals	5587.5	1	5587.5	1247.4	<0.001
4—Interaction	*22.6*	*1*	*22.6*	*5.04*	*0.044*
5—Error	53.7	12	4.5		
6—Total	6073.9	15			

a = two-way ANOVA of data presented in Table 2.38, b = two-way ANOVA of data presented in Table 3.5, SS = sum of squares, df = degree of freedom, MS = mean square (variance), F = Fisher's ratio

from hospital 2 (mean treatment A = 125.3 and mean treatment B = 135.8 mm Hg) were nearly equal to the overall mean results of the three hospitals (mean treatment A = 125.4 and mean treatment B = 135.7 mm Hg). Looking back to Table 3.6, we can quickly notice that removing hospital (2) from the analysis increased the variation among hospitals because the difference (variation) between the hospital (1) and the hospital (3) is more significant than the differences between the three hospitals.

Consequently, the SS of factor hospital increased from 88.3% (5587.8/6325.9) to as much as 92% (5587.5/6073.9) of the total variability. On the other hand, the SS of factor treatment decreased from about 10% (630.4/6325.9) to only 6.7% (410/6073.9) of the total variability. Consequently, removing hospital (2) increased the differences between hospitals and decreased the differences between treatments, resulting in more imbalance between the four subgroups of the second scenario than the six subgroups of the first scenario. Applying "Eq. 2.121", the interaction SS in the second scenario will equal 22.6 "Eq. 3.2". Note that because hospital 2 data were nearly equal to the

average values of the study, their removal was associated with a negligible reduction in interaction SS from 22.7 to only 22.6 (see Table 3.6). On the other hand, removing one hospital from the study decreased the hospital df (number of hospital −1 = 2−1 = 1) and the interaction df by 50%: from 2 to 1 (df of treatment × df of hospital = 1 × 1 = 1). Consequently, the variance of interaction (SS/df) will jump from 2.4 to as much as 5.04; (P = 0.044).

$$SS_{cr} = 4\,[(108 - 111.9 - 125.4 + 130.5)^2 \\ + (115.8 - 111.9 - 135.7 + 130.5)^2 \\ + (143 - 149.3 - 125.4 + 130.5)^2 \\ + (155.5 - 149.3 - 135.7 + 130.5)^2] = 22.6$$
(3.2)

Reporting Interaction

We can put this two-way interaction into words by saying that: the effect of treatment depends on the treating hospital. If we had included factor gender, the means pattern would now represent a three-way interaction between factors (treatment-hospital-gender). It would become more difficult to verbalize any assumptions. Suppose that females reacted better for treatment B than for treatment A; we may summarize that the two-way interaction between treatment and hospital was modified by gender. If we have a four-way interaction, we may say that the fourth variable changes the three-way interaction. A general way to express all interactions is to say that an effect is modified (qualified) by another effect. A comprehensive literature review permits suspecting and planning for interaction before the study. Interaction that is accidentally discovered after data collection and with no rationale will always be hard to explain [4, 5].

3.2.3   Testing Interaction Effects of Quantitative Variables: Analysis of Covariance (ANCOVA)

We have briefly discussed the idea of "controlling" for factors (i.e., qualitative variables). The inclusion of an additional factor(s) can reduce the residual SS; hence, increasing the power of the design to put into evidence a significant effect. We can extend the idea to the continuous variables, and when we include such continuous variables in the design, they are called covariates. Controlling for the effect of covariates is called analysis of covariance (ANCOVA) rather than analysis of variance (ANOVA). A covariance is included in a study if it is known to affect the outcome. Hence, unless controlled for, it can play the role of confounder in the study, i.e., confounding the relationship between the predictor and the outcome variable. *As such, ANCOVA can be seen as a way to control initial individual differences that were not (or could not be) randomized.* Introducing a covariate in the study must be based on a literature review and a clear rationale. Initially, the covariate is measured before the study and it must be statistically related to the outcome. As both covariate and outcome are continuous variables, we must measure their relationship before the study by Pearson's correlation coefficient.

3.2.3.1   One-Way ANCOVA

As in ANOVA, the "one-way" part of one-way ANCOVA refers to the number of independent variables included in the model. While one-way ANOVA compares the main effect of one independent variable, one-way ANCOVA is an extension in which we measure the main effect after adjusting the dependent variable for the differences associated with the covariate. Put it this way; it compares subgroup means after removal of the noise associated with the covariate or, put it another way as if all subjects had the same level covariate [4–6].

The Example

A researcher was interested in determining the effect of two oral hypoglycemic regimens in patients with type II diabetes mellitus. Sixty patients were equally randomized between the treatment groups (A and B) and a control group C. The judgment criterion was HbA1C measured after three months. The researcher expected that any reduction in HbA1C would also depend on the participant's initial HbA1C level. Hence, he used the pre-treatment HbA1C as a covariate when comparing the post-treatment concentrations. The researcher ran a one-way ANCOVA to compare the post-treatment HbA1C among the three groups with the pre-treatment HbA1C as a covariate. Data are shown in Table 3.7. Note that the table includes two more pieces of information that will not be used in this section but later on: regular physical activity as a second predictor (see Sect. 3.2.3.2) and measuring CRP as an additional outcome variable (see Sect. 3.2.4.1).

The Play of Covariance

In our example, we wanted to study the effect of both: the independent qualitative variable (treatment variable) and the numeric covariate ("x"; pre-treatment Hb A1C) on the outcome numeric variable ("y"; post-treatment HbA1C). As previously shown, the relation between two numerical variables ("x" and "y"; pre-and post-treatment HbA1C, in our example) can be studied by simple linear regression, which fits a

Table 3.7 One-way ANCOVA: Hb A1C pre-treatment and post-treatment values in three groups of patients receiving treatment A, treatment B or control

Treatment	Pre-Hb A1C	Post-Hb A1C	Exercise	CRP	Treatment	Pre-Hb A1C	Post-Hb A1C	Exercise	CRP
Control	8.00	8.00	0.00	3.00	A	7.50	6.70	1.00	2.71
Control	8.00	8.00	0.00	4.00	A	6.60	6.00	1.00	3.41
Control	7.00	7.00	1.00	2.50	A	6.00	5.50	0.00	3.67
Control	7.00	7.00	1.00	3.00	A	8.00	7.00	0.00	3.15
Control	7.00	7.00	1.00	4.00	A	8.00	7.00	0.00	3.54
Control	7.10	7.00	0.00	3.00	A	8.00	7.00	0.00	3.49
Control	6.00	6.00	1.00	3.00	A	8.00	7.00	0.00	3.06
Control	6.10	6.00	0.00	3.57	A	6.50	5.80	1.00	2.76
Control	8.00	7.40	1.00	3.00	A	7.00	6.00	0.00	3.03
Control	8.00	7.40	1.00	3.35	A	7.00	6.00	1.00	3.27
Control	7.50	7.00	0.00	3.00	B	7.00	6.00	0.00	2.00
Control	7.00	6.50	0.00	4.00	B	7.00	6.00	0.00	3.00
Control	7.00	6.50	1.00	2.50	B	7.00	6.00	0.00	2.00
Control	6.50	6.00	1.00	3.00	B	7.00	6.00	1.00	2.50
Control	6.60	6.00	1.00	4.00	B	7.00	6.00	1.00	3.00
Control	8.00	7.00	0.00	3.00	B	8.00	6.70	0.00	2.50
Control	8.00	7.00	0.00	3.00	B	8.00	6.70	1.00	2.50
Control	7.00	6.00	0.00	3.57	B	7.50	6.30	0.00	2.00
Control	7.00	6.00	0.00	3.00	B	7.50	6.30	1.00	2.50
Control	7.00	6.00	1.00	3.35	B	6.00	5.00	1.00	2.00
A	7.00	7.00	0.00	2.51	B	6.00	5.00	1.00	2.00
A	7.00	7.00	1.00	3.52	B	6.00	5.00	1.00	3.00
A	7.20	7.00	0.00	2.69	B	8.00	6.50	0.00	2.00
A	7.20	7.00	0.00	2.79	B	8.00	6.50	0.00	2.50
A	7.50	7.00	0.00	3.47	B	8.00	6.50	0.00	3.00
A	7.30	6.70	1.00	3.19	B	7.50	6.00	0.00	2.50
A	7.30	6.70	1.00	2.93	B	7.50	6.00	0.00	2.50
A	6.50	6.00	1.00	3.57	B	7.50	6.00	1.00	2.00
A	6.50	6.00	1.00	2.69	B	6.30	5.00	1.00	2.50
A	7.50	6.70	1.00	3.35	B	7.50	5.00	1.00	2.00

Pre and Post = pre-treatment and posttreatment values of Hb A1C, Exercise values 1 and 0 are indicator of patients being assigned or not to daily physical exercise. CRP = C-reactive protein measured after treatment

straight line to the x–y pairs of data (see Sect. 2.6.2.1). A good estimation of the relation between x and y is the coefficient of variation (r square), simply the squared value of the simple correlation coefficient. The coefficient of variation expresses the amount of variation of the outcome "y" that is supposed to be due to the covariate "x" effect.

Removing the variability that was explained by "x" (R^2) from the total variation of "y" (S_t^2) results in a smaller residual (unexplained) variance of "y" (S_r^2) "Eq. 3.3". *If the correlation* between pre and post-test results is substantial, then we can achieve a large reduction in the error SS. This occurs because in the F test we compute the ratio of the between-group variance over the error variance. If the latter becomes smaller due to the explanatory power of "x", then the overall F value will become larger. This shows how the introduction of significantly related covariates can make our test more powerful (i.e., more sensitive).

$$S_r^2 = S_t^2 - \left(1 - R^2\right) \qquad (3.3)$$

On the other hand, *One-way ANOVA fits a mean to each group, and hence, combining both simple regression and ANOVA techniques fits a straight line to each group of x–y data, such that the regression slopes of those lines are all equal.* To put it simpler, all conditions have to be verified on all levels of the predictor variable (treatment) [4–6].

The Procedure [6–10]

The procedure is complicated, with many assumptions to be made and many hypotheses to be tested. Out of the ten assumptions made, four need to be verified by the products of the analysis itself, and hence, the technique can be outlined in six steps:

1. Verification of the validity of the study design
2. Verification of the validity of the covariance
3. Execution of the analysis
4. Verification of the validity of the products of the analysis
5. Evaluation of the gain achieved by using the covariance over simple ANOVA
6. Calculation of the adjusted means and performing post-hoc-analysis of any statistically significant predictor with >2 classes.

1. **Verification of the Study Design**

There are four assumptions related to study design, and hence, we can verify them during the preparation period. A continuous outcome variable and a continuous covariate related to the outcome (covariant), as proven by a significant correlation coefficient r. A categorical independent variable of two or more groups and independence of the observations. The latter means that there is no relation between observations made in a particular category of the predictor or between the categories themselves. Our example verifies those four assumptions, with a correlation coefficient r value of 0.699; P < 0.001.

2. **Verification of Covariance Validity**

The covariate has to correlate with the outcome. Otherwise, we should not investigate its effect on the outcome in the first place. On the other hand, the covariate should be independent of (not related to and not interacting with) the predictor variable; otherwise, it will overshadow the predictor's effect outcome. Put it this way; we have to show dependence between the outcome variable and covariance but independence between the latter and the predictor variable. Technically, we have to show linearity between the covariance and the outcome at all independent variable levels (three in our example) and the absence of interaction between the covariance and the independent variable. We can verify the linear relation by plotting the pre-treatment and post-treatment HbA1C paired measures for each of the three groups (see Fig. 3.1). As shown, there is a linear relationship between the pre-and post-treatment values at the three levels of the predictor variable, with respective R^2 values of 0.669, 0.733, and 0.661 for treatment A, treatment B, and control groups (Fig. 3.1). In absence of linearity, the researcher can try to modify or replace the covariate or modify the levels of the predictor variable; otherwise, the researcher has to abort the technique.

We can verify the independence between the covariate and the predictor variable by showing no statistically significant interaction between both variables (pre-test Hb A1C and treatment). IBM-SPSS can calculate the interaction

Fig. 3.1 One-way ANCOVA: testing linearity on each level of the grouping variable. Treatment A = dark circles and continuous line, treatment B = gray circles and interrupted line, controls = open circles and dotted line, $R^2 = 0.669$, 0.733, and 0.661

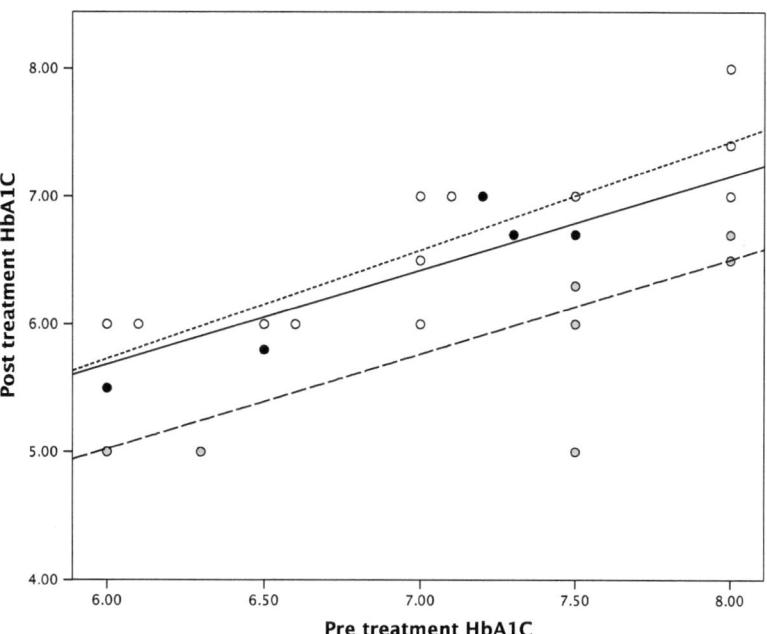

- We click on "Analyze" and request "Univariate analysis" from the "General linear model"
- We shift the (post-treatment HB A1C) to the "dependent variable" box, the (treatment group) to the "fixed factor" box, and the (pre-treatment Hb A1C) to the "covariate" box.
- We click on "Model" and change it from "full factorial" to a "*custom*" model. We highlight both the covariate and the factor and click on the arrow below "interaction" to test their interaction only. We click on "Continue" then "OK" to execute the analysis.

For our example, the predictor and the covariate were independent as verified by a statistically non-significant interaction; (P = 0.77) (Table 3.8). A significant interaction violates the assumption of independence, and we should not proceed with the covariate. Note that in this table, we are only concerned with the line denoting interaction between the predictor, and the covariate and all the other results should be discarded from the report. The proper execution of ANOVA itself will be performed in the following step.

Table 3.8 One-way ANCOVA: testing interaction between independent variable and covariance

Source	SS	df	Mean square	F	P value
Corrected model	21.3[a]	5	4.26	36.1	<0.001
Intercept	0.295	1	0.295	2.49	0.12
Treatment	0.039	2	0.019	0.164	0.849
HbA1C-pre	13.6	1	13.6	115.2	<0.001
*Treatment * Hb A1C-pre*	*0.62*	*2*	*0.031*	*0.263*	*0.77*
Residual	6.37	54	0.118		
Corrected total	27.66	59			

a = $R^2 = 0.783$ (Adjusted $R^2 = 0.756$)

3. Execution of ANCOVA

- We can re request a "Univariate analysis" form the "General linear model" but unlike when we tested for linearity, we keep the default "*full factorial model*".
- We click on "Save" and choose to save "predicted values" and "standardized residuals".
- We click on "Options" and request to acquire "Descriptive statistics", "Estimates of effect size", "Homogeneity tests". We shift the factor (groups) from the "Factors and Factor interactions" box to the "Display means for" box. We choose to "Compare main effects" and "Bonferroni" for "Confidence interval adjustment". We click on "Continue" then on "OK" to execute the analysis.

4. Verification of the Remaining Assumptions from the Products of the Analysis

Verifying the validity of a test after execution of the analysis itself may not seem coherent. However, we will not be surprised when we know that what we verify is the product of the analysis rather than the raw data.

The first assumption is that the outcome variable has to be approximately normally distributed for each category of the independent variables. We can test the normality of the standardized residuals of post-treatment Hb A1C across the three categories of the independent variable (treatment A, treatment B, and control) by the Shapiro Wilk test (see Sect. 1.4.3.3). A statistically non-significant result ($P > 0.05$) is needed to confirm normality. Otherwise, we can normalize data by an appropriate transformation (see Sect. 1.4.4). Concerning normality of residuals, ANCOVA is a robust test unless there is a substantial violation, with small sample size and unequal groups. In our example, only treatment B patients deviated from normality, and we carried on the analysis without data transformation.

The second assumption is the homoscedasticity of error variances in each group, which means that variances have to be homogeneous across all categories of the predictor variable. We can verify homoscedasticity by plotting the standardized residuals against the predicted values for each of the three categories (Fig. 3.2). If there is homoscedasticity, the standardized residuals (errors of prediction), will be equal across the predicted values. We will see that the paired

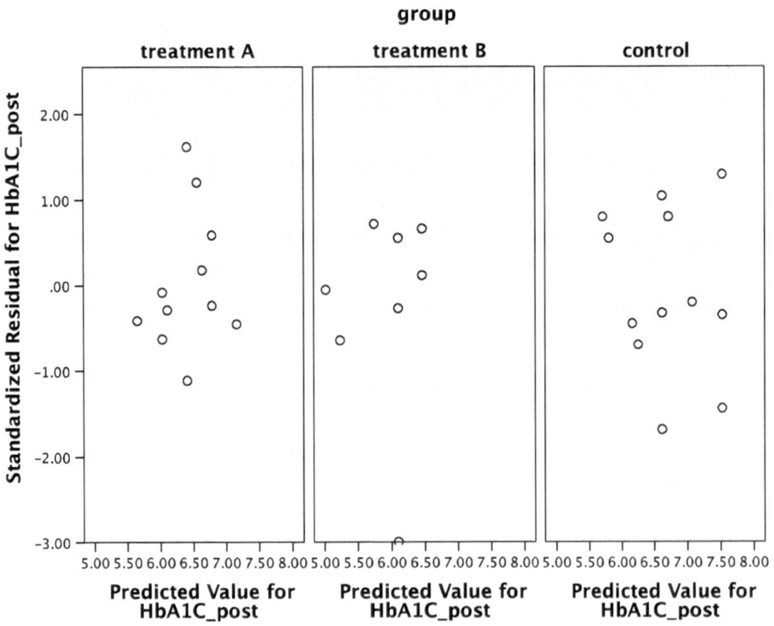

Fig. 3.2 One-way ANCOVA: testing homoscedasticity of error variances within each of the three categories of the predictor variable

measures of each of the three scatterplots will exhibit no particular pattern and will be approximately constantly spread (in the y-axis) across the predicted values (in the x-axis). The spread of points should be similar in the y-axis for each of the three scatterplots. Otherwise, we may attempt the transformation of the outcome variable.

The third assumption to be tested is that the variance of the residuals is equal for all groups of the predictor variable. Levene's test can verify the equality of variance, and the null hypothesis is that the error variance is equal among all groups. The test statistics is an F ratio with df (1, 2) equal to the number of groups minus one and the total sample size minus the number of groups, i.e., df (2, 57). In our example, our F value = 1.88 and a P-value = 0.162. As in our example, a statistically non-significant test means no significant difference between the residual variances of the three groups.

Finally, ANCOVA assumes the absence of significant outliers. As we usually request the software to save residuals, verifying that none of the standardized residuals is larger or smaller than three standard deviations. In our example, we have a single outlier with a standardized residual value of −3.38. There are numerous methods to deal with outliers, including data

transformation, especially in the absence of normality, removal, or running the analysis with and without the outlier and then testing whether there will be a significant difference.

5. **Testing the Significance of the Covariance**

Table 3.9 shows the result of a regular one-way ANOVA, with a statistically significant grouping variable (F = 10.23 and P-value < 0.001) and a residual variance of 0.357. Table 3.10 shows the result of execution of ANCOVA by step number 3. Note that after adjustment for pre-treatment HbA1C by one-way ANCOVA (Table 3.10), the residual variance was reduced by two-thirds from 0.357 to only 0.115 because of the substantial amount of variation explained by the covariate (F = 121.2; P < 0.001). This reduction improved the model sensitivity to show the effect of predictor from an F value of 10.23 (P = 0.001) to a much higher F value of 33.651 and a significantly lower P-value of < 0.001.

6. **Calculation of Adjusted Means and Post-hoc Analysis**

Adjusted Means

The test calculates the adjusted means (Table 3.11). Their standard error is the common

Table 3.9 One-way ANOVA: testing group effect

Source	SS	df	Mean square	F	P value
Treatment	*7.3*	*2*	*3.65*	*10.23*	*<0.001*
Within groups	20.35	57	0.357		
Total	27.66	59			

SS = sum of squares, df = degree of freedom

Table 3.10 One-way ANCOVA: testing adjusted group effect

Source	SS	df	Mean square	F	P value	η^2
Corrected model	21.23	3	7.07	61.6	<0.001	0.767
Intercept	0.298	1	0.298	2.56	0.113	0.044
HbA1C_pre	13.92	1	13.92	121.23	<0.001	0.684
Treatment	*7.723*	*2*	*3.864*	*33.65*	*<0.001*	*0.55*
Residual	6.43	56	0.115			
Corrected total	27.66	59				

SS = sum of squares, df = degree of freedom, η^2 = partial Eta-squared, a = R^2 = 0.767 (Adjusted R^2 = 0.755)

Table 3.11 One-way ANCOVA: non-adjusted and adjusted means of post-treatment Hb A1C

Group	N	Non-adjusted means (Sd)	Adjusted means (Se)	95% CI of the difference
Treatment A	20	6.55 ± 0.517	6.57 ± 0.076	6.41 to 6.72
Treatment B	20	5.92 ± 0.52	5.91 ± 0.076	5.76 to 6.06
Control	20	6.74 ± 0.667	6.74 ± 0.076	6.39 to 7.06

Non-adjusted values are presented as mean (Sd), adjusted values are presented as mean (Se), N = number of patients, CI = confidence interval

Table 3.12 One-way ANCOVA: post hoc-analysis with Bonferroni correction

Compared groups	N	Mean of the difference	Se of the difference	P value
Treatment A versus treatment B	20	0.657	0.107	<0.001
Treatment A versus control	20	−0.177	0.107	0.311
Treatment B versus control	20	−0.835	0.107	<0.001

Values are post-treatment Hb A1C

standard error calculated from the residual variance (0.115) of one-way ANCOVA (Table 3.10). We apply the usual formula: Se is the square root of the variance divided by sample size = square root of 0.115/20 = 0.076.

Post-hoc Analysis

ANCOVA is an omnibus test, which points to the presence of a difference but does not indicate where it comes from? A statistically significant predictor with >2 classes is an indication for post-hoc analysis. Table 3.12 shows the post-hoc results, calculated by the Bonferroni method. Note the statistically significant difference between treatment B and treatment A and control ($P < 0.001$). The adjusted means of treatment A and control group were comparable ($P > 0.05$). Figure 3.3 shows the analysis flowchart of one-way ANCOVA.

Interpretation of the Results

Sixty diabetic patients were equally randomized to receive treatment A, B, or control. A one-way ANCOVA was conducted to compare the effectiveness of three oral treatment modalities on post-treatment HbA1c, adjusted on the pre-treatment value of the latter. The covariate significantly correlated with the outcome ($r = 0.699$; $P < 0.001$), and all assumptions of ANCOVA were verified (the ten assumptions can be reported). The study showed a statistically

significant adjusted mean treatment effect (Eta-squared = 0.55; $P < 0.001$). Further post-hoc analysis (means and Sd of values can be reported) showed a statistically significant superior effect of treatment B over treatment A ($P < 0.001$) and control ($P < 0.001$). The adjusted mean effects of Treatment A and control were comparable ($P = 0.31$).

What Should Be Reported

We have to report non-adjusted and adjusted descriptive statistics (Table 3.11). Assumptions of ANCOVA have to be reported as being verified or data being transformed. We have to report inferential statistics, with F ratios, df and P-values (Table 3.10). We have to include $R^2 = 0.767$, adjusted $R^2 = 0.755$, effect size: partial $\eta^2 = 0.55$ and results of post-hoc analysis (Table 3.12).

3.2.3.2 Two-Way ANCOVA

Let us take an example; we are studying the effects of drug therapy (first predictor: treatment A or B) and salt restriction (second predictor: yes or no) in lowering blood pressure in the hypertensive patient (outcome), adjusted for the patient's age (covariate). ANCOVA begins by adjusting the outcome on the covariate, i.e., adjusting the patient's blood pressure on his age. Then it continues like a two-way ANOVA but using the adjusted outcome. The critical step is testing whether there is an interaction between

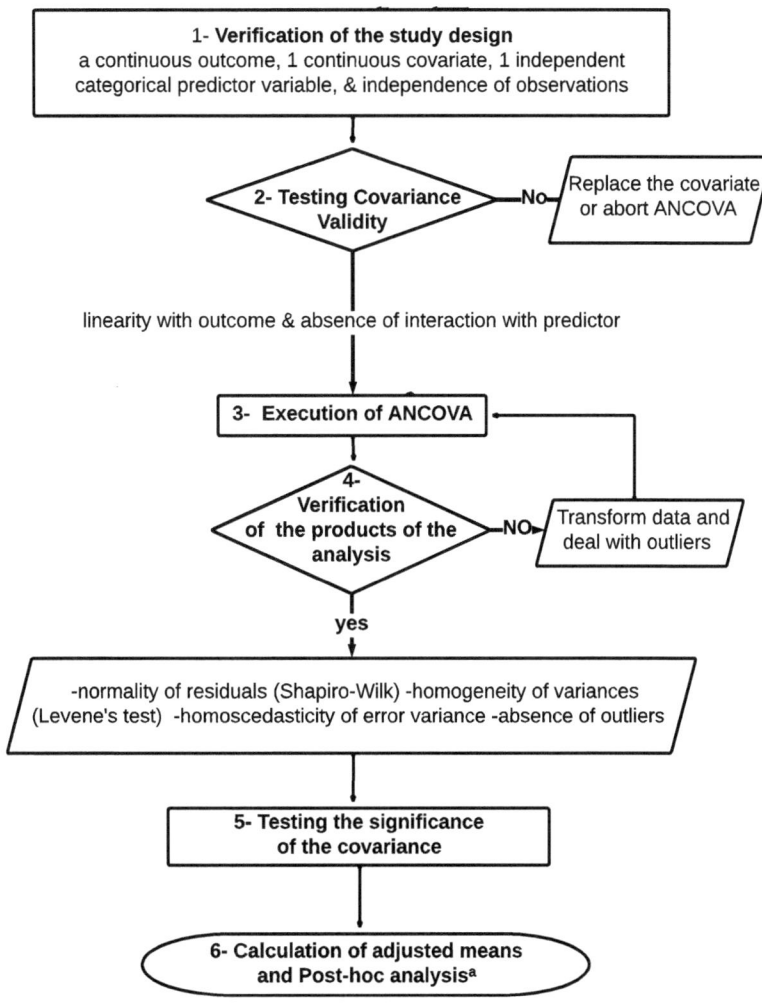

Fig. 3.3 One-way ANCOVA: the analysis flowchart, a = In case of a statistically significant factor with >2-class

the two predictors, followed by evaluating the effect of each predictor on outcome. The presence or absence of interaction dictates how it evaluates the predictors.

Suppose there is no interaction between treatment and salt restriction (the two predictors) on blood pressure (outcome). In that case, we can analyze the separate "main effect of each predictor" on the outcome, adjusted for age. On the other hand, an interaction means that patients on each combination of predictors will react differently from those following other combinations. For example, the blood pressure of patients receiving treatment A will do better with salt restriction, while patient's blood pressure on treatment B will not be affected by the salt restriction. Consequently, in the presence of a statistically significant interaction on the outcome, we cannot report the main effect of each predictor but the separate "simple result of each combination" because the combinations can react differently. Finally, we perform a post-hoc analysis to compare the effects of any statistically significant predictor with ≥ 2 classes.

The Example

Suppose that in our previous example, we were equally interested to see whether the physical activity will affect the post-treatment HbA1C levels (see Table 3.7). We now have two categorical predictors in this second scenario: treatment and exercise. We still have one continuous outcome

(HbA1C_post), and one continuous covariate measured before the outcome and is known to correlate with it (HbA1C_pre). One categorical predictor (treatment) has three levels (treatment A, treatment B, and placebo), and the other one (exercise) has two levels (doing exercise or not). Consequently, the 60 patients will be equally distributed among six groups (combinations): patients on treatment A with or without exercise, patients on treatment B with or without exercise, and controls on exercise and controls without exercise.

As "exercise" (second independent variable) is expected to moderate the effect of the treatment (first independent variable) on the post Hb A1C (outcome), it can also be called a moderator variable. The research question would be: does exercise influence the adjusted treatment effects? If this is true, would there be a statistically significant difference in treatment effects between those performing and those not performing physical activity?

The Procedure [6–10]

The procedure can be seen as an extension of one-way ANCOVA, but the calculations are modified to consider the two predictors. We start by verifying the ten assumptions of ANCOVA as before, including the execution of the analysis in the middle of the verification process to confirm those assumptions requiring the products of the analysis itself (see Sect. 3.2.3.1). The assumptions must be verified on the six combinations produced in our example. The number of combinations is the product of the number of classes of the two variables.

Once all assumptions are verified, the usual turning point is to find whether there is an interaction between the two predictors and the covariate, which can overshadow the effect of the former on the outcome. Unlike one-way ANCOVA, we have two predictors; hence, we create a new variable formed of both predictors (grouping variable). The number of classes of the grouping variable is the number of all possible combinations of the two independent variables (six in our example). We test the interaction between the "grouping variable" and the covariance, called dual interaction [10].

In the absence of a statistically significant dual interaction, we can report the adjusted main effect of each predictor on the outcome. In the presence of a statistically significant dual interaction, we have to report the adjusted simple effects of each combination of predictors on the outcome. Finally, post-hoc analysis has to be performed for statistically significant predictors of more than two categories.

1. **Verification of the Study Design**

As in one-way ANCOVA, we can verify the first four assumptions concerning the suitability of the study design during the preparation of the study itself. The predictors are ≥ 2 class categorical variables, outcome, and covariate are continuous variables known to be related. Observations are independent, meaning that there is no relation between observations made in a particular category of the predictor nor between the categories themselves (see Sect. 3.2.3.1).

2. **Arranging Data Combinations**

Unlike the one-way ANCOVA, we have two predictors, and, in our example, we have six possible combinations. All assumptions should be tested across all possible combinations and not across the individual categories of the two predictors. Using the command "compute" of the software, we can create a 6-class grouping variable [10] that we will simply name "group". The latter combines both predictors, and hence, we can use it to test all assumptions.

3. **Testing Covariance Validity**

As in one-way ANCOVA, the next step is to verify the validity of the covariance; i.e., it should be dependent on the outcome but independent from the predictor for the reasons explained before. Dependence between covariate and outcome can be tested by visualizing a linear relation between the covariance and the outcome, across "the 6-class grouping variable", with the calculation of the relevant R^2 values. Each calculated coefficient of variation (R^2) expresses how much the covariate explains the outcome in this particular combination; i.e., in each of the six categories of the grouping variable. As in one-way ANCOVA, a violation of linearity can be remedied by data transformation.

The second assumption can be primarily verified by visualizing that the six regression slopes of covariate effect on outcome are all parallel. However, formal statistical testing of independence between covariance and predictors is equally needed. We will repeat the same step performed in one-way ANCOVA and request a "custom univariate analysis" aiming only to test whether there is a statistically significant interaction between the covariate and the six combinations; i.e., the grouping variable "group".

- We click on "Analyze", "General linear Model" and "Univariate".
- We shift the (HbA1C_post) to the "dependent Variable" box, the (HbA1C_pre) to the "Covariate" box and the (six-class grouping variable) to the "Fixed Factors" box. No other variables are used in this temporary model.

- We click on the "Model" option to change it from the default "Full factorial" to a "Custom" model to test covariate, predictor and their interaction only. We click on "Continue" and then on "OK" to execute the analysis.

A statistically significant interaction is a serious alarm that the assumptions of two-way ANCOVA are seriously violated for being unable to separate the effects of the two predictors. We have to terminate two-way ANCOVA. As shown in Table 3.13, there was no statistically significant interaction (P = 0.841), and we can proceed with two-way ANCOVA. As in one-way ANCOVA, this model was just a side-way to calculate whether there is an interaction between the grouping variable (variable combining the effects of both predictors) and the covariance and, we have to build another conventional full factorial model to execute and analyze two-way ANCOVA properly (Table 3.14), which is shown in the following next step number 4.

Table 3.13 Two-way ANCOVA: testing between-subjects effect

Source	SS	df	Mean square	F	P value
Corrected model	21.62[a]	11	1.965	15.6	<0.001
Intercept	0.327	1	0.0327	2.6	0.113
HbA1C_pre	9.03	1	9.03	71.7	<0.001
Group	0.176	5	0.035	0.2791	0.922
*Group*HbA1C_pre*	*0.257*	*5*	*0.051*	*0.41*	*0.841*
Residual	6.04	48	0.126		
Corrected total	27.66	59			

SS = sum of squares, df = degree of freedom, a = R^2 = 0.782 (Adjusted R^2 = 0.732)

Table 3.14 Two-way ANCOVA: testing adjusted effects

Source	SS	df	Mean square	F	P value	η^2
Corrected model	21.36[a]	6	3.56	29.69	<0.001	0.772
Intercept	0.365	1	0.365	3.08	0.85	0.055
HbA1C_pre	10.94	1	10.94	92.1	<0.001	0.0.635
Treatment	*7.715*	*2*	*3.857*	*32.46*	*<0.001*	*0.551*
Exercise	*0.04*	*1*	*0.04*	*0.339*	*0.563*	*0.006*
*Treatment*exercise*	*0.098*	*2*	*0.049*	*0.413*	*0.664*	*0.015*
Residual	6.29	53	0.119			
Corrected total	27.66	59				

SS = sum of squares, df = degree of freedom, η^2 = partial Eta squared, a = R^2 = 0.772 (Adjusted R^2 = 0.747)

4. **Execution of ANCOVA**

Only after excluding a dependence between the predictors and the covariate can we execute the analysis and test the other assumptions using the products of the analysis itself. We will describe the steps using the IBM-SPSS statistical software version 24 for MAC.

- We click on "Analyze", then "General Linear Model" then "Univariate". In the main window, we shift the (HbA1C_post) to the "dependent Variable" box, the (HbA1C_pre) to the "Covariate" box and (treatment) and (exercise) to the "Fixed Factors" box. Unlike when we tested for homogeneity of regression slopes, we keep the default full factor model.
- To test the four remaining assumptions, we click on "Save" and we choose to save predicted values and standardized residuals, studentized residuals, leverage values, and Cook's distance. We click on "Continue" to return to the main window.
- We click on "Options" and we choose to acquire the "Descriptive statistics", "Effect size estimates", "Homogeneity tests". We shift both predictors (treatment) and (exercise) and, their interaction (treatment*exercise) to the "Displaying means for" box, click "Compare main effects" and choose "Bonferroni" for "Confidence interval adjustment" of the inflated P-value by multiple comparisons.
- Although we will decide whether there is a significant dual interaction by formal statistical testing (Table 3.14), we can request a profile plot to have a preliminary idea about interaction. In addition, the plot visualizes the overall patterns of adjusted means across the levels of each predictor. Conventionally, the researchers request to view the pattern of change of the moderator variable (second independent) across the primary independent variable, which is achieved by moving the former to the separate lines box and the latter to the horizontal axis [8]. Laerd statistics advised to request two schemes by

interchanging the positions of the two predictors (Figs. 3.4 and 3.5) [10]. The first will give the adjusted marginal estimates of means of outcome (Hb A1C_post) for patients belonging to each category of y (e.g., patients following treatment A, treatment B, or control), according to their x category (e.g., patients exercising or not). The second will give the other side of the coin, the estimated marginal mean values of outcome for patients exercising and those not exercising, according to the treatment received. This suggestion is based on the fact that regressing variable x on variable y is different from those obtained when y is regressed on x (see Sect. 2.6.2.1). We click on "Plots" and shift (treatment) to the "horizontal axis" box and (exercise) to the "separate lines" box and we click "Add" to shift the plot (treatment*exercise) to be lower box of execution. We repeat the process by alternating the positions of the variables on the x and y axis and, we click "Add" to create the second plot (exercise*treatment). We click "Continue" to return back to the main window.
- As such, the model will produce the post-hoc analysis of the main effects of type of treatment and exercise but not their interaction. Another point suggested by the same authors is to add a short syntax file to execute this analysis from within ANCOVA [8]. For those unfamiliar with the procedure, a syntax file contains the command lines for the software to perform a certain analysis. In IBM-SPSS, the user can open a syntax file by clicking on the "Paste" button at the bottom of the main window of any requested analysis. It shows the commands lines given by the program and all what we have to do is to modify those lines [10].
- Before clicking on the final "OK" button to execute the analysis, the researcher can click on the "Paste" button and look for the following line:
/EMMEANS=TABLES(diet*exercise)WITH (pretreatment_HbA1C=MEAN).

Fig. 3.4 Two-Way ANCOVA: effect of exercise on type of treatment received profile plot. Black circles represent patients on exercise and open circles represent patients not following exercise

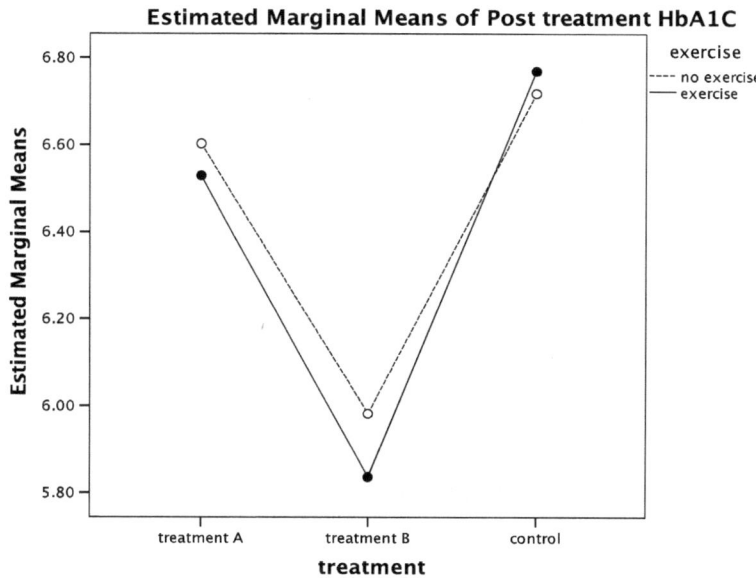

Covariates appearing in the model are evaluated at the following values: Pre treatment HbA1C = 7.1950

Fig. 3.5 Two-Way ANCOVA: effect of type of treatment received on exercise profile plot. Black circles represent patients tretament A, gray circles represent patients on treatment B and open circles represent controls

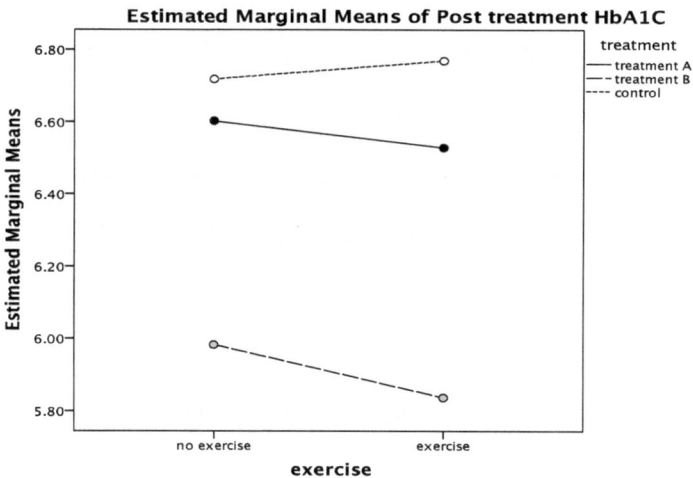

Covariates appearing in the model are evaluated at the following values: Pre treatment HbA1C = 7.1950

- We leave a space at the end of the line and we type COMPARE(diet)ADJ(BONFERRONI).
- The complete line becomes as follows:/ EMMEANS=TABLES(diet*exercise)WITH (pretreatment_HbA1C=MEAN) COMPARE (diet)ADJ(BONFERRONI).

- We copy the line we just completed and past it as a new line after replacing (diet) with (exercise).
- We click on run all to execute the program.

Note that there is a space before COMPARE and a space before ADJ and, we should not place a point at the end of any line and. Step by step details of applying this macro with screen shots are provided by acquiring a Laerd statistics premium account [10].

5. Verification of the Remaining Assumptions from the Products of the Analysis

We have four more assumptions to verify. *The first three are homoscedasticity, homogeneity of variances, and normality of outcome.* They are all tested likewise as we did for one-way ANCOVA but across the six combinations of the two predictors. Hence, homoscedasticity is tested graphically by plotting the standardized residuals against the predicted values for each of the six categories, homogeneity of variances is assumed by a statistically non-significant Levene's test, and normality is verified both graphically and formally by a statistically non-significant Shapiro Wilk test. The latter can be achieved after splitting the main file into the 6-combinations subfiles and applying the explore option on each subfile separately.

Finally, *data has to be tested for the absence of outliers and other unusual forms,* namely high leverage and influential points. They can be all a major source of bias, and hence, they have to be evaluated and dealt with, whether by data transformation or by removal or running the analysis with and without, and test whether there will be a significant difference. If the post-treatment HbA1C scores are normally distributed, we have them to lie within three standard deviations, and hence, a larger or smaller score has to be considered an outlier. Outliers are identified by simply checking the saved studentized values requested upon model execution for scores larger than (+3Sd) or (−3Sd).

Similarly, we must verify the saved leverage values, each measuring how much extreme its independent "x" value [11]. As a rule of thumb, leverage values are expected to be <0.2, values between 0.2 and 0.5 are risky, and values above 0.5 are dangerous and have to be dealt with. On the other hand, influential points can be identified by consulting the requested Cook's distances. As a rule of thumb, cases with a Cook's distance

above one should be investigated, and, if not important, they can be removed [12].

The results of verification in our example

In our example, homoscedasticity was verified graphically. Variances were shown to be homogeneous, with a statistically non-significant Levene's test (P = 0.114). After file splitting, the studentized residual values were tested for normality by the Shapiro Wilk test. With the exception of the subgroup of patients receiving treatment B and exercising, all other subgroups did not show a significant difference from normality. The maximum cook's distance recorded in our example was 0.05, the maximum leverage value was 0.08 and, only one case had a studentized residual >−3 (−3.38).

6. Testing the Statistical Significance of the Dual Interaction

The key turning point is testing the statistical significance of the dual interaction between the two predictors and the outcome. Interaction is primarily judged visually by examining the profile plots and formally showing a statistically non-significant dual interaction with the covariate. Figures 3.4 and 3.5 show the requested profile plots. Parallel plots favor the absence of interaction, while non-parallel or even crossing plots favor the reverse. *Interaction is ordinal if the plots are just non-parallel and disordinal for crossing plots.* To get the full picture, we have to look at both plots [10]. For our example, there is a large difference between patients receiving treatment B and those receiving treatment A or controls. With exercise, the adjusted post-treatment Hb A1C decreases in proportion in patients on treatment but does not have the same effect in controls and may even slightly increase. There is a nearly perfect parallel relation between treatments A and B profiles but post-treatment adjusted Hb A1C of controls is not parallel (ordinal interaction) and is even gently crossing (disordinal interaction). Although the results shown in ANCOVA Table 3.14 confirmed the overall absence of interaction (P = 0.664), seeing is always more impressive than reading.

In the case of a statistically significant dual interaction, the main effects (the effect of either predictor while ignoring the other) are definitely misleading, especially in the presence of disordinal interaction, i.e., contradictory effects across the different levels of each predictor. However, in the presence of ordinal effect, i.e., proportional but not contradictory interaction (non-crossing lines in Figs. 3.4 and 3.5), reporting main effects is controversial and a matter of judgment [13]. Nevertheless, and in all cases with significant interaction, we have to report individual adjusted simple effects of each level of both predictors.

In absence of a statistically significant dual interaction as in our example, we can report the main effects as well as the simple effects of the different groups made by our two predictors. Concerning factor treatment, we have three treatment groups (patients receiving treatment A, patients receiving treatment B, and control group); each will be individually analyzed for the effect of exercising or not. Concerning the factor exercise, we have two groups only (patients on exercise and patients who do not exercise); each will be individually analyzed for the type of treatment he is receiving (treatment A, treatment B, or placebo). Note that in the absence of a statistically significant interaction, the five individual simple effects are supposed to be equal.

7A. Calculation of Adjusted Main Effects and Post-hoc Analysis

Table 3.14 shows a statistically non-significant interaction (P = 0.664), and hence, we can predict the adjusted main effects of each predictor, averaging on the other one.

1. Adjusted Main Treatment Effect

For our example, there was a statistically significant main treatment effect on the outcome, adjusted for the covariate: $F(2,53) = 32.46$; $P < 0.001$. Put it this way: there was a statistically significant difference between the treatment effects, adjusted for the pre-treatment HbA1C and regardless of whether the patients were exercising or not.

There is a large difference between patients receiving treatment B and those receiving treatment A or controls. With exercise, adjusted post-treatment Hb A1C decreases in proportion in patients on treatment but does not have the same effect in controls and may even slightly increase. There is a nearly perfect parallel relation between treatments A and B profiles but post-treatment adjusted Hb A1C of controls is not parallel (ordinal interaction) and is even gently crossing (disordinal interaction).

The adjusted means of treatment outcomes (post-treatment Hb A1C scores) are reported in Table 3.15, compared to the non-adjusted means. The effect size of factor treatment was estimated as partial eta-squared of 0.551. In other words, 55.1% of the outcome variable (post treatment Hb A1C scores) can be explained by the effect of the treatments. As the variable treatment has three categories, we had to perform a post-hoc analysis. As shown in Table 3.16, there was a statistically significant difference between adjusted results reported with treatment B and both treatment A and control (P < 0.001). Results of treatment A and control were comparable (P = 0.328).

Table 3.15 Two-way ANCOVA: non-adjusted and adjusted means of post-treatment Hb A1C for factor treatment

Group	N	Non-adjusted means (Sd)	Adjusted means[a] (Se)	95% CI of the difference
Treatment A	20	6.55 ± 0.52	6.57 ± 0.077	6.41 to 6.72
Treatment B	20	5.92 ± 0.598	5.91 ± 0.077	5.755 to 6.04
Control	20	6.74 ± 0.67	6.74 ± 0.077	6.589 to 6.89

Non-adjusted values are presented as mean (Sd), adjusted values are presented as mean (Se), N = number of patients, CI = confidence interval, a = covariates evaluated at a pre-treatment Hb A1C = 7.195%

Table 3.16 Two-way ANCOVA: post hoc-analysis of adjusted factor treatment with Bonferroni correction

Compared groups	N	Mean of the difference	Se of the difference	P value
Treatment A versus treatment B	20	0.656	0.109	<0.001
Treatment A versus control	20	−0.177	0.109	0.328
Treatment B versus control	20	−0.834	0.109	<0.001

Values are post-treatment Hb A1C

Table 3.17 Two-way ANCOVA: non-adjusted and adjusted means of post-treatment Hb A1C for factor exercise

Group	N	Non-adjusted means (Sd)	Adjusted means[a] (Se)	95% CI of the difference
No exercise	30	6.62 ± 0.599	6.43 ± 0.066	6.3 to 6.57
Exercise	30	5.19 ± 0.71	6.38 ± 0.066	6.25 to 6.51

Non-adjusted values are presented as mean (Sd), adjusted values are presented as mean (Se), N = number of patients, CI = confidence interval, a = covariates evaluated at a pre-treatment Hb A1C = 7.195%

2. *Adjusted Main Exercise Effect*

On the other hand, the adjusted factor exercise was not statistically significant (P = 0.563), with a very small effect size of only 0.006 (Table 3.14). The estimated adjusted post-treatment Hb A1C are shown in Table 3.17, compared to the unadjusted means. Note that even if the exercise variable was formed of more than two levels, post-hoc analysis must not be performed because of the absence of a statistically significant effect of the variable "exercise".

7B. **Adjusted Simple Effects and Post-hoc Analysis**

This section is based upon the hypothetical assumption that there is a statistically significant dual interaction; hence, it is only considered for the purpose of demonstrating the calculations.

Analysis of the Different Scenarios

When the two-way (dual) interaction term is statistically significant, it indicates that the adjusted effect that one predictor has on the outcome depends on the level of the other independent variable and vice versa. Suppose that the dual interaction of our example was statistically significant, we have to consider that the differences in Hb A1C % resulting from participants following a particular treatment depends on whether they were exercising or not. At the same time, the differences in Hb A1C % resulting from

exercising (or not exercising) participants are dependent upon the type of treatment they are following. Consequently, the analysis will be based upon keeping one of the predictors constant, while looking for the effect of the other predictor on the outcome. For our example, we keep the exercise constant (disregard the exercise) and investigate the three groups of patients receiving treatment A, treatment B or the control. Each group is then analyzed separately to test the significance of the difference between those exercising and those not exercising. Playing the same tune, we disregard the type of treatment and investigate the two groups of patients (exercising and not exercising patients) and then perform post-hoc analysis for each group to investigate the significance of the difference between the three different types of treatments. Put it simpler; we have to test three simple main effects of treatment; each being formed of two levels (exercising or not). Meanwhile, we have to test the two simple main effects of exercise, each being tested for the three levels of treatment (treatment A, treatment B, or placebo). Note that in all cases, we are comparing the adjusted means of post-treatment HbA1C levels and not the ones that have been observed.

The number of simple effects is the number of classes in both categories; hence, we will study five simple effects. The x-axis of Fig. 3.4 shows the three types of treatments: treatment A, treatment B, and placebo. The y-axis represents the estimated marginal means for each treatment for exercising patients (black circles) and patients not following exercise (open circles). The vertical distance between every two circles represents the effect of exercise in each type of treatment. In conclusion, Fig. 3.4 shows the three simple adjusted main effects of the three treatment groups. Playing the same tune, Fig. 3.5 shows the estimated simple main effects of the remaining two groups: those exercising and those not following exercises, as placed on the x-axis. At each level, the vertical distances between the black circles, gray circles, and open circles indicate the differences between patients following treatment A, treatment B, or placebo, respectively. Table 3.18 shows the estimated adjusted means for the combinations of type of treatment and exercise.

1. Analysis of Two Simple Treatment Effects

A simple univariate analysis of patients without exercise shows a statistically significant effect of type of treatment, $F_{(2,53)} = 13$, P-value < 0.001, and partial Eta squared (η^2) $= 0.33$. The second

simple univariate analysis of patients on exercise equally shows a statistically significant effect of type of treatment, $F_{(2,53)} = 19.6$, P-value < 0.001, and partial Eta squared (η^2) $= 0.426$.

Table 3.19 shows the post-hoc analysis of exercise results for the three levels of the treatment effects, performed separately for the patients following exercise and those not on exercise. As shown, there was a statistically significant superior effect between patients receiving treatment B and other patients receiving treatment A ($P = 0.001$) or placebo ($P < 0.001$). The treatment effects of patients on treatment A and controls were comparable ($P = 0.377$). The result was the same, whether patients were following exercises or not.

2. Analysis of Three Simple Exercise Effects

Once more, we must not analyze the simple effects of exercise because the main variable (exercise) was not statistically significant in the first place; however, we forward it here for the purpose of demonstrating the calculations. We perform three separate univariate analyses for

Table 3.18 Two-way ANCOVA: estimated adjusted means according to treatment and exercise

Type of treatment	On exercise	No exercise
Treatment A	6.53 ± 0.11	6.6 ± 0.11
Treatment B	5.84 ± 0.112	5.98 ± 0.113
Control	6.77 ± 0.11	6.72 ± 0.11

Covariates evaluated at a pre-treatment Hb A1C = 7.195%

Table 3.19 Two-way ANCOVA: post hoc-analysis of simple adjusted effect of factor treatment with Bonferroni correction

Compared groups	N	Mean of the difference	Se of the difference	P value
Exercise group				
Treatment A versus treatment B	20	0.692	0.154	<0.001
Treatment A versus control	20	−0.24	0.154	0.377
Treatment B versus control	20	−0.932	0.154	<0.001
No exercise group				
Treatment A versus treatment B	20	0.62	0.155	0.001
Treatment A versus control	20	−0.115	0.154	1
Treatment B versus control	20	−0.736	0.155	<0.001

Values are post-treatment Hb A1C

Fig. 3.6 Two-way
ANCOVA flow chart.
a = number of combinations:
the product of the number of
classes of the two categorical
preditor variables, b = high
leverage and enfluencial
points, c = adjusted main
effects can additionally be
reported in presence of
interaction with ordinal
effect, d = reported for each
class of the two categorical
predictor variables

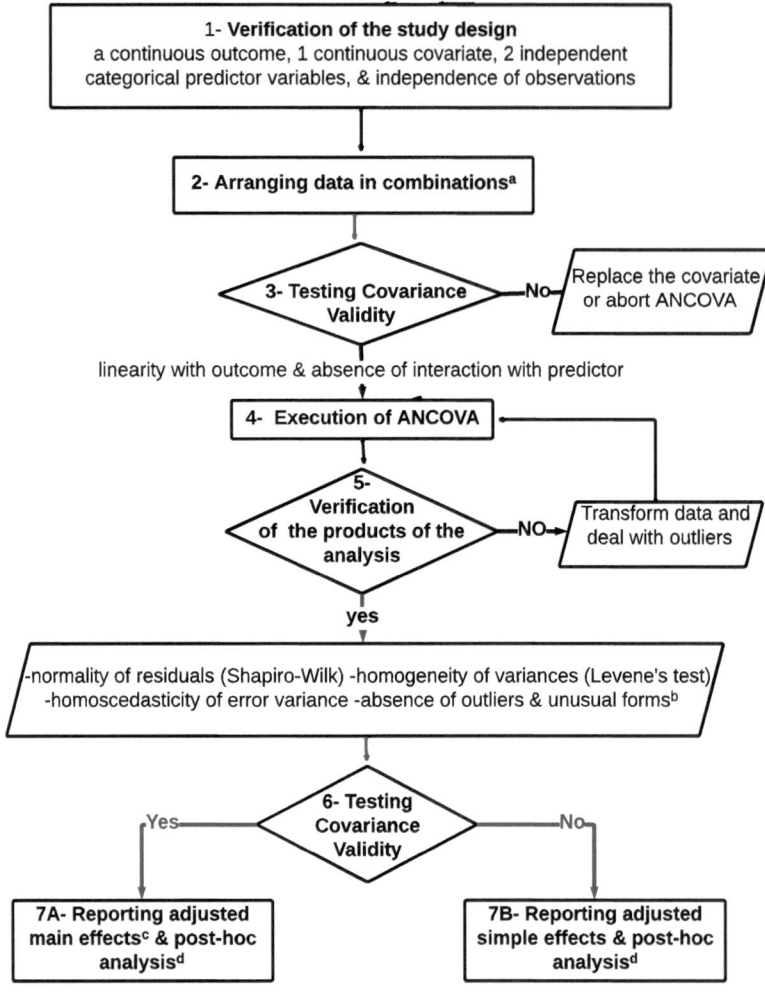

patients following treatment A, patients follow-ing treatment B and controls. As expected, there is no effect of exercise when considered sepa-rately in each group. The respective F (1,53) ratios were 0.22, 0.98, and 01, the P- values were 0.64, 0.37 and 0.75 and, the partial Eta squared values were (η^2) of 0.004, 0.015 and 0.002. Figure 3.6 shows the two-way ANCOVA anal-ysis flowchart.

Interpretation of the Results

Sixty diabetic patients were equally randomized to receive treatment A, B, or control. A two-way ANCOVA was conducted to compare the effec-tiveness of three oral treatment modalities and whether the patients were exercising or not on post-treatment HbA1C adjusted on the pre-treatment value of the latter. The covariate sig-nificantly correlated with the outcome (r = 0.699; P < 0.001), and all assumptions of two-way ANCOVA were verified (the ten assumptions can be reported). There was no statistically significant dual interaction between the two predictors and the outcome. The study showed a statistically significant adjusted mean treatment effect (Eta-squared = 0.55; P < 0.001). Further post-hoc analysis (means and Sd of val-ues can be reported) showed a statistically sig-nificant superior effect of treatment B over treatment A (P < 0.001) and control (P < 0.001). The adjusted mean effects of Treatment A and control were comparable (P = 0.31). On the other hand, the adjusted factor exercise was not statistically significant (P = 0.563), with a very small effect size of only 0.006.

What Should be Reported

We have to report non-adjusted and adjusted descriptive statistics. Assumptions of ANCOVA have to be registered as being verified or attained by data transformation. We have to report main effects in the absence of a statistically significant dual interaction but report simple main effects in its presence. Reporting both main and simple main effects is a matter of judgment, except in the presence of a statistically significant disordinal dual interaction, for being confusing and even not reasonable. In all cases, we have to include F ratios, df and P-values, R^2 and adjusted R^2, effect size (partial η^2), and results of any performed post-hoc analysis.

3.2.4 Multivariate ANOVA and ANCOVA (MANOVA and MANCOVA)

All examples discussed so far have involved only one dependent variable. In the case of having more than one outcome, many researchers tend to perform separate ANOVA (or ANCOVA) to test the effect of the set of predictors on each outcome, independently from the other. Unfortunately, such approach ignores the bias induced by the inflated risk of error due to the repeated testing of the same data [7]. The correct approach is to perform a multivariate ANOVA (MANOVA) or multivariate ANCOVA (MANCOVA).

Even though the computations become increasingly complex, the logic and nature of the calculations do not change when there is more than one outcome (dependent) variable at a time. ANOVA (or ANCOVA) tests the hypothesis of whether predictors significantly affect the single outcome variable in question; MANOVA tests whether predictors significantly affect a "joint distribution" of outcome variables in question or a joint distribution adjusted on the covariate(s), in case of MANCOVA [4–6].

In case of a statistically significant effect of predictors on the joint distribution of outcome variables, we will be tented to find where the difference came from by doing an independent analysis for each outcome and then proceeding as in a single outcome ANOVA procedure (see Sect. 3.2.1.2). The calculations of MANOVA and MANCOVA are too complicated to be performed by hand and, commercially available statistical packages (such as IBM-SPSS) can include both techniques under a general multivariate linear model. In this section, we will detail one-way MANOVA as an example of the procedure.

3.2.4.1 One-Way MANOVA

The Example

We will give a simple variant of the previous test. The investigator already tested the effect of one categorical predictor (type of treatment: A, B, and control) on a single numerical outcome (post-treatment Hb A1C). The investigators were interested in evaluating the patients' improvement in serum post-treatment Hb A1C and the well-known inflammatory marker CRP. In that case, we have two predictors, and we hypothesize that both together are affected by the difference in the type of treatment. We could now perform a multivariate analysis of variance (MANOVA) to test this hypothesis. Besides post-treatment, Table 3.7 shows the CRP calculated for the 60 patients who were equally randomized between treatment A, treatment B, and control.

The Procedure [6–10]

In statistical terms, ANOVA tests the differences in means of the outcome variable (Hb A1C in our example) for various categories of the predictors (3 different treatments in our model). MANOVA tests the differences in the centroid (vector) of means of the multiple outcomes (both: Hb A1C and CRP) for various categories of the predictors.

The univariate F value of ANOVA compares the variance of the effect (explained variance) to the error variance (unexplained or residual variance). The multivariable F value of MANOVA compares the effect "variance/covariance matrix" and the error "variance/covariance matrix". Technically, the sums of squares are arranged in a simple scalar form in ANOVA but in a more complex matrix form in MANOVA, called the sums of squares and cross-products matrices (SSCP). The "covariance" is included in the matrix because the two numerical outcome measures (Hb A1C and CRP) are probably correlated, and we must take this correlation into account when performing the significance test.

In MANOVA (or MANCOVA), several variants of statistical tests verify the significance of the independent variable on the joint outcome made by the two dependent variables. Suppose the overall multivariate test (Pillai's trace, Wilks' lambda, Hoteling's trace, and Roy's largest root criterion with approximate F statistic) is significant. In that case, we can conclude that the respective effect of the independent variable (e.g., type of treatment) is significant. However, our next question would be, of course, whether only Hb A1C improved, only CRP improved, or both? After obtaining a significant multivariate test, we can examine the univariate F tests for each outcome to identify the specific variable responsible for the significant overall effect, like in a regular ANOVA or ANCOVA. The researcher needs to verify ten assumptions

- Four basic assumptions are related to the study design: the inclusion of two continuous dependent variables, one categorical predictor of >2-class, independent observations, and an adequate sample size. Verification can be performed during the preparation of the study
- The raw data's following four assumptions are verified: normality and absence of univariate outliers, exclusion of collinearity, linearity, and the absence of multivariate outliers. Verification has to wait till all data has been collected.
- The last two assumptions must be verified from the products of the multivariate analysis: homogeneity of variances and variance-covariance matrix. Verification has to wait till after the execution of MANOVA.

1. Verification of the Study Design

The first group of assumptions is related to the study design, and hence, it can be verified during the preparation of the study. Both outcomes should be continuous variables. The predictor is a categorical variable of 2-class or more. The observations should be independent, meaning there is no relation between observations made in a particular predictor category or between the categories themselves. Finally, the sample size should be adequate, with a minimum number of cases equal to the number of outcome variables in each category of the predictor variable. In our example, we have two outcome variables (Hb A1C and CRP), and hence, we have to have a minimum of two patients in each of the three treatment groups (treatment A, treatment B, and controls).

2. Verification of Normality and Absence of Univariate Outliers

Although a minimum sample size of 20 cases in each category of the predictor variable is suggested to assume normality [6], we have to test the normality of each outcome (Hb A1C and CRP) in each category of the predictor variable (treatment A, treatment B, and placebo). In IBM-SPSS, we can run the "explore" procedure, request "normality plots and tests," and plot "dependents together", shifting Hb A1C and CRP to the dependent list and the treatment to the factor list. In addition to verification of normality by a statistically non-significant Shapiro Wilk test (see Sect. 1.4.3.3), the generated boxplot detects outliers by circular dots (o) and extreme outliers by asterisks (*). The former represents cases >1.5 box lengths away from the edge of their box, and the latter is farther away >3 box lengths away. In the absence of normality, we can attempt to normalize data (see Sect. 1.4.4). The test is known to be robust for normality, and hence, unless the deviation was not extreme, we can proceed and report the incidents in the results.

In our example, Fig. 3.7 shows the distribution of both outcomes, across the categories of the predictor variable, without detecting any

Fig. 3.7 One-way MANOVA: distribution of outcomes (post-treatment HbA1C and CRP) across the categories of predictor variable (types of treatment: A, B and controls)

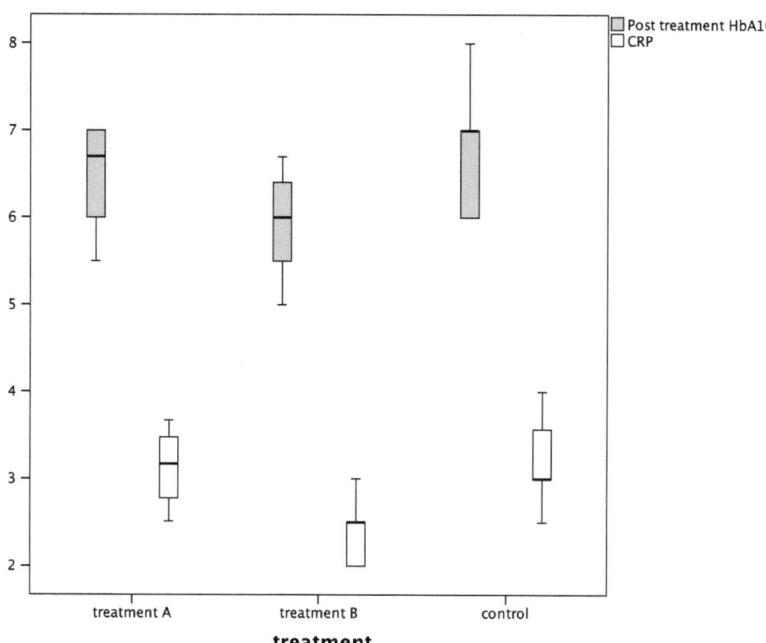

univariate outlier. On the other hand, the Shapiro Wilk test gave statistically significant results indicating that normality was breached. We decided to continue with the analysis with the observed data because the procedure is complicated enough to deviate the reader's attention to the many ways of dealing with the absence of normality (see Sect. 1.4.4). Moreover, MANOVA is known to be robust concerning normality provided that it is reported and, we just did.

3. Exclusion of Multicollinearity

Although both outcomes have to correlate with one another, an extreme correlation (multicollinearity), as indicated by a Pearson's correlation coefficient >0.9, violates the assumptions of MANOVA. In our example, Pearson's correlation coefficient calculated for Hb A1C and CRP was 0.3467, with a P-value = 0.007, indicating a moderate correlation between both variables and absence of collinearity. In the case of collinearity, the safest decision is to remove one of the variables and execute a regular ANOVA or to replace it with another variable.

4. Verification of Linearity

There should be a linear relationship between both outcomes for each category of the predictor variable.

- In IBM-SPSS, we can use the split file command to split the data file between the predictor categories (three treatment groups in our example).

We can then choose to create a scatter scatterplot matrix from the SPSS graph command. The software will plot the paired data of both outcomes (HbA1C*CRP) for each category of the predictor variable (treatment A, treatment B, and control). Linearity can be verified visually as a line passing through the center of the cloud of paired data. In the absence of linearity, we can attempt data transformation (see Sect. 1.4.4), remove one of the outcome variables or continue as such, knowing that breaching linearity will decrease the power of the test to detect a statistically significant effect. In our example, there was a linear relationship between HbA1C and CRP scores in patients receiving treatments A or

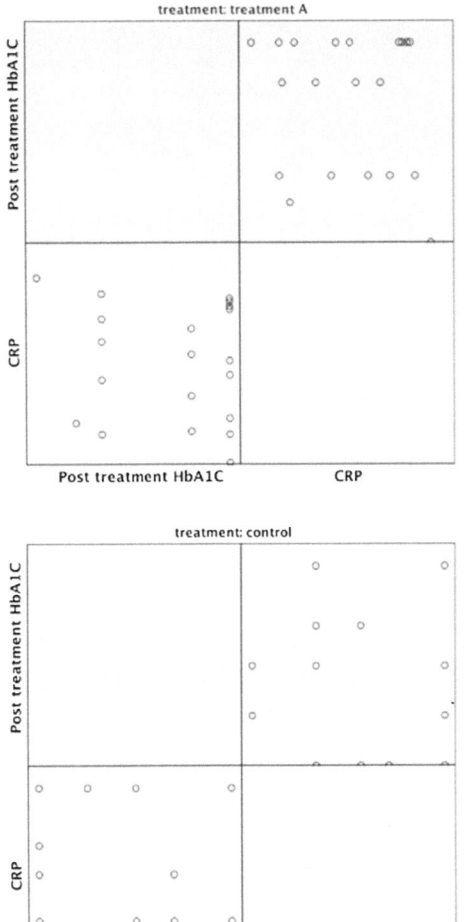

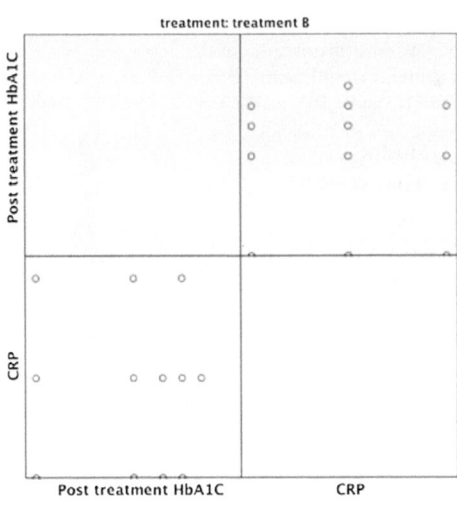

Fig. 3.8 One-way MANOVA. Verifying linearity of two outcomes (Hb A1C and CRP) across the categories of one predictor (type of treatment)

B. Still, it was difficult to assume linearity between both outcomes in the control group (Fig. 3.8).

5. **Verification on the Absence of Multivariate Outliers**

Univariate outliers are the usual cases of predictors that produce extreme values in each outcome. In IBM-SPSS, they can be visualized as circular dots or asterisks in a boxplot during testing normality. Outliers can be a significant source of bias for

causing extreme deviation of the mean and the Sd and have to be evaluated, dealt with, and reported (see Sect. 1.4.4). We did not have any univariate or extreme outliers (Fig. 3.7).

What is new here are cases of predictor variables producing unusual combinations of both outcome scores, i.e., *the multivariate outliers*, which can be detected by Mahalanobis distance. Unfortunately, IBM-SPSS does not offer the calculation from within the multivariate process. We have to use a sideway by giving each patient a serial number and requesting a linear regression [8, 10].

- We click on "Analyze", then "regression", then "linear" to open its main window.
- We shift the (Hb A1C) and (CRP) to the "independents" box and the (Patient number) to the "dependent" box. Note that the aim of giving each case a number was to tell the software where it should place the calculated distance. The test will regress both outcomes, which are now playing the role of predictors, to find (predict) the patient's number, which is now the outcome.
- We click on the "Save" option and check on calculating Mahalanobis distance. We click on "Continue" then on "OK" to execute the command.

The software calculates and saves the distance of each patient. A multivariate outlier is a case with a Mahalanobis distance that is at least equal or larger than a critical Chi-square value at a df equal to the number of outcome variables and an alpha level of 0.001. For our example with two outcomes, the corresponding critical value equals 13.82 and, the maximum calculated distance was 6.52. We can conclude that we did not find any univariate or multivariate outliers in our example.

- We have to unsplit the data file to continue the analysis.

6. Execution of MANOVA

We have to execute MANOVA to verify the remaining last two assumptions:

- We click on "Analyze", "General Linear Model", and then on "Multivariate" to open its main window.
- We shift the (Hb A1C) and (CRP) variables to the "Dependent Variables" box and the (type of treatment) to the "Fixed Factor(s)" box.
- We click on the "Post Hoc" button to open its window. We shift the variable (type of treatment) to the "Post Hoc Tests for" box. We

check on "Bonferroni" and click the "Continue" button to return to the main window.
- We click on "Options" to open its window. We shift (type of treatment) variable from the "Factor (s) and Factor interactions" box to the "Display Means for" box. We check on "Descriptive statistics", "Estimates of effect sizes" and "Homogeneity tests". We click on the "Continue" button and, finally, on the "OK" button in the main window to execute the analysis.

7. Verification of the Remaining Assumptions from the Products of MANOVA

Testing the Homogeneity of Variance–Covariance Matrices

To verify this assumption, we have to execute the analysis itself to produce the Box' M test for equality of covariance matrices of the outcome variables. The aim is to produce a statistically non-significant P-value, which can be interpreted as there is no sufficient evidence that the matrices differ; hence, the produced F tests can be assumed valid [14]. We have to note that the alpha limit of this test is 0.001 and not the usual 0.05. In our example, the P-value is much higher (0.74), and hence, we can conclude that this assumption was well met.

Testing the Homogeneity of Variances

MANOVA assumes equality of variances between the groups of the predictor variable (types of treatment) for each outcome variable (Hb A1C and CRP). In other words, Levene's test is performed twice to ensure that the variance of Hb A1C is equally distributed between the categories of the predictor variable and another time to ensure that the variance of CRP is equally distributed across the same categories. The procedure itself generates Levene's test, and hence, homogeneity is tested during the execution of the analysis. For our example, variance homogeneity was assumed for both Hb A1C: $F_{(2,57)}$, $P = 0.465$, and for CRP: $F_{(2,57)}$, $P = 0.412$.

8. Reporting and Interpreting the Results of MANOVA

We describe our results and give the observed means and standard deviation and the estimated marginal means, Se and 95%CI (Table 3.20). As shown, the mean post-treatment HbA1C and CRP scores of patients receiving treatment B are smaller than those receiving treatment A or placebo. The mean post-treatment HbA1C and CRP scores of patients receiving treatment A look to be comparable to those receiving placebo.

We report inferential statistics, starting with the main result of MANOVA, which answers whether the predictor is significant or not? The software usually executes several multivariate tests (Pillai's Trace, Wilks' lambda, Hoteling's Trace, and Roy's largest root criterion with approximate F statistic). Wilks' lambda is sometimes called the U statistic and is most commonly reported. Lambda ranges between 0 and 1, with values close to 0 indicating the group means different. Values close to 1 indicate the group means are not different (equal to 1 indicates that all means are the same). Pillai's Trace is a robust test that is recommended in the case of unequal sample size or when we assume a loss of power, as suggested by a statistically significant Box's M result. In our example, IBM-SPSS produces statistically significant treatment effect with Wilks' lambda value of 0.442,

$F (4, 112) = 14.139$, P-value < 0.001 and partial Eta squared $(\eta^2) = 0.336$.

9. Execution of Univariate ANOVA(s) and Post-hoc Analysis

A statistically significant multivariate test gives the green light to look for the source of variation, whether being due to Hb A1C or CRP or both, which can be answered by producing two univariate one-way ANOVA tests. Table 3.21 is an extract of the table produced by IBM-SPSS. We have omitted some of the less important lines and rearranged the table to read. A shown, there was a statistically significant treatment effect on both post-treatment Hb A1C and CRP (P < 0.001). The software equally calculated R^2, partial Eta squared (η^2) and adjusted R^2 values for both outcomes.

Post-hoc Analysis

Playing the same tune, a statistically significant univariate ANOVA test gives the green light for post-hoc analysis. Table 3.22 shows the multiple comparisons adjusted by the Bonferroni equation. As shown, Patients receiving treatment B showed significantly better results than those receiving treatment A or controls. The results of the latter two groups were comparable. These results applied to both outcomes, whether post-treatment Hb A1C or CRP. Figure 3.9 shows a simplified flow chart.

Table 3.20 One-way MANOVA: means of post-treatment Hb A1C and CRP for factor treatment

Outcome[a]	Predictor[b]	N	Mean	Sd	Se	95% CI of the difference
Hb A1C						
	Treatment A	20	6.55	0.52	0.134	6.29 to 6.82
	Treatment B	20	5.92	0.598	0.134	5.66 to 6.19
	Control	20	6.74	0.67	0.134	6.47 to 7
	Total	60	6.4	0.68		
CRP						
	Treatment A	20	3.14	0.36	0.91	2.96 to 3.3
	Treatment B	20	2.4	0.38	0.91	2.2 to 2.58
	Control	20	3.2	0.47	0.91	3.1 to 3.4
	Total	60	2.93	0.55		

a = dependent variable, b = independent variable, N = number of cases, Sd = standard deviation, Se = standard error

Table 3.21 One-way MANOVA: tests of between-subjects effects

Outcome[a]	Source of variation	SS	df	MS	F	P value
Hb A1C						
	Corrected model[b]	*7.3*	*2*	*3.65*	*10.23*	*<0.001*
	Residual	20.35	57	0.357		
	Corrected total	27.65	59			
CRP						
	Corrected model[c]	*8.45*	*2*	*34.22*	*25.39*	*<0.001*
	Residual	9.48	57	0.166		
	Corrected total	27.66	59			

a = dependent variable, SS = sum of squares, df = degree of freedom, MS = mean square (variance), b = R^2 = 0.264 (Adjusted R^2 = 0.238), c = R^2 = 0.471 (Adjusted R^2 = 0.453)

Table 3.22 One-way MANOVA: post hoc-analysis of effect treatment on post-treatment Hb A1C and CRP scores with Bonferroni correction

Outcome[a]	N	Mean difference	Se[b]	P value	95% CI[c]
Hb A1C					
Treatment A versus treatment B	20	0.63	0.19	0.005	0.16 to 1.09
Treatment A versus control	20	−0.185	0.19	0.995	−0.65 to 0.28
Treatment B versus control	20	−0.815	0.19	<0.001	−1.28 to −0.34
CRP					
Treatment A versus treatment B	20	0.74	0.129	<0.001	0.42 to 1.05
Treatment A versus control	20	−0.10	0.129	1	−0.42 to 0.21
Treatment B versus control	20	−0.84	0.129	<0.001	1.16 to −0.52

a = dependent variable, b = Se of the difference, c = confidence interval of the difference

What Should be Reported

We should report the descriptive statistics, including mean, Sd, 95% CI of each outcome variable, whether in total or across the categories of the predictor variable. Inferential statistics are of two parts. The first part is the result of MANOVA, pointing to whether there is a statistically significant difference between the groups of the predictor and both outcomes. In the case of a statistically significant MANOVA, the second part will be the unilateral ANOVA tests to see whether the difference came from one predictor or the other or both of them? A statistically significant univariate one-way ANOVA invites a post-hoc analysis, as usual.

3.2.5 Repeated Measures ANOVA (RMANOVA)

In medical studies, the patient is the focus of the research. He is the sample unit; hence, he should remain the unit of the analysis, even if several measurements were taken from the same patient. Treating the repeated measures and not the patients as the units of the analysis violates the basic rule of independence of observations and falsely increases the sample size, increasing the possibility of acquiring false positive results [15].

On the other hand, repeated observation in itself improves the statistical power of a study if the latter is analyzed correctly. The most straightforward approach is to collapse data taken

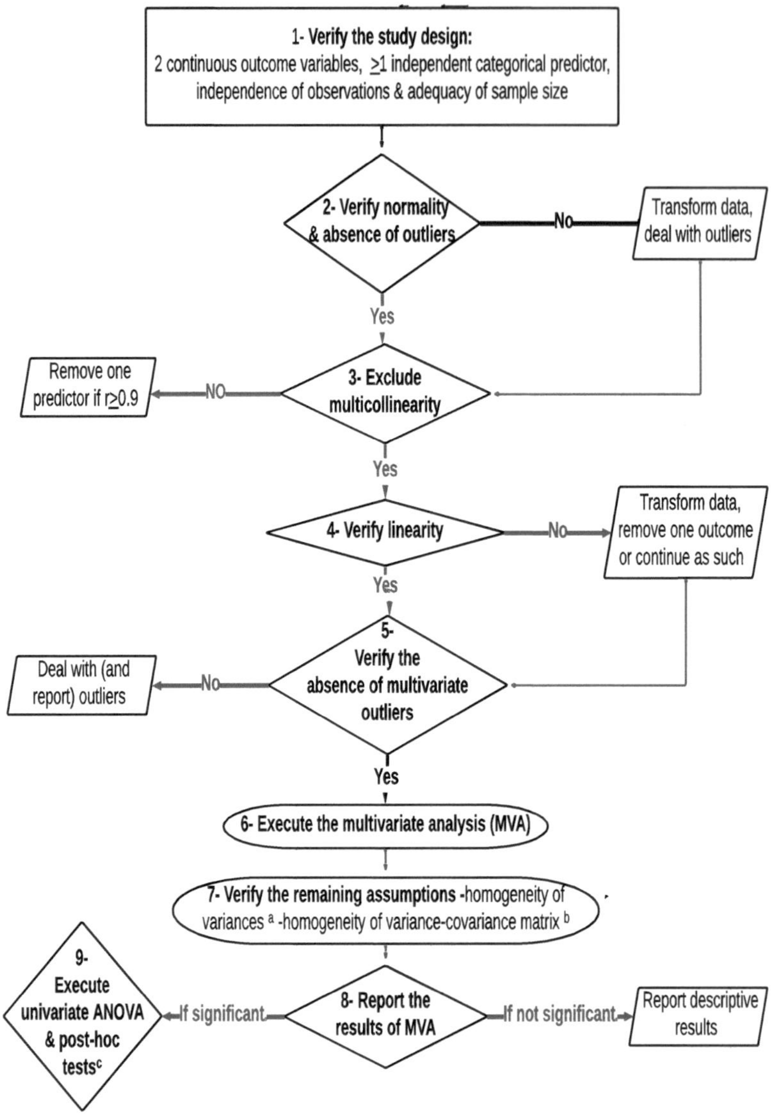

Fig. 3.9 One-way
MANOVA flowchart. a
= Levene's test, b = Box M
test, c = in case of a > 2-class
independent variable

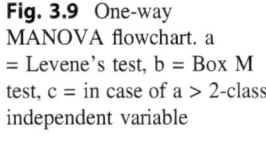

1- Verify the study design:
2 continuous outcome variables, ≥ 1 independent categorical predictor,
independence of observations & adequacy of sample size

2- Verify normality & absence of outliers —No→ Transform data, deal with outliers

Yes

Remove one predictor if $r \geq 0.9$ ←NO— **3- Exclude multicollinearity**

Yes

4- Verify linearity —No→ Transform data, remove one outcome or continue as such

Yes

Deal with (and report) outliers ←No— **5- Verify the absence of multivariate outliers**

Yes

6- Execute the multivariate analysis (MVA)

7- Verify the remaining assumptions -homogeneity of variances [a] -homogeneity of variance-covariance matrix [b]

9- Execute univariate ANOVA & post-hoc tests[c] ←If significant— **8- Report the results of MVA** —If not significant→ Report descriptive results

from the same individual into a summary measure. A good example is taking patients' blood pressure on several occasions, calculating the mean measurement for each patient, and then comparing those means as independent and non-inflated data. However, this simple approach cannot be used when data collected on different occasions have a prognostic value [15]. Comparing the means of three serial weight measurements of patients assigned to a weight reduction program or serial measurements of a biological marker of ischemia, such as troponin I,

ignores the prognostic value of those repeated measures and hence, is a mistake.

The repeated measures test the within-subjects variation either over time, as in the two previous examples, or under different conditions, such as measuring the weight of the same group of patients, once after following three different diet regimens for a week. In the first case, we test the effect time and the effect condition in the second case; always in one patient group. We have discussed the one-way repeated measures ANOVA design in Sect. 2.4.3.4.

On the other hand, a two-way repeated-measures ANOVA tests the effect of both independent variables: factor time and factor treatment, in the same group of patients. The latter is achieved by giving each patient one type of treatment and repeatedly measuring his weight over three weeks. The same patient is then given the other treatment, and we also measure his weight over another three weeks. Note that both independent variables (predictors) are categorical (k number of measurements and k types of treatment), testing the within-subject variation (in the same patient) and that the outcome is a continuous variable (weight measured in kgs.)

In addition, we can test the null hypotheses about any possible interaction between time (first predictor) and type of treatment (second predictor) on the outcome using the general linear model procedure. In case of the absence of a statistically significant interaction, we can separate the role of each predictor on the outcome, and we can test the separate main effect of each predictor on the outcome [4, 10, 13]. As usual, a statistically significant >2 classes predictor gives the green light for post-hoc analysis. In the presence of a statistically significant interaction, we can attempt to test each predictor's individual simple effects by running two one-way RMANOVA for each predictor variable (see Sect. 2.4.3.4), followed by post-hoc analysis, if indicated.

Note that we can also investigate the effects of constant covariates (e.g., the weight of the patient before the study) and covariate interactions (see Sect. 3.2.3). Finally, a model with more than one measure is sometimes called a doubly multivariable repeated measures model. The multiple continuous outcomes represent measurements of more than one variable for the different levels of the predictors. For example, we could have measured both weight and pulse rate several times on each subject.

3.2.5.1 Two-Way Repeated Measures ANOVA

Basic Assumptions

We will provide the example of two-way repeated measures, in which we will investigate the effect of two within-group predictors, with the repeated measurements of a single continuous outcome variable. The test necessitates the verification of six assumptions that can be outlined under two categories:

1. There are three assumptions related to the study design and can be verified before the analysis. A single continuous outcome (dependent) variable. Two predictors (independent variables, fixed factors), each is formed of 2 or more categories. Independence of observations which means that there is no relation between the observations made across the categories of each predictor or between observations made in different predictors.

2. The other three assumptions are the normal distribution of outcome, homogeneity of variances and absence of significant outliers across all possible combinations made by the two predictors. Those assumptions are verified using the products of the analysis and hence, they have to wait until the analysis is produced. The first assumption is normality of the studentized residuals of the analysis; which is verified by Shapiro Wilk test, as usual. RMANOVA is robust concerning normality but large deviation should be rectified by variable transformation (see Sect. 1.4.3.3). Another use of the studentized residuals is the verification outliers. Cases with $> \pm\ 3$ Sd are considered as being an outlier and should be delt with by transformation, removal or being kept and reported (see Sect. 3.2.3.2). Finally, the outcome variances across all combinations must be

equal, a condition that is known as sphericity and is usually tested by Mauchly's test [16], which is automatically produced by SPSS during the analysis. A statistically significant test statistics (M) means that sphericity is violated. However, the test is known to under estimate violations in small samples and over estimate it in large samples.

A Note on the Sphericity Assumption

The assumption of sphericity is crucial to apply RMANOVA for violation increasing type I error; i.e., the probability to conclude upon a statistically significant difference while it is not. The inflated P value can be counteracted by increasing the df of the used test statistics, which is the F ratio. The degree of sphericity itself is measured on a scale (ε) from 0 to 1 (100% sphericity); the (ε) is smaller than 1, the more sphericity is violated. On the other hand, SPSS recommends one of three suggested methods to estimate (ε): Greenhouse–Geisser, Huynh–Feldt and lower bound estimate, each test estimated its own Epsilon value. Multiplying the calculated df by an (ε) value < 1, decreases the df and hence, increases the critical value of F; i.e., it deflates the type I error that was inflated by violation of homogeneity of variances across the available combinations (sphericity). Lower bound estimate is too conservative and is not generally recommended, Greenhouse–Geisser is more conservative than Huynh–Feldt test, which is why it can be recommended for (ε) values less than 0.75 and Huynh–Feldt for larger values [7, 9, 10].

The Example

We organized a study to compare the effect of adopting low-dose warfarin of 5 mg/day or less versus a higher dose (>5 mg/day), as evaluated by measuring the patient's international normalized ratio (INR). Ten volunteers were randomized to either receive the low-dose or the high-dose first. Each dose was adopted for one week, and the INR was measured on Day 3, Day 5, and Day 7. The patient was then allowed a wash-out period of another week before shifting to the other regimen.

Table 3.23 shows the results obtained in the ten volunteers. As shown, the researcher acquired six measurements from each patient. There were six possible combinations of the two within-groups independent variables (predictors); i.e., the number of available combinations is the product of the multiplication of the number of categories of both predictors. Besides the assumptions related to the study design, assumptions related to data are normality, homogeneity of variances (sphericity), and absence of outliers. Statistically, we have to

Table 3.23 Two-way repeated measures ANOVA: the effect of low versus high dose warfarin on repeated INR measures

Patient ID	INR1-low dose	INR2-low dose	INR3-low dose	INR1-high dose	INR2-high dose	INR3- high dose
I	2.31	2.57	3.66	2.12	2.67	2.43
II	2.89	2.68	2.87	2.55	2.77	2.45
III	2.33	2.89	2.95	3.80	3.00	2.99
IV	3.20	3.45	3.12	3.05	3.12	3.23
V	2.88	3.12	3.18	2.55	2.95	2.45
VI	2.15	2.39	1.93	2.02	2.05	3.30
VII	2.06	2.14	2.00	1.77	1.98	3.98
VIII	2.30	1.87	2.00	1.77	2.00	3.98
IX	2.45	1.98	1.99	2.03	1.70	1.78
X	1.81	2.36	2.31	2.31	2.11	2.93

INR = international normalized ratio

verify those assumptions across the six categories of measurements.

The Procedure [7, 9, 10]

The procedure can be divided into two main parts: verification of assumptions, with the management of any violations and testing the results, with appropriate interpretation and proper presentation. Practically, we can carry out the procedure in six steps.

1. Verification of the Study Design

We had a single continuous outcome variable: INR units. Two categorical predictors, each being formed of 2 or more categories: two doses of treatment and three repeated measurements over time. Observations were independent. The three assumptions were verified during the preparation of the study.

2. Arranging Data Combinations and Execute the Analysis

Data has to be arranged in combinations, each represents the combined effects of the two independent variables; i.e., the INR measurement at the corresponding treatment dose. Hence, the number of combinations is the product of the K-classes of the two independent variables; six groups in our example. As usual, assumptions have to be verified, not in the two predictors but across the six combinations. In practice, data are arranged as six variables (columns); each representing a combination of the two predictors. Each row represents the six measurements acquired from each of the ten patients (Table 3.23). In our example, we uploaded the data to IBM-SPSS version 24 for MAC.

- We start by clicking on the "Analyze" button, then "General Linear Model," then "Repeated Measures," to open the "Repeated Measures Define Factors" window.
- We begin by giving a name to the "Within-Subject Factor Name" (treatment_type) and define the "number of levels" (2), and we click "Add" to shift it to the main box of the panel. We give a name to our second factor

(INR_levels) and "number of levels" (3) and click "Add" to shift it to the main box of the panel. We click on "Define," which will take us to the "repeated Measures" window.

- We have to shift the six blocks to the "Within-Subject Variables" box in this order (treatment_type, INR_levels): INR1_low dose, INR2_low dose, INR3_low dose, INR1_high dose, INR2_high dose, and INR3_high dose.
- We click on "Plots" and shift (INR_levels) to the panel "Horizontal Axis" and (treatment_type) to the "Separate Lines" box and then we click to "Add" the plot and click "Continue", which takes us back to the "Repeated Measures" window.
- We click on the "Save" button to request the creation and saving of the "Studentized residuals", which discover outliers and click on "Continue", which takes us back to the "Repeated Measures" window.
- We click to open the "Options" and shift both predictors (treatment_type) and (INR_levels) to the "Display Means" and request to "Compare main effects" by "Bonferroni" test. Finally, under "Display", we choose "Descriptive statistics" and "Estimates of effect size" and click on "Continue" to close this final window.
- As such, we are all set, and we click on the "OK" button to start getting our results.

3. Verification of Other Assumptions with the Products of the Analysis

Note that we have requested the software to calculate and to save six studentized values for each case (patient), corresponding to the six possible combinations in our example.

1. *Normality*

We begin by testing normality by clicking on the "Analyze" button, then on "Descriptive Statistics" then "Explore". We shift the six combinations to the "Dependent List" box. We click on "Plots" then request "Normality plots with tests". We can now verify that the outcome scores are normally distributed across the six combinations, as shown by non-statistically significant Shapiro

Fig. 3.10 Two-way repeated measures ANOVA: estimated marginal means of time by treatment

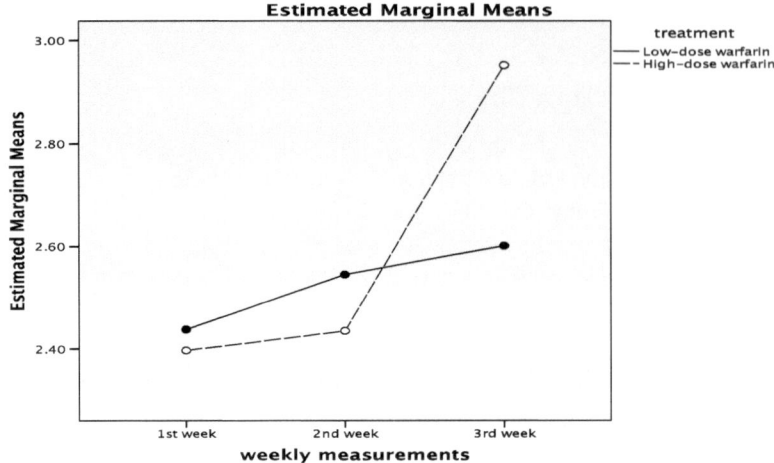

Wilk tests. None of the six combinations showed a significant deviation from normality in our example.

2. Absence of Outliers

We check on the absence of outliers by verifying that none of the cases had a studentized value larger than + 3sd or −3Sd. In our example, the largest studentized value was 2.34 and hence, we can conclude that we have no outliers.

3. Sphericity Assumption

IBM-SPSS automatically produces Mauchly's test for the predictors and their interaction. In our example, the test was statistically non-significant for both INR_levels (Chi-square = 5.24; P = 0.073) and interaction (Chi-square = 5.74; P = 0.057), and hence, we can use the produced F values for both (INR_levels; i.e., time) and (interaction), without any adjustment for the degree of freedom. Note that sphericity is assumed by default for any binomial variable and hence, the test was not produced for the factor treatment (low-dose versus high-dose warfarin).

4. **Testing Interaction Between Independent Variables**

Two-way repeated-measures ANOVA is mainly performed to see whether there is an interaction between the two predictors and the outcome. Hence, the key turning point is the presence or the absence of interaction. Figure 3.10 shows that INR measures tend to increase with time (INR_levels) and, the first two measures made while the patients were receiving either dose of warfarin are well parallel to one another. On the other hand, the third measurement of the INR of patients on high-dose warfarin crossed its counterpart low-measurement pattern. Although the figure suggests an interaction between treatment and time factors, interaction has to be verified by formal statistical testing. Table 3.24 shows the results of the within-subjects' effects in our example. There was no statistically significant interaction between treatment and time (treatment*time; P = 0.36). Hence, we can proceed and test the main effects of both predictors.

5A. **Calculation of Main Effects in Absence of Interaction**

There was a statistically significant effect of repeated measurements. In other words, measurements significantly varied over time, regardless of the treatment dose (P = 0.028). On the other hand, there was no statistically significant difference between the two doses of warfarin, regardless of the repeated measures (P = 0.615). Note that we have only reported the (uncorrected) df calculated under the assumption of sphericity. For all variables, their error fraction and interactions, IBM-SPSS produces the uncorrected as well as the corrected df of

Table 3.24 Two-way repeated measures ANOVA: the within-subjects effects

Source	SS	df[a]	MS	F	P value	η^2
Treatment	0.67	1	0.67	0.271	0.62	0.029
Error (treatment)	2.22	9	0.25			
Time	*1.44*	*2*	*0.72*	*4.4*	*0.028*	*0.329*
Error (time)	2.94	18	0.16			
*Treatment*time*	*0.62*	*2*	*0.31*	*1.1*	*0.36*	*0.107*
Error (treatment*time)	5.15	18	0.29			

SS = sum of squares, df = degrees of freedom, MS = mean square (variance), η^2 = partial Eta-squared, a = df calculated with sphericity being assumed

Table 3.25 Two-way repeated measures ANOVA: estimated marginal means of treatment, time and interaction of treatment and time

Predictor	Mean	Se	95% CI	Predictor[a]	Mean	Se	95% CI
Time							
1st week	2.42	0.142	2.1–2.74	Low-dose 1st week	2.44	0.135	2.13–2.74
2nd week	2.49	0.159	2.13–2.85	Low-dose 2nd week	2.54	0.159	2.18–2.9
3rd week	2.78	0.116	2.51–3.04	Low-dose 3rd week	2.6	0.199	2.15–3.1
Treatment				High-dose 1st week	2.40	0.2	1.95–2.85
–Low-dose	2.53	0.145	2.2–2.86	High-dose 2nd week	2.43	0.164	2.06–2.8
–High-dose	2.59	0.124	2.31–2.88	High-dose 3rd week	2.95	0.22	2.45–3.46

Se = standard error, CI = confidence interval of mean, (a) = interaction: time-dose

freedom as estimated by the Greenhouse–Geisser, Huynh–Feldt, and lower bound equations. It is up to the researcher to choose which one to present. In Table 3.24, we have only given the uncorrected df because sphericity was assumed, as indicated by the statistically non-significant Mauchly's test. Table 3.25 shows the estimated marginal means of both predictors: time, treatment, and their interaction.

Post-hoc Analysis

In absence of interaction and calculation of main effects (6A), the statistically significant time factor had three levels, and hence, we can proceed with the post-hoc analysis. On the other hand, factor treatment only has two levels; hence, both measurements can be compared by a paired student test. The results of those comparisons are presented in Table 3.26, and all are shown to be statistically non-significant.

5B. Calculation Simple Effects in Presence of Interaction

The presence of interaction means that the INR measurements in a patient following a particular warfarin dose depend upon the measurement time. The time of measuring INR depends upon the treatment dose. Consequently, we cannot separate the effects of the factor dose and the factor time, and hence, we have to analyze each one of them separately. In other words, we analyze the effect of treatment while ignoring the factor time and the effect of time while ignoring factor treatment. Ignoring the latter, we can perform two one-way RMANOVA: one for low-dose patients (INR1_lowdose, INR2_low dose, and INR3_low dose) and a separate one for the high-dose three subgroups of patients (INR1_high dose, INR2_high dose, and INR3_high dose).

Table 3.26 Two-way repeated measures ANOVA: post hoc-analysis of effect time with Bonferroni correction and paired student test comparing the two levels of factor treatment

Predictor[a]	Mean difference	Se[b]	P value	95% CI[c]
Time				
1st week versus 2nd week	−0.73	0.74	1	−0.29 to 0.145
1st week versus 3rd week	−0.359	0.157	0.144	−0.82 to 0.1
2nd week versus 3rd week	−0.287	0.138	0.2	−0.69 to 0.12
Treatment				
Low-dose versus high dose	−0.67	0.128	0.615	−0.357 to 0.223

a = independent variable, b = Se of the difference, c = confidence interval of the difference

Post-hoc Analysis

In case we have a significant effect of the time factor in low-dose patients, we can perform a post-hoc study to compare the 3-levels of measurement two-by-two. The same is done for the three groups following the high dose. Note that the analysis is done and reported separately in each of the two low dose and high dose subgroups.

Ignoring the repeated measures, and in the case of a 2-level predictor, as in the two treatment groups, we can compare the difference between the two levels (low dose vs. high dose cases) measured at each specific time point (1st week, 2nd week, and 3rd week) by a series of paired Student tests. The comparisons are done separately and reported individually for each time point. Because of the repeated comparisons made, it is better to apply a Bonferroni correction by raising the ceiling of the critical limit of alpha to the level of $alpha^n$, where n is the number of comparisons made (see Sect. 2.4.3.3). In case we have >2-class conditional factor, ANOVA becomes the procedure of choice to compare the multiple classes of the conditional factor, as measured at each specific time point. A post-hoc Bonferroni test will follow in case ANOVA produces a statistically significant effect, as usual. A simplified flow-chart of the main steps of the analysis is shown in Fig. 3.11.

The Interpretation

There is no statistically significant interaction between treatment dose and time of measurement, which paved the way to analyze the main effects of both predictors. We had a statistically significant effect of factor time (P = 0.028). INR measures tend to increase with time. However, there is no statistically significant difference between any two successive measurements. We could not put into evidence a statistically significant treatment effect (P = 0.62).

What Should be Reported

We have to report the descriptive statistics and the verified assumptions. In our example, INR measurements were normally distributed across all outcome combinations. We had no outliers, and sphericity was assumed. We have to report any method used for the normalization of data and how we dealt with an outlier. In the absence of sphericity, we have to report the variable of concern (a predictor or interaction), the equation used for correcting the df (Greenhouse–Geisser, Huynh–Feldt or lower bound estimate), the F ratio, df, and P-value.

In the absence of interaction, we should report the main effects of both predictors, with F ratio, df, and P values. A statistically significant predictor with >2 classes must undergo a post-hoc analysis with Bonferroni correction. We must report the results of the analysis with means of the differences, 95% confidence intervals, and P-values. In case of a statistically significant interaction, we have to report the simple effect of each predictor across the different classes of the other predictor. We have to perform post-hoc analyses when indicated. Reporting has to include the mean values (Sd), the means of the differences (Se), 95% CI, and the P-values.

Fig. 3.11 Two-way RMANOVA. Analysis flowchart. a = a minimum of 3 repeated measures and 2 conditions or treatments, b = the number of combinations is the product of the number of repetitions and the number of conditions, c = one-way repeated measures ANOVA (RMANOVA) to compare the repeated measures in each class of conditions or treatment variables, d = ANOVA or Student test to compare conditions or treatment variables for each repeated measure

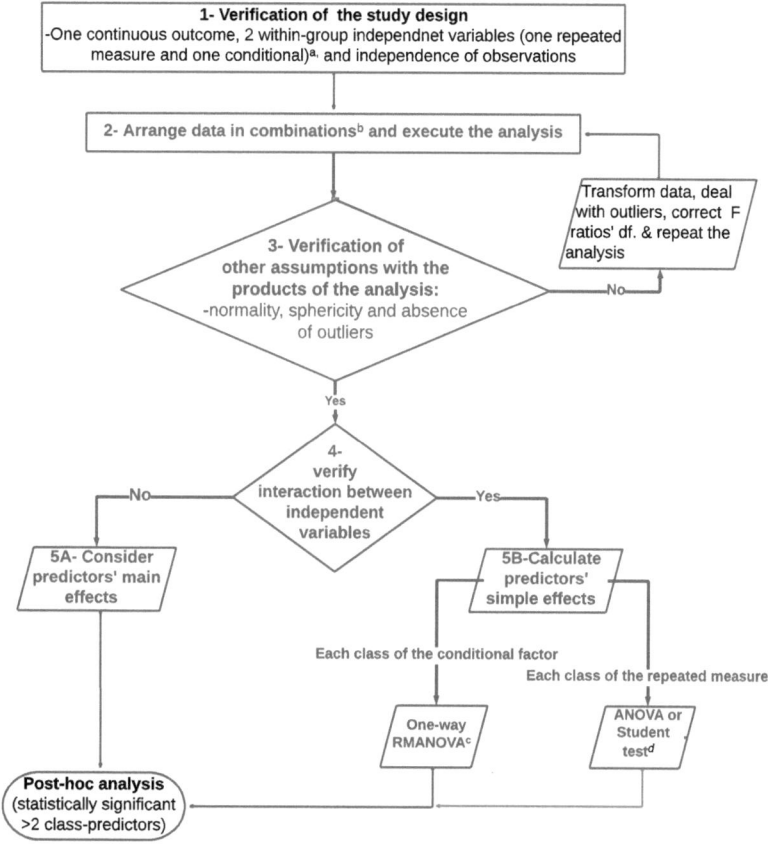

3.2.5.2 Two-Way Mixed ANOVA

We have shown that the primary aim of two-way RMANOVA is to test whether there is an interaction between the effects of two within-subject predictors (e.g., time and type of treatment) on a continuous outcome (dependent variable). Suppose that it was not possible to give the two treatments to the same group of patients, whether for a delayed residual effect of one of the treatments or one treatment being medical therapy and the other was surgery or else. The study will be carried out by acquiring the repeated measurements, which tests a within-subject variation, from two separate groups of patients, which tests a between-subjects variation. Such a mixed design is called a two-way mixed ANOVA. Here, we have two types of measurements within and in between and, mixing both types may be misleading. This is because the variability of measurements made on different subjects is usually much greater than the variability between measurements on the same subject, and we must take both kinds of variability into account.

Basic Assumptions [4, 7–10, 13, 17, 18]

Unlike the two-way repeated-measures ANOVA, we arrange variables in columns, as usual, i.e., one for the qualitative predictor (e.g., type of treatment) and one for each measurement made. However, from the point of view of the analysis, cases are arranged as combinations of both predictors. The number of all possible combinations is equal to the product of the classes of both predictors and, most importantly, assumptions must be verified across all combinations, which can also be called cells.

1. There are three assumptions related to the study design, which we can verify before the analysis: a single continuous outcome

(dependent) variable, two categorical predictors, and independence of observations. The first predictor splits the patients into two or more independent groups (the between-subjects variable). The second predictor is the repeated measure in each group (the within-subjects variable).

2. Normality and the absence of outliers can be verified from the row data after being collected.

3. However, we can only confirm the remaining three assumptions from the products of the analysis itself. Both homogeneities of variances and sphericity have been discussed. However, the homogeneity of covariance is the analog of homogeneity of variance between two groups. It warrants some explanations.

A Note on Homogeneity of Covariance and the Box M Test

In ANOVA, the significance of the effect of a variable is tested by the F ratio, which is based on comparing two variances: effect variance and error variance. The combined effect of two variables is based on comparing two matrices: the effect of the "variance/covariance matrix" and the error "variance/covariance matrix". The variance/covariance matrix displays the "variance and covariance" of the bivariate data set together. The "covariance" is included in the variability because the two variables are probably correlated, and we must take this correlation into account when performing the significance test. Put it in a simple term; it measures variability and mutual variability between data sets.

Box's M test usually tests the homogeneity of covariance, which verifies if two or more covariance matrices are equal. A statistically significant Box M value means that they are not equal and that the assumption of homogeneity of variance/covariance matrices is violated. The test is very sensitive to departures from normality and has very little power for small sample sizes and oversensitivity in large samples, which is why a particularly smaller critical alpha value of 0.001 is recommended [14, 18].

The Example

Oral anticoagulants are known to exhibit their therapeutic effect gradually over 3–4 days. A study was conducted to compare the patterns of anticoagulation achieved within 3–5 days of therapy in 30 patients who were randomly assigned to receive either low dose (<5 mg/day) or high dose of warfarin (>5 mg/day). Outcome was three repeated INR measures, made on Day 3, Day 5 and Day 7. Results are shown in Table 3.27.

The Procedure [6–10]

1. Verification of the Study Design

We verified the three assumptions related to the study design. We had a single continuous outcome (INR measure), two categorical predictors and independent observations. The first predictor (warfarin dose) split the patients into two independent groups and the second predictor was the repeated measure in each group.

2. Verification of Normality and Absence of Outliers

The data are uploaded to IBM-SPSS, as shown in Table 3.27. The Shapiro Wilk test can verify the normality of observed (row) data, and outliers can be visualized by requesting a boxplot diagram.

- In IBM-SPSS, we can click on the "Analyze" button, then on "Descriptive Statistics", then "Explore". We shift the three INR variables (INR 1, INR 2, and INR3) to the "Dependent List" and the (group) to "the Factor List".
- We click on "Plots" then request "Normality plots and tests" and request plotting "Dependents together". We verify that the three INR measures are normally distributed in both groups. In our example, the Shapiro-Wilk tests were not significant ($P > 0.05$), so normality was assumed.
- We can detect outliers by examining the boxplot diagram generated by the "Explore" procedure. In our example, we have detected

Table 3.27 Two-way mixed ANOVA: repeated INR measurements in 30 patients following either low dose or high dose warfarin therapy

Group	INR1	INR2	INR3
HDW	2.43	2.12	3.66
	2.31	2.57	2.67
	2.45	2.55	2.87
	2.99	3.80	2.95
	2.89	2.68	2.77
	3.23	3.05	3.12
	2.33	2.89	3.00
	3.20	3.45	3.12
	2.88	3.12	2.95
	2.45	2.55	3.18
	2.02	2.00	3.30
	2.39	2.39	2.15
	2.14	2.51	2.06
	1.87	2.43	2.30
	1.77	2.11	3.98
LDW	1.77	2.11	3.98
	1.98	2.99	2.45
	2.03	1.96	1.78
	2.31	3.34	2.93
	2.36	1.97	1.81
	2.20	2.30	3.40
	2.15	2.25	3.00
	2.00	3.00	2.40
	3.00	2.35	2.30
	2.40	2.40	3.30
	2.50	2.60	3.50
	2.15	2.80	2.90
	2.50	2.70	2.00
	2.60	3.20	2.90
	2.40	2.25	2.50

Values are repeated measures of INR at two days intervals: INR 1, INR 2 and INR 3. HDW = patients on high dose warfarin (>5 mg/day), LDW = patients on low dose warfarin (≤ 5 mg/day)

three outliers: the INR 3 measures of cases 13 and 15 and the INR 1 measure of case 24 (Fig. 3.12). As normality was assumed, we found no indication to manage those outliers by variable transformation. The three outliers were noted, and we continued the analysis. Note that both normality and absence of outliers could be also verified by examining the studentized residuals requested during the analysis.

Fig. 3.12 Two-way mixed ANOVA. Distribution of outcome (INR scores) across the grouping variable (high dose versus low-dose warfarin) circles represent outliers, numbers represent the oreder of the case in the list

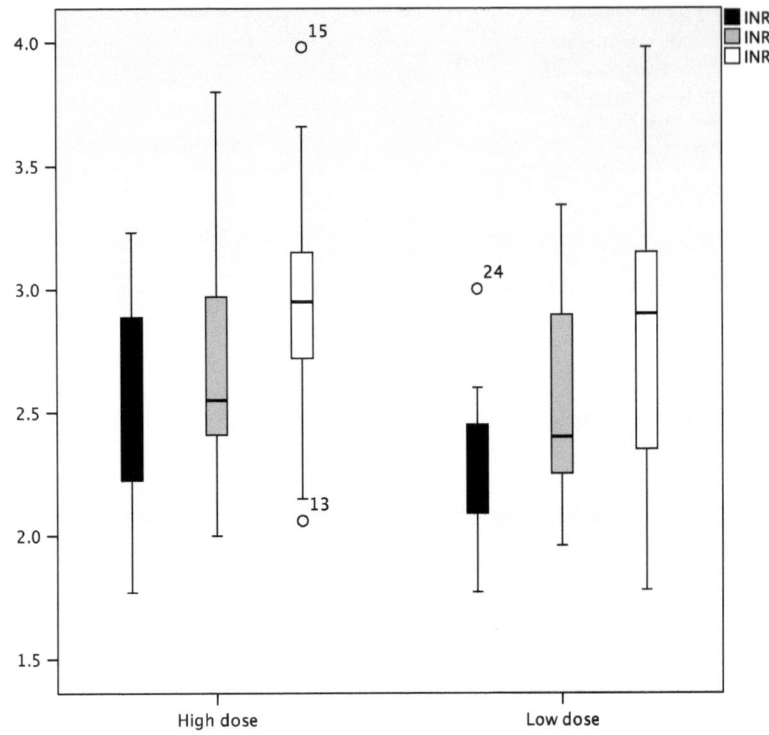

3. Execution of the Analysis

- We start by clicking on the "Analyze" button, then "General Linear Model," then "Repeated Measures," to open the "Repeated Measures Define Factors" window.
- We begin by giving a name to the "Within-Subject Factor Name" (INR) and define the "number of levels" (3), and we click "Add" to shift it to the main box of the panel. We click on "Define," which will take us to the "re-peated Measures" window.
- We shift our three INR measures (INR 1, INR 2, and INR 3) to the "Within-Subject Vari-ables" box. We shift our grouping variable (warfarin dose) to "the Factor List".
- We click on "plots" and shift (INR) to the panel "Horizontal Axis" box and (warfarin dose) to the "Separate lines" box and then we click to "Add" the plot and click "Continue" to return to the main window.

- We click on the "Save" button to request the creation and saving of the "Studentized Residuals", which discover outliers and click on "Continue" to return to the main window.
- We click to open the "Post Hoc" and shift the factor (warfarin dose) to the "Post Hoc Tests for" box and request "Bonferroni" correction. We click on "Continue" to return to the main window.
- We click to open the "Option" menu, shift (INR), (warfarin dose), and (Warfarin*INR) to the "Display Means for:" box and request "Compare main effects" by "Bonferroni cor-rection". Finally, we choose to "Display" the "Descriptive statistics", "Homogeneity tests", and "Estimates of effect size". We click on "Continue" to return to the main window. As such, we are all set and we click on the "OK" button to start getting our results.

As mentioned, from the point of view of the analysis, cases are arranged as combinations of both predictors and, the number of all possible combinations is equal to the product of the classes of both predictors. For our example, there are six possible combinations: HDW-INR1, HDW-INR2, HDW-INR3, LDW-INR1, LDW-INR2, and LDW-INR3. All remaining assumptions will be verified across all six (possible) combinations and using the products of the analysis.

4. **Verification of Other Assumptions with the Products of the Analysis**

1. Homogeneity of Variances

An important assumption is that the variance of outcome is equal across the groups (low dose and high dose warfarin groups) and IBM-SPSS automatically produces Leven's test to test this equality. A statistically significant test means that variances are not equal and the assumption was violated. In our study, there was no statistically significant difference between the variances of the outcome of both groups, across the three repeated INR measures. The respective F ratios $(1, 28)$ of the three measures (INR 1, INR 2, and INR 3) were 2.62, 0.023, and 1.5 and, the corresponding P-values were 0.117, 0.88, and 0.229. There is no remedy for the violation of this assumption.

2. Sphericity

Concerning sphericity, IBM-SPSS automatically produce Mauchley's test for the within-subject predictors (INR). In our example, Mauchly's M = 0.658, Chi-square = 11.287 and P = 0.004. Despite the very small P value, the result has to be considered as being statistically non-significant because the alpha level of this test is 0.001 due to its extreme sensitivity. Consequently, we can use the produced F values for (INR), without adjusting the degree of freedom. However, the test is also known to lack power in small samples, like ours, and hence, we prefer to use the Greenhouse–Geisser correction. The latter gives an Epsilon value of 0.745 and hence changing the df of our F ratio from F $(2, 56)$ to F $(2 \times 0.745, 56 \times 0.745) = F (1.49, 41.7)$. The corresponding P-values (0.002 and 0.005) were both statistically significant.

3. Homogeneity of the Covariance

Finally, the mixed ANOVA assumes homogeneity of covariances, which can be tested by the Box's test of equality of covariance matrices. The null hypothesis is that the observed covariance matrices of the outcome ae equal across the groups and hence, a statistically significant tests means that they are not equal and the assumption is violated. In our example, the test gave a statistically non-significant P value of 0.223. In the case the test was statistically significant, which means that both groups (patients receiving low dose warfarin and those receiving high dose warfarin) and hence, it becomes safer to perform two separate one-way repeated measures ANOVA, one for each group of the categorical variable.

5. **Testing Interaction Between the Predictors and the Outcome**

A main indication of the two-way mixed ANOVA is to see whether there is interaction between the two predictors and the outcome and hence, the key turning point is the presence or absence of interaction. Figure 3.13 shows that INR measures tend to increase with time and, the three measures are parallel to one another. Although the figure suggests the absence of interaction, yet it has to be verified by formal statistical testing.

Table 3.28 shows the results of the within-subjects' effects in our example. Although the P value of our Mauchly's test did not reach the limit of statistical significance of 0.001, yet we preferred to apply the Greenhouse–Geisser correction. Nevertheless, whether the F ratio was corrected or not, there was no statistically significant interaction between treatment and time (INR*warfarin; P value = 0.95 and corrected P value = 0.91) and hence, we can proceed and test main effects of both predictors.

Fig. 3.13 Two-way mixed ANOVA:estmated marginal means of three repeted INR measures in patients assigned to high dose and low dose warfarin

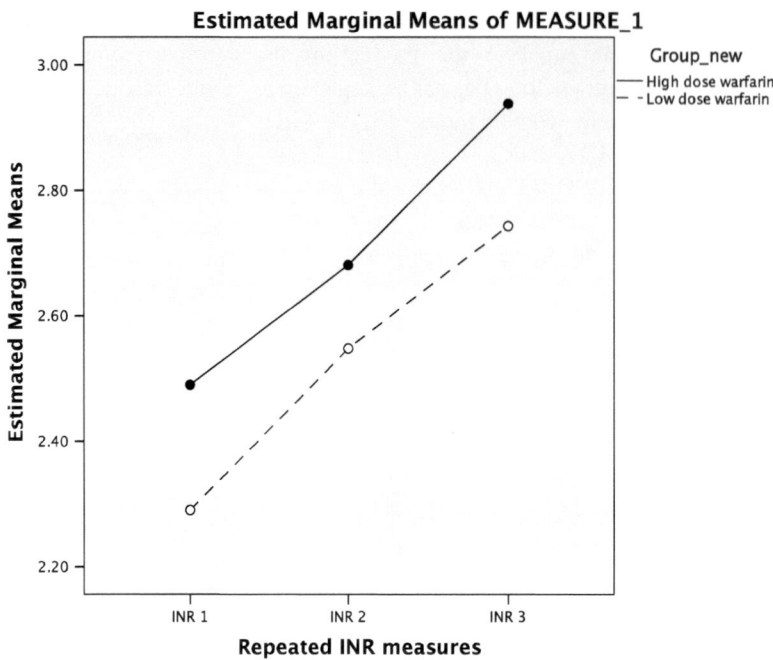

Estimated Marginal Means of MEASURE_1

Table 3.28 Two-way mixed ANOVA: the within-subjects' effects

Source		SS	df	MS	F	P value	η^2
INR	Sphericity assumed	3.05	2	1.53	7.12	0.002	0.203
	Greenhouse–Geisser	*3.05*	*1.49*	*2.05*	*7.12*	*0.005*	*0.203*
INR*warfarin	Sphericity assumed	0.21	2	0.01	0.048	0.95	0.002
	Greenhouse–Geisser	*0.21*	*1.49*	*0.014*	*0.048*	*0.91*	*0.002*
Error (INR)	Sphericity assumed	12	56	0.214			
	Greenhouse–Geisser	12	41.7	0.29			

SS = sum of squares, df = degrees of freedom, MS = mean square (variance), η^2 = partial Eta-squared

6A. Calculation of the Main Effects in the Absence of Interaction

The Within-Subject Main Effect

There was a statistically significant effect of repeated measurements. In other words, measurements significantly varied over time, adjusted for the treatment dose: P-value 0.002 and corrected P-value = 0.005. Table 3.29 shows the estimated marginal means of INR measurements and post-hoc analysis with Bonferroni correction. There was a statistically significant difference between INR 1 and both INR2 and INR 3. INR 2 and INR 3 were comparable.

The Between-Subject Main Effect

Table 3.30 shows the between-subject main effect of warfarin dose. There was no statistically significant drug dose effect: F (1, 56), P = 0.08) and η^2 = 0.08. Estimated mean INR (Sd) in patients on high dose warfarin (2.7 ± 0.08) was higher than that of patients on low dose warfarin (2.5 + 0.08) and the respective 95% CI were 2.54 to 2.87 vs. 2.36 to 2.69. However, the difference was not statistically significant.

Table 3.29 Two-way mixed ANOVA: estimated means of INR and post-hoc analysis with Bonferroni correction

INR	Mean	Se	95% CI	Bonferroni	Mean difference	Se	P value	95% CI
INR 1	2.39	0.071	2.25–2.53	(1 vs. 2)[a]	−0.225	0.77	0.021	−0.42 to 0.028
INR 2	2.62	0.086	2.44–2.79	(1 vs. 3)[b]	−0.451	0.133	0.006	−0.79 to −0.112
INR 3	2.84	0.107	2.62–3.06	(2 vs. 3)[c]	−0.226	0.138	0.339	−0.579 to 0.126

Se = standard error, CI = confidence interval, a = INR 1 versus INR 2, b = INR 1 versus INR 3, c = INR 2 versus INR 3

Table 3.30 Two-way mixed ANOVA: the between-subjects main effect (warfarin dose)

Source	SS	df	MS	F	P value	η^2
Intercept	615.5	1	615.5	2141.4	<0.001	0.987
Warfarin dose	0.699	2	0.699	2.41	0.13	0.08
Error (INR)	12	56	0.214			

SS = sum of squares, df = degrees of freedom, MS = mean square (variance), η^2 = partial Eta-squared

6B. Calculation the Simple Effects in the Presence of Interaction

The presence of interaction means that the measured INR (outcome variable) in a patient following a particular warfarin dose (the between-group variable) is dependent upon the time of measurement (the within-group variable) and vice versa. Consequently, reporting the main effects can be misleading because we cannot separate the effects of both predictors. Hence, we can only analyze the simple effect of each of them on the outcome while ignoring the other. The analysis technique depends on whether the predictor is a between-group or a within-group variable.

The Between-Subjects Simple Effects

The difference between a "main effect" of the between-group variable on the outcome and the "simple effect "is that in the former, we analyze the effect of the between-group variable, across all categories of the within-group variable; while a simple effect performs a separate and independent analysis, at each category of the within-group variable. The interaction between "the between-" and "the within-group" variables can bias any main evaluation across all categories. In our example, we will evaluate the effect of

"warfarin dose" separately on each INR level: INR 1, then INR 2, then INR 3. We can report and conclude on each comparison separately, with no attempt to link them or report the main conclusion.

In the case of a two-class predictor, we can compare the mean scores observed at each category of the within-group variable by the unpaired test of Student. In our example, the mean (Sd) of INR 1 in the 15 patients on high-dose warfarin (2.49 ± 0.46) was higher than that of the other 15 patients following low-dose warfarin (2.29 ± 0.3); P = 0.169. Similarly, the means and Sd of INR 2 (2.68 ± 0.5) and INR 3 scores in the patients on high dose warfarin (2.93 ± 0.51) were higher than those observed in patients following low-dose warfarin (2.55 ± 0.44; P = 0.45) and (2.74 ± 0.64; P = 0.37). In conclusion, the mean scores observed with high-dose warfarin were higher but not statistically different than their counterparts observed in patients on low-dose warfarin. Kindly refer to Sect. 2.4.1.2 for more details on the unpaired test of Student (see Sect. 2.4.1.2), including calculation of effect size. In the case of a K-class between groups variable, we perform a one-way ANOVA, including calculation of effect size, followed by a post-hoc test with Bonferroni correction if indicated (see Sect. 2.4.3.1).

The Within-Subjects Simple Effects

The analysis of the simple effects of the within-group variable will not be the same for the dependence between the repeated measures. It will be simply a repeated measure analysis performed for each level of the between-group variable. In our case, we will have to perform two separate repeated measure analyses, one for patients following high dose warfarin and the other for those following low dose warfarin. We can report and conclude on each comparison separately, with no attempt to link them or report the main conclusion.

In IBM-SPSS, we do not need to make two different data sheets, one for the repeated measures acquired in patients on high dose warfarin and the other for the repeated measures acquired in patients on low dose warfarin. It is sufficient to go to "data", then request "split file" according to the grouping variable (warfarin dose). Afterward, any analysis will be performed and presented for each group until we un-split the file again.

In our example, we can split the file into one containing the three repeated measures in patients on high-dose warfarin and the other containing the three repeated measures in patients on low-dose warfarin. We need to

execute the analysis only once to get the results of the analysis of the two separate files because of the split request that we performed. Following the same steps mentioned in "the execution of the analysis" under "the use of a statistical software package" in Sect. 2.4.3.4; the software will perform two separate one-way repeated measures analyses, one for each warfarin dose. Note to use the proper name of the variable, which is "INR" in our current example and not "dose", of course.

The conditions of application have been previously verified for all data and subgroups. Hence, we will be contented by presenting the simple within-subject effects assuming sphericity and the estimated means and post-hoc analysis. Table 3.31 shows the results of simple effects calculated for the two levels of dosing. As shown, there was a statistically significant effect of repeated measurements in patients on high ode warfarin (P = 0.031) but not in patients on low dose warfarin (P = 0.052). Table 3.32 shows the estimated marginal means of outcome scores, Se, and 95% confidence intervals.

Finally, Table 3.33 shows the post-hoc analysis, which should only be performed for patients on high-dose warfarin who have an omnibus statistical significance. We wished to further find out from which pairs the difference came.

Table 3.31 Two-way mixed ANOVA: simple effects of within-subject variable

Warfarin dose	Source	SS	df[a]	MS	F	P value	η^2
High dose	*INR*	*1.52*	*2*	*0.76*	*3.94*	*0.031*	*0.22*
	Error (INR)	5.39	28	0.193			
Low dose	INR	1.55	2	0.776	3.29	0.052	0.19
	Error (INR)	6.6	28	0.236			

SS = sum of squares, df = degrees of freedom, MS = mean square (variance), η^2 = partial Eta-squared, a = df calculated with sphericity being assumed

Table 3.32 Two-way mixed ANOVA: estimated marginal means of INR

Warfarin	INR	Mean	Se	95% CI
High dose	INR 1	2.49	0.118	2.24–2.74
	INR 2	2.68	0.13	2.4–2.96
	INR 3	2.94	0.134	2.65–3.22
Low dose	INR 1	2.29	0.078	2.12–2.46
	INR 2	2.55	0.114	2.30–2.79
	INR 3	2.74	0.166	2.39–3.1

Se = standard error, CI = confidence interval of mean

Table 3.33 Two-way mixed ANOVA: post hoc-analysis of effect INR (time) with Bonferroni correction

Warfarin	Paired comparison	Mean difference	Se	P value	95% CI
High dose	INR 1 versus INR 2	−0.191	0.81	0.098	−0.411 to 0.028
	INR 1 versus INR 3	−0.449	0.177	0.072	−0.93 to 0.033
	INR 2 versus INR 3	−0.257	0.198	0.644	−0.79 to −0.28
Low dose	INR 1 versus INR 2	−0.258	0.132	0.212	−0.616 to 0.1
	INR 1 versus INR 3	−0.453	0.199	0.117	−0.99 to 0.087
	INR 2 versus INR 3	−0.195	0.193	0.988	−0.72 to 0.33

Se = standard error of the difference, CI = confidence interval of mean

Unfortunately, there was no significant difference between any pairs after correcting the inflated P-value by the Bonferroni equation. The post-hoc analysis of patients on low-dose warfarin was done for instructive purposes and, it can only be reported as a part of descriptive statistics. Figure 3.14 shows the flow chart of the analysis.

Interpretation

There is no statistically significant interaction between warfarin dose and categories of INR measures (time) and hence, we can interpret the main effects of both variables. The INR measures significantly increase with time (P = 0.005).

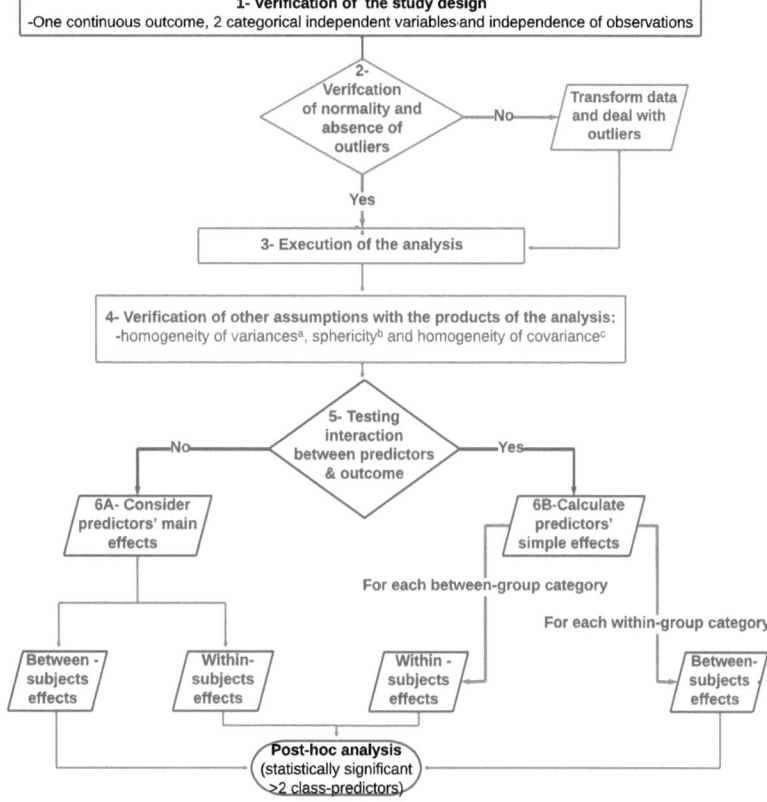

Fig. 3.14 Two-way mixed ANOVA flow chart, a = there is no remedy for the violation of this assumption, b = the df of F ratio has to be corrected accordingly, c = if the test is statistically significant, it is safer to make two separate one-way repeated measures ANOVA for each categorical predictor

Post -hoc analysis showed that the significant increase was between the first and the second and third measurements but not between the second and third measurements.

We can conclude that the INR measure is expected to increase significantly up to the 5th day of the beginning of treatment but not afterward. We can deduct that measuring INR after five days of the start of therapy can be a reliable measure of warfarin reaching significant activity, regardless of the given dose. On the other hand, the study could not put into evidence a significant difference between both doses, despite a higher INR score recorded in high-dose warfarin compared to low dose (P = 0.08).

What Should be Reported

We have to report the descriptive statistics and verify assumptions. In our example, we had normality of the distribution of INR measurements across all outcome combinations, no outliers, and sphericity for the interaction term. We have to report any method used to normalize data and how we dealt with an outlier. In the absence of sphericity, we have to report the variable of concern (a predictor or interaction), the equation used for correcting the df (Greenhouse–Geisser, Huynh–Feldt or lower bound estimate), the F ratio, df, and P-value.

In the absence of interaction, we should report the main effects of both predictors, with F ratio, df, and P values. With Bonferroni correction, a statistically significant predictor has to undergo a post-hoc analysis. The results should be reported with means of the differences, 95% confidence intervals, and P-values. In case of a statistically significant interaction, we have to report the simple main effect of the difference between each class of the first predictor across the different classes of the second predictors. Reporting includes the mean values (Sd), the means of the differences (Se), 95% CI, and P-values.

3.3 General Outlines of Multivariable Models [4–6, 13, 18–20]

3.3.1 Indications

There are five main indications for conducting a multivariable analysis. The first is to confirm the results of a conventional bivariate or adjustment analysis. The second indication is to evaluate the independent role of each predictor variable on the outcome, being adjusted for other variables in the study. Multivariable models quantify the effect of each predictor on outcome in a single number: the regression coefficient. Hence, the third indication is to measure and test the overall significance of the effect of the set of independent variables on the outcome. The regression coefficients of several independent variables (predictors) can then be used to create a risk score or a regression equation to predict the outcome. In other words, the fourth indication of multivariable analysis is to predict the outcome in future patients. Multivariable analysis can be beneficial in screening large databases, whereas bivariate analyses can be time-consuming and difficult to assimilate. Those are the five common indications of multivariable analysis It is recommended to begin look into the study data to see if we need to use a multivariable model? Does the question posed by the study lie within the five main indications? If the answer is negative, it is better to refrain. Many multivariable models need many prior demanding assumptions than simple bivariate analysis. If the answer is yes, it is now the time to know how this works.

3.3.2 Aim of the Model

It is essential to distinguish between two primary purposes for a model either to explain or to predict the outcome. In a predictive model, the researcher focuses mainly on whether the model can predict the outcome variable or not, rather than on the model's parameters. Consequently, the sample size is typically large, and the type of included variables is not essential as long as they predict the outcome.

On the other hand, an explanatory model is harder to design and mainly focuses on the model's parameters. The researcher has to examine the type and form of each included variable and how it influences the outcome. The number of included variables is typically small, and the researcher must examine and avoid confounders [2].

3.3.3 Selection of Predictors

Which Predictor to Include in the Model?

The choice of predictors is dependent upon many factors. First, models should include all theoretical risk factors and those shown in previous studies. In addition, researchers usually include statistically significant predictors in bivariate analysis. As long as the sample size permits, we can extend the inclusion to variables showing a near significance ($P < 0.1$). Second, the researcher has to avoid including highly similar variables because of variable inflation and reduction of variable tolerance (see Sect. 3.4.2.3) Finally, it is equally important to exclude extraneous ones. For example, diabetes is a known risk factor in patients with ischemic heart disease, and hence, it has to be included as a predictor of studying cardiac-related mortality. However, we should avoid including the same variable (diabetes) twice in the data set. Once, by identifying whether the patient is diabetic or not and, a second time, by recording his blood sugar in mg/dl or recording how many times the patient experienced diabetic coma. The result will be the inflation of the effect of diabetes itself on mortality and destabilization of the P-value (see Sect. 3.4). The researcher has to choose only one (the best) indicator of the same disease. On the other hand, introducing another variable that is known to be irrelevant to the outcome, such as the patient's social class in our example,

consumes sample size and overshadows part of the effect of other predictors in the model.

How Many Predictors Should we Include?

In general, 10–20 patients are required for each independent variable included in the model. The number is dependent upon the aim and the type of the model. While the researcher has to be cautious in selecting the predictors for an explanatory model, predictors are more welcomed in a predictive model as long as they can predict the outcome. If the outcome is an event (see Sect. 3.5) or time-to-event (see Sect. 3.6), the model's power is more related to the number of events rather than the number of patients. The variable's type and distribution are equally important; a quantitative variable introduced in the correct mathematical form is much more powerful than a qualitative outcome with considerable variability, especially when binary [2] (see Sects. 7.1.2 and 7.1.3).

An Algorithm for Selecting Predictors

The statistical software provides selection algorithms that can reduce the number of variables included in the model. In multiple regression, selection methods include standard, hierarchical, and statistical multiple regression. The former is the most commonly used, where all variables are introduced at once. Each variable is evaluated according to the "extra" predictive power it can offer over the other variables. In hierarchical selection, the researcher chooses the theoretical backgrounds of introducing the variables. The statistical multiple regression method is the most critical for allowing the software to manage the list on an exclusively statistical basis. In the forward stepwise variety, the variable with the strongest effect is introduced first. The introduction of less powerful variables continues until the predefined minimal critical limit is reached (e.g., $P < 0.1$). In the backward deletion variety, we begin with all variables in the model; then, variables are sequentially deleted, beginning with the weakest one. Stepwise regression is a dynamic compromise, where a variable is added or removed depending on whether it meets or loses a subset of specific statistical criteria [4, 8, 18].

Studying Interaction Effect

We have previously presented the role of ANOVA in testing the significance of interaction (see Sect. 3.2.1.2), where a third variable changes the effect of an independent variable on the outcome. For example, if we compare the amount of blood loss (outcome) following two different surgical procedures (predictor), the investigator wishes to know if the amount of blood loss depends upon the patient's preoperative hemoglobin level. On the other hand, the presence of a significant interaction between two predictor variables does not allow the researcher to evaluate the main effect of each variable on the outcome (see Sect. 3.2.5). Hence, it is recommended to limit studying interaction to the main and well-known risk factors to avoid the bias associated with the formation of multiple small subgroups [2]. Kindly refer to Sect. 3.2.5 for more information about the difference between the main and the simple study effects (see Sect. 3.2.5).

3.3.4 Model Selection

We will limit our discussion to three main multivariable methods in the medical literature: multiple regression, binary logistic regression, and Cox proportional hazard regression (Table 3.34). They have many mathematical similarities but mainly differ in the expression and format of the outcome variable [20].

Multiple Regression Analysis

The outcome is a continuous variable, such as the duration of hospital stay after surgery. The predictors can be either quantitative or qualitative variables. The effect of the latter is expressed as the beta coefficient, which measures how much the predictor influences the outcome. Each unit change in the predictor is expected to change the mean value of the outcome by a value equal to the beta coefficient.

Binary Logistic Regression

The outcome is a binary event, such as dead or alive, stroked or not, success or failure. Predictors can either be quantitative or qualitative variables. Their effect on the outcome is expressed in terms of the odds ratio. Each unit change in the predictor changes the odds of the outcome (the probability that the outcome occurs or not) by a value equal to the predictor's odds ratio. As the latter is skewed, all calculations are made in the log scale and then transformed into the regular scale for ease of presentation.

Cox Proportional Hazard

The outcome is the time-to-any event, such as death or hospital re-admission. The model's name is derived from the assumption that throughout the study, the hazard of developing the event is proportional between the groups (i.e., a constant hazard ratio). Predictors can either be quantitative or qualitative variables. Each unit change in the predictor changes the outcome's hazard (probability

Table 3.34 Common multivariable models

Outcome	Predictors	Model	Regression coefficient	Effect of each unit change in the predictor on the outcome
Continuous	Quantitative or qualitative	Multiple regression	Beta coefficient	Changes the mean of outcome by a value equal to beta coefficient
Binary	Quantitative or qualitative	Logistic regression	Odds ratio (OR)	Changes the log odds of the outcome by a factor equal to the predictor's OR
Hazard of the event	Quantitative or qualitative	Cox regression	Hazard ratio (HR)	Changes the log hazard of the outcome by a factor equal to the predictor's HR

that the event occurs at a particular time period) by a value equal to the predictor's hazard ratio. As the latter is skewed, all calculations are made in the log scale and then transformed into the regular scale for ease of presentation.

3.3.5 The Equations and Estimation of Regression Coefficients

Unlike bivariate analysis, only the general mathematical equations will be discussed, as those types of tests need long calculations and mathematical knowledge. They are usually executed with a statistical software package. All models are based upon the estimate of the regression coefficients (b_1, b_2, b_3,…b_j). Each represents the independent contributions of an independent variable to the prediction of the dependent or outcome variable (G). A number of independent variables (x_1, x_2, x_3…x_i) are related to the outcome variable via the multivariable equation that can be written as follows "Eq. 3.4":

$$G = b_0 + b_1 (x_1) + b_2 (x_2) + b_3 (x_3)\ldots\ldots + b_j (x_i) + epsilon$$

$$(3.4)$$

- G = a function of the outcome variable,
- b_j = regression coefficients (b_1, b_2, …, b_j), each indicating the effect of each x_i on the outcome,
- x_i = the predictor variables: x_1, x_2, …, x_i.
- b_0 = an intercept term included in the model (when all "x" values become zero),
- epsilon = an "error" term representing the amount by which any observed G deviates from the expected G.

If a particular b_j (regression coefficient) = 0, then the variable x_i has no effect on the outcome; a positive value indicates an increase in xi increases the outcome G; and negative values have the reverse effect. The function G is arranged in different mathematical forms:

1. In multiple regression, G is the outcome variable; e.g., the duration of hospital stays in days.

2. In binary logistic regression, G is the Odds of the outcome variable; i.e., the probability that the outcome (e.g., mortality) occurs or does not occur.

3. In Cox proportional hazards, G is the hazard of the outcome variable; i.e., the probability that the outcome (e.g., mortality) occurs during an interval of time, provided that the person was living at the beginning of the interval.

- The outcome variable (G), such as mortality, is produced by the combined effect of the predictor variables included in the model, plus a residual effect (unknown, error) that cannot be explained by any of the predictors included in the model (b_0). For example, a patient will die or develop stroke or else, even if he has no risk factors; i.e., the patient will still develop the event even if the predictors included in the model are absent or have no effect.
- The effect of each predictor (x) on the outcome is the product of (x) by its regression coefficient (b). Consequently, $G = b_0 + b_1x_1 + b_2x_2 + b_3x_3\ldots$. The question is how to calculate the b coefficient in each model and how this b coefficient changes (G).
- The b coefficient depends on the nature of the outcome (G), whether being a continuous variable (e.g., duration of hospital stays), binary event (e.g., mortality) or time to event (e.g., time to mortality).

1. In the case of a continuous outcome, each unit change of the predictor (increase or decrease), changes the outcome by an average value that is equal to the b coefficient calculated for this predictor. As example, if the b coefficient calculated for the effect of the patient's age (years) on the duration of ICU stay (days) equals 2; each year increase in the age of the patient increases his ICU stay by an average of two days.

2. In the case of a binary outcome (such as mortality), we need to know how the

predictor (e.g., age in years) will change (increases or decreases) the odds of mortality. The effect of the predictor (age in years) on the outcome (odds of mortality) is best expressed by the odds ratio between age and mortality. Consequently, the predictor is expected to change the odds of the outcome by a quantity that is equal to the OR between the predictor (age in years) and the outcome (mortality). Returning to our example, and provided that the OR calculated for age was 2, each year increase in the patient's age is expected to double the odds of mortality. Kindly remember that all OR calculations are made in the log scale and then the results are converted back to the regular scale for better presentation (see Sect. 1.8.2).

3. In the case of Cox regression analysis, the general outlines of the procedure are the same as in logistic regression however, the introduction of the time factor necessitated few modifications. One modification is the calculation of (b_0), which warrants some discussion and will be discussed later in Sect. 3.6. A second modification is the outcome itself (G), which had to change from being the odds of the event (yes/no) to become the hazard that the event occurs in a limited time period. Concordantly, the b coefficient had to change too, from being the OR between the predictor and the outcome to be their Hazard ratio (HR). Returning to our example, and provided that the HR calculated for age was 2, each year increase in the patients age is expected to double the hazard of mortality. Kindly remember that all HR calculations are made in the log scale and then the results are converted back to the regular scale for better presentation (see Sect. 1.8.3).

3.3.6   Evaluation of the Model

Model Fit

A good model fit is a model that accurately approximates the output when provided with unseen inputs. In other words, *the model is* *expected to fit the data obtained by other comparable studies*. Otherwise, the model would be of limited value [6]. There are many ways to calculate how the model fits the data.

In linear regression, we have previously shown that we can calculate the residuals by ANOVA as the difference between the observed (input) data and the (output) data produced by the models. As such, residuals can be thought of as estimation of the errors in the model (see Sect. 2.6.2.1). Consequently, large residuals (errors) suggest that the model does not fit the data. Large residuals may indicate that we did not include the correct variables or, that variables were not included in the appropriate form. The software output usually includes a complete section on the analysis of residuals. Residuals can equally be tested graphically in many ways; a standard test is to plot the standardized residuals against their predicted values. We expect residuals to be normally distributed, and hence, most residuals will lie between -3 and $+3$ Sd.

As we will show in a coming section, we cannot calculate residuals in logistic regression and investigators often use the Hosmer–Lemeshow goodness-of-fit test instead (see Sect. 3.5). This modified Chi-square test compares the number of observed (events) and (no events) to the corresponding expected numbers calculated by the model. The absence of a statistically significant difference between both likelihoods indicates model fit.

As in logistic regression, residuals cannot be technically calculated in Cox proportional hazard. How good the predictors fit in a Cox model is expressed as the difference between a model with intercept only and no predictors (0 model), and the model with all predictors being on board (full model). The reader is kindly invited to review Sect. 3.6 for more details (see Sect. 3.6)

The Power of the Model

How much the model can predict the outcome is an important question. We have previously shown that R^2 expresses how much one continuous predictor variable influences a continuous outcome (see Sect. 2.6.2.1). In multiple regression, we can calculate an adjusted R^2 to express how much the set of predictor variables explain or predict the outcome. Being a proportion, it will always vary between 0 (the set of variables has no effect on outcome) and 1 (the set of variables explain or predict the outcome fully) (see Sect. 3.4.6).

As will be explained later, residuals cannot be calculated in logistic regression; hence, R^2 cannot be computed. Statisticians have invented multiple pseudo-R-squared coefficients, such as Negelkerke's R^2 and McFadden's pseudo R^2 to assess how much the variables explain the model (see Sect. 3.5.6). In addition, the statistical software automatically calculates the sensitivity, specificity, and overall accuracy of the model; describing how well the results are in conformity with the uploaded data. In case of a quantitative outcome, the researcher can assess the overall predictive value of the model by constructing a ROC curve, whether over all or selected cut-off values [2] (see Sect. 1.9.4.3).

Reliability of the Model

The predictive ability of a model can be tested if a new set of data can predict the outcome, as efficiently as the original set. Playing the same tune, the explanatory ability of the model is evaluated by the new data set producing the same predictors and coefficients. A major threat to reliability is a small sample size or a small number of events in the case of logistic or Cox regression analysis. The low power will widen and hence, decrease the reliability of our confidence intervals, and the model is said to be an "overfitting model". The problem of an "underfitting model" is the other side of the coin. A study can have a large enough number of events per independent variable. However, the association estimates between a risk factor and an outcome may still be inaccurate if the risk factor is rare [6].

Resampling Methods

As it is always hard to collect new data for testing the model, alternative methods have been reported, including split-group, Jackknife and bootstrap. In the former, the researcher splits his data set in two halves, one used to construct the model and the other to test it. The Jackknife procedure involves resampling after sequentially deleting each case once; hence it is a leave-out more than a resampling procedure. Bootstrap is more demanding than Jackknife and more precise. It involves resampling with replacement of the previously selected persons so that each time it assesses a different sample and produce a different result [4, 21].

3.4 Multiple Regression Analysis [4–6, 13, 18–20]

The general purpose of multiple regression is to learn more about the relationship between several independent variables and an outcome variable. We will discuss the case with more than one outcome variable at the end of this section. As an example, a cardiologist may record for each of his patients with ischemic heart disease the number of cigarettes smoked per day, type and degree of obesity, life style (sedentary yes or no), presence of diabetes mellitus, family history of ischemic heart disease, mean diastolic blood pressure, etc....

The next step would be to investigate how he can use this information to interpret when a particular patient may need a coronary intervention in the next coming years. Most importantly, which one of those variables is the best predictor for the need of intervention, so as to work on it more vigorously than others. For example, one might learn that the number of cigarettes and age are better predictors than the family history or presence of diabetes. Hopefully, multiple regression can permit the formation of a regression equation that could predict the quantitative outcome event (number of stenting procedures) from the significantly associated independent predictors (number of smoked cigarettes, age in years, etc....).

3.4.1 Introduction: Simple Versus Multiple Linear Regression

The Simple Linear Regression

Multiple linear regression is an extension of simple linear regression discussed before. We advise the reader to go back to the section on simple linear regression and carefully revise the given basic information before proceeding in this section (see Sect. 2.6.2). In short, simple regression involves only two interrelated variables: one independent "x" and one outcome variable "y". Hence, the relationship between data can be visualized in a simple scatter plot graph. These variables may, for example, represent age in years (predictor) and the number of coronary stents needed (outcome), respectively. Each point in the plot represents one patient, the respective patient's age, and the number of stents performed. The goal of linear regression procedures is to fit a line through the points to minimize the squared deviations (distances) of the observed points from that line. In other words, to make the regression line representative of all points.

The regression line is defined by the simple regression equation "Eq. 2.90": $y = b_0 + b_1 x_1$. In full text, the "y" variable can be expressed in terms of a constant (b_0) and a slope (b_1) times the "x_1" variable. The constant, also known as intercept, is the value of y when x = 0. The slope is the regression coefficient or B coefficient. For example, the number of coronary stents may best be predicted as: $b_0 + b_1 * x_1$. Thus, knowing that $b_0 = 1$, $b_1 = 0.02$. and the patient's age = x_1 = 50; would lead us to predict that we expect to deliver two coronary stents in a 50 years old patient ($y = 1 + 0.02*50 = 2$).

The Multiple Linear Regression

In addition to the estimation of how much each predictor contributed to the outcome, the multivariable case allows us to examine the model's overall fit or how much the set of multiple predictors explains the outcome. In the case of multiple predictors, the regression line cannot be visualized in the two-dimensional space, but can be computed just as easily (via a statistical computer package; the computations are actually quite complex). For example, suppose in addition to age, we had additional predictors (e.g., presence of diabetes mellitus, family history of ischemic heart disease). In that case, a linear equation adding the effects of all predictors produces the outcome "Eq. 3.5":

$$y = b_0 + b_1 x_1 + b_2 x_2 + b_3 x_3 \ldots + b_i x_i \quad (3.5)$$

where "y" is the outcome variable, x_1, x_2, x_3, ..., x_i are the independent predictor variables, b_1, b_2, b_3.., b_i are the regression coefficients expressing the effect of each independent predictor on the outcome and, (b_0) is a constant or model intercept (value of "y" when all other variables are zero).

The Interpretation of Coefficient b

The sign of coefficient b indicates the direction of the effect of the predictor variable (x) on the outcome (y). Suppose that one of the predictors $(\times 1)$ is the patient's age in years and (y) is the duration of hospital stay after surgery in days. A positive b indicates that the older the patient, the longer he is expected to stay after surgery. A negative b indicates that older patients are expected to stay less than younger patients, and a (b coefficient) value of (0) indicates that the patient's age is unrelated to the duration of hospital stay.

On the other hand, the magnitude of b gives the expected average outcome for a given predictor value. Suppose that b equals 0.1; a patient who is 20 years old is expected to stay two days after surgery (20 years x 0.1 = 2 days), on average. Kindly note the following:

1. Each value is calculated on its own scale; i.e., age is calculated in years, and hospital stay is calculated in days.
2. The calculated (y) is the expected average.
3. The duration of hospital stay of this particular patient will be produced by summing all other $(b_2 x_2, b_3 x_3, \ldots)$ values calculated for other predictor variables such as the patient's gender and the duration of surgery; to which we have to add the intercept of the equation (b_0).

3.4.2 The Basic Assumptions

We have to satisfy ten assumptions, four are related to the study design (see Sect. 3.4.2.1); hence they can be taken care off during the preparation of the study. The other six assumptions are verified with the products of the analysis (see Sects. 3.4.2.2 to 3.4.2.5), and hence, we have to execute the analysis in the middle of the verification process (see Sect. 3.4.5.2).

3.4.2.1 Assumptions Related to the Study Design

Four assumptions have to be verified during the preparation of the study: one continuous outcome, two or more predictor variables (continuous, binomial, or categorical), independence of observations, and a randomized sample of adequate sample. Most authors recommend that one should have at least 10 to 20 times as many observations for each predictor included in the model. As we have previously shown, it is of utmost importance to decide which variables should be introduced in the model (see Sect. 3.3.3). In addition, qualitative variables having less than 5 cases per category weakens the model, and they have to be collapsed, or the variable is removed. An ordinal outcome can be treated as a continuous variable and, categorical or binomial variables can be coded or transformed into dummy numerical variables. For example, a dichotomous variable (diabetic/non-diabetic) can be coded into 1 for diabetics and 0 for non-diabetics. Class I, II, III, and IV can be coded as 1, 2, 3, and 4 (see Sect. 1.2.1). Although data independence may be net and clear, such as acquiring one information from different patients, formal statistical testing is necessary to exclude autocorrelation (serial correlation) of residuals, which violates the assumption of the independence of observations (see Sect. 3.4.2.4).

3.4.2.2 Individual and Collective Linearity Between the Predictors and the Outcome Variable

It is evident from its name that multiple linear regression assumes that the relationship between the outcome variable and each independent variable should be linear. In other words, the increase (or decrease) of the value of each independent variable is associated with a proportionate increase (or decrease) of the corresponding value of the outcome variable. A minimum correlation coefficient r of 0.3 is required to include a predictor in the model. We can test linearity between each individual quantitative predictor and outcome by requesting simple partial regression plots.

Collective linearity of all predictors and the outcome variable can be visualized by plotting the studentized residuals of regression (x-axis) against the unstandardized predictive values of outcome (y-axis). Fortunately, multiple regression procedures are not greatly affected by minor deviations from this assumption. However, if curvature in the relationships is evident, one may consider transforming the dependent and/ or the independent variable or using other nonlinear regression options.

3.4.2.3 Absence of Multicollinearity Among Predictors

Multi co-linearity is the undesirable situation where the correlations among the independent variables are strong. One should determine how much those independent variables are linearly related. The independent contribution of each variable is unstable (inflated) by the presence of the other correlated variable in the model. The solution is to choose one variable and exclude the other. As a rule of thumb, a correlation coefficient $r \geq 0.7$ between predictors indicates multiple collinearities and gives a red signal to exclude one of the two variables from the model.

Tolerance

The tolerance of an independent variable is the proportion of its variance not accounted for by other independent variables. It is an indicator of how much it contributes to the model. Consequently, a variable with a very low tolerance contributes little to a model and can cause computational problems. As a rule of thumb, a minimum tolerance of 0.1 is required to include a predictor in the model. As R^2 is the amount of variation in one variable due to another variable, tolerance will be equal to $1 - R^2$. If we remove the outcome from the model and regress predictor (A) on predictor (B), tolerance of (A) will be equal to 1 minus the calculated R^2.

Variance Inflation Factor (VIF)

The other side of the coin is the variable inflation factor (VIF), which indicates how much the effect of one variable is inflated by the other and, as a rule of thumb, the maximum tolerated VIF is 10. Otherwise, the predictor is better excluded from the model. Note that VIF is the reciprocal of tolerance, and hence, both tests verify the same assumption.

3.4.2.4 Analysis of Residuals for Normality, Autocorrelation, Independence, and Homoscedasticity

The Residuals of the Model

As previously mentioned in the section on simple linear regression, the aim of the regression model is to calculate a reliable estimate of the outcome variable (y) for any given value of the predictor variable (x) (see Sect. 2.6.2). However, there will be always a difference between the observed outcome used to create the model and the expected outcome calculated by the model itself; i.e., the residual values. The latter can be seen as the error of the model; hence, the smaller the residuals, the better is the value of the model itself [12].

Normality

By normality we mean the normal distribution of the outcome variable or, otherwise, the normal distribution of the residuals of the model. The normal distribution of residuals implies that the data set is random, and hence, the results of the model are stable and they can be generalized on a wide range of values. There are many ways to check normality [7, 10]. We can produce a histogram (with the normal curve superimposed) for the standardized residuals. The mean and Sd of the curve should be around the values expected in the normal distribution, i.e., a mean of 0 and an Sd of 1. We can produce a confirmatory normal P–P plot of standardized residuals against the expected cumulative probabilities. If the residuals are normally distributed, they should "approximately" align along the diagonal line. An alternative is a normal Q–Q plot of the studentized residuals to show the alignment of points along the diagonal line. Although the test is robust concerning normality, a significant violation can be corrected by data transformation that includes the outcome, the predictor variables or both.

Detection of Outliers

Residual statistics equally indicate outliers, as cases with more than (+3Sd) or (−3Sd) of standardized residuals (see Sect. 3.4.2.5). Outliers are a major source of bias and they have to be carefully analyzed, managed and reported (see Sects. 3.4.5.7 and 7.2.2).

Absence of Autocorrelation: The Durbin-Watson Test

The analysis of residuals permits us to verify an important assumption, autocorrelation (serial correlation) between adjacent cases. The statistical software package usually generates the Durbin-Watson statistics to test this assumption. In brief, autocorrelation refers to the degree of correlation of the same variables between two successive time intervals. Put it simply, the successive observations taken from one patient are usually correlated, while those taken from two different patients should not. For example, measuring the blood pressure of a subject at a certain time is expected to be correlated with his previous measurement, while the blood pressure of two different persons is not expected to be correlated. The test measures the autocorrelation between the linear regression residuals of observations; supposed to be acquired from different persons and should not be autocorrelated [22].

The test statistics range from 0 to 4, and a value around 2 is satisfactory. Nevertheless, the procedure of multiple linear regression with IBM-SPSS, tests the statistical significance of the latter and, a statistically non-significant test is required to assume the absence of dependence of cases or observations in the data file. A statistically significant test is a red signal that data are not suitable for the multiple regression analysis. We can check out the statistical significance by consulting the Durbin-Watson significance tables, which present a lower level (LL) and an upper level (UL) of the critical limit [23]. A Durbin Watson value towards 0 indicates positive autocorrelation. A value towards 4 indicates a negative one and a value of 2 indicates no autocorrelation. As a rule of thumb, values between 1.5 and 2.5 are good.

Homoscedasticity

Finally, homoscedasticity can be visualized graphically testing whether the variance remains stable along the whole line of best fit or not? Plotting the studentized residuals (as a measure of the variance) against the unstandardized predicted values (as a measure of change of values as one moves along the line of best fit). A specific pattern indicates violation of the random distribution of residuals; which should be equal, except for a change that is due to a random error. If violated, it can be corrected by many ways including data transformation, running a regression with robust standard errors [24, 25] or using other test such as weighted least square regression.

3.4.2.5 Absence of Outliers, High Leverage and Influential Points

We have previously defined outliers, data with high leverage, and influential points (see Sect. 3.2.3.2). We can detect outliers in multiple linear regression analysis by requesting case-wise diagnostics or studentized deleted residuals. The former shows the standardized residual value of each observation and, if outcome scores are normally distributed, we have to expect them to lie within (±) three standard deviations. Consequently, a larger or smaller score in absolute value has to be considered an outlier. Similarly, we can verify the requested studentized values for any value larger than (+3Sd) or (−3Sd).

As a part of the analysis, we can request to calculate and save the leverage values for each observed (x) value of the predictor. A leverage value measures how much extreme is (x), in relation to other values [11]. As a rule of thumb, leverage values are expected to be <0.2, values between 0.2 and 0.5 are risky, and values above 0.5 are dangerous and have to be dealt with.

Finally, a data point is influential if it unduly influences any part of regression analysis, such as the predicted responses, the estimated slope coefficients, or the hypothesis test results. We can identify influential points by consulting the requested Cook's distances. As a rule of thumb, cases with a Cook's distance above 1 should be investigated and, if not important, they can be removed [12]. Outliers, high leverage and influential points can all be a major source of bias, and hence, they have to be evaluated and dealt with, whether by data transformation or by removal or running the analysis with and without and test whether there will be a significant difference.

3.4.3 The Example

Sixty polytraumatized patients were managed surgically in a tertiary trauma center. Bivariate analysis showed that the duration of surgery (r = 0.986; P < 0.001), the amount of blood loss (r = 0.94; P < 0.001) and a motorcycle accident (MCA) (t = −3.6; P = 0.001) were related to the duration of ICU stay in days. The three variables were introduced into a multiple regression model to detect the independent predictors of the duration of ICU stay. Data are shown in Table 3.35.

Table 3.35 Outcome of surgery in 60 polytraumatized patients

Case number	Age[a]	Gender	Motorcycle accident	Duration of surgery[b]	Amount of blood loss[c]	ICU stay[d]	Hospital mortality
1	20.00	Female	No	20.00	100.00	5.00	Alive
2	30.00	Female	No	30.00	150.00	6.00	Alive
3	49.00	Female	No	40.00	190.00	6.00	Alive
4	30.00	Male	No	60.00	300.00	6.00	Alive
5	10.00	Male	No	80.00	400.00	7.00	Alive
6	40.00	Male	No	90.00	400.00	7.00	Alive
7	39.00	Male	Yes	100.00	800.00	8.00	Dead
8	20.00	Male	Yes	110.00	600.00	9.00	Dead
9	20.00	Male	No	140.00	500.00	8.00	Alive
10	10.00	Male	No	150.00	500.00	9.00	Alive
11	25.00	Male	No	180.00	1000.00	10.00	Aalive
12	30.00	Male	No	20.00	100.00	5.00	Alive
13	17.00	Male	No	30.00	150.00	5.00	Alive
14	20.00	Male	No	40.00	190.00	6.00	Alive
15	25.00	Male	No	60.00	300.00	6.00	Alive
16	40.00	Male	No	80.00	400.00	7.00	Alive
17	30.00	Male	No	90.00	400.00	7.00	Alive
18	20.00	Male	No	100.00	500.00	8.00	Alive
19	30.00	Male	No	110.00	600.00	8.00	Alive
20	32.00	Male	No	140.00	500.00	9.00	Alive
21	80.00	Male	No	150.00	800.00	9.00	Alive
22	60.00	Male	Yes	180.00	1000.00	10.00	Dead
23	20.00	Male	No	20.00	100.00	5.00	Alive
24	30.00	Female	No	30.00	150.00	6.00	Alive
25	20.00	Female	No	40.00	190.00	6.00	Alive
26	35.00	Male	No	60.00	300.00	6.00	Alive
27	30.00	Male	Yes	80.00	1000.00	7.00	Dead
28	22.00	Male	Yes	90.00	800.00	7.00	Dead
29	20.00	Male	Yes	100.00	500.00	8.00	Dead
30	20.00	Male	No	110.00	400.00	8.00	Alive
31	30.00	Male	No	140.00	400.00	9.00	Alive
32	34.00	Male	No	150.00	800.00	9.00	Alive
33	20.00	Male	Yes	180.00	1000.00	10.00	Alive
34	42.00	Female	No	20.00	100.00	5.00	Alive
35	70.00	Female	No	30.00	150.00	5.00	Alive
36	20.00	Female	No	40.00	190.00	6.00	Alive
37	60.00	Female	No	60.00	300.00	6.00	Alive
38	35.00	Male	Yes	80.00	400.00	7.00	Dead

(continued)

Table 3.35 (continued)

Case number	Age[a]	Gender	Motorcycle accident	Duration of surgery[b]	Amount of blood loss[c]	ICU stay[d]	Hospital mortality
39	41.00	Male	Yes	90.00	400.00	7.00	Dead
40	20.00	Female	Yes	100.00	500.00	8.00	Dead
41	19.00	Female	Yes	110.00	600.00	8.00	Dead
42	9.00	Male	No	140.00	500.00	9.00	Alive
43	30.00	Male	No	150.00	800.00	9.00	Alive
44	20.00	Male	No	180.00	1000.00	10.00	Alive
45	40.00	Male	No	110.00	600.00	8.00	Alive
46	20.00	Male	No	140.00	500.00	9.00	Alive
47	23.00	Male	No	150.00	800.00	9.00	Alive
48	44.00	Female	No	180.00	1000.00	10.00	Dead
49	20.00	Male	No	20.00	100.00	5.00	Alive
50	59.00	Female	Yes	30.00	150.00	6.00	Dead
51	20.00	Male	No	40.00	190.00	6.00	Alive
52	30.00	Male	No	60.00	300.00	6.00	Alive
53	30.00	Male	No	80.00	400.00	7.00	Alive
54	20.00	Male	No	90.00	400.00	7.00	Alive
55	20.00	Male	No	100.00	500.00	8.00	Alive
56	20.00	Male	No	110.00	600.00	8.00	Alive
57	24.00	Male	No	140.00	500.00	9.00	Alive
58	66.00	Male	No	150.00	800.00	9.00	Alive
59	30.00	Male	No	180.00	1000.00	10.00	Alive
60	20.00	Male	No	20.00	100.00	5.00	Alive

a = age in years, b = duration of surgery in minutes, c = amount of blood loss in milliliters, d = duration of ICU stay in days

3.4.4 Designing the Model

A main question is about the predictor variables introduced in the model: which variable to introduce and how many? Most of the researchers agree that we have to have 20 subjects for each predictor variable included in the model, and hence, which variable to introduce will be governed by this limit? The researchers usually preliminary multiple regression with a series of bivariate analyses. Ideally, we can introduce all variables that were significantly related to the preliminary analysis outcome. If the sample size permits, we can extend the level of inclusion up to those predictors with a larger P-value, usually 0.1. As any individual study is only one sample of the vast population, it seems logical to include predictors that were related to the outcome in the reliable literature, even if they did not reach the level of statistical significance in our study. On the other hand, we have to exclude extraneous predictors as well as highly similar variables (see Sect. 3.4.4).

Whether the model is used to explain or predict the outcome has to be taken into consideration. The primary aim of a predicate model is accuracy, and hence we have the aim to introduce as many "promising variables" as we can.. On the other hand, "redundant variables" weakens the explanatory model, and a cautious mathematical assessment of predictors is more important. The statistical software provides

Table 3.36 Multiple regression analysis: results of bivariate analysis of the duration of ICU stay in 60 polytraumatized patients

Age	Surgery duration[a]	Blood loss[b]	Gender	MCA	Mortality
r = −0.025	r = 0.98	r = 0.869	−Females: 6.38 ± 1.4 −Males: 7.68 ± 1.5	−Yes: 7.27 ± 1.6 −No: 7.91 ± 1.2	−Yes: 7.27 ± 1.6 −No: 7.91 ± 1.2
P = 0.85	P < 0.001	P < 0.001	P = 0.008	P = 0.21	P = 0.21

Values are presented as correlation coefficient r or mean ± standard deviation of the duration of ICU stay in days, a = duration of surgery in minutes, amount of blood loss in ml., MCA = motorcycle accident

selection algorithms that can reduce the number of variables included in the model. We have briefly reported the different methods of selection (see Sect. 3.3.3) and, the interested reader may refer to Tabachnick and Fidell for more details [6]. In our example, we will use the default standard method "enter", where all variables are introduced in one step together.

Table 3.36 shows the bivariate analysis results between the duration of ICU stay in days and other study outcomes. As we have a total of 60 patients, only the three statistically significant variables, namely the duration of surgery in minutes, the amount of blood loss in milliliters, and gender will be introduced in the multivariable analysis.

3.4.5   Verification of the Assumptions [6–10]

We will use IBM-SPSS version 24 for MAC to verify data and interpret the results.

3.4.5.1   The Study Design

The four assumptions related to study design are usually verified during the preparation of the study (see Sect. 3.4.2.1). We have one continuous outcome (dependent variable): the duration of ICU stays in days. We have three predictors (independent variables); two continuous variables (time of surgery and amount of blood loss), and one categorical variable (gender) that includes >5 cases per category. Observations are independent. The total sample size is 60 patients is sufficient to include the three predictors in the

analysis. Data are uploaded to the software, as shown in Table 3.35. The products of the analysis verify the remaining assumptions.

3.4.5.2   Execution of the Analysis

- We start by clicking on "Analyze" then request "Regression" and "linear" to open the main window. We shift the (ICU stay) to the "Dependent" section". We shift (the duration of surgery), (the amount of blood loss), and (gender) to the independent list section marked as "Block 1 of 1".

- We click on "Statistics", and we request: "regression Coefficients estimates and confidence intervals at 95%", "Model fit", "R squared change", Descriptive" statistics, "Part and partial correlations" and "collinearity diagnostics". Under "Residuals", we request "Durbin-Watson" statistics and Casewise diagnostics". We can keep "outliers outside" 3 standard deviations or change it to 2.5 or 2. We click on continue to close this window.

- Returning to the main window, we click on plots to open its window. Under the "standardized Residual Plots" we request "Histogram", "Normal probability plot", and to "Produce all partial plots". We click on "continue" to close this window.

- We click on "Save", and we request saving of: "the unstandardized predicted", "the unstandardized residuals", "the standardized residuals", "the studentized residuals" and the "studentized deleted residuals", Cook's distance, and "leverage values". We click on "OK" to execute the analysis.

3.4.5.3   Independence of Observations

The first assumption to verify is the independence of observations. A Durbin-Watson test result between 1.5 and 2.5 is generally accepted as a rule of thumb. However, our result is >2 (2.372), and hence, it suggests an unusual negative collinearity. To check our results in Durbin-Watson tables, we have to subtract it from 4 (2.372–4 = 1.628, in absolute value). For a sample size of 60 patients and three regressors, the tables show an upper and lower limit of 1.48 and 1.689 and, an absolute value within those two limits has to be considered as being doubtful. An absolute value below the lower limit (<1.48) indicates significant collinearity. A value above the upper limit (>1.689) indicates the absence of multicollinearity. Our value looks doubtful, and we will benefit from the doubt and continue the analysis, provided that we note this finding in the results section.

3.4.5.4   Linearity

Linearity is verified graphically, whether individual linearity between each predictor and outcome or collective linearity between all predictors and outcome. The qualitative variable (MCA in our example) is excluded from this test,

of course. The individual linearity was requested during the analysis and is verified by plotting each predictor (x-axis) against the outcome (y-axis). We can assume linearity between the duration of surgery and the ICU stay (Fig. 3.15) and to a less extent between the amount of blood loss and the ICU stay (Fig. 3.16). After excluding the (MCA) qualitative variable, we can visualize collective linearity between both predictors and outcome by requesting a scatter plot through the "Graphs" procedure of IBM-SPSS. We can assume linearity between the "unstandardized predictive value" and the "studentized residuals" of the outcome (Fig. 3.17).

3.4.5.5   Homoscedasticity

Homoscedasticity can be defined as the variance being equal along all predicted outcome values. We mean the variability of the residuals or the errors by the variance. Put it simpler, regardless of the duration of ICU stay; we expect a constant error in the calculation, which would be nearly the same whether the patient stayed for just one day, two days, or any number of days. In other words, we expect that any calculated error is random and does not have a special trend in relation to a specific ICU stay duration. As

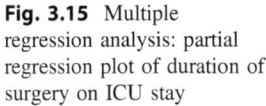

Fig. 3.15 Multiple regression analysis: partial regression plot of duration of surgery on ICU stay

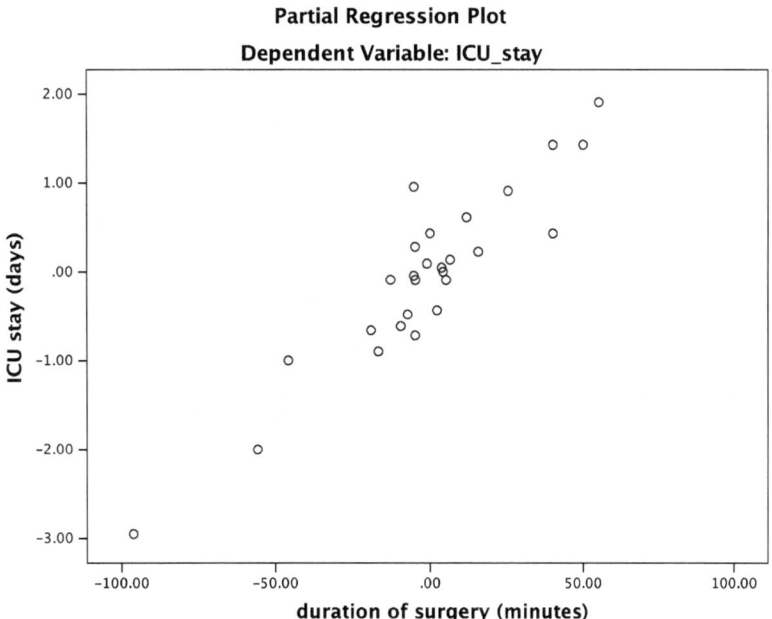

Fig. 3.16 Multiple regression analysis: partial regression plot of the amount of blood loss on ICU stay

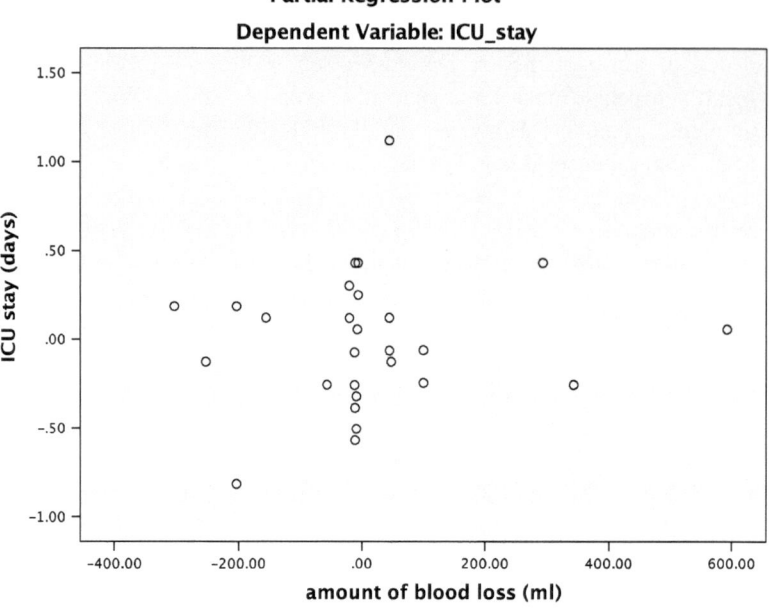

Fig. 3.17 Multiple regression analysis: regression plot of unstandardized predictive values on the studentized residuals

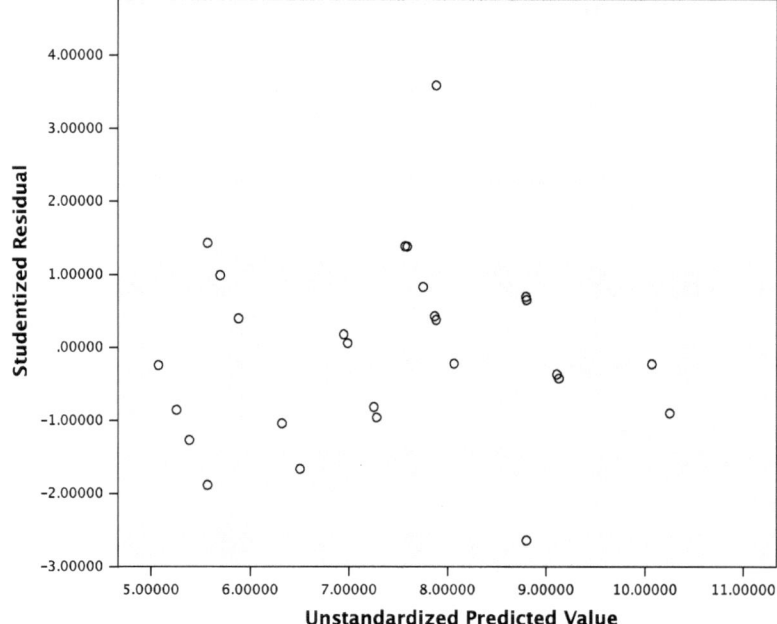

shown in Fig. 3.17, the range of the dots that represent those errors tends to be constant across the outcome (across the different ICU durations). In case the scatter plot takes the shape of a funnel or a double funnel (a butterfly), it indicates heteroscedasticity; i.e., errors tend to increase or decrease across the predicted values. Homoscedasticity can be formally tested by Breusch-Pagan and Koenker tests, which can be downloaded as a part of an IBM-SPSS macro to test homoscedasticity [16]. We have to note that the violation of homoscedasticity will not affect

Table 3.37 Multiple regression analysis: regular versus robust standard errors of regression coefficients

Model	Source of variation	Unstandardized B	Se	Standardized beta	t	P value	CI 95%
Regular	Constant	4.633	0.1		46.199	<0.001	4.43 to 4.83
	Duration of surgery	0.031	0.002	0.988	17.56	<0.001	0.027 to 0.034
	Amount of blood loss	0.000014	0.0007	0.0003	0.223	0.824	−0.001 to 0.001
	Gender	0.183	0.107	0.048	1.7	0.092	−031 to 0.398
Robust	Constant	4.633	0.1128		41.7	<0.001	4.4 to 4.86
	Duration of surgery	0.031	0.0016	0.9879	19	<0.001	0.0276 to 0.0341
	Amount of blood loss	0.000014	0.0003	0.0123	0.25	0.8023	−0.0005 to 0.0006
	Gender	0.183	0.1114	0.048	1.64	0.1053	−0.0398 to 0.4064

Regular model = regular output of multiple linear regression, Robust model = robust standard error in case of heteroscedasticity

the calculated regression coefficients but their standard errors and hence, the 95% CI and the calculated P values.

Heteroscedasticity can be cured by calculating robust standard errors; which correct the 95% confidence intervals and the statistical significance of the regression coefficients. The calculations can be easily executed by downloading one of two freely available SPSS macros written by Andrew Hayes [15] and Ahmed Daryanto A [16]. Although we have verified the homoscedasticity of our data as suggested by a statistically non-significant Breusch-Pagan (P = 0.835) and Koenker tests (P = 0.9312), yet we have calculated the robust standard errors by Andrews Hayes macro, just for demonstrative purposes, but they will not be used. Table 3.37 shows an extract of IBM-SPSS output for the calculated "unadjusted" regression coefficients, standard errors and CI at 95%, alongside Hayes "adjusted" values. Although robust standard errors are usually larger than conventional ones, they can be smaller than a traditional standard error, whether due to sampling error or because a study with a small sample size has originally inflated the latter [15].

3.4.5.6 Exclusion of Multicollinearity

Multicollinearity is tested first by examining the correlation coefficient r calculated between predictors themselves and the degree of tolerance and variance inflation factors. In our example, there was a statistically significant high correlation between the duration of surgery and the amount of blood loss (r = 0.886, P < 0.001). R^2 equals 0.7849, which means that about 78.5% of the variation of one variable is explained by the other. However, the tolerance and variance inflation factors (VIF) for the duration of surgery were 0.211, and 4.737 and those for the amount of blood loss were 0.219 and 4.56, all being well distant from the critical limit of tolerance (≤ 0.1) and VIF (≥ 10).

3.4.5.7 Checking on Outliers, High Leverage and Influential Points

- Part of the procedure was to request IBM-SPSS to produce "a case-wise diagnostic table" that reveals extreme cases with "standardized residuals" more than + 3Sd or −3Sd, so as the researcher can deal with those outliers. In case there are no outliers, IBM-SPSS does not produce the table. In our example, the software has shown that case number 8 had a standardized residual value of 3.548. Another way is to examine the saved column of "studentized residuals" and remove cases with >+3SD or >−3d, in absolute value. In our example, the same case had a high studentized residual of 3.59, of course. The case was left and reported.

- Checking on the saved column of leverage values, we had a single case (case number 27) with a high leverage value of 0.34645. The case was left and reported.
- The highest calculated Cook's distance was 0.13373 and hence, none of our cases can be considered as being influential (Cook's distance >1).

3.4.5.8　Normality

Normality is checked out graphically by several ways requested from the program during the construction of the model. Figure 3.18 shows the histogram with the superimposed normal curve. Note the normal distribution of the standardized residuals, with a mean of zero and a standard deviation of nearly 1 (0.974). Figure 3.19 is a P–P

plot, showing the points "approximately aligned" along the diagonal line, which verify the assumption of "approximate normality of residuals". Another method is to request a normal Q-Q plot of studentized residuals. Plotting observed to expected values can show the points approximately aligned along the diagonal line, verifying the required near-normal distribution of the residuals.

3.4.6　Model Evaluation

The value of the model is dependent upon its ability to answer three main questions.

How well are the data fitted in the model? So that the collection of the predictors explained a significant part of the outcome. What is the value of the independent role of each predictor included in the model? Can we use the model to predict the outcomes of future studies?

3.4.6.1　The Model Summary

The R Square

While the Pearson's correlation coefficient r is an indicator of the strength of the linear relation between the observed and the predicted scores of

Fig. 3.18 Multiple regression analysis: Histogram with superimposed normal curve

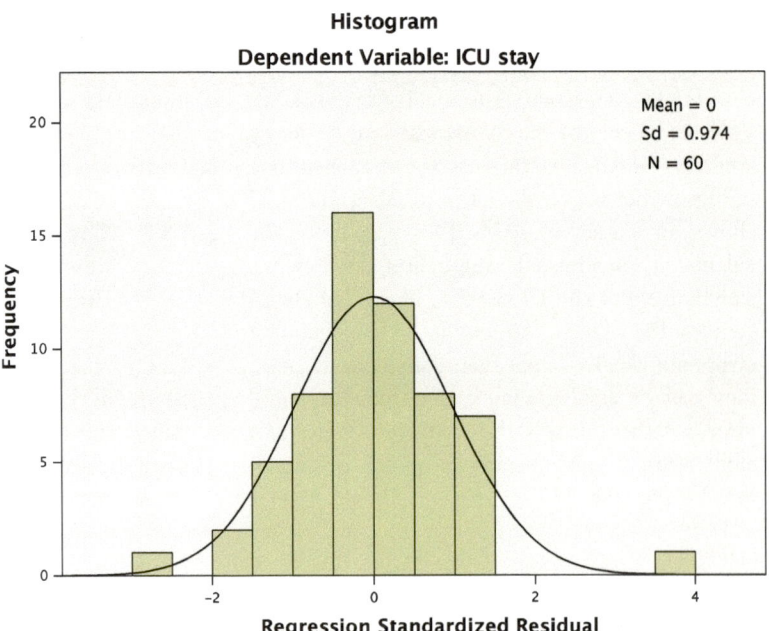

Fig. 3.19 Multiple regression analysis: P-P plot

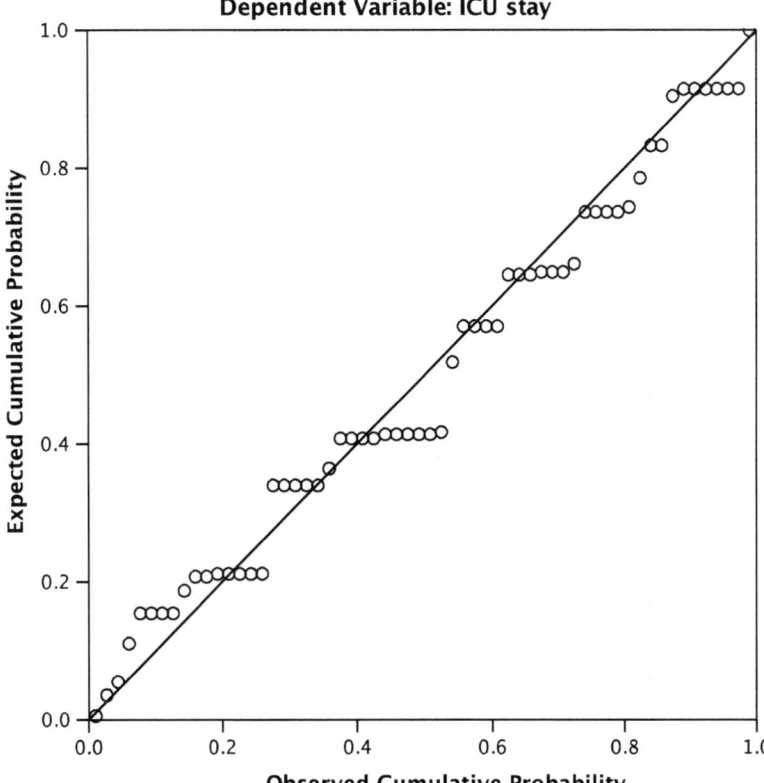

Normal P-P Plot of Regression Standardized Residual
Dependent Variable: ICU stay

the outcome variable, R-squared (R^2) is a reliable indicator of the proportion of variation in the outcome that is explained by the set of predictor variables; i.e., by the model itself. In other words, it is a good indicator of how well the model fits the data. The value of R^2 ranges from 0 to 1, expressing the proportion of variation in the outcome due to the independent variables. When presented as a percentage, it is called the coefficient of variation. Ideally, we would like to explain most if not all of the original variability. An R-square close to 1 indicates that the variables in the model have explained almost all outcome variability [6].

In our example, R-square equals 0.963 (Table 3.38); then we know that the variability of the outcome values around the regression line is 1–0.963 times the original variance; in other words, we have explained 96.3% of the original variability, and are left with 3.7% residual variability. Put it another way, 96.3% of the variability in ICU

stay can be explained by all variables included in the model (constant + duration of surgery + amount of blood loss + gender). The part remaining unexplained is the residual variability in the model (Table 3.39), which is why the following formula calculates R^2 "Eq. 3.6".

$$R^2 = 1 - \frac{Residual\ SS}{Total\ SS} = 1 - \frac{5.551}{148.400} = 0.963$$

(3.6)

The Adjusted R Square

R^2 express the amount of variation in the outcome variable explained by (due to) the predictor variables in the model. Adding more predictors to the model, reduces the amount of unexplained (residual) variability, and hence, R^2 increases. In general, the variability of any sample is larger than the variability of the population form which the sample is drawn (see Sect. 1.3.4.1).

Table 3.38 Multiple regression analysis: model summary[a]

R	R Square	Adjusted R Square	Se	R square change	F change	df1, df2	Significance of F change	Durbin Watson
0.981[b]	0.963	0.961	0.3148	0.963	480.344	3, 56	<0.001	2.372

a = dependent variable ICU stay, b = predictors = constant, duration of surgery, amount of blood loos, gender

Table 3.39 Multiple regression analysis: ANOVA[a]

Source of variation	Sum of squares	df	Mean square	F ratio	P value
Regression	142.849	3	47.616	480.344	<0.001[b]
Residual	5.551	56	0.099		
Total	148.400	59			

a = dependent variable ICU stay, b = predictors = constant, duration of surgery, amount of blood loos, gender

Consequently, adjusted R^2 was suggested as a remedy to reduce the inflated part of explained variability R^2, so as to better fit the variability in the population [6]: "Eq. 3.7".

$$Adjusted\ R^2 = 1 - \frac{Residual\ MS}{Total\ MS}$$
$$= 1 - \frac{Residual\ SS/df_{residual}}{Total\ SS/df_{total}}$$
$$= 1 - \frac{5.551/56}{148.4/59} = 0.961 \quad (3.7)$$

The Analysis of Variance

ANOVA calculates the overall significance of regression (the constant + duration of surgery + amount of blood loss + gender), as shown in Table 3.39. Remember that ANOVA is an omnibus test, and hence, it does not mean that every variable in the model is statistically significant but the overall model. Put it another way, at least one of the regression coefficients is statistically significant from (0). The individual significance of each regression coefficient will be dealt with in Sect. 3.4.6.2.

3.4.6.2 Interpreting the Regression Coefficients

Table 3.37 shows estimates of regression coefficient beta, standard error of beta, standardized coefficient beta, t-value of beta, and two-level

significance of t. The confidence intervals of those coefficients are given at the 95% level. The reader is requested to refer back to Sect. 2.6.2.1 to understand the difference between unstandardized B and standardized beta coefficients. The unstandardized coefficient is commonly termed as "B coefficient", the standardized coefficient as "coefficient beta". In brief, the B coefficient quantifies the effect of the predictor on the outcome and is used to test whether this effect is statistically significant or not, but it cannot be compared to the effect of the B coefficients of other predictors on the outcome because they are usually calculated in different scales. The B coefficient was standardized "coefficient beta" so that we could compare the effects of different predictors on the outcome. For example, the B coefficient of the duration of surgery was smaller (0.031) than that calculated for gender (0.183), which may give the false impression that gender has a larger impact on the outcome than the duration of surgery. Now looking at the beta coefficients (standardized values), the beta coefficient of the duration of surgery is more than 20 times that of gender, which explains why the duration of surgery was significantly related to outcome, with an extremely small P-value < 0.001, while gender was not (P = 0.092). The reader is requested to refer back to Sect. 2.6.2.1 for more details on the meaning of both coefficients (see Sect. 2.6.2.1).

For our example, the B coefficient of the duration of surgery equals 0.031, and it can be interpreted as follows: each minute increase in the duration of surgery increases the average ICU stay by 0.031 days. Put it simpler, each hour increase in the duration of surgery increases the average ICU stay by nearly two days (0.031 day × 60 = 1.86 days); all other variables in the model held constant. A negative B coefficient would mean that an increased duration of surgery would shorten ICU stay. What does the 95% CI tell us? It tells us that the average increase in ICU stay will not always be 1.86 days, but it is expected to vary between 1.62 (0.027 × 60) and 2.04 (0.034 × 60) days in 95% of the cases. The effect of the amount of blood loss on ICU stay was non-conclusive; the 95% CI was (−0.001 to +0.001). It means that each liter of blood loss can sometimes increase and other times decrease the patient's average ICU stay by one day, with all other variables in the model kept constant (P = 0.824).

The interpretation of the dichotomous variable is somehow different and depends upon which is the reference category. We have coded the reference value as 0 (e.g., female) and the other value as 1 (male). The B coefficient indicates the difference between the two categories. In our example, a male patient is expected to stay on an average of 0.183 days more than a female patient. Put it simpler, on average, a male is expected to stay nearly 4.4 h more than a female, with all other variables in the model being kept constant. The 95% CI tells us that this prediction is not conclusive because it bypasses the null (0), and, hence, a male can stay 0.74 h less (−0.031 × 24 h) and up to 9.5 h more than a female patient (0.398 × 24 h), with all other variables in the model, kept constant.

3.4.6.3 Prediction of the Outcome: The Regression Equation

An important aim of multiple regression is to construct a regression equation that we can use to predict the outcome when fed with the appropriate information. However, our example opens the unsettled debate about whether statistically non-significant variables, such as gender and amount of blood loss, should be included in the equation or not? There is no straightforward answer to this question. We favor including statistically non-significant variables whenever they are making sense or have a large regression coefficient, with narrow variation (Se), especially if other studies reported them. After consulting the relevant literature, it is up to the researcher to weigh all those factors and make his own decision. In our study, including the amount of blood loss in the prediction of ICU stay does make sense; what is against is the minimal non-significant effect of this variable. On the other hand, gender has a larger "mathematical" influence, but we cannot see how it influences ICU stay. For demonstrative purposes, we will just include both variables in the equation "Eq. 3.8".

$$ICU\ stay = 4.633 + (0.031)\ surgery\ duration$$
$$+ (0.000014)\ amount\ of\ blood\ loss + (0.183)\ Gender$$

$$(3.8)$$

As the average ICU stay, duration of surgery and amount of blood loss were: 7.4 ± 1.58 days, 93.3 ± 50 min and 473 ± 283 ml; let us calculate the expected ICU stay for a female person who was operated upon for 90 min and lost about 500 ml of blood. The average ICU stay of such person is expected to be: $4.4774 + (0.031) \times 90 + (0.000014) \times 500 + (0.183) \times 0 = 7.43$ days. A male patient's expected ICU stay is 0.183 days more, about 4.4 h.

Calculation of a 95% CI of Outcome

IBM-SPSS provides the opportunity to calculate an interval of confidence at 95% for the outcome variable through the syntax option [10].

- We click on "Analyze" then choose the "General Linear Model" and "Univariate" analysis.
- We shift (the duration of ICU stay) to the "Dependent Variable" box and the three predictors (duration of surgery, amount of blood loss and gender) to the "Covariate(s)" box.
- We click on the "Paste" button to open the syntax file. We can note that the last line in the syntax shows: /DESIGN = Gender

Fig. 3.20 Multiple
regression analysis flow chart.
a = Durbin-Watson test,
b = individual and collective
linearity, c = in case of
heteroschedacity robust
standard error regression
coefficients are calculated,
d = outliers, high leverage
and influential points

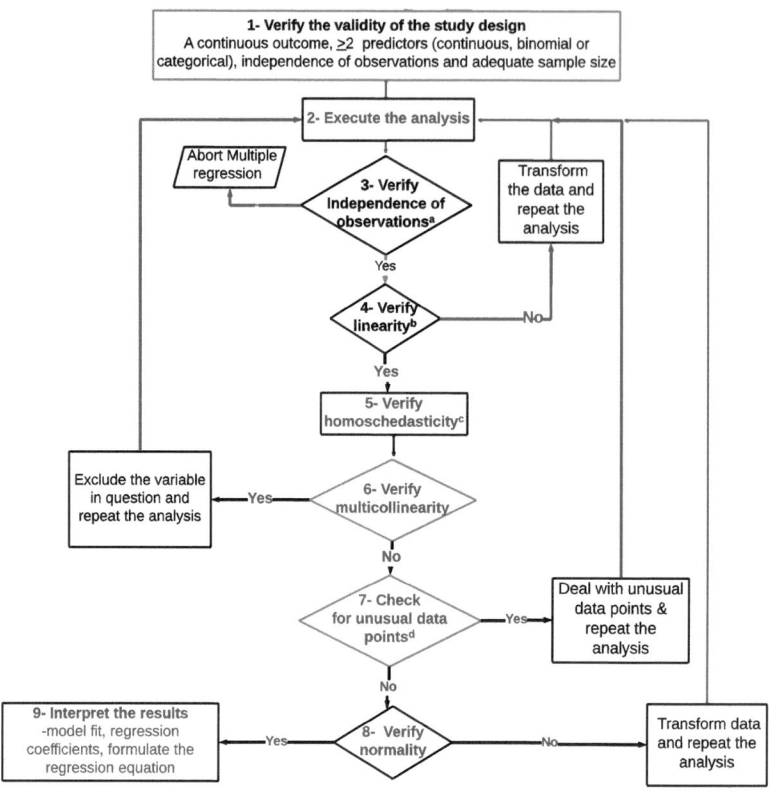

duration_of_surgery blood_loss. We insert one line before: /LMATRIX = ALL 1 0 90 500

Note that the semicolons are not typed and the typed line should not end with a dot. This line means that we request a matrix (/LMATRIX) that includes all the information (ALL) in the regression equation, including the intercept (1), ninety minutes duration of surgery (90), female gender (0), amount of blood loss (500).

- We click on "Run" and then "ALL".

The software produces the estimated mean ICU stay for a female patient who spent 90 min in surgery and lost 500 ml of blood = 7.442 days, Se = 0.093 days, and 95% CI = 7.256 – 7.629 days. The interpretation of the result is as follows: a female patient who passed 90 min in surgery and has lost about half a liter of blood is expected to stay about one week in the ICU

(7.443: 7.256–7.629 days). We can repeat the syntax for other surgery durations, different amounts of blood loss, and male patients. Figure 3.20 shows the flow chart of the procedure.

3.4.7 What Should Be Reported

- The descriptive statistics, mean (Sd) and number (%).
- The results of bivariate analysis.
- The variables introduced in the model and how they were selected.
- The verification of the assumptions, including independence, linearity, normality, homoscedasticity, and absence of collinearity. We have to report outliers, high leverage, or influential points, and how they were dealt with?.
- The results of the analysis have to be fully reported, including overall significance, R^2 and adjusted R^2.

- The significance of individual predictors, B coefficients and 95% CI.
- The model significantly predicted the ICU stay (7.4 ± 1.58 days), $F_{(3,56)} = 480.344$, $P < 0.001$, $R^2 = 0.963$ and adjusted $R^2 = 0.961$. Only the duration of surgery (93.3 ± 50.8 min) added significantly to the model; B coefficient 0.031, Se = 0.002; $P < 0.001$.
- Finally, we should report the effect size and basis of sample size calculation (see Sects. 4.11.1 and 4.11.2).

3.4.8 The Case of Multiple Outcome Variables

Returning to the previous example and suppose that in addition to the ICU stay, the researcher equally wants to know the effect of the studied predictors on other factors, such as the total medical expenses. Regression analysis can give such information by providing an overall evaluation of the impact of independent variables on several outcome variables. The model can specify the role of each independent variable on each outcome and outcome combination.

We have previously shown that the methods used for the analysis of variance in the multivariate analysis include Pillai's trace, Wilk's lambda, Hoteling's trace, and Roy's largest root criterion with approximate F statistic (see Sect. 3.2.4). After an overall F test has shown significance, post hoc tests are used to evaluate differences among specific means. The post hoc multiple comparison tests are performed for each dependent variable separately. The statistical package usually provides analysis of variance as well as estimates of parameters for each outcome variable. The required assumptions that have to be checked out, include normal distribution of the outcome variables and equality of the variance–covariance matrices in the population; however, analysis of variance is robust to departures from normality. To check assumptions, statistical packages usually use tests of homogeneity of variances such as (Box's M) or examine residuals and residual plots.

3.5 Binary Logistic Regression Analysis [4–6, 26–29]

3.5.1 Introduction: The Linear Versus the Logistic Regression

The main indication of binary logistic regression is to predict (or explain) the presence or absence of a binary outcome based on a set of qualitative and quantitative predictor variables. The procedure is most valid in case of a true category, such as living and dead rather than being based on a cut-off value of a continuous variable, such as mild and moderate hypertension. In that case, we should consider using linear regression to take advantage of the richer information and the limited variability offered by the continuous variable itself (see Sect. 7.1.2).

Binary logistic regression is similar to a multiple linear regression model but is technically derived to suit a binary outcome. A main difference is the outcome variable that can only acquire one of two values, yes (1) or no (0), and nothing in between. Consequently, we cannot fit a straight line across the cloud of paired data, as we did in multiple regression. The statisticians had to follow certain technical maneuvers to linearize the relationship between the predictor and the outcome variables. Suppose that the development of an adverse event is related to the level of a specific biomarker. The researchers will not know the patient's probability of developing the adverse event at a particular biomarker level and not just yes or no. Table 3.40 shows the results of a fictitious study calculating the number of patients who developed MI, with the corresponding level of a known biomarker of myocardial ischemia. The curve will be most probably S-shaped for the usual low probability to develop the event at the low level of biomarker and the very high probability at the high level

Table 3.40 Logistic regression analysis: the proportion of myocardial infarction (MI), according to the level of biomarker of ischemia

Biomarker level	0.1	0.2	0.3	0.4	0.5	0.6	0.7	0.8	0.9	1
Number of events	1	3	5	19	19	31	83	45	47	99
Sample size	100	50	50	100	50	50	100	50	50	100
Proportion of events	0.01	0.06	0.1	0.19	0.38	0.62	0.83	0.90	0.94	0.99

Fig. 3.21 Logistic regression: S-shaped correlation between the proportion of myocardial infarction (MI) and the level of biomarker of ischemia

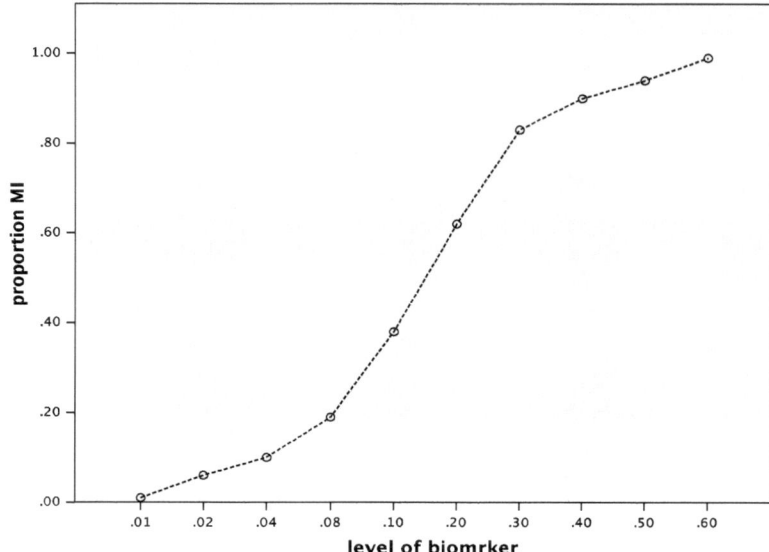

(Fig. 3.21). To predict the probability of developing MI with good accuracy, we have to have a straight linear relation. Linearity will provide a good estimate of MI at each measured level of biomarker and other unmeasured points as well, provided that those points were within the study limits.

We have previously shown that the logarithmic transformation of biological variables is an effective tool to achieve normalization (see Sect. 1.4.4). As we need to know the probability for a patient presenting with a particular biomarker level to develop MI, we will be interested in calculating the odds of the event. The odds equal P/1-P, and its logarithmic value (logit P) is normally distributed, and hence, it will straighten the S-shaped curve "Eq. 3.9". Plotting the normalized logit P against the biomarker levels allows an accurate prediction of the event across the whole biomarker range (Fig. 3.22),

calculation of a standard error and a 95% confidence interval. The linearized regression curve permits the estimation of a B coefficient and testing the statistical significance of its effect. Like in multiple regression, we will be able to calculate the amount of variation in the outcome that is due to the predictors, effect size, and estimates of outcome to be applied in future studies [28].

$$Logit\ (P) = In\left(\frac{P}{1-P}\right) \qquad (3.9)$$

3.5.1.1   Variable Transformation

Figure 3.23 shows the results of biomarker measurements in a small group of 17 patients, 7 out of whom (41%) developed myocardial infarction (MI). The right-hand side shows the results of regressing the binomial variable (1 = MI, 0 = no MI) on the six biomarker levels,

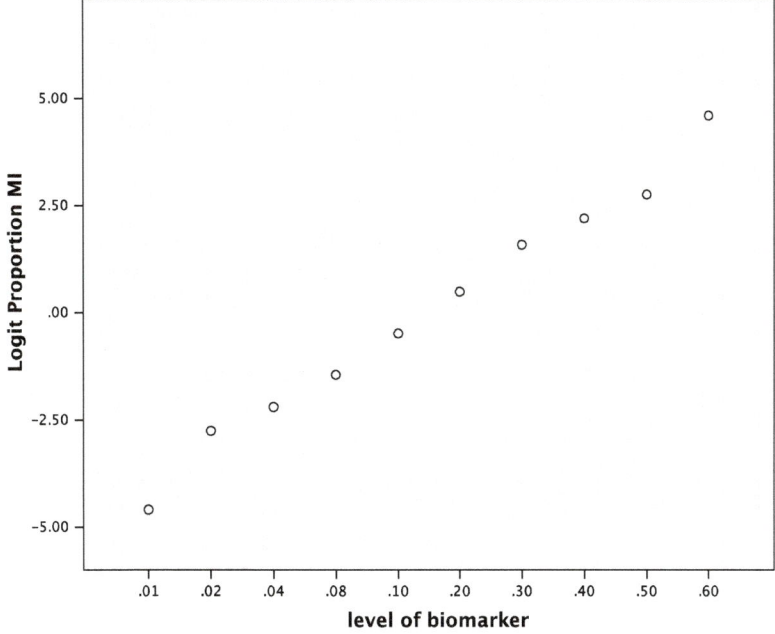

Fig. 3.22 Logistic regression analysis: linear correlation between the Logit of the proportion of myocardial infarction (MI) and the level of biomarker ischemia

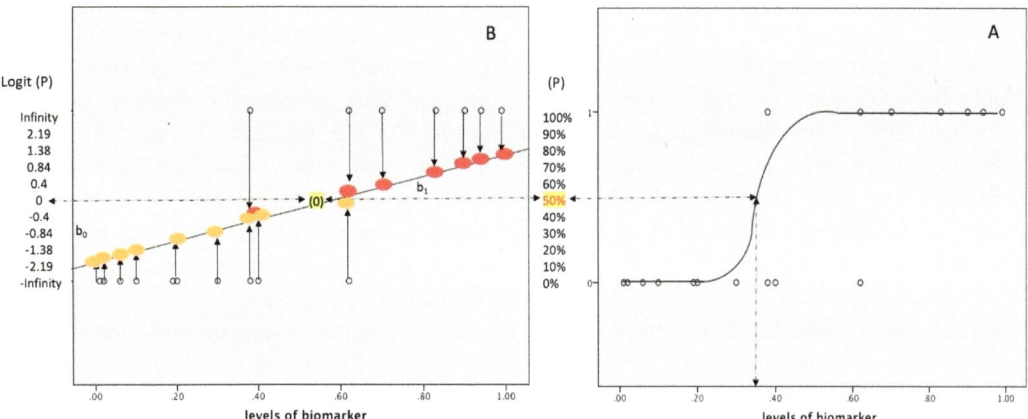

Fig. 3.23 Logistic regression analysis: transforming the binomial values into log odds. Open circles = observed data, closed circles = transformed data

measured in ng/ml. As cases were either infarcted or not, and nothing in between, it was impossible to fit a straight line passing by (or at equidistant of) the 18 pairs, as in linear regression. The line had to jump from one level (e.g., no MI) to the other (presence of MI); producing an S-shaped curve.

We begin by creating a continuous probability scale from 0 to 100% in the distance between 0 (no MI) and 1 (MI), along the y-axis. Raising an ascending arrow from a particular biomarker level on the x-axis, will hit the S-shaped curve to reflect the corresponding probability of MI on the y-axis. Theoretically, a patient presenting with a biomarker level of 0.35 ng/ml will have a 50% chance to develop MI, provided that the curve shown is a good fit for the data (Fig. 3.23A). Another higher point, e.g., a case presenting with a biomarker value of 0.4 ng/ml, will have an 80% probability of developing MI and, hence, a 20% probability of not developing MI. In other words, the case is four times more likely to develop than not develop the event, and hence, the probability scale (P) is better changed into an odds scale (P/1−P).

3.5.1.2   Normalization

Table 3.41 shows the transformation of the probability scale into the odds scale, using the simple equation: odds = P/(1−P) "Eq. 1.23". The odds answer the logistic question and express the tightness of the relation between the predictor (measure) and the outcome (event). However, we have previously shown that the odds are not normally distributed but can be normalized by being transformed into the logarithmic values, (Log odds = Logit P) (see Sect. 1.8). Kindly examine Table 3.41 and note that the center of the probability scale (0.5 = 50%) gives an equivalent logit P of (0). Unlike the odds, you can quickly note the bilaterally symmetrical distribution of Logit (P), on either side of the null; reflecting a good sign of normality. The values on the right side of the center (0) are just a mirror image of those on its left side.

3.5.1.3   The Linear Logistic Curve

The logarithmic transformation of the binomial distribution of the event, into a proportion, then into the odds and finally into the log odds (Logit P), has normalized the outcome and transformed the S-shaped logistic curve (Fig. 3.23A) into a straight linear curve (Fig. 3.23B). The 17 paired data can now be reflected on the curve. Each one

of the 17 paired data points on the S-shaped logistic curve on the right side is pushed to its equivalent point on the straightened linear curve on the left side. As such, data is normally distributed. Hence, we can calculate a mean and a standard deviation and assign a 95% confidence interval with the same characteristics as any normally distributed variable. As in the usual linear regression, the linearized logistic regression curve makes an angle with the horizon (b_1). The beta coefficient reflects the effect of the predictor on the outcome and, intercepts the y-axis at a point (b_0), which is the constant of the regression equation. Now we will move forwards to explain some technical differences between the linear and the logistic regression; including how to find the best fitting curve, how to evaluate its usefulness and how to calculate the coefficients for predictors?

3.5.1.4   The Best Fitting Curve

Remember how the simple regression line was made (see Sect. 2.6.2.1). We positioned the line in the center of the data points so as to minimize the squared differences between all points and the line itself (the least squares method). We rotated the line and recalculated the squared differences between data points and the line itself (the residuals). We repeated the rotation and the recalculations until we found the line the smallest residuals: this is the line that best fitted our data. Those residuals will be also used to calculate how much the regression model explains the outcome (R^2) (see Sect. 2.6.2.1).

Now moving to the logistic regression, the logistic regression line cannot be positioned in the same way because the logarithmic transformation has pushed the data points away into infinity (Fig. 3.23B). Yes, into infinity, because of the log of (1) and (−1) equal positive and negative infinity. Remember that the "true" positions of outcome are still 1 (MI) and 0 (no

Table 3.41 Logistic regression analysis: transformation of probability (P) into Odds and Logit P

Probability P	0%	10%	20%	30%	40%	50%	60%	70%	80%	90%	100%
Odds: P/(1 − P)	0	0.11	0.25	0.43	0.66	1	1.5	2.33	4	9	0
Logit P		$-\infty$	*−2.19*	*−1.38*	*−0.84*	*−0.4*	*0*	*0.4*	*0.84*	*1.38*	*2.19*	$+\infty$

MI) and that the log values are just "a transformation of calculation" and not a true change of the position of the outcome. As the data points are present in infinity, the distance between them and the line (i.e., the residuals) will be equal to infinity too. Consequently, the least square method cannot position the logistic regression line, and we cannot calculate a "true R^2".

The best position of the logistic regression curve is the one that maximizes the likelihood of the event. In other words, the best position is the one which permits that an arrow departing upwards from the x-axis (a particular biomarker level) will hit the curve, and it is then reflected towards the y-axis to land on the most correct probability that "the patient will develop the event" or "he will not develop the event".

To find the line of best fit, we "re transform" the normalized data points shown in Fig. 3.24B into the probability scale and "shift them back" to the S-shaped logistic curve (Fig. 3.24A), using "Eq. 3.10". For example, for a patient whose log-odds (Logit P) equals 0.4, his probability of developing MI is 60% P, and hence, the probability not to have MI is 40%. Note that a patient with logit P = (−0.4) has the reverse probabilities (see Table 3.41) [28].

$$P = \frac{e^{log(odds)}}{1 + e^{log(odds)}} \qquad (3.10)$$

The next step is to calculate the likelihood for each back-transformed data point repositioned on the logistic curve (Fig. 3.24A). The likelihood for "a patient who developed the event" equals the predicted probability (P) on the y-axis. The likelihood for "a patient who did not develop the event" equals (1 − P). The likelihood ratios of the seven patients who developed the event (dark circles) is equal to the corresponding (P) on the y-axis, and the likelihood ratios of the ten patients who did not develop the event (light circles) is equal to (1 − P). The maximal likelihood ratio is the product of all those ratios and reflects this curve's maximal likelihood value.

Remember how we found the best fitting line in multiple linear regression. We repeatedly rotate the line and recalculate the residuals until we found the line with the smallest residuals. In logistic regression, we keep on shifting the logistic curve in a new position, and we recalculate the log odds on the linearized curve as in (Fig. 3.24B). Then we shift back the log odds data from the linear curve to the original logistic curve, as probabilities (Fig. 3.24A) to recalculate the likelihood ratios of each data point and, multiply all likelihood ratios to produce the maximum likelihood ratio of the second curve. We keep repeating this process until we find the best fitting curve that gives the maximum likelihood ratios. Many statisticians prefer to calculate the loglikelihood ratio and not the

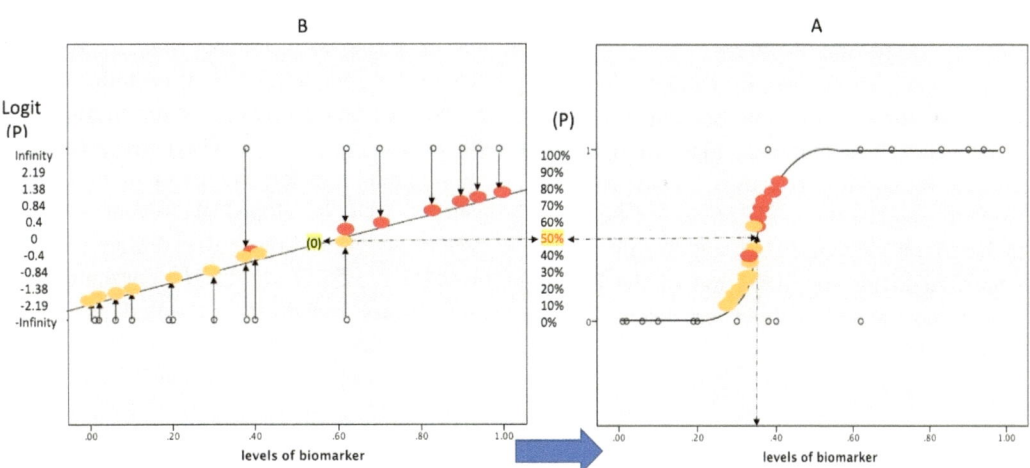

Fig. 3.24 Logistic regression analysis: projecting the transformed log odds values on the logistic curve

likelihood ratios themselves, which will end in the same conclusion as the curve which maximizes the likelihood ratio is the same one that maximizes their log values. We cannot execute those multiple calculations manually, and we need a statistical software package to perform the analysis. For our example, IBM-SPSS shows that the maximum loglikelihood was (-4.188),

3.5.1.5 Estimation of Coefficients and Testing Significance

Like in linear regression, the now "linearized best fit curve" of logistic regression intercepts the y-axis at a constant point (b_0), which represents the value of outcome in case there are no predictors and, it has a slope (b_1) that represents the effects of the predictor on the outcome (Fig. 3.23). Note that those coefficients and all calculations are in the log-odds scale. As in linear regression, the Wald χ^2 statistics are used to test the significance of individual coefficients in the model = (coefficient/Se)^2. Each Wald statistic is compared with a χ^2 distribution with 1 degree of freedom. The reliability of Wald statistics is questionable, particularly for small samples. For data that produce large estimates of the coefficient, the standard error is often inflated, resulting in a lower Wald statistic. Therefore, the explanatory variable may be incorrectly assumed to be unimportant in the model. Likelihood ratio tests are generally considered to be superior [28].

3.5.1.6 Calculation of Pseudo R^2, Effect Size and P-value

As previously mentioned, we cannot calculate an R^2 as in linear regression because we cannot calculate residuals in the first place for data being pushed to infinity. However, there are many ways to evaluate the model. Cox and Snell's R^2 is based on the log-likelihood for the model, compared to the log-likelihood of the baseline model, i.e., model without predictor variables [30]. However, the theoretical value is smaller than 1 (i.e., smaller than 100%), even in perfect models, and hence, it cannot be a reliable replacement of R^2. Negelkerke's R^2 is an adjusted version to cover the full scale from 0 to1 [31]. McFadden's pseudo R^2 is another suggestion that

is supposed to be similar to the usual calculated R^2 in linear models [32].

Calculation of R^2

Let us refresh our memory on how linear regression calculates R^2 and the P-value from the residuals. In brief, we square the residuals around the best fit line and we sum them up (SS_{fit}); this is the best model (Fig. 2.7). We square the sum of the residuals around the worst fitting line (SS_{mean}), the horizontal line passing by the mean of the y-axis (Fig. 2.6). R^2 compares the measure of the good fit with the measure of bad fit = ($SS_{mean} - SS_{fit}$) / (SS_{mean}) (Fig. 2.8) and, it can be rewritten as: ($SS_{total} - SS_{error}$) / (SS_{total}) "Eq. 2.93 ". Being a proportion out of a total, the value of R^2 is always between 0 and 1. Put it simpler, R^2 is the proportion of variation that is removed or explained by regression (see Sect. 2.6.2.1).

Calculation of McFadden's Pseudo R^2

The logistic regression coefficient is also the result of comparing two models, a measure of a good fit and a measure of a bad fit, which cannot be the residuals that are now placed at infinity "Eq. 3.11". A measure of good fit is the likelihood ratio calculated for the best fit logistic regression line (LL_{fit}) that reflects the effect of the predictor on the outcome. The worst fit will be the likelihood ratio calculated for the outcome, regardless of the predictor, i.e., calculated from the overall probability of the event (Fig. 3.25). For our example, the overall probability = number of events/total number = 7/17 = 0.41. We project our data along this worst fitting line and we calculate the likelihood of the overall probability: $LL_{overall\ probability}$. The latter is calculated by summing the log-likelihood ratios of the 7 patients who developed the event [=7 × log 0.41 = -6.24] and those who did not [10 × log (1−0.41) = -5.27] = (-11.51). For our example, McFadden's pseudo R^2 = $-11.51-(-4.188)/-11.51 = 0.636$; which is the effect size too. The P value is calculated by a chi-square test, where 2 ($LL_{fit} - LL_{overall\ probability}$) = Chi-square value with df = difference in the number of parameters in the two models. In the former, we have to calculate two estimates (slope of y-axis and the

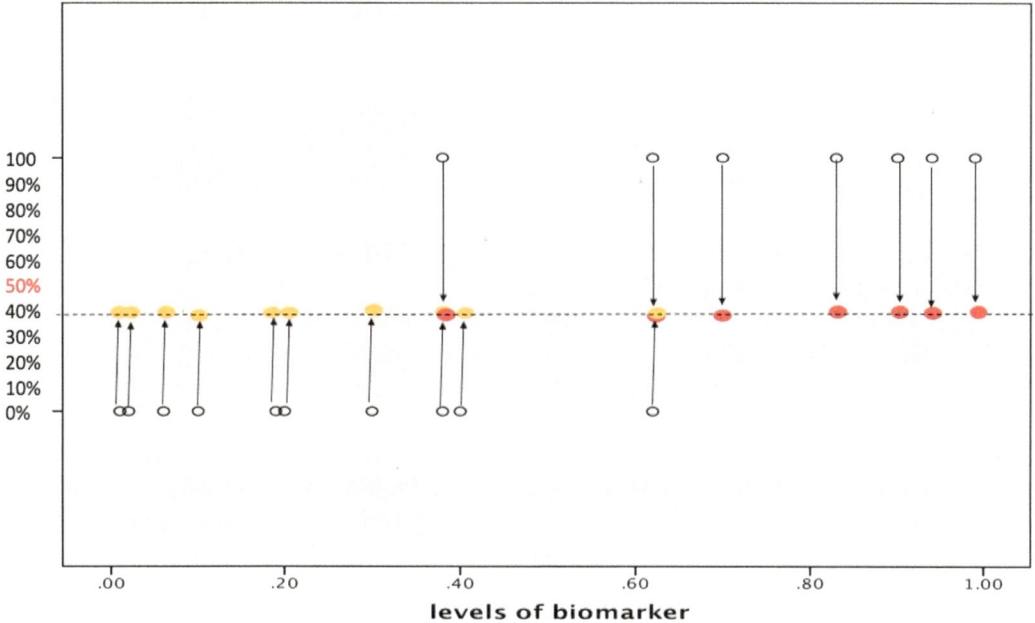

Fig. 3.25 Logistic regression analysis: the worst fitting line. Open circles = observed data, closed circles = data projected on the worst fitting line

intercept), while in the latter, we have to estimate the y-axis only, and hence, df = 2–1 = 1 df. In our example, the chi-square equals 2 (–4.188 – (–11.51)) = 14.6; P < 0.001.

$$R^2 = \frac{LL_{overall\ probability} - LL_{fit}}{LL_{overall\ probability}} \quad (3.11)$$

3.5.1.7 The Logistic Regression Equation

Provided that we have multiple predictors (x_1, x_2, x_3,... x_i), exerting their effects on the outcome by the coefficient (b_1, b_2, b_3,... b_i), we can construct the logistic regression equation as a modification of multiple regression "Eq. 3.12". Despite the apparent similarity, we have to note that the distribution is binomial, and the maximum likelihood ratio estimates the constant parameter (a) and the predictors (b).

$$Logit\ (P) = a + b_1 x_1 + b_2 x_2 + b_3 x_3 + \ldots + b_i x_i \quad (3.12)$$

3.5.1.8 Interpretation of the Results: The Odds Ratio

Because the predictor variable x increases by one unit from x to x + 1, the odds of the outcome change from ($e^a\ e^{bx}$) to ($e^a\ e^{b(x+1)}$) = ($e^a\ e^{bx}\ e^b$). The odds ratio (OR) is therefore ($e^a\ e^{bx}\ e^b$)/($e^a\ e^{bx}$) = e^b. Put it this way; the OR is the exponential of coefficient beta "Eq. 3.13". When the predictor is binary too, OR is the OR of one category, compared to the other.

$$OR = e^b \quad (3.13)$$

3.5.1.9 Prediction of the Probability of the Outcome

The model can be used to calculate the predicted probability of the event (P) for a given value of the predictor (x), corresponding (b) and a constant (a). For example, in the case of one predictor, P can be calculated by the following formula "Eq. 3.14":

$$P = \frac{e^{(a+bx)}}{1 + e^{(a+bx)}} \quad (3.14)$$

3.5.1.10 The Case of a Qualitative or a Discrete Predictor Variable

Suppose that in our example, the predictor is not the level of the biomarker in ng/ml but rather a biomarker that gives either a positive or negative result? In the case of a qualitative predictor, what will change from what we have just explained is how the coefficients will be estimated. Table 3.42 shows the distribution of myocardial infarction and discriminative test results, as applied to our example.

We have previously shown that the logistic regression coefficient is the result of comparing two models, a measure of a good fit and a measure of a bad fit. After transforming the probability of MI into log-odds MI, the measure of bad fit is log-odds MI, calculated for the negative test = log (1/8) = log (0.125), and it represents the constant (b_0). The measure of good fit is what improved in the model by the test being positive or the log odds MI, calculated for a positive test = log (6/2) and, the B coefficient is the difference between the two logs (b_1). As the difference between two logs is equal to their ratio, (b_1) will be equal to the log of the OR, which tells us, on the log scale, how much the change in predictor (the test is positive or negative) changes (increases or decreases) the odds of outcome (MI). In our example, the logs of OR (b_1) = log (3/0.125) = 3.178 and hence, OR = 24.

Uploading our data to IBM-SPSS confirms the results performed manually and provides the Se, Wald value, and P-value of 1.339, 5.637, and

0.018 for the qualitative test. With an OR 24 (1.74 to 330.8). The interpretation is as follows: there is a statistically significant positive relationship between a positive test and MI; a positive test increases the odds of MI 24 times, compared to a negative test (P = 0.018).

3.5.2 The Basic Assumptions

The logistic regression analysis is less demanding than multiple regression. We have to satisfy seven assumptions, four of which are related to the study design (see Sect. 3.5.2.1); hence they are usually verified during the preparation of the study. In IBM-SPSS version 24, checking on linearity between the outcome and the predictor variables (see Sect. 3.5.2.2) and exclusion of multicollinearity between predictors are executed outside the main analysis (see Sect. 3.5.2.3). On the other hand, abnormal data points are verified by the product of the analysis itself after being executed (see Sect. 3.5.2.4).

3.5.2.1 Assumptions Related to the Study Design

We have to verify four assumptions during the preparation of the study, concerning the outcome, the predictor variables, the observations and the sample size. The outcome variable should be dichotomous. Independent predictor variables can be quantitative or qualitative. If qualitative, they should be dummy or indicator coded, with mutually exclusive categories. If quantitative, they can be discrete or continuous. As in regression, observations have to be independent, and the minimum required number is 10–15 observations per each predictor variable introduced in the equation.

Table 3.42 Logistic regression analysis with one discrete predictor

	Negative test	Positive test	Total
Myocardial infarction	1	6	7
No myocardial infarction	8	2	10
Total	9	8	17

3.5.2.2   Linearity Between the Quantitative Predictors and the Logit of the Outcome

By looking to "Eq. 3.12" we can see that logistic regression assumes a linear relationship between (logit P) and the predictors (x). A change (increase or decrease) in a predictor is expected to induce a concomitant change in the logit of the outcome. This linearity has to be valid for the full range of the continuous predictors but is not necessary for the qualitative predictors.

The Box-Tidwell Test

There are several methods to test for a linear relationship between the continuous independent variables and the logit of the dependent variable. The Box-Tidwell is a two-step approach that transforms each continuous predictor into its natural log value and adds the interaction term (predictor*natural log) to the regression equation [14]. Linearity is verified whenever the interaction term is statistically non-significant [9]. This setting applies the Bonferroni correction for the inflated value due to multiple testing. Consequently, the critical P value to reject the null hypothesis (to reject linearity) will be equal to 0.05/number of variables in the model [6]. For example, suppose we have three variables in the model. In that case, we can reject the linearity of a particular predictor variable if the P-value of its interaction term is equal to 0.0125 or smaller.

As we cannot compute the log of zero or negative values, predictors with such values must be initially manipulated to have a minimum value of one. Suppose the name of the original variable is Score and that x is its actual non-transformable minimum (x = zero or a negative value).

- We click on "Transform" then "Compute" and suggest a new name for the variable in the "Target Variable" box.
- In the "Numeric Expression" box, we type: 1 + abs(x) + Score. We click "OK" to execute the transformation.

Note that we do not type the semicolons, x was put between brackets and, there are no spaces in the command. The command means that the software has to add to Score (the original variable) the number 1 plus the minimum original value in the absolute scale. Now we become ready to apply the two steps of the Box-Tidwell approach.

3.5.2.3   Absence of Multicollinearity

Multi co-linearity is the undesirable situation where the correlations among the independent variables are strong, and one should determine how much those independent variables are linearly related to one another. The independent contribution of each variable is unstable (inflated) by the presence of the other correlated variable in the model. The solution is to choose one variable and exclude the other.

Multicollinearity is tested in the same way as in regression. As a rule of thumb, a correlation coefficient $r > 0.7$ alarms possible multiple collinearities that can be confirmed in multiple ways, including low tolerance (<0.1) or high variance inflation factor (>10) (see Sect. 3.4.2.3).

3.5.2.4   Absence of Outliers, High Leverage and Influential Points

We have previously defined outliers, data with high leverage, and influential points (see Sect. 3.2.3.2). As in linear regression, data with unusual points negatively affect the regression equation that is used to predict the outcome from the independent variables. In IBM-SPSS, those points are identified by requesting Casewise diagnostics and dealt with, as we have shown in linear regression (see Sect. 3.4.2.5).

3.5.3   The Example

We will continue with the same example used in linear regression, which showed that the duration of ICU stay was significantly related to the period of surgery. There were 12 mortalities among the 60 patients, and the researchers were interested in investigating the sample for possible independent predictors of mortality (Table 3.35).

3.5.4 Designing the Model

The reader is requested to refer back to multiple regression analysis to get the general information about the design regarding how variables are introduced in the model (see Sect. 3.4.3). We usually introduce variables that were found to be statistically significant on bivariate analysis. We can extend our inclusion to those predictors with a P-value between 0.05 and 0.1 and to predictors that were found by others to be statistically significant. Qualitative variables with less than 5 cases per category weaken the model and, they are better avoided, or we can collapse categories, if possible. In total, the researcher can introduce one variable for each 10–15 cases included in the study in logistic regression.

Table 3.43 shows the results of bivariate analysis. The amount of blood loss and motorcycle accidents were significantly related to mortality, and hence, we will include those two variables in the analysis.

3.5.5 Verification of the Assumptions [6–10]

We will use IBM-SPSS version 24 for MAC to verify data and interpret the results.

3.5.5.1 The Study Design
The four assumptions related to study design are usually verified during the preparation of the study. We have one binary outcome (dependent variable), which is mortality. We have two predictors (independent variables); one continuous variable (amount of blood loss) and one categorical variable (motorcycle accident) that includes > 5 cases per category. Observations are independent. The total sample size is 60 patients is sufficient to include the two predictors. Data are uploaded to the software, as shown in Table 3.35.

3.5.5.2 Linearity Between the Quantitative Predictors and the Logit of Outcome
We begin by the first step of Box-Tidwell procedure and transform the continuous variable (amount of blood loss) into its natural log value.

- We click on "Transform then "Compute".
- We suggest a name for the new predictor (e.g., Ln amount) in the "Target Variable" box.
- In the "Numeric Expression" box, we type: Ln [amount of blood loss] and click "OK". We can return to the data view to verify that the new variable was created (Ln amount).

The second step involves the execution of the logistic regression procedure just to verify the linearity of the logit of outcome across all levels of the continuous predictor variable.

Table 3.43 Logistic regression analysis: results of bivariate analysis of mortality in 60 polytraumatized patients

	Age	Female gender	MCA	Blood loss[a]	Surgery duration[b]	ICU stay[c]
Survivors (n = 48)	29.18 ± 14.8	9 (69.2%)	1 (8.3%)	430.2 ± 271.2	90.6 ± 52.9	6.25 ± 1.65
Mortalities (n = 12)	34.1 ± 14.9	4 (30.8%)	11 (91.7%)	645.8 ± 275.9	104.2 ± 41.2	7.91 ± 1.2
P value	0.312	0.271	<0.001	0.017	0.414	0.21

Values are presented number (%) or mean ± Sd. as correlation coefficient r or mean ± standard deviation of the duration of ICU stay in days, MCA = motorcycle accident, a = amount of blood loss in ml, b = duration of surgery in minutes, c = ICU stay in days

- We click on "Analyze" then "Regression" then "Binary Logistic".
- We open the main window and shift (mortality) to the "Dependent" box and three variables (motorcycle accident), (amount of blood loss) and the interaction term (Ln amount* amount of blood loss) to the "Covariates" box.
- We click on "Categorical" to open the "Define Categorical Variables" window and shift (motorcycle accident) to the "Categorical Covariates" box.
- We click "Continue" then "OK" to execute the analysis. We scroll down along the many results and verify that our interaction term was statistically non-significant (P = 0.855); which is all that we need to know from this "quick" analysis.

3.5.5.3 Exclusion of Multicollinearity

Unfortunately, IBM-SPSS does not allow verification of multicollinearity between predictors from within the logistic regression analysis procedure. One simple solution is to request a multiple regression analysis using the same predictors, where the program routinely calculates the correlation coefficient r, Tolerance, and Variance inflation factor (VIF). Continuous predictors should not be highly correlated, and as a rule of thumb, correlation coefficient r must be below 0.7. A variable with low Tolerance (<0.1) and high VIF (>10) indicates the presence of multicollinearity with another variable and should be dealt with (see Sect. 3.4.5). Multicollinearity will not be tested in our example as the model includes only one continuous predictor variable.

3.5.5.4 Execution of the Analysis

- We click on "Analyze" then "Regression" then "Binary Logistic" to open the "logistic Regression" window. We shift (mortality) to the "Dependent" box and the (amount of blood loss) and (motorcycle accident) to the "Covariates" box.

- We click on "Categorical" to open the "Define Categorical Variables" window and shift (motorcycle accident) to the "Categorical Covariates" box. As motorcycle accident was coded as (0, 1) for (no, yes), we have to make sure to change the "indicator" from being "last", which is the default in SPSS, to "first" and click "change" then "continue" to close this window.
- Click on "Options" to open its window and request "Classification plots", Hosmer-Lemeshow goodness-of-fit", "Casewise listing of residuals" and "Outliers outside 2 Std. dev"., "CI for exp(B) 95%", and click "Continue" to close the window.
- Click to open the "Save" window and request "Probabilities", Cook's distance", "Leverage values", "Studentized" Residuals and "Standardized" residuals. Click "Continue" then "OK" to generate the output of the analysis.

3.5.5.5 Checking on Outliers, High Leverage and Influential Points

- Part of the procedure was to request IBM-SPSS to produce a "Case Wise List" that reveals cases with "standardized residuals" more than + 3Sd or −3Sd, so as the researcher can deal with those outliers. In case there are no outliers, IBM-SPSS does not produce the table, which was our case.
- Cases 33 and 48 had a high Cook's distance of 2.5.
- Checking on the saved column of leverage values, we had a case (case number 50) with a high leverage value of 0.294. All three cases were left and reported.

3.5.6 Model Evaluation

The model's value depends on its ability to answer three main questions: how well are the data fitted in the model so that the collection of predictors explains a significant part of the outcome? What is the value of the independent role of each predictor included in the model? Can we use the model to predict the outcomes of future studies?

3.5.6.1   The Model Summary

The Hosmer–Lemeshow (H–L) Goodness of Fit

The main aim of a logistic regression model is to predict the probability of the event to occur for a particular patient, i.e., the expected probability of the event. The H–L test classifies the patients according to their expected probabilities into ten groups (g) of approximately equal size. For each group of size (n), there is a number of patients who already developed the event (observed events) and others who did not (observed non-events). For each group, the test calculates the predicted number of events (expected events) and, the predicted number of non-events (expected non-events). A regular Pearson's Chi-square test is then applied to compare the observed to the expected counts and, the calculated difference is verified in Chi-square value, at 8 (g-2) df. It is clear that the larger is the difference between what was observed in the study and what is expected by the model, the less likely data are fit in the model. As many goodness-of-fit tests, a statistically significant result means that our data does not fit in the model, and a statistically non-significant result means that we do not have enough evidence that data do not fit but it does not confirm that they do. Consequently, the test has low power in small studies, i.e., not being able to collect evidence of non-fitting due to a small sample size. Among other things, the test has been largely criticized for being largely dependent on the number of groups (g), the number of covariates and the unstable effect of interaction [27].

IBM-SPSS calculates H–L test upon request and presents the H–L contingency table, with observed and calculated (expected) number of events in the ten groups. In our example, the calculated chi-square value was 7.683 and the corresponding P value was 0.465 and hence, we can assume that there is no enough evidence that it is a poor fit.

The Omnibus Test for Model Coefficients

IBM-SPSS begins by calculating a (*Step 0 model*) that does not include any predictor but just the constant. IBM-SPSS present this step in a table entitled "Variables in the equation". The aim is just to create a benchmark to show how much the inclusion of the predictors will improve the model later on.

The omnibus tests of model coefficients (*Step 1 model*) test the statistical significance of the model after including the two predictors besides the constant. The test is a modified Chi-square comparing the results obtained before to those obtained after including the two predictor variables. At 3 df, the resulting large chi-square value of 43.8 is highly significant; $P < 0.001$. How should we interpret this result? Being an omnibus test, it does not mean that the two predictors and the constant have significant shares in explaining the outcome, which will be assessed by analyzing the regression coefficients of each predictor. It only means that at least one of the predictors (and maybe more than one) significantly explains the outcome.

The Model Summary

BM-SPSS produces two pseudo R2 coefficients in a "Model Summary" table. In our study, the software calculated Cox and Snell's R^2 value of 0.518 and Negelkerke's R^2 value of 0.819. As mentioned earlier, Negelkerke's R^2 is an adjusted version of Cox and Snell's R^2, and hence, it is more likely to be presented. The result suggests that the model (motorcycle accident + amount of blood loss + intercept) explained 81.9% of the variability in mortality. The software does not allow the calculation of McFadden's R^2 from within the binary logistic interface, but it is obtained by default in multinomial logistic regression. We can request the latter and shift (mortality) to the "Dependent" box, (motorcycle accident) to the "Factors" box, and the (amount of blood loss) to the "Covariates" box and click "OK". The output provides the three pseudo R2 variants, including McFadden's R^2 value of 0.729, meaning that the model explained 72.9% of mortality.

3.5.6.2 Interpretation of the Regression Coefficients

Table 3.44 shows the variables used in the equation, their B coefficient and Se, the Wald test used for interpreting the statistical significance, the calculated P-value, the odds ratio (Exp B) and its 95%CI. The interpretation is as follows, a one-unit change (increases or decreases) in the predictor changes (increases or decreases) odds of the event by an amount that is equal to the odds ratio (OR). In our example, having a motorcycle accident increases (for having an OR > 1) the odds of mortality by 433 times, which is huge. The increase in the odds varies between nearly 25 and 7485 times (P < 0.001). On the other hand, the amount of blood loss did not significantly contribute to mortality (P = 0.562). A one ml. increase in the amount of blood loss increases the odds of mortality by 0.002% (OR = 1.002; 95 CI = 0.996–1.007). Put it another way, each one liter (1000 ml.) increase in the amount of blood loss doubles the odds of mortality. Remember that we can always change the odds into the risk Odds/(1+Odds) and hence, each 1 L of blood loss increases the risk of mortality by 66%. However, this increase is not statistically significant (P = 0.562). In the case of a motorcycle accident, the risk of mortality is almost certain 99.77% [433/(433+1); P < 0.001.

3.5.6.3 Prediction of the Outcome

Classification Tables

We have already requested and saved the expected probability of the outcome. If the expected probability is better than chance (>50%), the software classifies as being expected to occur and otherwise as not expected. Consequently, we can calculate sensitivity (Sn), specificity (Sp), and the overall percentage accuracy (TAC) for the model.

Table 3.45 shows the observed events (or no events) and the expected events (or no events) predicted by the analysis. Sensitivity (Sn) can be defined as the proportion of cases that were correctly predicted as dead (having the event) among observed mortalities (11/12 = 91.7%). Specificity (Sp) can be defined as the proportion of cases that were correctly predicted as alive (free from the event) among living cases (47/48 = 97.9%). The percentage accuracy in classification (TAC) = (11 + 47) / (12 + 48) = 96.7%.

Furthermore, we can deduct the positive predictive value (PPV) of the model, which is the proportion of correct diagnosis among all those diagnosed as having the event (true positive + false positive) = 11/(11 + 1) = 91.7%. Equally, we can deduct the negative predictive

Table 3.44 Logistic regression analysis: the coefficients of regression

	B	Se	Wald	df	P value	Exp B	95% CI Exp B
Motorcycle accident	*6.072*	*1.46*	*17.3*	*1*	*<0.001*	*433.7*	*24.8–7484.7*
Amount of blood loss	0.002	0.003	0.336	1	0.562	1.002	0.996–1.007
Constant	−4.593	1.759	6.916	1	0.009	0.010	

B = Beta coefficient = Log Odds, Se = standard error of B coefficient, Wald = Wald Chi-square statistics, Exp B = Exponent value of Beta coefficient = Odds ratio (OR)

Table 3.45 Logistic regression analysis: the classification tables

	Predicted alive	Predicted dead	Correct percentage
Observed alive	47	1	97.9 (specificity)
Observed dead	1	11	91.7 (sensitivity)
Overall percentages			96.7

The cut value is 0.5

Fig. 3.26 Logistic regression
analysis flowchart. H–L
test = Hosmer–Lemeshow
test

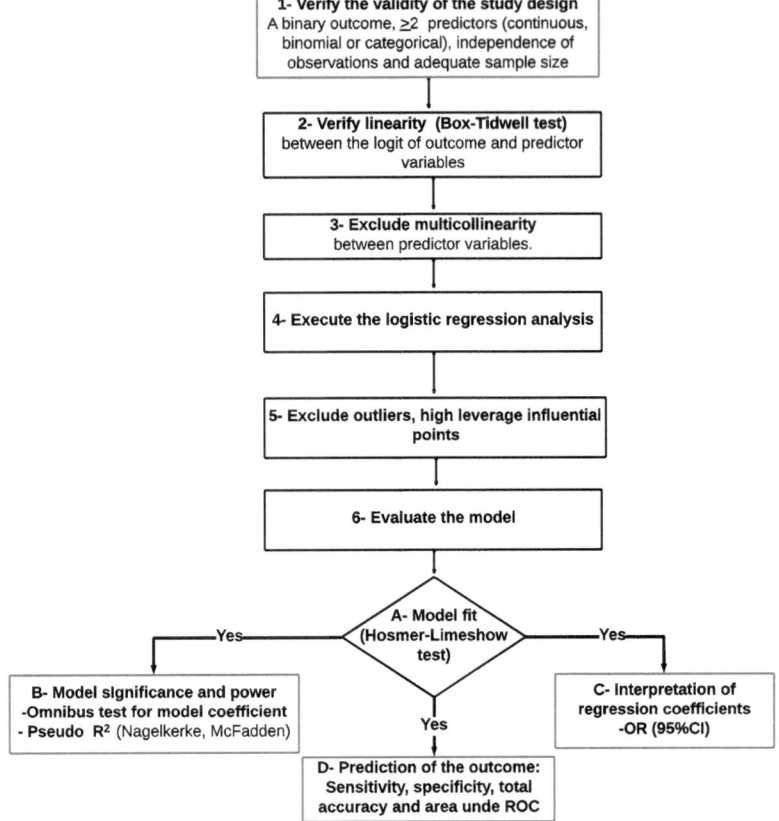

value (NPV) of the model, which is the proportion of correct diagnosis among all those diagnosed as being alive (true negative + false negative) = 47/(47 + 1) = 97.9%. Kindly note that the exact similarity between the calculated Sn and PPV and between the Sp and NPV is just a coincidence. On the other hand, in the case one of the predictors is a quantitative variable and, instead of calculating a single sensitivity and specificity point, we can produce a ROC analysis to evaluate the usefulness of the predictor across a whole spectrum of Sn and Sp (see Sect. 1.9.4.3). Figure 3.26 shows the flow chart of the model.

3.5.7 What Should Be Reported

- The descriptive statistics, as mean (Sd) and numbers (%).
- Results of bivariate analysis results.

- Variables included in logistic regression analysis and reasons behind inclusion or exclusion of some variables.
- The verifications of assumptions, including testing linearity between the logit of the outcome and the dependent predictor variables, verifying the absence of collinearity between predictors, and whether there were any unusual points. We have to report any applied corrections or remedies.
- How data fit the model and test used. The significance of logistic regression, with χ^2 and P-values.
- The percent variation of the outcome, as Negelkerke's R^2 or McFadden's R^2.
- The independent predictors detected by the model, with OR, 95% CI, and P-values.
- The classification tables with Sn, Sp, PPV, NPV, TAC, and AUC-ROC analysis when performed.

- Finally, we should report the effect size and basis of sample size calculation (see Sects. 4.10.1 and 4.10.2).

3.6 Cox Regression Analysis

3.6.1 Introduction: Life Tables Versus Cox Regression Analysis

Like Kaplan–Meier and actuarial analysis, Cox regression is a method for modeling time-to-event data in the presence of censored cases. For example, do men and women have different risks of developing lung cancer based on the number of cigarettes smoked per day? We cannot answer the question by simply regressing (studying the effect of) gender and the number of cigarettes (predictors) on the development of lung cancer (outcome).

First, there is the problem of censoring, such as cases lost to follow-up, that we explained in the chapter on the analysis of time-related events (see Sects. 2.7.2 and 2.7.3). In addition, the outcome variable of interest (developing lung cancer) is most likely not normally distributed, which is a serious violation of an ordinary regression. Moreover, by the end of the study, not all patients will develop the event and hence, we have to calculate an estimate for those patients [33]. We have previously shown that life tables, whether Kaplan–Meier or actuarial analysis can handle the censored cases correctly and provide survival (or event-free) estimates at specific time periods [34] (see Sect. 2.7). Although the researcher can compare estimates among patients' groups by the log-rank test [35] or one of its derivates (see Sect. 2.7.4), yet he cannot investigate the effect of covariates on survival; which is a question of regression. Cox regression analysis was designed to cover up for this advantage [36]. In other words, Cox regression improves the estimates of survival probabilities and cumulative hazards by considering the effect of the predictors, whether being a factor or a covariate. Moreover, it does not only calculate and test the statistical significance of

the individual impact of each predictor but supply estimates of power analysis to calculate sample size for future studies [37] (see Sects. 4.9.1.2 and 4.9.2.2). However, assuming that Cox regression analysis is a superior substitute of life tables analysis is wrong. Cox regression does not provide life tables; i.e., it does not tell the important information which is the probability of having (or being free from) the event, at a specific time period. Hence, we usually have to complement a Cox regression analysis with the more descriptive Kaplan Meier or actuarial analysis.

We have previously shown how to calculate cumulative survival from the probability of the event (see Sect. 2.7.2). The cumulative probability of survival (CP) at a particular interval is the product of the survival probability (SP) and the CP of the preceding interval. For example, suppose that a disease is known to have a high a constant annual hazard mortality of 40% (0.4) in diabetic patients. The cumulative probability of survival for the next seven years will be equal to 0.6, 0.6^2, 0.6^3, 0.6^4, 0.6^5, 0.6^6, 0.6^7 = 60%, 36%, 22%, 13%, 8%, 5%, 3%. Non-diabetic cases have a lower constant annual hazard mortality of 20% (0.2) and hence, their respective cumulative survival rates are 0.8, 0.8^2, 0.8^3, 0.8^4, 0.8^5, 0.8^6, 0.8^7 = 80%, 64%, 51%, 41%, 33, 26%, 21%. As shown in Fig. 3.27, despite the constant hazard rate (parallel dotted lines), the survival rates cannot be linear but make two nearly parallel curves. Kaplan Meier calculates and displays the successive cumulative survival rates for the two groups. Cox regression assumes that the difference between the hazard rates remains constant (proportional), and hence, it took its name: Cox proportional hazard regression. Although it is not calculated as straightforward as it looks, yet anytime throughout the hazard of mortality in diabetic patients is twice that on non-diabetic cases (i.e., the hazard ratio), regardless of the cumulative survival probability at that time. This ratio reflects the effect of diabetes on survival.

In some studies, however, the validity of the proportionality assumption may be questionable. For example, when we analyze the effect of age on patients' survival after surgery, it is likely,

Fig. 3.27 Cox regression analysis: the hazard rate and the cumulative survival

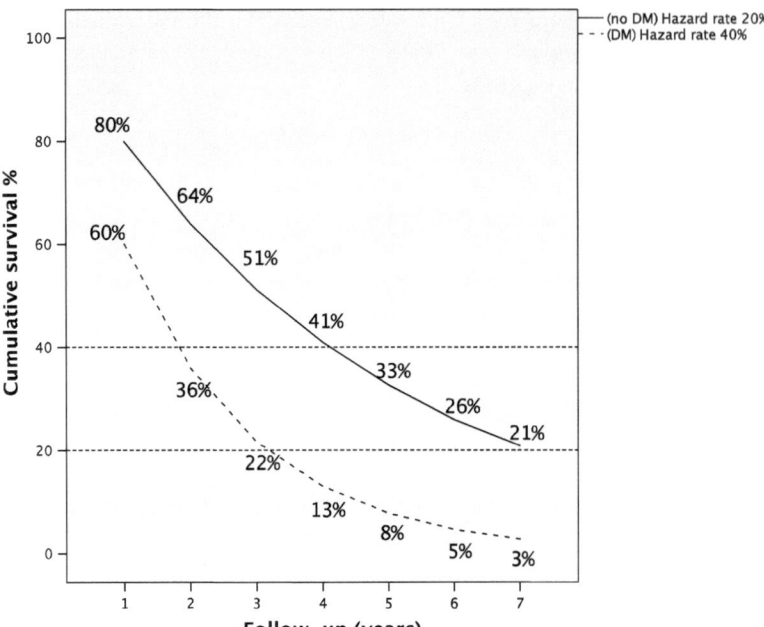

that age is a more important predictor of risk immediately after surgery than after recovery. In other words, early postoperative mortality is expected to be higher among older individuals, while late postoperative survival is expected to be irrelevant with the patient's age. The impact of such a covariate is dependent on time and hence, they are now called time-dependent covariates permitting the model to account for the varying hazard ratio [2]. We thought that the mathematical complexity of Cox regression analysis with a time-dependent covariate might be beyond the scope of this book.

The analysis retains the same three main assumptions of time to event analysis that have been previously discussed (see Sect. 2.7.1). In brief, we have to assume that censored patients will have the same prognosis as those still followed in the study, and hence, we should always investigate if censoring was not related to the event of concern. The second assumption is that the event really happened and is not just being discovered at the specified time. Hence, follow-up has to be as meticulous and as complete as possible. Finally, we have to assume that patients have to have the same prognosis, whether they have been censored or not and, regardless of their

follow-up duration and when they were recruited for the study [33, 36–40].

3.6.2   The Basic Assumptions [36–40]

Cox regression analysis is demanding, and the researcher has to verify seven delicate assumptions before executing the analysis. Six assumptions can be verified and arranged for during the preparation of the study (Sect. 3.6.2.1). The last important assumption is the proportionality of hazard and is the key element to execute the analysis (see Sect. 3.6.2.2). Otherwise, the researcher has to shift to the more demanding Cox regression analysis with time-dependent covariate.

3.6.2.1   Assumptions Related to the Study Design

- The event status should consist of two mutually exclusive and collectively exhaustive states: event and censored. There should be independence between censoring and the event. We have to minimize or better avoid left censoring (patients developing the event before the beginning of the study), with a nearly similar amount of censoring in compared groups. The latter is essential to perform a log-rank test as part of a complementary Kaplan Meier analysis.

- The time variable should be quantitative, clearly defined, and precisely measured.
- The predictor variables can be either categorical or continuous (covariates).
- The observations should be independent.
- The sample size has to be adequate and the reader is requested to refer to chapter four for sample size calculation (see Sect. 4.9.2.2).
- During the study, there should be no secular trends, such as a change in disease pattern, risk factors, the appearance of a new treatment, new study methods, or the introduction of any element that can bias our judgment. Secular trends are mostly due to prolonged time of recruitment or extended follow-up periods.

3.6.2.2 Proportionality Assumption

Before going through this section, the reader is advised to refer to chapter one to review the definition of the hazard, types of hazard estimation, and hazard ratio (see Sect. 1.8.3.2). Let us revise some definitions. The hazard rate h(t) is defined as the rate of the event at time t, provided that the patient was alive at that time or beyond. Put it this way; it is the rate of the event that will occur in the next coming minute, provided that the person was free till that minute; i.e., The hazard function is instantaneous. The cumulative hazard at a time (t) is the risk of the event to occur between time 0 and time t, and the survivor function at time t is the probability of surviving to time (t) [38]. The hazard ratio (HR) is the ratio between two hazards and, in Cox regression analysis, the HR, and not the hazard itself, is assumed to be constant over time.

Cox proportional hazard regression analysis is a combination of 2 techniques: survival analysis and regression analysis. The idea of the analysis is to divide the effect of time into a series of repeated observations over specific time intervals in a way that, for example, each year lived by a member of the sample constitutes an observation. We calculate the corresponding series of probabilities of new cases developing the event of interest in all observations. Finally, we average the probabilities to obtain an overall reference survival curve called the baseline hazard function [$h_0(t)$]. Cox proportional hazard assumes that the basic hazard function is time-dependent and free to vary (to increase or decrease) as time goes by [39]. As the time to an event does not follow a normal distribution, this part of the Cox model is called the non-parametric component of Cox regression.

The second part of the model calculates the effect of predictors (explanatory variables) on the annual risk of experiencing the event through regression analysis. Each variable is associated with a regression coefficient that measures its effect on the annual risk of developing the event. The model assumes that the hazard to develop the event due to a particular predictor is unrelated to time. In other words, the ratio between the hazard to develop the event due to the presence of one predictor (e.g., in the treatment group) and the hazard to develop the event in its absence (e.g., in the control group) is constant (proportional), at all times [39]. This part of the model is the parametric component: a regression analysis weighting the effect of each predictor on the outcome as the adjusted HR. As outcome will be the combination of the effects of an "averaged" baseline hazard and the individual effect of each predictor, a change in outcome can be explained by the change in hazard ratio. As such, Cox regression is often described as being a semi-parametric procedure.

Before going through the equation, the reader is advised to refer back to logistic regression because both techniques have many similarities. Kindly revise why we had to transfer the binary event into a probability, then into odds and why we adopted the logarithms of the odds in the calculations instead of the odds themselves. We will adopt the same demarche in Cox regression analysis. In short, we will transform the binary outcome into probability to calculate a particular probability percent to develop the event, and not just yes or no, in concordance with the observed change on the scale of the predictor variable. We then changed the probability into hazard because the hazard answers the study question: what are the odds to have or not to have the outcome? We transform the "non-linear" hazard into a "linear" log-hazard to predict an "accurate" log-hazard value for each corresponding value of the predictor variable, as we do in linear regression. The resulting "accurate log-hazard" can be converted back to the easily expressed and more understandable hazard scale.

On the other hand, we have shown that the Exp. of b coefficient of logistic regression is the OR, and hence, a one-unit change in predictor changes the odds of the outcome by a value that is equal to the odds ratio of the predictor (see Sect. 3.5.1). Synonymously, the hazard ratio is the Exp. of the beta coefficient in Cox regression. A one-unit change in predictor changes the hazard of the outcome by a value equal to the hazard ratio of the predictor. As an example, if the HR associated with the presence of diabetes mellitus is (2) and the event is mortality after surgery, being diabetic doubles the hazard of mortality, compared to a non-diabetic patient.

The model calculates the hazard rate of the event (h), at a given time (t) and for the given values of the predictor variables for the respective case $(x_1, x_2, x_3,..., x_i)$ by the equation "Eq. 3.15":

$$h(t), (x_1, x_2, x_3, \ldots, x_i) = h_0(t) * \exp^G \quad (3.15)$$

The left side of "Eq. 3.15" denotes the resultant hazard, given the respective time to event (t) and the values of the covariates $(x_1, x_2, x_3, ...x_i)$. The right side of the equation shows that the hazard is the product of the baseline hazard $[h_0(t)]$ and the exponential value of (G) "Eq. 3.16". The baseline hazard is the hazard when all independent variable values are equal to zero. In other words, it is the synonym of the constant in the regression equation, which leaves us with the term (G) to be explained.

$$G = b_1x_1 + b_2x_2 + b_3x_3 + \ldots + b_jx_i \quad (3.16)$$

(G) describes the effect of predictors on the outcome by a regular regression equation: the sum of the product of each variable (x) by its regression coefficient "Eq. 3.16". Where $b_{1,2,3, \ldots, j}$ are the regression coefficients indicating the impact of $x_{1,2,3, \ldots i}$ predictor variables on the outcome. Note that the b coefficients shown in "Eq. 3.16" are log-hazard and not hazard, which permitted the addition of their effects $(b_1x_1 + b_2x_2 + \ldots)$. Consequently, we transferred G to "Eq. 3.15" as $(\exp^G)$. Both equations "Eqs. 3.15 and 3.16" can now be combined into "Eq. 3.17".

$$h(t), (x_1, x_2, x_3, \ldots x_m) = h_0(t) * \exp^{b_1x_1, b_2x_2, b_3x_3, \ldots b_jx_i} \quad (3.17)$$

Finally, let us see now see how we calculate HR? We have already assumed that the baseline hazard $[h_0(t)]$ is an average and is hence, the same for all study individuals. Suppose that we have only one predictor variable for two individuals (x_1) and (x_2), for an example, being diabetic or not. The hazard ratio of those two individuals will be calculated by "Eq. 3.18", which clearly shows (HR) is a function of only the difference in the respective regression variables (difference between being diabetic or not = effect diabetes). It is independent of the baseline hazard.

$$HR = \frac{h_i(t), x1}{h_j(t), x2} = \frac{h_0(t) * e^{x_1}\beta}{h_0(t) * e^{x_2}\beta} = e^{(x_1-x_2)\beta} = e^{(\Delta x)\beta}$$

$$(3.18)$$

3.6.3 The Example

We will continue with the same example used in linear and logistic regression, which showed that the duration of ICU stay was significantly related to the duration of surgery and that mortality was significantly associated with the type of accident, with the victim riding a motorcycle. There were 12 mortalities among the 60 patients; all died in the ICU, while the other 48 survivors have left the hospital. The researchers wanted to know the predictors of time to mortality, and hence, Cox regression was the analysis of choice? We have already uploaded the data shown in Table 3.35 to IBM-SPSS.

3.6.4   Designing the Model [6, 7, 37]

SPSS commands for analyzing Cox regression are very similar to those used for logistic regression, and the main difference is how to interpret the coefficients. In addition, we will perform a Kaplan Meier analysis to obtain survival tables.

3.6.5   Verification of the Assumptions

3.6.5.1   The Study Design

- We had two mutually exclusive event states: mortality or censored.
- The time variable was quantitative: the duration of follow-up in ICU, calculated in days, was clearly defined and precisely measured.
- We had two mutually exclusive categorical predictor variables: gender and motorcycle accident and three continuous variables: age in years, duration of surgery in minutes, and amount of blood loss in ml.
- Observations were independent and the sample size was judged as being adequate.
- Due to the nature of the study, we did not have any left-censored cases lost to follow-up or secular patterns.

3.6.5.2   Execution of a Complementary Kaplan–Meier Analysis

It is not mandatory to perform a Kaplan Meier analysis, which will not help in evaluating the effect of multiple predictors; however, it provides life tables and a visual check on the proportionality assumption. The procedure was described in detail in Sect. 2.7.2, and hence, we will be satisfied here by performing a complimentary quick analysis:

- We click on "Analyze" then "Survival," and we choose "Kaplan-Meier" to open the main window of the analysis. We shift (mortality) to the "Status" box and click on "Define event" to open its window. We type the code given to mortality (1) and click "Continue" to return to the main window.

- We shift the (duration of ICU stay) to the "Time" box and the factor (motorcycle accident) to the "Factor" box. We have chosen the latter because it was shown to be significantly related to mortality in bivariate analysis.
- We click on "Compare Factor" and then choose the "Test statistics": "Log-rank" test, and we click on "Continue" to return to the main window.
- We click on "Options" and choose "Survival tables", "Mean and median survival", and "Survival" "Plots". By clicking on "Continue" we become all set for the analysis and click "OK".

The overall mean survival was 9.336 ± 1.93 days (95% CI; 8.9 to 9.7 days). The 12 patients who were not involved in a motorcycle accident showed significantly better survival than the other 48 patients ($75 \pm 21.7\%$ versus $8.33 \pm 8\%$; $P < 0.001$). The median survival of the 12 patients who experienced a motorcycle accident was 8 ± 3.75 ($7.26 - 8.73$) days. On the other hand, we could not calculate a median value for the 48 patients who did not experience a motorcycle accident because only one case did develop the event. Figure 3.28 shows parallel survival curves, which visually verifies the proportionality assumption.

3.6.5.3   Verification of the Proportionality Assumption

- Besides the eyeball check of Kaplan Meier curves, we can verify the proportionality assumption of a categorical predictor variable (e.g., treatment groups) by requesting a log minus log plot and confirming that the lines are parallel. In IBM-SPSS, we begin by clicking on "Analyze", then "Survival", then on "Cock's regression" to open its main window.
- We shift the (ICU stay) to the "Time" box and (mortality) to the "Status" box. We click on "Define Event" to enter the "Single value" (1) and click on "Continue".

Fig. 3.28 Cox regression
analysis: the Kaplan Meier
curves

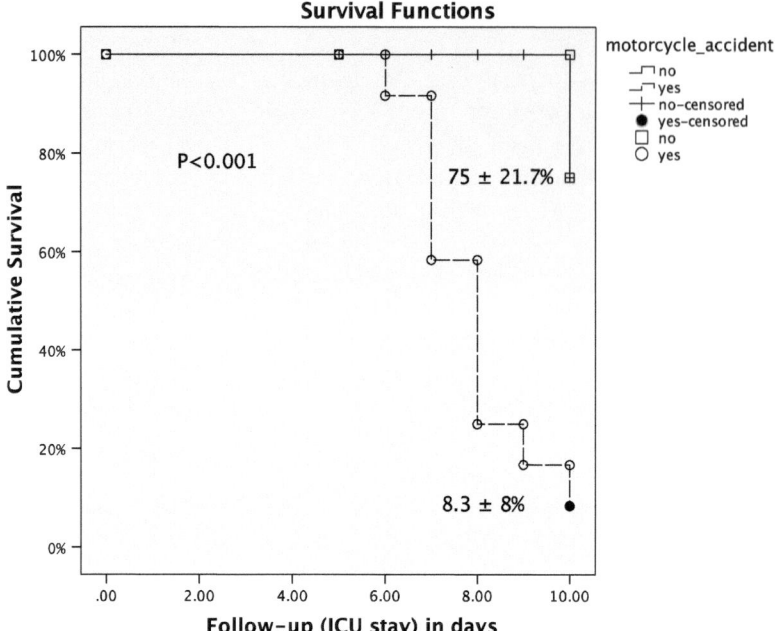

- We shift the binomial predictor to the "Strata" box, we click on "Plots" and request a "log minus log" from the "Plot type", and then we click on "OK". The curves are produced, and we can inspect whether they are parallel or not?

- On the other hand, we can check the proportionality assumption of a continuous predictor by formal statistical testing. The idea is simple and bright. The regression model is mended to estimate the value of a (y) outcome, given an (x) predictor and, subtracting the "y-estimate" from the "y-observed" gives the residual error of the regression. Flipping the concept on its head by estimating x for a given y and subtracting that estimate from the observed x gives the residuals for the predictors or Schoenfeld residuals [27]. The proportionality assumption is verified when there is no interaction between the predictor and time; i.e., the predictor does not vary with time. In IBM-SPSS, we click on "Analyze", then "Survival", then on "Cock's with time-dependent covariate" to open its main window. We shift the

Time[T_] variable to the "Expression for T_COV_" box, then we multiply it by the predictor variable in question, e.g., surgery_-duration, by clicking on (*) then the variable name (surgery_duration). It will look like this: T_*surgery_duration. We click on the "Model" button to open the "Cock's analysis main window", where we will find the new variable that we have just created. We shift both the new variable (T_COV_) and the old variable (surgery_duration) to the "Block 1 of 1" box. We shift the (ICU stay) to the "Time" box, and (mortality) to the "Status" box. We click on "Define Event" to enter the "Single value" (1) and click "Continue". The output will contain the table entitled "variables in the equation" and shows that the P-value of the interaction term (T_COV_) is not significant. In our example, the P-value was 0.883; which verified the proportionality assumption. Unfortunately, we must repeat the same process for each continuous predictor (age and amount of blood loss) to verify that they are not dependent on time.

3.6.5.4 Execution of the Cox Regression Model

- In IBM-SPSS, we begin by clicking on "Analyze", then "Survival", then on "Cock's regression" to open its main window.
- We shift the (ICU stay) to the "Time" box and (mortality) to the "Status" box. We click on "Define Event" to enter the "Single value" (1) and click on "Continue."
- We shift the predictors (age, gender, amount of blood loss, surgery_ duration, and motorcycle accident) to the "Block 1 on 1" box.
- We click "Categorical" to ensure the coding of our variables: 0 for females and no motorcycle accident and 1 for males and motorcycle accident. We change the indicator from the SPSS default "last" to "first," and we click on "Change" then on "Continue", which takes us back to the main Cox regression window.
- We click on "Plots" and choose "Survival" and "Hazard" and separate lines for categorical variables such as (gender) and (motorcycle accident). We click on "Continue," which takes us back to the main window.
- We click on "Save" and choose to save "Survival function" and "Hazard function," and we click on "Continue" to return to the main window.
- We click on "Options" and check on the (95% confidence interval of expB). We click on "Continue" to go back to the main window and finally click on "OK" to execute the analysis.

3.6.6 Model Evaluation

3.6.6.1 The Model Summary

We have previously mentioned that the usual model fit by least of squares could not be applied for binary outcomes and the best fitting curve was the one achieving the maximum likelihood ratios (see Sect. 3.5.1). Deviance is a term used to describe the difference between two models: the model with intercept only and no predictors (0 model) and the model with all predictors being

on board (full model). The difference (deviance) expresses how good the predictors fit in the model? We have previously shown that statisticians prefer to use the log-likelihood ratios, and the goodness of fit statistics for those models is calculated as -2 log-likelihood ratio [26, 27]. The difference (deviance) is then tested against a chi-square distribution with degrees of freedom equal to the difference between the old and new models' degrees of freedom.

In our example, SPSS showed a (-2log-likelihood) of (77.097) for model (0) and (32.666) for the full model. The statistical significance of the difference (44.431) was checked out in the Chi-square table at 5 df (5 predictors + 1 constant $-$ 1); $P < 0.001$.

3.6.6.2 The Individual Contribution of the Predictors

The regression coefficients predict the hazard of the event. A positive coefficient indicates a positive relationship between the predictor and the hazard of the event, which means that higher values are associated with a higher mortality hazard. A negative coefficient indicates a negative relationship between the predictor and the hazard of the event. Higher values are associated with a smaller hazard of mortality [6, 38].

The calculated HR ratio is interpreted as follows: "a unit change" in the predictor "changes the hazard of the outcome" by an average amount equal to the calculated HR. For example, a study has shown that age calculated in years and male gender were independent predictors of mortality, with respective hazard ratios of 1.1 and 1.5. The interpretation is as follows: there is an average 10% increase in the hazard of mortality, relative to each one-year increase in age or, the expected hazard is 1.1 times higher in a person who is one year older than another, holding other predictors constant. The expected mortality hazard is 1.5 times higher in men than women, holding all other predictors constant. The model equally calculates the 95% confidence intervals of HR, and the reader is advised to refer to Sect. 1.8.7 for the accurate interpretation of those intervals.

Table 3.46 shows the results of our example; both the duration of surgery and a motorcycle

Table 3.46 Cox proportional regression analysis: the coefficients of regression

	B	Se	Wald	df	P value	Exp B	95% CI Exp B
Age	0.047	0.037	1.610	1	0/204	1.048	0.975–1.127
Gender	−1.627	0.987	2.717	1	0.099	0.197	0.028–1.360
Duration of surgery	*−1.21*	*0.052*	*5.392*	*1*	*0.02*	*0.886*	*0.801–0.981*
Amount of blood loss	0.001	0.002	0.163	1	0.686	1.001	0.997–1.004
Motorcycle accident	*2.345*	*1.095*	*4.59*	*1*	*0.032*	*10.438*	*1.221– 89.220*

B = Beta coefficient = Log hazard, Se = Standard error of B coefficient, Wald Chi-square statistics, Exp B = Exponent value of Beta coefficient = Hazard ratio (HR)

accident significantly explained the variation in mortality. The duration of surgery had a negative effect on outcome; i.e., longer duration of surgery was associated with a significant decrease in the hazard of mortality, in the sense that one minute increase in the duration of surgery decreased the hazard of mortality by about 11%, with all other variables being kept constant. The decrease varied between 1.9–19.9%; P = 0.02. Remember that surgery had a significant positive effect on the duration of ICU stay (i.e., it prolonged the follow-up duration). Hence, it delayed the onset of mortality (see Sect. 3.4.6). A motorcycle accident was previously shown to increase mortality (see Sect. 3.5.6). It has a significant positive effect on the outcome. The risk of mortality in a patient who had a motorcycle accident is ten times that of another case who was not involved in such an accident; all other variables being kept constant (1.2 to 89 times; P = 0.032). Figure 3.29 shows the Cox regression analysis flowchart.

3.6.7   What Should Be Reported

- The descriptive statistics and results of survival tables analysis, with mean and median survival, standard errors and 95% confidence intervals.

- Verification of assumptions related to the study design; the method used to verify the proportionality assumption.
- The overall significance value of the model, with Chi-square and P-values.
- Table of hazard coefficient, with standard error, results of Wald statistics, P-value, hazard ratios, and 95% confidence intervals.
- Plots of survival or hazard rates and log minus log plot if performed.
- Finally, we should report the effect size and basis of sample size calculation (see Sects. 4.9.1 and 4.9.2).

Cox regression analysis can be seen as the control of predictor variables in survival analysis through regression or the introduction of the temporal factor in regression analysis. The idea is that one technique will fill the gap of the other. namely the factor time missing in the logit model, which neglect the information contained in the censored cases. In the survival technique we mis the effect of explanatory variables and splitting the sample into multiple small samples is a source of bias and we cannot calculate the interaction

Fig. 3.29 Cox regression anlysis flow chart, a = secular trends should be maintained (avoided) throughout the analysis

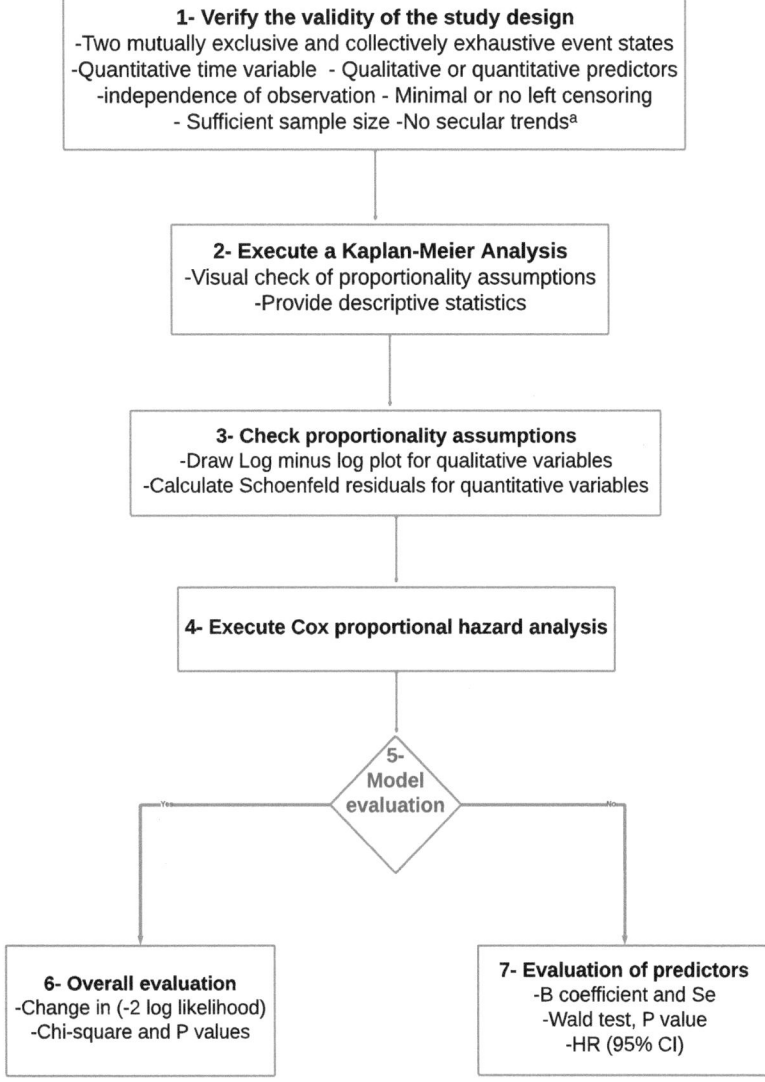

1- Verify the validity of the study design
-Two mutually exclusive and collectively exhaustive event states
-Quantitative time variable - Qualitative or quantitative predictors
-independence of observation - Minimal or no left censoring
- Sufficient sample size -No secular trends[a]

2- Execute a Kaplan-Meier Analysis
-Visual check of proportionality assumptions
-Provide descriptive statistics

3- Check proportionality assumptions
-Draw Log minus log plot for qualitative variables
-Calculate Schoenfeld residuals for quantitative variables

4- Execute Cox proportional hazard analysis

5- Model evaluation

Yes

No

6- Overall evaluation
-Change in (-2 log likelihood)
-Chi-square and P values

7- Evaluation of predictors
-B coefficient and Se
-Wald test, P value
-HR (95% CI)

References

1. Hidalgo B, Goodman M. Multivariate or multivariable regression? Am J Public Health 2013; 103:39–40. https://doi.org/10.2105%2FAJPH.2012.300897.

2. Katz, M H. Multivariable analysis: A primer for readers of medical research. Ann Intern Med. 2003;138 (2003): 644-650. https://doi.org/10.7326/0003-4819-138-8-200304150-00012.

3. Laplanche A, Com-Nougue C, Flamant R. Methodes statistiques appliquées a la recherche Clinique. Paris: Flammarion-Medecine-Sciences. 1987. http://bdsp-ehesp.inist.fr/vibad/index.php?action=getRecordDetail&idt=52329.

4. Armitage P, Berry G. Statistical Methods in Medical Research. 4th ed. UK: Blackwell publishing; 2002.

5. Rosner B. Fundametals of biostatistics. 4th ed. Belmont, California: Duxbury Press; 1995.

6. Tabachnick BG, Fidell LS. Using Multivariate Statistics. 6th ed. Boston, MA: Pearson Education; 2013.

7. IBM SPSS Advanced Statistics 24. https://people.math.aau.dk/~rw/Undervisning/PhDMixedModels/Material/IBM_SPSS_Advanced_Statistics.pdf. Copyright IBM Corporation 1989, 2016. Assessed June 202.

8. Pallant J. SPSS survival manual. A step-by-step data analysis using IBM SPSS. 6th ed. Berkshire, England. Open University press. McGraw-Hill Education; 2016.

9. Field A. Discovering statistics using IBM SPSS statistics. 5th Ed. Los Angeles: Sage publications; 2018. https://us.sagepub.com/en-us/nam/discovering-statistics-using-ibm-spss-statistics/book260423.

10. Laerd Statistics. SPSS Statistical tutorials and software guides. Lund Research Ltd. 2018. https://statistics.laerd.com/; Accessed 15 Aug 2021.

11. Chatterjee S, Hadi AS. Influential observations, high leverage points, and outliers in linear regression. Statist Sci. 1986;1(3):379–93. https://doi.org/10.1214/ss/1177013622.

12. Cook RD, Weisberg S. Residuals and influence in regression. 2nd Ed. New York-London: Chapman and Hall; 1982. https://hdl.handle.net/11299/37076.

13. Howell DC. Statistical methods for psychology, 7th ed. Canada: Wadsworth Cengage Learning; 2010.

14. Box GEP, Tidwell PW. Transformation of independent variables. Technometrics 1962; 4:531–50. https://www.jstor.org/stable/1266288.

15. Altman DG, Bland JM. Units of analysis. BMJ. 1997;314:1874. https://doi.org/10.1136/bmj.314.7098.1874.

16. Mauchly JW. Significance Test for Sphericity of a Normal n-Variate Distribution. Annals Math Stat. 1940;11(2): 204–9. http://www.jstor.org/stable/2235878.

17. O'Brien RG, Kaiser MK. MANOVA method for analyzing repeated measures designs: An extensive primer. Psychol Bull. 1985; 97(2): 316–33. https://doi.org/10.1037/0033-2909.97.2.316.

18. Hahs-Vaughn DL. Applied multivariate statistical concepts. 1st ed. New York: Routledge; 2016. https://doi.org/10.4324/9781315816685.

19. Concato J, Feinstein A, Holford T. Review: the risk of determining risk with multivariable models. Annals Internal Med. 1993;118(3):201–10.

20. Campbell MJ. Statistics at square two. 2nd ed. Blackwell Publishing: India, BMJ Books; 2006.

21. Rodgers JL. The Bootstrap, the Jackknife, and the randomization test: a sampling taxonomy. Multivar Behav Res. 1999;34(4):441–56. https://doi.org/10.1207/S15327906MBR3404_2.

22. Durbin J, Watson GS. Testing for serial correlation in least squares regression I. Biometrika 1950;37:409–28. https://www.jstor.org/stable/2332391; Accessed Nov 2021.

23. Durbin-Watson significance tables. https://www3.nd.edu/~wevans1/econ30331/Durbin_Watson_tables.pdf. Accessed 10 May 2021.

24. Hayes AF. RLM version 1.02. In Darlington RB, Hayes AF editors. Regression analysis and linear models: concepts, applications, and implementation. New York: The Guilford Press; 2017 https://www.processmacro.org/index.html Accessed Jan 2022.

25. Daryanto A. Tutorial on heteroskedasticity using heteroskedasticityV3 SPSS macro. Quantit Methods

26. Cox DR, Snell EJ. The analysis of binary data, 2nd ed. London: Chapman and Hall; 1989. https://doi.org/10.1201/9781315137391.

27. Hosmer DW, Lemeshow S. Applied logistic regression, 2nd ed. New York: John Wiley and Sons; 2004. https://doi.org/10.1002/sim.1236.

28. Bewick V, Cheek L, Ball J. Statistics review 14: logistic regression. Crit Care. 2005;9(1):112–8. https://doi.org/10.1186/cc3045.

29. Allison PD. Logistic regression using SAS: theory and application. 2nd ed. North Carolina: Kindle edition; 2012.

30. Cox DR, Snell EJ. A general definition of residuals. J Roy Stat Soc. 1989;30(2): 248–75. https://www.jstor.org/stable/2984505. Accessed 2 Feb 2022.

31. Nagelkerke NJD. A note on a general definition of the coefficient of determination. Biometrika. 1991;78 (3):691–2. https://doi.org/10.1093/biomet/78.3.691.

32. McFadden D. Quantitative methods for analyzing travel behavior of individuals: Some recent developments. In Cowles foundation for research in economics at Yale University. 1977. https://cowles.yale.edu/sites/default/files/files/pub/d04/d0474.pdf. Accessed 2 Feb 2022.

33. Altman DG, Bland JM. Time to event (survival) data. BMJ. 1998;317(7156):468–9. https://doi.org/10.1136/bmj.317.7156.468.

34. Kaplan EL, Meier P. Nonparametric estimation from incomplete observations. J Am Stat Assoc. 1958;53:457–81.

35. Bland JM, Altman DG. The logrank test. BMJ. 2004;328:1073.

36. Cox DR. Regression models and life-tables. J Roy Stat Soc Ser B (Methodol). 1972;34(2):187–202.

37. Abd Elhafeez S, D'Arrigo G, Leonardis D, Fusaro M, Tripepi G, Roumeliotis S. Methods to analyze time-to-event data the Cox regression analysis. Oxid Med Cell Longev. 2021;2021 Article ID1302811, p. 6. https://doi.org/10.1155/2021/1302811.

38. Luke DA, Homan SM. Time and change: using survival analysis in clinical assessment and treatment evaluation. Psychol Assess. 1998;10:360–78. https://doi.org/10.1037/1040-3590.10.4.360.

39. Wright RE. Survival analysis. In Grimm LG, Yarnold PR editors. Reading and understanding more multivariate statistics. Washington DC: American Psychological Association; 2000. p. 363–408. https://onesearch.library.rice.edu/permalink/01RICE_ INST/i8rmhu/alma991013709539705251.

40. Schoenfeld D. Partial residuals for the proportional hazards regression model. Biometrika. 1982;69 (1):239–41. https://doi.org/10.2307/2335876.

Psychol. 2020; 16(5), v8–v20. https://www.tqmp.org/Vignettes/vol16-5/v008/v008.pdf.

Abstract

The power of a study is its ability to put into evidence the treatment effect, as expected in the population (the effect size). Because statistical significance (P-value) depends upon the number of patients included in the study, a "too large" sample can put a "small or clinically irrelevant" effect size into evidence. A major pharmaceutical company can arrange for a mega trial only to favor the small effect of a newly invented treatment. On the other hand, many independent researchers have limited resources, arranging for studies that are "too small for their goals" and can easily miss "a substantial effect." These studies are not only a waste of time and resources but can be unethical for exposing the patients to the "potential harm" of a new treatment that missed approval. This chapter aims to help the biologist calculate an "adequate sample size" for his study.

Keywords

Effect size · Sample size · Non-inferiority studies · Equivalence studies · Reliability testing · Diagnostic accuracy

4.1 Introduction

Every clinical study has multiple outcomes, and the researcher has to decide which one will primarily answer his study question. The "primary outcome" is the outcome used to calculate sample size before the study's beginning and make conclusions by the end. On the other hand, the results of other "secondary outcomes" should always be considered observational, even in randomized controlled clinical trials and regardless of their statistical significance.

Once we settle on the primary outcome, the next step will be to pick up a sufficient sample from the population, which will have a good chance to unveil what we are looking for. How many patients we should include in the study depends on "the size of the effect of the primary outcome in the population of concern," which is known as the effect size (ES).

Besides ES, the researcher has to consider the two main risks omnipresent in any research: the primary and the secondary risk of error. The probability of rejecting a true null hypothesis (acquiring a false positive result) and failing to reject a false null hypothesis (acquiring a false negative result), respectively. We have previously shown that both risks can never be avoided but must be limited to universally accepted margins, founding a common platform for all researchers to discuss and compare their results fairly. Limiting the risks of error means more accurate results; however, it inevitably necessitates the inclusion of a sufficient sample size. This introductory section will focus on those two main points common for every study: estimation of effect size in the population of concern and calculation of a sample size that is sufficient to find this ES in his study, with the universally acceptable margins of error.

We dedicate the following sections to sample size calculation relevant to the type and the distribution of primary outcome and the statistical tests used for the analysis. Chapter 7 includes a closing section on how the researcher can "sculpt" the primary outcome of his study and maximize the chances of achieving a statistically significant result (see Sect. 7.1).

4.1.1 Estimation of the Effect Size

Once we identify the primary outcome, we have to estimate its magnitude and variability among the population, which is known as the "effect size" (ES). An (ES) of small magnitude and large variability will be hard to find. We should estimate effect size by an *extensive review of the literature*. In the absence of credible literature sources, the researcher must get a preliminary estimate by arranging a *pilot study*. Another way is *to postulate an ES* that would be clinically attractive and accepted by the medical community. For example, if we are studying a new drug to treat a non-curable disease, a 10% decrease in mortality can be considered an acceptable benefit as no effective drug exists. We do not recommend this postulation for being mainly based on the researcher's opinion and experience and carrying uncalculated risks of error.

4.1.1.1 The Magnitude

A researcher wants to prove that boys are significantly taller than girls. If boys are only a few millimeters taller than girls, he will have to examine hundreds of persons to ensure the presence of this slight difference, compared to the situation where all boys are twice as tall as girls. In such a case, a much smaller sample will be sufficient to convince us that boys are taller than girls. *Searching a room for an "ant" is much more difficult than looking for an "elephant".*

It is hard to miss the elephant at first sight, and no one will look for it twice, except by curiosity. On the other hand, the researcher looking for an "ant" is obliged to search as many times as the ant is small and invite others to assist him. The smaller is the "evidence" we are looking for (ant versus elephant), the larger our sample should be (number of times we have to look for the evidence).

4.1.1.2 The Variability

Although an effect size of large magnitude is supposed to be easily found and hence, requiring a small sample size; ES is not dependent on the magnitude alone but also, and to a large extent, on the variability. We are comparing two treatments: one giving complete cure in "every" patient and the other showing no benefit in "any" patient. How many successes and failures (sample size) will be necessary to convince us that the first treatment is superior to the second one? Only a few patients, of course. In real life, however, no treatment gives 100% cure, and, on the other hand, the use of a "weak" treatment or placebo is associated with a certain percentage of cure. Due to this "real-life variability", more cases will be needed to put into evidence the ES, compared to the first "utopic" situation of 100% success or failure rates. The use of every treatment is associated with the complete cure of some patients, the amelioration of others, and the failure in a few cases too.

The more is the variability of the response to the treatment, the more we have to increase our sample size to show the difference between both treatments. In conclusion, variability increases sample size, and the magnitude of the difference decreases it. As shown later during the application, the effect of variability is much more influential than the magnitude.

4.1.1.3 Effect Size Families

There is no single "universal" effect size, and ES is rather a name given to a family of indices that measure the magnitude and variability of the relationship between variables [1]. There are two leading families: the (d) family measuring the differences between observations, such as Cohen d, Hedges g and Cohen f. An example is measuring the effect of adopting/not adopting a specific diet (group 1/group 2) on the body weight by calculating the difference in body weight between groups 1 and 2 after a certain period.

The second is the (r) family measuring the proportion of variation in the dependent variable that could be related to (explained by) a particular predictor; including Odds ratio, relative risk (RR), Pearson correlation coefficient (r), and R squared (R^2). We can analyze the relationship between diabetes and myocardial infarction (MI) by the Odds ratio. The ratio between the proportion of diabetic patients with and without MI and, the proportion of the non-diabetic cases with and without MI. It expresses the tightness of the relation between diabetes mellitus and myocardial infarction.

Effect size indices are estimated from the sample, which is typically small and of high variability. Consequently, the drawn effect sizes are described as being *unstandardized effect sizes*, i.e., not considering the variability (the difference) between the sample and the population. Examples include Cohen ds, and Eta squared η^2. Researchers have created other "reduced" (deflated) indices to fit the population better. Hence, they are called *standardized effect sizes*. Examples include Cohen g and omega square ω^2. The following link is helpful to compute and exchange the different effect sizes [2, 3]. In the following sections, we will explain each one of those effect sizes, relevant to the type and the distribution of the primary outcome and the statistical test used for the analysis.

4.1.2 Choosing the Risks of Error

The primary risk of error is universally set to 5%, with very few exceptions, such as the case of a non-curable or a rare disease, where we are obliged to accept modest results. On the other hand, the secondary risk of error is a point of debate for being largely dependent on the available resources. The researcher has to ask himself: is it ethical to put patients at risk during the experiment without a fair chance to prove that the treatment is effective? In other words, is it ethical to arrange for an underpowered study?

On the other hand, we should not put too many patients at risk if we can find evidence with a much smaller sample. An overpowered study is unethical and a waste of time and resources. The researcher must follow the universally accepted guidelines to limit the two omnipresent risks of error associated with any study, i.e., adopting the 5% primary risk of error (see Sect. 1.5.1) and choosing between 10 and 20% secondary risk of error (see Sect. 1.7.4).

4.1.2.1 The Primary Risk of Error

All researchers have to expect that there is always this probability that the evidence detected by any study can be just a fluke. In order to protect society from our mistakes, there is this universal agreement to limit this probability error to a maximum of 5%, and researchers have no right to overcome this patient-protective siege, with only few exceptions. Although lowering this risk to 2% or even 1% seems to be more protective, it simply denies our patients the right to benefit from treatments that can be 98, 97, 96, and 95% effective, which would be unfair. It is worth noting that in particular situations, the primary risk of error can be increased to as much as 20% or more in clinical trials involving terminal diseases, where no other cure exists.

4.1.2.2 The Secondary Risk of Error

The primary risk of error is concluding upon evidence in the study that does not exist in the population. The secondary risk of error is the other side of the coin: missing the evidence in the study, despite that it exists in reality (in the population). The famous demonstrative example is the baby boys to baby girls' situation, given by Nisbett and colleagues, where the authors compared the ratios of baby boys to baby girls observed in two hospitals: a large and a small hospital [4]. If the expected baby boys to baby girls' ratio is 1:1, deviations will be more frequently observed in the small hospital. For example, suppose in the latter, only two babies are usually born daily. In that case, it can easily happen that both babies are boys (2:0) or girls (0:2). Missing the evidence (1:1 ratio) can be repeated for a couple of days, and nobody will be surprised: they are just two babies. On the other hand, if 100 babies are usually born each day in the larger hospital, it will be nearly impossible that they can be all-boys (100 boys and no girls) or all-girls (100 girls and no boys), even for a single day. *A small study can easily miss the reality (the evidence), and this probability decreases as the study grows larger.* In other words, *the power of the study is to match reality* by including a sufficient number of patients so as NOT to miss the evidence [4]. A study with a 20% secondary risk of error (β) means that a sufficient number of patients empowered this study to have an 80% chance of finding the evidence $(1 - \beta)$.

Missing the evidence is the researcher's main problem. He wasted his time and resources and failed to prove a "true" difference in the population simply because he did not arrange for a sufficient sample size to demonstrate it in his study. On the other hand, once the researcher reaches a positive conclusion, he throws the ball back to society: would the society accept his evidence or not? Returning to the baby boys and baby girls' situation, imagine that society does not know the boys to girls' ratio and has received "two different ratios", one from the small clinic and the other from the main hospital. Society will believe those issuing from the large study for having a smaller probability to deviate from (larger probability to match) reality.

The question will be about defining an acceptable limit for the secondary risk of error. Choosing a secondary risk of error of 20% is a midway compromise between the considerable 50% risk of missing the evidence and a "safety" 5% risk of giving our patients an ineffective treatment, i.e., the primary risk of error. Remember that a 50% risk of missing the

evidence is no better than tossing a coin, and hence, it is unacceptable. On the other hand, raising the ceiling of the secondary risk of error to as high as 5% inflates all sample sizes, depriving the community of the contribution of eminent researchers with limited financial resources. Society will equally lose the contribution of developing countries. A 20% secondary risk of error (80% power) appeared as a good compromise. This minimum is based on the idea that concluding a false positive effect is four times as serious as concluding a false negative one ($\beta = \alpha \times 4 = 0.05 \times 4 = 0.2$) [5].

4.1.3 The Direction of the Study

4.1.3.1 The Unilateral (One-Tail) Versus the Bilateral (Two-Tails) Study

Although the primary risk of error (α) is an implementation of the 5% universal limit and is followed by almost all investigators, its distribution depends on whether the study design is unilateral or bilateral. We have previously detailed the difference between the two designs (see Sects. 1.7.2 and 1.7.3). In brief, a basic study has two arms: treatment A and treatment B, procedure A, and procedure B, etc. Such study design is termed "bilateral" because the researcher is "looking into the two arms" to find out which is better: A or B. In consequence, there are two possible conclusions: A is better than B (A > B), or B is better than A (A < B) and hence, the accepted 5% risk to make a "wrong" conclusion (α) is equally split between those two possibilities; being (α/2) on each side (Fig. 1.12). By the end of the study, the researcher will eventually reach only one of the two conclusions.

On the other hand, if one of the two arms is a placebo, the researcher is not expecting and has no benefit to show that placebo is better than treatment. Another example is one arm containing patients with a risk factor (e.g., smokers), and the other includes patients without the risk factors (non-smokers). The researcher does not expect non-smokers to develop lung cancer more than smokers. This study design is termed as being "unilateral" because the researcher is looking to prove the superiority (or harm) of only one arm (treatment arm, arm with risk factor, etc.) over the other (an arm of a placebo, arm without risk factor, etc.). Consequently, the whole 5% of (α) is fully dedicated to that arm (Fig. 1.13). In other words, the whole risk of error (5%) is linked to the single possible conclusion of the unilateral study: treatment is effective compared to placebo, the risk factor is harmful, etc.… but never the reverse. Although placebo can theoretically be more effective than treatment, no study will conclude on this, simply because it is not looked for and not because it is impossible. In a unilateral study, we conclude upon a smaller difference between treatment and placebo than if the design was bilateral. Consequently, a unilateral design has the advantage of requiring a smaller sample size by about 20%. It is worth noting that using a unilateral design to compare two treatments for the benefit of declaring statistical significance with only ($\alpha/2$) is cheating.

4.1.4   Study Specific Factors

4.1.4.1   Factors Related to the Primary Outcome

Sample size depends upon the type of variable, whether being continuous (see Sects. 4.2 and 4.6, 4.7, and 4.8), binomial (see Sect. 4.3), categorical or ordinal (see Sect. 4.4), or time to event (see Sect. 4.9). Size also depends on its distribution being parametric or following other distribution than normal (see Sect. 4.2).

In general, comparing the patient to himself (see Sect. 4.5) or repeating the measurement (see Sect. 4.12) decreases variability and reduces sample size. On the other hand, sample size increases with the number of study groups and, specifically, the number of comparisons made (see Sect. 4.6). We will discuss the role of each factor and the statistical test used for the analysis in the appropriate section. Special sections are dedicated for sample size calculation in multi-variable analysis (see Sects. 4.10 and 4.11), non-inferiority and equivalence studies (see

Sect. 4.13), diagnostic accuracy (see Sect. 4.14), measuring agreement (see Sect. 4.15), and survey analysis (see Sect. 4.16).

4.1.4.2   Factors Related to the Secondary Outcomes and Post-Hoc Analysis

The researcher may believe that some of his secondary endpoints are important and merit to be put into evidence by the study. Hence, he empowers the study to support those secondary findings, which is different from considering a co-primary outcome. It simply means that the study was empowered to put the secondary outcome into evidence too, even with different study powers; e.g., 90% power for the primary outcome and 80% power for the secondary outcomes. The same can be applied for post-hoc analysis (see Sect. 4.6.2.2).

4.1.4.3   Interim Analysis

The methodology section should include the details of any suggested interim analysis. Interim can be defined as a temporary "situation" intended to be used to make decisions before reaching the desired final status. In clinical trials, an interim analysis is usually used to compare randomized arms at any time point before the end of a phase 3 trial. It provides many opportunities before recruitment is complete.

It provides the opportunity of re-assurance that the trial is going on as pre-planned, the re-evaluation of trial design, or the re-calculation of sample size. It may end by stopping the trial for proven efficacy or its inability to achieve study objectives (trial futility). Although several interim analyses can be performed at different timings, depending on the size and scope of the trial, a common choice is a single midway interim analysis.

Every time the data is analyzed, there is a 5% chance of making a Type I error if $\alpha = 0.05$. As the number of analyses increases, the chance of making a Type I also error increases. Hence, (α) is often adjusted by raising its ceiling from the usual 5% to a smaller value. In other words, instead of concluding statistical significance with a P-value of <0.05, we have to reach a smaller P-value to conclude primarily, e.g., <0.04, <0.03, <0.02, etc. We can look at it as a penalty for the repeated testing of our results against chance.

Pocock SJ suggested a conservative approach that raises the ceiling of (α) according to the number of analyses made, whether interim or final [6]. O'Brien and Fleming used a stricter alpha adjustment at interim, small adjustment at final [7], while Haybittle, Peto and collaborators uses a rigorous (α) adjustment at interim but no adjustment at final [8, 9]. In practice, if the main intention for interim analysis is to stop the trial prematurely for efficacy, Pocock SJ provides the comparatively smaller adjustment for interim analysis, which will be the procedure of choice. On the other hand, if the primary concern is about the significance of the final analysis, Haybittle-Peto method will be the procedure of choice for not making any adjustment at the final analysis. Regardless of the adopted approach, the sample size equation has to use the adjusted (α) value to calculate the number of patients necessary to perform each interim analysis and the final analysis. A table calculating sample size for different scenarios using the most common methods can be retrieved online [10].

Let us take the example used in the next section, where a unilateral study was organized to compare the observed difference in the incidence of bronchogenic carcinoma among smokers (10%) and non-smokers (3%) (see Sect. 4.3.1.1). Suppose that an interim midway analysis was pre-planned, and the investigators have chosen to adopt the Pocock procedure hoping to terminate the study at an earlier date. As the sample size equation includes the designated (α), they consulted the Z table to find the $Z_{1 - (\alpha)}$ of their newly adjusted (α): it increases from the usual 1.65 value of a unilateral study with ($\alpha = 5\%$) to 1.89 for a smaller adjusted ($\alpha = 0.0294$), as expected. Recalculating our new sample size using the adjusted (α), shows that we have to include 184 patients in each group instead of 153. In other words, the investigator has to increase his sample size by about 20% to perform one interim and one final analysis in order to conclude on the same usual 5%

primary risk of error if he had performed a single analysis. This is the penalty that he has to serve. The same result can be obtained by consulting an online calculator and plotting the two proportions, the usual 80% power, choosing a one-tail study, and the new adjusted ($\alpha = 0.294$) [11]. The interested reader is requested to postpone going through these calculations until after reading Sect. 4.3.

4.1.5 Sample Size Calculation

Although effect size is the "true effect" expected in the population of concern, this does not mean that we will find this effect in our study, simply because another factor is now introduced, sample size. The challenge will then be: can we arrange for enough patients to avoid type II error and reveal this effect size in our study or, will we miss it? Note that pharmaceutical companies arrange for mega trials to put into statistical evidence small differences between compared treatments (small effect size), which would be otherwise hidden if the study was carried out on a reasonable number of patients. On the other hand, we have to consider that the effect size shown in the literature, and upon which we calculated our sample size, could itself be just a fluke (type I error), and our study will always be prone to it.

It is logical that the more we would like to be more precise by decreasing our risks of error (whether primary or secondary), the more we have to increase our sample size. If α and β are the risks of error, $1 - \alpha$ and $1 - \beta$ reflect precision; sample size is directly proportional to $1 - \alpha$ and $1 - \beta$. Let us start with the primary risk of error. In a unilateral study, the researcher has planned to reach only one conclusion (treatment > placebo), and hence, he will finally face the whole 5% of (α) and precision $= 1 - \alpha$. In a bilateral study, the researcher will only reach one of two possible conclusions: either (A > B) or (B > A). Smaller risk of error ($\alpha/2$), i.e., better precision ($1 - \alpha/2$), invites an increase in sample size by about 20%. In all cases, the "overall universal" primary risk of error is 5%, regardless of the study being unilateral or bilateral. For more details on the unilateral and bilateral study designs, the reader is invited to refer back to Sects. 1.7.2 and 1.7.3.

The same rule applies to the secondary risk of error. The more we would like to be precise and not miss the evidence $(1 - \beta)$, the more we must include patients in our study. In practice, decreasing the secondary risk of error from the "usual" 20% to only 10% (increasing study power from 80 to 90%) increases our sample size by as much as 30%. A power of 95% is also used to evaluate new drugs in Phase III clinical trials, based on the inferences of confidence intervals.

Besides effect size, study design, and adopted risks of error, sample size calculation depends on the type and distribution of variables, the number of measurements made, and the statistical test used in the analysis. In the following sections, we will provide and explain the equations used for sample size calculation in different study scenarios, the relevant statistical software packages as well as the links to the freely available and tested online calculators.

4.1.5.1 A Basic Formula: The Magic Numbers [5, 12, 13]

Figure 4.1 summarizes graphically the components of sample size calculations in the case of a bilateral study comparing two means: (u_a and u_b). The red curve on the left side represents the null hypothesis (H_0) of no difference between both means ($u_a - u_b = 0$). This curve defines the type I error (α): only 5% of observed differences will lie at a distance of 2 standard errors from the reference point of having no difference between the observed means (point 0). This 5% is equally split between the two possibilities of any bilateral study ($u_a > u_b$ or $u_a < u_b$), forming two rejection areas (black triangles) on either side of the left curve ($2 \times \alpha/2$). The base of each triangle marks the critical limit of rejection. Looking to the black triangle on the right side, any observed difference that lies to the right of the critical limit has a very slim chance of being part of the null hypothesis. Hence, once we reach this point, the probability that the null hypothesis is true is rejected. As the normal distribution curve is bilateral and symmetrical, the same will apply to any observed difference that lies to the left side of the black triangle on the left.

On the other hand, the blue curve on the right side represents the alternative hypothesis, where the difference between both means is not equal to zero ($u_a - u_b = \delta$). The shaded part of the curve represents those observed differences that lie to the left of the critical limit marked by the left curve (the null hypothesis). Consequently, any

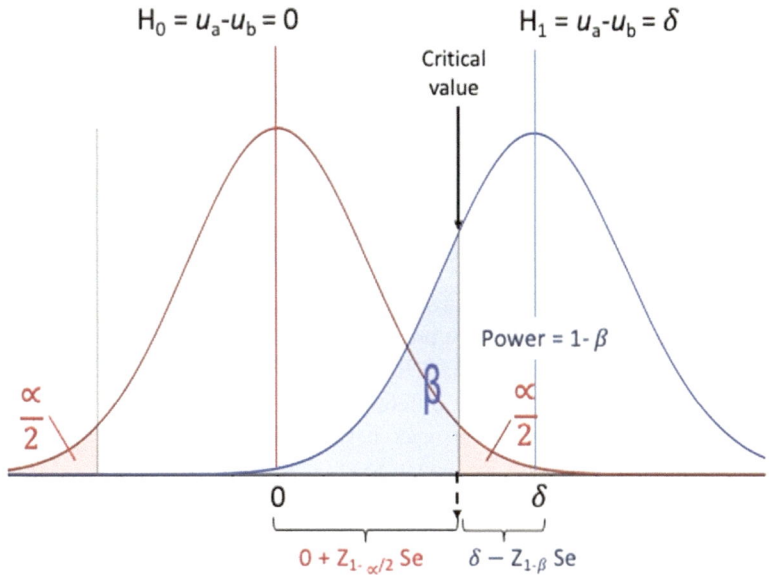

Fig. 4.1 The null and the alternative hypothesis of a bilateral study

$$H_0 = u_a - u_b = 0 \qquad H_1 = u_a - u_b = \delta$$

observed difference under the right curve (alternative hypothesis) that will lie at the same time to the left of the critical value has a >5% chance of being part of the null hypothesis. Hence, the latter cannot be rejected. This shaded part of the right curve represents the observations made under the alternative hypothesis, yet we still cannot reject the null hypothesis. In other words, the shaded area represents the type II error (β) or the probability that the observed difference under the alternative hypothesis does not have enough power to reject the null hypothesis. By deduction, the remaining (non-shaded area) of the right curve ($1 - \beta$) represents the power of the study.

The critical value defines the boundary between rejection and non-rejection regions. It is the point at which we have to decide between either keeping the null hypothesis and considering the observed difference may still be due to chance or rejecting the null hypothesis and accepting the alternative hypothesis that the difference is true. Note that we have one null hypothesis of strictly no difference between both means ($u_a - u_b = 0$). On the other hand, there are multiple alternative hypotheses ($u_a - u_b = \delta$), for the difference can acquire any possible value, whether larger or smaller than the null ($\delta < 0 > \delta$).

The process is dynamic, and the more the right curve moves away from the left curve, the study's power increases ($1 - \beta$), but the critical limit remains the same ($\alpha/2$). Although the critical limit on Fig. 4.1 is shown to be nearer to the alternative hypothesis than the null, the critical limit has to be exactly mid-way between both curves. In other words, the distance between the reference point of the left curve (0) and the critical limit has to be equal to the distance between the reference point of the alternative hypothesis (δ) and the critical limit.

Let us now define those two distances. Concerning the left curve, we have previously shown that the null hypothesis is rejected in a bilateral study whenever the observed difference touches the critical zone ($\alpha/2$). The distance between the null (0) and ($\alpha/2$) will be equal to $1 - (\alpha/2)$.

Remember that the way by which we can compare values is to standardize them, i.e., changing the raw values into their corresponding Z scores: how many standard errors (Se) is the value away from its reference points. In consequence, this standardized difference = $Z_{(1-\alpha/2)}$ Se. Playing the same tune, the standardized difference between the right curve's reference point (δ) and the critical limit = $Z_{(1-\beta)}$ Se. Now we can write down the basic equation used for sample size calculation "Eq. 4.1":

$$\delta = Z_{(1-\alpha/2)}Se + Z_{(1-\beta)}Se$$
$$= Se[Z_{(1-\alpha/2)} + Z_{(1-\beta)}] \qquad (4.1)$$

We can replace the Se by the standard deviation (Sd) divided by square root of sample size: Se = $Sd/\sqrt{n} = Sd\sqrt{1/n}$ and, provided that the two samples are of equal size (n), their common Se = $Sd\sqrt{1/n + 1/n} = Sd\sqrt{2/n}$ "Eq. 4.2". Squaring all values to have (n) and not $\sqrt{n}$ and, shifting (n) to the left side of the equation and (δ) to the right side; we get the basic equation to calculate sample size per group in case of a bilateral study comparing two groups "Eq. 4.3". The equation is valid as long as the two groups are equal in size and have equal variances. Remember that the latter does not mean strict equality but the absence of a statistically significant difference between the two variances. As (δ/Sd) is the standardized difference, i.e., the difference between the two treatments, in terms of standard deviation, the equation can be simplified by replacing (δ/Sd) with d "Eq. 4.3". In the case of a unilateral study, we can replace $Z_{(1-\alpha/2)}$ with $Z_{(1-\alpha)}$ "Eq. 4.4".

$$\delta = Sd\sqrt{\frac{2}{n}}[Z_{(1-\alpha/2)} + Z_{(1-\beta)}] \qquad (4.2)$$

$$n_{bilateral} = \frac{2[Z_{(1-\alpha/2)} + Z_{(1-\beta)}]^2}{\left(\frac{\delta}{Sd}\right)^2}$$
$$= \frac{2[Z_{(1-\alpha/2)} + Z_{(1-\beta)}]^2}{d^2} \qquad (4.3)$$

$$n_{unilateral} = \frac{2[Z_{(1-\alpha)} + Z_{(1-\beta)}]^2}{\left(\frac{\delta}{Sd}\right)^2}$$
$$= \frac{2[Z_{(1-\alpha)} + Z_{(1-\beta)}]^2}{d^2} \quad (4.4)$$

We have to consult the Z table to get the numerical values of the calculated Z scores (Statistical table 1: Z table). For $\alpha = 0.05$, $Z_{(1-\alpha/2)} = 1.96$ and $Z_{(1-\alpha)} = 1.65$. On the other hand, the respective numerical values of $Z_{(1-\beta)}$ for a 20% type II error = 0.84 and for a 10% type II error = 1.28. As example, adopting the usual 5% primary and 20% secondary risks of error (Fig. 4.2), the numerator of the equation shown above = 2 $[Z_{(1-\alpha/2)} + Z_{(1-\beta)}]^2 = 2$ $(1.96 + 0.84)^2 = 2$ $(2.8)^2 = 15.68$; which was approximated to 16 by Lehr "Eq. 4.5" [12]. Playing the same tune, the numerator in case of a unilateral study = 2 $[Z_{(1-\alpha)} + Z_{(1-\beta)}]^2 = 2$ $[1.65 + 0.84]^2 = 12.4$; which we can also approximate to 13 "Eq. 4.6". The numbers 16 and 13 can be thought of as being the magic numbers that give "a flash sample size", for a given standardized difference ($\delta/Sd = d$) or effect size.

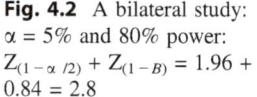

$$n_{bilateral} = \frac{16}{(\delta/Sd)^2} = \frac{16}{d^2} \quad (4.5)$$

$$n_{unilateral} = \frac{13}{(\delta/Sd)^2} = \frac{13}{d^2} \quad (4.6)$$

We can increase the number 16 to 21 or 26, concordance with a more powerful study of 90% or 95%. Now, the primary risk of error is almost always constant (5%). The secondary risk of error is usually one of four choices, 13 or 21 in a unilateral study and 16 or 21 in a bilateral study. By deduction, a more simplified equation for calculating sample size per group would be M/d^2 "Eq. 4.7". where M is a constant that can be approximated to either 13, 16, 21, or 26 depending upon the desired secondary risk of error and the direction of the study [13].

$$n = \frac{M}{d^2} \quad (4.7)$$

However, the equation may become more complicated if the variances (Var_1 and Var_2) and sample sizes are not equal (n_1 and n_2). In such a case, and provided that group 1 is the reference group, the Sd under the null hypothesis = $Sd\sqrt{1/n_1 + 1/n_2}$ and the Sd under the alternative hypothesis = $\sqrt{Var_1/n_1 + Var_2/n_2}$; which will increase the total sample size of the study. A simple equation to calculate sample size for two unequal groups will be given in Sect. 4.2.2.1.

4.1.5.2 The Non-centrality Parameter (ncp)

Despite the importance of effect size, the testing hypothesis requires sufficient statistical power to reject the null hypothesis, producing evidence

Fig. 4.2 A bilateral study: $\alpha = 5\%$ and 80% power: $Z_{(1-\alpha/2)} + Z_{(1-B)} = 1.96 + 0.84 = 2.8$

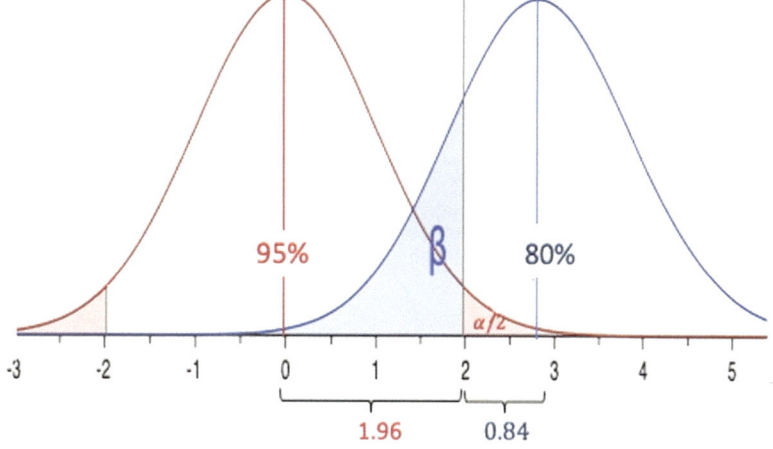

about treatment effect. Every statistical test (Student test, chi-square, test, ANOVA, etc.) has a characteristic distribution under the null hypothesis, i.e., if the null hypothesis is true. This distribution of probabilities is called the central distribution. As an example, Figs. 1.12 and 1.13 show the probabilities of a "central" Normal distribution, where there is a 5% chance to reject the null hypothesis while it is true. However, what if the null hypothesis is false? The distribution will change, of course, acquiring many possibilities in concordance with the degrees of change. Put it this way, the one central distribution observed under the null hypothesis is replaced by one of many possible non-centrality distributions under the alternative hypothesis [14].

Non-central distributions are multiple, representing the infinite possibilities of treatment effects. For example, an antihypertensive can decrease blood pressure by 1% of pre-treatment value, 2%, 3%, and up to infinite effects, compared to the single one central distribution of "no" treatment effect under the null hypothesis (0%). *The question is whether those possible "different" treatment effects will influence the central distribution "similarly"; the answer is straightforward, of course not.*

The non-centrality distributions apply to all distributions that can be approximated to the Normal distribution, such as Chi-square distribution, Student (t) distribution, and Fisher's (F) distribution. Figure 4.3 shows on the extreme left side the central Fisher's distribution when the null hypothesis is true. We can note on the right side four out of the infinite possibilities of the non-central distributions, in case the null hypothesis is false.

Lambda (λ) symbolizes the non-centrality parameter (ncp) designed to measure the degree of the null hypothesis being false. As shown in Fig. 4.4, the (ncp) reflects the difference (the distance) between the central t-distribution of (0) mean effect and the non-central t-distribution on the right side with a mean effect of (non-zero) that equals (λ-0). The more the non-central distribution moves to the left, the smaller will be λ. Note that β represents the risk that the test fails to demonstrate the evidence (the secondary risk of error). The remaining area under the alternative hypothesis $(1 - \beta)$ represents the power of the test (the ability to put into evidence a statistically significant difference). The (ncp) is directly proportional to power, and if (λ) = 0, the test will have zero power. On the other hand, the larger the difference between both distributions (large ncp), the more powerful the test is. In consequence, knowing the (ncp) allows power calculation for this t-test.

The (ncp) is close to effect size, expressing how wrong the null hypothesis is; however, they are not the same. Let us take the example of comparing two independent means by a Student test. In both parameters (ncp and effect size), the numerator of the equation is the difference between both means (u1 − u2) but the denominators are not the same.

Fig. 4.3 Central and non-central F distributions

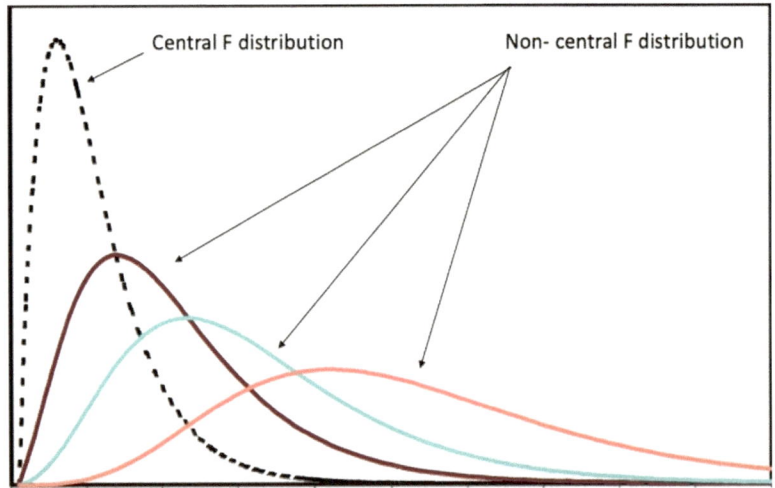

Central F distribution   Non- central F distribution

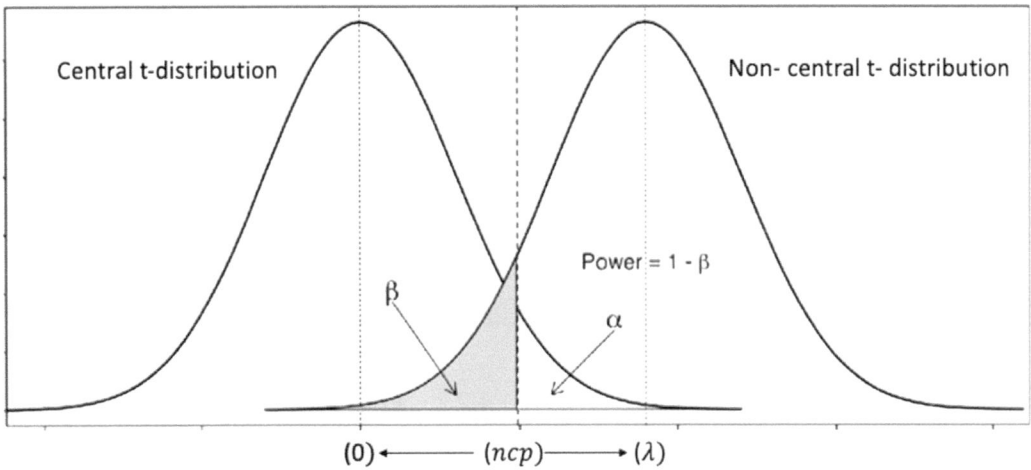

Fig. 4.4 The non-centrality parameter (λ)

As we will show later, the effect size Cohen ds expresses the difference between the two means of a normal distribution "Eq. 4.8" (see Sect. 4.2.1.1). When we calculate the effect size, we assume that we are still under the central distribution (i.e., the null hypothesis of no difference), and hence the difference between the two means is expressed in units of the within-groups variability; which is *a pooled standard error* derived from both "sister" variances of two means under the same central distribution.

On the other hand, ncp assumes that we have two different distributions: the central and the non-central. Consequently, the difference between the now two different means have to be expressed in units of the in between-groups variability, which is *the standard error of the difference* coming from the variances of two different groups "Eq. 4.9". The equations are shown below with u_a, n_a, Sa^2 and, u_b, n_b, Sb^2 is the mean, sample size and variance of groups (a) and (b); respectively. The reader can refer to Sect. 2.4.1.2 to have a detailed calculation of the pooled standard error and the standard error of the difference.

$$Cohen\ ds = \frac{(\mu_a - \mu_b)}{\sqrt{S^2_{pooled}}} \qquad (4.8)$$

$$\lambda = \frac{(\mu_a - \mu_b)}{\sqrt{\frac{S^2_a}{n_a} + \frac{S^2_b}{n_b}}} = d\sqrt{\frac{n_a \times n_b}{n_a + n_b}} \qquad (4.9)$$

As shown in Fig. 4.4, the non-centrality parameter (λ) depends on the power of the study: the more the two distributions are distant from one another, the more is the in-between group variability; the more (λ) increases and the study gains power. (λ) can be calculated from sample size and effect size "Eq. 4.9". On the other hand, effect size (ES) is inversely proportional to study power; the smaller is the effect size, the more we have to empower the study to find it. The relation between the three parameters, in case of comparison of two independent means, can be presented by the following equation "Eq. 4.10":

$$n = \frac{2\lambda^2}{d^2} \qquad (4.10)$$

where (n) is the sample size per group and (d) is the effect size. *In conclusion, the ncp can be seen as the ES calculated for a given power; i.e., for a given sample size.* As shown later, variations of this basic equation will be customized to different distributions and statistical tests. However, the basic relation between the three parameters will remain the same. Many statistical programs such as G*power are programmed with those non-central cumulative distributive functions to facilitate the computation of exact power (sample size) and provide the researcher with multiple power estimates, with every possible value of (λ). Instead of performing multiple power calculations for each specific effect size, the researcher can now "view" an entire power curve and "manipulate" the risks of the error to find the sample size that is most appropriate for his resources.

4.1.5.3 Power Calculation Software and Online Calculators

The following links are useful to compute and interchange the effect sizes [2, 12]. On the other hand, there are many available free sample size calculation software, whether online [11, 15–18], or can be downloaded such as G*power [19, 20]. The software can be freely downloaded for both MAC and Windows [21]. Tables for sample size calculation from effect size for the comparison of 2 groups or more are equally available online [22]. Those sources may use different estimates of effect size and different variations of sample size calculation formulae. Although those estimates and formula are interchangeable, we do not advise the "lay clinical" to play too much with the statistical formulae; the risk of making gross conversion errors can be huge.

4.2 Comparison of Two Independent Quantitative Variables: Student and Mann & Whitney Tests

A majority of medical studies involve the comparison of the outcome of treatments or procedures in two independent groups of patients to investigate which is the better treatment (A or B) or prove that a treatment is better than a placebo. In the case of a quantitative outcome, the two means (e.g., duration of therapy, drug dose, hospital stay, etc....) are usually compared by the unpaired test of Student. The Mann and Whitney test is the non-parametric alternative that is most commonly used whenever the quantitative

variable follows other distribution than normal. In a usual superiority study, sample size calculation is straightforward. It depends mainly on a comprehensive literature review to get a reliable estimate of the effect size, and the researcher usually adopts the 5% primary and the 20% secondary risks of error [23–25]. Sample size calculation for a paired design (see Sect. 4.5) or non-inferiority and equivalence studies (see Sect. 4.13) are discussed in separate sections.

4.2.1 Effect Size

4.2.1.1 Cohen ds

The Example

The normal mitral valve area in an adult is about 4 cm^2. Rheumatic fever can lead to valve stenosis requiring dilatation whenever the valve area is reduced to 1 cm^2 or less. Surgical dilatation was the classical approach, but researchers proposed to substitute this procedure with a less invasive percutaneous technique (valvuloplasty), and many studies were organized to compare both procedures.

Reviewing the literature showed that mean (Sd) of mitral valve area achieved in 200 hundred patients equally divided between surgery and valvuloplasty group were: 3.8 ± 0.6 cm^2 and 4.1 ± 1.1 cm^2, respectively. The researchers wished to calculate the sample size for a future study on the subject based on this published data. They will start by estimating appropriate effect size, adopt the usual primary and secondary risks of error and finally calculate the sample size for a bilateral study to find the better procedure: surgery or balloon valvuloplasty?

The Equation

Ideally, we can calculate the effect size (d) by dividing the difference between the two means (Δ) by the Sd of the population, which is usually not known, and the question is, where to get the best estimate of it? For the effect size Cohen ds, a common variance can be derived by pooling the variances of both groups (S^2_{pooled}) "Eq. 4.11". The best estimate for the Sd of the population will then be the square root of the pooled variance "Eq. 4.12".

$$S^2_{pooled} = \frac{S^2_1(n_1 - 1) + S^2_2(n_2 - 1)}{(n_1 + n_1 - 2)}$$
$$= \frac{0.6^2(99) + 1.1^2(99)}{(198)} = 0.785 \quad (4.11)$$

$$Cohen\ ds = \frac{\Delta}{\sqrt{S^2_{pooled}}} = \frac{(\mu_1 - \mu_2)}{\sqrt{S^2_{pooled}}} = \frac{(4.1 - 3.8)}{\sqrt{0.785}}$$
$$= 0.34$$
$$(4.12)$$

We can build a 95% CI around the effect size. The standard deviation Sd(d) can be calculated from effect size and sample size using Hedges and Olkin formula "Eq. 4.13" [26]. For our example, the 95% IC of Cohen's ds = 0.34 ± 1.96 (0.14) = 0.07 to 0.62; indicating a statistically significant ES for not bypassing the null (zero).

$$Sd(d) = \sqrt{\frac{n_1 + n_2}{n_1 \times n_2} + \frac{d^2}{2(n_1 + n_2)}} = 0.142$$
$$(4.13)$$

Cohen ds can be calculated online [2, 3]. It can be calculated from the t-value of Student's test and can be converted to biserial correlation coefficient (r) "Eq. 4.14" and "Eq. 4.15".

$$Cohen\ ds = t\sqrt{\frac{1}{n1} + \frac{1}{n2}} \quad (4.14)$$

$$r = \frac{d_s}{\sqrt{d^2_s + (N^2 - 2N)/n_1 n_2}} \quad (4.15)$$

Interpretation of Cohen ds

An effect size can be interpreted as the Z score of our result, indicating that *the mitral valve area of an average patient in the treatment group is 0.34 standard deviation above an average patient in the control group.* Consulting the Z table, a Z score of 0.34 corresponds to a probability of 63.3%. The result can be interpreted as follows: *the mitral valve area of an average patient in the treatment group exceeds the valve area of 63.3% of controls* [27].

It is worth noting that Cohen has given an arbitrary evaluation of Z values of 0.2, 0.5, and 0.8 as being indicators of small, medium, and large effect sizes. They can be interpreted as follows: an average patient in the treatment group is expected to show a treatment effect above 58%, 69%, and 79% of controls, respectively. Accordingly, our effect size can be described as being mild to moderate [27]. A point of crucial importance is that all these calculations of effect size and CI intervals are based upon the assumption of Normal distribution of the variables and equality of their variances.

4.2.1.2 Hedges g

Due to the inherent large variability of the small sample, Cohen ds overestimates the effect size of the population, which is why it is sometimes called the unstandardized effect size. Hedges and Olkin proposed a correction that is always recommended, especially for samples smaller than 20 cases [26]. Applying the correction to our example and substituting n1 and n2 by their values, Hedges g is calculated by multiplying Cohen ds by 0.996, giving a smaller (0.337) but a less biased effect size estimate "Eq. 4.16".

$$Hedges\ g = Cohen\ ds\left(1 - \frac{3}{4(n_1 + n_2) - 9}\right)$$
$$(4.16)$$

Hedges g can be directly calculated by the "Eq. 4.17". Note that while Cohen's ds is standardized with the pooled standard deviation of both groups, Hedges' g is standardized with the pooled sample size weighted standard deviation of both groups. In other words, it was designed to take the sample size into consideration.

$$Hedges\ g = \frac{(\mu_1 - \mu_2)}{\sqrt{\frac{S^2_1}{n_1} + \frac{S^2_2}{n_2}}} \quad (4.17)$$

4.2.1.3 *Glass* Δ

Glass Δ is another estimation of the effect size suggested for experimental studies, where there is a significant difference between the Sd of both groups. The Sd of the control is used as the sole estimate of the population: $(\mu_1 - \mu_2)/\sigma$. For our example, Glass Δ = $(4.1 - 3.8)/0.6 = 0.5$.

4.2.1.4 Non-parametric Effect Size

The Example

A researcher wishes to compare the effects of the duration of analgesia achieved with two analgesics (x) and (y) based on a small study that included only ten patients per group. The details of the study are provided in Sect. 2.5.1.1. A Mann and Whitney test showed Uyx = 69 and a statistically non-significant difference between both analgesics (Z = 1.44); P > 0.05 (see Sect. 2.5.1.1).

The Equation

The violation of parametric assumptions limits the value of Cohen's ds and other parametric effect sizes. Grisson and Kim suggested two suitable effect size for nonparametric data [28]. The test statistics (P_{ab}) is the probability that a score randomly chosen from a population (a) is greater (or smaller) than a score randomly chosen from a population (b); with (U) statistics being calculated by Mann and Whitney test and (n_1) and (n_1) are the numbers of scores in both population "Eq. 4.18" (see Sect. 2.5.1.1).

$$\widehat{P}_{ab} = \frac{U}{n_1 n_2} = \frac{31}{100} = 0.31 \qquad (4.18)$$

Interpretation of effect size

Kindly note that the two treatments in our example were given the symbols x and y (see Sect. 2.5.1.1) rather than the symbols a and b shown in the equation. In terms of the latter, we can conclude that there is a 31% chance that a random score chosen from "a" is smaller than a random score chosen from "b". Alternatively, there is a 69% chance that a random score from "b" is larger than a random score from "a". The non-parametric effect size can also be expressed as the coefficient

(r), calculated from the (z value) of the test and the total sample size (N) "Eq. 4.19". The coefficient r can then be interpreted according to Cohen's rules (large effect size) or better according to the previous reports in the literature. The same effect sizes can be applied to the non-parametric alternative of ANOVA: Kruskal and Wallis test.

$$r = \frac{z}{\sqrt{N}} = \frac{1.44}{\sqrt{20}} = 0.89 \qquad (4.19)$$

4.2.2 Sample Size

4.2.2.1 Normal Distribution: Comparison of Two Means

We have already presented the equations necessary for calculating sample size in the case of a bilateral "Eq. 4.3" and a unilateral study "Eq. 4.4". We have also presented the simple versions adopting the usual 5% primary risk of error and study power of 80% "Eqs. 4.5 and 4.6". The equations give the sample size per group (n), and the total sample size of the study (N) will be equal to (n) multiplied by the number of compared groups. The reader has to note some important points:

- As any statistical equation, we have to be free from the limitations of a specific scales and hence, all quantities involved are written in standardized values: the z values of $1 - \alpha$, $1 - \alpha/2$, $1 - \beta$ and, the standardized difference between the two proportions or means (d = Δ/Sd).

- The larger sample size calculated by the second equation (n) is due to the larger precision $(1 - \alpha/2)$ needed for a bilateral study compared to a unilateral design $(1 - \alpha)$.

- The more we would like to be more precise, the more we will need patients, and hence, $1 - \alpha$, $1 - \alpha/2$, $1 - \beta$ are placed in the numerator.

- Increasing the variability increases the sample size (Sd), while a larger difference (Δ) decreases (n) and hence, (n) is directly proportional to (1/d). Remember that variability is originally calculated in the squared scale as variance and not as Sd. Hence, we use (d^2) in the calculations and not (d); which indulges that all values in the equation are raised to the power of 2.

- As the primary risk of error is universal and constant at 5% and the secondary risk of error is usually chosen either as 10% or 20%, the quantities: $[2\ (Z_{1-\alpha} + Z_{1-\beta})^2]$ and $[2\ (Z_{1-\alpha/2} + Z_{1-\beta})^2]$ have a are more or less constant values (M). Consulting the Z table, the values of $(Z_{1-\alpha})$, $(Z_{1-\alpha/2})$ and $(Z_{1-\beta})$ are: 1.65, 1.96 and 0.84. In consequence, M = 12.4 and 17.1 for the respective secondary risks of error of 10 and 20% of a unilateral design. The corresponding values of M in the case of a bilateral design will be 15.7 and 21.

- The equation was found to be underestimating the sample size. It is advised to increase (n) by about 10% to compensate for this bias as well as for those patients expected to be lost during follow-up. It is worth noting that a larger percentage should be added in case of studies associated with a significant loss, such as cancer patients, studies involving extended periods of follow-up, or inability to access patients' information for any reason.

- After calculating the number of patients per group (n), the total number of patients in the study (N) will depend upon the number of comparisons made between the study groups and the balance between groups. The simplest scenario is the study comparing two equal groups of patients, and hence, the total sample size will be equal to 2n. In the case of a study formed by more than two groups, the number of patients per group (n) is calculated as usual (with the 10% raise), and the total number of patients of the study (N) will be a function of the number of comparisons (C) that will be made. For example, in a study of 4 groups that should be compared, six comparisons have to be made, and N = 6n. If one of the groups is a placebo and the others are three treatment groups, we may not be interested in comparing treatment groups to one another, and hence, we can be satisfied by making three comparisons only. In such a case, the total sample size is N = 3n.

- The next question would be: should we correct the sample size for the repeated comparisons? A straight forward answer is yes, we have to. For example, if we plan to make three comparisons in a bilateral study, the true α will not be 0.05, and, according to the Bonferroni equation, α has to be equal to $\alpha/3 = 0.0167$. In such case, $\alpha/2$ used in sample size calculation has to be changed from 0.025 to 0.0083, and hence, in order to conclude upon a difference at the usual 5% level, M $[2\ (Z_{1-\alpha/2} + Z_{1-\beta})^2]$ will be equal to 21 and not 15.7; producing a 30% increase in sample size per group.

- In the case where the study is formed of unequal groups and suppose that the number of patients in the group a (na) is expected to be (K) times the number of patients in group b (nb). We start by calculating the number of patients per group (n) as usual, then na and nb are calculated by "Eq. 4.20". Note that a balanced design is the most potent design.

$$na = \frac{n}{2} \times (1 + K); nb = \frac{n}{2} \times \left(1 + \frac{1}{K}\right) \quad (4.20)$$

The Example

We will base our analysis on the same example used for effect size calculation. In brief, a group of researchers wishes to compare surgical to balloon valvuloplasty, based on a previous study conducted on 200 patients equally divided between both groups. The mean (Sd) mitral valve area achieved was 3.8 ± 0.6 cm^2 in the valvuloplasty group versus 4.1 ± 1.1 cm^2 in the surgical group.

The Calculation

For a usual α of 5% and a β value of 20%, M equals 16 for a bilateral study aiming to show the best treatment. Effect size (Cohen ds) equals 0.34 "Eq. 4.12". The number of patients necessary to compare surgical to balloon valvuloplasty = M/d^2 = 16/(0.339)^2 = 139 patients per group.

In case the two groups were unequal and na (surgery group) equal 2 nb (balloon group) and the calculated (n) was 70; na = (70/2) x (1 + 2) = 105 patients and nb = (70/2) x (1 + 1/2) = 53 patients. As one can easily notice, the total sample size (158 patients) is larger than the one calculated in the case of equal groups (140 patients). A balanced group design is much more powerful (i.e., capable of showing a difference with the use of a comparatively smaller number of patients); than the unbalanced design. Finally, we should not forget to add to the calculated numbers the extra 10%.

Consulting Online Resources

Consulting an online calculator [15–18], gives nearly the same number: 138 patients per group. After adding the usual 10%, a total of 155 patients are needed per group to give the study an 80% power to put into evidence an effect size of 0.34. Several online calculators offer calculations for unequal groups [16–18]. Consulting an online table shows that a minimum of 130 patients per group is needed to put into evidence an effect size of 0.35 for the usual primary and secondary risks of error of 5% and 20%, respectively [22].

G*power Software

The G*power software is freely available for download [21]. It calculates the effect size, λ, and the sample size as well. Most interestingly, it provides the researcher with an entire power curve and tables for his convenience to explore the most suitable sample size for his resources. The software is user-friendly and provides a concise manual. After launching the software and opening the main window:

1. Check the "Test family" drop-down menu and select "t tests".
2. Check the "Statistical test" drop-down menu and select "Means: Difference between 2 independent means (two groups)"
3. Check "Type of power analysis" and select: "A priori: Compute required sample size-given α, power and effect size".
4. Under "Input parameters", check "Tail(s)" and select (Two). Leave "α err prob" as such (0.05). Select "Power (1-B err Prob)"; usually (0.8). Define the "Allocation ratio N2/N1); (1) in case of two equal samples. Fill in the

effect size if previously known (0.0339 in our example) and skip directly to step 6.
5. If the effect size is unknown, click on "Determine" to open the effect size side drawer. Provide the mean and Sd of the first group (4.1) and (1.1) and, mean and Sd of the second group (3.8) and (0.2). In case of unequal groups, provide the mean of each group and the Sd within each group. Click on "Calculate and transfer to main drawer" to close this side drawer and transfer the calculated effect side to the main window.
6. Verify your choices: two-tailed study, effect size d = (0.339), α = (0.05), power = (0.8), allocation ratio = (1). Click on "Calculate" to get the reveal the output parameters on the right side of the drawer.
7. Verify the output parameters: (λ = 2.8), (critical t = 1.96), (df = 274); total sample size − 2 = 276 − 2 = 274, sample size per group (138 patients) and (actual power = 0.8).
8. In case we would like to make any change, such as changing the allocation ratio, we just make the change in the "input parameters" and click on "Calculate" again to get the change done in the "Output parameters". There are three more buttons in the main window that offers three important information: 'Protocol of power analysis", Central and non-central distribution" and "x–y for a range of values".
9. Check on the "Protocol of power analysis" it keeps the dated records of all input and output parameters. We can use them to verify the decisions made and choose the best option. We can copy the file and save it to our own records.
10. Check on the "Central and non-central distributions" to visualize a graphic presentation of the null and alternative hypothesis, with the critical t values for the corresponding degree of freedom. The plot can be printed or saved to a file.
11. Check on the "x–y for range of values" to open another side drawer, which offers a tabulated as well as a graphical display of a large range of two chosen values among total sample size, effect size, α, and study power. The plots can be printed or saved to a file.

Verification of the Calculation

The conditions necessary for applications of the equations have to be verified: normality of distribution and equality of variance. In the case of a quantitative outcome, the sample's mean (e.g., mean mitral valve area in our example) is supposed to follow a normal distribution with a minimum sample size of 30 patients per group. Fortunately, a normally distributed variable usually verifies the second condition, which is the equality of variances, i.e., the absence of a statistically significant difference between both variances. It is worth insisting that although the inclusion of a minimum of 30 patients per group will permit the use of those formulae, it will not be sufficient to reach a statistically significant difference between compared groups. We have demonstrated that more than five times this number (138 patients per group) is necessary to achieve such a goal.

Power Calculation for a Given Sample Size

We have calculated sample size from effect size, α, and study power. We can compute the power of given sample size, α, and effect size by simple algebra. In our example, the researchers were eager to know whether the authors of the published manuscript put a good power in their study to detect the evidence or, their achieved results were mainly due to chance? We know that the minimum acceptable study power is 80% and the question is whether the previous authors respected this limit or not? Although controversial, we favor calculating the power of published manuscripts before considering their results. We have to be cautious while examining significantly underpowered or overpowered studies.

Online calculators and power software offer the possibility of simple power calculation. In G*power software [21]. we can repeat the previous 11 steps, except step number 3, where we will choose "Post hoc: Compute achieved power-given α, sample size, and effect size" from the drop-down menu of "Type of power analysis". Concordantly, in step number 4, we will upload the sample size per group of the study in question (100), instead of the study power. Finally,

clicking on "Calculate" will show that $\lambda = 2.39$ and a study that was definitely underpowered to detect the evidence: 66.47% only! Kindly compare how sample size affects (ncp) calculated in both studies "Eq. 4.21" and "Eq. 4.22"

$$\lambda_{input\ study} = \frac{(4.1 - 3.8)}{\sqrt{\frac{1.1^2}{100} + \frac{0.6^2}{100}}} = 2.4 \qquad (4.21)$$

$$\lambda_{output\ study} = \frac{(4.1 - 3.8)}{\sqrt{\frac{1.1^2}{138} + \frac{0.6^2}{138}}} = 2.8 \qquad (4.22)$$

What Should be Reported

We must clearly define the primary outcome upon which sample size will be calculated and the previous studies, with references from which we have estimated effect size. We have to report the statistical test used for the comparison, the limit of alpha, the desired study power, the equation used for calculation, and the used software if any.

4.2.2.2 Other Distributions Than Normal

The Wilcoxon-Mann–Whitney test (or U-test) is the nonparametric alternative of the test of Student. The test comes in rescue in small studies and is mainly used when data follow other distributions than normal. It is based on substituting numerical values by ranks like all parametric tests. According to the central limit theorem, ranks follow a normal distribution (see Sect. 2.5.1.1).

The Example

We will use the same example of comparing surgery results to balloon valvuloplasty in patients with rheumatic mitral stenosis, aiming to demonstrate the difference between the parametric and the non-parametric approach to sample size calculation.

The Equation

Al-Sunduqchi and Guenther have shown that we can use a modified approach to sample size calculation in the case of a two-tailed Student test (n). The proposed method can be applied to a small sample of normally distributed data and for data following other distributions than normal. The adjusted sample size (n_i) is the product of the originally calculated sample size (n) multiplied by an index (W) "Eq. 4.23". The value of (W) depends upon the distribution of the data in question, being equal to 2/3, 9 /π^2, π/3 for Laplace, logistic (double exponential), and normal distribution, respectively [29]. The respective new sample size per group (ni) for n = 138 patients will equal 92, 126, and 145 patients per group. Note that (π) is a constant that equals 3.14.

$$n_i = nW \qquad (4.23)$$

G*power Software

1. Check the "Test family" drop-down menu and select "t tests".
2. Check the "Statistical test" drop-down menu and select "Means: Wilcoxon-Mann–Whitney test (two groups)".
3. Check "Type of power analysis" and select: "A priori: Compute required sample size-given α, power and effect size".
4. Under "Input parameters", check "Tail(s)" and select "Two". Leave "α err prob" as such (0.05). Select "Power (1-B err Prob)"; type (0.8), which is the usual power. Define the "Allocation ratio N2/N1) and type (1), in case of two equal samples. Select the "Parent distribution" and choose (Normal, Laplace, logistic, or min ARE). Fill in the effect size if previously known (0.339 in our example) and skip directly to step 6.
5. If the effect size is unknown, click on "Determine" to open the effect size side drawer. Provide the mean and Sd of the first group (4.1) and (1.1) and, mean and Sd of the second group (3.8) and (0.2). In case of unequal groups, provide the mean of each group and the Sd within each group. Click on "Calculate and transfer to main drawer" to close this side drawer and transfer the calculated effect side to the main drawer.

6. Verify your choices: two-tailed study, parent distribution, effect size d = 0.339, α = 0.05, power = 0.8, allocation ratio = 1. Click on "Calculate" to get the reveal the output parameters on the right side of the drawer.
7. Verify the output parameters. If we have chosen a parent "normal distribution," ncp, df, and critical t values are those calculated for a test of Student. On the other hand, the required sample size is much larger, pointing to the amount of power lost with real data being substituted by ranks. It is worth noting that this loss of power is very more acceptable than the biased alternative of applying a parametric test when it should not be. By changing the suggested parent distribution of our data, we can easily verify that the calculated sample sizes are well concordant with the simple formula suggested by Al-Sunduqchi and Guenther.
8. Steps from 8 to 11 are the same as when comparing two normally distributed means (see Sect. 4.2.2.1).

4.3 Association of Two Independent Binary Variables: Chi-Square and Fisher's Exact Tests

The significance of the association between two binary qualitative variables is primarily verified by Chi-square or Fisher's exact test (see Sect. 2.3.1).

4.3.1 Effect Size [28]

4.3.1.1 Cohen d and Cohen h
The Example

A study was designed to analyze the role of tobacco in cancer lung. A literature review has shown that the incidence of cancer in smokers (Pa) is 10% and in non-smokers (Pb) is as low as 3%.

The Equation

The effect size (d) is calculated as the standardized difference between proportions = Δ/Sd. However, several formulae calculate the difference between two proportions (Δ). The simplest is to multiply their difference (Pa-Pb) in decimals by the square root of 2, i.e., by 1.4. In our example, (Δ) = (0.1 − 0.03) × 1.4 = 0.099. The variability in the population is usually unknown, and we have to estimate it from the sample itself. The variance of a proportion among two groups a and b = Pa(1 − Pb) + Pb (1 − Pa) = 0.1(1 − 0.03) + 0.03 (1 − 0.1) = 0.124. The standard deviation (Sd) is the square root of the variance = 0.35 and hence, the effect size = d = Δ/Sd = 0.099/0.35 = 0.28 "Eq. 4.24".

$$Cohen\, d = \frac{\Delta}{Sd} = \frac{(Pa - Pb)\sqrt{2}}{\sqrt{Pa(1 - Pa) + Pb(1 - Pb)}}$$
$$= \frac{0.099}{0.35} = 0.283$$

$$(4.24)$$

Cohen suggested the arcsin transformation of independent binomial proportions to normalize data. Arcsin is the inverted sin of a value and can be directly calculated online [30]. Note that the larger effect size will produce a smaller sample size "Eq. 4.25".

$$Cohen\, h = \emptyset_a - \emptyset_b$$
$$= 2\arcsin(\sqrt{Pa}) - 2\arcsin(\sqrt{Pb})$$
$$= 0.295$$

$$(4.25)$$

4.3.1.2 Phi (φ)

The first letter of the Greek alphabet was used to symbolize the effect size of the association of 2 binomial (2 classes) qualitative variable. An example is testing the association between diabetes (being diabetic or not) and hypertension (being hypertensive or not). (χ^2) is the Chi square value calculated by the Chi-square test and N is the total sample size "Eq. 4.26" (see Sect. 2.3.1).

$$\varphi = \sqrt{\frac{\chi^2}{N}}$$

$$(4.26)$$

4.3.1.3 Cramer's V (Φc)

Cramer's V is equally calculated from Chi-square value and total sample size "Eq. 4.27". However, unlike Phi, Cramer's V can measure the effect size for a multiple-class qualitative variable. An example is to test the association between a 2-class qualitative variable (being diabetic or not) and a 4-class qualitative variable (having severe hypertension, moderate hypertension, mild hypertension, or normotensive). K is the smallest number of classes, which equals 2 in our example. Although the result of both effect sizes is identical, the fact that the use of Phi is restricted to binomial proportions; Cramer's V is the preferred reported measure of effect size for any Chi-square test, regardless of the two variables being binomial or multinomial (see Sect. 2.3.1).

$$\varphi_C = \sqrt{\frac{\chi^2}{N(K - 1)}}$$

$$(4.27)$$

4.3.1.4 Relative Risk (RR)

The relative risk has been discussed before (see Sect. 1.8.2). In brief, the risk is the probability of developing an event. The relative risk (RR) in clinical studies is the ratio between the risk of developing the event in the treatment group and the risk of developing the event in the control group. The interpretation of the RR is simple and straightforward. A relative risk of 1 means no difference between the treatment and the control groups, a RR > 1 indicates higher risk, and an RR < 1 indicates a lower risk in the treatment group than the control group. Such a straightforward and causal interpretation makes the relative risk the choice outcome in clinical trials.

View its skewed distribution; we cannot calculate the 95% CI of the RR. It has to be normalized through logarithmic transformation. We calculate the 95% CI of log RR and then antilog its lower and upper limits to get the 95% CI of RR itself [31] (see Sect. 1.8.7.1). The calculation of the RR, the 95% CI, the Z, and P-values can be automatically generated by many freely available online calculators [32].

4.3.1.5 Odds Ratio (OR)

The odds ratio has been discussed before (see Sect. 1.8.2). In brief, the odds are the number of times that the event of interest occurs to the number of times it does not. The odds ratio is the ratio between two odds: the odds in the treatment group and the odds in the control group. The odds ratio reflects the tightness of the relation between the two binomial variables, regardless of the direction of the study; which makes Odds ratio a perfect outcome to describe observational studies that are not meant to analyze causality. Note that a ratio can never be zero and the null of any ratio = 1. Hence, an Odds ratio >1 means that the relationship is positive (the increase of one variable increases the other), and an Odds ratio <1 means a negative relationship between both variables.

Although the sample odds ratio has a skewed distribution, its logarithmic value has an approximately normal distribution, permitting to assign a 95%CI of log OR (see Sect. 1.8.7.2). The standard error of the log odds ratio is estimated as the square root of the sum of the reciprocals of the four frequencies [33]. Note that all those calculations of Odds ratio, its 95%CI, and Z and P values are generated once we upload the four frequencies to an online calculator [32].

The odds (patients with the event/patients without the event) will always be larger than the risk (patients with the event/all patients) "Eq. 1.23". Consequently, the OR is expected to overestimate the effect size, especially in cases of high prevalence and an unbalanced number of events between the compared groups [34]. We have previously reported that the odds ratio can be interpreted as the relative risk up to a prevalence of 10% (Sect. 1.8.2). In the context of clinical trials and systematic reviews, Altman and Dicks extended the limit to less than 20% [34].

4.3.1.6 Number Needed to Treat (NNT)

We have previously discussed the number needed to treat (see Sect. 1.8.7.4). In brief, the NNT is the number of patients we have to treat, either to prevent the occurrence of one adverse event or to get a single benefit (saving one life, for example). Mathematically, the NNT is the reciprocal of the absolute risk reduction. The NNT is a very important number to decision-makers; the larger is the effect treatment, the smaller will be the NNT and, in concordance, the budget that has to be assigned for the management of this disease.

Altman suggested expressing the NNT as NNT benefit (NNTB) for a positive number to treat and NNT harm for a negative on (NNTH) [35]. The NNTB and NNTH can be deducted from the Odds ratio and the risk of the event in the experimental group (Risk) "Eqs. 1.53 and 1.54" or, by consulting an online calculator [32].

The NNT is like the arithmetic mean. Its statistical significance can be evaluated by building a 95% CI around that mean. As the NNT is the reciprocal of the ARR, the upper and lower limits of the former 95% confidence interval are just the reciprocal values of the latter. Consequently, a 95% CI of the ARR that includes (0) gives a reciprocal 95% CI of NNT that includes infinity (see Sect. 1.4.2.7). The calculation of the NNT, its 95% CI as well as the Z and P-values can be made online [32].

4.3.1.7 Cluster Design [36]

Patients may be distributed to either treatments or procedures as groups or clusters. As example, patients can be randomized according to their geographic distribution or hospitals of management, etc.... The unit is no more the individual patient but the group of patients belonging to each district or receiving treatment in a particular hospital. Variability will not be only between different hospitals but within the same hospital as well. Compared to individual patient randomization in which the variance is between patients only (S^2), the variance is now formed of two components: the intra-cluster variance (Sw^2) which is the variance between the individuals' values and their mean value within each cluster (hospital) and, the variability between clusters themselves (Sc^2). Assuming that (Sw^2) is the same for all clusters and (m) is the number of patients in each cluster, the intra-cluster variance = Sw^2/m. In consequence, the total variance = $[Sw^2/m + Sc^2]$. We can use the usual equation to calculate sample size per group $(n = M/d^2)$ but substitute the d^2 of the equation with the "cluster d^2". Consequently, the resulting (n) would be the number of clusters (and not the number of patients) required in each treatment group "Eq. 4.28".

$$Cluster\ d^2 = \frac{\Delta^2}{\left(S_W^2/m + S_C^2\right)} \quad (4.28)$$

If the patient was our unit of analysis, the number of clusters would equal the number of patients, and cluster design will have no effect $(Sw^2 = 0)$. The more we would like to include patients per cluster, the more cluster design will have an effect $(Sw^2 > 0)$; increasing total variability, which per rule inflates sample size. Consequently, the total number of patients calculated in cluster randomization is always larger than that calculated for simple randomization. The proportion between the two numbers is always > 1 and is called the design effect. A design effect of 1.3 means our sample size will be inflated by 30% to maintain the same power of the study if simple randomization is used. An illustrative example is given by Kerry and Bland [36].

Intra-cluster Correlation Coefficient (r_{icc})

The intra-cluster correlation coefficient (r_{icc}) is another way to summarize the relationship between the two components of variance in a cluster design and to express the design effect "Eq. 4.29". If there is no effect design, such as if the cluster is formed by only one patient or many patients who give "the same reading"; $Sw^2 = 0$ and $r_i = 1$; reflecting a perfect theoretical correlation between readings within clusters. The intra-cluster correlation coefficient (r_{icc}) is usually small due to large intra-cluster variations

(Sw^2), compared to variations between clusters (Sc^2).

$$r_{icc} = \frac{S_C^2}{\left(S_C^2 + S_W^2\right)} \quad (4.29)$$

Donner (D) Design Effect

Donner suggested another way to present cluster design effect, derived from the number of patients per cluster (m) and the r_{icc} "Eq. 4.30". Once more, if the cluster is formed of only one patient, D = 1 and there is no design effect, compared to D = 2, which means that twice as many subjects are required to keep the same study power as a trial where patients were randomized individually.

$$D = 1 + (m - 1)r_{icc} \quad (4.30)$$

4.3.2   Sample Size

4.3.2.1   Difference Between Two Independent Proportions

The Example

We will calculate the sample size to show the significance of the association of smoking with bronchogenic carcinoma. Studies have shown that as much as 10% of smokers have bronchogenic carcinoma, compared to only 3% of non-smokers. The study will have a unilateral design as there would be no point in proving that smoking is protective from bronchogenic carcinoma.

The Equation

As the primary risk of error is universal and constant at 5% and the secondary risk of error is usually chosen 20%, M = 12.4 and sample size per group (n) = M/d^2 = $12.4/(0.098/0.345)^2$ = 153. We have to add an extra 10%. Hence, the number of patients necessary to demonstrate that tobacco is a statistically significant risk factor in developing bronchogenic carcinoma is 170 patients per group.

The continuity correction of a binomial distribution

Calculations involving sample size and power for a qualitative variable were achieved by approximating the binomial distribution to the Normal distribution. By default, any approximation invites imprecision, and hence, mathematical corrections were then made to improve those approximations: the continuity correction (see Sect. 1.4.2.4). A "larger" corrected sample size can be retrieved online [18] or calculated by using G*power software [21]. The question is whether to apply the continuity correction or not. The answer is simple; the continuity correction is applied whenever the expected number of cases in the smallest subgroup of patients is less than 5. The latter is the subgroup of non-smokers who are expected to develop bronchogenic carcinoma, and the expected number of cases just exceeds the limit ($170 \times 3\% = 5.1$ cases). Hence, we are not obliged to apply the correction.

Consulting Online Resources

We have to expect limited variations in the results of sample size calculation of a binomial variable, which may be due to the adopted effect size (Cohen d or Cohen h) and whether a continuity correction was applied or not? We must pay attention to those two elements when calculating or reporting our sample size. Some online resources use the same uncorrected equation that we have just used to compare two proportions, producing a sample size of 153 patients per group [11]. Others give both uncorrected (153 patients) and corrected sample size per group (182 patients) [18]. G*power software provides various options, as we will show in a moment [21]. Nevertheless, and in all cases, we have to increase the calculated sample size by 10%. If we expect a long follow-up period or a significant loss of subjects, this 10% has to be raised, as guided by a comprehensive literature review.

G*Power Software

1. Check the "Test family" drop-down menu and select "z tests".

2. Check the "Statistical test" drop-down menu and select "(Proportions: the difference between two independent proportions)".

3. Check "Type of power analysis" and select: "(A priori: Compute required sample size—given risks of error and effect size)".

4. Under "Input parameters", check "Tail(s)" and select (One). Select (Two) in case of a bilateral study design.

5. Check on "α err prob," and we usually leave it as such (0.05).

6. Check on "Power (1-B err Prob)" and type (0.8), which is the default power of a majority of studies.

7. Check "Allocation ratio N2/N1" and type (1) in case of two equal samples.

8. Check "Proportion p2" and type (0.1), which is the proportion of smokers with lung cancer.

9. Check "Proportion p1" and type (0.03), which is the proportion of non-smokers with lung cancer.

10. Click on "Options" to open a side window, permitting computational and input options. The former includes: "Use continuity correction" and or "Use arcsin transform" in computation. The latter includes keeping the input as such "Use two proportions p1/p2" or "Use Cohen effect size index h" to normalize data. The options include making a "Plot normal distribution (instead of z). We click on Ok, which takes us back to the original window.

11. In case we have taken the option to "Use Cohen effect size index h", we will note that the "Proportion p2" box is replaced by an "Effect size h" box. We type our calculated Cohen h value (0.295) and click "OK".

12. The "Output parameters" include the "Critical z value": 1.65 for one-tail and 1.96 for 2-tails study, "Sample size group 1", Sample size group 2", "Total sample size", "Proportion P2", and the "Actual power" of the test. The calculated sample size per group depends upon our computational choices taken in the "Options" menu. Regardless, the input was made using the two proportions or Cohen h index. The maximum sample size per group is calculated using the continuity correction

(180 patients), the smallest is when requesting an arcsin transformation (142 patients). A smaller sample was produced when both requests were made (169 patients). If no transformation was requested, the calculated sample size would be similar to the one made by hand, i.e., 153 patients per group. We have to be careful about the choices we make during calculation as well as during reporting.

13. The remaining steps are the same as the final four steps from 8 to 11 in case of comparing two normally distributed means (see Sect. 4.2.2.1).

Verification of the Calculations

In the case of a qualitative variable, we have to calculate the proportions of the presence (p) and absence (q) of outcome (cancer lung in our example) in the respective patient groups of smokers (group a) and non-smokers (group b). The second step is calculating sample size per group (n) for smokers and non-smokers by the equation: (na and nb). The third step is to check whether the binomial variable follows an approximately normal distribution or not. Normality is verified whenever nap, naq, nbp, and nbq are all at least equal to 5. In the given example with two equal groups (na = nb = 170 patients), the respective numbers are all above 5: nap = 17, naq = 153, nbp = 5.1, and nbq = 164.9. It is sufficient to verify that the smallest percentage is above 5 (nbp = 170 × 3% = 5.1).

4.3.2.2 Odds Ratio and the Relative Risk

The Example

Binary outcomes are not always presented as proportions but sometimes as relative risk or Odds ratio; both are deductible from one another or the proportions. Returning to our example, where Pa (0.1) and Pb (0.03) are the proportions of cases developing cancer lung among smokers and non-smokers, respectively. The Odds of

having/not having cancer lung among smokers = Pa/(1 − Pa) = 0.1/0.9 = 0.111. Similarly, the Odds of having/not having cancer lung among non-smokers 0.03/0.97 = 0.03. The Odds ratio is the ratio between those 2 Odds = 0.111/0.03 = 3.6, reflecting the tightness of the relation between smoking (risk factor) and cancer lung (the disease).

The Equation

An approximate formula for calculation of sample size from Odds ratio was given by Campbell and colleagues, where (p) is the common proportion of the two groups; p = (Pa + Pb)/2 [24]. We will present the equation for calculating sample size in the case of unilateral study design "Eq. 4.31". The same equation can be used for a bilateral design after replacing (α) with ($\alpha/2$).

$$n = \frac{2\left(z_{1-\alpha} + z_{1-\beta}\right)^2}{(log\, OR)^2 p(1-p)}$$
$$= \frac{2(1.64 + 0.84)^2}{(1.28)0.065(1 - 0.065)} = 160 \quad (4.31)$$

In case of unequal groups with Pa = K Pb, it may be easier to use the nearly similar formula; with ($z_{1-\alpha/2} = 1.96$) in a bilateral design and, ($z_{1-\alpha} = 1.64$) in a unilateral design "Eq. 4.32" [37]. We will present the equation for a unilateral design. As applied to our study on the relation between smoking and bronchogenic carcinoma, K = 1 indicating equal sample sizes "Eq. 4.33".

$$n = \frac{\left(z_{1-\alpha} + z_{1-\beta}\right)^2}{(log\, OR)^2} \left(\frac{1}{k\, pA(1-pA)} + \frac{1}{pB(1-pB)}\right)$$
$$(4.32)$$

$$n = \frac{(1.64 + 0.84)^2}{(log\, 3.6)^2}$$
$$\left(\frac{1}{1 \times 0.1(1 - 0.1)} + \frac{1}{0.03(1 - 0.03)}\right) = 172$$
$$(4.33)$$

Consulting Online Resources

We can consult an online calculator for the sample size required to investigate the association between smoking and bronchogenic carcinoma [17] The result matches that acquired by hand using "Eq. 4.31"; i.e., 172 patients per group. We have to be careful with some online calculators which do not ask the user whether the study design is unilateral or bilateral. In such a case, the design is usually bilateral by default and, we have to change alpha to 10% in case we are planning for a unilateral design [17, 18]:

1. From the side menu of the online calculator sample-size.net [18], we choose to calculate "Proportions-sample size" to open its window.
2. We define "alpha" (0.1), "Beta" (0.2), the proportion of subjects in group 1; i.e., the sample size of group 1 patients to total sample size "q1" (0.5), the risk in the control group "P0" (0.03), and the risk in the exposed group "P1" (0.1) and, we click "Calculate"
3. The calculator gives the Odds ratio (3.59), relative risk (3.33), sample size per group with (182 patients), and without continuity correction (153 patients).

4.3.2.3 Cluster Design

Sample size calculation for a cluster design can be made online [38]. We will use the same example, where the investigators wished to analyze the association between smoking and lung cancer (see Sect. 4.2.2.1). Previous calculations have shown a minimum of 153 patients is required for the study to have an 80% power to prove that the prevalence of cancer is 10% among smokers and 3% among non-smokers. The researchers decided to carry on the study in 10 hospitals (clusters), and they would like to know the average number of patients they have to include per hospital. In addition to the variability between hospitals (Sc^2), they have to consider and eventually add to it, the variability within each hospital (Sw^2). Reviewing the literature has shown that the intraclass correlation, i.e., correlation of in-between hospitals

variability and total variability ($r_i = Sc^2/(Sc^2 + Sw^2)$) was 0.01.

1. We type the input parameters: "Proportion 1%" (3), "Proportion 2%" (0.1), "Power %" (80), "Ratio n2/n1" (1), Alpha risk % (5), and we choose the direction of the study "One-sided test."
2. We choose "Cluster sampling design," and we type: the "Intraclass correlation" (0.01), "Number of clusters" (10), or Number of observations per cluster (we leave it blank). We click on "Calculate".

The output parameters include 153 patients per group, regardless of cluster design, nearly the same given by the simplified equation and other software. Considering cluster design, with a minimum number of ten clusters (hospitals), we have to have an average of 44 cases per hospital. The total sample size was raised from 306 to 440 patients, equally divided between smokers and non-smokers. The cost of cluster design is a 43% increase in sample size to maintain the same power of the study if simple randomization was used. The cost of the design can be expressed as $D = 1 + (44–1)\ 0.01 = 1.43$; indicating a 43% increase.

4.4 Categorical and Ordinal Variables: Chi-Square Tests of Independence and Goodness of Fit

We have previously discussed the Chi-square tests (see Sect. 2.3.1). In brief, those tests are used to compare the patterns of distribution of two qualitative variables (Chi-square test of independence) or the distribution of one qualitative variable to a theoretical distribution (Chi-square of the goodness of fit). In the latter case, the null hypothesis states no difference between the observed and the theoretical values. Alternatively, the probability that both distributions match is as small as 5%. Hence, we can reject the null hypothesis and conclude that the observed distribution is significantly different from the theoretical one. The Chi-square test for independence is the most common. It tests the independence between two qualitative variables, nominal, ordinal, or one of each kind. The null hypothesis is that the distributions of both variables are independent. The alternative hypothesis is an association (dependence) between both distribution variables (see Sect. 2.3.1.2).

Both tests calculate the difference between what we have observed and what is expected under the null hypothesis (χ^2 value). The larger the latter, the smaller the probability of the null hypothesis is true. Once this probability drops to just 5% or smaller, we reject the null hypothesis and adopt the alternative hypothesis of statistical significance.

4.4.1 Effect Size

4.4.1.1 Cramer's V (φc)

The Example

A study was conducted to test the significance of the association between gender (male, female) and the degree of hypertension (mild, moderate, and severe). Data are shown in Table 4.1. The calculated (χ^2) is shown in the "Eq. 4.34" value. The larger is the (χ^2) value. The more is the association between the two variables, and hence, Cramer's V was suggested to measure the size of this association (effect size) from the calculated (χ^2) value. For a total sample size (N = 36 cases) and with (K = 2) being the smaller number of classes of the two variables; Cramer's V = 0.21 "Eq. 4.35"; reflecting a small effect size according to the usual interpretations of Cohen [39]. As (χ^2) can take any value

between zero and infinity, Cramer's V will range between 0 and +1 and, like (χ^2) itself, it cannot be negative for being issued from squared values.

$$\chi^2 = \frac{(9 - 7.5)^2}{7.5} + \frac{(6 - 7.5)^2}{7.5} + \frac{(6 - 6)^2}{6}$$
$$+ \frac{(6 - 6)^2}{6} + \frac{(3 - 4.5)^2}{4.5} + \frac{(6 - 4.5)^2}{4.5} = 1.6$$
(4.34)

$$\varphi_C = \sqrt{\frac{\chi^2}{N(K - 1)}} = \sqrt{\frac{1.6}{36(2 - 1)}} = 0.21$$
(4.35)

4.4.1.2 Cohen W

Cohen proposed to express the effect size from the difference between observed (Po) and expected proportions (Pe) "Eq. 4.36", rather than the observed (O) and expected counts (E) used to calculate (χ^2) value "Eq. 2.1" [39]. Table 4.1 shows the six observed proportions (% of total): 25% females with mild hypertension, 16.7% males with mild hypertension, 16,7% females with moderate hypertension, 16.7% males with moderate hypertension, 8.3% females with severe hypertension, and 16.7% males with severe hypertension. As patients were equally distributed between both genders, we expect equal proportions of males and females (50%:50%) in each of those categories (mild, moderate, and severe hypertension). For example, 41.7% of patients with mild hypertension have to be equally distributed: 20.8% in each gender; however, the observed proportions were different: 25% females and 16.7% males. In fact, the respective six expected proportions should can be obtained by dividing each total category by 2: 0.417/2 = 0.208; 0.333%/2 = 0.167; 0.25/2 = 0.125.

Table 4.1 Sample size calculation: testing the independence between gender and the degree of hypertension

	Males	Females	Total
Mild hypertension	9 (25%)	6 (16.7%)	15 (41.7%)
Moderate hypertension	6 (16.7%)	6 (16.7%)	12 (33.3%)
Severe hypertension	3 (8.3%)	6 (16.7%)	9 (25%)
Total	18 (50%)	18 (50%)	36 (100%)

Values are presented as numbers (%)

Table 4.2 Sample size calculation: the cumulative odds ratio

Hypertension	na	nb	Pa	Pb	Ca	Cb	OR
Mild	9	6	0.5	0.33	0.5	0.33	2
Moderate	6	6	0.33	0.33	0.83	0.66	2.4
Severe	3	6	0.16	0.33	1	1	–
Total	18	18	1	1			

N, p, and c represent numbers, proportions, and cumulative proportions of females (A) and males (B); respectively. OR = odds ratio

Cohen W is calculated as the sum of standardized squared differences between observed and expected proportions. The larger is (W), the more is the dependence between the two variables (gender and hypertension). Like Phi (φ), Cohen W can also be calculated from (χ^2) and total sample size (N) "Eq. 4.36". Applying "Eq. 4.36" on our example gives an effect size of 0.212 "Eq. 4.37".

$$Cohen\ w = \sqrt{\sum \frac{(P_o - P_E)^2}{P_E}} = \sqrt{\frac{X^2}{N}} \quad (4.36)$$

Cohen W

$$= \sqrt{\begin{array}{c} \frac{(0.25-0.208)^2}{0.208} + \frac{(0.167-0.208)^2}{0.208} + \frac{(0.167-0.167)^2}{0.167} + \frac{(0.167-0.167)^2}{0.167} + \\ \frac{(0.083-0.125)^2}{0.125} + \frac{(0.167-0.125)^2}{0.125} = 0.212 \end{array}}$$

$$(4.37)$$

4.4.1.3 Cumulative Odds Ratio

We have shown how to express effect size as Odds ratio calculated for a binary outcome from the two proportions: Pa and Pb: OR=Pa (1 − Pb)/Pb(1 − Pa). Campbell and colleagues have demonstrated that it is better to use the cumulative proportions in an ordered categorical design with more than two categories rather than the proportions themselves [24]. In other words, OR will be the probability of a subject being in a given category or lower in one group, compared to the other group members. If c_1, and c_2 are the cumulative proportions in group 1 and group 2, at the given order; OR can be calculated with the following formula "Eq. 4.38":

$$Cumulative\ OR = \frac{C_1/(1-C_1)}{C_2/(1-C_2)} = \frac{C_1(1-C_2)}{C_2(1-C_1)}$$

$$(4.38)$$

Let us take the example of testing the independence of the degree of hypertension and the patient's gender. As shown in Table 4.2, mild hypertension is the first category in its order, and hence, their cumulative proportions (Ca and Cb) are equal to the respective proportions (Pa and Pb = 0.5 and 0.33). On the other hand, Ca in patients with moderate hypertension = (Pa in mild hypertension + Pa in moderate hypertension) = 0.5 + 0.33 = 0.83 and Cb in patients with severe hypertension = 0.33 + 0.33 = 0.66. As shown, the cumulative proportion of the last category of the order will always be equal to 1 in both groups (Table 4.2).

As OR will differ from one category to the other (2 in mild hypertension and 2.4 in moderate hypertension, in our example) and, unlike in the binary outcome, there are multiple OR(s); reflecting the second fact that proportions are also different from one category to the other. All this "valuable information" would have been simply lost if the outcome was reduced to the binomial situation, e.g., mild to moderate versus severe hypertension. This valuable information is the strength of an ordered categorical design that makes it more powerful than a binomial outcome. In our example, OR is the mean of the two Odds ratios = (2 + 2.4)/2 = 2.2, compared to the relatively smaller ES calculated by Cramer's V (0.21) or Cohen W (0.212).

4.4.2 Sample Size

4.4.2.1 Independence from Odds Ratio

View the presence of different proportions across categories and the need to calculate several (OR)s, the equation to calculate sample size from cumulative OR is complex in its original form and hence, Campbell and colleagues suggested a simple equation as well as Tables for sample size calculation and different study powers "Eq. 4.39" [24].

$$n = \frac{3M}{(\log OR)^2} \qquad (4.39)$$

The equation is based upon the "pragmatic" assumptions that the mean proportions are roughly equal, the mean OR(s) are more or less constant, and that the number of categories >5. In the case of a smaller number of categories, the calculated sample size per group (n) has to be multiplied by the factors: 1.042, 1.067, 1.125, and 1.333; in case we have only 5, 4, 3, and 2 categories; respectively. M represents the "more or less constant" weight of the risks of error calculated for a unilateral $[2 \ (Z_{1-\alpha} + Z_{1-\beta})^2]$ and bilateral study $[2 \ (Z_{1-\alpha/2} + Z_{1-\beta})^2]$. M equals 12.4 for a unilateral study with an 80% power and 17.1 for the larger 90% power. In the case of a bilateral study, the respective values of (M) are 15.7 and 21 [13].

Returning to our example: for a mean OR of 2.2 $[(2 + 2.4)/2 = 2.2]$, a bilateral design with power of 80% and $\alpha = 5\%$; M = 15.7 and n = 1.125{3 × 15.7/(log 2.2)2} = 85 patients per group. We have to note that if there were only two categories, (n) would have been multiplied by 1.333, instead of 1.125, and a larger sample of 98 patients has to be included in each group; which means that we had to increase our sample size by about 30%.

Going further and comparing "mild" to "combined moderate and severe" cases, i.e., transforming our ordered categorical outcome into a binary variable. The OR = (9/9)/(6/12) = 2. With the usual risks of error, the sample size will be equal to 130 patients per group. In other words, if we decide to lose the information that the treatment effect differs according to different outcome categories, we have to recruit as many as 50% more patients. The researcher has to answer the important

question: does the additional power achieved by the ordered categorical design (the smaller sample size) overweight the risk associated with the many pragmatic assumptions that have to be made to calculate the cumulative odds ratio? If the answer is yes, we have to be sure that the categories are clinically meaningful, provided that the assumptions made (constant OR and equality of proportions across categories) are nearly verified.

4.4.2.2 Independence from Cohen's (W)

G*power software does not calculate directly sample size for K-class Chi-square for independence. We need to calculate the non-centrality parameter (λ) first.

1. Check the "Test family" drop-down menu and select "χ^2 tests".
2. Check the "Statistical test" drop-down menu and select "Generic χ^2 test".
3. Check "Type of power analysis" and select: "Sensitivity: Compute noncentrality parameter -given α, and power".
4. Under "Input parameters", heck on "α err prob" and we usually leave it as such (0.05).
5. Check on "Power (1-B err Prob)" and type (0.8), which is the default power of a majority of studies.
6. Check "Df" and type (2), which is the degrees of freedom = number of classes of the first variable minus one multiplied by the number of classes of the second variable minus one = 2–1 × 3–1 = 2.
7. Click on "Calculate" to execute the analysis.
8. The output parameters include the critical χ^2 value (5.99) for 2 df and, the noncentrality parameter ($\lambda = 9.634$). The following equation calculates the total sample size (N) "Eq. 4.40":

$$N = \frac{\lambda}{(Cohen\,W)^2} = \frac{9.634}{(0.212)^2} = 214 \quad (4.40)$$

4.4.2.3 Goodness of Fit

We start by calculating effect size Cohen (w) as the sum of the differences between observed and expected proportions, squared and standardized by being divided by the expected differences as usual. We will give a binomial example for simplicity, but the test equally applies to multinomial (ordinal) data. A researcher wants to examine whether an observed distribution of 32 baby boys (41%) and 46 baby girls (59%) born at a particular year period fits the theoretical 50/50 proportion of gender among newly born. The 78 newly born were expected to be 39 baby boys (50%) and 39 baby girls (50%). Chi-square test goodness of fit shows a statistically non-significant difference Chi-square value of 2.51 "Eq. 4.41". Cohen W can be calculated either from the Chi-square value and the total sample size or, from the individual proportions "Eq. 4.42".

$$\chi^2 = \frac{(32-39)^2}{39} + \frac{(46-39)^2}{39} = 2.51 \quad (4.41)$$

$$
\begin{aligned}
Cohen\,W &= \sqrt{\frac{X^2}{N}} = \sqrt{\frac{2.51}{78}} \\
&= \sqrt{\sum \frac{(P_o - P_E)^2}{P_E}} \\
&= \sqrt{\frac{(0.41-0.5)^2}{0.5} + \frac{(0.59-0.5)^2}{0.5}} \\
&= 0.18
\end{aligned}
$$

$$(4.42)$$

We can follow the same steps of Sect. 4.4.2.2 to calculate ncp (λ) from the usual primary (5%) and secondary risks (20%) of error. However, in the goodness of fit model, the degree of freedom is equal to the number of cells (observed boys, expected boys, observed girls, and expected girls) minus one = 4–1 = 3. The noncentrality parameter (λ) = 10.92 and the total sample size (N) = (λ)/(Cohen W)^2 = 337 patients.

In addition, G power software offers the mean to calculate sample size for the goodness of fit Chi-square directly.

1. Check the "Test family" drop-down menu and select "X^2 tests".
2. Check the "Statistical test" drop-down menu and select "goodness of fit: Contingency tables".
3. Check "Type of power analysis" and select: "Compute required sample size—given α, power and effect size".
4. Under "Input parameters", check on "α err prob", and we usually leave it as such (0.05).
5. Check on "Power (1-B err Prob)" and type (0.8), which is the default power of a majority of studies.
6. Check on "Df" and type (3). The df equals the number of cells minus one.
7. Type the "Effect size W" if known (0.212) and click on "Calculate" to execute the analysis. Otherwise, click on "Determine" to open the effect size drawer.
8. Determine the "Number of cells" (4), type the two observed proportions "p(H0)": (0.41) and (0.51) and the two expected proportions "p(H1)" (0.5) and (0.5). Click "Calculate and transfer to main window" to compute "Effect size W" (0.1829) and transfer it to the main window.
9. The "Output parameters" include the non-centrality parameter (λ) = 10.9, the critical X^2 value (7.81), the total sample size (326), and the "Actual power" (0.80).
10. The remaining steps are the same as the final four steps from 8 to 11 in case of the comparison of two normally distributed means (see Sect. 4.2.2.1).

4.5 Paired Analysis

4.5.1 Paired Student Test

Comparing the patient to himself (or to a matched control), removes (or at least reduces to a minimum) the variability between subjects. Hence, it empowers the analysis and reduces the required sample size. This gain of power has two sources: arithmetic and statistic. The arithmetic gain is obvious that the same patient will be used twice, and hence if N is the total sample size for an independent two groups study, only N/2 patients will be required for a paired design [5].

The statistical gain is based on the fact that the variability of the response of one individual to the two treatments is theoretically less than when the two treatments are given to two different individuals. The patients' response to 2 different treatments of the same disease is expected to be less variable than the response of two different patients to the same treatments. The response of the two treatments is expected to correlate with each other when given to the same patient. The more they correlate, the more we gain in power for the well-known inverse relationship between sample size and variability. When comparing two unpaired or paired means, statistical software routinely expresses this correlation between both measurements as correlation coefficient "r". The more "r" is positive and approaching 1, the more we gain from the cross-over design as we will have to include fewer patients, compared to the situation if the same trial was conducted on two independent groups. The value of "r" is either looked for in the literature or calculated from data; otherwise, it would not be unreasonable if we included N/2 patients from the start.

4.5.1.1 Effect Size: Cohen dz

The Example

Let us take the example of a study conducted to compare the duration of pain relief with two analgesics (a) and (b) in patients with chronic arthritis. A review of the literature has shown that the mean (Sd) duration of pain relief after analgesic (a) and (b) were: 4.1 ± 1.1 and 3.8 ± 0.6 h. Note that those are the same data that we have previously used to calculate sample size to compare two independent means (with different variable names). In the unpaired design set, the analysis showed an effect size of 0.34, a non-centrality parameter (λ) of 2.8, and a minimum sample of 138 patients per group is required to give the study an 80% power, with the usual primary risk of error of 5% (see

Sect. 4.2.1.1). Let us now use the same data to calculate (λ) and total sample size (N) for a paired design to appreciate the gain produced.

The Equation

According to Cohen, the effect size of a paired design is expressed as the standardized mean of the difference (Cohen dz) [39]. The mean of the difference (M_{diff}) is simply the difference between both means, standardized by being divided by the Sd of the difference "Eq. 4.43". The more the response of the same patient to one treatment positively correlates with his response to the second treatment, the more it reduces the variability. Such "covariation" depends on the variability (Sd) of the two treatments and their correlation (r). Consequently, the covariation is the product of the three components. Put it this way; the quantity [r*Sda*Sdb] is the covariance of variables a and b [Cov_{ab}]; which is the amount of correlation that is expected to be reduced from the total variability $[(Sda)^2 + (Sdb)^2]$. The covariation represents the gain achieved by the paired design, and it has to be removed from the total variability "Eq. 4.43".

The quantities u_a, u_b, and M_{diff} are the mean values of treatment a, treatment b, and the difference between both treatments. Sd_a, Sd_b, Sd_{diff}, and (r) are the standard deviation of treatment a, standard deviation of treatment b, the Sd of the difference, and the positive correlation coefficient r between the two measurements. Most statistical software produces correlation coefficient r when calculating the Student test and supposing that r was equal to 0.4, the Sd_{diff} will be equal to 1.02 and Cohen dz = 0.294. If the correlation coefficient was not measured, the quantity [r*Sda*Sdb] would be equal to zero; the Sd_{diff} will be larger (1.253); reducing effect size to 0.239. As per rule, the smaller the effect size, the larger will be the sample size, and hence, we are all interested in looking for the value of r and introducing it in our equation. As in the case of Cohen ds of unpaired design, Cohen dz can be calculated from the paired (t) value and total sample size (N). Cohen ds and Cohen dz are themselves interchangeable "Eq. 4.44".

$$Cohen\,d_z = \frac{M_{diff}}{Sd_{diff}} = \frac{\mu_a - \mu_b}{\sqrt{Sd_a^2 + Sd_b^2 - 2rSd_aSd_b}}$$

$$= \frac{4.1 - 3.8}{\sqrt{1.1^2 + 0.6^2 - 2(0.4) \times 1.1 \times 0.6}}$$

$$= 0.294$$

$$(4.43)$$

$$Cohen\,d_z = \frac{t}{\sqrt{N}} = \frac{Cohen\,d_s}{\sqrt{2}} \qquad (4.44)$$

4.5.1.2 Sample Size

As previously noted, G*power software can also calculate effect size, λ and sample size. Most interestingly, it provides the researcher with an entire power curve and tables for his convenience to explore the most suitable sample size for his resources.

1. Check the "Test family" drop-down menu and select "t tests".
2. Check the "Statistical test" drop-down menu and select "Means: Difference between 2 dependent means (matched pairs)"
3. Check "Type of power analysis" and select: "A priori: Compute required sample size-given α, power and effect size"
4. Under "Input parameters", check "Tail(s)" and select (Two). We would choose one-tail if we compare a treatment to a placebo. Leave "α err prob" as such (0.05). Select "Power (1-B err Prob)"; usually (0.8). Fill in the effect size if previously known (0.294 in our example) and skip directly to step 6.
5. If the effect size is unknown, click on "Determine" to open the effect size side drawer. Choose between calculating effect size "From differences" or "From group parameters". In the former case, provide "Mean of the difference" (0.3) and "SD of the difference" (1.02). In the latter case, provide "Mean group 1" (4.1), "Mean group 2" (3.8), SD group 1" (1.1), "SD group 2" (0.6), and "correlation between groups (0.4). Click "Calculate and transfer to the main window".
6. Verify your choices in the main window: two-tailed study, approximate effect size

d = (0.3), α = (0.05), power = (0.8). Click on "Calculate" to show the output parameters on the right side of the drawer.

7. Verify the output parameters: "Noncentrality parameter λ" (2.84), "Critical t" (1.98), "Df" (N − 1 = 92); "Total sample size N" (93), and "Actual power" (0.8).
8. The remaining steps are the same as the final four steps from 8 to 11 in case of the comparison of two normally distributed means (see Sect. 4.2.2.1).

Variations of the Calculation

The reader is advised to apply those variants himself to "appreciate" their effects on the outcome. A negligible difference is produced between calculating effect size from differences (0.3) or from group parameters (0.294), which may be due to the effect of approximation. The difference in total sample size is small: 90 versus 93 patients. On the other hand, neglecting the covariance decreases the effect size to 0.24. The price of neglecting this valuable information will be a 50% increase in the total sample size, which is enormous. On the other hand, comparing treatment to placebo by a one-tailed design usually reduces any sample size by about 20%.

Finally, the following formula expresses the relationship between the effect size (Cohen dz), the non-centrality parameter, and the total sample size (N) "Eq. 4.45":

$$N = \frac{\lambda^2}{(Cohen\,d_Z)^2} \qquad (4.45)$$

4.5.2 Paired Wilcoxon-Sign-Rank Test

The Wilcoxon signed-rank test (or T-test) is a nonparametric alternative to the paired test of Student used when we are not confident about data being normally distributed. The test is based on substituting numerical values by ranks, which have a normal distribution according to the central limit theorem.

4.5.2.1 Effect Size: Grisson and Kim and Correlation Coefficient R

The Example

We will use the same example reported in Sect. 2.5.1.3. A study was conducted to compare the duration of pain relief associated with the use of two analgesics, A and B. Ten patients were randomized to either receive treatment A for one week followed by treatment B for another week or the reverse, with a suitable wash-out period. In brief, analgesic A provided significantly longer periods of pain relief than analgesic B. Positive ranks were 32, negative ranks were 4, and Z score was 1.96. Two patients did not show any preference, and hence, data were available for eight patients only. Due to the small sample size, we have checked on the T-rank tables, which showed that our smaller calculated sum (N = 4) was larger than the critical sum (=3) figured in the table. Hence, the result was judged as being statistically non-significant (see Sect. 2.5.1.3).

The violation of parametric assumptions limits the value of Cohen's dz as an appropriate effect size. As the test is based upon comparing positive and negative differences of paired values, Grisson and Kim suggested reporting the probability that a random value has a positive difference (n+) from all calculated paired differences (N) "Eq. 4.46" [28]. In our case, a value (duration of pain relief) drawn at random from patients receiving analgesic (A) has a 75% chance to be larger than another random value drawn from patients receiving analgesic (B). We can also deduct another effect size r from the calculated Z score and total sample size (N) "Eq. 4.47". Whichever the chosen effect size, we have to remove the two cases that gave no preferences from the calculations.

$$PS_{dep} = \frac{n+}{N} = \frac{6}{8} = 0.75 \qquad (4.46)$$

$$r = \frac{z}{\sqrt{N}} = \frac{1.96}{\sqrt{8}} = 0.693 \qquad (4.47)$$

4.5.2.2 Sample Size: Al-Sunduqchi and Guenther

We have previously shown that Al-Sunduqchi and Guenther suggested a modified approach from the one used to calculate sample size in the case of a one-tailed Student test [29]. This approach can be applied to a small sample of normally distributed data and for data following other distributions than normal. The originally calculated (N) is adjusted by being multiplied by the index (W), which is equal to 2/3, $9/\pi^2$, $\pi/3$ for Laplace, Logistic (double exponential), and normal distribution, respectively (see Sect. 4.2.2.2).

The Example

In order to show the loss of power associated with a non-parametric test, we will take the same example used with the paired Student test (see Sect. 4.5.1.2). In brief, a study was conducted to compare pain relief associated with the use of two analgesics in patients with chronic arthritis. A total sample size of 93 patients was required to give the study an 80% power to find a significant difference between both analgesics.

Suppose the researchers have decided to use the non-parametric Wilcoxon-sign rank test instead of the paired test of Student. According to Al-Sunduqchi equation and, assuming that the duration of pain relief is normally distributed, the calculated sample size for a paired t-test has to be multiplied by $\pi/3$, giving a total sample size of 98 patients [29].

G*power software

G*power software gives the same sample size. We will proceed as if we are calculating sample size for a paired Student's test (see Sect. 4.5.1.2), except in step 6, where we have to define the parent distribution of our data as being normal, Laplace, or logistic.

1. Check the "Test family" drop-down menu and select "t tests".
2. Check the "Statistical test" drop-down menu and select "Means: Wilcoxon signed-rank test (matched pairs)".

3. Check "Type of power analysis" and select: "A priori: Compute required sample size-given α, power and effect size".
4. Under "Input parameters", check "Tail(s)" and select (Two). We would choose one-tail if we compare a treatment to a placebo. Leave "α err prob" as such (0.05). Select "Power (1-B err Prob)"; usually (0.8). Fill in the effect size if previously known (0.294 in our example) and skip directly to step 6.
5. If the effect size is unknown, click on "Determine" to open the effect size side drawer. Choose between calculating effect size "From differences" or "From group parameters". In the former case, provide "Mean of the difference" (0.3) and "SD of the difference" (1.02). In the latter case, provide "Mean group 1" (4.1), "Mean group 2" (3.8), SD group 1" (1.1), "SD group 2" (0.6), and "correlation between groups (0.4). Click "Calculate and transfer to the main window".
6. Define the "Parent distribution" of data, choose (normal).
7. Verify your choices in the main window: two-tailed study, normal distribution, effect size d = (0.295), α = (0.05), power = (0.8). Click on "Calculate" to show the output parameters on the right side of the drawer.
8. Verify the output parameters: "Noncentrality parameter λ" (2.84), "Critical t" (1.98), "Total sample size N" (98), and "Actual power" (0.8).
9. The remaining steps are the same as the final four steps from 8 to 11 in case of comparing two normally distributed means (see Sect. 4.2.2.1).

4.5.3 McNemar's Test

McNemar's test is applied to verify the independence of the distribution of two binomial variables, whether being observed in the same group of patients or in two matched groups.

4.5.3.1 Effect Size: Odds Ratio

The Example

A study was conducted to compare two antidepressants (A and B) given simultaneously to a group of 80 patients. The second treatment was only given after a sufficient wash-out period to ensure the absence of any residual effect of the first treatment on the results of the second one. The outcome was patient satisfaction tested as yes (1) or no (2). Seventy patients agreed (87.5%), whether as being satisfied with both treatments (52 patients; $P_{11} = 65\%$) or not satisfied with either treatment (18 patients; $P_{22} = 22.5\%$). The point of research is the remaining ten patients with disconcordant results ($P_{disc} = 12.5\%$): seven patients were satisfied with the treatment (A) but not with treatment B ($P_{12} = 8.8\%$). In comparison, only three patients reported the reverse ($P_{21} = 3.8\%$) and the question is whether such disagreement is significant or not?

The Equation

Under the null hypothesis, there should be no difference in patients' preferences to either treatment ($P_{12} = P_{21}$). In other words, the odds of a patient being satisfied with treatment A and not satisfied with treatment B should be equal to the odds of the patient being not satisfied with treatment A but satisfied with treatment B. Consequently, the ratio of those two odds (OR) should be equal to 1.

In our example, the respective observed proportions were 0.088 and 0.038, and the Odds ratio was equal to 2.315. In other words, the odds (let us say the probability) for a patient to be satisfied with the first treatment and not the second is more than twice the reverse (Odds) probability. It looks like patients are more satisfied with treatment A and the question is whether such observation is significant or not? This is what the McNemar test is about.

The effect size is expressed as odds ratio (P_{12}/P_{21}). Knowing the proportion of disconcordant pairs (P_{disc}) and the difference between the two proportions ($P_{diff} = P_{12} - P_{21}$), the odds ratio can be also expressed as in "Eq. 4.48":

$$OR = \frac{\left(P_{diff} + P_{disc}\right)}{\left(P_{diff} - P_{disc}\right)} \qquad (4.48)$$

The verification of the calculation shows: $P_{diff} = 0.088 - 0.038 = 0.05$, $P_{disc} = 0.125$, $OR = (0.05 + 0.125)/(0.05 - 0.125) = 2.315$. Although the effect size considers only disconcordant pairs (yes/no and no/yes patients), the proportion of concordant pairs has to be known too ($1 - P_{disc} = 1 - 0.125 = 87.5\%$, in our study) in order to calculate the total sample size of the study, which includes both: concordant (yes/yes and no/no) and disconcordant (yes/no and no/yes) patients.

According to Greenland [40], variance paired log OR = $(a + b)/ab = (3 + 7)/3 \times 7 = 0.476$ and hence, its square root, the Se of Log OR in our example = 0.69. The 95% CI of our Log OR $(0.84) \pm 1.96 (0.69) = -0.5$ to 2.19 and, their anti-log lower and upper limits are: 0.61 and 8.96. A 95% confidence interval bypassing 1 is non-significant, the Z value of Log OR = Log OR/Se Log OR = 1.2; hence P > 0.05. We can conclude that there was no statistically significant difference between the effect of either antidepressant.

4.5.3.2 Sample Size: Machin Formula, Schork & Williams Formula

Let us now calculate the appropriate sample size to put into evidence the calculated effect size (OR = 2.315). Adopting the usual 5% primary and 20% secondary risks of error and a bilateral study design, the total sample size (N) can be calculated using the approximate formula of Machin and colleagues "Eq. 4.49" [41]. We present the formula of a two-tailed study. In the case of a one-tail study, we have to replace $Z_{1-\alpha/2}$ with $Z_{1-\alpha}$, as usual.

$$N = \frac{\left\{Z_{1-\alpha/2}(OR+1) + Z_{1-\beta}\sqrt{(OR+1)^2 - (OR-1)^2 P_{disc}}\right\}^2}{(OR-1)^2 - P_{disc}}$$

$$(4.49)$$

Knowing that $Z_{1-\alpha/2} = 1.96$, $Z_{1-\alpha} = 1.65$, $Z_{1-\beta} = 0.84$ for a study power of 80% as in our example and = 1.28 for a 90% power, OR = 2.315, $P_{disc} = (P_{12} + P_{21})/(P_{11}/P_{22}) = 0.125$; total sample size (n) = 392 for bilateral study and 296 for a unilateral study. A more exact formula was suggested by Schork and colleagues, which gives a larger sample size by about 10%. [42].

The Use of G*Power Software

1. Check the "Test family" drop-down menu and select "Exact".
2. Check the "Statistical test" drop-down menu and select "Proportions: Inequality, two dependent groups (McNemar)".
3. Check "Type of power analysis" and select: "A priori: Compute required sample size-given α, power and effect size".
4. Under "Input parameters", check "Tail(s)" and select (Two). We would choose one-tail if we compare a treatment to a placebo. Leave "α err prob" as such (0.05). Select "Power (1-B err Prob)"; usually (0.8). Fill in the effect size: "Odds ratio" (2.315). Fill in "Prop disconcordant pairs" (0.125). Click on "Calculate".
5. Verify the "Output parameters": "Noncentrality parameter λ" (2.84), "Critical t" (1.98), "Df" (N − 1 = 89); "Total sample size (392), "Actual power" (0.8), "Actual α" (0.044), "Proportion p12" (0.0873). "Proportion p21" (0.0377). If we choose a one-tail study, the total sample size will be reduced to only 296 patients.
6. The remaining steps are the same as the final four steps from 8 to 11 in case of comparing two normally distributed means (see Sect. 4.2.2.1).

The Use of Online Calculator

Connor and colleagues have suggested a pretty similar formula using P_{disc} (proportion of disconcordant pairs = 0.125 in our example) and P_{diff} (proportions of the difference between disconcordant pairs = 0.05 in our example) "Eq. 4.50" [43].

$$N = \left[\frac{Z_{1-\alpha/2}\sqrt{P_{disc}} + Z_{1-\beta}\sqrt{P_{disc} - P_{diff}^2}}{P_{diff}} \right]^2$$

$$(4.50)$$

The test is available online, and the researcher has just to introduce P_{12} and P_{21} (0.088 and 0.038 in our example), define his primary risk of error, the direction of the study (0.05 for a bilateral study and 0.1 for a unilateral study) and the study power (80% in our example). The software calculates P_{disc} and P_{disc} in the background and just reveals the required sample size: 393 patients for a bilateral study and 310 patients for a unilateral design [17].

4.6 Comparison of Multiple Means: One-Way ANOVA

Analysis of variance (ANOVA) is the test of choice to compare multiple means. The outcome is a continuous variable (e.g., duration of hospital stays) that has to be normally distributed among groups (e.g., patients subjected to different types of surgery). The aim is to prove that the mean outcome is dependent on groups, and by deduction, groups are called independent variables or predictors of outcome. In our example, the duration of hospital stay after surgery is usually due to (is dependent on) the cumulative effect of many variables such as type of surgery, age of the patient, associated disease, the occurrence of complications, etc. ANOVA can partition, analyze and test the statistical significance of the role of each of those predictors on the outcome.

Remember that the variance (S^2) is computed as the sum of squared deviations of individual values from their mean (SS), divided by the degrees of freedom (sample size-1). Thus, given a certain n, the variance is a function of (SS). ANOVA partitions the total variability of the duration of hospital stay (the total sum of squares; SS_{total}) into a series of SS_{effect} due to: type of surgery, patient age, associated disease or complications and, a residual variability that remains unexplained ($SS_{residual}$).

The larger is the proportion of an individual (SS_{effect}) to the total SS (SS_{total}), the more is the importance of the role of this individual variable on the outcome. This proportion is called: the Eta squared $\eta^2 = (SS_{effect}/SS_{total})$ and is a good estimate of the effect size of the impact of the independent variable on the outcome. On the other hand, a part of (SS_{total}) will always remain unexplained by any of those factors and is called the residual or error variability ($SS_{residual}$ or SS_{error}) that needs to be explained by introducing other variables in the model. Sample size calculation will follow the same steps as before, including estimating the proper effect size, choosing a unilateral or bilateral study design, adopting the primary and secondary risks of error, and finally, sample size calculation.

4.6.1 Effect Size

There are several ways to measure the effect size in ANOVA, including Eta squared, partial Eta squared, Omega squared, Cohen f, and intra-class correlation coefficient (see Sect. 2.4.3) [25].

4.6.1.1 Eta Squared η^2

Eta squared η^2 is the proportion between the variability due to the predictor and the total outcome variability (SS_{effect}/SS_{total}); hence, it represents how much the predictor explains the outcome.

The Example

Consider the following data set in Table 4.3 recording the duration of pain relief after surgery among three groups of patients. Fifteen patients were equally randomized among three groups, each receiving a different analgesics Ketorolac (A), morphia (B), or placebo (C). Let us see how ANOVA analyses variability in terms of SS (Table 4.3).

1. *Calculation of the total variability (SS_{total})*

The duration of pain relief differs among the 15 patients, as expected. Although this variability can be logically due to the type of analgesic received, other factors could intervene, of course. We begin by calculating the overall variability

Table 4.3 Sample size calculation: pain relief following three analgesics (one-way ANOVA)

Pain relief	Treatment A	Treatment B	Treatment C	Overall
I	6	3	1	
II	6	3	1	
III	8	4	2	
IV	8	4	2	
V	7	4	1	
Mean	7	3.6	1.4	4
SS-within group (error)	4	1.2	1.2	6.4
SS-between group (effect)				79.6
SS total				86

I, II, III,IV, and V represent the five patients in each treatment group A, B and C. Values in the table are durations of pain relief in hours

among the 15 patients. The overall mean duration of pain relief (Grand mean = u) can be easily calculated by summing all 15 durations and getting the average = 4 h. The overall variability can then be expressed as $SS_{total} = [(6 - 4)^2 + (6 - 4)^2 + (8 - 4)^2 + (8 - 4)^2 + (7 - 4)^2 + (3 - 4)^2 + (3 - 4)^2 + (4 - 4)^2 + (4 - 4)^2 + (4 - 4)^2 + (1 - 4)^2 + (1 - 4)^2 + (2 - 4)^2 + (2 - 4)^2 + (1 - 4)^2] = 86$. This represents the total variability (change) in outcome (duration of pain relief) due to type of analgesic received + other factors that we should look for, e.g., patient age, gender, duration of surgery, etc. These other factors would be responsible because patients receiving the same analgesic will respond differently.

2. *Calculation of the residual variability (SS_{error}) or (SS_{within})*

All group A patients received the same analgesic (ketorolac); however, their response varied between 6 and 8 h; with a within-group sum of squares = $[(6 - 7)^2 + (6 - 7)^2 + (8 - 7)^2 + (8 - 7)^2 + (7 - 7)^2] = 4$. This within-group variability is also observed among patients of other groups. The within-group variability for B and C patients were 1.2 and 1.2. The sum of the within-group variabilities = 4 + 1.2 + 1.2 = 6.4. Note that this within-group sum of squares (SS_{within}) has nothing to do with the treatment effect, which is why it is also called the residual variability,

i.e., the part of variability that remains unexplained by the treatment. It is also called "error variability" because it can be attributed to an error in measurement (SS_{error})."

3. *Calculation of the in-between group variability (treatment effect)*

If SS_{total} represents the total variability (total change in the dependent variable) due to the effect of known as well as unknown predictors and, if $SS_{residual}$ represents the effect of variables other "other than" treatments; SS_{effect} of analgesics is calculated by simple deduction of $SS_{residual}$ from SS_{total} = 86–6.4 = 79.6. In our example, effect size = SS_{effect}/SS_{total} = 0.926 "Eq. 4.51". In other words, the difference in effect between the groups of analgesics explains about 93% of the outcome; which is substantial.

$$\eta2 = \frac{SS_{effect}}{SS_{total}} \qquad (4.51)$$

4. *Calculation of variance (mean square) and F ratio*

The variance is called the mean square (MS) because it is calculated by dividing the "sum" of squares (SS) by a number derived from the "sample size" (df). The within-group MS = 6.4/12 = 0.533 and, the treatment MS = 79.6/2

= 39.8 = 74.625. The latter is the F ratio, which is significantly larger than the critical value tabulated in the F table at df (2, 12); $P < 0.001$ (see Sect. 2.4.3.1).

4.6.1.2   Partial Eta Squared $\eta_P{}^2$

Although Eta squared is a measure of the effect of analgesics on the outcome, whenever other independent variables are included in the model, such as the effect of patient's gender or age, those variables will explain more of the residual variability. Hence, η^2 is automatically increased. A better estimation of effect size in the ANOVA model, including more than one predictor, will be achieved by adjusting $\eta_P{}^2$ (reducing the overestimated effect size) by adding SS_{error} to the dominator of the equation "Eq. 4.52".

$$\eta P^2 = \frac{SS_{effect}}{SS_{total} + SS_{error}} \qquad (4.52)$$

4.6.1.3   Omega Squared ω^2

Omega squared ω^2 was suggested to improve η^2, which measures the variance in the sample but not in the population. As the variability in any sample is larger than the variability in the population—especially with small samples—η^2 will always overestimate the effect size. In an attempt to move beyond a particular study sample to the population from which the sample was drawn, ω^2 was designed to express a more predictable effect size, whenever the study is repeated. We have to note that the equation is limited to in-between subject analysis, with equal sample sizes in each cell (subgroup) "Eq. 4.53".

$$\omega 2 = \frac{SS_{effect}\left(df_{effect} \times MS_{error}\right)}{SS_{total} - MS_{error}} \qquad (4.53)$$

Applying this formula to data presented in Table 4.3 gives a smaller but less biased effect size: $\omega^2 = [79.6 - (2 \times 0.533)]/(86 - 0.533) = 0.918$ The larger is the sample, the more it will be representative of the population, and the gap between η^2 and ω^2 will eventually decrease.

4.6.1.4   Cohen f

Cohen f "Eq. 4.54" is an extension of Cohen's ds "Eq. 4.8" used to express the effect size of the difference between two means [39]. For the presence of more than two groups, the numerator, which was just the difference between the two means, it is now replaced by the average of the squared differences between the individual group means (u_j = 7, 3.6 and 1.4) and the grand mean (u = 4); with K being the number of groups (=3). The denominator represents the common standard deviation that can be estimated from previous studies or can be calculated as the square root of pooled variance derived from the sample itself "Eq. 4.55". Applying the formula to our example gives a pooled variance of 0.533 "Eq. 4.56" and a huge effect size of 3.16 "Eq. 4.57".

$$Cohen f = \sqrt{\frac{(\mu_k - \mu)^2/k}{S_{pooled}^2}} \qquad (4.54)$$

$$S_{pooled}^2 = \frac{S_1^2(n_1 - 1) + S_2^2(n_2 - 1) + \ldots + S_k^2(n_k - 1)}{(n_1 + n_2 + \ldots + n_k) - k} \qquad (4.55)$$

$$S^2 pooled = \frac{1^2(4) + 0.547^2(4) + 0.547^2(4)}{(5 + 5 + 5) - 3}$$
$$= 0.533 \qquad (4.56)$$

$$Cohen f = \sqrt{\frac{\left[(7-4)^2 + (3.6-4)^2 + (1.4-4)^2\right]/3}{0.533}} = 3.16 \qquad (4.57)$$

It is worth noting that all previously reported effect sizes are approximately interchangeable using "Eq. 4.58".

$$Cohen f = \sqrt{\eta^2/(1 - \eta^2)}$$
$$= \sqrt{\eta P^2/(1 - \eta P^2)}; \eta^2 = f^2/(1 + f^2) \qquad (4.58)$$

4.6.2 Sample Size

We have previously noted different derivatives of sample size calculation formulae in concordance with how effect size was estimated and whether ncp is known or has to be calculated. The reader must be cautious when using different online calculators or when executing calculations by hand. In general, we follow the usual process by defining the effect size (ES), either found in previous studies or calculated by hand as shown above or by one of the many available software, such as G power. Sample size can be also looked for online in special tables [22].

4.6.2.1 Sample Size for a Given Power

1. Check the "Test family" drop-down menu and select "F tests".
2. Check the "Statistical test" drop-down menu and select "ANOVA: Fixed effects, omnibus, one-way".
3. Check "Type of power analysis" and select: "A priori: Compute required sample size-given α, power and effect size".
4. Under "Input parameters", leave "α err prob" as such (0.05). Select "Power (1-B err Prob)"; usually (0.8). Type the "Number of groups" (3). Fill in the effect size if previously known (3.16) and skip directly to step 6.
5. If the effect size is unknown, click on "Determine" to open the effect size side drawer. "Select procedure" either (effect size from means) or effect size from variances. Type the "Number of groups| (3), Type the "SD within each group", which is the square root of S^2 pooled (0.73). Along with the "Group" number (1, 2, 3), type the "Mean" (7, 3.6, 1.4) and "Size" (5, 5, 5). Click on "Calculate and transfer to main window" to calculate effect size (3.155).
6. Verify your choices in the main window: Cohen effect f = (3.155), α = (0.05), power = (0.8) and "Number of groups" (3). Click on "Calculate" to show the output parameters on the right side of the drawer.
7. Verify the output parameters: "Noncentrality parameter λ" (59.75), "Critical F" (9.55), "Numerator df" (number of groups $-$ 1 = 3 $-$

1 = 2); "Denominator df" (total number of patients – number of groups = 6–3 = 3); "Total sample size" (6), and "Actual power" (0.964).
8. The remaining steps are the same as the final four steps from 8 to 11 in case of comparing two normally distributed means (see Sect. 4.2.2.1).

Interpretation of the Results

Before interpreting the results of the calculation, we have to repeat that, throughout this book, we insisted upon using "small examples", whenever hand calculation was feasible. The small sample allows the reader to follow the calculations and better understand them. However, it usually stops short of fulfilling all the conditions necessary for applying some statistical tests. We were not able to do both: using a large sample that fulfills the requirements of normality, as an example, and at the same time, expecting that the non-statistician will follow the lengthy calculations. We have chosen to use the small and easy example and, at the same time, fully describe any missing condition of application. What we are presenting here is an illustrative example. We were able to follow the calculations, knowing that we needed a larger sample to validate the results. The rules of ANOVA are quite rigid concerning normality and equality of variances. It usually requires a larger sample, and the conditions of application have to be checked out before the analysis (see Sect. 2.4.3.1).

Nevertheless, this min-example can be interpreted as follows: provided that the data used in the calculations of effect size (Table 4.3) fulfills the requirements of ANOVA, we can assume that the calculated effect size reflects that of the population. We can use any of the effect sizes shown above since they are all interchangeable. Note that we are not always obliged to calculate ES ourselves, but we can use what was calculated by other reliable sources.

The second step is to define our primary and secondary risks of error and to upload our data to the power software of our choice. For the usual risks of error, the results show that we need to include a total of 6 patients to give our study an 80% power to put into evidence such a large effect size.

4.6.2.2 Post-Hoc Power Calculation

A part of the software output was "the actual power of the study". The actual study is the original study that included a larger sample of 15 patients and, being a larger study, it had a 96.4% power to put into evidence the same effect size. In other words, the software calculated the power of the original study that included 15 patients (96.4%). However, as we requested a smaller power (80%), it was calculated that six patients were enough to give any future study this smaller desired power. Another point in the output window was the calculated ncp parameter ($\lambda = 59.76$), and the question would be is it the ncp of the original study that included 15 patients and had 96.4% power to detect Cohen f of 3.16 or, it is the ncp of the future study that we plan to conduct with s smaller number of cases (=6) a and limited power (=80%)?

The Noncentrality Parameter of the Original Study

Both Effect size and noncentrality parameter express the deviation of the sample from what is expected under the null hypothesis. We have shown that effect size can be expressed as the proportion of total variability explained by treatment effect (SS_{effect}/SS_{total}). The ES of data presented in Table 4.3 = 79.6/86 = 0.926. The conclusion is that treatment is responsible for about 93% of variability detected in the whole study. On the other hand, Kirk has defined the noncentrality parameter (λ) as a measure of the degree to which a null hypothesis is false, and hence, it can be expressed as the odds of variability explained by treatment (SS_{effect}) to that remaining unexplained (MS_{error}) "Eq. 4.59" [12]. The more the probability that the null hypothesis is false, the larger (λ) will be. In our example, ncp of the original study = 79.6/0/0.533 = 149.

$$\lambda = \frac{SS_{effect}}{MS_{error}} \qquad (4.59)$$

Another way to calculate (λ) is to use the original data presented in Tables 4.3. While Cohen's f was calculated as the average of the in-between

group variability (differences), λ is the sum of those differences "Eq. 4.60" and "Eq. 4.61".

$$\lambda = \frac{n(\mu_k - \mu)^2}{S^2_{pooled}} \qquad (4.60)$$

$$\lambda = \frac{5\left[(7-4)^2 + (3.6-4)^2 + (1.4-4)^2\right]}{0.533}$$
$$= 149 \qquad (4.61)$$

Note the difference between the two equations derived from the same data: Cohen F expresses an average of the effect treatment "Eq. 4.57" and (λ) expresses the sum of treatment effect "Eq. 4.61". As the difference between the sum and the average is the number of patients, it becomes quite logical to calculate the total sample size (N) by simply dividing the sum by the average "Eq. 4.62". Note that: a) all differences were calculated in standardized values as usual b) Cohen's f had to be raised to the same squared scale as λ and, c) verifying the calculation gives the total sample size (N) of data of the original study, presented in Table 4.3. N = 149/3.16^2 = 15 patients.

$$N = \frac{\lambda}{Cohen f^2} \qquad (4.62)$$

The Noncentrality Parameter of the Planed Study

As previously mentioned, we have only one central distribution but many non-central distributions (λ) depending upon the adopted primary and secondary risks of error. In other words, each study will have its own (λ). In concordance, each study will have its own sample size too. We have calculated the λ value ($\lambda = 149$) and total sample size (N) of input study = (λ/Cohen f^2) = 15 patients. Let us now use the same equations to calculate (λ) and (N) for the future study, with the same effect size. The λ value of the output study is much less (about 2/5) for the smaller study power (sample size). Despite that, both studies are each composed of 3 groups, n (sample size per group) equals 2 and not 5, as in the input study. The λ value for the output study will be 59.75 "Eq. 4.63", and its required total sample size   N = $(\lambda/f^2) = (59.75/3.1^2) = 6$ patients. These were also the values calculated by G power software output.

$$\lambda = \frac{2\left[(7-4)^2 + (3.6-4)^2 + (1.4-4)^2\right]}{0.533}$$
$$= 59.75$$

$$(4.63)$$

Power Analysis Using G*Power Software

The software permits the calculation of power for a given sample size.

1. Check the "Test family" drop-down menu and select "F tests".
2. Check the "Statistical test" drop-down menu and select "ANOVA, Fixed effects, omnibus, one-way".
3. Check "Type of power analysis" and select: "Post hoc: Compute archived power-given α, sample size, and effect size".
4. Under "Input parameters", leave "α err prob" as such (0.05). Type "Total sample size" (15) and "Number of groups" (3). Fill in the effect size if previously known (3.155 in our example) and skip directly to step 6.
5. If the effect size is unknown, click on "Determine" to open the effect size side drawer. "Select procedure" either (effect size from means) or effect size from variances. Type the "Number of groups| (3), Type the "SD within each group", which is the square root of S^2 pooled (0.73). Along with the "Group" number (1, 2, 3), type the "Mean" (7, 3.6, 1.4) and "Size" (5, 5, 5). Click on "Calculate and transfer to main window" to calculate effect size (3.155).
6. Verify your choices in the main window: Effect size f (3.155), α = (0.05), total sample size (15), and the number of groups (3). Click on "Calculate" to get the reveal the output parameters on the right side of the drawer.
7. Verify the output parameters: "Noncentrality parameter λ" (149.3), "Critical F" (3.88),

"Numerator df" (number of groups $- 1 = 3 - 1 = 2$), "Denominator df" (total sample size – number of groups = 15–3 = 12) and "Power" (1).

8. The remaining steps are the same as the final four steps from 8 to 11 in case of comparing two normally distributed means (see Sect. 4.2.2.1).

Interpretation of the Results

Because of the large ES (=3.15), including 15 patients has given the original study 100% power to detect such a large (ES). For a future (output) study, a total sample size of 6 patients will be sufficient to give such study the requested 80% power to detect this quite large ES.

4.7   Simple Correlation: Pearson's Correlation Coefficient R

In the general meaning of the term, correlation describes the association between two quantitative variables (x and y). As a crude approximation, the correlation between the two variables can be considered linear if the value of one variable increases (or decreases) by a more or less "steady amount", in response to a unit change of the other variable. Statisticians have more accurate definitions and tests for linearity, of course.

The Example

Figure 2.4 shows the correlation between the duration of surgery in minutes and the amount of blood loss in ml in ten polytraumatized patients. Each data point on the scatter plot represents both information collected from the same patient. We can visualize a linear association by taking a ruler and fitting a straight line by eye to the data points on the graph, passing through as many points as possible and minimizing the distances from others: the trend line. The correlation coefficient r expresses how data fit this line: from no correlation (r = 0) to perfect 100% correlation (r = 1). In our example, both variables correlated positively. On the other hand, two variables can correlate negatively when the increase in one variable is associated with a decrease in the other variable. A well-known example is the number of cigarettes smoked per day and life expectancy in years. Consequently, r can acquire any value between +1 and −1; reflecting the strength and direction of the relation between x and y. More details are given in Sect. 2.6.1.1.

4.7.1 Effect Size

4.7.1.1 Fisher's Transformation

Fisher remarked that the distribution of the correlation coefficient r becomes extremely skewed, especially when r lies in the neighborhood of +1, even in large samples. As such, r may be unsuitable to express the variability in the population (i.e., to be used as effect size) and, hence, he suggested normalizing the sampling distribution of Pearson's correlation coefficient r by transforming it into the normal distribution "Eq. 4.64". In other words, he transforms the r score into a Z score [44].

If (x) and (y) are two normally distributed variables, with correlation r and the (x, y) pairs being measured independently, they will follow an approximately normal distribution. Like any other normal distribution, it can be described by its mean value and its standard error. The mean is a normalized r (Z_r), and the standard error equals ($1/\sqrt{N} - 3$), where N is the total number of pairs. Consequently, we gain all the advantages of a normal distribution and became able to:

- Create a confidence interval around r (r ± 1.96 Se).
- Check its statistical significance by consulting the Z table.
- Compare the correlation coefficients of two independent samples.
- Calculate a normalized effect size "Eq. 4.64".

In our example, r = 0.887 and, using Fisher's transformation, $Z_r = 1.09$, the Se = $1/\sqrt{9}$ = 0.333, and the 95%CI = 1.09 (±1.96) 0.333 = 1.74 to 0.437. The Z score can be back transformed to r by "Eq. 4.65".

$$Z_r = \frac{1}{2} \log\left[\frac{(1+r)}{(1-r)}\right] \qquad (4.64)$$

$$r = \frac{\exp 2z - 1}{\exp 2z + 1} \qquad (4.65)$$

4.7.2 Sample Size

4.7.2.1 A Simple Equation

There are several methods for sample size calculation. One commonly used method is based on Fisher's normalization of Pearson's correlation coefficient "Eq. 4.66" [45]. The interested reader can return to May and Looney for details of the equation and sample size charts, with informative examples [46]. As usual, the total sample size (N) is directly proportional to the risks of error and inversely proportional to effect size (C); which represents the normalized r. The present calculations are based on the usual 5% risk of error and a bilateral study design with 80% power. In a unilateral design, $Z_{1-\alpha/2}$ (1.96) will be replaced by $Z_{1-\alpha}$ (1.65). If the researcher is interested in increasing the power of the study from 80 to 90%, he has to increase $Z_{1-\beta}$ from (0.842) to (1.28), as usual.

$$N = \left(\frac{Z_{1-\alpha/2} + Z_{1-\beta}}{C}\right)^2 + 3 \qquad (4.66)$$

The reader can easily verify that approximately seven patients (6.6) are needed to give his study an 80% power to detect a significant positive correlation (r = 0.887) between the duration of surgery and amount of blood loss, with the usual primary risk of error of 5%.

G*Power Software

1. Check the "Test family" drop-down menu and select "Exact".
2. Check the "Statistical test" drop-down menu and select "Correlation: Bivariate normal model".
3. Check "Type of power analysis" and select: "A priori: Compute required sample size-given α, power and effect size".

4. Under "Input parameters", check "Tail(s)" and select (Two). Leave "α err prob" as such (0.05). Select "Power (1-B err Prob)"; usually (0.8). Leave the "Correlation p H0" as such (0), unless previous studies have shown that it is >0. Click on "Options" to choose between two methods of "Computation": "use exact distribution if N<" or "use large sample approximation (Fisher Z)". Take the first option if you have a small sample size of less than ten cases and otherwise take the second option. Click "OK".

5. If the effect size is unknown, click on "Determine" to open the effect size side drawer. Type R^2, which is simply the squared value of r. Click "Calculate and transfer to the main window".

6. Verify your choices in the main window: two-tailed study, correlation p H1 = (0.887), correlation p H0 = (0), α = (0.05), power = (0.8). Click on "Calculate" to get the reveal the output parameters on the right side of the drawer.

7. Verify the output parameters: "lower critical Z value" (−1.96), "upper critical Z value" (1.96), "Total sample size" (7), and "Actual power" (0.8).

8. The remaining steps are the same as the final four steps from 8 to 11 in case of comparing two normally distributed means (see Sect. 4.2.2.1).

Verification of the Calculation

The sample size calculated by the software is the same as the one calculated by the approximate formula shown above, i.e., seven patients in total.

4.8 Simple Linear Regression

In bivariate correlation, the coefficient of correlation "r" measures the strength of the mutual relation between the two variables (x) and (y). A single equation can then express the mutual relation. In regression, however, the change of one variable is dependent upon the other. The first can then be called the dependent or outcome variable, and, by deduction, the latter is called the independent or predictor variable. Unlike the unique "r" in correlation, the "influence" of the predictor (x) on the dependent variable (y) is expressed by the regression coefficient of (x) function (y), called the B coefficient. In order to measure or express the effect of "y" on "x", we have to calculate a different regression coefficient of (y) function (x), i.e., another B coefficient. In consequence, there will be two different equations: one to deduct (x) from a known (y) and the other to calculate (y), in case (x) is defined (see Sect. 2.6.2.1).

4.8.1 Effect Size

4.8.1.1 The B Coefficient

We have previously discussed simple regression in Sect. 2.6.2.1, and hence, we will give a briefing. Let us take the example of studying the effect of the duration of surgery on the amount of postoperative blood loss (Table 2.25). As shown in Fig. 2.5, each point on the scatter plot represents the amount of blood loss related to a particular surgery duration. Under the null hypothesis, the amount of blood loss is unrelated to the duration of surgery, and hence, the patient is expected to lose the same amount of blood, regardless of the duration of surgery. Consequently, a line joining all those pairs of points will be strictly horizontal. However, it was well noticed that the longer is the duration of surgery, the more patients will lose blood, and hence, the line joining those pairs of data will concordantly incline away from the horizon, forming a slope (P_0) (Fig. 2.5). The slope (P_0) reflects the effect of surgery duration on the amount of blood loss (Fig. 2.5). The B coefficient is just the standardized value of this slope (P_0), and, in our example, it is equal to 0.804 (Table 2.29).

4.8.2 Sample Size

4.8.2.1 A Simple Equation

Remember that we have to deal with the two components of effect size: its magnitude and its variability. Under the null hypothesis, the regression line is horizontal; hence, its slope (P_0) = 0. The magnitude of the effect of x on y can be calculated as the product of the variation of (S_x) multiplied by the slope (P_0). The larger is the magnitude of the effect $[(P_0) S_x]$, the smaller is the required sample size. On the other hand, the more is the variability of the effect (standard deviation of regression = $S_{regression}$), the more we need patients to put the effect size into evidence. We have previously reported the equation to calculate the Sd of regression from the variance of outcome (S_y), the variance of (S_x), and the slope (P_0) "Eq. 2.97".

All we have to do now is choose our risks of error and upload the equivalent standardized values: i.e., $(Z_{1 - \alpha/2} = 1.96)$ in case of a bilateral study or $(Z_{1-\alpha} = 1.65)$ if the study was unilateral. We usually choose between 80% or 90% power with the corresponding $(Z_{1 - \beta})$ values of 0.84 and 1.28. We present the equation for a bilateral study and the usual 80% power "Eq. 4.67". The interested reader can return to Dupont and Plummer for more mathematical details [47].

$$N = \frac{(Z_{1-\alpha/2} + Z_{1-\beta}) Sd_{regression}}{PoSd_x}$$
$$= \frac{(Z_{1-\alpha/2} + Z_{1-\beta}) \sqrt{(Sd_y)^2 - (P_0)^2 (Sd_x)^2}}{PoSd_x}$$
(4.67)

The equation may look terrifying, yet it follows the same basic rule: sample size is proportional to the variability $(Sd_{regression})$, which is why the latter is the denominator of the equation and, is inversely proportional to the magnitude of the effect $[(P_0) Sd_x]$, which is why it takes numerator's position, together with the usual indices of precision for a bilateral study; i.e., $(Z_{1 - \alpha/2})$ and $(Z_{1-\beta})$.

The Example

For example, a study was conducted to examine the effect of the duration of myocardial ischemia during coronary artery bypass grafting (CABG) on the total operative time, both measured in minutes. Previous studies have shown that the respective standard deviations of both measurements were: 37.8 and 92.3 min, and the correlation coefficient r was 0.49. The researchers wanted to arrange for a study that can prove that

each minute of myocardial ischemia increases the operative time by about 20%, i.e., $Sd_x = 37.8$, $Sd_y = 92.3$, and $P_o = 1.2$. Applying "Eq. 4.67", we can calculate the Sd of regression "Eq. 4.68" and then the total sample size "Eq. 4.69". Whether we used the equation or consulted an online calculator [48], we can verify that we need to include 25 patients in our study to have an 80% power to detect this 20% difference, with the usual 5% primary risk of error.

$$Sd_{regression} = \sqrt{92^2 - 1.2^2 \times 37.8^2} = 80 \quad (4.68)$$

$$N = \left[\frac{(1.96 + 0.84) \times 80}{37.8 \times 1.2} \right]^2 = 25 \quad (4.69)$$

G*Power Software

1. Check the "Test family" drop-down menu and select "t tests".
2. Check the "Statistical test" drop-down menu and select "Linear bivariate regression: One group, size of slope".
3. Check "Type of power analysis" and select: "A priori: Compute required sample size-given α, power and effect size".
4. Under "Input parameters", check "Tail(s)" and select (Two). Leave "α err prob" as such (0.05). Select "Power (1-B err Prob)"; usually (0.8). Leave "Slope H0" as such (0). Fill in the three required information: "Slope H1" (1.2), "Std dev x" (37.8), and "Std dev y" (92.3) if known and skip directly to step 6
5. If one of the last three required information, "Slope H1, Std dev x, or Std dev y" is missing, click on determine to find it. Upload "r" (0.49) and the two known values to find the missing one. Remember Po = r(Sy/Sx) "Eq. 2.81". Click "Calculate and transfer to the main window".
6. Verify your choices in the main window: two-tailed study, α = (0.05), power = (0.8), Slope H0 = 0, Slope H1 = 1.2, Std dev x = 37.8, and Std dev y = 92.3. Click on "Calculate" to get the reveal the output parameters on the right side of the drawer.
7. Verify the output parameters: "Noncentrality parameter λ" (2.93), "Critical t" (2.059), "Df"

(N − 2 = 27); "Total sample size N" (27), and "Actual power" (0.8).

8. The remaining steps are the same as the final four steps from 8 to 11 in case of comparing two normally distributed means (see Sect. 4.2.2.1).

4.9 Time to Event

A distinguishing feature of time-related data is that the event probably will not have occurred for all patients at the end of the follow-up period. Censoring can occur when the patient is lost to follow up or experience a competitive event like being dead, whether from other diseases or in an accident. We do not know whether the censored patients would develop the event or not. The second point is that patients are usually recruited over time but followed up till a fixed date, and hence, patients are not followed for the same period of time. Because of censoring and unequal follow-up durations, not all patients will be at the same risk of experiencing the event. Hence, special statistical tests were suggested to consider those points during the analysis [49].

The analysis of time to events has been discussed before (see Sect. 2.7 and 3.6). In brief, time-related events are usually observed with the actuarial or Kaplan–Meier methods and analyzed by the simple (bivariate) Log-rank test or through the hazard ratio (HR) calculated with (the multivariate) Cox regression analysis. Among the basic assumptions of those two tests: patients have to have the same prognosis regardless of their participation times and whether they were being censored or not. Before proceeding, we urge the reader to review Sects. 1.8.3.2, 2.7 and 3.6.

4.9.1 Effect Size

4.9.1.1 The Hazard Rates

For survival analysis in clinical trials comparing two treatments, the hypothesis of interest could be comparing the hazard rates or the median survival times. Since the time-to-event is assumed to be exponentially distributed (occurring at constant rate), the hazard rate determines the median survival time (λ). As a result, comparing median survival times is equivalent to comparing hazard rates. Lachin proposed sample size calculation for two survival rates by comparing their respective hazard rates: $\lambda 1$ and $\lambda 2$ [50]. Under the null hypothesis, there should be no difference between both hazard rates $H_0 = (\lambda 1 - \lambda 2) = 0$. The alternative hypothesis (H_1) is that the difference is not equal to 0.

4.9.1.2 The Hazard Ratio

The effect size can also be expressed as the hazard ratio (HR) or the Log HR in a Cox regression model [51]. Under the null hypothesis, the hazard of the event of interest (mortality in our example) at a particular time (t) in one group (h1) is equal to that in the second group (h2). Assuming that this hazard (risk) is proportional (constant) at all times, the hazard ratio at a certain time (HR = h1/h2) is equal to 1, for all times (t).

4.9.2 Sample Size

Regardless of the method used to predict effect size, and as per rule, the sample size is directly proportional to the risks of error ($Z_{1-\alpha/2} + Z_{1-\beta}$); a quantity that equals 2.8 for the usual risks: $\alpha = 5\%$ and 80% power. In the case of a unilateral design, $\alpha/2$ is substituted by the whole α, and this quantity will be equal to 2.49, giving a smaller sample size by about 20%.

4.9.2.1 The Exponential Method

Lachin and Foulkes suggested a model to compute sample size for the Log-rank test comparing survival, under the assumption of proportional hazards [52]. The study time (T) is divided into the accrual time (T_0) and follow-up time ($T_0 - T$). The former is the time during which we recruit the patients for the study. The latter is the time of follow-up and no patient recruitment. The hazard rates of group 1 and group 2 are denoted as λ_1 and λ_2. The survival is assumed to have an exponential distribution ($1 - e^{-\lambda x}$), where λ is the average event rate and x is the follow-up duration. The following formula calculates the variance of survival in each group ($\sigma^2 \lambda_i$) "Eq. 4.70":

$$\sigma^2(\lambda_i) = \lambda_i^2 \left(1 + \frac{e^{-\lambda_i T} - e^{-\lambda_i (T - T_0)}}{\lambda_i T_0} \right)^{-1}$$

(4.70)

Under the null hypothesis, there should be no difference between both hazard rates: $H_0 = (\lambda_1 - \lambda_2) = 0$. The alternative hypothesis is that the difference is not equal to 0, of course. If K is the proportion between the two groups: n_1 and n_2, with $n_2 = Kn_1$; "Eq. 4.71" calculates the sample size of group 2 (n_2):

$$n_2 = \frac{\left(Z_{(1-\alpha/2)} + Z_{(1-\beta)} \right)^2}{(\lambda_1 - \lambda_2)^2} \left[\frac{\sigma^2(\lambda_1)}{k} + \sigma^2(\lambda_2) \right]$$

(4.71)

Although the equation looks complicated, it follows the same basic formula of sample size calculation. The sample size (n) is directly proportional with variability (σ^2) and precision $(Z_{1-\alpha/2} + Z_{1-\beta})$ and, indirectly proportional to large survival difference $(\lambda_1 - \lambda_2)$, as usual.

The Example

A study was designed to compare the progression-free survival of patients with lymphocytic leukemia who received conventional chemotherapy or a new biological treatment. The total duration of the study (T) was three years and the accrual period (T_0) was one year; hence, the follow-up period $(T - T_0)$ was two years. Previous studies have shown that the progression hazard rates of group 1 and group 2 were: 1 and 2 patient-years; respectively. The data were substituted in "Eq. 4.70" to produce the variances of survival in the first "Eq. 4.72" and the second group "Eq. 4.73".

$$\sigma^2(\lambda_1) = 1^2 \left(1 + \frac{e^{-1x3} - e^{-1(3-1)}}{1x1} \right)^{-1} = 0.97$$

(4.72)

$$\sigma^2(\lambda_2) = 2^2 \left(1 + \frac{e^{-2x3} - e^{-2(3-1)}}{1x1} \right)^{-1} = 3.94$$

(4.73)

The question was how many patients were needed to give the study an 80% power to find a statistically significant difference between both groups, with the classic primary risk of error of 5%. Substituting the data in "Eq. 4.71" produces a sample size of about 39 patients per group "Eq. 4.74".

$$n_2 = \frac{(1.96 + 0.84)^2}{(2 - 1)^2} \left[\frac{0.97}{1} + 3.94 \right] = 38.5$$

(4.74)

4.9.2.2 Cox Proportional Hazard Model

We start by calculating the number of events (ne) required to show a significant difference between both groups. Then, we calculate the total sample size.

Calculation of the Number of Required Events

The number of required events depends on the proportions of patients in each group (P1 and P2), the risk of experiencing the event in one group compared to the other (HR = hazard ratio), the assigned risks of error and the direction of study. Using the example of testing a new treatment for bronchogenic carcinoma, with an expected survival benefit of 50%; the HR = 0.5. For the usual primary risk of error (α) of 5%, a bilateral study with planned 80% power, the number of events can be calculated by the same usual logic. The more we would like to be precise $[(Z_{(\alpha/2)} + Z_{(\beta)})^2]$ and the smaller the effect size $[P_1 P_2 (log_{HR})^2]$, the more events $[n_e]$ are needed "Eq. 4.75". Applying the equation to our example, ne = (2.8)²/0.5*0.5 (log 0.5)² = 65 events

$$n_e = \frac{\left(Z_{(\alpha/2)} + Z_{(\beta)} \right)^2}{P_1 P_2 (log_{HR})^2 (1 - R^2)}$$

(4.75)

The Role of Interim Analysis

Suppose we would like to test part of our data by interim analysis. In that case, we have to compensate for the inflated (α) by multiplying the number of calculated events for a bilateral study by the suggested correction made by Pocock [53]. For an 80% power, the calculated number of events should be multiplied by 1.11, 1.17, 1.20, and 1.23 in the case of 2, 3, 4, and 5 planned (final + interim) analysis. The respective factors for a 90% power are 1.1, 1.15, 1.18, and 1.21. Returning to our example, planning two additional intermediate analyses necessitates multiplying the calculated ne by 1.17 = 76 events.

The Role of Other Variables (Covariates)

Cox regression is a multivariable analysis aiming to show the role of other covariates on the outcome, which effect is denoted by R square (R^2). In order to consider this during the calculation of the number of events and eventually sample size, Hsieh and Lavori modified the equation; where R square is the proportion of variance explained by the multiple regression of the main variable of comparison (e.g., type of treatment) on the remaining covariates in the model. In our example, if the model shows an R^2 value of 0.2, the number of calculated events will increase from 65 to 81 events. The sample size will eventually increase proportionally [54].

Sample Size Calculation

The next step is to determine the number of patients who will experience those events during the study period "Eq. 4.76". Suppose that all patients will experience the event during one year (i.e., the probability of having the event is 100% = Pre = 1). It will be sufficient to enroll 65 patients and follow them up for one year; (ne/Pre = 65/1 = 65 patients). In a balanced two groups design, the total number of patients (N) can be directly calculated by dividing the total number of events (ne) by the probability of having the event (Pre), at this period (t). (Pre) is the average probability of having the event in both groups, per patient-year.

$$N = \frac{n_e}{Pr_e} \qquad (4.76)$$

Continuing our example, previous studies have shown that the rate of death with bronchogenic carcinoma = (λt) = ten patients/100 patient-year = 0.1 events/patient-year. The probability of being free from the event (to survive) = S_1, and by deduction, the probability of having the event (to die) = $1 - S_1 = Pr_{e1}$ "Eq. 4.77":

$$Pr_{e1} = (1 - S_1) = (1 - e^{(-\lambda x)}) = (1 - e^{(-0.1*1)})$$
$$= (1 - 0.905) = 9.5\%$$
$$(4.77)$$

Suppose that a new treatment was given to a comparable group of patients. Previous studies have shown that the new treatment decreases the hazard of mortality by 50%: HR = 0.5. The expected survival of group 2 patients at one year is S_2, and by deduction, the probability of having the event (to die) = $1 - S_2 = = Pr_{e2}$ "Eq. 4.78":

$$Pr_{e2} = (1 - S_2) = (1 - e^{(-\lambda HR)})$$
$$= (1 - e^{(-0.1*0.5)}) = (1 - 0.951) = 4.9\%$$
$$(4.78)$$

The average probability of having the event (Pr_e) is related to group proportions, and as both groups were equal, the proportions were 0.5 "Eq. 4.79".

$$Pr_e = (0.5 \times 9.5\%) + (0.5 \times 4.9\%) = 7.2\%$$
$$(4.79)$$

The total sample size (N) is then calculated by simply dividing the total number of required events (n_e) by the average probability of having the event (Pr_e) = 65/0.072 = 903 patients "Eq. 4.80". A number that has to be raised by at least 10% to compensate for censored patients. We have to note that this simple formula is quite valid for the calculation of number of events but it becomes highly approximate in calculating sample size. Note that total sample size for a bilateral study and 80% power can be directly calculated in one step by the following equation, including the inclusion of the effect of other covariates as expressed by R^2

$$N = \frac{\left(Z_{(1-\alpha/2)} + Z_{(1-\beta)}\right)^2}{Log\,HR^2 p_1 p_2 Pr_e\left(1 - R^2\right)} \quad (4.80)$$

The Use of Online Calculators

1. *Comparison of two survival curves*

An online calculator supported by Harvard school of public health can be used to verify the calculations made by hand [55]. We begin by choosing the "Significance level" (0.05), (two) "Sided" study, the duration of (1) "Accrual interval" (2), "Follow-up interval", (0.69) "Median time to failure in the group with the shortest time to failure in" (Years). Note that the median follow-up is calculated as: $\ln 2/\lambda = 0.69/1 = 0.69$ years. (0.8) "Power", and (2) "Minimal detectable hazard ratio (>1)". By clicking on the "Calculate" button, the online calculator gives the total sample size (80) "Total number of patients". The total number is nearly equal to that calculated by hand; i.e., 39 patients per group in "Eq. 4.74".

2. *Cox proportional hazard*

We are applying the example calculated by hand on the online calculator supported by the UCSF Clinical and translational science institute [18]. We begin by designing the limit of "α" (0.05), "β" (0.2), the proportion of subjects in the exposed group "q1" (0.5), the proportion of subjects in the un-exposed group "q0" (0.5), the hazard ratio "relative hazard RH = group 1/group 0" (0.5), and we click on "Calculate events" to get the number of events. The calculator produces the same number we calculated by hand "Total events needed = A/B" (65).

The second step is to calculate the sample size required to develop those 65 events. We have to introduce either the basic event rate "BER0" (0.1) or the median survival of Group 0 "ST0" (6.93) and the software automatically calculates the other. We introduce the duration of follow-up "FU" (1). Keeping a (0) censoring rate gives a total sample size of 903 patients, nearly identical to the one calculated by hand. Uploading a usual censoring rate of 0.3, gives us a much larger total sample size of 1043 patients.

Another calculator equally gives similar results [17]. Where all that is required is designing "Power $1 - \beta$" (0.8), "Type I error, α" (0.05), "Hazard ratio" (0.5), "Overall probability of the event" (0.072), "proportion of the sample in Group A" (0.5). However, none takes into consideration the effect of other variables. Fortunately, and as shown by Hsieh and Lavori, corrected sample size can be estimated by dividing the given sample by the quantity $(1 - R^2)$ [54].

4.10 Logistic Regression

Binary logistic regression has been discussed before (see Sect. 3.5). In brief, logistic regression is commonly used to analyze epidemiological studies to examine the relationship between possible risk factors and disease. In follow-up studies, it can predict the probability that a dichotomous outcome such as dead/alive is dependent upon or can be explained by one or more categorical or continuous variables such as gender, age, type of medication, duration of treatment, etc.… Let us start by the case of having only one independent variable ($\times 1$): the level of a particular biomarker of ischemia. The relation between the probability of myocardial infarction (MI) and the level of the biomarker is "S" shaped and not linear for the usual low probability to develop the event at the low level of biomarker and the very high probability at the high level (Fig. 3.21). The odds of the probability of MI [P/$(1 - P)$] follow the same S relation; however, its logarithmic value "log $P(1 - P)$" is linearly related to the biomarker; which facilitates the prediction of the event for a given biomarker level (Fig. 3.22). The slope that this "regression line" creates with the horizon reflects how much the biomarker can explain the event; the larger the angle, the more the biomarker can explain the occurrence of MI (Fig. 3.23).

Under the null hypothesis, the biomarker level is not related to the development of MI: the regression line is horizontal, and hence its slope (B_0) has a null value. Under the alternative hypothesis, the probability of MI is related to the level of the biomarker (x), and hence, the slope (B_1x) is an addition to (B_0). Remember that we use the logarithmic values of the odds (the log of the odds) to linearize the relation, and hence, $B_0 = Log P_0 (1 - P_0)$ and $B_1x = Log P_1 (1 - P_1)$. As the difference between two logarithmic values is equal to their ratio, the effect of the independent variable (B_1x) on the outcome variable is equal to the ratio between the two odds, i.e., their Log OR and, OR itself can be deducted as $e^{(BX)}$. With the introduction of other independents in the model $(x_2, x_3... x_i)$, the overall odds of the outcome variable become the function of their additive effects "Eq. 3.12". The reader is advised to refer to Sect. 3.5 for more details.

4.10.1 Effect Size: Log Odds Ratio

We have shown that the effect of the predictor variable (x) on the outcome variable (y) is calculated as Log OR. The latter can be looked for in the literature or calculated from the probabilities of the outcome event. As example, if (x) is the type of treatment and the literature shows that the probability of mortality among patients receiving treatment A (P1 = 15%), compared to (P2 = 10%) in patients receiving treatment B, the Odds ratio = (0.15/0.85)/(0.1/0.9) = 1.588 and log Odds ratio = 0.46. In the case of multiple predictor variables, the investigator has to decide the most important to calculate the effect size. The role of other variables on outcome has to be considered during sample size calculation by including R^2 in the equation [56]. R^2 is the proportion of variation in the outcome (x) due to other predictors in the model.

4.10.2 Sample Size

4.10.2.1 Large Sample Approximation Formulae

Hsieh and colleagues have presented "simple" formulae relating the sample size, risks of error, and the effect size (B) in two situations: when the predictor variable (x) is a normally distributed quantitative variable "Eq. 4.81" and when (x) is a binomial variable "Eq. 4.82" [56]. The presented equations are calculated for a bilateral design and, in case the design is unilateral $(1 - \alpha/2)$ has to be substituted by $(1 - \alpha)$, as usual.

In the case of a normally distributed quantitative variable, the effect size (B) = Log $[P_1(1 - P_1)/P_2(1 - P_2)]$. Where, P_1 is the probability that the event occurs at the mean value of the predictor (x) and, P_2 is the probability that the event occurs when (x) is 1 Sd above the mean.

$$N = \frac{\left(z_{(1-\alpha/2)} + z_{(1-\beta)}\right)^2}{P_1(1 - P_1)B^2} \quad (4.81)$$

In case (x) is binomially distributed (x = 0, 1), P_0 is the event rate when x = 0, P_1 is the event rate when x = 1, R is the proportion of the sample with x = 1, and P is the overall event rate given by $[P_1 R + P_0 (1 - R)]$ "Eq. 4.82".

$$N = \frac{\left(z_{(1-\alpha/2)}\sqrt{\frac{P(1-P)}{R}} + z_{(1-\beta)}\sqrt{P_0(1 - P_0) + \frac{P_1(1-P_1)(1-R)}{R}}\right)^2}{(P_0 - P_1)^2(1 - R)}$$
$$(4.82)$$

Demidenko E further modified the equation. Monte Carlo simulations have shown that the modified equation gives better sample size estimates and it is the one used by default in G power software [57]. Both equations are large-sample approximations and assume the normal distribution of covariates.

4.10.2.2 The Enumeration Procedure

G software proposes the more accurate but complicated enumeration procedure proposed by Lyles and colleagues, which provides power analysis for the Wald test and the Likelihood ratio test [58]. The maximum likelihood ratio is a way to find the population's parameters that are most likely to have generated our sample (see Sect. 3.5). G power software offers the choice to choose between the Wald test (see Sect. 3.5.6.2) or likelihood ratio for small samples of 30 patients or less (see Sect. 3.5.1.4).

If the model includes more than one predictor, we can correct the original sample size (N) to accommodate their possible effect on the outcome. The correcting factor is R^2, which is the proportion of variation of the outcome explained by other predictors in the model. The corrected sample size (Nc) can be calculated as in "Eq. 4.83" [56]. The more the importance of the other predictors on the outcome, as indicated by a large R^2, the more we have to increase the sample size.

$$N_c = \frac{N}{\left(1 - R^2\right)} \qquad (4.83)$$

The Use of G*power Software

We will begin by considering the simple case of including a single binomial variable (x) and using the default Demidenko procedure. In order to appreciate the effect of the nature of the covariate on sample size, we will then deal with (x) as a normally distributed quantitative variable. The third step will be to test the effect of considering other covariates in the model. Finally, we will terminate our exercise by appreciating the effect of applying the enumeration procedure. In order to avoid any confusion, the effect of each of the four steps will be evaluated separately. All calculations will be made using the usual 5% primary risk of error, 80% power, and a two-tailed study. Remember that choosing a one-tail study will reduce the calculated sample size by about 20%, as previously noted.

1. A single binomial predictor variable

Let us begin by calculating the sample size in the case of a single binomial variable. The outcome is the probability of adverse events (yes/no) after major surgery. A literature review has shown that diabetes increases this probability from 30 to 50%.

1. Check the "Test family" drop-down menu and select "z tests".
2. Check the "Statistical test" drop-down menu and select "Logistic regression".

3. Check "Type of power analysis" and select: "A priori: Compute required sample size-given α, power and effect size".
4. Check on "Options" to open the side drawer. Choose between "Input effect size as Odds ratio and Two probabilities", and as the probabilities are available in our example, we will choose the (Odds ratio). Choose between the two main procedures of "Computation: Use enumeration procedure or Use large sample approximation, with either Demidenko the recommended 2007 with variance correction or Hsieh et al. 1998". Choose Demidenko 2007. Click 'OK" to return to the main window.
5. Click "Determine" to open the effect size side drawer. Upload "Pr H1" (0.5) and "Pr H0" (0.3) to calculate odds ratio. Click on "Calculate and transfer to the main drawer".
6. Under "Input parameters", check "Tail(s)" and select (Two). Leave "α err prob" as such (0.05). Select "Power (1-B err Prob)"; usually (0.8). Check on "Pr H_0" (0.3), "Odds ratio" (2.3333). Upload "R^2 other X" when known, otherwise leave it as such (0). Check on "X distribution" and choose (Binomial) from the drop-down menu and maintain the default balanced design by keeping "x parm" = (0.5); i.e., 1:1 ratio of diabetic versus non-diabetic patients. Click on "Calculate".
7. Check the output parameters: "Critical z" (1.96), "Total sample size" (190), and "Actual power" (0.8).
8. The remaining steps are the same as the final four steps from 8 to 11 in case of comparing two normally distributed means (see Sect. 4.2.2.1).

The calculations can be verified by the simple equation suggested by Campbell and colleagues [24]. The equation gives sample size per group (n), knowing the OR and the common probability (P) of the two groups = (Pa + Pb)/2 = (0.3+ 0.5)/2 = 0.4; assuming a usual 5% primary risk of error and 80% power "Eq. 4.84" (see Sect. 4.3.2.2).

$$n = \frac{2(z_{1-\alpha} + z_{1-\beta})^2}{(log\ OR)^2 p(1-p)} = \frac{2(1.64 + 0.84)^2}{(2.333)^2 0.4(1-0.4)}$$
$$= 92\ patients$$

(4.84)

2. *A single normally distributed predictor variable*

We will follow the same steps as before, except step number 6, where we check on "X distribution" and choose (normal) from the dop-down menu and, we keep the default mean "xμ" and standard deviation "xσ" as (0) and (1). As previously noted on many occasions, the inherent variability of a quantitative variable is much less than that of a qualitative variable giving more power to the study evidenced by a considerable decrease in the calculated total sample size from 190 to only 67 patients.

3. *Including other covariates besides the main binomial predictor variable*

Returning to the binomial situation, the inclusion of other covariates in the calculation by signing a value of just 0.1 to R^2 increases our sample size from 190 patients to as many as 211 patients. The larger is R^2, the more we have to include patients to evidence the same effect size. The same procedure applies when the main predictor follows any other distribution, of course.

4. *Applying the enumeration procedure for the main binomial predictor variable*

We have decided to use the enumeration procedure whenever our sample size is smaller than 200 patients, but we can pick up any other cut-off point. We return to step number 4: the "Options" window, and select to activate the procedure instead of the large sample approximation. As mentioned, the default calculations use Wald statistics, but researchers are advised to use the more accurate likelihood ratio in case of a small sample <30 patients, which is not our case. No other changes are requested.

Now check step number 7: the "Output parameters". It shows the "non-centrality parameter" (7.86), "Critical Chi-square value" (3.84), "DF" (1), "Total sample size" (192), and "Actual power" (0.8). The more accurate enumeration procedure gives a larger sample size, as expected. If we return to step number 4 and choose to use the more accurate Likelihood ratio for the calculations, instead of the Wald statistics, a larger total sample size of 200 patients will be produced in step number 7.

4.11 Multiple Regression

Multiple regression uses a linear model to approximate the relationship between a dependent quantitative outcome variable (y) and one or more independent predictor variables (x1, x2…, xi), with (B1, B2…, Bi) being the regression coefficients that quantify the effect of covariates on the outcome "Eq. 3.5". Although interest focuses typically on the regression coefficients of each covariate, those covariates are usually not available during the planning phase, and little is known about their coefficients until after the analysis is run. We have previously noted that R^2 explains how much a variable (x) influences another variable (y). In multiple regression, the procedure uses the squared multiple correlation coefficient (R^2) to measure the effect size upon which the power analysis and sample size are based. (R^2) is the proportion of variation in the model explained by the covariates (predictors). Sampson and colleagues presented power analysis results for two approaches: conditional and unconditional, with the former being the most commonly used for the reasons that we will present by the end of this section [59, 60].

4.11.1 Conditional Fixed Factors Model

The model assumes that covariates (x) are fixed, and known predictors and that (R^2) represents the set of regression coefficients, which denotes the effect of those covariates (B) on the outcome (y). R^2 can then be written as: (R^2_{Y-B}). Under the null hypothesis, there is no effect of covariates on the model and hence, (R^2_{Y-B}) is equal to zero and the alternative hypothesis is that (R^2_{Y-B}) > zero. Note that R^2 is a squared value and cannot be negative, of course.

4.11.1.1 Effect Size (f^2)

The total variation (total variance) in the model is partly explained by the variance explained by predictors (Vs), and of course, there is always a part that will remain unexplained, which is called the residual or error variance (Ve). The larger is the (Vs), the more is the effect of the predictors on the model, and hence, effect size (f^2) can be expressed as the proportion: (Vs)/(Ve). As Vs + Ve = 1, and the effect of predictors will be expressed as an R^2 value, the proportion of variance explained (Vs) is equal to (R^2_{Y-B}) and, by deduction, the residual variance will be equal to $(1 - R^2_{Y-B})$. The following equation can calculate the effect size "Eq. 4.85":

$$f^2 = \frac{R^2_{Y-B}}{\left(1 - R^2_{Y-B}\right)} \qquad (4.85)$$

R^2 is a standard output of statistical software and is usually cited in relevant manuscripts. The freely available G power software gives the facility to compute R^2 from a matrix of biserial correlations between predictors and outcome as well as between predictors themselves. Finally, if the effect size is known, we can compute R^2 from the effect size "Eq. 4.86". According to Cohen, f^2 values of: 0.02, 0.15, and 0.35 can be considered as being small, medium, and large effect sizes. The equivalent R^2_{Y-B} values are: 0.02, 0.13 and 0.26.

$$R^2_{Y-B} = \frac{f^2}{\left(1 + f^2\right)} \qquad (4.86)$$

4.11.1.2 Sample Size

In general, we follow the usual process by defining the effect size (f^2), either found in

previous studies or calculated from R^2 by the above equation or by using a sample size calculator software, such as G power. The second step is to define study design (unilateral or bilateral), the primary risk of error, study power, number of predictors and, to upload that information to the software to calculate the noncentrality parameter (λ) and total sample size (N), as in "Eq. 4.87"

$$N = \frac{\lambda}{f^2} \qquad (4.87)$$

The Example

For example, we assume that the duration of hospital stay in days is predicted by a set of 5 variables (patient age, sex, duration of illness, uncontrolled diabetes, and type of surgery). Previous studies have shown that population $R^2 = 0.3$.

Calculation by G*Power Software

1. Check the "Test family" drop-down menu and select "F tests".
2. Check the "Statistical test" drop-down menu and select "linear multiple regression: Fixed model, R^2 deviation from zero".
3. Check "Type of power analysis" and select: "A priori: Compute required sample size-given α, power and effect size".
4. Under "Input parameters", leave "α err prob" as such (0.05), select "Power (1-B err Prob)"; usually (0.8), type the "Number of predictors" (5). Upload "Effect size f^2" if known and skip directly to step 6
5. Click on "Determine" to open the effect size (f^2) calculation window. We can calculate effect size either "From correlation coefficient R^2" or "From predictors correlation". Choosing the former, we just upload the know R^2, as in our case (0.3). By choosing the latter option, we must define the "Number of predictors" and click on "specify matrices". It opens another window to upload the set of biserial correlations "Corr between predictors and outcome" and "Corr between predictors themselves". We upload the values

of all correlation coefficients that we know, and we click "OK" to calculate and transfer the calculated R^2 to the effect size window. Regardless of the chosen option, this step is terminated by calculating and transferring the calculated f2 to the main window. Click on "Calculate and transfer to the main window".

6. Verify your choices in the main window: effect size f2 = 0.428, α = 0.05, power = 0.8, and number of predictors = 5. Click on "Calculate" to get the output parameters on the right side of the drawer.

7. Verify the output parameters: "Noncentrality parameter λ" (15.428), critical f value (2.533), "Numerator DF" (5) = number of predictors, Denominator Df (30) = total number of patients minus number of predictors – 1, "Total sample size" (36), and "Actual power" (80.16%).

8. The remaining steps are the same as the final four steps from 8 to 11 in case of comparing two normally distributed means (see Sect. 4.2.2.1).

Based on the relation between f^2 and other effect sizes, this test can be used to calculate sample size for comparing several means or biserial correlation. The relation between f^2 and effect size (d) of ANOVA is $f^2 = (d/2)^2$ and hence, the test can be used to calculate sample size for ANOVA, with replacement of the number of predictors by the number of NOVA groups -1. The test can also be used to calculate power for a univariate biserial correlation (r) by setting $R^2 = r^2$, calculating $f^2 = r^2/(1 - r^2)$ and setting the number of predictors to 1.

4.11.2 Unconditional Random Effect Model

Unlike the fixed factor model, this model assumes that (y) and (x) are not fixed, but random variables that have a joint multivariate normal distribution with a positive covariance matrix and hence, the vector (R^2_{Y-B}) of the sample used in the fixed model is replaced by the squared population multiple correlation coefficient (ρ^2_{yx}). Under the null hypothesis, there is no relation between covariates (x), and outcome (y), and hence, (ρ^2_{yx}) is equal to zero. The alternative hypothesis is that it is not, of course.

4.11.2.1 Effect Size

As $H_0(\rho^2_{yx})$ equals zero, the effect size is (ρ^2_{yx}) under the alternative hypothesis = $H_1(\rho^2_{yx})$. However, we have to note that to define the alternative hypothesis, we have to specify the null hypothesis as well. As an example, if a classic treatment has a (ρ^2_{yx}) of 0.1 and we want to prove that a new treatment is better, $H_0(\rho^2_{yx}) = 0.1$ and the alternative hypothesis $H_1(\rho^2_{yx}) \neq 0.1$. Being the equivalent of (R^2_{Y-B}) of the fixed model, $H_1(\rho^2_{yx})$ can be equally computed by nesting a covariance matrix from the set of biserial correlations between outcome variable (y) and predictors as well as between predictors themselves.

Being a random model of normally distributed variables, a second method to determine $H_1(\rho^2_{yx})$ is to use the observed R^2 (multiple correlations of variables in a sample) reported by previous studies to create a 95% confidence interval for (ρ^2_{yx}) (multiple correlations of variables in the population). The second step will be to choose a "suitable" cuts-off point for $H_1(\rho^2_{yx})$, within the limits of this confidence interval and, finally, to calculate sample size according to this choice.

The relation between effect sizes of fixed (f^2) and random (ρ^2_{yx}) models is expressed by "Eq. 4.88". In concordance, (ρ^2_{yx}) values of: 0.02, 0.13 and 0.26 are equivalent to f^2 values of: 0.02, 0.15 and 0.35; denoting Cohen's mild, moderate and large effect sizes; respectively. It is clear that the effect size of a fixed model is larger than that of a random model, and hence, it is more powerful to detect the evidence.

$$f^2 = \frac{\rho^2_{yx}}{(1 - \rho^2_{yx})} \qquad (4.88)$$

4.11.2.2   Sample Size

For simplicity, we will denote (ρ_{yx}^2) as ρ^2. After defining $H_1\rho^2$ $H_0\rho^2$ and the number of predictors, we have to define the direction of the study, the primary risk of error, and study power. We will use G Power software to apply the random model on the same example used in the fixed model to show the difference between the two models.

1. Check the "Test family" drop-down menu and select "Exact tests".
2. Check the "Statistical test" drop-down menu and select "Linear multiple regression: Random model".
3. Check "Type of power analysis" and select: "A priori: Compute required sample size-given α, power and effect size".
4. Under "Input parameters", check "Tail(s)" and select (Two). Leave "α err prob" as such (0.05). Select "Power (1-B err Prob)"; usually (0.8). Leave "$H_0\rho^{2}$" as such (0). Leave "$H_1\rho^{2}$" empty as it will be calculated soon. Type the "Number of predictors" (5).
5. Click on "Determine" to open the effect size H_1 ρ^2 calculation window. We can calculate effect size either "From confidence interval" or "From predictors correlation". By choosing the latter, we have to define the "Number of predictors" and click on "specify matrices", and carry on the same procedure for the fixed model. By choosing the former option, we have to upload the data of the study chosen from the literature; including "Total sample size" (36), "Number of predictors" (5), "Observed R^2 (0.3), "Confidence level" (0.95), and "CI position to use" (0.5). By clicking on "Calculate", the software produces the "CI lower ρ^{2}" (0), "CI upper ρ^{2}" (0.4776), "Statistical lower bound" (0.00213), "Statistical upper bound" (0.434), and "H_1 ρ^{2}" (0.2388). We click on "Calculate and transfer to the main window"
6. Verify the input parameters: two Tails, H_1 ρ^2 = 0.2388, H_0 ρ^2 = 0, α = 0.05, power = 0.8, and number of predictors = 5. Click on "Calculate" to execute the analysis.

7. Verify the output parameters: Total sample size (58), actual power (0.806), lower (0.015), and upper (0.213) critical R^2 limits.
8. The remaining steps are the same as the final four steps from 8 to 11 in case of the comparison of two normally distributed means (see Sect. 4.2.2.1).

The Interpretation

In order to get a statistically significant result in a bilateral design, R^2 has to be (<0.015) or (>0.213). As expected, choosing a one-tail study gives equivocal upper and lower R^2 critical limits and smaller sample size. Note that the sample size of a random model will always be larger than that of the fixed model, reflecting the inherent uncertainty and low power of the random model. If previous studies have shown that $H_0\rho^2$ is not equal to (0) but is equal to, let us say, 0.1. Changing $H_0\rho^2$ to its new value increases the total sample size to 198 cases. This result can be explained as follows: if a classic treatment already has an effect size of 0.2, the sample size should increase by nearly four-folds to maintain the same 80% power.

The Fixed Versus the Random Model

The critical question is: a random or a fixed model? The conditional fixed model is recommended for many reasons. By definition, regression analysis estimates the conditional expectation of (y), given that the values of the (x) variables are fixed and known, which are online with the model assumptions. Power calculations are based on the assumption of the residuals being normally distributed and of constant variance, conditions that already need to be fulfilled in regression analysis. The model uses R square as input, and R^2 is usually reported or can be easily computed. On the other hand, the random model is based on a special algorithm, necessitates that both (y) and (x) are normally distributed, uses (ρ^2) which is seldom reported and difficult to calculate and finally reduces power for the uncertainty of (x) values till the time of analysis.

4.12 Repeated Measures

4.12.1 Repeated Measures ANOVA (RMANOVA)

We have previously discussed One-way (see Sect. 2.4.3.4) and two-way repeated-measures ANOVA (see Sect. 3.2.5.1). In some conditions, several measurements can be taken from each patient, and treating each of those measurements (and not each patient) as a unit is a major source of bias. The patient is our sampling unit and not the measurement. In addition, the repeated measures as a "process" have a prognostic value itself. Recording the patient body weight on regular occasions during a diet regimen may show that patients lose significant weight at the beginning but can regain some weight by the end. ANOVA can test the significance of this "pattern" of "within-subjects variability". If the study is equally concerned with comparing two diet regimens and not only analyzing the within-subject variability of a single regimen, then a second partition: the "in-between groups variability", is created, which can be analyzed too. ANOVA can also partition and examine the possibility of interaction between repeated measurements and type of regimen "the within-between subject variability". In this section, we will calculate the sample size for these situations.

We are returning to the analyzing effect of taking multiple measurements instead of a single one. We have discussed sample size calculation in the case of a single measurement, whether recorded in 2 groups and compared by Student test (see Sect. 4.2.2) or in case of comparing the means of multiple groups by One-Way ANOVA (see Sect. 4.6.2). We have shown that the in-between groups' effect size (Cohen f) for ANOVA is an extension of (Cohen d) calculated for the Student test. The question is, what will the process of repeated measurements add to this? The answer is straightforward: it increases effect size by decreasing variability and empowers ANOVA. Remember some basic concepts: the means of values are always less variable than the

values themselves, and the more we add values (measurements), the more variability of their mean decreases. In this setting, Vickers AJ and colleagues have demonstrated that beyond four measurements or seven where baseline assessments are taken, the gain in power becomes of little value [61].

On the other hand, the gain of power is proportional to the number of measurements and the correlation between measures. If (n) is the number of patients per group, as calculated for a Student's test in case of a single measurement, Borm and colleagues have demonstrated that for repeated measurements, this number decreases in proportion to the correlation between measurements themselves (ρ) [62]. The number of patients per group in repeated measures ANOVA $= n (1 - \rho^2)$; which is why the software need to have (ρ) to calculate the size of the sample.

4.12.1.1 Effect Size: Within-Group, Between-Group and Interaction

We have previously shown that in the case of the ANOVA model with more than one predictor, partial eta squared (η_P^2) is a better estimation of predictor effects than eta squared (η^2). Although (η_P^2) can be easily calculated by hand, it is part of outputs of any statistical software. A simple transformation easily deducts effect size (Cohen f) too "Eq. 4.58".

The Within-Group Variability

Before proceeding, the reader is advised to revise Sect. 2.4.3.4. Let us start with the simple situation where we analyze the effect of repeated measurement in one group of patients: one-way repeated measures ANOVA. The total variability SS_{total} of such study is partitioned into a within-group sum of squares $SS_{effect\ (WG)}$ that can be explained by (due to) the repeated measurement and a residual part of variability that still needs to be explained SS_{error}. The repeated measurements effect size $\eta_P^2 = SS_{effect\ (WG)}/(SS_{total} + SS_{error})$ "Eq. 4.52".

The Between-Group Variability and Interaction

In the case where we are equally interested in comparing the patterns between patients' groups. A two-way (RMANOVA) calculates, in addition to the repeated measures effect, the between-groups variability $SS_{effect\ (BG)}$, the corresponding between groups: (η_P^2) and (Cohen f), as usual (see Sect. 3.2.5.1). Do we have to ask ourselves if there is any interaction between the two factors, i.e., a within-between group variability? ANOVA can answer this question in its way by calculating the sum of squares of interaction $SS_{effect\ (WG-BG)}$, its corresponding (η_P^2), and Cohen f too.

As shown in Sect. 2.4.3, the between-group effect size (Cohen f) can also be calculated from group means and standard deviations using the same equations "Eq. 4.54". Sample size calculation can then be tailored to the repeated measurements situation by considering the correlation between repeated measures (ρ), as indicated above. A repeated measures effect size W^2 can be derived from the F ratio, the numbers of repetitions (K), and the sample size (n) "Eq. 4.89" [63]

$$W^2 = \frac{(K-1)(F-1)}{(K-1)(F-1)nk} \qquad (4.89)$$

4.12.1.2   Sample Size

We follow the usual procedure by finding or calculating Cohen's f from previous studies, defining the study direction, the risks of error and uploading this information to a suitable sample size calculator such as G power software. Different scenarios have to be taken into consideration. Suppose the question is about calculating sample size to put into evidence a statistically significant effect for the repeated measurement per se. In that case, the sample size will be calculated from repeated measurement Cohen's f. On the other hand, if the investigator is also willing to put into evidence an effect group or interaction, sample sizes will be equally calculated from the respective effect sizes of between groups and interactions. *The investigator has to pick up the largest calculated sample size that will give sufficient power to demonstrate the statistical significance of the effect sizes that he is willing to uncover.*

In addition, the software will need to know the correlation between measurements and whether sphericity is assumed? We have previously shown the importance of the correlation between measurements (ρ) in empowering the study and decreasing sample size. Some statistical software such as SPSS incorporates (ρ) within the calculated partial eta squared (η_P^2), and hence, we do not need to add (ρ) again. G power software will remove the (ρ) button whenever we indicate that the uploaded (η_P^2) was calculated as in SPSS. Otherwise, (ρ) should be looked for in the literature and then uploaded to be used in the calculations. *If (ρ) is unknown, the researcher is advised to calculate all effect sizes (within, between, and interaction) directly from (η_P^2), as calculated by SPSS.*

A main assumption of repeated measures ANOVA is that the variances of the difference between all possible pairs of within-subjects levels are equal, which is known as sphericity. Statistical software usually uses Mauchly's test to investigate whether data violates sphericity or not? A statistically significant result means that sphericity has been violated and must be corrected. The test statistics indicating sphericity is defined as (ε), and a value of 1 means that sphericity has been assumed. *Several corrections have been suggested, and Garden E recommended that when $(\varepsilon) > 0.75$, the Huynh–Feldt correction can be applied, and when $(\varepsilon) < 0.75$ or nothing is known about sphericity, the more conservative Greenhouse–Geisser correction becomes the test of choice* [64]. Both corrections are standard outputs of SPSS and other statistical software. Note that sphericity evaluates the within-subject measurements. Hence, it has to be checked and corrected for the within-group and the within-between group variabilities and does not concern the between-group variability. We advise the reader to refer to Sects. 3.2.5.1 and 3.2.5.2 for more details about sphericity.

The Example

Patients with mechanical cardiac valves follow a life-long oral anticoagulation regimen. Although warfarin is the drug of choice, it takes between 2 to 4 days to reach its therapeutic level, defined by an international normalized ratio (INR) between 2.5 and 3.5. A researcher wished to study the pattern of INR change (within-group variability) and to compare the response between males and female patients (between groups variability) during the first week of initiation of therapy, as well as the possibility of interaction. Three INR measurements were planned to be made: one pre-treatment and two post-treatment measures, with an interval of 3 days between samples. In order to calculate sample size, the required information was taken from SPSS outputs of a comparable study that included 159 patients; 49 males (30.8%) and 110 females.

Sample Size for Within-Group Effect

One-Way Repeated Measures ANOVA

We will begin by analyzing the repeated measure (One-way RMANOVA), without considering gender effect or effect interaction. Besides the desired primary (0.05) and secondary risks of error (0.8), we must verify the information needed to calculate the sample size. We need to know or to calculate effect size (f), number of groups (2), number of measures (3), correlation among measures (unless partial eta squared was calculated by SPSS), and non-sphericity correction when violated. In our example, SPSS showed a statistically significant difference from sphericity: Mauchly's $W = 0.42$; $P < 0.001$. As the Epsilon (ε) value was less than 0.75, we can adopt the given Greenhouse–Geisser corrected (ε) value (0.633), as well as its corresponding effect size η_P^2 (0.283). We can consult G*power software to calculate the sample size based on this information.

1. Check the "Test family" drop-down menu and select "F tests".
2. Check the "Statistical test" drop-down menu and select "ANOVA, Repeated measures, within factors".
3. Check "Type of power analysis" and select: "A priori: Compute required sample size-given α, power and effect size".
4. Under "Input parameters", leave "α err prob" as such (0.05). Select "Power (1-B err Prob)"; usually (0.8), type "Number of groups" (2), "Number of measures" (3), "non-sphericity correction" (0.633). Leave "Effect size F" as it will be calculated. Click on "Options" and choose "Effect size specification" (as in SPSS) to indicate that correlation was included in the calculation of effect size made by SPSS. Once done, the box of "Correlation among repeated measures" will disappear.
5. Click on "Determine" to open the effect size calculation window. Choose between "Direct" and type the partial eta squared given by SPSS (0.283) or calculation "from variances": "variance explained by special effect" and "error variance", if known. Click on "Calculate" to produce "effect size f" (0.628). Click on "Calculate and transfer to main window" to close the drawer.
6. Verify the "input parameters" including Effect size = 0.628, $\alpha = 0.05$, Power = 0.8, number of groups = 2, number of measures = 3, non-sphericity correction = 0.633 and click on "Calculate" to execute the analysis.
7. Verify the "output parameters": "Noncentrality parameter λ" (=9.99), critical f value (=3.92) for the corresponding degrees of freedom (numerator df = 1.266; denominator df = 25.32), total sample size (22) and actual power of the test (0.83).
8. The remaining steps are the same as the final four steps from 8 to 11 in case of comparing two normally distributed means (see Sect. 4.2.2.1).

Interpretation of the Result

View the large ES, a total sample size of 22 patients will have an 80% power to put into evidence a statistically significant change among the three repeated INR measurements, with a usual 5% primary risk of error.

Two-Way Repeated Measures ANOVA

We have just calculated sample size for the within-group variability, in the case of one-way ANOVA, using η_P^2 to calculate the effect size. We will repeat the analysis after introducing the variable gender. A property of η_P^2 is that it changes when other variables are introduced in the model to reflect better the corresponding change in variability, which is why η_P^2 was created in the first place. Introducing the in-between group variable (gender) in the analysis changes the corrected Greenhouse–Geisser (ε) from 0.633 to 0.624 and reduces η_P^2 from 0.283 to 0.267. Uploading those "new" values in G power software decreases Effect size (f) from 0.628 to 0.60 and hence, increases the total sample size from 22 to 24 cases; which is almost higher by 10% from what has been previously calculated by one-way repeated measures ANOVA.

Interpretation of the Result

View the large ES, a total sample size of 24 patients will have an 80% power to put into evidence a statistically significant change among the three repeated INR measurements, controlling for the factor gender, with a usual 5% primary risk of error.

Sample Size for Between-Group Effect

The next step will be to repeat the calculations after adding the between-groups (gender) and interaction between the within and between grouping variables (INR*gender). Remember that sphericity is only tested for the within-group variable (INR repeated measures) and interaction (INR*gender) but not for the between-group variable (gender). Moreover, sphericity is assumed by default for any two-class variable. On the other hand, the software produced a statistically significant effect size η_P^2 of (0.052) for the grouping variable gender; P < 0.001.

1. Check the "Test family" drop-down menu and select "F tests".
2. Check the "Statistical test" drop-down menu and select "ANOVA, Repeated measures, between factors".

3. Check "Type of power analysis" and select: "A priori: Compute required sample size-given α, power and effect size".
4. Under "Input parameters", leave "α err prob" as such (0.05, select "Power (1-*B* err Prob)"; usually (0.8), type "Number of groups" (2), and "Number of measures" (3). Leave "Effect size F" as it will be calculated. Click on "Options" and choose "Effect size specification" (as in SPSS) to indicate that correlation was included in the calculation of effect size made by SPSS.
5. Click on "Determine" to open the effect size calculation window. Select one of two procedures: calculate "Effect size from variance" or "Effect size from means", which depends upon the available information we have. Calculating "Effect size from means" necessitates having: "mean of each group", "size of each group", the "number of groups", "Sd within each group", "Number of measures", and "correlation among repeated measures". On the other hand, calculating "Effect size from variances" can be "Direct" by η_P^2 (0.052) or calculated from: "Variance explained by special effect", "Error variance". Number of groups", and "Total sample size". Regardless of our choice, this step terminates by clicking on "Calculate" to produce "effect size f" (0.234). Click on "Calculate and transfer to main window" to close the drawer.
6. Verify the "input parameters" including Effect size = 0.234, α = 0.05, Power = 0.8, number of groups = 2, and number of measures = 3. Click on "Calculate" to execute the analysis.
7. Verify the "output parameters": "Noncentrality parameter λ" (8), critical f value (3.9) for the corresponding degrees of freedom (numerator df = 1), denominator df (146), total sample size (148), and actual power of the test (0.8).
8. The remaining steps are the same as the final four steps from 8 to 11 in case of comparing two normally distributed means (see Sect. 4.2.2.1).

Interpretation of the Result

View the small ES, a total sample size of 148 patients will have an 80% power to put into evidence a statistically significant difference between both genders, with a usual 5% primary risk of error.

Sample Size for Effect Interaction

The introduction of the between-group variable (gender) and interaction (INR*gender) in the analysis confirmed the absence of sphericity, with a statistically significant Mauchly's test: W = 0.399; P < 0.001. Consequently, the new proposed Greenhouse correction for the repeated measure (0.624), the corresponding effect size η_p^2 of INR measures (0.267), and the η_p^2 of interaction (INR*gender) (0.0082) will be used in the calculations. The new analysis confirmed the large significant effect of the repeated measures (P < 0.001) while the interaction was non-significant (P = 0.28). We have shown a statistically significant effect of gender and calculated the appropriate sample size to put it into evidence (148 patients).

On the other hand, there was no statistically significant interaction between measures and gender. In other words, the measures change over time, regardless of being acquired from a male or a female patient. We will proceed and calculate the sample size required to put such a small interaction effect into evidence, just for a demonstrative purpose.

1. Check the "Test family" drop-down menu and select "F tests".
2. Check the "Statistical test" drop-down menu and select "ANOVA, Repeated measures, within-between factors".
3. Check "Type of power analysis" and select: "A priori: Compute required sample size-given α, power and effect size".
4. Under "Input parameters", leave "α err prob" as such (0.05), select "Power (1-*B* err Prob)"; usually (0.8), type "Number of groups" (2), "Number of measures" (3), "non-sphericity correction" (0.624). Leave "Effect size F" as it will be calculated. Click on "Options" and

choose "Effect size specification" (as in SPSS) to indicate that correlation was included in the calculation of effect size made by SPSS. Once done, the box of "Correlation among repeated measures" will disappear.

5. Click on "Determine" to open the effect size calculation window. Choose between "Direct" and type the partial eta squared given by SPSS (0.008) or calculation "from variances": "variance explained by special effect" and "error variance", if known. Click on "Calculate" to produce "effect size f" (0.0898). Click on "Calculate and transfer to main window" to close the drawer.
6. Verify the "input parameters" including Effect size = 0.0898, α = 0.05, Power = 0.8, number of groups = 2, number of measures = 3, non-sphericity correction = 0.624 and click on "Calculate" to execute the analysis.
7. Verify the "output parameters": "Noncentrality parameter λ" (8.41), critical f value (3.55) for the corresponding degrees of freedom (numerator df = 1.248; denominator df = 1043.3), total sample size (838), and actual power of the test (0.8).
8. The remaining steps are the same as the final four steps from 8 to 11 in case of comparing two normally distributed means (see Sect. 4.2.2.1).

Interpretation of the Results

View the small ES, a considerable sample size of 838 patients will have an 80% power to put into evidence a statistically significant interaction effect, with a usual 5% primary risk of error.

4.12.2 Friedman Test

Friedman test is the non-parametric alternative of one-way repeated measures ANOVA, and it has been discussed elsewhere (see Sect. 2.5.2.2). The test is mainly indicated whenever the quantitative outcome variable does not follow a normal distribution or is normally distributed but has been observed in a small sample. In concordance with

RMANOVA, Friedman's test assumes that the repeated measurements are performed at equal intervals and are independent within each group.

4.12.2.1 Effect Size: Kendall W Coefficient of Concordance

The Example

We have reported the example of testing the efficacy of an antihypertensive drug over time by measuring the diastolic blood pressure repeatedly in 15 individuals on three different occasions: before treatment, one month, and three months after treatment (K = 3). Cases were chosen at random from a population of patients with chronic hypertension. Measurements were independently made and recorded (Table 2.24). Like many non-parametric tests, the test of Friedman uses the ranks rather than the raw values to calculate the statistics. The test calculates the mean ranks of the (k) repeated measures made over time or, the conditions made for matched groups of patients. Under the null hypothesis, the mean ranks of the three measures are equal, while under the null hypothesis, they are not. The calculated "Fr" or Friedman's Q statistics can be approximated to a Chi-square value at k − 1 degrees of freedom, provided that the number of patients (n) is at least 15. Otherwise, the significance of the value of Friedman Q can be checked out in special Q tables [65]. In our example, our Friedman's Q value calculated by hand was 17.5; P < 0.001. Uploading our data to SPSS gives a slightly higher Chi-square value of 18.4 (P < 0.001) (see Sect. 2.5.2.2).

The Equation

We cannot calculate effect size directly from Friedman's test, but it can be derived from Z statistics using pairwise comparison of only two measures by a Wilcoxon sign rank test (see Sect. 4.5.2). For example, we can compare measurements made before treatment to those acquired after one month. Effect size can be estimated by the PSdep index proposed by Grisson and Kim or by correlation coefficient r

(see Sect. 4.5.2.1). The sample size can be calculated by the equation proposed by Al-Sunduqchi and Guenther (see Sect. 4.5.2.2). The process can be repeated to compare each of those two measurements to the measurement made after three months and, finally, adopt the highest calculated sample.

A better alternative is to consider benefiting from Kendall W, a test designed to look at the agreement between subjects (see Sect. 2.10.4.4). The test calculates a measure of agreement (W) that varies from 0 to 1 and, hence, is a good indicator of effect size. Testing data presented in Table 2.24 with Kendall W can show how much the three repeated measurements had the same ranks in all subjects. The higher W, the more it indicates how much the three measures agree. Kendall W can be seen as a normalized Freidman's test, and the latter can be seen as the other side of the coin; i.e., is there a difference between subjects? Both tests give the same Chi-square statistics that are tested at the same df (number of measurements minus one) to eventually end by producing the exact P-value (P < 0.001), of course.

In conclusion, the calculated Kendall W can be used as an effect size for both tests. In our example, uploading the data shown in Table 2.24 to SPSS and requesting Kendall W statistics gives a high Kendall W value of 0.614 and the same statistically significant Chi-square value of 18.4; P < 0.001. The reader can refer back to Sect. 2.10.4.4 for the details of executing a Kendall W analysis. On the other hand, we can directly calculate effect size (W) from Freidman's Q statistics, total sample size, and the number of measurements (k) by the following equation "Eq. 4.90":

$$W = \frac{Fr_Q}{N(K-1)} = \frac{17.5}{15(3-1)} = 0.614 \quad (4.90)$$

4.12.2.2 Sample Size

May and Looney provided several methods for sample size calculation based on the methods used in the case of Pearson's correlation coefficient r. The authors provided helpful charts and illustrative examples [46]. One method is to apply Fisher's Z transformation "Eq. 4.64" to normalize Kendall W. Normalizing our Kendall W (0.614), produces a normalized Fisher's value (C) of (0.715). Based on previous studies, which showed that the sample variance could be estimated as: $0.437/(n - 4)$ [45], May and Looney suggested calculating the total sample size as in "Eq. 4.91". In our example, we need to include nearly 11 patients, provided adopting the usual 5% primary risk of error and a study power of 80%.

$$N_{Fr} = 0.437 \left(\frac{Z_{1-\alpha/2} + Z_{1-\beta}}{C} \right)^2 + 4 \quad (4.91)$$

4.13 Non-inferiority and Equivalence Studies

A bilateral superiority study comparing two treatments (ua and ub) aims to prove that one treatment is superior to the other. The null hypothesis (H_0) is that both treatments are equal "Eq. 4.92", and the alternative hypothesis (H_1) is that they are not "Eq. 4.93".

$$H_0 = \mu_a - \mu_b = 0 \quad (4.92)$$

$$H_1 = \mu_a - \mu_b \neq 0 \quad (4.93)$$

Unlike the classic superiority clinical study, a non-inferiority study usually aims to prove that a new treatment is "no more worse" than the classic treatment by a small amount that we can neglect or overlook. Hence, we may declare that the new treatment is not inferior to the classic one. This "negligible" amount is called the non-inferiority margin (δ). The non-inferiority margin has to be both: clinically relevant and statistically significant. The first is the choice of the concerned medical community. The second can be chosen as the lower inferiority margin of the 95% CI when the classic treatment was compared to placebo. In other words, the new treatment should always behave better than placebo.

Let us give some explanation: although we can "disregard" that the new treatment is somewhat inferior to the classic one, the new treatment should not be as or more inferior than placebo, when the latter was compared to the classic treatment; in other words, the new treatment has to behave better than placebo, of course. For example, suppose previous studies have shown that the 95% confidence interval of the success rate of classic treatment compared to placebo was "2–10%". In that case, the least acceptable inferiority of the new treatment should always be "below 2%". Otherwise, it will be comparable to (as inferior as) the placebo.

The null hypothesis is that the new treatment is "more worse" than the classic treatment by an amount $>(\delta)$; i.e., >2% in our example "Eq. 4.94". The alternative hypothesis or what we want to prove is that the new treatment is non-inferior to classic treatment by less than < (δ). i.e., <2% "Eq. 4.95". The latter is called the non-inferiority margin (δ). Note that ($\geq$) means new treatment is "equal or more worse" than classic treatment, despite the sign being positive or negative. In concordance, (<) denotes being less worse than classic treatment, despite the sign. The null (H_0) and the alternative hypothesis (H_1) of comparing the mean effect of a new treatment (μT) to the classic or reference treatment (μR) can be written as follows:

$$H_0 = \mu_T - \mu_R \geq \delta \quad (4.94)$$

$$H_1 = \mu_T - \mu_R < \delta \quad (4.95)$$

On the other hand, an equivalent study aims to prove that the difference between both: the new treatment (T) and the reference (classic) treatment (R) "is no more worse" (<δ) in favor of either treatment. An equivalence study is usually carried on as two non-inferiority studies. Hence, to declare equivalence, we have to reject each component of the null hypothesis; a procedure known as the two one-sided tests (TOST). The components of the null H0: "Eq. 4.96" and "Eq. 4.98" and the alternative hypothesis H1 of an equivalent study: "Eq. 4.97" and "Eq. 4.99" can be written as such:

$$H_{01} = \mu_T - \mu_R \leq \delta_1 \qquad (4.96)$$

$$H_{11} = \mu_T - \mu_R > \delta_1 \qquad (4.97)$$

and,

$$H_{02} = \mu_T - \mu_{Rr} \geq \delta_2 \qquad (4.98)$$

$$H_{12} = \mu_T - \mu_R < \delta_2 \qquad (4.99)$$

Equivalence will be concluded only after rejecting both hypotheses; which will be itself finally equivalent to "Eq. 4.100"

$$H_1 = \delta_1 < \mu_T - \mu_R < \delta_2 \qquad (4.100)$$

Other Suggested Non-inferiority Limits

Knowing that an odds ratio of 1 means no difference between the odds, an odds ratio of 1.25 was suggested as a non-inferiority limit. The FDA suggested a 20% difference as an acceptable equivalence limit for bioequivalence studies. As noted, the non-inferior and the two components of the equivalence studies have all unilateral designs. In a non-inferiority study, the whole α is confined to the only possible conclusion that the new treatment is "no more worse" than the classic treatment. In the two-unilateral equivalence study, α is confined to the only possible conclusion at a time; treatment (T) is not inferior to reference treatment (R) and that the latter is not inferior to (T) as well. We will provide a few examples for sample size calculations and, for other cases, the reader can return to Stein-Chung Chow and colleagues for more complete information [25].

4.13.1 Comparison of 2 Means

4.13.1.1 Effect Size

In a regular superiority study, the effect size is the standardized difference between the two means (Cohen ds). In the non-inferiority situation, the two means are supposed to only differ by the margin of error (δ). In case we assume that there is still a difference between the treatments' effects and that (μT − μR) equals a value (ε); the

latter has to be added to (δ) "Eq. 4.101". For example, suppose (δ) is estimated to be 10%, and we still believe that the new treatment will be "worse" than the classic treatment by another 1%. In that case, the accepted margin of non-inferiority will be 11% instead of 10%. We will then follow the routine procedure, expressing the effect size (d_{NIF}) as the standardized combined difference of (ε) and (δ). In many studies, however, authors suggest no true difference between treatments and d_{NIF} will be the standardized difference of (δ).

$$d_{NIF} = \frac{(\mu_T - \mu_R) - \delta}{\sqrt{S^2_{pooled}}} = \frac{\varepsilon - \delta}{\sqrt{S^2_{pooled}}} \qquad (4.101)$$

In equivalence studies, the effect size (d_{Eq}) is the standardized difference of (δ-ε) "Eq. 4.102". Unlike the NIF study, the equivalence limit is removed from the difference. If the authors suggest no true difference between treatments, Cohen d_{NIF} will be resumed to the standardized difference of (δ). We must note that small changes in the equivalence margin can cause significant changes in the required sample size to achieve the same power.

$$d_{Eq} = \frac{\delta - (\mu_T - \mu_R)}{\sqrt{S^2_{pooled}}} = \frac{\delta - \varepsilon}{\sqrt{S^2_{pooled}}} \qquad (4.102)$$

4.13.1.2 Sample Size

After choosing the usual primary and secondary risks of error, the equation of sample size calculation per group for a non-inferiority study (n_{NIF}) is the same as any other routine unilateral study "Eq. 4.103".

$$n_{NIF} = 2(z_{1-\alpha} + z_{1-\beta})^2 / d_{NIF}{}^2 \qquad (4.103)$$

On the other hand, as the common approach to test equivalence is through 2 one-sided tests, larger sample size is needed (n_{Eq}) to prove equivalence, compared to that calculated for a non-inferiority study, for the same (δ) value. This is achieved by increasing $Z_{(1-B)}$ to $Z_{(1-B/2)}$ "Eq. 4.104".

$$n_{Eq} = 2(z_{1-\alpha} + z_{1-\beta/2})^2 / d_{Eq}^2 \qquad (4.104)$$

We should be careful about including any true difference between our compared treatments in the calculations. In the case of a non-inferiority study, we have to enlarge the effect size so as to include (ε), which decreases our calculated sample and makes it easier to prove non-inferiority. *Unlike the NIF study, the presence of a true difference between treatments makes it harder to prove that both are equivalent.* Taking the same example shown above: if we choose an equivalence limit of 10% and we know that both treatments already differ by 1%, we are actually looking for a 9% difference only, which decreases our effect size and hence, enlarges our sample. *The equation gives the sample size per group, and we have to add the usual extra 10% with all calculations.*

Non-inferiority Study

A trial was designed to test non-inferiority of a new analgesic compared to the standard therapy. The primary outcome was the duration of pain relief in hours, with (δ) 30 min and an anticipated standard deviation of 60 min "Eq. 4.105", assuming a one-sided type I error rate of 5% and 80% power. The investigators thought there was no true mean difference between the treatments "Eq. 4.106".

The calculations showed that we need to include 50 patients per group (a total of 100 patients) to provide the study with an 80% power to show that the lower limit of the one-sided 95% confidence interval (or equivalently the 90% two-sided confidence interval) lies above the non-inferiority limit of half an hour.

$$d_{NIF} = \frac{\varepsilon - \delta}{\sqrt{S_{pooled}^2}} = \frac{0 - 30}{60} = -0.5 \qquad (4.105)$$

$$n_{NIF} = \frac{2(z_{1-\alpha} + z_{1-\beta})^2}{d_{NIF}^2} = \frac{2(1.65 + 0.84)^2}{-0.5^2} = 50$$
$$(4.106)$$

Now consider that there was a true difference (ε) between both treatments of about 10 min; this will increase the difference that we are looking for by about one-third from 30 to 40 min "Eq. 4.107", decreasing our sample size to 28 patients per group "Eq. 4.108". Note that (ε) is not removed from (δ) but is added to it.

$$d_{NIF} = \frac{\varepsilon - \delta}{\sqrt{S_{pooled}^2}} = \frac{-10 - 30}{60} = -0.666$$
$$(4.107)$$

$$n_{NIF} = \frac{2(z_{1-\alpha} + z_{1-\beta})^2}{d_{NIF}^2} = \frac{2(1.65 + 0.84)^2}{-0.666^2} = 28$$
$$(4.108)$$

Equivalence Study

The same authors also considered if it is better to prove that both treatments are equivalent, using the same equivalence limit of 30 min (δ) and the standard deviation of 60 min. Equally, they assumed a one-sided type I error rate of 5% and 80% power and the absence of a true difference between treatments "Eq. 4.109". Although we will still be targeting the same NIF limit, more patients will be needed to reject the two null hypotheses. A total of 138 patients (69 patients per group) are needed to give the study an 80% power to show that the limits of a two-sided 90% confidence interval will exclude a difference in means of more than 30 min "Eq. 4.110".

$$d_{Eq} = \frac{\delta - \varepsilon}{\sqrt{S_{pooled}^2}} = \frac{-30 - 0}{60} = 0.5 \qquad (4.109)$$

$$n_{Eq} = \frac{2(z_{1-\alpha} + z_{1-\beta/2})^2}{d_{Eq}^2} = \frac{2(1.65 + 1.28)^2}{-0.5^2}$$
$$= 69$$
$$(4.110)$$

Now consider a true difference between both treatments of about 10 min (ε). The latter will decrease the difference that we are looking for by about one-third from 30 to 20 min only (δ-ε) "Eq. 4.111"; increasing our sample size to a total of 310 patients (not shown), equally distributed between both groups. Note that, unlike the NIF study, the true difference (ε) is removed from the NIF limit (δ) and is not added to it.

$$d_{Eq} = \frac{\delta - \varepsilon}{\sqrt{S^2_{pooled}}} = \frac{-30 - (-10)}{60} = -0.333 \tag{4.111}$$

Consequently, a true difference decreases the sample size of the NIF study (narrows the gap between the two treatments). However, it increases the sample size of an equivalence study (widens the gap between the two treatments).

Online Calculators

The presented sample size calculations can be verified by checking the freely available online calculators [17, 66]. Suppose an online calculator does not discriminate between (δ) and (ε). In that case, we have to add both of them as one number and take care of when to add and when to subtract any basal difference from the non-inferiority limit.

4.13.2 Comparison of Two Proportions

4.13.2.1 Effect Size

In a routine superiority study, the effect size (d) is the standardized difference between two proportions. In order to normalize data, Cohen has also suggested the arsenic transformation of binomial proportions: Cohen h (see Sect. 4.3.1.1). In the non-inferiority study, both treatments are supposed to only differ by the non-inferiority margin (δ) standardized by the standard error of the reference treatment (p_R). We have previously shown that the standard error of a binomial variable with a proportion (p_R) is equal to the square root of the quantity [p_R (1 − p_R)] "Eq. 4.112" (see Sect. 1.4.2.4).

$$d_{NIF} = \frac{\delta}{\sqrt{p_R(1 - p_R)}} \tag{4.112}$$

On the other hand, if we believe that there is a difference between both proportions p_T and p_R, with ε = ($p_T - p_R$), the effect size will be the standardized difference between the two proportions "Eq. 4.113" (see Sect. 1.4.2.7). In case of an equivalence study, the effect size is calculated as in "Eq. 4.114"

$$d_{NIF} = \frac{(p_T - p_R) - \delta}{\sqrt{p_T(1 - p_T) + p_R(1 - p_R)}} \tag{4.113}$$

$$d_{Eq} = \frac{\delta - (p_T - p_R)}{\sqrt{p_T(1 - p_T) + p_R(1 - p_R)}} \tag{4.114}$$

4.13.2.2 Sample Size from Proportions

After defining the effect size and choosing the usual primary and secondary risks of error, the equation of sample size calculation per group for a non-inferiority study (n_{NIF}) is the same as for a routine unilateral study. The primary risk of error is totally dedicated to this one possibility, which is achieved by the equation implying ($Z_{1-\alpha}$) and not ($Z_{1-\alpha/2}$) of a bilateral study "Eq. 4.115". In the case of an equivalence study, the routine approach is to perform two one-sided studies: one to prove that new treatment is not inferior to classic treatment and the other to prove that the latter is not inferior to the new treatment. Consequently, a larger sample size is needed (n_{Eq}) to prove equivalence, compared to that needs to prove non-inferiority, for the same (δ) value, which is achieved through increasing the power of the equation by implying ($Z_{1-B/2}$) instead of (Z_{1-B}) "Eq. 4.116".

We should be careful when including any true difference between compared treatments (ε) in the calculations. The true difference (ε) is added to (δ) in the case of a non-inferiority study, but it is subtracted from (δ) in the case of an equivalence study, all being in absolute values. The reader is invited to follow our working example to eliminate any confusion.

$$n_{NIF} = \left(z_{1-\alpha} + z_{1-\beta}\right)^2 / d_{NIF}^2 \qquad (4.115)$$

$$n_{Eq} = \left(z_{1-\alpha} + z_{1-\beta/2}\right)^2 / d_{Eq}^2 \qquad (4.116)$$

Non-inferiority Study

An antibiotic is known to be 85% effective in preventing postoperative wound infection. A non-inferiority study was designed to compare it with a new therapy, considering a 10% difference as being not important. The authors supposed that the new treatment is 65% effective, and hence, the difference between both cure rates (20%) should be added to the suggested 10% to declare non-inferiority "Eq. 4.117".

A total of 50 patients (25 patients per group) are required to be 80% sure that the upper limit of a one-sided 95% confidence interval (or equivalently a 90% two-sided confidence interval) will exclude a difference in favor of the standard group of more than 10% "Eq. 4.118".

$$d_{NIF} = \frac{(0.65 - 0.85) - (0.1)}{\sqrt{0.65(1 - 0.65) + 0.85(1 - 0.85)}}$$
$$= -0.5$$

$$(4.117)$$

$$n_{NIF} = (1.65 + 0.84)^2 / -0.5^2 = 25 \qquad (4.118)$$

Suppose we assume that both antibiotics are thought to be equally effective. In that case, the difference that we will look for will be only the 10% non-inferiority margin "Eq. 4.119", and as per rule, our sample size will increase to 158 patients per group "Eq. 4.120". The same online calculator can verify the same results.

$$d_{NIF} = \frac{(-0.1)}{\sqrt{2 \times 0.85(1 - 0.85)}} = -0.198$$

$$(4.119)$$

$$n_{NIF} = (1.65 + 0.84)^2 / 0.198^2 = 158 \qquad (4.120)$$

Equivalence Study

The same authors also considered proving that both treatments are equivalent, using the same assumptions as before and implying $(Z_{1-B/2})$ in

the equation; sample size increases to 307 patients per group. Note that, unlike a non-inferiority design, the 10% non-inferiority margin (δ) has to be uploaded as (+10% = 0.1), in order to be "subtracted = removed" from the "negative difference" between both proportions: "Eq. 4.121" and "Eq. 4.122".

$$d_{Eq} = \frac{0.1 - (0.85 - 0.65)}{\sqrt{0.65(1 - 0.65) + 0.85(1 - 0.85)}}$$
$$= \frac{-0.1}{0.6} = -0.167$$

$$(4.121)$$

$$n_{Eq} = (1.64 + 1.28)^2 / 0.167^2 = 307 \qquad (4.122)$$

If both groups are expected to have the same proportions of success (85%) "Eq. 4.123", the only difference remaining is the equivalence rate, and hence, the sample size will decrease to only 219 patients per group "Eq. 4.124".

$$d_{Eq} = \frac{\delta}{\sqrt{2 p_R (1 - p_T)}} = \frac{-0.1}{\sqrt{2 \times 0.85(1 - 0.85)}}$$
$$= -0.198$$

$$(4.123)$$

$$n_{Eq} = (1.64 + 1.28)^2 / -0.198^2 = 219 \quad (4.124)$$

Online Calculators

Sample sizes can be verified by checking one of the online calculators: [17, 66]. We have to be careful when using different online calculators, not because they give different results but because of the difference in the ways by which data is uploaded. Concerning [17]; we have to upload the 10% non-inferiority margin (δ) as (−0.1) to be "added" to the "negative difference" between both proportions, in favor of reference treatment.

4.13.2.3 Sample Size from Odds Ratio Non-inferiority Study

We have previously discussed sample size calculation from Odds ratio for a routine superiority study (see Sects. 4.3.1.5 and 4.3.2.2). The example given concerned the relation between smoking and the development of bronchogenic carcinoma. The recorded respective proportions of bronchogenic carcinoma among smokers and non smokers were: 10 and 3%, with an Odds ratio of 3.6. Assuming a unilateral design with the usual risks of error, the calculated sample size was 172 patients per group.

In order to note the effect of non-inferiority and equivalence study design on sample size, we will use the exact figures and the same online calculator [17]. Suppose that those rates of 10 and 3% are the efficacy rates obtained by two treatments, and a 2% difference was suggested as being an acceptable limit of non-inferiority. As we are looking for non-inferiority, δ has to be "added" to log OR ($1.28 + 0.02 = 1.3$), producing an odds ratio of 3.69 and a total of 334 patients, equally distributed between both groups "Eq. 4.125" and "Eq. 4.126". The same online calculator can verify the results [17, 66].

$$n_{NIF} = \frac{(z_{1-\alpha} + z_{1-\beta})^2}{(log\ OR - \delta)^2} \left(\frac{1}{kp_T(1 - p_T)} + \frac{1}{kp_R(1 - p_R)} \right)$$

(4.125)

$$n_{NIF} = \frac{(1.65 + 0.84)^2}{(1.28 - (-0.02))^2} \left(\frac{1}{0.1 \times 0.9} + \frac{1}{0.03 \times 0.97} \right)$$
$$= 167$$

(4.126)

Superiority Study

Suppose that we are looking to prove superiority by a certain margin, $\delta > 0$, and hence it has to be "subtracted" from log OR by calculating: log OR $- (\delta)$. In such case, effect size effect will be equal to log OR $- (\delta) = 1.28 - (0.02) = 1.26$, and a total of 356 patients equally distributed between both groups (178 patients per group) will be needed to give the study an 80% power to detect the effect size presumed. Compared to the non-inferiority design, the smaller is the effect size, the more significant is the calculated sample size, as per the general rule.

Equivalence Study

Supposing that the investigators wanted to put into evidence the equivalence of both treatments, the same authors also considered proving that both treatments are equivalent, using the same assumptions as before and implying ($Z_{1-B/2}$) in the equation; sample size increases to 246 patients per group. Unlike the non-inferiority design, the 2% non-inferiority margin (δ) has to be uploaded as ($+2\% = 0.02$), in order to be "removed" from the "negative difference" between both proportions "Eq. 4.127" and "Eq. 4.128".

$$n_{Eq} = \frac{(z_{1-\alpha} + z_{1-\beta/2})^2}{(\delta - log\ OR)^2} \left(\frac{1}{kp_T(1 - p_T)} + \frac{1}{kp_R(1 - p_R)} \right)$$

(4.127)

$$n_{Eq} = \frac{(1.65 + 1.28)^2}{(0.02 - 1.28)^2} \left(\frac{1}{0.1 \times 0.9} + \frac{1}{0.03 \times 0.97} \right)$$
$$= 246$$

(4.128)

If both treatments are thought to be equivalent with P = 10%, OR will be equal to 1 and hence, Log OR equals 0. Being the equivalence limit of an OR of 50%, δ will be equal to 0.5. The calculated sample size jumps to 761 patients per group to compensate for the smaller effect size and the double unilateral design "Eq. 4.129" and "Eq. 4.130".

$$n_{Eq} = \frac{(z_{1-\alpha} + z_{1-\beta/2})^2}{(0.5)^2} \left(\frac{1}{kp_T(1 - p_T)} + \frac{1}{kp_R(1 - p_R)} \right)$$

(4.129)

$$n_{Eq} = \frac{(1.65 + 1.28)^2}{(0.5)^2} \left(\frac{1}{0.1 \times 0.9} + \frac{1}{0.03 \times 0.97} \right) = 761$$

(4.130)

Online Calculators

The result can be verified by checking on an online calculator [17, 66].

4.13.3 Time to Event Analysis

4.13.3.1 Calculation of Effect Size: Hazard Rates and Hazard Ratio

In the routine superiority study, the effect size could be expressed as the difference between 2 survival rates ($\lambda1 - \lambda2$), hazard ratio (HR), or the Log HR in a Cox regression model (see Sect. 4.9.1). *In the non-inferiority design, the non-inferiority margin δ is practically "added" to log HR by calculating: log HR $- (-\delta) = $ log HR $+ \delta$. The resulting increase in the size of the difference that the investigator is looking for decreases the required sample size. On the other hand, and as previously mentioned, the presence of a true difference between compared treatments makes it harder to prove equivalence for δ being "removed" from effect size: log HR $- (\delta) = $ log HR $- \delta$. The resulting decrease in effect size increases sample size by default. The same rules apply when the effect size is expressed as the difference between 2 survival rates ($\lambda1 - \lambda2$). The non-inferiority margin (δ) is added to effect size in non-inferiority, making it easier to achieve. However, it is removed from effect size in the case of equivalence design, rendering achievement harder.

4.13.3.2 Calculation of Sample Size: Exponential and Cox Proportional Hazard Methods

After defining the effect size, sample size calculation proceeds as usual by adopting a unilateral design for the non inferiority study and a TOST design for the equivalence study. In both cases, the primary risk of error is totally dedicated to the single available conclusion and is expressed in the calculations as ($z_{1-\alpha}$). In addition, the 2 one-sided test (TOST) procedure of the equivalence study implies the consideration of ($Z_{1-\beta/2}$) - instead of ($Z_{1-\beta}$)—for the usual 80% power.

Exponential Method (Lachine and Foulkes)

The method has been explained in Sect. 4.9.2.1. In short, effect size is expressed as the standardized difference between the two hazard rates

($\lambda1 - \lambda2$). The variance (σ^2) is design independent "Eq. 4.131" and sample size is calculated for one group (n_2), from which (n_1) is deducted from the proportion K = n1/n2.

The usual modifications will then be made to effect size by "adding" (δ) in case of non-inferiority and "removing" (δ) in case of equivalence study and, adopting a unilateral design in case of non-inferiority and TOST in case of equivalence. In order to clarify the modified calculations, we present the equations for sample size calculation in case of superiority (n_{2Sup}) "Eq. 4.132", non-inferiority (n_{2NIF}) "Eq. 4.133" and equivalence (n_{2Eq}) designs "Eq. 4.134".

$$\sigma^2(\lambda_i) = \lambda_i^2 \left(1 + \frac{e^{-\lambda_i T} - e^{-\lambda_i(T-T_0)}}{\lambda_i T_0}\right)^{-1}$$
(4.131)

$$n_{2Sup} = \frac{\left(Z_{(1-\alpha/2)} + Z_{(1-\beta)}\right)^2}{(\lambda_1 - \lambda_2)^2} \left[\frac{\sigma^2(\lambda_1)}{k} + \sigma^2(\lambda_2)\right]$$
(4.132)

$$n_{2NIF} = \frac{\left(Z_{(1-\alpha)} + Z_{(1-\beta)}\right)^2}{(\lambda_1 - \lambda_2 - \delta)^2} \left[\frac{\sigma^2(\lambda_1)}{k} + \sigma^2(\lambda_2)\right]$$
(4.133)

$$n_{2Eq} = \frac{\left(Z_{(1-\alpha)} + Z_{(1-\beta/2)}\right)^2}{(\delta)^2} \left[\frac{\sigma^2(\lambda_1)}{k} + \sigma^2(\lambda_2)\right]$$
(4.134)

The Example

Reviewing the example of comparing progression-free survival in two equal groups of patients with lymphocytic leukemia, who are either receiving conventional chemotherapy or a new biological treatment. The total duration of the study was three years and the follow-up period (T − T0) was two years. Previous studies have shown that the progression hazard rates of group 1 and group 2 were: 1 and 2 patient-years; respectively. The researchers accepted a non-inferiority margin of 20%. The question was how many patients are needed to give the study 80% power, with the usual 5% primary risk of error. Applying the above equations to our data gives a sample size of about 22 patients per group "Eq. 4.135". Note that (δ) was practically added to effect size and, in the case the authors will be interested in putting into evidence 20% superiority margin, (δ) would be removed from effect size, increasing the sample size to 48 patients per group (not shown). if we assume that $\lambda 1 = \lambda 2$ and an acceptable δ margin of 0.5, the sample size needed to achieve equivalence will be 67 patients per group "Eq. 4.136".

$$n_{NIF} = \frac{(1.65 + 0.84)^2}{(2 - 1 - (-0.2))^2}[0.97 + 3.94] = 22$$

(4.135)

$$n_{Eq} = \frac{(1.65 + 1.28)^2}{(-0.5 - 0)^2}[0.97 + 0.97] = 67$$

(4.136)

Cox Proportional Hazard Method

The method has been explained in Sect. 4.9.2.2. The effect size is expressed as Log Hazard ratio (HR) that can be derived from Cox regression analysis. The usual modifications will then be made to the effect size by "adding" (δ) in case of non-inferiority and "removing" (δ) in case of equivalence study. We will adopt a unilateral design in case of non-inferiority and TOST in case of equivalence, as usual. In order to clarify the modified calculations, we present the equations for sample size calculation in case of superiority (N_{Sup}) "Eq. 4.137", non-inferiority (N_{NIF}) "Eq. 4.138", and equivalence (N_{Eq}) designs "Eq. 4.139". Note that this equation gives the total sample size. Kindly refer to Sect. 4.9.2.2 for more details.

$$N_{Sup} = \frac{\left(Z_{(1-\alpha/2)} + Z_{(1-\beta)}\right)^2}{Log\,HR^2 p_1 p_2 Pr_e (1 - R^2)}$$

(4.137)

$$N_{NIF} = \frac{\left(Z_{(1-\alpha)} + Z_{(1-\beta)}\right)^2}{(Log\,HR - \delta)^2 p_1 p_2 Pr_e (1 - R^2)}$$

(4.138)

$$N_{Eq} = \frac{\left(Z_{(1-\alpha)} + Z_{(1-\beta/2)}\right)^2}{(\delta)^2 p_1 p_2 Pr_e (1 - R^2)}$$

(4.139)

The Example

We are reviewing the example outlined in Sect. 2.7.4, where a new treatment was suggested to increase the survival of patients with bronchogenic carcinoma by 50%, compared to the reference treatment. The overall event rate was 7.2%. The investigators wished to calculate sample size with an 80% power to prove that the new treatment is not worse than the standard therapy by more than 10% ($\delta = 0.1$), with a conventional (α) of 5%. Applying the given equation gives a sample size of 548 patients, providing equal allocation "Eq. 4.140". An online calculator can verify the result [17].

$$N_{NIF} = \frac{(1.65 + 0.84)^2}{[Log\,0.5 - (-0.1)]^2 0.5 \times 0.5 \times 0.072} = 548$$

(4.140)

If the investigators were concerned about proving the equivalence of the two treatments and using the same parameters as above, 1350 patients would be necessary "Eq. 4.141". On the other hand, if both treatments were thought to be equal (HR = 1), 1900 patients would be necessary to prove that the difference between treatment effects will respect an equivalence margin of 0.5 "Eq. 4.142". Note the significant sample size change, in concordance with the increased (δ). An online calculator can verify the results [17].

$$N_{Eq} = \frac{(1.65 + 1.28)^2}{[(-0.1) - Log\,0.5]^2 0.5 \times 0.5 \times 0.072} = 1350$$

(4.141)

$$N_{Eq} = \frac{(1.65 + 1.28)^2}{(-0.5 - 0)^2 0.5 \times 0.5 \times 0.072} = 1900$$

(4.142)

4.14 Diagnostic Accuracy

Although the diagnosis of a disease has to be made by a gold-standard test, the latter is usually replaced by a simpler, more reachable, or less expensive diagnostic test. Consequently, evaluating the accuracy of a diagnostic test is fundamental to measuring its credibility. Despite the numerous studies testing diagnostic accuracy, sample sizes calculations are rarely reported. Researchers often decide about the sample size arbitrarily either for their convenience or from the previous literature [67]. Measures of diagnostic accuracy have been discussed before (see Sect. 1.9). This section will consider sample size calculation for three indices, namely, sensitivity, specificity, and area under the receiver operating curve.

4.14.1 Sensitivity and Specificity

Sensitivity (Sn) and specificity (Sp) are just proportions. Sn is the proportion of true positive (TP) in diseased patients [true positive + false negative (FN)]. Sp is the proportion of true negative (TN) in healthy cases or controls [true negative + false positive (FP)]. Consequently, if we are looking to calculate the sample size necessary to establish the Sn or the Sp of a new diagnostic test, we will use the simple equation of calculating sample size for a proportion. On the other hand, if we wish to compare the accuracy of a particular test to a reference or fixed value, we will use the general equation of comparing a proportion to a reference value. Finally, if we compare the Sn or the Sp of two separate tests, we will use the equation to calculate sample size for comparing two independent proportions. If both tests were performed in the same subject, we would use the equation to calculate sample size for comparing two dependent proportions.

The Role of Prevalence (P)

A second point is the role of prevalence (P) in sample size calculation. *Calculation of Sn and Sp are independent of prevalence.* We assume that the patient's condition is known when the test is performed. In other words, we calculate Sn in patients who are already known to have the disease and Sp in normal controls. *The (P) acquires its importance when we lack a prior diagnosis*, as when calculating Sn and Sp in a sample of the population that includes both cases and controls and, we do not know which is which? In such a case, we have to include the prevalence in calculating sample size [68, 69]. Once the diagnosis is made, the (P) will lose its importance as calculation of (Sn) will be limited to known patients, and, the calculation of (Sp) will be limited to known controls. In this section, we will keep using the capital letter (P) to indicate the prevalence in the distinction of the small letter (p) that will be used to indicate a proportion.

Always in this section, we will adopt a bilateral study, the usual 5% primary risk of error and an 80% study power and hence, the respective Z values will be $Z_{1 - \alpha/2} = 1.96$ and, $Z_{1 - B} = 0.84$. The researcher can adopt other alternatives, such as $Z_{1 - \alpha} = 1.65$ in case of a unilateral study and $Z_{1 - B/2} = 1.28$ for a 90% power. All calculated sample sizes have to be increased by a minimum of 10% to compensate for the dropouts.

4.14.1.1 Establishing Sensitivity or Specificity with a Known Disease State

If we know whether the examined subjects are cases or controls, sample size calculation of either Sn or Sp will be simply the calculations made for a proportion (p) "Eq. 4.143". The latter will be the (Sn) when calculated among known disease cases and Sp if calculated among known controls without the disease. We will follow the usual procedure, starting with the researcher reviewing the literature to estimate (p). This is followed by assigning an additional estimate of precision or a margin of error (d) around which he expects the proportion in the sample (p) to fluctuate around the population's proportion. Finally, the researcher has to choose the primary risk of error α (usually 5%) to give the result an appropriate confidence level $(1 - \alpha)$, usually 95% [69, 70].

$$N_p = \frac{\left(Z_{(1-\alpha/2)}\right)^2 p(1 - p)}{d^2} \quad (4.143)$$

We have previously given the example of testing the diagnostic accuracy of a new digital sphygmomanometer versus the golden standard mercury sphygmomanometer (Table 1.12). The study has shown that the new instrument has an Sn of 80% and an Sp of 95%. Based on those results, we wish to calculate sample size to establish those results, with 5% precision (d) and 95% confidence $(Z_{1 - \alpha/2})$. In "Eq. 4.143", we replace $(Z_{1 - \alpha/2})^2$ by $(1.96)^2$ and (d^2) by $(0.05)^2$. Whether we wish to calculate sample size for Sn or Sp, we replace (p) by 0.8 or by 0.95, producing a total sample size of 246 or 73 subjects. We have to add the extra routine 10% dropout rate. The calculations can be easily verified online, using many freely available links [16, 71].

4.14.1.2 Establishing Sensitivity or Specificity with an Unknown Disease State

If we intend to calculate Sn, Sp, or both in a mixed but unmarked population of diseased and healthy subjects, we have to consider the prevalence of the disease (P). *The smaller is (P), the more we have to include patients if the study's primary aim is Sn and, the less we need patients if the study's primary aim is Sp.* The denominator of "Eq. 4.143" is modified by adding (P) to calculate sample size for Sn "Eq. 4.144" and $(1 - P)$ in case we are calculating Sp "Eq. 4.145" [68]. Finally, we will adopt the larger calculated sample size whenever the aim is to calculate both indices. Tables of sample sizes calculated for different values of Sn, Sp, (P), and precision are available in many resources [68, 69]

$$N_{Sn} = \frac{\left(Z_{(1-\alpha/2)}\right)^2 Sn(1 - Sn)}{d^2 \times P} \quad (4.144)$$

$$N_{Sp} = \frac{\left(Z_{(1-\alpha/2)}\right)^2 Sp(1 - Sp)}{d^2 \times (1 - P)} \quad (4.145)$$

Applying the equation on population 2 in the example given in Table 1.12 gives a total sample size of 1230 cases "Eq. 4.146" in the case we wish to calculate sample size to establish Sn. The same equation gives a total sample size of 92 cases to establish an Sp of 95% (not shown). Note that those are the total numbers of subjects, and the ratio of cases to controls will be equal to $P/(1 - P)$. For example, out of the total number of 1230 subjects necessary to establish 80% sensitivity, we need a minimum of 246 cases (20%) and 984 controls (80%). We have to add the extra 10% to compensate for the dropouts. Calculations can be verified online [16, 71].

$$N_{Sn} = \frac{(1.96)^2 0.8(1 - 0.8)}{0.05^2 \times 0.2} = 1230 \quad (4.146)$$

4.14.1.3 Testing Sensitivity or Specificity of a Test

Suppose that in the previous example, the researchers had a predetermined Sn of 0.7, and they wished to prove that the test has a higher Sn of 0.8. How many patients should they include in the study to prove this 10% difference, adopting the same 5% precision and giving their results the same 95% confidence level. The equation is used in calculating the sample size to compare a theoretical proportional (P_0) to an observed proportion (P_1) "Eq. 4.147". *By now, the researchers usually know the condition of the patients; they do not have to include the prevalence in the equation. Otherwise, it would be included in the denominator as before.* Nevertheless, the difference between the two proportions $(P_1 - P_0)$ follows an approximately normal distribution. Adopting the usual 5% primary risk of error, a bilateral study of np (154) cases per group will have an 80% power to show a statistically significant difference of 10% between both proportions "Eq. 4.147". Calculations can be verified online [16, 71].

$$n_p = \frac{\left[\left(Z_{(1-\alpha/2)}\right)\sqrt{P_0(1-P_0)} + \left(Z_{(1-\beta)}\right)\sqrt{P_1(1-P_1)}\right]^2}{(P_1 - P_0)^2}$$

$$= \frac{\left[1.96\sqrt{0.7 \times 0.3} + 0.84\sqrt{0.8 \times 0.2}\right]^2}{(0.8 - 0.7)^2} = 154$$

(4.147)

4.14.1.4 Comparing Sensitivity or Specificity of Two Independent Tests

The other side of the coin is the researchers comparing the Sn or the SP of two tests. Sample size calculation will follow the general formula of comparing two independent proportions; adopting the larger "variance of the difference". As each test has its variance, the variance of the difference is the sum of the variances of both tests (see Sect. 1.4.2.7).

Suppose that the researchers wished to compare the Sn acquired by the digital sphygmomanometer ($P_1 = 0.8$) with the Sn acquired with a different sphygmomanometer ($P_2 = 0.7$). Pc is the common average proportion (0.75), provided that an equal number of patients will be subjected to each test. We calculate sample size by replacing $Z_{(1-\alpha/2)}$ by 1.96, $Z_{(1-\beta)}$ by 0.84, Pc by 0.75, P1 by 0.8 and P2 by 0.7 in "Eq. 4.147". Despite comparing the same 10% difference between both proportions, the researchers needed to include 294 cases to compensate for the higher variation due to independence "Eq. 4.148" [16, 71]. Note that n_p is the calculated sample size per group, and hence in case the two groups are equal, the total sample size will be 588 subjects, to which we have to add the extra 10% to compensate for the expected dropout.

$$n_p = \frac{\left[\left(Z_{(1-\alpha/2)}\right)\sqrt{2P_c(1-P_c)} + \left(Z_{(1-\beta)}\right)\sqrt{P_1(1-P_1) + P_2(1-P_2)}\right]^2}{(P_1 - P_2)^2}$$

$$= 293$$

(4.148)

4.14.1.5 Comparing Sensitivity or Specificity in a Paired Design

Table 4.4 shows the results of comparing the sensitivity of two tests on the same subject. Unlike the unpaired design, the question is not about comparing two proportions (sensitivities) to see the more sensitive test. The question is about the accuracy, i.e., testing the new test's accuracy by showing how the results are concordant with those acquired with the golden standard. Table 4.4 shows the results acquired from a group of 100 diseased cases examined by both the gold standard and the diagnostic test in question. The concordant proportions are the proportion of yes/yes (a) and the proportions of no/no (d).

In our example, the overall proportion of concordant results ($Pr_{conc} = a + d = 65 + 15$) is 80 and 20% of the results were disconcordant (Pr_{disc} c + b = 15 + 5). There is no point that a diagnostic test indicates the presence of the disease, while it was proved to be absent by the gold standard and vice versa. *Consequently, the study question is about how much both tests disagree.* In other words, was the 20% overall rate of disagreement ($Pr_{disc} = 0.2$) significantly different between both tests? The proportion of disagreement between the two tests was 5% (Pb) versus 15% (Pc), and their OR = 0.3333. *For simplicity of calculations, we have replaced OR = Pb/Pc = 0.3333 in the equation by OR = Pc/Pb = 3; which gives the same result.*

Under the null hypothesis, Pb is equal to Pc, and their ratio equals 1. After designing α and β are type I and type II error rate probabilities, the researcher can calculate sample size by many equations, the simplest being an approximate equation suggested by Machin and colleagues [41], which has been given before "Eq. 4.49".

$$N = \frac{\left[1.96(3+1) + 0.84\sqrt{(3+1)^2 - (3-1)^2 \times 0.2}\right]^2}{(3-1)^2 \times 0.2}$$

$$= 156$$

(4.149)

Table 4.4 Sample size calculation: comparing sensitivity (paired design)

Gold standard				
Diagnostic test		Yes	No	Total
	Yes	65 (a)	5 (b)	70
	No	15 (c)	15 (d)	30
	Total	80 (a + c)	20 (b + d)	100 (N)

N = total number of patients with documented disease

The equation included the proportion of disconcordant cases (Pr_{disc}) to account for the proportion of concordant cases in the calculation. In other words, it calculates the size of the whole sample that is expected to include concordant and disconcordant cases, of course. The equation presented as for a bilateral study and hence, in case of a unilateral design, $[(Z_{(1-\alpha/2)})=1.96]$ is replaced by $[(Z_{(1-\alpha/2)}) = 1.65]$. Moreover, we will adopt a usual 80% power and hence, $[(Z_{(1-\beta)}) = 0.84]$ will be replaced by $[(Z_{(1-\beta)}) = 1.28]$, in case of adopting a 90% power. Compared to the larger sample size needed in the unpaired study "Eq. 4.148", the researcher needs a much smaller number of patients to put into evidence the same difference between both tests "Eq. 4.149". The calculations can be verified either online [72] or by using G*power software [21]. Applying the continuity correction gives a larger sample size of 165 patients by both the software and the online calculator. A more exact and complex formula was designed by Schork and Williams and is the one used by PASS sample size software [42].

What Should be Reported

As an example of what should be reported: a sample size of 150 subjects has an 80% power to detect a difference of 10% between two diagnostic tests whose sensitivities are 0.7 and 0.8. The procedure uses a two-sided McNemar test with a significance level of 0.05. The prevalence of disease in the population is 20%, and the proportion of discordant pairs is 20%. A minimum of 10% should increase the sample size to account for dropouts.

4.14.2 ROC Analysis

We have previously discussed the idea behind the analysis of a ROC (see Sect. 1.9.4.3). In short, plotting Sn on the y-axis and 1-Sp on the x-axis enables the probability of each paired data point to be true positive (having the disease) or false positive (being healthy). Repeating the same interpretation of all data points plots the whole spectrum of probabilities. The size and shape of the area formed under this plot (curve) express the overall diagnostic performance of the test. Consequently, it helps to choose the cut-off values that best serve its main purpose, whether for screening or confirmation of the disease, and it allows comparing the performance of different tests.

4.14.2.1 Estimating Accuracy Index

The area under the ROC estimates the accuracy of the diagnostic test. Table 1.10 shows the results of measuring the fasting blood sugar in 30 diabetic patients and 30 normal controls. Data analysis by IBM-SPSS statistical software showed a large area under the curve of 0.91, and the question is what is the required sample size that can put into evidence this AUC, with acceptable precision (d = 5%) and a 95% level of confidence? The sample size depends on the variability of the index, and there are multiple parametric and non-parametric methods to calculate the variance of AUC.

We will use the parametric method based on binormal assumption [73]. The equation looks complicated but mainly consists of constants, with only one variable to calculate: (a). The latter is the cumulative inverse normal function of the AUC. In other words, it is the Z score corresponding to the AUC (0.91, in our example). Many calculators can produce it, but a simpler way is to consult the Z table. The AUC is the probability shown by the table, and hence, we look for the probability of 0.91 and find the corresponding Z score for this probability. The corresponding Z score is calculated by adding the marginal values of the probability, i.e., adding the head of the corresponding column and raw. Put it another way, instead of the usual procedure, i.e., checking for the probability of a given Z score, we will simply check for the Z score for a given probability (AUC). For our example, the Z score (inverse cumulative probability) = 1.34 and (a) is calculated by multiplying it by the square root of 2; a = $1.34\sqrt{2} = 1.895$. Some tables directly give the inverse cumulative standard distribution, which must be multiplied by $\sqrt{2}$ to get (a) [74]. Equation 4.150 calculates the variance of the AUC (0.062), assuming samples of equal size "Eq. 4.150". Equation 4.151 calculates the total sample size for a bilateral study, with 95% confidence $(1 - \alpha/2)$ and 5% precision (d) "Eq. 4.151".

$$Var\,AUC = (0.0099 \times e^{\left(-\frac{a^2}{2}\right)} \times (6a^2 + 16)$$
$$= (0.0099 \times e^{\left(-\frac{1.895^2}{2}\right)}$$
$$\times (6 \times 1.895^2 + 16)$$
$$= 0.062$$

$$(4.150)$$

$$N = \frac{(Z_{(1-\alpha/2)})^2 Var\,AUC}{d^2} = \frac{1.96^2 \times 0.062}{0.05^2} = 95$$

$$(4.151)$$

4.14.2.2 Testing Accuracy of a Quantitative Diagnostic Test

If the researcher wishes to test the accuracy of a new test with AUC_1 to a predetermined AUC_0, the sample size calculation will be a variant of that used to test a predefined Sn or Sp index to that of a new method "Eq. 4.147". For a bilateral study, the required sample size per group to detect a statistically significant difference between both areas $(AUC_1 - AUC_0)$ can be

calculated by "Eq. 4.152", on the assumption that we have as many patients as controls. The predetermined AUC_0 (Var AUC_0) is 0.8 (0.07) and the suggested AUC_1 (Var AUC_1) is 0.9 (0.06). Replacing $Z_{(1-\alpha/2)}$ and $Z_{(1-\beta)}$ by 1.96 and 0.84 in "Eq. 4.152"; the required sample size will be 73 patients per group.

$$n = \frac{\left[(Z_{(1-\alpha/2)})\sqrt{Var\,AUC_0} + (Z_{(1-\beta)})\sqrt{Var\,AUC_1}\right]^2}{(AUC_1 - AUC_0)^2}$$

$$(4.152)$$

4.14.2.3 Comparing Accuracy of Two Independent ROC Curves

If the researcher wishes to compare the AUC acquired by two diagnostic tests (AUC_1 to AUC_2), the sample size calculation will be a variant of that used to compare Sn (or Sp) of two independent diagnostic tests "Eq. 4.148". The difference will be calculating the common $[AUC_c]$ as the average of $[AUC_1 + AUC_2]$. In the equation, we replace the variabilities of the common proportion $[2P_c(1 - P_c)]$, of the first $[P_1(1 - P_1)]$, and the variability of the second proportion $[P_1(1 - P_1)]$ by the variabilities of the common AUC $[2Var\,AUC_c]$, of the first AUC $[Var\,AUC_1]$ and the variability of the second AUC $[Var\,AUC_2]$ "Eq. 4.153". In all cases, variance AUC is calculated using the same equation "4.150" after calculating the constant (a) as the product of the inverse cumulative probability of the corresponding AUC and $\sqrt{2}$. Hand calculations are lengthy and can be easily performed by statistical software: [32, 75] or checked out in in the freely available ready-made tables [69, 76].

$$n = \frac{\left[(Z_{(1-\alpha/2)})\sqrt{2Var\,AUC_c} + (Z_{(1-\beta)})\sqrt{Var\,AUC_1 + Var\,AUC_2}\right]^2}{(AUC_1 - AUC_2)^2}$$

$$(4.153)$$

4.14.2.4 Comparing Accuracy of Two Dependent ROC Curves

It is generally accepted that the paired design is much more powerful than the unpaired situation.

The researchers may wish to compare the accuracy of two diagnostic tests when performed on the same patient. The reader is invited to revise the section on correlation to appreciate that when the variability of paired data (x, y) is not only dependent on the variability of x and y but also on their covariance Cov (x, y). Consequently, the equation to calculate sample size is the same as for the independent situation, except that the common variation should not be only deducted from both variables but from their covariation too. In the equation, the common variation used in "Eq. 4.153" $[2Var\ AUC_c]$ is replaced by $[2Var_{H0}(AUC_1 - AUC_2)]$ "Eq. 4.154", which expresses variabilities of both AUC as well as their coverability "Eq. 4.155" [69]. It is clear that hand calculation becomes more demanding and is better performed by statistical software: [32, 75] or checked out in the freely available ready-made tables [69, 76].

$$N = \frac{\left[(Z_{(1-\alpha/2)})\sqrt{2Var_{H0}(AUC_1 - AUC_2)} + (Z_{(1-\beta)})\sqrt{VarAUC_1 + VarAUC_2}\right]^2}{(AUC_1 - AUC_2)^2}$$

$$(4.154)$$

$$Var_{H0}(AUC_1 - AUC_2)$$
$$= nVar(AUC_1) + nVar(AUC_2) - 2nCov(AUC_1, AUC_2)$$

$$(4.155)$$

4.15   Measuring Agreement

Measuring agreement has been discussed before (see Sect. 2.10). In brief, it refers to the degree of concordance between two or more measurements, whether made by different methods, repeated by the same method, or reproduced by different operators. In short, measuring agreement is mainly about reliability and if one method can replace the other? Following the elimination of a systematic bias, choosing the measure of the agreement depends upon the study material, the predictor, and the outcome variables. The study material is usually the patients themselves or patients-related material,

such as tissue samples or radiological documents. The predictor variable is the evaluated set of different tests, experimental conditions, or raters. The outcome is what is being measured, and it can be binomial, such as having or not having the disease, a categorical variable, or a quantitative variable, such as the change in body weight, blood sugar, or else.

4.15.1   Qualitative Outcome

4.15.1.1   Cohen's Kappa

Cohen's Kappa measures agreement between two predictors on a binomial or categorical outcome or one predictor evaluating the same material twice. It can equally measure agreement between two groups of predictors, provided that each group gives a single joint decision. As agreement can be due to chance (Pc), we measure the proportion of agreement (Pa) over and above (Pc). Cohen's Kappa calculates the difference between the observed and expected measures (Pa-Pc), standardized by being related to a perfect agreement from which the part that can be due to chance (Pc) has been removed; i.e., (1 − Pc). Hence, Kappa (K) = (Pa-Pc)/(1 − Pc) "Eq. 2.127". The result is a proportion of "genuine" agreement above what can be due to chance. Being a proportion, K ranges between −1 and +1; with a (0) value indicating no agreement at all and up to a Kappa of 1 indicating perfect agreement (see Sect. 2.10.3.1).

We will use the example previously presented in Sect. 1.10.3.1, showing the agreement between MSCT and coronary angiography (CA) on whether coronary stents are re-stenosed after percutaneous angioplasty. The calculations showed a statistically significant substantial agreement between both tests: Kappa (95% CI) = 0.695 (0.52–0.87): P < 0.001 (see Sect. 2.10.3.1). Table 4.5 shows the number of cases in which both procedures agree on a positive (d11) or a negative finding (d00). Cases of disagreement are indicated as (d10, d01). The proportions of agreement (π_A) and disagreement

Table 4.5 Sample size calculation: Cohen Kappa

	CA (ISR)	CA (patent stent)	Total
MSCT (ISR)	18 (d_{11})	3 (d_{01})	21
MSCT (patent stent)	7 (d_{10})	52 (d_{00})	59
Total	25	55	80 (N)

MSCT = multislice CT, CA = coronary angiography, ISR = in-stent restenosis, d_{11} = number of cases in which both MSCT and CA agree on the positive finding, d_{00} = number of cases in which both MSCT and CA agree on the negative finding, d_{10} = and d_{01} = number of cases in which both MSCT and CA disagree on the finding, N = total number of cases

(π_D) are 87.5% and 12.5%, respectively "Eq. 4.156".

$$\pi_A = \frac{d_{00} + d_{11}}{N} = \frac{52 + 18}{80} = 0.875 \; and, \pi_D$$
$$= \frac{d_{10} + d_{10}}{N} = \frac{7 + 10}{80} = 0.125$$
$$(4.156)$$

The study question is not about what both measures agree upon but on the proportions of disagreement (π_D). In the case where Kappa (K) is known, Machin and colleagues have demonstrated that sample size can be calculated as in "Eq. 4.157" [41]. (π_D) is the proportion of disagreement, (d^2) is type II error, which is usually set to 0.2 (=0.84) to give the study an 80% power to detect (k). $Z_{(1-\alpha/2)}$ is the probability value belonging to the normal distribution, with α being the type I error (5%) that is usually set to $\alpha/2$ for a bilateral study (=1.96) or, less commonly, to α for a unilateral study (=1.65). For our example (Table 4.5), with a 12.5% disagreement (π_D), a total sample of 460 subjects (n_k) give a bilateral study an 80% power to detect a Kappa value that is equal to 0.695.

$$n_k = \frac{4\left(Z_{(1-\alpha/2)}\right)^2 (1-k)}{d^2} \left[(1-k)(1-2k) + \frac{k(2-K)}{2\pi_D(1-\pi_D)} \right]$$
$$(4.157)$$

4.15.1.2 A General Formula

If Kappa is unknown, we can calculate sample size for an agreement statistic, based on the proportion of disagreement (π_D) [41]. The calculation follows the general rules of calculating sample size for a proportion "Eq. 4.143" (see Sect. 1.14.1.1). $Z_{(1-\alpha/2)}$ is the probability value belonging to the normal distribution, with α being

the type I error (5%) that is usually set at $\alpha/2$ for a bilateral study or, less commonly, at α for a unilateral study. Type II error is represented as (d) and is set to 0.2 to give the study the usual 80% power. The proportion used in the equation is that of disagreement (π_D), calculated as the sum of disagreements ($d_0 d_1$, $d_1 d_0$) to the total number of cases (N). The variation of the proportion will be the usual $P(1 - P) = \pi_D(1 - \pi_D)$. As such, we are all set for sample size calculation. Adopting the previous example used in Sect. 4.15.1.1, the researcher needs to include a total of 43 cases to detect 12.5% possible disagreement between the two raters "Eq. 4.158".

$$N = \frac{4\left(Z_{(1-\alpha/2)}\right)^2 \pi_D(1 - \pi_D)}{d^2}$$
$$= \frac{4 \times 1.96^2 \times 0.125(1 - 0.125)}{0.2^2} = 43$$
$$(4.158)$$

4.15.2 Quantitative Outcome

4.15.2.1 Intra-class Correlation Coefficient (ICC)

Intraclass correlation coefficient (ICC) was discussed before (see Sect. 2.10.4.3). ICC can measure reproducibility and repeatability in paired numerical data acquired from 2 or more predictors. When first proposed by Fisher, ICC assumed that diagnostic tests follow a one-way repeated measures ANOVA [77]. The total variability in the model (σ_{total}^2) is partitioned into the repeated measures of the same subject by different raters or tests (σ_{within}^2) and, the variability between the different subjects $(\sigma_{between}^2)$. ICC will be the ratio between the latter and the total variability

"Eq. 2.148" Being a proportion out of a total, ICC will vary between 0 (no agreement) and 1 (perfect agreement), being a proportion out of a total. The model further developed with time to answer more questions, such as a two-way ANOVA model, equally accounting for the effect of the predictors (raters, tests, instruments, conditions) replications or repetitions and possible interaction. Variations also included whether study material and predictors are fixed or chosen at random and whether the analysis shows consistency between measurements or absolute agreement [78].

In order to calculate the sample size for his future study, the researcher has to review the literature to define the expected ICC (ρ). After setting the type I (α) and type II errors (d^2), Machin and collaborators proposed "Eq. 4.159" to calculate sample size for (K) number of raters [41]. The usual setting includes a (d^2) of $(0.2)^2$ to give the study an 80% power, $Z_{(1-\alpha/2)}$ of 1.96 for a bilateral study or, less commonly, a $Z_{(1-\alpha)}$ of 1.65, in the case the study was unilateral. Bonnet suggested that the calculated sample size is equally valid for three ANOVA models of ICC and for measurement reliability for consistency or absolute agreement (see Sect. 2.10.4.3) [79, 80].

We will apply the equation on the example shown in Table 2.50, comparing the agreement between two mercury sphygmomanometers (A and B). We can upload our data to SPSS-IBM statistical software and request a two-way ANOVA analysis. The output results are shown in Table 2.50, from which we can calculate an ICC equal to 0.967 "Eq. 2.150". Now suppose that another researcher wishes to repeat the analysis based on the results of this study. For K = 2, $Z_{(1-\alpha/2)} = 1.96$, d = 0.2 and $\rho = 0.967$; the researcher will need to include only four patients for his study, after accounting for the usual 10% increase for the expected dropouts

$$N_{ICC} = 1 + \frac{8\left(Z_{(1-\alpha/2)}\right)^2 (1-\rho)^2 [1+(K-1)\rho]^2}{k(K-1)d^2}$$

$$(4.159)$$

The Eq. 4.160 is another formula for sample size calculation based upon the number of raters (K), the value of ICC when the null hypothesis is true (R_0), and the expected ICC under the alternative hypothesis (R_1) "Eq. 4.160". Both ICC values are better to be looked for in the literature than to be postulated by the researchers. The values (θ_0) and (θ_1) represent the odds of (R_0) and (R_1) and, (C_0) is then deducted from (k), (θ_0) and (θ_1) "Eq. 1.61" [81–83]. The equation has the advantage of assuming a degree of initial agreement before the study. If there is no initial agreement between the raters, (R0) will be equal to zero. In such a case, (θ_0) will be equal to zero too and hence, (C_0) = (1)/(1 + $k\theta_1$).

$$N_{ICC} = 1 + \frac{2\left(Z_{(1-\alpha)} + Z_{(1-B)}\right)^2 k}{(\ln C_0)^2 (K-1)} \quad (4.160)$$

$$C_0 = \frac{1+k\theta_0}{1+k\theta_1}; \theta_0 = \frac{R_0}{1-R_0}; \theta_1 = \frac{R_1}{1-R_1}$$

$$(4.161)$$

We will apply the equation on our example, with (R_0) = zero and (R_1) = 0.967, (θ_1) = 29.3 and (C_0) = (1)/(1+ 2 × 29.3) = 0.0168. The equation gives an equal number of 3 patients that should be raised to four cases to account for the usual 10% increase for the expected dropouts "Eq. 4.162". Consulting an online calculator gives similar results [71]

$$N_{ICC} = 1 + \frac{2(1.96+0.84)^2 2}{(\ln 0.0168)^2 (2-1)} = 3 \quad (4.162)$$

4.15.2.2 Kendall Correlation Coefficient (W)

We have previously discussed the Kendall coefficient of concordance (W). In brief, Kendall's W is a measure of the agreement among multiple predictors measuring several quantitative or semiquantitative variables following other distributions than normal. Kendall W is the proportion of variation between raters and the maximal possible variation of perfect agreement. The more is the agreement, the larger this proportion will be (see Sect. 2.10.4.4). We have taken the example of five raters ranking ten manuscripts, and the resulting W was 0.76 indicates substantial agreement between raters. We have also shown that coefficient W can be used to calculate another effect size, Spearman's rank correlation (r_s) = 0.7 (see Sect. 2.10.4.4).

May and Looney provided several methods for sample size calculation based on those used to calculate sample size for Pearson's correlation coefficient r, [46]. One method is to apply Fisher's Z transformation on Kendall W coefficient, yielding an approximately normally distributed coefficient C "see Eq. 4.64" (see Sect. 4.7.1.1). For a Kendall W value of 0.76, the normalized Z value "C" = 0.996. Assuming the usual 5% type I error and 80% study power, the required total sample size is eight cases (manuscripts) "see Eq. 4.91".

4.16 Survey Analysis

4.16.1 Introduction

In the following lines we will discuss sample size calculation for a clinical survey conducted to answer a question or to take a decision related to our main area of concern; i.e., the comparative clinical study. A survey or a pilot study can supply estimates of variability or effect size necessary to calculate sample size of a future study, in case those estimates are unreliable or missing from the literature. In absence of hypothesis to test, the size of the study is determined by how accurately we would like to answer the study question. We have previously discussed that we can estimate the proportion of the population from that of the sample with a certain degree of confidence, provided that the sample is large, and hence, permitting the normal approximation of the binomial distribution. We are 95% confident that the proportion of the population (which is what we are looking for in the survey) lies within about 1.96 Se from that of

the sample. The 1.96 Se is the expected margin of error (ME) between our sample proportion (p) and that of the population "Eq. 4.163".

$$95\% \, CI = p \pm 1.96 \sqrt{\frac{p(1-p)}{N}} = p \pm ME \tag{4.163}$$

Looking the other way round, and applying simple algebra, we can estimate the sample size (N), which can provide us with the desired margin of error (ME) and 95% level of confidence (the Z value corresponding to the 95% probability) "Eq. 4.164".

$$N = p(1-p)\left(\frac{1.96}{ME}\right)^2 \tag{4.164}$$

We can calculate the sample size for any desired confidence level (e.g., 90% or 99%) by replacing 1.96 with the Z value corresponding to this level of confidence. In short, sample size can be estimated whenever we define: the margin of error that we can accept (ME), the level of confidence that we would like to give to our results, and the expected variability of our data: p(1 − p). *Once we understand the inputs of the equation, we can manipulate them to produce a "reasonable" sample size.* A sample within our limits that answers the study question.

4.16.2 Factors Regulating Sample Size Calculation

4.16.2.1 Level of Confidence

Generally speaking, a sample must be representative of the aimed population. Although the larger the sample, the more likely it will achieve this goal, the sampling method is the main support for representativeness. A randomized sample remains the best method for drawing safe scientific conclusions. Nevertheless, we will present a method to calculate the sample size of a clinical survey based upon the three factors indicated above. The more we want to be confident that our sample is representative of the population, the more we have to increase the sample size. If (α) denotes our sampling error, i.e., the accepted risk that the sample miss-matches the population; $(1 - \alpha)$ will be the degree of confidence in this sample. Most of the investigators choose a primary risk of error of 5%, assigning a level of confidence of 95% to the sample. As previously shown, the latter is expressed in terms of Z score. The Z score of $\alpha = 0.05$ is equal to 1.96 and, if α was chosen to be 10% (i.e., the confidence level of 90%), the calculated Z score would be equal to 1.65, etc.…

4.16.2.2 Variability of Outcome

The sample size is directly proportional to the outcome variability in the population of concern. If all patients receiving a particular treatment either get healed (or die), there will be no point in testing the efficacy of such miraculous treatment (or deadly poison) on many patients. Because patients' response to "any treatment" is variable, we have to study its effect on a group of patients. The more the effect is expected to vary from one patient to another, the more we are obliged to increase our sample size. In statistical terms, in the case of a qualitative outcome, the variance of a proportion is expressed as p $(1 - p)$, where p = proportion of presence and $(1 - p)$ = proportion of absence of studied variable or its effect in the population. Variability of a quantitative variable is expressed by (σ^2); which is the squared standard error of the population of concern.

4.16.2.3 Margin of Error

The third predictor of sample size is the margin of error (ME) that we can tolerate between our sample and the population of concern. The ME reflects imprecision, and hence, it is inversely proportional to the sample size. The more we want to be precise, the more we must include patients in our survey. (ME) has to be suggested by the investigator. It can be set to (0.05) in case of proportions and to the level 5–10% of the mean value in case of a quantitative outcome.

4.16.3 Sample Size Calculation

4.16.3.1 Infinite or Unknown Population

The respective sample size (N) calculation formulae for qualitative and quantitative outcomes are shown above "Eqs. 4.165 and 4.166". Where; N = sample size, Z = the Z score for the chosen confidence level $(1 - \alpha)$, p = proportion of outcome of interest, $(1 - p)$ = proportion of the absence of the outcome, σ_2 = variance of a quantitative variable, ME = margin of error. If p is not known, we have to maximize our sample size by choosing the highest variability p(1 − p), which corresponds with a proportion of 50% and a variance of $(0.5 \times 0.5 = 0.25)$. Any smaller or higher proportion will give a smaller variance. According to the pathology and follow-up duration, the calculated (N) is usually augmented by 10–20% to compensate for follow-up loss.

$$N = p(1 - p)\left(\frac{Z}{ME}\right)^2 \qquad (4.165)$$

$$N = \sigma^2\left(\frac{Z}{ME}\right)^2 \qquad (4.166)$$

4.16.3.2 Known Population

In case we estimate the population size (Np), a modification (can) be applied to the given equation, which reduces sample size in absolute numbers, yet it increases in proportion due to the limited size of the population of concern. Where; N = sample size, Z = Z score for the chosen confidence level $(1 - \alpha)$, p = proportion of outcome of interest, $(1 - p)$ = proportion of the absence of outcome, σ_2 = variance of a quantitative variable, ME = margin of error, α = primary risk of errors, Np = known population size. "Eq. 4.167" and "Eq. 4.168" can be used to calculate sample size for a qualitative and quantitative outcome, respectively.

$$N = \frac{Z^2[p(1 - p)]\left(N_p/N_p - 1\right)}{\left(ME + Z^2\sigma^2\right)\left(N_p - 1\right)} \qquad (4.167)$$

$$N = \frac{Z^2 \sigma^2 \left(N_p / N_p - 1\right)}{\left(ME + Z^2 \sigma^2\right)\left(N_p - 1\right)} \qquad (4.168)$$

The Examples

A study was conducted to implement, monitor, and evaluate the Mission program in Assiut University Hospital. The population was considered as being infinite. Preliminary studies showed that the proportion of STEMI (elevation of ST-segment in ECG of patients with myocardial infarction) was 40% (0.4) among adult cardiac patients presenting with chest pain. How many patients should we include in our study so the sample would represent the population of interest? Our accepted sampling error (α) was 5% (0.05) and hence z ($1 - \alpha$) = 1.96. Applying "Eq. 4.164", we need to include 369 patients in our study "Eq. 4.169", to whom we have to add the usual 10% increase.

$$N = 0.4 \times (1 - 0.4) \times \left(\frac{1.96}{0.05}\right)^2 = 369$$
$$(4.169)$$

Another example for a quantitative outcome: a comparative clinical study was planned to compare outcomes of CABG (coronary artery bypass grafting) 4 h after STEMI to conventional medical therapy in a newly well-equipped rural hospital. Although the ICU (intensive care unit) stay after STEMI could be looked for in the literature. Yet, investigators thought they had to estimate more specific figures reflecting hospital circumstances and working environments. Consequently, a pilot survey analysis was first conducted to measure the mean duration of ICU stays after STEMI. The population was also considered as being infinite. The procedure to calculate the sample size for the survey was as follows: first, we have to estimate the variation of outcome measure (σ) in the population of concern. The latter can be found in the literature or checked in hospital files or previous studies. The literature review showed that the mean and standard deviation of ICU stay after STEMI was 46 ± 20 h and hence, $\sigma^2 = 20^2 = 400$. The

second step is to define an acceptable margin of error (ME) between our sample and the population. It was suggested that a (ME) of ± 10 h would be acceptable; i.e., the mean ICU stay of the sample (which is still unknown and have to be demonstrated by the study) will be estimated within a limit of ± 10 h of that of the population of concern (46 h); i.e., between 36 and 56 h. Note that this ME is >20% of the reported mean (46 h). Finally, we have to choose the confidence level that we are quean to give to our results, usually 95% and, we apply "Eq. 4.166". The latter shwed that we have to include 16 patients in our study "Eq. 4.170".

$$N = 20^2 \times \left(\frac{1.96}{10}\right)^2 = 16 \qquad (4.170)$$

The conclusion of the researcher will be as follows: provided that the duration of ICU stay in the population varies by 20 h, we will be 95% confident that a sample of 16 patients will represent this variability with a margin of error of 10 h; i.e., between 10 and 30 h. Isn't this a very wide and hence, imprecise margin? In order to be more precise, a second researcher from the same institution suggested a smaller ME of 5 h (around 10% of the mean duration reported by the literature: 46 h). Hence, he calculated a larger sample of 62 cases. Although the new sample size will be about four times that calculated by the first researcher, the conclusions will be more precise. We are assuming that the duration of ICU stay in the population varies around 10 h. In that case, we will be 95% confident that the duration of ICU stay in a sample of 62 patients will vary between 15 and 25 h, hence enclosing the truth much more tightly than the first suggestion. Most importantly, using this new smaller variability to calculate sample size for the "future study", will reduce sample size and the researcher's time and money.

Looking the other way round and suppose that the institution supported the second researcher, but he could not recruit the 62 patients and did only recruit 16. After terminating his study with 16 patients only, what confidence level should we assign to his results? The equation can be simply re-ordered to calculate Z, given n and σ "Eq. 4.171"

$$Z = \sqrt{\frac{ME^2 \times N}{\sigma^2}} = \sqrt{\frac{5^2 \times 16}{20^2}} = 1 \quad (4.171)$$

Consulting the Z table, a Z score of 1 is equivalent to a high α value of 0.3 and hence, a significant drop of our level of confidence to only 70%. A steep price to pay in the case where we fail to attain a high precision (low ME) with inadequate patient resources.

Online Calculators

After the designation of ME, $1 - \alpha$, and p, calculation of sample size (N) can be easily performed online using one of many freely available calculators, such as [84]. The default values given by the interface of the software is: ME = 5%, confidence level = 95%, infinite population size = 20,000, p = 50% and n = 377. These numbers represent a "usual situation": the researcher assumes that the population is infinite, suggests a commonly used 5% margin of error, but as he does not have a previous idea about the value of (p) in the population and hence, he maximizes his chances by assigning the largest possible variance to his proportion. The reader can "verify" that the highest pq is obtained by the 50% proportion (pq = 0.5 × 0.5 = 0.25; 0.4 × 0.6 = 0.24; 0.3 × 0.7 = 0.21; etc.). Applying the above equation gives the default: sample size of 377 patients. As advised, (N) should be increased by a minimum of 10%, giving a round number of 400 patients. Not surprisingly, many surveys set sample size of 400 patients to provide a reasonable 5% ME and 95% confidence interval in an infinite population with unknown variance (pq). The researcher is advised to search the literature for N and p and be more precise by suggesting smaller ME, if possible. Another interesting facility is given in the lower table, where we can estimate what would be our ME or confidence interval, with changing sample size, a handy facility for researchers, especially those with limited resources.

References

1. Sullivan G, Feinn R. Using effect size - or why P value is not enough. J Grad Med Educ. 2012;4(3):279–82. https://doi.org/10.4300/JGME-D-12-00156.1.
2. Becker LE. Effect size calculator. University of Colorado, Colorado Springs. 1999. https://www.uccs.edu/lbecker/. Accessed 7 Mar 2022.
3. Lenhard W, Lenhard A. Computation of effect sizes. Psychometrica. 2016. https://www.psychometrica.de/effect_size.html. Accessed 7 Mar 2022.
4. Nisbett RE, Fong GF, Lehman DR, Cheng PW. Teaching reasoning. Science. 1987;238:625–31. https://doi.org/10.1126/science.3672116.
5. Laplanche A, Com-Nougue C, Flamant, R. Méthodes statistiques appliqués a la recherché clinique. 1st ed. Paris: Médecines-Sciences Flammarion;1987. http://bdsp-ehesp.inist.fr/vibad/index.php?action=getRecordDetail&idt=52329.
6. Pocock SJ. Clinical trials: a practical approach. Chichester, New York: John Wiley & Sons;1983. https://doi.org/10.1002/bimj.4710270604.
7. O'Brien PC, Fleming TR. A multiple testing procedure for clinical trials. Biometrics. 1979;35(3):549–56. https://doi.org/10.2307/2530245.
8. Haybittle JL. Repeated assessment of results in clinical trials of cancer treatment. Br J Radiol. 1971;44(526):793–7. https://doi.org/10.1259/0007-1285-44-526-793.
9. Peto R, Pike MC, Armitage P, Breslow NE, Cox DR, Howard SV, Mantel N, McPherson K, Peto J, Smith PG. Design and analysis of randomized clinical trials requiring prolonged observation of each patient. I. Introduction and design. Br J Cancer. 1976; 34 (6):585–612. https://doi.org/10.1038/bjc.1977.1.
10. Frequentist methods: O'Brien-Fleming, Pocock, Haybittle-Peto. Design and analysis of clinical trials. Penn State Eberly college of science. 2022. https://online.stat.psu.edu/stat509/lesson/9/9.5. Accessed 2 Feb 2022.
11. Rollin B. Inferences for proportions: comparing two independent samples. In: Department of statistics. Faculty of Science, The University of British Columbia. https://www.stat.ubc.ca/~rollin/stats/ssize/. Accessed 2 Feb 2022.
12. Lehr R. Sixteen S-squared over D-squared: a relation for crude sample size estimates. Stat Med. 1992;11: 1099–102. https://doi.org/10.1002/sim.4780110811.
13. Schwartz, D. Méthodes statistiques a l'usage des médecins et des biologists, 3rd ed. Paris: Médecines-Sciences Flammarion;1969. http://bdsp-ehesp.inist.fr/vibad/index.php?action=getRecordDetail&idt=85872
14. Kirk RE. Experimental design volume 2. Research methods in psychology. Handbook in psychology, second ed. Wiley Online library;2012. https://doi.org/10.1002/9781118133880.hop202001. Accessed 7 Mar 2022.
15. Rollin B. Inferences for means: comparing two independent samples. Department of statistics,

Faculty of Science, The University of British Columbia. https://www.stat.ubc.ca/~rollin/stats/ssize/n2.html. Accessed 7 Mar 2022.

16. Sergeant, ESG. Epitools Epidemiological Calculators. Ausvet. https://epitools.ausvet.com.au/samplesize?page=SampleSize (2018). Accessed 7 Mar 2022.

17. HyLown Consulting LLC, Atlanta, GA. Overview of power and sample size.com calculators. 2013–2021. http://powerandsamplesize.com/Calculators/. Accessed Mar 2022.

18. Kohn MA, Senyak J. Sample size calculators [website]. UCSF CTSI, 20 Dec 2021. https://www.sample-size.net/. Accessed 07 Mar 2022.

19. Faul F, Erdfelder E, Lang A-G, Buchner A. G*Power 3: a flexible statistical power analysis program for the social, behavioral, and biomedical sciences. Behav Res Methods. 2007;39:175–91. https://doi.org/10.3758/bf03193146.

20. Faul F, Erdfelder E, Buchner A, Lang A-G. Statistical power analyses using G*Power 3.1: tests for correlation and regression analyses. Behav Res Methods. 2009;41:1149–60. https://doi.org/10.3758/BRM.41.4.1149.

21. Faul F, Erdfelder E, Lang A-G, Buchner A. G*power 3.1.9.3. Statistical power analysis for MAC and Windows. Heinrich Heine Dusseldorf University. 2009. https://www.psychologie.hhu.de/arbeitsgruppen/allgemeine-psychologie-und-arbeitspsychologie/gpower.html. Accessed Mar 2022.

22. Stat tools: sample size for differences in measurements between unpaired groups tables. The Chinese University of Hong Kong. 2017. http://www.obg.cuhk.edu.hk/ResearchSupport/StatTools/SSizUnpairedDiff_Tab.php. Accessed 7 Mar 2022.

23. Florey Ch. Sample size for beginners. BMJ. 1993; 306:1181–4. https://doi.org/10.1136/bmj.306.6886.1181.

24. Campbell MJ, Julious SD, Altman G. Estimating sample sizes for binary, ordered categorical, and continuous outcomes in two group comparisons. BMJ. 1995;311:1145. https://doi.org/10.1136/bmj.311.7013.1145.

25. Chow S-C, Wang H, Shao J. Sample size calculation in clinical research. Chapman and Hall CRC biostatistics series. Sample size calculations in clinical research, 2nd ed. Boca Raton, FL: Taylor & Francis Group;2008. https://doi.org/10.1201/9781584889830.

26. Hedges L, Olkin I. Statistical methods for meta-analysis. 1st ed. New York: Academic; 1985.

27. McGraw KO, Wong SP. A common language effect size statistic. Psychol Bull 1992; 111:361–5. https://doi.org/10.1037/0033-2909.111.2.361.

28. Grissom RJ, Kim JJ. Effect size for research: univariate and multivariate applications, 2nd ed. New York, NY: Routledge;2012. https://doi.org/10.4324/9780203803233.

29. Al-Sunduqchi MS. Statistics. Ph.D. dissertation under the direction of William C. Guenther, Dept. of Statistics, University of Wyoming, Laramie, Wyoming. 1990.

30. Georgiev GZ. Arcsin Calculator. Giga calculator. 2017–2022. https://www.gigacalculator.com/calculators/arcsin-calculator.php. Accessed 07 Mar 2022.

31. Altman DG. Practical statistics for medical research, 1st ed. New York. Chapman and Hall/CRC;1990. https://doi.org/10.1201/9780429258589.

32. MedCalc software Lt. SciStat.com online. 2021. https://www.scistat.com. Accessed 9 Oct 2021.

33. Bland JM, Altman DG. Statistics notes: the odds ratio. BMJ. 2000;320:1468. https://doi.org/10.1136/bmj.320.7247.1468.

34. Altman DG, Deeks JJ. Odds ratios should be avoided when events are common. BMJ. 1998; 317:1318. https://doi.org/10.1136/bmj.317.7168.1318.

35. Altman DG. Confidence intervals for the number needed to treat. BMJ. 1998;317:1309–12. https://doi.org/10.1136/bmj.317.7168.1309.

36. Kerry MS, Bland JM. Sample size in cluster randomization. BMJ. 1998;316:549. https://doi.org/10.1136/bmj.316.7130.549.

37. Hansheng W, Shein-Chung C, Gang L. On sample size calculation based on odds ratio in clinical trials. J Biopharm Stat. 2002; 12:471–83. https://doi.org/10.1081/bip-120016231.

38. Glaziou P. Sampsize project. Source Forge 2005. http://sampsize.sourceforge.net/iface/s1.html#comp. Accessed 8 March 2022.

39. Cohen J. Statistical power analysis for the behavioral sciences, 2nd ed. Hillsdale, NJ: Lawrence Erlbaum Associates Publishers;1988. https://doi.org/10.4324/9780203771587.

40. Greenland S. Modern epidemiology. 2nd ed. Philadelphia, PA: Lippincott Williams & Wilkins; 1998.

41. Machin D, Campbell M, Fayers P, Pinol A. Sample size tables for clinical studies, 2nd ed. Malden, MA: Blackwell Science;1997.

42. Schork M, Williams G. Number of observations required for the comparison of two correlated proportions. Commun Stat-Simul Comput.1980; B9(4):349–57. https://doi.org/10.1080/03610918008812161.

43. Connor RJ. Sample size for testing differences in proportions for the paired-sample design. Biometrics. 1987;43(1):207–11. https://doi.org/10.2307/2531961.

44. Fisher RA. Frequency distribution of the values of the correlation coefficient in samples of an indefinitely large population. Biometrika. 1915;10(4):507–21. https://doi.org/10.2307/2331838.

45. Fieller EC, Hartley HO, Pearson ES. Tests for rank correlation coefficients. Biometrika. 1957; 44:470–81. https://doi.org/10.2307/2332878.

46. May JO, Looney SW. Sample size charts for Spearman and Kendall coefficients. J Biom Biost 2020; 11:2. https://doi.org/10.37421/2155-6180.2020.11.440.

47. Dupont W, Plummer WD. Power and sample size calculations for studies involving linear regression. Control Clin Trials. 1998;19:589–601. https://doi.org/10.1016/S0197-2456(98)00037-3.

48. Sample size calculator: simple linear regression. Center of clinical research and biostatistics. The Chinese University of Hong Kong. 2017. https://www2.ccrb.cuhk.edu.hk/stat/epistudies/reg1.htm. Accessed 8 March 2022.

49. Altmann DG, Bland JM. Statistics notes: time to event (survival) data. BMJ. 1998;317:468–9. https://doi.org/10.1136/bmj.317.7156.468.

50. Lachin J. Introduction to sample size calculation and power analysis for *clinical* trials. Control Clin Trials. 1981;2:93–113. https://doi.org/10.1016/0197-2456(81)90001-5.

51. Schoenfeld DA. Sample-size formula for the proportional-hazards regression model. Biometrics. 1983;39:499–503. https://doi.org/10.2307/2531021.

52. Lachin J, Foulkes M. Evaluation of sample size and power analysis of survival with allowance for nonuniform patient entry, losses to follow-up, noncompliance and stratification. Biometrics. 1986;42:507–16. https://doi.org/10.2307/2531201.

53. Pocock SJ. Group sequential methods in the design and analysis of clinical trials. Biometrika. 1977;64 (2):191–9. https://doi.org/10.1093/biomet/64.2.191.

54. Hsieh FY, Lavori PW. Sample-size calculations for the Cox proportional hazards regression model with nonbinary covariates. Control Clin Trials. 2000; 21 (6):552–60. https://doi.org/10.1016/S0197-2456(00)00104-5.

55. Schoenfeld DA. Find statistical considerations for a study where the outcome is a time to failure. Dschoenfeld@parteners.org. 2001. http://hedwig.mgh.harvard.edu/sample_size/time_to_event/para_time.html. Accessed 8 Mar 2022.

56. Hsieh FY, Bloch DA, Larsen MD. A simple method of sample size calculation for linear and logistic regression. Stat Med. 1998;17(14):1623–34. https://doi.org/10.1002/(SICI)1097-0258(19980730)17:14%3C1623::AID-SIM871%3E3.0.CO;2-S.

57. Demidenko E. Sample size determination for logistic regression revisited. Stat Med. 2007;26:3385–97. https://doi.org/10.1002/sim.2771.

58. Lyles RH, Lin HM, Williamson JM. A practical approach to computing power for generalized linear models with nominal, count, or ordinal responses. Stat Med. 2007;26:1632–48. https://doi.org/10.1002/sim.2617.

59. Sampson AR. A tale of two regressions. Am Stat Assoc. 1974;69:682–9.

60. Gatsonis C, Sampson AR. Multiple correlation: exact power and sample size calculations. Psychol Bull. 1989;106:516–24. https://doi.org/10.1037/0033-2909.106.3.516.

61. Vickers AJ. How many repeated measures in repeated measures designs? Statistical issues for comparative trials. BMC Med Res Methodol. 2003;3:22. https://doi.org/10.1186/1471-2288-3-22.

62. Borm GF, Fransen J, Lemmens AJG. A simple sample size formula for analysis of covariance in randomized clinical trials. J Clin Epidemiol. 2007;60:1234–8. https://doi.org/10.1016/j.jclinepi.2007.02.006.

63. Keppel G, Wickens TD. Design and analysis: a researcher's handbook, 4th ed. Upper Saddle River, NJ: Pearson Prentice Hall;2004.

64. Girden ER. ANOVA: repeated measures. Newbury Park, CA: Sage;1992. https://doi.org/10.4135/9781412983419.

65. Lee PM. Statistical tables. Q tables of Friedman's test. The University of York. 2005. https://www.york.ac.uk/depts/maths/tables/friedman.pdf. Accessed 13 Nov 2021.

66. Power calculators. Sealed envelope Ltd. 2018. https://www.sealedenvelope.com/power/. Accessed 19 Feb 2022.

67. Bachmann LM, Puhan MA, Gerben R, Bossuyt PM. Sample size of studies on diagnostic accuracy: literature survey. BMJ. 2006;332:1127–9. https://doi.org/10.1136/bmj.38793.637789.2F.

68. Buderer NMF. Statistical methodology: I. Incorporating the prevalence of disease into the sample size calculation for sensitivity and specificity. AEM. 1996; 3(9):895–900. https://doi.org/10.1111/j.1553-2712.1996.tb03538.x.

69. Tilaki KH. Methodological review. Sample size estimation in diagnostic test studies of biomedical informatics. J Biomed Inform. 2014; 48:193–204. https://doi.org/10.1016/j.jbi.2014.02.013.

70. Arifin WN. Introduction to sample size calculation. Edu Med J. 2013;5(2):e89–96. https://doi.org/10.5959/eimj.v5i2.130.

71. Arifin WN. Sample size calculator (web). 2022. https://wnarifin.github.io/ssc/ss1prop.html. Accessed 8 March 2022.

72. Sample size calculator for comparing paired proportions. Statulator 2014. University Saint Malaysia. https://statulator.com/SampleSize/ss2PP.html. Accessed 8 March 2022.

73. Obuchowski NA. Sample size calculation in studies of test accuracy. Stat Methods Med Res. 1998; 7:371–92. https://doi.org/10.1177/096228029800700405.

74. Table 5. Normal distribution-inverse cumulative distribution function. Statistical tables for students. Bar-Ilan University. https://faculty.biu.ac.il/~shnaidh/zooloo/library/normal.3.pdf. Accessed 8 Mar 2022.

75. StataCorp. Stata statistical software: release 16. College Station, TX: StataCorp LLC;2019.

76. Obuchowski NA. Sample size tables for receiver operating characteristic studies. AJR. 2000; 175:603–8. https://doi.org/10.2214/ajr.175.3.1750603.

77. Fisher RA. Statistical methods for research workers. Edinburgh: Oliver and Boyd;1954. https://doi.org/10.1002/qj.49708235130.

78. Morgan CJ, Aban I. Methods for evaluating agreement between diagnostic tests. J Nucl Cardiol. 2016; 23:511–3. https://doi.org/10.1007/s12350-015-0175-7.

79. Bonett DG. Sample size requirements for testing and estimating coefficient alpha. J Educ Behav Stat. 2002; 27(4):335–40. https://doi.org/10.3102/107699860 27004335.

80. Temel G, Erdogan S. Determining the sample size in agreement studies. Marmara Med J. 2017; 30:101–12. https://doi.org/10.5472/marumj.344822.

81. Shrout PE, Fleiss JL. Intraclass correlations: uses in assessing rater reliability. Psychol Bull. 1978; 86:420–8. https://psycnet.apa.org/doi/10.1037/0033-2909.86.2.420.

82. Walter SD, Eliasziw M, Donner A. Sample size and optimal designs for reliability studies. Stat Med. 1998; 17(1):101–10. https://doi.org/10.1002/(SICI) 1097-0258(19980115)17:1%3C101::AID-SIM727% 3E3.0.CO;2-E.

83. Winer BJ, Brown DR, Michels KM. Statistical principles in experimental design, 3rd ed. New York: McGraw-Hill;1991.

84. Sample size calculator. Raosoft. 2004. http://www.raosoft.com/samplesize.html. Accessed 8 Mar 2022.

Abstract

A detailed protocol design is far beyond the scope of this book, even for our primary concern: the generic comparative clinical study. The reader can refer to numerous sources for protocol guidelines of much better quality and more complete documentation [1–6]. This chapter will only review the essential items of the protocol focusing on the statistical methods necessary to design the study and analyze the results. We aim to help the reader implement the basic statistical knowledge provided in the first four chapters to improve his research protocol.

Keywords

Study designs · Primary endpoints · Randomization · Stratification · Blinding · Analysis population

5.1 Background and Rationale

The researcher must satisfy several factors to upgrade a research idea to become a research question. The idea must be novel, whether to confirm or refuse previous findings or provide new results. The research question is formulated after completing the bibliographic review of the subject. Its value is mainly dependent upon the existing body of evidence, the comparison of benefits and harms, and the scientific and ethical justification of the study. The background section should include the results of previous studies and clarify the gap of knowledge required to be bridged. The researcher has to provide references to back up his arguments and support his expectations.

5.2 Objectives

A single reachable aim is always better than multiple ones, which can pose difficulties in conditioning the study, contradictions in the analysis, and false interpretations. The researcher must be satisfied by one primary objective, such as the incidence of stroke, and not include a co-primary goal, even if it seems related, such as mortality. No treatment is one-hundred percent effective nor safe, and hence, which medicine should he recommend if one of the compared treatments showed higher mortality while the other showed a higher rate of stroke? Choosing between both conditions is hard for the physician and the patient. We must be satisfied with one main objective. As many as we wish to demonstrate, we can have multiple secondary purposes.

Another solution is to group clinically related objectives into composite outcome, usually, a score, which we can compare among the patients' groups. An example is the MACE score (Major adverse cardiac events), which combines myocardial infarction, coronary revascularization, stroke, need for hospitalization, and cardiac mortality into a single score [7]. As such, the score is a single variable reflecting the deterioration of the patient due to his heart condition. Only after the score shows a statistically significant difference among patient groups can we safely investigate the significant effect of each component. We have to be careful when dealing with the secondary subgroups or post-hoc analysis. Unless properly managed, those procedures inflate the risk of error and may lead to false interpretations. The reader is requested to refer to Sect. 4.1.4 to appreciate study related factors.

5.3   Study Design

Any study has to be properly designed to permit adequate analysis. In case the researcher or the reviewers are unsatisfied by the results of the analysis, the researcher can easily repeat it as long as the study design permits. On the other hand, the design is permanent. *A poor design has no remedy*. Most of the studies involves one or more input variables, output variables and covariates. The former are supposed to have an effect on the latter, while covariates are analyzed for their ability to modify this effect. Input variables can be the given treatments or the compared procedures. The output variable is usually an event or a time-to-event, such as cure, hospital discharge, or mortality. It can be also a quantitative variable such improvement of systolic pressure, blood sugar, or duration of hospital or ICU stay. Covariates are the risk factors that can improve or worsen the outcome variable, such as the age of the patient, his gender, and the associated disease.

A prospective study follows the patients from the input till the occurrence of the outcome, while retrospective studies take the reverse route. Although being costly, prospective studies are much more informative than the latter because the researcher has all the time to prepare for his study in advance. On the other hand, *retrospective studies are handier but suffer from many inherent points of weakness* such as missing data that cannot be retrieved, unequal study groups and lack of initial comparability [8–12]. The main bulk of the literature is made by those outlined variants and many more. However, the summit of the evidence is the prospective controlled randomized clinical trial, and the most standard type is the parallel-group, two-arm superiority trial with a 1:1 allocation ratio.

5.3.1   The Formulation of the Study

The researcher has to define whether the study will be unilateral or bilateral. A unilateral study is a one-way trial aiming to demonstrate the effectiveness of a treatment as compared to a placebo, the importance of a risk factor, or else. The bilateral study aims to demonstrate whether the difference is in favor of either treatment modalities or methods of investigation. The reader is requested to revise the role of the study direction in testing the hypothesis (see Sects. 1.7.2 and 1.7.3) and in sample size calculation (see Sects. 4.1.3 and 4.1.5).

5.3.2   Number of Study Groups and Number of Effectuated Comparisons

The researcher must define whether the study will be conducted on two or more patient groups. In the case of multiple groups, a statistically significant ANOVA or Chi-square test does not mean that every two groups are significantly different from one another. The researcher needs to add a post-hoc analysis. We have previously shown that *the number of comparisons, rather than the number of groups per se, is behind the subsequent inflation of the primary risk of error*. The researcher has to keep the number of comparisons to the minimum required and adjust the primary risk of error accordingly (see Sect. 2.4.3.3).

5.3.3 The Classic Parallel Groups Versus Other Designs

Although many trials have a parallel-group design in which treatment and control are allocated to different individuals, a *matched design* reduces variability by allocating the compared treatments between matched pairs. The latter can be different individuals matched for the same study-related risk factors, such as age and gender, and relevant associated diseases. It can also indicate paired body parts, such as ears or arms, where the same patient receives one treatment (e.g., one type of lotion) on each side (e.g., each arm). The patient can act as his own control if he receives the two compared treatments *sequentially*, with a suitable washout period in between so that the effect of the first order treatment does not influence the second order treatment.

A *cross-over design* can be achieved by randomizing the patients into two groups. One group can receive treatment A first, then treatment B (Group AB), while the second group receives treatment B first, then treatment A (Group BA). Each patient acts as his control, reducing variability and sample size. However, extreme caution has to be taken in calculating the washout period between the two treatments. During the analysis, the researcher has to ensure the absence of a statistically significant difference between the results of group AB and group BA. Otherwise, he has to discard the results of all second-order treatments, whether treatment A or B. Instead of empowering the study, a poorly studied washout period can result in a major loss of power and hence, the inability of the study to put into evidence a treatment effect [10, 13].

The reader is requested to review special sections related to the paired design of qualitative data (see Sect. 2.3.2), normally distributed quantitative data (see Sect. 2.4.1.3), and data following other distributions than normal (see Sect. 2.5.1.3). He is equally requested to revise which test to choose (see Sect. 2.8.3) and calculate the relevant sample size (see Sect. 4.5).

5.3.4 Design Framework: Superiority, Non-inferiority, Equivalence or Pilot Study

Unlike the classic superiority clinical study, a non-inferiority study aims to prove that a new treatment is "no more worse" than the classic treatment by a small acceptable non-inferiority margin ($<\delta$). On the other hand, an equivalent study aims to prove that the difference between both: new treatment (T) and reference treatment (R) is "no more worse" than ($<\delta$) in favor of either treatment. Being a non-inferiority or an equivalence study has to be shown in the title and included in the abstract. The reader is invited to refer to Sect. 1.4.2.8 to interpret their confidence intervals and to Sect. 4.13 for correct sample size calculation. On the other hand, in the absence of literature resources, a pilot study is mended to gather preliminary information on a new subject before launching a full-scale clinical study.

5.3.5 Allocation Ratio

A balanced design (1:1 ratio) is much more powerful than unequal allocation ratios. The more the design is unbalanced, the more we have to increase the total number of patients in the study. The unequal allocation may be needed for many reasons, such as a costly or unavailable treatment or ethical concerns if one of the treatments is potentially more harmful than the other treatment. The reader is invited to refer to "Eq. 4.20" to calculate the sample size in each group according to the (K) ratio between both groups (see Sect. 4.2.2.1).

5.4 Methods

5.4.1 Study Endpoints

The study endpoints, also called study outcomes or the judgment criteria of the study results. An ideal outcome should be "valid, reproducible, relevant to the target population, and responsive to changes in the studied health condition" [12]. Statistically, an outcome has to be computable so as to calculate an average value, a standard error, and create a confidence interval. The latter permits the identification of the corresponding values in the population of concern to compare our results with others and extrapolate our findings to future patients; which are the descriptive, comparative and predictive values of the interval of confidence (see Sects. 1.4.2 and 7.1.2.8).

Outcomes can measure benefit or harm and can generally be divided into primary and secondary outcomes. *We have to note when, how and by whom each outcome will be harvested and analyzed* [8]. For example, in a study comparing the efficacy of two anti-rejection regimens after cardiac transplantation, a cardiac muscle biopsy was routinely performed 15 days after transplantation and then every two months for the first year. Biopsy was also indicated whenever clinical signs of rejection (the latter have to be clearly defined). Biopsy was planned to be performed by a single cardiologist (who ignores the specific type of regimen followed by the patient) in the operating theater and under strict aseptic conditions (that must also be described). The type of biopsy catheter, the size and number of punches, and the method of handling the specimen must be specified. The latter should be sent to the pathology laboratory within a definite period. The process of specimen examination should be detailed, and the doctor responsible for the trial must receive the results within a defined time. Supplementary anti-rejection drugs must be named and defined, whether to be given in case of clinical suspicion or to wait till receiving the laboratory results and for how long.

5.4.1.1 Primary Outcome

The primary outcome incarnates the aim of the study. It is the one upon which we calculate the sample size before the beginning of the study and the one upon which we conclude by its end. It is advisable to have *a single primary outcome* rather than more than one to prevent confusion whenever one outcome favors the first treatment and, in contrast, the other favors the second one.

Another alternative is to define a set of clinically related outcomes; expressed in a single numerical score. Those *composite outcomes* are criticized when the individual components have significantly different event rates or clinical weights, whether for the patient or the clinician (see Sect. 5.2).

Choosing the primary outcome is extremely important and has to be discussed on the clinical as well as the statistical level. We have previously shown that variability is the principal adversary in achieving statistical significance. Hence, we have to *pick up the primary outcome with the smallest variability*. The inherent variability of a qualitative outcome can be enormous, and, unfortunately, it is usually hidden from the lay physician. As a rule of thumb, a single continuous primary outcome with a small variability (standard deviation) can have the highest chance of achieving statistical significance compared to outcomes of different scales. *The clinician must have decent basic statistical knowledge to "sculpt" his primary outcome to "achieve" a statistically significant result* (see Sect. 7.1.2). Otherwise, he should seek the help of a professional statistician.

5.4.1.2 Secondary Outcomes

All other outcomes are considered as being secondary. They are usually not considered during a sample size calculation, and *their results are always seen as being just observational, even in prospective randomized controlled studies*. However, they merit the same attention from the researcher: when chosen, as harvested, and during the analysis. We have to remember that *reliable secondary outcomes are the solid foundation of future studies*.

5.4.2 Assignment of Interventions

5.4.2.1 Allocation Sequence Generation: Randomization

In order to evaluate a particular treatment effect, the studied groups of patients have to be initially comparable before the beginning of the study so that the difference in the results collected after the study can be attributed to the evaluated treatment modality. However, strict initial comparability among the studied groups is theoretically impossible due to individual variability. Consequently, it is always advisable to randomize patients and, hence, confining to hazard their fair distribution among the compared groups. *Hazard has no benefit in selecting straightforward patients to drug therapy and leaving complex cases to surgeons; internists do have such a benefit.* By doing so, results may conclude that surgery is more hazardous to patients, while the truth was that the two groups were non-comparable from the start and hence, could not be compared at the end.

A question arises: does hazard (randomization) distribute the patients into comparable groups? The answer is not always but most probably, as demonstrated by the following example. Suppose we ask a blind man to pick up, twice, ten balls (representing the two groups of patients) from a basket containing 500 red balls and 500 white balls (representing the population from which our studied patients originate). Although the chance to pick up five red balls and five white balls at both times (i.e., two strictly comparable groups of patients) is low, getting only red balls or only white balls is much lower. His chance to get, in each group, a number of red balls or white balls around five is the most probable. Hence, by randomization (the effect of hazard or the blind picking up of ball samples), we have the highest probability of constituting comparable groups of patients before the beginning of the study, which will only differ later on, after the study, by the effect of the studied variable. One must note that the more balls he picks up each time—e.g., 20 or 30 balls instead of 10 balls—the more chance he has to have at the end more proportionate red and white balls, which is an additional point of strength in including more patients in the study [8]. Remember the example of baby boys and baby girls given in the previous chapter (see Sect. 4.1.2.2).

One has to mention that although we have used the word hazard to explain the randomization, it does not mean haphazard. *Randomization* *means that each patient has an equally fair chance to be allocated to any treatment group* and only hazard who decides which patient will be allocated to a particular group.

Another critical reason for randomizing, is the credibility of the statistical analysis. All statistical tests assume that compared groups are created at random; hence, *the absence of randomization questions the validity of the results of statistical tests.* Unfortunately, many among us do not appreciate this fundamental concept.

Simple Randomization

It is like tossing a coin in case of two treatments. Random numbers can be generated by a computer and are displayed in freely available tables and multiple internet resources [8, 14]. Each column of a randomization table includes the same series of numbers; e.g., from 1 to 9. However, the numbers are arranged randomly in each column. Hence, the sequence of numbers differs from one column to the other. Table 5.1 is an example of a randomization table, where a series of numbers (from 1 to 9) are arranged haphazardly. The randomization process starts by picking any number in one of the columns and proceeding downwards till the bottom of the column. We then shift to the head of the following column and proceed as before, until every patient is assigned one number. As numbers are randomly distributed, patients will be randomized too.

Suppose we want to compare the incidence of thromboembolic events associated with three anticoagulation regimens: A, B, and C. We wish to equally randomize 18 patients with mechanical cardiac valves between the three treatment groups. As we would like to form 3 equal groups of patients (A, B, and C), we will divide the numbers (1–9) equally between the three groups and assign any three numbers to each group. The numbers assigned must be chosen independently from their sequence in the randomization table (the hazard play). Hence, we have to assign the numbers before looking at the table [8]. In our example, we have chosen the numbers 1, 2, and 3 to group A patients, 4, 5, and 6 to group B and the numbers 7, 8, and 9 to group C patients.

Table 5.1 Randomization table (9 elements)

5[a]	5	6	7	1	4	3	8	3	6
4	1	2	8	2	7	1	9	2	8
9	3	3	2	9	8	8	2	6	1
7	9	7	4	3	5	5	1	5	3
1	6	9	6	5	6	9	4	9	2
6	4	4	3	6	2	4	7	1	4
8	7	8	1	7	1	2	3	8	9
3	2	1	9	4	3	6	6	7	7
2	8	5	5	8	9	7	5	4	5

The table shows the numbers from 1 to 9, randomly arranged in each column. [a]= the first number to begin with, chosen haphazardly. We proceed in the column from top to bottom then we shift to the top of the following column and proceed as before. We stop when every patient has been assigned to a number. As numbers are arranged randomly, patients will be randomized too.

Then, we look at the table and haphazardly choose any number, to begin with (at the site of * in our example). We note the sequence of the following 18 numbers in a downwards direction (going downwards along the same column). Once a column has been used, we move to the next column to the right, and so on. The sequence of numbers in the first column is 5, 4, 9, 7, 1, 6, 8, 3, and 2. We continue by moving to following column on our right side: 5, 1, 3, 9, 6, 4, 7, 2, and 8. As such, we have chosen the sequence of our 18 cases. If we had more patients to randomize, we would continue by the next column to the right and so on until all patients are randomized. Returning to our example, the sequence of random numbers (5, 4, 9, 7, 1, 6, 8, 3, 2, 5, 1, 3, 9, 6, 4, 7, 2, and 8) is equal to a randomization sequence list of B, B, C, C, A, B, C, A, A, B, A, A, C, B, B, C, A, and C.

Hence, in recruiting the patients for the study, the first patient will be confined to group B, the second to group B, the third to group C, the fourth to group C, the fifth to group A, and so on. If we need to form only two groups of patients (A and B), one can omit any number among the nine numbers of the randomization table, let us say the number 9. Then assign the numbers 1, 2, 3, and 4 to group A; the numbers 5, 6, 7, and 8 to group B. Then, we proceed as before, without considering the number 9 in the table as if it does not exist. The sequence of numbers will be: 5, 4, 7, 1, 6, 8, 3, 2, 5, 1, 3, 6, 4, 7, 2, and 8; and the randomization list will be B, A, B, A, B, B, A, A, B, A, A, B, A, B, A, and B. On the other hand, sometimes, we may need to randomize patients in a 2:1, 3:1, or any other ratio. For example, if we need to randomize two groups of patients (A and B) while having twice as many patients in one group (e.g., group A) as the other, we can assign the numbers 1, 2, 3, 4, 5, and 6 to group A and the numbers 7, 8, and 9 to group B [8].

Blocked Randomization

Simple randomization has the disadvantage of creating unequal trial arms sizes. Hence, blocked randomization was suggested to ensure such balance, at the least. Blocks are small and balanced with predetermined group assignments. The block size must be multiple of the number of groups; e.g., with two treatment groups, block size of either 4, 6, or 8. After block size has been determined, all possible balanced combinations of assignment within the block are calculated; e.g., AABB, ABAB, ABBA, etc... The researcher (or the computer software) will randomly choose one of those sequences to assign four subsequent patients to the treatment groups. In our example, the maximum imbalance we can get is two patients per group; e.g., AABB or BBAA.

However, balance improvement comes with the cost of reducing the unpredictability of the sequence. A person running the trial and knowing the block size can deduce the next allocation.

For example, if we used a block of (4), the group of the fourth patient can always be deducted after knowing the groups of the first three patients in the block. A remedy is to choose different blocks (e.g., a block of 4 and a block of 6) and then randomly choose the sequence of using either block. Hence, the observer cannot guess which is the following sequence because he does not know which block (4 or 6) is actually in use.

Another disadvantage of blocked randomization is its inability to balance the baseline characteristics, especially in small trials [14, 15]. Consequently, it cannot ensure the equal distribution of important covariates that can influence the primary outcome (prognostic variables) across the treatment groups, which opens the door for stratified randomization. Block randomization can be efficiently executed online by numerous software [16, 17].

Stratified Randomization

Stratification is considering (neutralizing) a prognostic factor during randomization. Recalling the example of comparing the prophylactic effect of three oral anticoagulation regimens, A, B, and C, in preventing thromboembolic complications shown in Table 2.3 (see Sect. 2.3.1.2). It is well known that monoleaflet prosthetic cardiac valves have higher thromboembolic rates than bileaflet valves. Suppose during randomization, valve type was not considered. In that case, it can easily happen that monoleaflet valves concentrate in one group and causes more thromboembolic events, which will be wrongly attributed to the received anticoagulation regimen and thus, biasing the study's result.

The solution is to separate patients with monoleaflet valves from patients with bileaflet valves before randomization, i.e., to form two separate randomization lists, instead of one. Each list is then randomized between the three treatment groups, hence ensuring that a comparable number of each valve type is randomized between the three treatment groups, neutralizing the effect of the risk factor. Whenever a trial is multi-center, it is advisable to stratify on the factor center to minimize center-related bias. Other stratification factors include diabetes, smoking, obesity,

hypertension, or any other factor that is suspected to affect the studied disease.

Another advantage of stratification is that it clarifies during the analysis the prognostic role of the stratification variable on the results. The researcher can analyze the individual effect of those factors and tests their statistical significance (see Sect. 2.9). For example, the analysis can show that monoleaflet valves may need a different anticoagulation therapy than bileaflet valves.

Disadvantages of stratification include over stratification, the creation of many subgroups, and imbalances due to incomplete blocks. In other words, stratification can be a source of bias by creating too small groups for randomization. Remember that stratification means that we have multiple small lists instead of having one large randomization list. By default, each of the former is less representative of the population than the larger (mother) list, just for being smaller. Hence, it is usually advisable to stratify on a limited number of factors, one or two. Moreover, the assignment can be predicted if nonvarying, small blocks are used, especially when blinding is not feasible [14, 15].

Covariate Adaptive Randomization: Minimization

Minimization aims to ensure balance in the trial arms by balancing important baseline characteristics that are potential outcome predictors, i.e., covariates. The first participant is randomized, and then for each subsequent participant, the treatment is allocated to minimize the imbalance in the selected factors between groups at that time is identified. Once the balance is achieved, we can go back and randomize patients. Minimization can also be described as dynamic randomization and is a valid alternative to ordinary randomization. It has the advantage, especially in small trials, that there will be only minor differences between groups in those variables used in the allocation process. However, the procedure may be complex, especially when several predictors are considered, and is best performed with the aid of software [18]. Another disadvantage is that we are only interfering in the known risk factors and not the rest, for being unknown, of course.

5.4.2.2 Allocation Concealment and Implementation

The implementation of the allocation sequence necessitates the concealment of that sequence until implemented. Put it this way; it aims to prevent participants, recruiters, and all personnel involved in the study from knowing or correctly guessing the group of the next participant until it is done. It is sometimes confused with blinding, which means that either the patient, the investigator or both do not know the treatment that has been allocated [19].

The protocol should describe the mechanism of concealment, such as centralized assignment or locally, by using sealed envelope that have to be opaque and numbered sequentially. The trial has to designate the personnel responsible for generating randomization, enrolling participants, and assigning participants to intervention. Every effort should be made to separate the personnel involved in assigning a particular patient to one group and from those implementing such an assignment [8].

5.4.3 Blinding (Masking)

Unfortunately, the comparability of the studied groups does not end with successful randomization. The latter only may provide the initial comparability of the study groups. Comparability, however, should be maintained throughout the study. Whenever a drug is compared to a placebo and patients receiving the latter become informed, they will stop using this (false) treatment. A simple blind study in which the patient ignores the nature of his treatment can solve the problem.

On the other hand, a physician can assign to a particular patient (who appears to him as being severely ill) the treatment he believes in, instead of the newly tested treatment. This will bias the initial comparability and, consequently, the study's results. A double-blind study, in which both patients and doctors ignore the treatment type, is a better guarantee for the maintenance of comparability. The condition becomes more complicated whenever the outcome is highly subjective to the observer's opinion, experience, and mode of preference for a particular type of treatment, such as radiological pictures and the shape of a residual scar. Blind evaluation of the judgment criteria (outcome), in which the physician evaluating the result ignores the type of treatment given to the patient, ensures comparability maintenance. Blinding can extend to data analysts and manuscript writers. It is better to describe the ways used for achieving blinding and specifying the involved personnel in detail rather than just describing the study by a non-informative term, such as being a single or double-blinded study [20].

5.5 Study Population and Samples

The population from which the patients will be chosen has to be defined; so that the other researchers can extrapolate the result of the study to similar populations. On the other hand, the studied group of patients (the sample) has to be demonstrated by clear criteria that will allow the inclusion or exclusion of a particular patient in the study.

5.5.1 Study Settings

The design has to identify the centers, hospitals, communities, and countries where the study will occur, with specified dates. Identification of the environmental and infrastructural settings may help assess the future applicability of the study results.

5.5.2 Inclusion Criteria

The Patients

Patients' Demographics

The researcher has to clearly define the demographic characteristics of patients, including limits of age, gender, social class, geographical distribution, and any special demographics related to the disease, such as family history in ischemic heart disease and parental consanguinity in congenital malformations.

The Clause of Ambivalence

Each patient has to be fit to receive either treatment, and only hazard (randomization) decides which type of treatment a particular patient will receive. For example, medical and surgical treatments cannot be compared when some of the patients, by definition, are not candidates for surgery, and in others, medical treatment is considered insufficient.

The Informed Consent

The patients have to sign an informed consent if required. The consent has to be well explained to the patients. It has to be written in a language that the patient (or the patient's guardian) can understand. It has to be tested before the study and approved by an independent committee.

The Disease

Clinical Forms of the Disease

The studied clinical form of the disease has to be well defined with references to main literature, society guidelines or other documented resources. An example is type IIb Hodgkin's disease, stage IV chronic ischemia of the lower limbs. Remarkable characteristic clinical findings have to be noted.

Complementary Investigation

The complementary laboratory, radiological or other forms of investigations are essential to remove any doubt about the diagnosis. For example, we cannot include controlled diabetic patients without specifying the exact laboratory limits of controlling blood sugar. Suppose a study was conducted to compare the results of balloon versus surgical dilatation in patients with severe stenosis of the mitral valve. The patients were included in the study after confirming the absence of a left atrial thrombus by a transesophageal echocardiographic examination. The results of this study cannot be extrapolated on comparable patients but examined by transthoracic echocardiography.

Risk Factors and Associated Diseases

The presence or absence of a specific risk factor may change the type of management and the patient's prognosis. For example, the actual knowledge indicates that balloon dilatation and stenting of coronary artery stenosis (PTCA) have a poor prognosis in diabetic patients. On the other hand, the results of surgery in diabetic and non-diabetic cases are comparable. Ignoring this Information can be a major source of bias if the study compares surgery to PTCA.

The presence of an associated disease may equally change the medical decision. For example, moderate aortic insufficiency per se is not a surgical indication. However, if a patient with moderate aortic insufficiency is scheduled for coronary artery bypass grafting, the aortic valve must be dealt with during surgery. The impact of such "*prognostic factors*" and the investigations necessary for their diagnosis have to be clearly defined, and all Information has to be reinforced with recent valid references.

5.5.3 Exclusion Criteria

It is insufficient to rely on patients not fulfilling our inclusion criteria to exclude them from the study automatically. The key in preparing scientific research is to plan almost everything, leaving minimal gaps for surprises emerging during the study, the latter being a source of significant bias. On the other hand, *the exclusion criteria are not the reverse of the inclusion criteria.* We cannot indicate that we will include patients operated upon electively and then mention that emergency cases have to be excluded. Such exclusion criterion is just a piece of redundant information.

The exclusion criteria could be defined as those criteria that the patient would have been included in the study if they were not present. For example, we can indicate that we will include diabetic patients, whether insulin-dependent or following oral hypoglycemics. As tested before the study, the exclusion criterion would be diabetic patients with HbA1C above 6%. The meaning is that a particular diabetic patient would have been included if his HbA1C level was below 6%.

The Patients

Patient-related Exclusion Criteria

The researcher must clearly define the demographic characteristics of excluded patients, such as pregnant females, patients with uncontrolled diabetes mellitus, and else. In addition to patients refusing to participate in the study from the start, we have to remove patients refusing to sign the consent. *It is better to exclude hesitant patients and patients who cannot be followed up regularly* for various reasons, such as being non-cooperative, non-intelligent, or coming from distant localities.

The Disease

Clinical   Forms   and   Complementary Investigations

The excluded clinical forms and the investigation necessary for their diagnosis have to be defined in detail.

Risk Factors and Associated Diseases

Associated diseases affecting the course of the studied disease and the investigation necessary for their diagnosis have to be discussed in the protocol. For example, in a study comparing medical versus surgical treatment in stage II ischemia of lower limbs, diabetic patients were excluded due to the poor surgical outcome of such patients. Diabetes mellitus had to be confirmed by defined laboratory figures. If patients were not investigated for diabetes before the study (by ignoring this exclusion criterion in the protocol), a major bias would then occur.

5.5.4   Study Timeline

The researchers have to present a schematic diagram of the study scenario, starting from initial eligibility screening to study closeout. The main corners include the schedule of enrolment, interventions, assessments, participants' visits, and the procedures and assessments performed at

each visit. The researcher is advised to plan carefully his study, to think ahead and to be prepared by a full protocol. He must be well organized and have to keep records, and plan for the study for longer than he thinks and it always does [5, 6, 8].

5.5.5   Follow-Up

The researchers have to survey all patients similarly from the beginning to the end of the study. A standard error is surveying controls or patients receiving a placebo lightly, assuming nothing will happen. The organizer has to arrange the detailed follow-up schedule, including the follow-up place, the timings, the persons in charge, examinations and investigations that must be performed, and data they need to collect [5, 6, 8].

5.5.5.1   Patients Who Become Illegible

We should discuss in detail the solutions for the discovery, after randomization and beginning of the trial, that some of the patients were or became illegible. For example, to discover that a patient was or became diabetic, although people with diabetes were excluded in this particular study. The researcher has to plan whether the patient will be kept or not?

An acceptable solution is to keep those patients as long as their percentage remains small (up to 10%). The reason is that their exclusion disrupts randomization, which is the pillar of initial comparability among groups. However, a higher percentage can raise questions about the extrapolation of results on similar populations, i.e., non-diabetic patients, and hence, the whole study will be in question.

5.5.5.2   Patients' Discontinuation, Withdrawal or Crossing-Over

Patients may not respect the protocol by neglecting their treatment, totally or partially. Moreover, some patients may cross over to another group, i.e., patients randomized in one group but received the treatment of the other group. Those two types of protocol disrespecting must be reported and carefully analyzed concerning their numbers and, most importantly, their distribution among the study groups. *As a general rule, they are accepted as long as they represent no more than 10% of the total sample size and are equally distributed among groups* [8]. A significantly higher rate in one group than the others have to be thoroughly investigated. For example, in a double-blind study, a significantly higher withdrawal (or cross-over) rate among the placebo group may point to the study being unmasked. Hence, patients will discontinue (or change) the "useless" treatment. On the other hand, higher discontinuation among the treatment group may point to more complications or side effects of a newly investigated treatment. *Following the rule of thumb, "once randomized, always analyzed,"* those cases are usually not removed from the study; however, it raises many questions about how they should be analyzed.

A significant source of bias is making the decision case by case, and a general rule has to be detailed in the protocol well before the beginning of the study. The researchers have to decide whether those who discontinued or withdrew from the study should be *counted "as last seen", as "a success", or "a failure".* This decision can be taken regardless of the patient group. The researcher can decide to apply *"the rule of maximum bias"* by counting the patient receiving a placebo (or classic treatment) as a success and the one receiving the (new) treatment as a failure [8]. Equally, the researchers have to decide in advance whether the patients crossing over to another group will be *analyzed as pre-planned (counted in their original group) or according to the received treatment (counted in the actual group)* [8, 10]. Both procedures are explained in the statistical analysis section (see Sect. 5.8.1).

5.5.5.3 Patients Lost to Follow-Up

Patients can be lost to follow-up at different times and for many reasons. Patients may disappear after randomization and just before the beginning of the treatment. Others may receive the treatment but disappear before collecting the outcome. The researchers can adopt one of three alternatives. Exclude them from analysis if their percentage is small (up to 10%) and they are more or less equally distributed among the studied groups. This choice is not recommended in randomized studies because it breaches the randomization process. The second alternative is to consider all these patients a success or a failure, regardless of their study group. Finally, we can apply the rule of maximum bias by choosing the unfavorable side for the new treatment modality, i.e., a failure if they belong to the group receiving the new treatment and success for those belonging to the other group. The last two options are more suitable for randomized studies. The researcher is requested to report the causes and percentages of these problematic cases and the adopted solutions [5, 6, 8].

5.6 Treatments and Interventions

5.6.1 Studied Treatments and Interventions

The intervention in each group should be described in full detail to allow implementation by health care providers, evaluation by systematic reviewers and policymakers, and replication by other researchers. In case of comparing treatments, the protocol has to indicate the generic and manufacturer names and the detailed composition and pharmacokinetics. It has to specify the treatment dose, frequency, and route of administration. Any necessary precaution, such as giving the treatment over a certain period, dilution is a special fluid, and patient's position during administration have to be specified in detail, with complete references. The common complications and side effects have to be listed, and the methods that can be used to prevent and manage them, with references too. All necessary examinations, drugs or investigations that may be needed before, during or after administration of the treatments have to be defined in detail. Placebo and standard care should take the same definition as active treatments.

In case of comparing equipment, the researchers have to provide the full equipment details, including the scientific background, the manufacturer's name, country of origin and serial numbers, precautions before, during, and after its use, the probability of false results, and how they can be avoided. The protocol should include a clear strategy promoting patients' adherence to the intervention and a detailed procedure if a modification of intervention is needed in response to the participant's request or potential harm [5, 6, 8].

5.6.2　Associated Treatments and Interventions

The protocol must indicate the complete list of authorized and non-authorized treatments; a common bias is to focus on the former and neglect the latter. The researchers must address both equally, with complete information regarding the indications, contraindications, doses, administration methods, and substitutes. The researchers must specify the expected complications and side effects and how each can be managed [5, 6, 8].

Associated treatments have to be equally discussed in detail before the study. The researchers must have a vision of which associated treatment could be needed in a specific study [8]. For example, a study comparing two antimitotic agents is expected to focus on the associated use of pain killers and medications used to manage expected complications such as gastrointestinal upset, anemia, and depression. The researchers should also address some commonly used over-the-counter medications. For example, a study was designed to compare the use of two anticoagulants in preventing thromboembolic events in patients with atrial fibrillation. The patients were not allowed to take aspirin in case of simple headache; for being known to increase the probability of anticoagulant-related bleeding. Paracetamol is safe and can be used instead, and it was specifically added to the allowed medication list.

5.7　Data Management

5.7.1　Data Collection and Storage

The protocol has to include the assessment plans, collection, and coding of baseline data and study outcomes. Duplicate hard copies and electronic recordings are recommended and must be planned and tested in advance. Details should include a full description of methods, instruments, involved personnel, collection schedule, and data preservation. The protocol should also include management of cases of non-adherence and non-retention, as well as ways of handling missing data [8].

5.7.2　Data Monitoring and Auditing

Adverse Events

The researchers have to plan for collecting, assessing, recording, reporting, and managing *expected major and minor adverse events.* *Unexpected events* have to be collected and reported separately.

Interim Analysis

An interim analysis is usually pre-planned in studies of long durations or expected serious side effects. The protocol has to define the timing of the analysis, the personnel in charge who will become unblinded, and the guidelines for managing results. A trial can be stopped because of serious side effects, even when statistically non-significant. On the other hand, we can terminate a study once we achieve a statistically significant net benefit. A trial can be stopped for futility if interim analysis shows that the observed benefit is so slim to reject the null hypothesis by the end of the study. Interim analysis may be used to modify the trial by recalculating the sample size, changing the proportion of participants in study arms, and modifying the inclusion or exclusion criteria [21]. For more details on the interim analysis, the reader can refer to Sect. 4.1.4.3.

Data Monitoring Committee

The researchers of large multicentric trials or long durations can create an independent data monitoring committee (DMC) to oversee the trial and advise data management. The members and charter of DMC have to be defined in the study's protocol, together with the exact role and responsibilities and, most importantly, the independence of the DMC from the steering committee and sponsors [5, 6].

Auditing

Auditing involves periodic independent verification of the whole process and suggesting corrective action when necessary. Audits can be performed separately on each part of the process or collectively on individual centers. The procedure has to be pre-planned, with the designation of involved personnel, roles and responsibilities. The chair and members of the auditing committee have to be independent of the steering committee and sponsors.

5.8 Statistical Methods

5.8.1 Population for the Analysis

5.8.1.1 Intention to Treat Analysis

To conclude a statistically significant difference at the end of the study, we have to have comparable groups at the beginning of the study, which is primarily achieved by randomization. In respecting this initial comparability, all patients are analyzed as randomized, regardless of the treatment received or protocol adherence. Most randomized clinical trials follow this intention to treat analysis [8].

5.8.1.2 Modified Intention to Treat and Per Protocol Analysis

Modified intention to treat excludes data from patients discovered to be ineligible after randomization, who did not follow treatment long enough as they should be, or who deviated from the protocol for one reason or another. The definition is somehow subjective and varies between studies. Finally, in the per-protocol analysis, patients are analyzed according to the treatment they have already received, regardless of their original randomization group. This approach is mainly applied to evaluate adverse events so that the absence or occurrence of harm is not attributed to a treatment that was never received [8].

Superiority Versus Non-inferiority Study

In a regular superiority study, all factors are working to dilute differences between the new treatment and the placebo. In contrast, in a non-inferiority study, we are motivated to demonstrate that the new and standard treatments are more or less equal (non-inferior). If poorly designed or conducted, the non-inferiority study can greatly enhance the risk of missing the evidence and approving a useless alternative whose inadequacies could not be detected. Hence, analysis based on intention to treat, which is desirable in a superiority study for its tendency to dilute differences, can increase type I error in the non-inferiority study. On the other hand, the per-protocol analysis may also become questionable in case of significant non-compliance. Pocock suggests performing and comparing both methods in non-inferiority studies [13].

5.8.2 Statistical Hypothesis

The researchers have to explain the conceptual framework of the trial design, whether being a *regular superiority study or a non-inferiority or equivalence trial*. A bilateral superiority study comparing two treatments aims to prove that one treatment is superior to the other. The null hypothesis is that both treatments are equal, and the alternative hypothesis is not. Unlike the classic superiority clinical study, a non-inferiority study usually aims to prove that a new treatment is "no more worse" than the classic treatment by a small amount that we can neglect, i.e., the non-inferiority margin (δ). On the other hand, an equivalent study aims to prove that the difference between both: new treatment (T) and reference treatment (R) "is no more worse" ($<\delta$) in favor of either treatment (see Sect. 4.13).

5.8.3 Statistical Analysis

5.8.3.1 Descriptive and Inferential Analysis

The statistical methods for data description have to be outlined in detail for all variables. Quantitative variables have to be tested for normality (see Sect. 1.4.3), and researchers have to use the proper measure of variable dispersion (see Sect. 1.3.4). Any method used for variable transformation must be explained in detail, with references (see Sects. 1.4.4 and 7.2.4). The researchers are urged to calculate the 95% confidence intervals of their results to display the limits of variation expected in the population of concern. Kindly refer to Sect. 1.4.2 to correctly calculate various confidence intervals (see Sect. 1.4.2).

The researcher must specify the main type of analysis for the primary outcome, whether by intention to treat or per protocol. The same measures are used for secondary outcomes. The protocol should outline the statistical tests used for analyzing primary and secondary outcomes. The conditions necessary to use each statistical test have to be verified before the analysis and not left to chance. The reader is requested to revise those conditions as outlined in Chaps. 2 and 3.

The researcher has to designate the P-value of statistical significance, usually 5% or less. However, clinical trials are characterized by the multiplicity of comparisons, inflating the primary risk of error that must be appreciated and adequately adjusted, and reported (see Sect. 2.4.3.3).

5.8.3.2 Interim and Subgroup Analysis

Intermediate analyses performed before completing data collection are indicated in the case of studies of long durations as well as those in which one of the treatments has severe possible side effects. Moreover, the researcher's curiosity may urge him to look for the statistical significance of his results before completing his work. An interim analysis is permissible on two conditions; the first is planning in the protocol. The second is to appreciate the risk of error from repeating a statistical test. Armitage and colleagues have calculated such risk as follows: suppose (N) is the total necessary number of patients, and it is decided to carry out an intermediate analysis with a smaller number (n). To maintain the usual risk of error (P = 0.05), the new P* of the intermediate analysis can be calculated according to the proportion N/n [22].

For example, if N/n = 2 (analyzing only half of the necessary number), we should arrive at a P* value of 0.029 to consider that our test was statistically significant at the least accepted degree of significance of 0.05. Similarly, a P* value of 0.022 is necessary for concluding the statistical significance of only 0.05 if we performed the analysis on only one-third of patients. A much higher P* value of 0.018 or even up to 0.1 is needed if the analysis only included one-fourth or one-tenth of the necessary number of patients; respectively [22].

On the other hand, unless pre-planned before the study, subgroup analysis may become problematic for being underpowered, especially when subgroups are based on variables measured after randomization [23]. The reader is invited to revise the measures of post hoc analysis (see Sect. 2.4.3.3).

5.8.3.3 Adjusted Analysis

An adjusted analysis is sometimes indicated to account for imbalances between study groups or accounts for a known prognostic variable (see Sect. 2.9). The main analysis should be identified when both unadjusted and adjusted analyses are intended. As with subgroup analyses, adjustment variables based on post-randomization data rather than baseline data can be a significant source of bias [24].

5.8.3.4 Analysis of Repeated Measures

In studies where there are repeated observations done on the same person, whether on different parts of the individual or the same part but repeated over time- sometimes we forget that the individual—and not the parts—is still the unit of analysis [25]. Doing so will lead to two main statistical errors. The violation of the widespread assumption that data should be independent. In other words, as if the two groups of data were taken from two independent groups of persons and not from a single group of persons. The second is sample inflation, like analyzing blood pressure measurement from the two arms of a single patient as being two observations, which may lead to spurious statistical significance [25]. In well-designed studies, and as will be shown in the concerned chapter, the repeated measure ANOVA takes into account the multiplicity and is provided by most statistical software (see Sects. 2.4.3.4 and 3.2.5.1).

5.8.3.5 Sequential Analysis

Sequential analysis is indicated whenever the studied disease is rare, e.g., cancer gall bladder. It consists of grouping patients in pairs; each patient receives one of the designed treatments. The difference between treatments (e.g., days of survival) obtained in each pair is cumulated on the following one till a statistically significant result is obtained, and the study can be stopped [26].

5.8.3.6 Handling of Missing Data

All studies have missing data, and the main problem is whether those misses have a special pattern other than being random rather than the volume of these data. Trials have to define how to deal with missing data and any planned methods for imputation. Methods of multiple imputations are complex but are preferred to single imputation methods such as adopting baseline data, last observation, mean value, etc. Sensitivity analyses are highly recommended to assess the robustness of trial results under different methods of handling missing data [27]. Imputation can be executed by IBM-SPSS or other statistical software packages. More information on handling missing data is outlined in a coming section (see Sect. 7.2.3).

5.8.4 Sample Size Determination

Sample size calculation is a cornerstone in study design and is usually the leading budget player. Detailed information on sample size calculation is outlined in Chap. 4. In brief, to achieve the primary outcome, the researcher has to define the number of participants he intends to include in the study, according to the effect size, the study design, and the adopted risks of error.

5.8.4.1 Choosing the Effect Size

The researcher usually begins by reviewing the literature for the appropriate effect size for his study. The choice of effect size depends upon many factors, including study design, type, distribution of primary outcome, and the used statistical test (see Sect. 4.1.1).

The Parallel Groups Superiority Design

Clinically appreciated indices of effect size include relative risk, odds ratio, hazard ratio, number needed to treat (see Sect. 4.3.1), correlation coefficient (see Sect. 4.7.1), and cumulative odds ratio (see Sect. 4.4.1.3).

Other indices may be clinically less appealing. However, they are potent estimates of the expected outcome effect on the population of interest. Measurements of effect size used to compare two quantitative variables by the unpaired test of Student, or the non-parametric Mann–Whitney test, includes Cohen's ds, Hedges g, Glass delta, and the non-parametric P_{ab} (see Sect. 4.2.1). Effect sizes used to test the significance of the association of two qualitative variables include Cohen h, Phi, Cramer's V, and Cohen W (see Sects. 4.3.1 and 4.4.1). Effect size used to compare multiple means by one-way ANOVA include Eta squared η^2, partial eta-square η_P^2, omega squared w^2, and Cohen F (see Sect. 4.6.1). The hazard rate and hazard ratio can be used to compare time to event studies (see Sect. 4.9.1). Beta coefficient, F^2, and Log odds ratio are the respective outputs of linear regression (see Sect. 4.8.1), multiple regression (see Sect. 4.11.1), and logistic regression analysis (see Sect. 4.10.1).

The Cluster Design

Patients may be distributed to either treatments or procedures as groups or clusters. The unit is no more the individual patient, and variability will be between different clusters and within the same cluster. The variance is now formed of two components, and both must be included in the cluster effect size calculation (Cluster d^2). Other suggested effect size includes the intra-cluster correlation coefficient (r_i) and Donner (D) design effect (see Sect. 4.3.1.7).

The Paired Superiority Design

We have previously shown that using the patient as his own control is a much more powerful test than the unpaired design. Besides the arithmetic gain in power, because each patient will be used twice, the statistical gain is due to the reduced variability by an amount equivalent to the expected correlation between the responses of the same patient to the two different treatments. Appropriate effect sizes include Cohen dz (see Sect. 4.5.1.1) used to compare two normally distributed quantitative variables by the paired Student test. The P_{ab} effect size is the non-parametric alternative used to compare quantitative variables following distributions other than normal (see Sect. 4.5.2.1). The odds ratio can be used to estimate effect size in the case of a paired qualitative outcome variable usually tested by McNemar's test (see Sect. 4.5.3.1).

The Repeated Measures

Partial eta-square η_P^2 effect size is a routine output of repeated measures ANOVA performed by most statistical software. Another repeated measure effect size W^2 can be derived from the F ratio, numbers of repetitions, and sample size (see Sect. 4.12.1.1). In the case of repeated quantitative variables following other distributions than normal, the Kendall W coefficient of concordance can be used to express effect size that is usually compared by the non-parametric test of Friedman (see Sect. 4.12.2.1).

The Non-inferiority and Equivalence Design

In non-inferiority and equivalence studies, the two treatments are not supposed to differ by no more than the accepted non-inferiority margin. Hence, indices of effect size used in the superiority study have to be adjusted accordingly. In the case of a non-inferiority study, any other true difference between the classic and new treatment is removed from the effect size, while it is added to the effect

size in the case of an equivalence study. The standard approach to test equivalence is through 2 one-sided tests, and hence, larger sample size is needed to prove equivalence compared to that calculated for a non-inferiority study for the same (δ) value. This is achieved by increasing $Z_{(1-B)}$ to $Z_{(1-B/2)}$ (see Sects. 4.13.1.1, 4.13.2.1, and 4.13.3.1).

Diagnostic Accuracy

Sensitivity and specificity are measures to test the diagnostic accuracy of a qualitative outcome. They are just proportions, and hence, indices of effect sizes are those of proportions. We have previously demonstrated effect sizes used to establish an observed sensitivity or specificity with a known (see Sect. 4.14.1.1) or unknown disease state (see Sect. 4.14.1.2). We have also calculated effect size to test the sensitivity or specificity of a particular test (see Sect. 4.14.1.3) and to compare sensitivity or specificity in the unpaired (see Sect. 4.14.1.4) and in the paired design (see Sect. 4.14.1.5).

In the case of quantitative measurement, ROC analysis provides the opportunity to test the overall accuracy of a diagnostic test. The area under the curve is a good estimate of effect size expressing an index of accuracy (see Sect. 4.14.2.1), to test the accuracy of a specific test (see Sect. 4.14.2.2) and to compare two independent (see Sect. 4.14.2.3) or dependent diagnostic tests (see Sect. 4.14.1.4).

Measuring Agreement

Measuring agreement refers to the degree of concordance between two or more measurements, whether made by different methods, repeated by the same method, or reproduced by different operators (see Sect. 2.10). In qualitative outcomes, the effect size is usually expressed as Cohen's Kappa (see Sect. 4.15.1.1).

In the case of a quantitative outcome, the effect size can be expressed as intraclass correlation coefficient for the normally distributed variable (see Sect. 4.15.2.1) and as Kendall W correlation coefficient for quantitative variables following other distribution than normal (see Sect. 4.15.2.2).

5.8.4.2   The Risks of Error

The researchers have to define the adopted primary and secondary risk of errors and explain the reasons behind any deviation from the usual values, i.e., 5% for the former and 20% for the latter (see Sects. 1.5.1, 1.7.4, 4.1.2). Although a smaller primary risk of error, such as 1%, may appear to be safer for the patients, it will deprive them of getting treatments with high margins of benefit between 96 and 98%, which will be unfair. On the other hand, the common pitfall is undermining an inflated risk of error associated with interim analysis, repeated analysis, and subgroup analysis. First, all those additional analyses must be pre-planned in the protocol. The researchers should appreciate the inflated risk of error, and the P-value has to be adjusted accordingly (see Sects. 2.4.3.3, 4.1.2.1, 4.6.2.2, 5.7.2, and 5.8.3.2).

The power of a study is based upon the ability to extend its results to a comparable population. Setting the secondary risk of error at 0.2 (20%) means that the study has 80% power to detect the evidence, provided that the latter exists. The price of empowering the study to 90% is steep, necessitating an increased sample size of about 30% (see Sects. 1.7.4 and 4.1.2.2). On the other hand, a larger secondary risk of error may be permissible in the case of serious or fatal diseases and absent effective treatment.

5.8.4.3   The Direction of the Study

Every new treatment is primarily tested versus placebo or standard care in which patients do not receive a "real treatment." A one-sided or one-tailed study is not concerned with looking to the other side of the coin and seeing whether the placebo is better than the new treatment (see Sects. 1.7.2 and 1.7.3). Consequently, the whole primary risk of error is shifted to the only possible conclusion: the new treatment is effective (and safe). Being of limited precision for neglecting the possible superiority of placebo, the researchers will conclude upon a smaller difference. Hence, they will need about 20% fewer patients than in the bilateral situation (see Sect. 4.1.3).

5.9   Study Documentations

1. Study title. A descriptive title identifies the study design, population, and interventions.
2. Study registration with the trial identifier (or application) and name of the registry.
3. Protocol version with number and date.
4. Name and contact information for the trial sponsor and funders.
5. The researchers have to designate the main responsible for the study. A steering committee and an independent data monitoring committee can be designated in large studies, with clear roles, guidelines, and responsibilities. They have access to the randomization codes of a blind study and the power to decode them when indicated. The protocol has to specify those indications in details and define the action plan in each case.
6. The protocol must identify every participant's name, affiliations, and roles in study design, protocol writing, data collection and management, data analysis, writing reports, and publication.
7. Name of participating centers and coordinating center, if any. Names, duties, and responsibilities of the persons in charge in each center.
8. A list of all dates indicating when the patients are examined for legibility and when they will be randomized. When the study begins and when it ends and, in between, the dates of follow-up schedule. The specific dates of meetings of different committees and, finally the date of data analysis [8].
9. A road map and datasheet for the study visits indicate data collected during each visit, place and dates of the visits, and persons in charge.
10. If a questionnaire is used to collect data, and unless it has been implemented in similar trials, it has to be preliminary tested on few cases before the beginning of the study. In general, the questions should be easy to read and have a straightforward interpretation. The reader can refer to the review of

Edwards P for the guidelines of the optimal design and administration [28].
11. A complete list of references.
12. Tracked dated protocol amendments.

5.10 Study Ethics

1. Ethical approval: research ethics approval by the institutional ethics committee and review board, with number and date of demand and approval, when available.
2. The informed consent from potential participants or authorized surrogates ensures that they understand the research, possible advantages, and drawbacks and agree to participate voluntarily. Additional consent provisions for collection and use of participant data and biological specimens, if required.
3. Confidentiality of data. The protocol has to show how the patients' information will be obtained and kept securely, with a limited number of personnel having data access for study purposes.
4. Declaration of interest. All personnel must declare any competing or conflict of interest between their own or institutional interests and their assigned responsibilities. All financial and non-financial ties have to be declared and updated throughout the study period and till results are published.

5.11 Data Sharing and Publication

1. Access to data. The protocol should identify the participants who can access data and describe any restrictions.
2. Dissemination policy to communicate the results to participants, reports to health authorities, and databases.
3. Granting authorship on the final trial report.

5.12 Appendices

1. Model consent form.
2. Model questionnaire form.
3. Plans for collection, laboratory evaluation, and storage of any biological specimen, if required, with measures to keep confidentiality.

References

1. Schwartz D, Lellouch J. Explanatory and pragmatic attitudes in therapeutical trials. J Chronic Dis. 1967;20:637–48. https://doi.org/10.1016/0021-9681 (67)90041-0.
2. Schulz KF, Altman DG, Moher D. CONSORT 2010 Statement: updated guidelines for reporting parallel group randomised trials. BMJ 2010;340:c332. https://doi.org/10.1136/bmj.c332.
3. Juszczak E, Altman DG, Hopewell S, Schulz K. Reporting of multiarm parallel-group randomized trials: extension of the CONSORT 2010 statement. JAMA. 2019;321:1610–20. https://doi.org/10.1001/jama.2019.3087.
4. Kwakkenbos L, Imran M, McCall SJ, McCord KA, Frobert O, Jemkens LG, et al. CONSORT extension for the reporting of randomized controlled trials conducted using cohorts and routinely collected data (CONSORT-ROUTINE): checklist with explanation and elaboration. BMJ 2021;373:n857. https://doi.org/10.1136/bmj.n857.
5. Chan A-W, Tetzlaff JM, Altman DG, Laupacis A, Gøtzsche PC, Krleža-Jerić K, et al. SPIRIT 2013 Statement: defining standard protocol items for clinical trials. Ann Intern Med. 2013;158:200–7. https://doi.org/10.7326/0003-4819-158-3-201302050-00583.
6. Chan A-W, Tetzlaff JM, Gøtzsche PC, Altman DG, Mann H, Berlin J, et al. SPIRIT 2013 explanation and elaboration: guidance for protocols of clinical trials. BMJ. 2013;346:e7586. https://doi.org/10.1136/bmj.e7586.
7. Choi BG, Rha SW, Yoon SG, Choi CU, Lee MW, Kim SW. Association of major adverse cardiac events up to 5 years in patients with chest pain without significant coronary artery disease in the Korean population. JAMA. 2019;8:e010541. https://doi.org/10.1161/JAHA.118.010541.
8. Laplanche A, Com-Nougue C, Flamant R. Comparaison de deux traitements. Méthodes statistiques appliqués a la recherché clinique. 1st ed. Paris. Médecines-Science: Flammarion; 1987. http://bdsp-

ehesp.inist.fr/vibad/index.php?action=getRecordDe-tail&idt=52329.

9. Campbell MJ, Machin D. Medical statistics: a common sense approach. 2nd ed. Chichester: Wiley; 1993.

10. Swinscow TDV. Statistics at square one. 9th ed. London: BMJ Publ. Group; 1997. https://doi.org/10.1002/(SICI)1097-0258(19971130)16:22%3C2629::AID-SIM698%3E3.0.CO;2-Z.

11. Pocock SJ. Clinical trials: a practical approach. Chichester, New York ed: Wiley; 1983. https://doi.org/10.1002/bimj.4710270604.

12. Prescott RJ, Counsell CE, Gillespie WJ, Grant AM, Russell IT, Kiauka S, et al. Factors that limit the quality, number and progress of randomized controlled trials. Health Technol Assess. 1999;3:1–143. https://doi.org/10.3310/hta3200.

13. Senn SJ. The design and analysis of crossover trials. 2nd ed. Chichester: Wiley; 1982.

14. Altman DG, Bland JM. How to randomise. BMJ 1999;319:703–4. https://www.bmj.com/content/319/7211/703.1.

15. Schulz KF, Grimes DA. Generation of allocation sequences in randomized trials: chance, not choice. Lancet. 2002;359:515–9. https://doi.org/10.1016/s0140-6736(02)07683-3.

16. Create a randomization list. In: Sealed envelope Ltd. 2018. https://www.sealedenvelope.com/simple-randomiser/v1/lists. Accessed 18 March 2022.

17. Randomly assign subjects to treatment groups. In: GraphPad Prism. 2022. https://www.graphpad.com/quickcalcs/randomize1/. Accessed 18 March 2022.

18. Altman DG, Bland JM. Treatment allocation by minimization. BMJ. 2005;330(7495):843. https://doi.org/10.1136/bmj.330.7495.843.

19. Schulz KF, Grimes DA. Allocation concealment in randomised trials: defending against deciphering. Lancet. 2002;359:614–8. https://doi.org/10.1016/s0140-6736(02)07750-4.

20. Devereaux PJ, Manns BJ, Ghali WA, Quan H, Lacchetti C, Montori VM, et al. Physician interpretations and textbook definitions of blinding terminology in randomized controlled trials. JAMA. 2001;285:2000–3. https://doi.org/10.1001/jama.285.15.2000.

21. Kairalla JA, Coffey CS, Thomann MA, Muller KE. Adaptive trial designs: a review of barriers and opportunities. Trials. 2012;13:145. https://doi.org/10.1186/1745-6215-13-145.

22. Armitage P, McPherson K, Rowe BC. Repeated significance tests on accumulative data. JRSS 1969;132:235–44. https://dokumen.tips/documents/repeated-significance-tests-on-accumulating-data.html.

23. Hirji KF, Fagerland MW. Outcome based subgroup analysis: a neglected concern. Trials. 2009;10:33. https://doi.org/10.1186/1745-6215-10-33.

24. Rochon J. Issues in adjusting for covariates arising post randomization in clinical trials. Drug Inf J. 1999;33:1219–28. https://doi.org/10.1177/009286159903300425.

25. Altman DG, Bland JM. Statistics notes: units of analysis. BMJ. 1997;314:1874. https://doi.org/10.1136/bmj.314.7098.1874.

26. Armitage P. Sequential medical trials: some comments on F.J. Anscombe's paper. JASA 1963; 58:384–7. https://doi.org/10.1080/01621459.1963.10500852.

27. Berger VW. Conservative handling of missing data. Contemp Clin Trials. 2012;33:460. https://doi.org/10.1016/j.cct.2012.02.008.

28. Edwards P. Questionnaires in clinical trials: guides for optimal design and administration. Trials. 2010;11:2. https://doi.org/10.1186/1745-6215-11-2.

Abstract

It is well acknowledged that the information acquired from a large body of evidence, based on combining multiple studies, is more useful and less biased than what can be acquired by a single work. However, like any other clinical study, the quality of the meta-analysis results depends on the selected material and the adopted methods. The analysis relies on choosing a computable effect size that can answer the research question and combining the effects of different studies in a fixed or more realistic random-effects model that considers the variability between studies. Whether related to subgroups or risk factors, true variability can be further illuminated by moderator analysis. A major concern will be whether there was a publication bias or other inclinations related to the literature being full of small studies producing clinical effects disproportionate to their small size. The heterogeneity of the study material and the multiplicity of the methods implicate conducting a sensitivity analysis throughout the study to ensure that the results are robust and can be safely applied to the population.

Keywords

Hand meta-analysis · Meta-analysis models · Meta-analysis heterogeneity · Subgroups meta-analysis · Meta regression · Small-study effects

6.1 Introduction

6.1.1 From Narrative to Systematic Review

Three decades ago, the usual procedure of obtaining a global view on a particular subject was to confine the whole mission to an expert in the field. The expert's role was to formulate the research question, review the literature, pick up the relevant manuscripts, summarize the finding and provide the medical community with a conclusion. It is clear that this approach suffered from significant limitations and was full of flows.

First, the whole process is subjective, depending on the reviewer's experience and personal opinions. Moreover, in the pre-internet era, not all the literature was available to everyone, and not all new information was available at all times, as nowadays. The net result is that two recognized experts can reach different and sometimes opposing conclusions. Besides subjectivity, the whole process usually lacks transparency. Consequently, it lacks an essential corner in any scientific work: repeatability. A third limitation was the lack of a statistical evaluation of the conclusion, which opened the door for unclear and even divergent interpretations of the same result. By the beginning of the nineties, the narrative review was unable to cope with the rapid increase of available information, the escalating development of newer treatments, the increasing patients' demands for shorter and more efficient therapy and the hope of prolonged life expectancy.

In response to those demands, the literature review had to change from relying on the quality of the person in charge (the expert reviewer) to the quality of the adopted methods used for reviewing. The reviewing process became more institutional rather than personal. Consequently, a systematic and transparent approach was needed to define the rules concerning where and how the study material was obtained, studied, and analyzed. The researcher had to define the approached databases, registers, and other sources, including websites, organizations, citation manager, and unpublished data. He must define the publication periods, and adopt keyword combinations and publication language. He had to present the inclusion and exclusion criteria, filter the studies, and the methods of critical appraisal used to ensure the quality of the selected manuscripts. He must present and classify reports assessed for legibility and those excluded with reasons. The transparency of the procedure largely overweighs and inevitably remains potential selection bias. The net result is

that the informed reader can now examine and judge each step's quality from the beginning till the end of the reviewing process. The PRISMA 2020 statement provides an updated guideline for identifying, selecting, appraising, and reporting systematic reviews [1]; the meta-analysis is the key element to evaluate the results.

6.1.2 Why Do We Need Meta-Analysis?

It is well acknowledged that large prospective randomized clinical trials (RCT) provide a solid answer to a particular research question. However, the results usually have different magnitudes and sometimes different directions. Table 6.1 shows the results of three studies comparing the duration of pain relief achieved with two analgesics A and B. The first study showed statistically significant superiority of treatment A compared to treatment B (P < 0.001). The second study was non-conclusive (P < 0.2), while the third study showed that treatment B was the one that showed a significantly superior effect (P = 0.02). The question was how to deal with a bunch of not only variable but contradictory results? The disadvantage of multiple clinical trials is that the outcome of each study stands alone, and we can either take it if significant or leave it when non-significant! Unfortunately, the results of multiple trials are not always in harmony, and this open circle is not closed by doing more studies. The more we do studies, the more the piles of positive and negative conclusions increase, and the more we become confused.

Table 6.1 From randomized controlled trials to meta-analysis

Study	Analgesic A	Analgesic B	Difference (A–B)	P value
1	10 ± 3	8 ± 3	2 ± 0.4	0.001
2	10 ± 1	9.5 ± 3	0.5 ± 0.4	>0.2
3	9 ± 3	10 ± 3	-1 ± 0.4	0.02
...			...	
Total			1.5 ± 0.86	

Values are mean $\pm$ standard deviation of pain relief calculated in hours

The meta-analysis provided an exit from this dilemma by only considering the result achieved in each study but not the conclusion made. In our example, provided that the studies were carried out in comparable groups and conditions, we can sum the three results, calculate an average value and measure the variability between the studies. As the conclusions (P values) can neither be summed nor averaged and are the main source of confusion, we disregard this confusing part. Returning to our example; the calculated differences were 2 ± 0.4, 0.5 ± 0.4, and -1 ± 0.4 h. Their mean value (1.5 ± 0.86 h) indicates that the average duration of analgesia provided by treatment A in the three studies is one and half times that achieved by treatment B. In other words, we replace the three contradictory results with a meaningful one.

Moreover, this one meaningful result is based on all studies, including the non-significant result of study number 2. In other words, we do not disregard any study for giving a small effect, as long as it fulfills the required inclusion and exclusion criteria. The next step will be to create a 95% CI for the final result and test its statistical significance. Put it this way, instead of rushing to the statistical significance of each study and getting three contradictory P values; we delayed the test till after getting the average final result of all studies and calculating only the last P-value. As such, meta-analysis helps us *improve precision* that many small studies cannot provide and, it has much more to give. It can help us *settle controversies* from apparently conflicting studies. Moreover, it can *pose new questions, generate new hypotheses, and open new research horizons.*

6.1.3 Types of Meta-Analysis

There are different methodological approaches to meta-analysis. Hunter and Schmidt classified meta-analysis methods into three categories. Purely descriptive methods, methods limiting the analysis to sampling error and finally, methods extending the analysis to consider any possible distorting artifact [2].

6.1.3.1 Descriptive Meta-Analysis
Gene V. Glass was the founding father in 1976 [3]. He suggested that the observed variabilities in the effect size are true; hence, they should be taken at face value without paying too much attention to statistical significance [4]. Despite the more refinements introduced, such as limiting the study to only one effect size or related outcomes and inviting more quality assessment, such purely descriptive meta-analysis is rarely adopted nowadays [2].

6.1.3.2 Methods Focusing on Sampling Error
Before categorizing, we have to briefly define the two main models of meta-analysis: the fixed and the random. The former assumes that the studies issue from the same population, and hence, any observed difference is due to a sampling error (see Sect. 6.2.4.1). On the other hand, the more realistic random model suggests that the studies represent various subpopulations. Hence, some of the observed differences are true, reflecting different subpopulations or risk factors (Sect. 6.2.4.2).

Researchers have advocated numerous methods, and we will present some common examples. We must note that these methods are not always alternatives to one another, and each has its advantage and disadvantages.

- Some methods are for general use. They can analyze qualitative and quantitative data and provide both fixed and random models. In this setting, the method proposed by Hedges and colleagues [5–8] is much more in use than the binomial effect size display (BESD) suggested by Rosenthal and Rubin [9]. Some reports claim that both methods give similar results [10], while others point out that the latter produces distorted results when proportions are away from 50% [11].
- Mantel–Haenszel [12] and Peto one-step approach [13] are good examples of methods with limited use. Both methods can only analyze binomial data of a fixed model. Despite the limited indications, they are known to work well in the case of rare events and small studies (see Sect. 6.2.6.3).

- The third category represents the other side of the coin: the exclusive random "barebone method" developed by Hunter and Schmidt [2]. It applies to qualitative and quantitative effect sizes but has different variability and heterogeneity estimates from the other methods described above. The authors have further developed their technique into a complete psychometric analysis extending the source of bias beyond sampling error. We will discuss the barebone analysis as an introduction to psychometric meta-analysis (see Sect. 6.3).

6.1.3.3   Psychometric Meta-Analysis (Hunter and Schmidt)

No study is methodologically perfect, and hence, studies will always yield unperfect results. For example, studies involving continuous data cannot include the whole range of measurements because of the limited sample size. Due to the limited range, their effect size will be smaller (attenuated). Attenuation of effect size can also be produced by dichotomizing the continuous scale or by an error in the measuring instrument itself. Hunter and Schmidt thought of these methodological imperfections as artifacts in the study design. Limiting the question of bias to sampling error as suggested by other methods is incorrect. The authors proposed that a complete list of artifacts be identified and corrected before the meta-analysis [2]. We will discuss their technique separately (see Sect. 6.3).

The Method Adopted in the Actual Review

The two most widely used meta-analysis methods are those proposed by Hunter and Schmidt [2] and the method suggested by Hedges and colleagues [5–8]. Our review will focus on the latter for being simple, understandable by most researchers, applicable to a large variety of effect sizes, and providing both fixed and random effect models. However, we will outline the other methods of calculation that are of everyday use within specific indications, namely the binomial effect size display (BESD) of Rosenthal and Rubin, the Mantel and Haenszel odds ratio, the one-step Peto approach, and the barebone technique (see Sect. 6.2.6.3). Finally, we will briefly discuss the psychometric meta-analysis separately (see Sect. 6.3).

6.2   Stages of Meta-Analysis

The steps of performing meta-analysis are the same as any other research in biology, except that the unit of analysis is not the patients but the studies already completed. Cooper and Hedges have suggested five-stages guidelines for the process: the problem formulation stage (see Sect. 6.2.1), the data collection (see Sects. 6.2.2), the data evaluation (see Sect. 6.2.3), the data analysis and interpretation (see Sects. 6.2.4, 6.2.5, 6.2.6, 6.2.7, 6.2.8, 6.2.9, 6.2.10, 6.2.11), and the public presentation stage (see Sect. 6.2.12) [14]. In our review, the fourth stage of the data analysis and interpretation section involved eight steps:

1. Choosing between a fixed and random-effects model (see Sect. 6.2.4).
2. Managing the reported effect size estimates, selecting an effect size of choice and converting other reported effect sizes. Requesting unpublished data from authors and calculating the unreported effect size. Normalizing selected effect sizes if needed and weighting all effect sizes by inverse variance or other weighing methods (see Sect. 6.2.5).
3. Calculating an average primary weighted effect size for the meta-analysis, its Se, 95% CI, and P-value (see Sect. 6.2.6).
4. Analyzing the heterogeneity of the meta-analysis studies, expressing the heterogeneity percent, and testing its statistical significance (see Sect. 6.2.7).
5. Subgroup analysis (see Sect. 6.2.8).
6. Analyzing the effect of one or more moderator variables on effect size: meta-regression (see Sect. 6.2.9).
7. Assessment of publication bias (see Sect. 6.2.10).
8. Sensitivity analysis to test the robustness of the model (see Sect. 6.2.11).

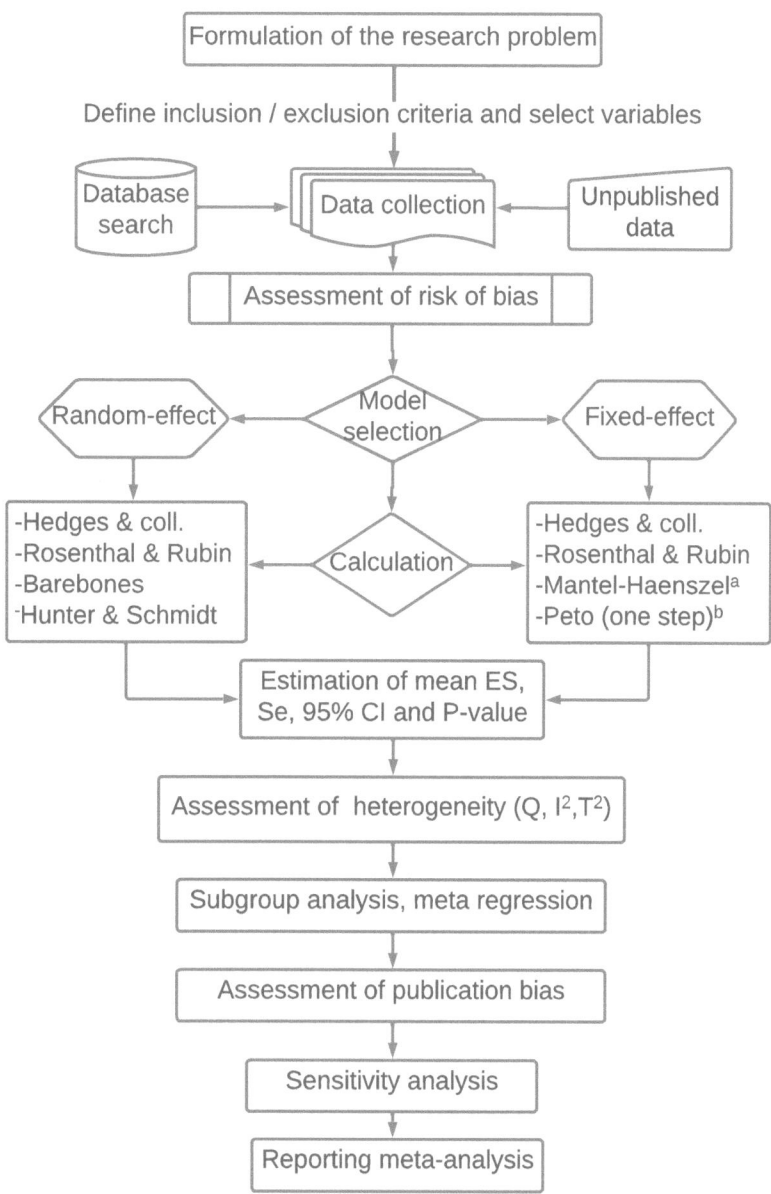

Fig. 6.1 Flow chart of meta-analysis. a = combines odds ratio, risk ratio and risk difference; b = combines odds ratio only, preferred with uncommon events observed in small equal group

Figure 6.1 is a flowchart of the main steps of the meta-analysis (Fig. 6.1). We draw the reader's attention that going through the details of each stage is far beyond the scope of our book. We will follow our main aim, which is to focus on the statistical considerations from the biologists' perspective, namely the data analysis, interpretation, and reporting methods (see Sects. 6.2.4, 6.2.5, 6.2.6, 6.2.7, 6.2.8, 6.2.9, 6.2.10, 6.2.11, 6.2.12).

6.2.1 Formulation of the Problem

This first stage includes three main tasks: formulate the research question, define the inclusion and exclusion criteria, and select all variables collected during the data reviewing process.

Formulation of the research question

The research idea must be formulated appropriately into an answerable research question that can fill an actual knowledge gap. An ideal research question should be feasible, interesting, novel, ethical, and relevant (FINER) [15]. For a question about the effect of a treatment or an intervention, the PICO approach is usually used to describe the population of the study (P), the proposed treatment or intervention (I), the type of comparator (C), and the outcome measure (O). Hence, the approach can be used to develop the research question [16].

Definition of inclusion and exclusion criteria

The next task is to define the inclusion and exclusion criteria of the research units or the studies that we intend to include in the meta-analysis. The essential criteria are those concerning the study design, the population, the type of treatment or intervention, and the study outcomes. In short, the requirements related to the study design include the type of study, whether a clinical trial or an observational study, a prospective or retrospective analysis, or else (see Sect. 5.2). The population criteria must define the relevant patients' demographics, the full description of the disease, and the associated risk factors (see Sect. 5.3). The treatment or interventional type usually includes one or two treatment groups (see Sect. 5.4). The meta-analyst may include other criteria such as the study settings, the periods of the study, the publication language, and the study economics.

Definition of the Collected Variables

The third task is to select and define all the variables we intend to collect during the study besides the effect size. Those variables may include patients' demographics, factors related to the disease, risk factors, factors related to the treatments or interventions, investigations, and secondary outcomes. On the one hand, those variables help define the population of the actual study and the future population that can benefit from the study outcomes. On the other hand, they provide the basis for subgroup analysis and study validity. All researchers have to revise and approve the complete protocol of the meta-analysis before the beginning of the study. They

must keep in mind that well-planned research can always be re-analyzed but not the reverse. The researchers can check on the actual ongoing research in the field and register their study on a specialized database [17].

6.2.2   Data Collection

The researchers have to define the consulted electronic databases, such as the web of science and PubMed, the keywords, the years of publication, and the study language. They have to define the number of screened manuscripts and the number of manuscripts retrieved for each publication type. In time, the search is extended beyond the selected manuscript, both forward and backward. On one hand, they can track authors who cited the selected manuscript to identify new articles. On the other hand, they may track authors appearing on the reference list of the selected manuscript to get older articles. Search can extend beyond the electronic database by selectively hand-searching the electronic library of relevant journals not included in the consulted databases.

We have previously mentioned that the power of meta-analysis is to benefit from statistically non-significant data to build a conclusion based upon all results, whether significant or non-significant (see Sect. 6.1.2). By deduction, not including the non-significant results weakens the meta-analysis. Unfortunately, researchers are usually reluctant to send their statistically non-significant studies to journals. Reviewers tend to reject those negative studies, and editors are not enthusiastic about publishing them if accepted. Consequently, the literature is full of significant findings, but negative results exceptionally see the light [18]. As unpublished data are kept because they have a smaller effect size, a meta-analysis relying only on publications inflates the effect size. Consequently, the researchers can extend the search to universities and research centers, meetings, and websites of relevant scientific societies, and can personally contact selected authors for their unpublished data.

Finally, the researchers must report their search methods to ensure the included studies' quality and similarity [1].

6.2.3 Assessment of Risk of Bias

Bias is a systematic error, such as always confining the old treatment to sick patients and the new treatment to relatively healthy patients. The result is that the new treatment will give better results on average compared to the old treatment. In other words, it leads to a systematic change in the magnitude and sometimes the direction of the studied effect, jeopardizing the validity of the whole study. Bias is not imprecision, which is a random effect, such as the imprecise measuring of treatment effect that is sometimes in favor of one treatment and other times in favor of the other. The net result is a more or less balanced average. Bias can result from the meta-analyst themselves for the absence of the results of the studies that they did not include in the meta-analysis.

Risk of bias assessment is also called quality assessment or critical appraisal. The meta-analysts have to check every study included for bias, which can be in every step, starting with the study design and up to making conclusions. Among the many tools for assessing the risk of bias, many researchers recommend Cochrane RoB 2 for risk assessment in randomized and non-randomized clinical studies, qualitative studies, economics studies, and overviews.

In short, this new update defined five domains for bias, including the randomization process, deviations from the intended interventions, missing the outcome data, bias in measuring the outcome, and in reporting the results. Each domain is investigated to examine whether the author's selection or decision has biased the outcome. For example, the randomization process is checked for bias in the random generation, allocation concealment, and the absence of baseline difference between groups [19].

Each of the five domains is evaluated by a series of signaling questions, a judgment algorithm, a free text box to justify responses, and an option to predict (and explain) the likely direction of the bias. Finally, an overall risk of bias is addressed the same as for the five primary domains. Bias assessment has to be reported clearly in the review and reflected in the analysis and the conclusions. A study is judged to have a high risk of bias when having a single high risk of bias in one domain or concerns in multiple domains [19].

6.2.4 Choosing the Model

6.2.4.1 The Fixed-Effect Model

The fixed model implies that all the selected studies are samples drawn from the same population, and hence, the estimated effect size will be fixed (the same) across all samples (studies). The fixed model assumes that the only source of bias is the sampling error (the within-study variability), a usually limited small variation associated with taking several samples from the same population. The confidence interval created around the average effect size will be narrow due to the limited variability; hence, increasing type I error or the probability to report a false positive result. In other words, *the fixed model increases the risk of concluding upon a statistically significant effect size while it is untrue* [20].

6.2.4.2 The Random Effects Model

The random model implies that, besides the within-study variability, there is an additional variability between studies because each study estimates a different mean within the grand population. Put it this way; the samples are drawn from a super-population, and each one is drawn from a different mean. The total variability is the sum of both sampling error and the variability between the studies (T^2). *The additional source of variability makes the confidence intervals wider* [2] *and reduces the chances of concluding upon a significant effect size.* In a random-effects model, the study effect sizes are assumed to represent a random sample from a particular distribution of these effect sizes. Hence, the description is being random effects (multiple) model, in contradiction to the fixed effect (unique) model [3]. There are numerous methods of calculations, which will be discussed along with testing heterogeneity (see Sect. 6.2.7). Note that the null hypothesis is that the average effect size is the same across the subpopulations. The alternative hypothesis is that the average effect sizes are significantly different from each other.

6.2.4.3 The Mixed Effects Model

We can include one or more independent qualitative or quantitative predictors in a fixed or a random-effects model to explain part of the effect size (see Sects. 6.2.8 and 6.2.9). For example, we can include the patient's age or gender and analyze their individual or combined effect on the duration of pain relief of two analgesics. The predictor variable is called the moderator and the procedure is called moderator analysis. The procedure permits explaining part of the variability that was initially suggested as being only random (before introducing the moderator variable in the model) to be at least partially due to (influenced by) the moderator variable. We can calculate an average effect size for each category of the grouping qualitative variable (e.g., males versus females) or for a cut-off point on the continuous scale of the moderator variable (e.g., effect treatment at a certain age in years). Most interestingly, we can calculate the proportion of variability that has been reduced by the moderator variable and test its statistical significance, which reflects the importance of the effect of the moderator variable on the effect size.

6.2.4.4 Which Model to Choose?

Choosing to adopt a fixed or random effect model depends on the assumptions made about the population and the types of inferences we wish to make from the meta-analysis. A fixed-effect model may suit studies limited to a well-defined small population sector, and any inferences will also be limited to this sector. Hence, all roads lead to a random effect model. On one side, meta-analysis usually involves real-world data with variable population parameters. Prospective randomized controlled trials are generally multicenter and include many subgroups, even if they are well-defined. On the

other hand, trialists wish to expand the benefit of their studies to all patients; pharmaceutical companies want to generalize their inferences unconditionally to compensate for the significant expenses. A fixed model cannot satisfy the needs of either party.

One additional point is the risk associated with adopting the inappropriate model, i.e., analyzing fixed data by a random model, as opposed to the risk associated with analyzing random data by the fixed approach. A fixed model assumes that all studies come from the same population, and hence, the only difference between the studies is the variability within the studies (Se^2). The random model assumes studies come from different subpopulations, and hence, an additional source of variation is the variability between studies themselves, reflecting the variability between the subpopulations (T^2); i.e., the variability of a random effect model = $Se^2 + T^2$. The main difference in calculation between the two models is the variability, which is equal to (Se^2) in the fixed-effect model and ($Se^2 + T^2$) in the random-effects model. If data are fixed (i.e., perfectly homogenous), the calculated T^2 will be equal to zero. Hence, even if analyzed by a random effect model, the computed variability = $Se^2 + T^2 = Se^2 + 0 = Se^2$; which is the variability of the fixed-effect model. In other words, the analysis results will be the same, whether we requested a fixed or a random model, and the meta-analyst has nothing to lose by asking for a random analysis for fixed data, provided that data is truly homogenous.

On the other hand, *the consequences of applying fixed-effects methods to random-effects data will be dramatic*. Instead of calculating a random variability composed of ($Se^2 + T^2$), only the (Se^2) part will be calculated, inflating type I error from the usual 5% to as much as 11–28% [20]. In conclusion, the debate of whether choosing a random or a fixed model is more theoretical than practical implications, and a random effect model has to be always calculated. The reason is that even if population effects are constant and the authors wish to limit inferences on the same fixed population, methodological variations across studies alone will cause variation in study outcomes, questioning the pertinence of fixed-effects models in general [2].

6.2.5 Managing the Effect Size Estimates

Let us remember a primary aim of the meta-analysis: to calculate an average effect size that will be more representative of the population than that provided by any single study, which is far from being a one-step approach. First, we have to review all reported effect sizes and choose the effect size of choice that eases the calculation and suits the presentation. We have to compute the effect size for those studies that did not report an estimate and convert different estimates to our effect size of choice.

We need to combine the effect sizes reported by all studies and create a mean effect size and a standard error to describe the variability around this mean. However, some effect sizes such as Person's correlation coefficient, odds ratio, and relative risk are not normally distributed, and hence, we cannot directly compute a reliable mean and, most importantly, a reliable standard error. Those effect sizes must be normalized first for computation and then reconverted to their original scales for presentation.

The following fundamental step is to weigh the effect size of each study, usually by its inverse variance, giving more weight to large studies with small variability and lowering the pitch of smaller ones. The weighted effect size can be combined to create a more reliable mean effect and standard error. The work of Rosenthal on meta-analysis procedures provides an excellent classic source to understand and convert effect sizes to one another [21]. Effect sizes can also be calculated or converted through online links [22, 23].

6.2.5.1 The Effect Size Families

The reader is requested to refer to chapter four to explain those most commonly used effect sizes. In short, there are two leading effect size families: the (d) family measuring raw or standardized differences between observations and the (r) family measuring the proportion of variation

in the dependent variable that could be related to (explained by) a particular predictor (see Sect. 4.1.1.3). The most commonly used effect size among the d family are Cohen d (see Sect. 4.2.1.1) and Hedges g (see Sect. 4.2.1.2), with some investigators preferring to calculate the unstandardized raw differences.

The most commonly used effect sizes among the r family include Pearson's correlation coefficient r (see Sect. 4.7), odds ratio (see Sect. 4.3.1.5), relative risk (see Sect. 4.3.1.4), and hazard ratio (see Sect. 4.9.1.2). Besides Pearson's correlation coefficient, which examines the relationship between two continuous variables, other correlation coefficients include the biserial, point biserial, and rank-biserial correlations. The biserial and point biserial correlations are the relationship between a continuous variable and a ranked or dichotomous variable. The rank-biserial correlation is between a ranked and a dichotomous variable [24]. Unlike Person's and biserial correlation, how other measures are included in the meta-analysis depends on whether the dichotomy was true, such as males and females, or artificially induced by taking a particular cut-off point on a scale. The true dichotomy can be seen as a true difference between two groups, i.e., an original true d-effect size. Consequently, a true point biserial correlation (r_{AB}), such as the correlation between the patient's height (A) and gender (B), can be calculated from the standardized difference between the body weights of males and females (d), with known proportions (p and $1-p$) "Eq. 6.1" [25]. In the case of a false dichotomy, the relationship between variables is of an original continuous nature, and effect size d has to be transformed to point biserial correlation first then to biserial correlation [2].

$$r_{AB} = \frac{d}{\sqrt{1/[1-(1-p)]+d^2}} \tag{6.1}$$

The Effect Size of Multivariable Analysis

The previously discussed effect sizes measure the direct relationship between two variables. However, an effect size originating from the multivariable analysis depends not only on the relationship between two variables (the predictor and the outcome) but also on the effect of other variables (predictors) in the multivariable analysis. Unless all studies included in the meta-analysis employ the same multivariable technique, we must *approximate the beta coefficient (β) originating from a multivariable study to the correlation coefficient* before being added to a series of r values originating from the regular bivariate analysis. The equation is dependent upon whether (β) has a nonnegative ($\lambda = 1$) or a negative value ($\lambda = 0$) "Eq. 6.2" [26].

$$r = 0.98\beta + 0.05\lambda \qquad (6.2)$$

6.2.5.2 Selecting an Effect Size

Once all observed effect sizes have been collected from different studies, the meta-analyst may wonder about choosing the best effect size for the meta-analysis. Borenstein and colleagues advised reviewing the collected studies' summary statistics for the most commonly reported effect size. The researcher has to look for other available data such as proportions, means, and standard deviation to evaluate if he can compute the missing effect sizes. If data is not available, the meta-analysts can call on authors to send their raw data, which should be the final resort [3]. On the other hand, some studies may report different effect sizes across different measures of the same outcome. Rosenthal suggested calculating an average effect size across all measures of the same outcome within a study [21].

As we write to publish, the potential reader has to have a role in this decision. Readers in psychology have the habit and preference for correlation (r-type) effect size indicators and standardized mean differences [3, 27]. On the other hand, readers in other specialties may appreciate the outcomes of clinical trials and observational studies, such as the risk ratio, hazard ratio, and odds ratio [3]. We have to make it easier for the reader to go through the discussion section. *Going from odds ratios to relative risks may be smooth, but jumping between standardized mean differences and risk ratios or*

Pearson's r may be more difficult to assimilate for many readers. Our point of view of the ideal effect size is the easiest to understand by the reader on the subject, provided clinical relevance and statistical correctness.

6.2.5.3 Converting Among Effect Size Estimates

Researchers have the opportunity to express the effect size with different indices, even when studying the same subject. For example, the effect of a particular treatment on a binomial outcome, some researchers may express their results in terms of odds ratio, while others may prefer to report the relative risk. The meta-analyst has to be able to convert either index to his own effect size of choice, e.g., the risk difference or else. A more demanding conversion would be if the meta-analyst wishes to include a study that expresses the effect size in correlation coefficient or standardized mean of the difference. Moreover, some researchers do not report an effect size at all, and hence, the meta-analyst has to use the reported data to calculate the missing effect size. There are numerous simplified sources for calculation and conversion of effect sizes [27, 28] and free online calculators [22, 29] and convertors [23]. There is no point in repeating those equations, especially since most of the simple resources are freely available. However, we have to draw the readers' attention to a few basic rules. First, we can combine studies using different metrics, provided that this is the only main difference between those studies. Second, *the SMD is at the heart of conversion*, and hence, we can convert a binomial ES or a correlation to SMD and the reverse. However, converting a binomial ES to r must pass by SMD first.

6.2.5.4 Creation of a Reliable Variance

As early as 1928, Fisher noticed that the population value of correlation coefficient r gets further and further away from zero as the distribution of r sampled from the population becomes more and more skewed, and it has to be corrected [30]. Other biases were found in the standardized mean of the difference (SMD) when used in small samples [28], and Hedges' g was suggested to improve the bias. In addition, we have previously shown that the skewed nature of the odds ratio (see Sect. 1.8.2.2), the relative risk (see Sect. 1.8.2.1), and the hazard ratio (see Sect. 1.8.3.1) do not permit the calculation of a reliable Se. Consequently, effect size calculations using those ratios are made in the log scale (see Sect. 1.8.7) and then converted back to the usual scale for the final presentation. Put it another way; we weight effect sizes by the inverse variance. Hence, we need to have a reliable variance, which is polishing about: creating a stable and reliable variance.

6.2.5.5 Weighing by Inverse Variance

To perform a meta-analysis, we need to combine the effect sizes of different studies and calculate a mean effect size. We cannot simply sum the means of various studies as if they all have the same importance. We have to give more weight to important and precise studies and less weight to other studies not fulfilling these criteria. The debate is about importance and precision; we have to decide which study is more important and more precise and, hence, is more representative of the population. Although Rosenthal and DiMatteo urged researchers to give more weight to methodologically sound studies [24], a more objective approach is to look for a numerical expression of representativeness rather than a subjective evaluation. In this setting, the most commonly used weighting factor is the inverse variance and, less commonly, the artifact multiplier proposed by Hunter and Schmidt, both of which will be discussed separately (see Sects. 6.2.5.5 and 6.3.2).

Let us revise what is the variance (S^2)? It expresses the average variation of a particular variable in a study, such as the duration of pain relief in hours or the relative risk of developing a new episodes of tuberculosis after BCG vaccination. The variance is calculated as the sum of variation (sum of squares = SS) divided by the degree of freedom (sample size $- 1 =$ n $- 1$). Hence, the variance expresses two important pieces of information in a single number: the total variability within the study (SS) and the sample size (n $- 1$). A small (S^2) means that the study is of large size, has a small variability, or both. As

the aim of any study is to represent the population and, as the latter has the largest size and the smallest variability, the smaller the variance of a study, the more it is representative of the population. Consequently, it has to have a more significant role in the meta-analysis, which is looking to estimate the effect size in the population (ES), and vice versa. Dividing the effect size of every study by its variance (ES/S^2) inflates the effect size of studies with smaller variability and (or) larger sample size and attenuates the ES of studies with larger variability and (or) or small sample size [25]. In other words, it inflates the effect size of studies that are more representative of the population and attenuates the ES of other studies studies that are not and hence, the computed average ES will be more representative to that of the population. Dividing effect size by the variance is the same as multiplying the effect size of each study by its inverse variance, from which we deduct the name of the technique: weighting the effect size by inverse variance.

Fixed effect model

In conclusion, the effect sizes observed in the different studies cannot be simply added to one another and then get the average effect size by dividing their sum by their number. Instead, the effect sizes of included studies have to be weighed before being summed, giving more importance to those studies with a larger chance to represent the population: i.e., studies with smaller variances. The weighting factor of each study will be its inverse variance. W = 1/Se^2. The weighted effect size (WES_i) of a particular study (i) is the product of its effect size (ES_i) and its inverse variance $(1/Se_i^2)$ "Eq. 6.3".

$$WES_i = ES_i \times \frac{1}{Se_i^2} \qquad (6.3)$$

Random effects model

In the case of a random model, another element of variability has to be added to the meta-analysis, which is the variability between the studies (T^2). In other words, the weighted effect size $(W^R ES_i)$ of each study (i) included in a random-effects model will be the product of its effect size (ES_i) and the reciprocal value of the sum of the variability within the study (Se_i^2) and in-between studies variance (T^2) "Eq. 6.4". There are different methods to estimate (T^2) that will be discussed in the section on testing homogeneity (see Sect. 6.2.7.3)

$$W^R ES_i = ES_i \times \frac{1}{Se_i^2 + T^2} \qquad (6.4)$$

6.2.6 Estimation of a Mean Effect Size, Se, 95% CI and P Value

The basic aim of the meta-analysis is to compute two estimates: the mean and standard error of underlying population effects from the collection of studies addressing the same research question with the least bias possible. We have reached a critical intermediate stage regarding the previously described five stages of a meta-analysis [14]. We are now ready to produce the two desired estimates, which permit the creation of a 95% CI of the estimate and testing its statistical significance.

By this point, the meta-analysis can answer two critical questions. What is the extent of the effect size in the main population of interest, which is the general descriptive part of the meta-

analysis? The second question is whether the effect size is statistically significant or just due to chance; which is the inferential part of the analysis? We have to admit that the meta-analysis should not stop at this point. Like any other biological study, we have "to shake" those main results. We test their homogeneity, robustness, and internal and external validity, which we will discuss in the following sections (see Sect. 6.2.7 to Sect. 6.2.11). Moreover, what we will report here should not replace the main full report given at the end of this chapter (see Sect. 6.2.12).

6.2.6.1 How Does Meta-Analysis Work: Can We Do It by Hand?

Before going through the details, let us perform a generic example of the meta-analysis by hand, not by computer software, to test how it works. We will give a simple example to show how the meta-analysis benefits from the data provided by all studies included in the model to better estimate the effect size.

The Fixed-Effect Model

Table 6.2 shows three sets of meta-analyses: I, II, and III. For simplicity, we will only present the minimum amount of data necessary for the calculations; assuming a fixed model effect. Afterward, we will show the changes associated with a random-effects model.

Table 6.2 The power of meta-analysis: a mini-example

Meta-analysis	Studies	ES	n	Se^2	W	WES	Mean $\pm$ Se	95% CI
(I)	A	0.5	50	0.083	12	6		
Summary	–	*0.5[a]*	*50[b]*	*0.083[c]*	*12[d]*	*6[e]*	*0.5 ± 0.29*	*−0.07 to 1.07*
(II)	A	0.5	50	0.083	12	6		
	B	0.5	50	0.083	12	6		
Summary	*A + B*	*0.5[a]*	*100[b]*	*0.04[c]*	*24[d]*	*12[e]*	*0.5 ± 0.2*	*0.1 to 0.9*
(III)	A	0.5	50	0.083	12	6		
	B	0.5	50	0.083	12	6		
	C	0.5	50	0.083	12	6		
Summary	*A + B + C*	*0.5[a]*	*150[b]*	*0.028[c]*	*36[d]*	*18[e]*	*0.5 ± 0.17*	*0.16 to 0.84*

ES = effect size; n = sample size; Se^2 = variance; W = weighing method for effect size = $1/Se^2$; WES = weighed effect size = Wx ES; A, B, and C = study ID; Meta-analysis I, II, and III = three independent meta-analysis: (I) includes study A only, (II) includes studies A + B, (III) includes studies A + B + C. Values of summaries of the three meta-analyses are presented in italics; a = mean ES of the meta-analysis, b = total number of cases, c = variance, d = total weights, e = total weighed effect sizes of the meta-analysis

Meta-analysis I

Meta-analysis I included only one study: study A, carried out in 50 patients, reported mean numeric effect size (ES) of 0.5 and a variance (Se^2) of 0.083. Given that the study has fulfilled the inclusion and exclusion criteria, we will weigh its ES by the inverse variance, $W = 1/Se^2$. In our example, $W = 1/Se^2 = 1/0.083 = 12$, and the weighted effect size of study A (WES) will be equal to: $12 \times 0.5 = 6$. Note that meta-analysis I included only one study; hence, the total weight of meta-analysis I will be 12 ($\Sigma W = 12$), and the total weighed effect size will be 6 ($\Sigma WES = 6$).

Summary of meta-analysis I

Putting study A aside and reporting the summary of meta-analysis I. Meta-analysis I included only one study (study A), the mean ES of the meta-analysis (M_{meta}) equals the total weighted effect size divided by the total weight $= \Sigma WES/\Sigma W = 12/6 = 0.5$ "Eq. 6.5". As the weight is equal to the inverse variance, the meta-analysis variance will be simply the reciprocal value of the total weight $= 1/\Sigma W = 1/12 = 0.083$. The Se of the meta-analysis is the square root of its variance $= 0.29$. The 95% CI of the effect size of meta-analysis I = mean ES ± 1.96 Se $= 0.5 \pm 1.96 (0.29) = -0.07$ to 1.07 "Eq. 6.6". A simple Z test calculates the statistical significance of the effect size of the meta-analysis: P is non-significant for the Z score being below the critical limit of 1.96 "Eq. 6.7".

$$M_{meta} = \frac{\sum WES}{\sum W} = \frac{6}{12} = 0.5. \qquad (6.5)$$

$$95\% \text{ CI} = M_{meta} \pm 1.96(Se_{meta})$$
$$= 0.5 \pm 1.96(0.29) = -0.07 \ to \ 1.07 \qquad (6.6)$$

$$Z = \frac{M_{meta}}{Se_{meta}} = \frac{0.5}{\sqrt{0.083}} = 1.73. \qquad (6.7)$$

The calculations of the meta-analysis summary are shown in italics in Table 6.2. As meta-analysis I is formed by study A only, its effect size will be the effect size of study A. Consequently, the interpretation of the summary of the meta-analysis is as follows: the effect size can be negative (-0.07) or positive (1.07), and hence, the effect size is statistically non-significant, which is quite logical for being based on a single statistically non-significant study (study A).

Figure 6.2 shows the forest plot for meta-analysis I. It shows the summary of Study A and the summary of the meta-analysis at the bottom. Both summaries are identical for the meta-analysis being formed of study A only. The mean ES of the meta-analysis ($M_{meta} = 0.5$), variance of the meta-analysis ($Se^2_{Meta} = 0.083$) and its 95% confidence intervals (-0.07 to 1.07) are shown in grayed rectangles (Fig. 6.2).

Meta-analysis II

Meta-analysis II is a second analysis that was done independently from meta-analysis I after adding a replica of study A: study B. Both studies have the same sample size, same ES and same variance, a condition that perfectly fits with a fixed-effect model.

Summary of meta-analysis II

The summary of the meta-analysis II is shown in italics in Table 6.2 and at the bottom of Fig. 6.3. Meta-analysis II included two studies; the mean ES of the meta-analysis (M_{meta}) equals the total weighed effect size of the two studies divided by their total weight $= 0.5$ "Eq. 6.8". The variance of the meta-analysis is the reciprocal value of the total weight $= 0.04$ "Eq. 6.9" and hence, its Se $= 0.2$ "Eq. 6.10". The 95% CI of the effect size of meta-analysis II $= 0.1$ to 0.9, which is a statistically significant effect size for excluding the null "Eq. 6.11". A simple Z test calculates the exact degree, giving a Z score (2.5) that is larger than the critical value shown in Z table (1.96); P = 0.0124 "Eq. 6.12".

$$M_{meta} = \frac{\sum WES}{\sum W} = \frac{6+6}{12+12} = 0.5. \qquad (6.8)$$

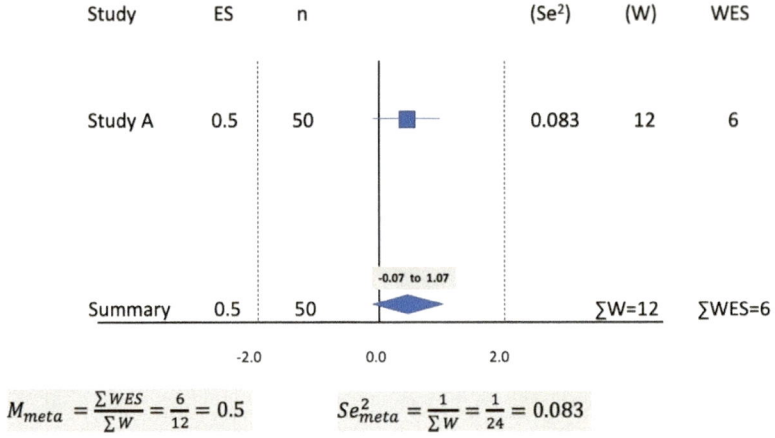

$$M_{meta} = \frac{\sum WES}{\sum W} = \frac{6}{12} = 0.5 \qquad Se^2_{meta} = \frac{1}{\sum W} = \frac{1}{24} = 0.083$$

Fig. 6.2 Forest plot of meta-analysis I: fixed effect model. ES = effect size; n = sample size; Se² = variance; W = weighting method for effect size = 1/Se²; WES = weighted effect size = Wx ES; M_{meta} = mean ES of the meta-analysis; ΣWES = sum of weighted ES, ΣW = sum of weights; Se²$_{meta}$ = variance of the meta-analysis

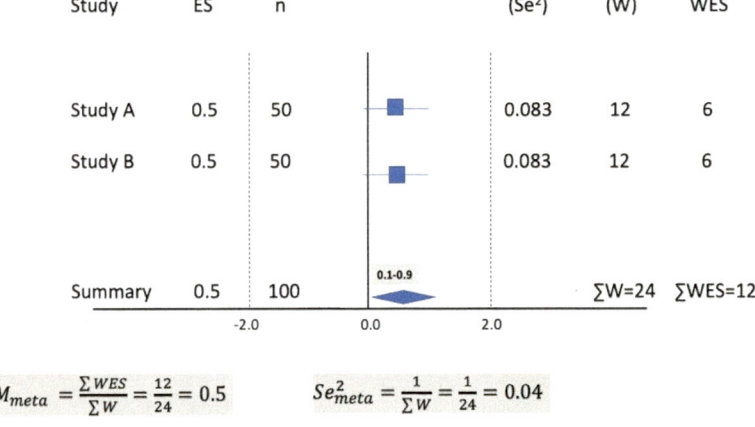

$$M_{meta} = \frac{\sum WES}{\sum W} = \frac{12}{24} = 0.5 \qquad Se^2_{meta} = \frac{1}{\sum W} = \frac{1}{24} = 0.04$$

Fig. 6.3 Forest plot of meta-analysis II: fixed effect model. ES = effect size; n = sample size; Se² = variance; W = weighting method for effect size = 1/Se²; WES = weighted effect size = Wx ES; M_{meta} = mean ES of the meta-analysis; ΣWES = sum of weighted ES, ΣW = sum of weights; Se²$_{meta}$ = variance of the meta-analysis

$$\text{Var}_{meta} = \frac{1}{\sum W} = \frac{1}{12+12} = 0.04 \qquad (6.9)$$

$$Se_{meta} = \sqrt{\text{Var}_{meta}} = \sqrt{0.04} = 0.2 \qquad (6.10)$$

$$95\% \text{ CI} = M_{meta} \pm 1.96(Se_{meta})$$
$$= 0.5 \pm 1.96(0.2) = 0.1 \; to \; 0.9 \quad (6.11)$$

$$Z = \frac{M_{meta}}{Se_{meta}} = \frac{0.5}{0.2} = 2.5. \qquad (6.12)$$

This is the power of the meta-analysis: cumulating weighed ES from every study included and delaying the conclusion to the final result. Note that the 95% CI of each of the two studied is non-significant when calculated alone, as shown in the summary of meta-analysis I. The key element is the reduction of variance, associated with the increase in sample size: the variance of the larger meta-analysis II (0.04) is less than half that of meta-analysis I (0.083). Remember that the variance is the mean variability (SS/n−1), which is why the variance is also called the mean square (see Sect. 1.3.4). Provided that studies come from the same population, the more we include patients (adding study B to study A), the smaller will be the mean variability (variance) and, hence, the narrower will be the 95% CI.

Meta-analysis III

Meta-analysis III is a third analysis done independently from the two previous ones, after adding another replica: study C. The three studies (A, B, and C) have the same sample size, same ES, and same variance.

Summary of meta-analysis III

We report the summary of the meta-analysis III, as shown in italics in Table 6.2 and at the bottom of Fig. 6.4. Meta-analysis III included three studies, the mean ES of the meta-analysis (M_{meta}) = 0.5 "Eq. 6.13". The variance of the meta-analysis is the reciprocal value of the total

weight = 0.028 "Eq. 6.14", and hence, its Se = 0.17 "Eq. 6.15". The 95% CI of the effect size of meta-analysis III = 0.16 to 0.84 "Eq. 6.16". The Z score = 2.94; which is higher than the critical limit in Z table (1.96); P = 0.0033 "Eq. 6.17".

$$M_{meta} = \frac{\sum WES}{\sum W} = \frac{6+6+6}{12+12+12} = 0.5. \tag{6.13}$$

$$Var_{meta} = \frac{1}{\sum W} = \frac{1}{12+12+12} = 0.028 \tag{6.14}$$

$$Se_{meta} = \sqrt{Var_{meta}} = \sqrt{0.08} = 0.17 \tag{6.15}$$

$$\begin{aligned} 95\% \ CI &= M_{meta} \pm 1.96 \, (Se_{meta}) \\ &= 0.5 \pm 1.96(0.17) = 0.16 \, to \, 0.84 \end{aligned} \tag{6.16}$$

$$Z = \frac{M_{meta}}{Se_{meta}} = \frac{0.5}{0.17} = 2.94. \tag{6.17}$$

We do not need to repeat that the ES of any of the three studies alone is statistically non-significant. Empowering the research by cumulating the weighed ES of multiple comparable studies reduces the variability and improves precision.

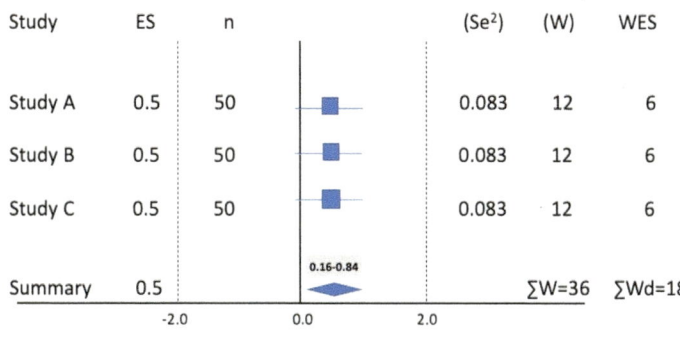

$$M_{meta} = \frac{\sum WES}{\sum W} = \frac{18}{36} = 0.5 \qquad Se_{meta}^2 = \frac{1}{\sum W} = \frac{1}{36} = 0.028$$

Fig. 6.4 Forest plot of meta-analysis III: fixed effect model. ES = effect size; n = sample size; Se^2 = variance; W = weighting method for effect size = $1/Se^2$; WES = weighted effect size = Wx ES; M_{meta} = mean ES of the meta-analysis; $\sum WES$ = sum of weighted ES, $\sum W$ = sum of weights; Se^2_{meta} = variance of the meta-analysis

The Random-Effect Model

The random model implies that, besides the within-study variability (Se^2), there is an additional variability between studies (T^2) because each estimates a different mean within the grand population. The total variability is the sum of both sampling error and the variability between the studies ($Se^2 + T^2$) "Eq. 6.18". Due to the increased total variability, the random model appears to be less precise than the fixed model but is more accurate, reflecting the true effect size in the population. We will apply the random effect model on meta-analysis III. Suppose that the between-study variability is equal to the within-study, the total variability of each study (Var_i) will be equal to the sum of both variabilities = 0.166 "Eq. 6.18". Consequently, the weighing inverse variance ($W_i = 1/0.166 = 6$) "Eq. 6.19″ and the weighted effect size ($WES_i = 0.5 \times 6 = 3$) will both be smaller than those calculated for a fixed model "Eq. 6.20".

$$Var_i = Se^2 + T^2 = 0.083 + 0.083 = 0.166 \tag{6.18}$$

$$W_i = \frac{1}{Se^2 + T^2} = \frac{1}{0.166} = 6 \tag{6.19}$$

$$WES_i = ES \times \frac{1}{Se^2 + T^2} = 0.5 \times \frac{1}{0.166} = 3 \tag{6.20}$$

The mean ES of the meta-analysis (M_{meta}) = sum of all weighted effect sizes divided by the total weights = 0.5 "Eq. 6.21". The variance of the meta-analysis is the reciprocal value of total weights = 1/18 = 0.055 "Eq. 6.22" and the Se is its square root value = 0.234 "Eq. 6.23". The 95% CI = 0.04 to 0.96 "Eq. 6.24". The random model gives a wider confidence interval and hence a less precise but more realistic estimation of ES. As expected, the calculated Z value is smaller than that calculated for the fixed model III and the P value is larger (P = 0.033); which increases the chances of type II error "Eq. 6.25". Figure 6.5 shows the forest plot graphic presentation.

$$M_{meta} = \frac{\sum WES}{\sum W} = \frac{3+3+3}{6+6+6} = 0.5 \tag{6.21}$$

$$Var_{meta} = \frac{1}{\sum W} = \frac{1}{6+6+6} = 0.055 \tag{6.22}$$

$$Se_{meta} = \sqrt{Var_{meta}} = \sqrt{0.055} = 0.234 \tag{6.23}$$

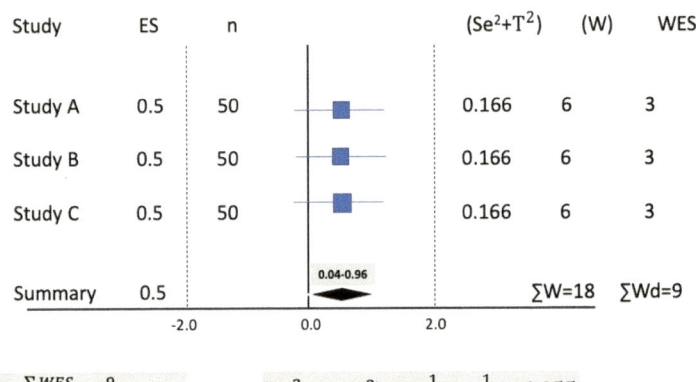

$$M_{meta} = \frac{\sum WES}{\sum W} = \frac{9}{18} = 0.5 \qquad (Se^2_{meta} + T^2) = \frac{1}{\sum W} = \frac{1}{18} = 0.055$$

Fig. 6.5 Forest plot of meta-analysis III (random-effect model). ES = effect size; n = sample size; T^2 = between-study variance, Se^2 = within-study variance; W = weighing method for effect size = $1/(T^2 + Se^2)$; WES = weighted effect size = Wx ES; M_{meta} = mean ES of the meta-analysis; $\sum WES$ = sum of weighed ES, $\sum W$ = sum of weights, ($Se^2_{meta} + T^2$) = variance of the meta-analysis

$$95\% \ \mathrm{CI} = \mathrm{M}_{meta} \pm 1.96 \,(\mathrm{Se}_{meta})$$
$$= 0.5 \pm 1.96(0.234) = 0.04 \,to\, 0.96$$
$$(6.24)$$

$$Z = \frac{M_{meta}}{\mathrm{Se}_{meta}} = \frac{0.5}{0.234} = 2.13. \qquad (6.25)$$

Graphic presentation: the forest plot

Meta-analyses are usually illustrated using a forest plot. Examples appear in Figs. 6.2, 6.3, 6.4 and 6.5. The forest plot is the graphic presentation of the weighted effect size of each study included plus a summary of weighted effect size estimate for the whole meta-analysis. Each estimate is presented as a block centralized along a horizontal line. The size of the block is proportional to weight assigned to the study and the arms represent the lower and upper 95% CI of the estimate. Estimates are usually placed in the order they were cited in the text and the block indicating the summary is usually placed at the bottom and has a unique shape, usually a diamond, for easier identification [31]. The plot usually shows the study ID, including author name and year of publication, effect size, sample size, weight proportion (study weight/total weights), indicators of heterogeneity (Q-statistics, P-value, and I2), and the P-value of the weighted summary.

Note that the confidence interval depicts the range of intervention effects compatible with the study's result. The larger the block and the narrower the confidence interval, the more weight is given to the study. As shown in Figs. 6.4 and 6.5, the blocks of the three studies are of equal size, reflecting the equal weights given to each of them for being of similar size and equal variance [31].

6.2.6.2 Calculation of Individual Effect Sizes

In this section, we will present the most commonly used effect sizes, whether expressing correlation (Pearson's correlation coefficient), proportions (odds ratio, relative risk, and hazard ratio), or unpaired and paired differences (unstandardized and standardized means of the

differences and Hedges g). We will give one detailed example for each category, as other members of the same category are calculated similarly, except for a few details, which will be noted too. We will discuss each example under the two main assumptions: the fixed and random-effects models. We will provide a detailed example for Pearson's correlation coefficient (see Sect. 6.2.6.2.1), unpaired standardized mean of the difference (see Sect. 6.2.6.2.4), and relative risk (see Sect. 6.2.6.2.8).

The procedure is the same, regardless of the effect size category. If necessary, we start by polishing the effect size to create a reliable standard error. The next step is to weigh the effect size with inverse variance and combine the weighted effect sizes of all clinical studies to compute a mean value and a standard error and create a 95% CI. A simple Z test verifies the statistical significance of the effect size. Calculations are lengthy but straightforward and usually performed by dedicated software. As an example, we will present and explain all the necessary equations and then polish and weigh the effect size of the first included study. The calculations of the remaining studies will be precisely the same. The next step will be calculating the total weights, total weighted means, and mean effect size. The same will be applied to calculate the standard error. We will verify the results by dedicated software, generating the forest plot.

Another point is the calculation of the variance between studies (Tau-squared: T^2) used to weigh the effect size in a random-effects model. Several methods are used to produce (T^2), and in our book, we adopt the most commonly used and easiest method proposed by DerSimonian and Laird. In the actual section, we will only give the value of (T^2) provided by the software to avoid interrupting the flow of effect size calculations. We will give the details of (T^2), whether calculated by DerSimonian and Laird method or else separately (see Sect. 6.2.7.3).

Many dedicated and few general statistical software are capable of performing a meta-analysis. Paid software offers a free trial for a limited period, such as the dedicated

Comprehensive meta-analysis, STATA, and the recent 28th version of IBM-SPSS software. Commonly recommended free software includes RevMan of Cochran collaboration (RevMan) and software-based upon R-programing such as the metafor package [32], Jamovi [33], JASP [34] and OpenmetaAnalyst [35]. RevMan is an excellent complete program for performing systematic reviews and meta-analyses. As the main aim of this section is limited to the calculations of meta-analysis, using RevMan necessitates the discussion of too many details before reaching those calculations, which can complicate our main aim. The excellent metafor package necessitates knowledge of R-programing, which is beyond the scope of this book. We were left with the simple software that goes directly to the calculations and does not necessitate any back knowledge of R-programing it-self, namely Jamovi [33], JASP [34], and OpenmetaAnalyst [35]. It may not be the perfect approach, but we thought that it best suits our primary audience: the young researcher and the interested busy biologist. Both are pretty easy to use and hardly need any learning curve.

Pearson Correlation Coefficient r
Polishing and Normalizing r

In case the correlation coefficient r is being used as an effect size, the slight positive bias can be first corrected (deflated) "Eq. 6.26". The corrected r (rc) or, (r) itself when used as such, is then normalized using Fisher's r to Z transformation "Eq. 6.27" (see Sect. 2.6.1.1). We calculate the variance of Z as the reciprocal value of the sample size minus three $(1/n-3)$ "Eq. 6.28". We remind the reader that the normalized correlation coefficient (variance of Z) used here to weigh Z is not the same as the variance of the correlation coefficient r itself, which is calculated by a totally different equation "Eq. 2.85".

$$r_c = r - \left[\frac{r - (1 - r^2)}{2(n - 3)}\right] \quad (6.26)$$

$$Z = \frac{1}{2}\log\frac{1 + r_c}{1 - r_c} \quad (6.27)$$

$$\mathrm{Var}\, Z = \frac{1}{n - 3} \quad (6.28)$$

Weighing the Normalized r (Z)

The normalized r (Z) is then weighted by the reciprocal value of the total variance: the variance of Z in a fixed model (W) "Eq. 6.29" or, the reciprocal value of the sum of the variance of z and (T^2) in a random-effects model (WR) "Eq. 6.30". We repeat the calculation of weighted ES for all the studies included in the meta-analysis.

$$WZ_i = Z_i \times \frac{1}{Var_{zi}} \quad (6.29)$$

$$W^R Z_i = Z_i \times \frac{1}{Var_{zi} + \mathrm{T}^2} \quad (6.30)$$

Calculating the Mean Effect Size

The mean effect size of the meta-analysis itself (Mean Z) can now be calculated as the sum of weighted effect sizes for the (i) studies ($\sum W_i Z_i$), divided by the sum of weights ($\sum W_i$) "Eq. 6.31". The Se of the mean effect size (Se_Z) is the square root of the reciprocal value of the sum of weights "Eq. 6.32". W is substituted with WR in the random-effects model as in "Eq. 6.30".

$$\mathrm{Mean}\, Z = \frac{\sum W_i Z_i}{\sum W_i} \quad (6.31)$$

$$\mathrm{Se}\, Z = \sqrt{\frac{1}{\sum W_i}} \quad (6.32)$$

Calculating the 95% CI and P value

As usual, we calculate a 95% CI of (Mean Z) "Eq. 6.33" and test its statistical significance by the Z equation "Eq. 6.34". The effect size is statistically significant whenever the produced z score is ≥ 1.96. We have to be careful in appreciating the difference between (Z) as the normalized Fisher's value of correlation coefficient r (see Sect. 4.7.1.1) and the z score used for testing the statistical significance of any normally distributed value (see Sect. 1.4.1).

$$95\% \ CI = \text{M}ean \ Z \pm 1.96 \ (\text{Se } Z) \quad (6.33)$$

$$z \ score = \frac{\text{Mean } Z}{\text{Se } Z} \quad (6.34)$$

Converting r to the Original Scale

In order to report the results, the normalized r (Z), as well as the upper and lower limits of the 95% CI, are then converted back to r, using "Eq. 6.35" (see Sect. 2.6.1.1).

$$r = \frac{e^{2z_r} - 1}{e^{2z_r} + 1} \quad (6.35)$$

Some statisticians omit the first step of correcting r "Eq. 6.26" and go straight to normalizing r by Fisher's transformation [3]. Hunter and Schmidt have a different approach to r that does not include normalization nor weighing by inverse variance [2] (see Sect. 6.3).

A Working Example

1. *The fixed effect model*

A meta-analysis was conducted to assess the correlation between the duration of surgery and the amount of blood loss. The meta-analysis combined the results of five studies, all expressing the effect size in terms of Pearson's correlation coefficient. For training purposes, we will first calculate the effect size assuming a fixed model effect (Table 6.3) and then repeat the calculations adopting random model effects (Table 6.4). For simplicity, we will omit the step of polishing r [36], which had a trivial effect in our example anyway.

- Calculation of the weighted effect size of individual studies

We will begin with the first study (study A) and calculate Fisher's normalized r (Zi)

"Eq. 6.36", then the variance of Z (Var Zi) "Eq. 6.37". We weight the effect size by the inverse variance (Wi), then we calculate the weighted effect size as the product of normalized Z by the inverse variance (WiZi) "Eq. 6.38". We repeat the calculations for the remaining four studies (not shown).

$$Z_i = \frac{1}{2}\log\frac{1+r}{1-r} = \frac{1}{2}\log\frac{1+0.1}{1-0.1} = 0.1 \quad (6.36)$$

$$Var \ Z_i = \frac{1}{n_i - 3} = \frac{1}{50 - 3} = 0.021 \quad (6.37)$$

$$W_i Z_i = Z_i \times \frac{1}{Var \ Z_i} = 0.1 \times \frac{1}{0.021} = 4.7 \quad (6.38)$$

- Calculation of the mean effect size and the standard error

We calculate the mean effect size (Mean Z) as the sum of the weighted effect sizes divided by the sum of weights "Eq. 6.39", and we calculate its Se (Se Z) as the square root of the reciprocal value of the sum of weights "Eq. 6.40".

$$\text{Mean } Z = \frac{\sum W_i \ Z_i}{\sum W_i} = \frac{238}{465} = 0.51 \quad (6.39)$$

$$\text{Se } Z = \sqrt{\frac{1}{\sum W_i}} = \sqrt{\frac{1}{465}} = 0.046 \quad (6.40)$$

- Creation of the 95% CI and testing statistical significance

As usual, we can assign a 95% CI around (mean Z) "Eq. 6.41" and test the statistical significance of Z by dividing the mean by its Se "Eq. 6.42".

$$\begin{aligned} 95\% \ CI &= \text{Mean } Z \pm 1.96 \ (Se \ Z) \\ &= 0.51 \pm 1.96 \ (0.046) \\ &= 0.423 - 0.604 \end{aligned} \quad (6.41)$$

$$z \ score = \frac{0.51}{0.046} = 11.1; P < 0.001 \quad (6.42)$$

Table 6.3 Pearson's correlation coefficient: the duration of surgery and the amount of blood loss, fixed effect model

Study ID	n_i	r_i	Zi	Var Zi	Wi	WiZi
A	50	0.1	0.1	0.021	47	4.7
B	80	0.2	0.2	0.013	77	15.4
C	100	0.4	0.42	0.01	97	40.7
D	200	0.6	0.69	0.005	197	136
E	50	0.7	0.87	0.021	47	41
Total				0.07	465	237

n_i = sample size, r_i = Pearson's correlation coefficient, Zi = Fisher's normalized correlation coefficient, Var Zi = variance of Zi, Wi = weighting factor (inverse variance), WiZi = weighed normalized correlation coefficient

- Conversion of the normalized values to the original scale for presentation

Finally, we need to convert the normalized r and the lower and upper limits of the 95% CI into the original scale for proper interpretation. Equation 6.43 shows the result of converting the mean r value "Eq. 6.43". There was a statistically significant positive correlation between the amount of blood loss and the duration of surgery; the mean r was 0.47 (0.40 and 0.54); (P < 0.001).

$$r = \frac{e^{2z} - 1}{e^{2z} + 1} = \frac{e^{2 \times 0.51} - 1}{e^{2 \times 0.51} + 1} = \frac{2.77 - 1}{2.77 + 1} = \frac{1.77}{3.77}$$
$$= 0.47$$

(6.43)

- Graphic presentation: the forest plot

Figure 6.6 shows the forest plot of the fixed-effect model (Fig. 6.6). Depending upon the software, values can be displayed in the normalized scale, as in our example or in the usual scale of r. Note that Q, I^2, and other indices of heterogeneity will be explained separately (see Sect. 6.2.7).

2. *The random effects model*

We will repeat the same calculations, assuming a random-effects model (Table 6.4). Note that the effect size is weighted by the reciprocal value of the total variance formed of the sum of the study's variance and the variance between the

studies. As will be shown later, the variability between studies (T^2) can be calculated by different methods, and the one adopted in this chapter is the one that is the most commonly used (DerSimonian and Laird). In our example, we will be satisfied by giving the result of (T^2), which is equal to 0.072. The calculation details are presented elsewhere (see Sect. 6.2.7.3).

- Calculation of the weighted effect size of individual studies

Returning to Study A, the weighted effect size of a random model is calculated by the following equation "Eq. 6.44":

$$W_i^R Z_i = Z_i \times \frac{1}{Var_{zi} + T^2} = 0.1 \times \frac{1}{0.021 + 0.072}$$
$$= 10.75$$

(6.44)

- Calculation of the mean effect size and the standard error

We repeat the calculations for the remaining four studies (not shown). We calculate the mean effect size (Mean Z^R) as the sum of the weighted effect sizes divided by the sum of weights "Eq. 6.45" and its Se (Se Z^R) as the square root of the reciprocal value of the sum of weights "Eq. 6.46".

$$\text{Mean } Z^R = \frac{\sum W_i^R Z_i}{\sum W_i^R} = \frac{26.7}{58.46} = 0.46 \quad (6.45)$$

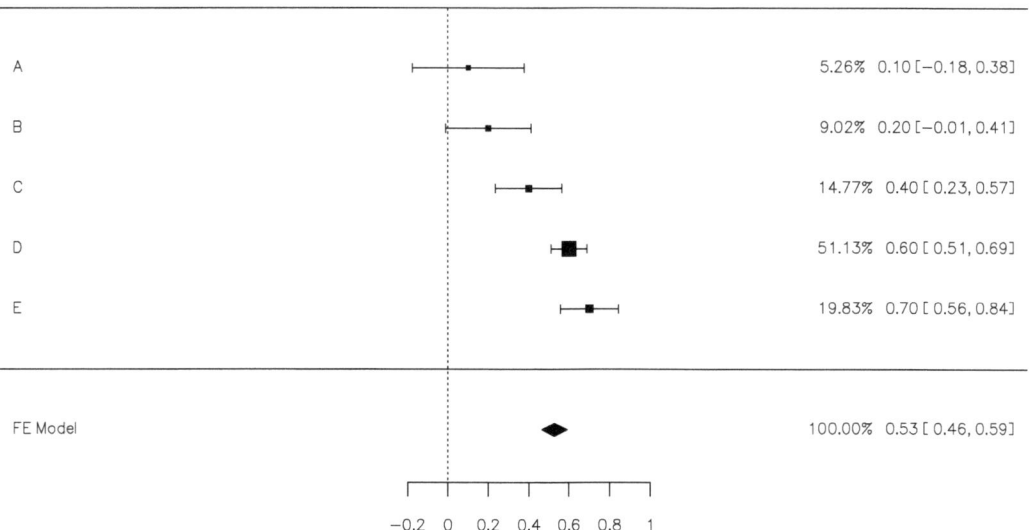

Fig. 6.6 Forest plot: Pearson's correlation coefficient relating the amount of blood loss and the duration of hospital stay, fixed effect model (FE). Values (95% CI) are presented as normalized Fisher's values. Q = 28.48, df = 4, P < 0.001, I^2 = 85.96%

Table 6.4 Pearson's correlation coefficient: the duration of surgery and the amount of blood loss random effects model

Study ID	n_i	r_i	Z_i	Var $Z_i + T^2$	W_i^R	$W_iZ_i^R$
A	50	0.1	0.1	0.021 + 0.072	10.75	0.96
B	80	0.2	0.2	0.013 + 0.072	11.76	2.35
C	100	0.4	0.42	0.01 + 0.072	12.2	5.1
D	200	0.6	0.69	0.005 + 0.072	13	8.97
E	50	0.7	0.87	0.021 + 0.072	10.75	9.35
Total				0.07 + 0.072	58.46	26.7

n_i = sample size, r_i = Pearson's correlation coefficient, Zi = Fisher's normalized correlation coefficient, Var Zi = within-study variance of Zi, T^2 = Tau-square variance between studies, W_i^R = weighting inverse variance of random model, $W_iZ_i^R$ = weighed normalized correlation coefficient of random model

$$Se \; Z^R = \sqrt{\frac{1}{\sum W_i^R}} = \sqrt{\frac{1}{58.46}} = 0.13 \quad (6.46)$$

- Creation of the 95% CI and testing statistical significance

As usual, we can assign a 95% CI around (Mean Z) "Eq. 6.47" and test the statistical significance of Z by dividing the mean by its Se (Se Z) "Eq. 6.48".

$$95\% \; CI \; Z^R = Mean \; Z^R \pm 1.96 \; (Se \; Z^R)$$
$$= 0.46 \pm 1.96 \, (0.13) \quad (6.47)$$
$$= 0.204 - 0.718$$

$$z \, score = \frac{0.46}{0.13} = 3.52; P < 0.001 \quad (6.48)$$

- Conversion of the normalized values to the original scale for presentation

Finally, we need to convert the normalized r and the lower and upper limits of the 95% CI into the original scale for proper interpretation. Equation 6.49 shows the result of converting the mean r value "Eq. 6.49". There was a statistically significant positive correlation between the amount of blood loss and the duration of surgery; the mean r was 0.43 (0.20 and 0.62); (P < 0.001). As expected, the CI of a random model is broader than that of a fixed-effect model, reflecting more uncertainty.

$$r = \frac{e^{2z} - 1}{e^{2z} + 1} = \frac{e^{2 \times 0.46} - 1}{e^{2 \times 0.46} + 1} = \frac{2.51 - 1}{2.51 + 1} = \frac{1.51}{3.51}$$
$$= 0.43$$

$$(6.49)$$

- Graphic presentation: the forest plot

Figure 6.7 shows the forest plot of the random-effects model (Fig. 6.7), with the values being expressed in terms of normalized r (Z). Note that Q and I2 and other indices of heterogeneity will be explained separately (see Sect. 6.2.7).

Unstandardized (Raw) Mean of the Difference: Unpaired Design

A good indication of using the raw difference between two means is when all studies included in the meta-analysis use the same continuous scale. In case of two studies with mean values μ_a and μ_b, variances S^2_a and S^2_a and of sample size n_a and n_b; the difference between the two means is simply equal to: $\mu_a - \mu_b$ "Eq. 6.50". The calculation of the variance of the difference is dependent upon whether the two populations are assumed to have equal variances or not. Assuming equality of variances, we calculate a pooled variance first "Eq. 6.51" that is then used to estimate the variance of the difference "Eq. 6.52". In cases both variances are assumed to be significantly different from one another, we calculate the variance of the difference directly from both variances "Eq. 6.53". In either case, the Se of the difference is the square root of the calculated variance "Eq. 6.54", as usual.

$$d = \mu_a - \mu_b \qquad (6.50)$$

$$S^2_{pooled} = \frac{S^2_a(n_a - 1) + S^2_b(n_b - 1)}{(n_a + n_b - 2)} \qquad (6.51)$$

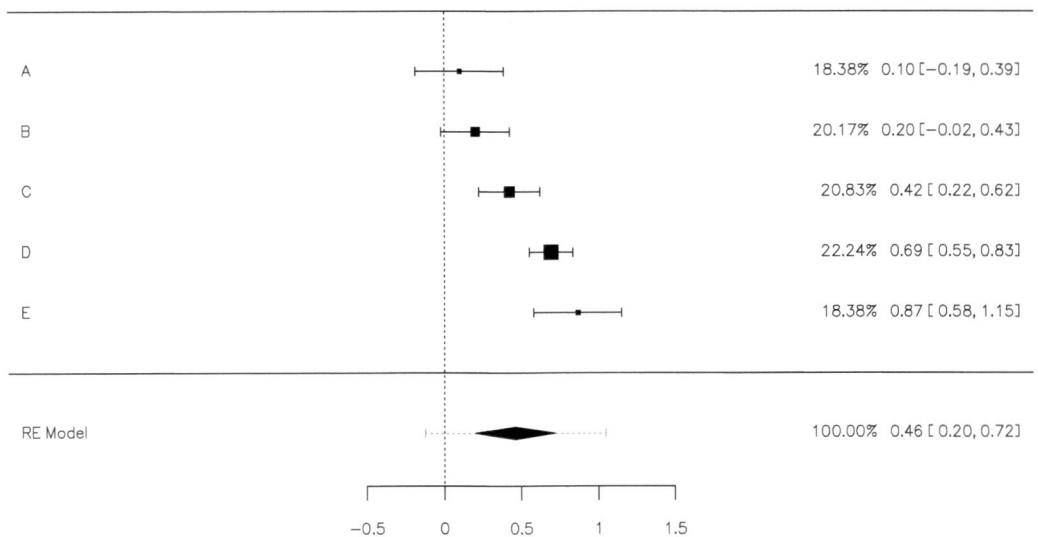

A		18.38% 0.10 [−0.19, 0.39]
B		20.17% 0.20 [−0.02, 0.43]
C		20.83% 0.42 [0.22, 0.62]
D		22.24% 0.69 [0.55, 0.83]
E		18.38% 0.87 [0.58, 1.15]
RE Model		100.00% 0.46 [0.20, 0.72]

−0.5   0   0.5   1   1.5

Fig. 6.7 Forest plot: Pearson's correlation coefficient between the amount of blood loss and the duration of hospital stay, random effect model (RE). Values and 95% CI are presented as normalized Fisher's values. Q = 28.48, df = 4, P < 0.001, I^2 = 85.96%

$$\text{Var d} = S^2_{pooled} \frac{n_a + n_b}{n_a \times n_b} \quad (6.52)$$

$$\text{Var d} = \frac{S^2_a}{n_a} + \frac{S^2_b}{n_b} \quad (6.53)$$

$$\text{Se d} = \sqrt{\text{Var d}} \quad (6.54)$$

- Calculation of the weighted effect size of individual studies

In a fixed-effect model, we calculate the weighted effect size of each study by multiplying the effect size (d) by the weighting factor, which is the inverse variance (W = 1/Var) "Eq. 6.55". In a random-effects model, the weighting factor is the reciprocal value of the sum of the study's variance and the variance between studies. $W^R = 1/(\text{Var} + T^2)$ "Eq. 6.56". We repeat the calculations for all the included studies.

$$Wd_i = d_i \times \frac{1}{\text{Var d}} \quad (6.55)$$

$$W^R d_i = d_i \times \frac{1}{\text{Var d} + T^2} \quad (6.56)$$

- Calculation of the mean effect size and the standard error

As in the general equation, we compute the average unstandardized mean difference by dividing the summed weighted effect sizes by the

sum of weights (sum of inverse variances) "Eq. 6.57". The Se of the difference is the square root of its variance "Eq. 6.58". In the random-effects model, we substitute W with W^R

$$Mean\ d = \frac{\sum W_i\ d_i}{\sum W_i} \quad (6.57)$$

$$Se\ d = \sqrt{\frac{1}{\sum W_i}} \quad (6.58)$$

- Creation of the 95% CI and testing statistical significance

We follow the same procedure, construct a 95% CI around the calculated mean "Eq. 6.59", and test its statistical significance by the Z equation, as shown in the general approach "Eq. 6.60". A Z score $\geq$ 1.96 denotes a statistically significant effect size.

$$95\%\ CI = Mean_d \pm 1.96(Se_d) \quad (6.59)$$

$$Z\ score = \frac{Mean\ d}{Se\ d} \quad (6.60)$$

A Working Example

1. *The fixed effect model*

Table 6.5 shows the results of six studies included in a fixed-effect model meta-analysis comparing the duration of hospital stay between minimally invasive and conventional open-heart

Table 6.5 The row mean difference between the durations of hospital stay following minimally invasive and conventional open-heart surgery, fixed effect model

Study	Na	Ma	Sda	Nb	Mb	Sdb	d	Vard	W	Wd	Wd^2
A	60	7	1.1	60	12	1.5	−5	0.057	17.4	−86.96	435
B	65	7	1.2	65	10	1.2	−3	0.044	22.7	−68.2	204
C	100	6	0.5	100	8	2	−2	0.042	23.5	−47.1	94
D	200	6	0.5	200	8	2.1	−2	0.023	42.9	−85.83	172
E	50	9	1	50	7	3	2	0.2	5	10	20
F	90	5	2	90	11	3.1	−6	0.15	6.66	−40	240
Total									118.2	−317	1165

Na and Nb, Ma and Mb, Sda and Sdb = sample size, mean and standard deviation of hospital stay in group a and group b patients. Vard = variance of the difference, W = the weighing unit (inverse variance), Wd = weighted difference, Wd^2 = W × d^2

surgery. The effect size was the row mean of the difference.

- Calculation of the weighted effect size of individual studies

The effect size is weighted by the inverse variance. For example, the weighed effect size of manuscript A is computed as in "Eq. 6.61". We repeat the calculations for the other five manuscripts (see Table 6.5)

$$W_i d_i = d_i \times \frac{1}{Var_{di}} = -5 \times \frac{1}{17.4} = -86.96$$
$$(6.61)$$

- Calculation of the mean effect size and the standard error

We repeat the calculations for the other five manuscripts (see Table 6.5), and the mean effect size is computed as the sum of weighted differences divided by the sum of weights "Eq. 6.62". The Se is the square root of the reciprocal value of the sum of weights "Eq. 6.63".

$$Mean\ d = \frac{\sum W_i d_i}{\sum W_i} = \frac{-317}{118.16} = -2.69 \quad (6.62)$$

$$Se\ d = \sqrt{\frac{1}{\sum W_i}} = \sqrt{\frac{1}{118.16}} = 0.092 \quad (6.63)$$

- Creation of the 95% CI and testing statistical significance

The 95% CI of the difference is calculated by assigning 1.96 Se on either side of the mean "Eq. 6.64". A usual Z test tests the statistical significance of the difference "Eq. 6.65". In conclusion, the mean hospital stays of patients benefiting from minimally invasive techniques

were significantly shorter than those calculated after conventional surgery; P < 0.001.

$$\begin{aligned} 95\%\ CI &= Mean\ d \pm 1.96\ (Se\ d) \\ &= -2.69 \pm 1.96\ (0.092) \\ &= -2.867\ to\ -2.51 \end{aligned} \quad (6.64)$$

$$z\ score = \frac{-2.69}{0.092} = -29.2 \quad (6.65)$$

- Graphic presentation: the forest plot

The forest plot of the study is shown in Fig. 6.8. Note that Q and I^2 and other heterogeneity indices will be explained separately (see Sect. 6.2.7).

2. *The random effect model*

Table 6.6 shows the results of a random effect model, the weighing variance ($Var d^R$) is the sum of both: the within-group variance shown in Table 6.5 (Vard) and the between-group variances (T^2). As previously noted, (T^2) can be calculated by different methods and the one adopted in this chapter is the most commonly used method proposed by DerSimonian and Laird (DerSimonian and Laird). In our example, (T^2) was equal to 3.37, but the calculation details will be presented separately (see Sect. 6.2.7.3).

- Calculation of the weighted effect size of individual studies

Returning to Study A, the weighed effect size of a random model is calculated as in "Eq. 6.66". We repeat the calculations for the other five manuscripts (see Table 6.6)

$$\begin{aligned} W_i^R d_i &= d_i \times \frac{1}{Var\ d_i + T^2} = -5 \times \frac{1}{3.42} \\ &= -1.46 \end{aligned} \quad (6.66)$$

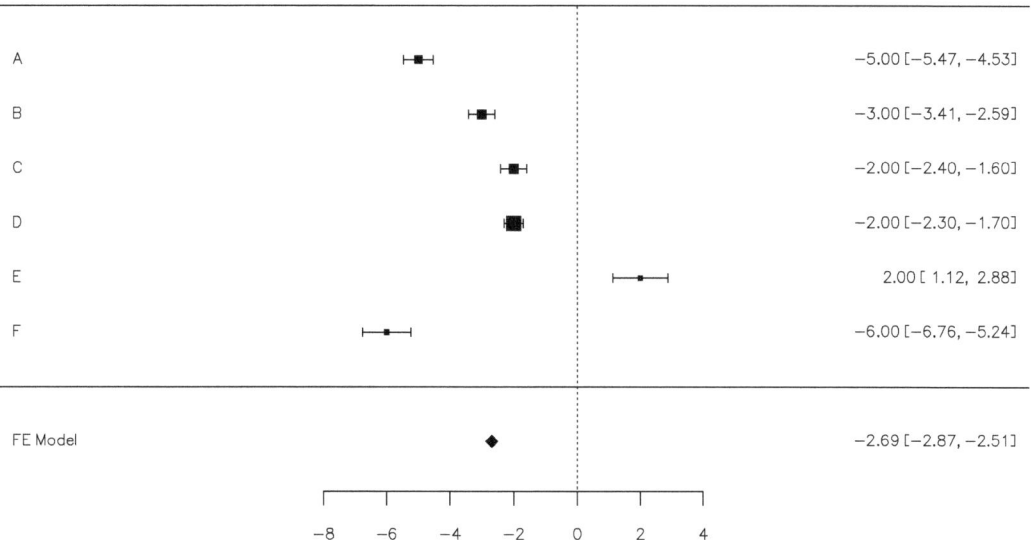

Fig. 6.8 Forest plot: the row mean difference of hospital stays (95% CI), fixed effect model (FE) Q = 308.7, df = 5, P < 0.001, I^2 = 98.38%

Table 6.6 The row mean difference between the durations of hospital stay following minimally invasive and conventional open-heart surgery, random effects model

Study	Na	Ma	Sda	Nb	Mb	Sdb	d	Vard^R	W^R	Wd^R
A	60	7	1.1	60	12	1.5	−5	3.42	0.29	−1.46
B	65	7	1.2	65	10	1.2	−3	3.41	0.29	−0.88
C	100	6	0.5	100	8	2	−2	3.41	0.29	−0.57
D	200	6	0.5	200	8	2.1	−2	3.39	0.29	−0.57
E	50	9	1	50	7	3	2	3.57	0.28	0.56
F	90	5	2	90	11	3.1	−6	3.52	0.28	−1.7
Total									1.72	4.62

Na and Nb, Ma and Mb, Sda and Sdb = sample size, mean and standard deviation of hospital stay in group a and group b patients, Vard^R = variance of the difference for the random model = within group variance plus variance between groups (T^2 = 3.37), W^R = the weighing unit of random model (1/Vard^R), Wd^R = weighted difference for the random model, W^{R}d^2 = W^R × d^2

- Calculation of the mean effect size and the standard error

The average effect size is calculated as the sum of weighted differences divided by the sum of weights "Eq. 6.67". The Se is the square root of the reciprocal value of the sum of weights "Eq. 6.68".

$$Mean\ d^R = \frac{\sum W_i^R d_i}{\sum W_i^R} = \frac{-4.62}{1.72} = -2.68$$

$$(6.67)$$

$$Se\ d^R = \sqrt{\frac{1}{\sum W_i}} = \sqrt{\frac{1}{1.72}} = 0.76 \quad (6.68)$$

- Creation of the 95% CI and testing statistical significance

The 95% CI of the difference is calculated by assigning 1.96 Se on either side of the mean difference "Eq. 6.69". Note that all calculations are executed with the larger random model variance ($Vard^R$). The mean value does not change much but the confidence interval is much wider. A usual Z test tests the statistical significance of the difference "Eq. 6.70". In conclusion, the mean hospital stays of patients benefiting from minimally invasive techniques were significantly shorter than those calculated after conventional surgery; P < 0.001.

$$95\%\ \ CI = Mean\ d^R \pm 1.96\left(Se\ d^R\right)$$
$$= -2.68 \pm 1.96\ (0.76)$$
$$= -4.17\ to\ -1.19 \tag{6.69}$$

$$Z\ score = \frac{-2.68}{0.76} = -3.54 \tag{6.70}$$

- Graphic presentation: the forest plot

The forest plot of the study is shown in Fig. 6.9. Note that Q, I^2, and T^2 and other heterogeneity indices will be explained separately (see Sect. 6.2.7).

Unstandardized (Raw) Mean Difference: Paired Design

In case the patient was compared to himself, as in pre-to-post studies, as well as in the case of a matched group design, the magnitude of the effect size depends on the correlation between both measurements (see Sect. 2.4.1.3). Suppose two measurements with mean values μ_a and μ_b, variances S^2_a and S^2_a, standard deviations of S_a and S_b, and sample sizes n_a and n_b. The estimates of the average paired difference ($Mean_{dp}$), and the variance of the difference (Var_{dp}) is calculated by "Eq. 6.71" and "Eq. 6.72". Note that the variance in the equation depends on the presence of a positive correlation between the paired measurements. The Se of the difference is the square root of the variance "Eq. 6.73," and the 95% CI of the paired difference is calculated by assigning 1.96 Se on either side of the mean "Eq. 6.74".

$$Mean\ d_p = \mu_a - \mu_b \tag{6.71}$$
$$Var\ d_p = \left(S^2_a + S^2_b\right) - 2 \times r \times S_aS_b \tag{6.72}$$
$$Se\ d_p = \sqrt{Var\ d_p} \tag{6.73}$$
$$95\%\ \ CI = Mean\ d_p \pm 1.96\left(Se\ d_p\right) \tag{6.74}$$

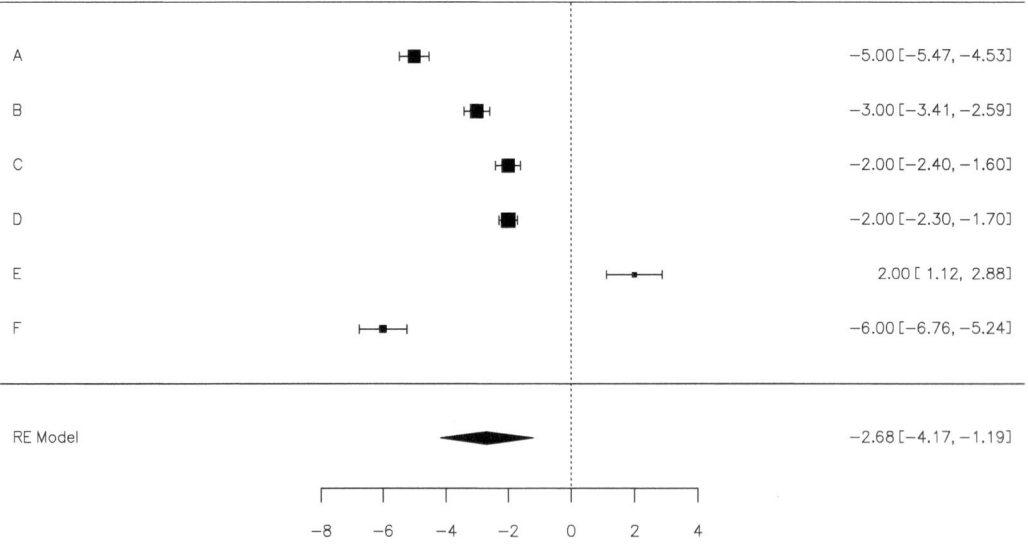

A	−5.00 [−5.47, −4.53]
B	−3.00 [−3.41, −2.59]
C	−2.00 [−2.40, −1.60]
D	−2.00 [−2.30, −1.70]
E	2.00 [1.12, 2.88]
F	−6.00 [−6.76, −5.24]
RE Model	−2.68 [−4.17, −1.19]

Fig. 6.9 Forest plot: the row mean difference of hospital stay (95% CI), random effect model (RE). Q = 308.7, df = 5, P < 0.001, T^2 = 3.37. I^2 = 98.38%

Standardized Mean of the Difference (SMD): Unpaired Design

In the case of a quantitative outcome, the effect size is usually calculated as Cohen ds or hedges g. Note that Cohen ds was initially described to express the standardized difference between the means of the population. However, it is commonly used to express the difference between the means (μ_1 and μ_2) of two samples (n_1 and n_2), standardized by the pooled Se "Eq. 6.75". The latter is calculated from both groups' variances and sample sizes "Eq. 6.76" (see Sect. 4.2.1.1).

$$Cohen\ ds = \frac{(\mu_1 - \mu_2)}{\sqrt{S^2_{pooled}}} \qquad (6.75)$$

$$S^2_{pooled} = \frac{S^2_1(n_1 - 1) + S^2_2(n_2 - 1)}{(n_1 + n_2 - 2)} \qquad (6.76)$$

- Calculation of the weighted effect size of individual studies

In a fixed-effect model, the effect size of each study has to be weighted by the inverse variance (W = 1/Var_d), calculated by squaring both sides of "Eq. 4.13" presented in Sect. 4.2.1.1 "Eq. 6.77". In a random effect model, the weighing unknit (W^R) is the reciprocal value of the sum of the within-study variability (Var_d) and in the variability between study (T^2). In either model, the effect size is weighted by being multiplied by the appropriate inverse variance "Eqs. 6.78" and "6.79."

$$Var\ d_i = \frac{n_1 + n_2}{n_1 n_2} + \frac{d^2}{2(n_1 + n_2)} \qquad (6.77)$$

$$Wd_i = d_i \times \frac{1}{Var\ d_i} \qquad (6.78)$$

$$W^R d_i = d_i \times \frac{1}{Var\ d_i + T^2} \qquad (6.79)$$

- Calculation of the mean effect size and standard error

The weighted effect size is calculated for each study included in the meta-analysis. As in the general equation, the mean SMD is computed as the sum of weighted SMD divided by the sum of all weights (sum of inverse variances) "Eq. 6.80". The Se of the mean effect size is the square root of the variance "Eq. 6.81". In random effects model, W is substituted with W^R.

$$Mean\ d = \frac{\sum W_i\ d_i}{\sum W_i} \qquad (6.80)$$

$$Se\ d = \sqrt{\frac{1}{\sum W_i}} \qquad (6.81)$$

- Creation of the 95% CI and testing statistical significance

We follow the same procedure and construct a 95% CI around the calculated mean ES (mean ± 1.96 $\sqrt{Var_d}$) "Eq. 6.82" and test its statistical significance by the Z equation "Eq. 6.83", as shown in the general approach. A Z score >1.96 denotes a statistically significant effect size.

$$95\%\ CI = Mean\ d \pm 1.96\ (Se\ d) \qquad (6.82)$$

$$z\ score = \frac{Mean\ d}{Se\ d} \qquad (6.83)$$

Hedges g

In the case of small sample size (small number of manuscripts), Hedges and Olkin suggested that Cohen's (ds) overestimates the difference, and hence, it has to be corrected (deflated) by being multiplied by a factor (J) "Eq. 6.84". Equally, the variance of Cohen d "Eq. 6.85" can be corrected by being multiplied by (J^2). The reason is that Cohen d was essentially described for the population and not for the samples. As we calculate the sample parameters, it seems more logical to use and report the corrected Hedges g. We have to note that the equation to calculate the term (J) is an approximation of what was reported by Hedges and Olkin, and there are other different variations of the equation, such as replacing the denominator $4(n_1 + n_2) - 9$ by $4(n_1 + n_2) - 1$ or $4(n_1 + n_2 - 2)$ and up to disregarding (J^2) for being always very near to unity [3]. Borenstein and colleagues suggested that in practice those differences are usually minor and negligible [3].

$$H\,edges\,g = Cohen\,ds \times J$$
$$= ds\left(1 - \frac{3}{4(n_1+n_2)-9}\right) \quad (6.84)$$

$$Var\,g = Var_d \times J^2$$
$$= Var_d\left(1 - \frac{3}{4(n_1+n_2)-9}\right)^2 \quad (6.85)$$

The rest is similar to what we have just presented before. We proceed as usual by calculating the effect size for each of the studies included in the meta-analysis. The new effect size must be weighed by the inverse variance in the fixed model (W) and by the reciprocal value of the sum of the inverse variance of the study plus the variance between studies (T^2) in the random-effects model (W^R). We calculate the mean ES as the sum of all weighted effect sizes, divided by the sum of weights, and the Se of the effect size as the square root of the inverse sum of weights. We construct the usual 95% CI around the mean ES and test its statistical significance by a Z test: Z = mean ES/Se, which should produce a minimum value of 1.96 to declare a statistically significant effect size.

Standardized Mean of the Difference (SMD): Paired Design

In matched group or pre-post scores studies, the effect size is Cohen dz, calculated from the standardized mean of the differences between a series of two paired measures of mean values u_1 and u_2, standard deviations Sd_1 and Sd_2 and correlation coefficient r "Eq. 6.86". The equation clearly shows that the more the two measures positively correlate, the larger the ES is (see Sect. 4.5.1.1). We calculate the effect size variance as in "Eq. 6.87".

$$Cohen\,d_z = \frac{M_{diff}}{Sd_{diff}} = \frac{\mu_1 - \mu_2}{\sqrt{Sd_1^2 + Sd_2^2 - 2rSd_1Sd_2}} \quad (6.86)$$

$$Var\,d_z = \left(\frac{1}{n} + \frac{d_z^2}{2n}\right)2(1-r) \quad (6.87)$$

The ES of each study is weighted (W) by the reciprocal of its variance ($1/Var_{dz}$) in a fixed-effect model "Eq. 6.88", to which we have to add (T^2) in random-effects model (W^R) "Eq. 6.89". We calculate the weighted effect size for each study included in the meta-analysis.

$$Wd_z = d_z \times \frac{1}{Var\,d_z} \quad (6.88)$$

$$W^R d_i = d_i \times \frac{1}{Var\,d_z + T^2} \quad (6.89)$$

We complete the procedure by calculating the average effect size as the sum of all weighted ES divided by the sum of weights. The Standard error is the square root of the reciprocal value of the sum of weights. As usual, we construct a 95% CI and test its statistical significance by the Z equation.

In the case of a small number of studies, we can correct Cohen dz and its variance as we did in the case of unpaired design. The denominator of the correction factor (J) has to be changed by changing the degrees of freedom from ($n_1 + n_2$) to ($n - 1$) "Eqs. 6.90" and "6.91". The remaining of the procedure is as before.

$$H\,edges\,g = dz \times J = dz\left(1 - \frac{3}{4(n-1)}\right) \quad (6.90)$$

$$Var\,g = Var\,d_z \times J^2 = Var\,d_z\left(1 - \frac{3}{4(n-1)}\right)^2 \quad (6.91)$$

The Odds Ratio

We have pointed out that the odds ratio, the relative risk (see Sect. 1.8.2), and the hazard ratio (see Sect. 1.8.3) are not normally distributed. Converting those ratios into the logarithmic scale allows for the calculation of a proper Se, creating

Table 6.7 Calculation of the risk and the odds

	Event (+)	No event (−)	Total
Treatment group	(a)	(b)	(a + b = n_t)
Control group	(c)	(d)	(c + d = n_c)
Total	(a + c)	(b + d)	N

(a) and (b) = number of cases with events and number of cases without events in the treatment group, (c) and (d) = number of cases with events and number of cases without events in the control group, (n_t) and (n_c) = total number of cases in the treatment group and in the control group. N = total sample size

a 95% CI and testing the statistical significance of the effect size (see Sect. 1.8.7). The odds ratio is the ratio between the odds of having/not having the event in the treatment group and the same odds in the control group = ad/cb (see Table 1.4) "Eq. 6.92". As the OR is not following a normal distribution, calculations are usually made on the logarithmic scale. The variance of the log OR_i of a study (i) equals the sum of the four reciprocal values "Eq. 6.93" (see Table 6.7).

$$OR = \frac{ad}{cb} \qquad (6.92)$$

$$Var_i = \frac{1}{a} + \frac{1}{b} + \frac{1}{c} + \frac{1}{d} \qquad (6.93)$$

- Calculation of the weighted effect size of individual studies

The weighting factor (W) is the inverse variance of log OR in the fixed-effect model "Eq. 6.94". In the random effect model, the weighting factor (W^R) is the reciprocal value of the sum of the variance of log OR and the variance between studies (T^2). The weighted effect size (WES) is the product of log OR and the appropriate variance: (W) in the case of a fixed effect model "Eq. 6.94" and (W^R) in the case of a random effect model "Eq. 6.95".

$$WES_i = Log_{OR} \times \frac{1}{Var\,Log_{OR}} \qquad (6.94)$$

$$WES_i^R = Log_{OR} \times \frac{1}{Var\,Log_{OR} + T^2} \qquad (6.95)$$

- Calculation of the mean effect size and the standard error

We calculate the mean effect size of the meta-analysis (mean ES) as the sum of all weighed Log OR divided by the sum of all weights "Eq. 6.96", its Se is the square root of the reciprocal value of the sum of weights "Eq. 6.97"; all being calculated in the log scale. In the random-effects model, W is substituted with W^R.

$$Mean\ ES = \frac{\sum W_i\,Log_{ORi}}{\sum W_i} \qquad (6.96)$$

$$Se\ ES = \sqrt{\frac{1}{\sum W_i}} \qquad (6.97)$$

- Creation of the 95% CI and testing statistical significance

We can assign a 95% CI to our effect size by placing 1.96 Se on either side of the mean "Eq. 6.98". The statistical significance of the effect size is tested using the Z score by the usual equation by dividing the Log weighed OR by the Log Se; a Z score ≥ 1.96 points to a statistically significant effect size "Eq. 6.99".

$$95\%\ CI\ ES = Mean\ ES \pm 1.96\ (Se\ ES) \qquad (6.98)$$

$$Z\ score = \frac{Mean\ ES}{Se\ ES} \qquad (6.99)$$

- Conversion of the log value to the original scale for presentation

The Log OR and the upper and lower borders of the 95% CI of Log OR are back-transformed to the original scale for presentation "Eq. 6.100".

$$95\%\ CI\ (OR) = e^{LL\,95\%CI\,(\log OR)}\ to\ e^{UL\,95\%\,CI\,(\log OR)} \tag{6.100}$$

The Relative Risk

The relative risk is the proportion between the risk in the treatment group and the risk in the control. It is not normally distributed and has to be converted into the logarithmic scale to proceed with the calculation of a reliable Se and a 95% CI. In a meta-analysis, all the calculations are precisely similar to those performed with the odds ratio. In the fixed-effect model, the weighting factor (W) is the inverse variance $(1/\log RRi)$. In the case of a random effects model, the weighting factor (W^R) will be the reciprocal value of the sum of the variability within the study and the variability between studies T^2. However, the only difference is the equation used to calculate the relative risk itself "Eq. 6.101" and its variance "Eq. 6.102" (see Table 6.7).

$$RR_i = \frac{a}{n_t}\Big/\frac{c}{n_c} \tag{6.101}$$

$$Var_i = \frac{1}{a} + \frac{1}{c} + \frac{1}{a+b} + \frac{1}{c+d} \tag{6.102}$$

- Calculation of the weighted effect size of individual studies

We calculate the weighted effect size (WES) for each study by multiplying the effect size by (W) in a fixed-effect model "Eq. 6.103" and by (W^R) in a random-effects model "Eq. 6.104".

$$WES_i = Log\,RR_i \times \frac{1}{Var\,Log_{RRi}} \tag{6.103}$$

$$WES_i^R = Log\,RR_i \times \frac{1}{Var\,Log_{RRi} + T^2} \tag{6.104}$$

- Calculation of the mean effect size and the standard error

We calculate the mean effect size of the meta-analysis (mean ES) as the sum of all weighed Log RR divided by the sum of all weights "Eq. 6.105". The variance is the reciprocal value of the sum of weights "Eq. 6.106", and the standard error is the square root of variance "Eq. 6.107".

$$Mean\ ES = \frac{\sum W_i\,Log_{RRi}}{\sum W_i} \tag{6.105}$$

$$Var\ ES = \frac{1}{\sum W_i} \tag{6.106}$$

$$Se\ ES = \sqrt{\frac{1}{\sum W_i}} \tag{6.107}$$

- Creation of the 95% CI and testing statistical significance

We can assign a 95% CI by placing 1.96 Se on either side of the mean "Eq. 6.108," all being calculated in the log scale. In the random-effects model W is substituted with W^R. We can test the statistical significance of the effect size by a simple Z test "Eq. 6.109" and a Z score ≥ 1.96 points to a statistically significant effect size.

$$95\%\ CI\ (ES) = (Mean\ ES)\ \pm 1.96\ (Se\ ES) \tag{6.108}$$

$$Z = \frac{Mean\ ES}{Se\ ES} \tag{6.109}$$

- Conversion of the log value to the original scale for presentation

The Log RR and the upper and lower borders of the 95% CI of log RR are back-transformed to the original scale for presentation "Eq. 6.110".

$$95\% \ CI \ (RR) = e^{LL \, 95\% CI \, (\log RR)} \ to \ e^{UL \, 95\% \ CI \, (\log RR)}$$

(6.110)

A Working Example

We will present data extracted from the study of Colditz and colleagues on the efficacy of the BCG vaccine in the prevention of Tuberculosis [37]. The vaccine has been shown to significantly reduce the rate of new cases by around 50%. Table 6.8 shows part of the results of the analysis of 13 manuscripts included in their study: the number of events and the total number of patients in vaccinated (group A) and control groups (group B), the relative risk calculated in each study as well as the upper and lower limits of the 95% confidence interval. The authors equally reported the effect of several quantitative and qualitative moderator variables on vaccine efficacy, including the effect of climate and latitude. The analysis of the effect of those moderator variables will be discussed in the relevant sections (see Sects. 6.2.8 and 6.2.9).

1. *The fixed effect model*

We will begin by assuming a fixed-effect model. Calculations will be made from scratch, using the crude data presented in Table 6.8: the number of patients with and without the events in the vaccinated and the control groups.

- Calculation of the weighted effect size of individual studies

We will present the steps of the calculation of the first clinical study (Aronson 1948). The analysis of the other 12 manuscripts will be similar. The first step is to calculate the odds ratio "Eq. 6.111" and convert it to the log scale "Eq. 6.112". We have to compute the variance of the odds ratio "Eq. 6.113" to get the weighting factor, which is the inverse variance (W = 1/Var). We compute the weighted effect size of Aronson's study by multiplying his log odds ratio with his inverse variance "Eq. 6.114".

$$RR_i = \frac{na}{Na} \Big/ \frac{nc}{Nc} = \frac{4}{123} \Big/ \frac{11}{139} = 0.41 \quad (6.111)$$

Table 6.8 The relative risk: evaluation of the efficacy of the BCG vaccine

Study[a]	na	Na	nb	Nb	RR	LL	UL	L	C
Aronson 1948	4	123	11	139	0.41	0.13	1.26	44	c
Ferguson 1949	6	306	29	303	0.21	0.09	0.49	55	c
Rosenthal 1960	3	231	11	220	0.26	0.07	0.92	42	c
Hart 1977	62	13,598	248	12,867	0.24	0.18	0.31	52	c
Frimodt 1973	33	5069	47	5808	0.8	0.52	1.25	13	h
Stein 1953	180	1541	372	1451	0.46	0.39	0.54	44	c
Vandiviere 1973	8	2545	10	629	0.2	0.08	0.5	19	h
Madras 1980	505	88,391	499	88,391	1.0	0.89	1.15	13	h
Coetzee 1968	29	7499	45	7277	0.63	0.39	0.99	27	h
Rosenthal 1961	17	1716	65	1665	0.25	0.15	0.43	42	c
Comstock 1974	186	50,634	141	27,338	0.7	0.57	0.89	18	h
Comstock 1969	5	2498	3	2341	1.56	0.37	6.53	33	h
Comstock 1976	27	16,913	29	17,854	0.98	0.58	1.66	33	h

[a] = name of the first author and year of publication, na and nb = number of cases with event in vaccinated and control groups a and b, Na and Nb = total number of patients in vaccinated and in control groups, RR = relative risk, LL and UL = lower and upper limits of the 95% interval of confidence, L = latitude, C = climate, c = cold, h = hot

$$ES_i = \log 0.411 = -0.89 \qquad (6.112)$$

$$\text{Var } ES_i = \frac{1}{na} + \frac{1}{nc} + \frac{1}{Na} + \frac{1}{Nb}$$
$$= \frac{1}{4} + \frac{1}{11} + \frac{1}{123} + \frac{1}{139} = 0.356$$
$$(6.113)$$

$$WES_i = Log\, RR_i \times \frac{1}{Var\, Log\, RR_i}$$
$$= -0.89 \times \frac{1}{0.356} = -2.49 \qquad (6.114)$$

We can calculate the standard error of the effect size (Se ES) as the square root of the variance "Eq. 6.115", which gives us the advantage of calculating a 95% CI for the weighted effect size of Aronson's study "Eq. 6.116". The conversion of the effect size and the upper and lower limits of the 95% confidence interval into the original scale facilitates the presentation of the result "Eq. 6.117". Concluding solely upon Aronson's study gives a confusing result. The relative risk (RR) can vary from 0.13 to 1.26, which means that the BCG vaccine can sometimes have a

protective effect (RR < 1) but can be harmful (RR > 1).

$$\text{Se } ES_i = \sqrt{\text{Var } ES_i} = \sqrt{0.356} = 0.597$$
$$(6.115)$$

$$95\% \ CI\ ES_i = ES_i \pm 1.96\,(\text{Se } ES_i)$$
$$= -0.89 \pm 1.96\,(0.597)$$
$$= -2\ to\ 0.23 \qquad (6.116)$$

$$RR_i\,(95\%\ CI) = 0.41(0.13\ to\ 1.26) \quad (6.117)$$

Table 6.9 shows the calculations for the 13 studies included in the meta-analysis. Calculations are lengthy but straightforward and hence, they are usually performed by a computer software package. Note that all calculations are made in the log scale.

- Calculation of the mean effect size and the standard error

We compute the mean effect size of the meta-analysis itself (mean ES) by dividing the sum of the weighted effect sizes of the 13 manuscripts

Table 6.9 The relative risk: evaluation of the efficacy of the BCG vaccine, analysis of a fixed effect model

Study	ES	Var	W	WES	WES^2	W^2
Aronson 1948	−0.89	0.33	3.07	−2.73	2.43	9.43
Ferguson 1949	−1.59	0.19	5.14	−8.15	12.92	26.41
Rosenthal 1960	−1.35	0.42	2.41	−3.25	4.38	5.80
Hart 1977	−1.44	0.02	49.98	−72.04	103.85	2497.50
Frimodt 1973	−0.22	0.05	19.53	−4.25	0.92	381.32
Stein 1953	−0.79	0.01	144.80	−113.83	89.48	20,967.51
Vandiviere 1973	−1.62	0.22	4.48	−7.27	11.78	20.11
Madras 1980	0.01	0.004	252.40	3.02	0.04	63,704.64
Coetzee 1968	−0.47	0.06	17.72	−8.32	3.90	313.99
Rosenthal 1961	−1.37	0.07	13.69	−18.78	25.75	187.52
Comstock 1974	−0.34	0.01	80.57	−27.34	9.28	6491.07
Comstock 1969	0.45	0.53	1.88	0.84	0.37	3.53
Comstock 1976	−0.02	0.07	14.00	−0.24	0.005	196.13
Total			609.7	−262.3	265.1	94,804.9

ES = effect size (Log relative risk), Var = variance within the study, W = weight of the effect size = inverse variance, WES = weighed effect size = W × ES, WES^2 = WES × ES, W^2 = W × W by the sum of weights "Eq. 6.118" and the (Se ES) as the square root of the reciprocal value of the sum of weights "Eq. 6.119"; all being calculated in the logarithmic scale.

$$\text{Mean ES} = \frac{\sum W_i \, Log_{RR_i}}{\sum W_i} = \frac{-269}{625} = -0.43 \tag{6.118}$$

$$\text{Se ES} = \sqrt{\frac{1}{\sum W_i}} = \sqrt{\frac{1}{625}} = 0.04 \tag{6.119}$$

- Creation of the 95% CI and testing statistical significance

We calculate the 95% CI of the Log RR of the fixed-effect model by assigning 1.96 Se on either side of the mean "Eq. 6.120". We assess its statistical significance (Z test) by dividing the Log RR by its Se "Eq. 6.121" and check the degree of significance in the Z table. The vaccine was associated with a significant reduction in the risk of developing the disease ($P < 0.001$).

$$\begin{aligned} 95\% \;\; CI(ES) &= \text{MeanES} \pm 1.96 \, (\text{SE ES}) \\ &= -0.43 \pm 1.96 \, (0.04) \\ &= -0.51 \; to -0.35 \end{aligned} \tag{6.120}$$

$$Z = \frac{\text{Mean ES}}{\text{Se ES}} = \frac{-0.43}{0.04} = -10.6; P < 0.001 \tag{6.121}$$

- Conversion of the log value to the original scale for presentation

Finally, we convert the log RR (-0.43) and the upper and lower limits of the 95% CI (-0.51 and -0.35) into their original scale for better interpretation when presented in "Eq. 6.122". The vaccine was associated with a significant decrease in the risk of developing the disease: the relative risk of vaccinated cases was about two-thirds of that calculated for normal controls.

$$RR \; (95\% \; CI)_{fixed \, model} = 0.65 (0.6 \; to \; 0.7) \tag{6.122}$$

- Graphic presentation: the forest plot

Figure 6.10 shows the forest plot, with the values being presented in the logarithmic scale as produced by the Jamovi software package [33]. Other software, such as Open meta [35] may present the confidence intervals after being converted into the relative risk itself, which may be more informative. The indices of heterogeneity, such as Q, I^2, df, and P-value, have to be presented on the plot. Those indices' meaning and interpretation will be discussed separately (see Sect. 6.2.7).

2. *The random effects model*

We will repeat the same calculations, assuming a random-effects model. The effect size is weighted by the total inverse variance formed by the sum of the study's variance and the variance between the studies (T^2). We will denote this total variance that includes T^2 as (Var^R) to differentiate it from a fixed model's variance that assumes that $T^2 = 0$. In our example, T^2 was equal to 0.31, and the calculation details will be presented separately (see Sect. 6.2.7.3).

- Calculation of the weighted effect size of individual studies

Returning to the first study by Aronson 1948, the effect size ($ES_i = -0.89$) was previously calculated in "Eq. 6.112". Assuming a random-effects model, the weighting factor for this study is the reciprocal value of the total variance (Var^R) "Eq. 6.123". The weighted effect size (WES) is calculated by multiplying the effect size in log scale by the inverse variance "Eq. 6.124". The produced effect size is smaller than the one calculated for a fixed effect model because of the larger variance.

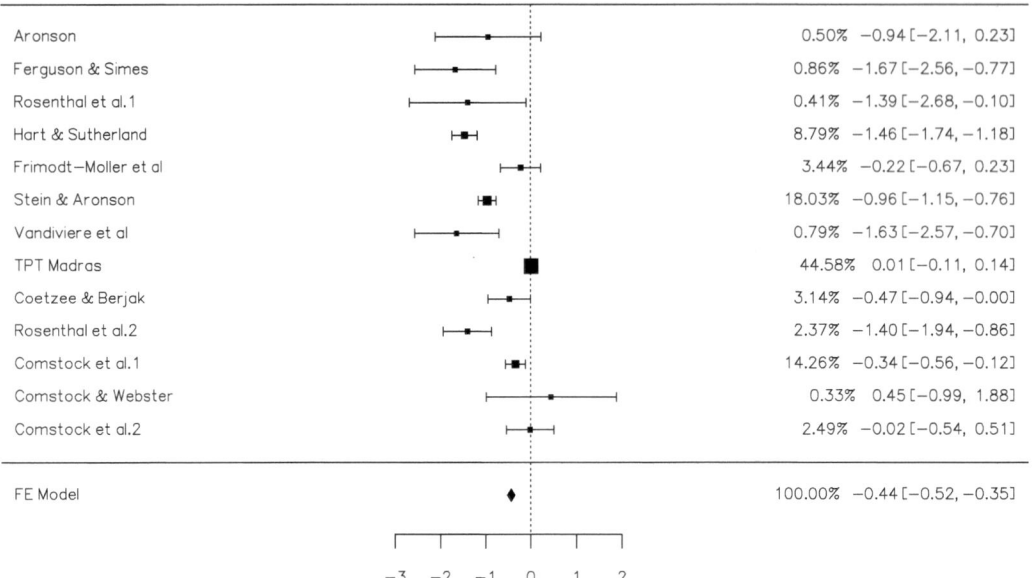

Fig. 6.10 Forest plot: the relative risk of BCG vaccine, fixed effect model (FE). Values (95% CI) are presented in the logarithmic scale, Q = 152.2, df = 12, P < 0.001, I^2 = 92.12%

$$Var_i^R = Var\ log_{RR_i} + T^2 = 0.33 + 0.31 = 0.63 \tag{6.123}$$

$$WES_i^R = Log\ RR_i \times \frac{1}{Var^R}$$
$$= -0.89 \times \frac{1}{0.33 + 0.31} = -1.39 \tag{6.124}$$

The Se of the effect size is the square root of the new (larger) variance "Eq. 6.125". Hence, it is larger than the one calculated for a fixed-effect model. We can assign a 95% CI for the result of this study by placing 1.96 Se on either side of the logarithmic value of the relative risk "Eq. 6.126". We can convert the log values to get the relative risk and the upper and lower limits of the 95% CI of Aronson's study, assuming a random model "Eq. 6.127". Table 6.10 shows the results of the calculations made for the 13 studies.

$$Se\ ES_i^R = \sqrt{Var_i^R} = \sqrt{0.64} = 0.8 \tag{6.125}$$

$$95\%\ CI\ ES_i = ES_i \pm 1.96\left(Se\ ES_i^R\right)$$
$$= -0.89 \pm 1.96\ (0.8)$$
$$= -2.46\ to\ 0.68 \tag{6.126}$$

$$RR_i\ (95\%\ CI)^R = 0.41(0.08\ to\ 1.97) \tag{6.127}$$

- Calculation of the mean effect size and the standard error (random model)

We compute the mean effect size of the meta-analysis itself (Mean ES) by dividing the sum of the weighted effect sizes of the 13 manuscripts by the sum of weights "Eq. 6.128" and its Se as the square root of the reciprocal value of the sum of weights "Eq. 6.129"; all being calculated in the logarithmic scale and using the new larger variance of the random effect model.

$$Mean\ ES^R = \frac{\sum W_i^R\ Log_{RRi}}{\sum W_i^R} = \frac{-22.28}{31.36} = -0.71 \tag{6.128}$$

Table 6.10 The relative risk: evaluation of the efficacy of the BCG vaccine, analysis of a random effects model

Study	ES	Var	Var^R	W	WES	WES^2	W^2
Aronson 1948	−0.89	0.33	0.63	1.58	−1.40	1.25	2.49
Ferguson 1949	−1.59	0.19	0.50	1.99	−3.15	5.00	3.96
Rosenthal 1960	−1.35	0.42	0.72	1.38	−1.86	2.51	1.91
Hart 1977	−1.44	0.02	0.33	3.05	−4.39	6.34	9.29
Frimodt 1973	−0.22	0.05	0.36	2.78	−0.61	0.13	7.75
Stein 1953	−0.79	0.01	0.31	3.18	−2.50	1.96	10.08
Vandiviere 1973	−1.62	0.22	0.53	1.88	−3.05	4.95	3.55
Madras 1980	0.01	0.004	0.31	3.21	0.04	0.00	10.28
Coetzee 1968	−0.47	0.06	0.36	2.74	−1.29	0.60	7.53
Rosenthal 1961	−1.37	0.07	0.38	2.62	−3.60	4.94	6.89
Comstock 1974	−0.34	0.01	0.32	3.12	−1.06	0.36	9.74
Comstock 1969	0.45	0.53	0.84	1.19	0.53	0.24	1.42
Comstock 1976	−0.02	0.07	0.38	2.64	−0.05	0.00	6.95
Total	−9.63			31.36	−22.39	28.28	81.83

ES = effect size (Log relative risk), Var = variance within the study, Var^R = total variance = Var + T^2 = Var + 0.31, W = weight of the effect size in a random model = inverse Var^R, WES = weighed effect size = W × ES, WES^2 = WES × ES, W^2 = W × W

$$Se\ ES^R = \sqrt{\frac{1}{\sum W_i^R}} = \sqrt{\frac{1}{31.36}} = 0.179 \tag{6.129}$$

- Creation of the 95% CI and testing statistical significance

We calculate the 95% CI of the Log RR of the random effect model by assigning 1.96 Se on either side of the mean "Eq. 6.130". We assess its statistical significance (Z value) by dividing the Log RR by its Se "Eq. 6.131". A Z score ≥ 1.96 indicates a statistically significant effect size. The vaccine was associated with a significant reduction of the risk of developing the disease (P < 0.001), for the log values being negative (reduction on the log scale) and excluding zero.

$$95\%\ CI\ ES = \text{Mean}\ ES^R \pm 1.96\left(Se\ ES^R\right)$$
$$= -0.714 \pm 1.96\,(0.179)$$
$$= -1.06\ to - 0.36 \tag{6.130}$$

$$Z = \frac{-0.71}{0.179} = -4; P < 0.001 \tag{6.131}$$

- Conversion of the log value to the original scale for presentation

Finally, we convert the log RR (−0.714) and the upper and lower limits of the 95% CI (−1.06 and −0.36) into their original scale for better interpretation when presented "Eq. 6.132". The vaccine was associated with a significant decrease in the risk of the development of the disease: the relative risk of vaccinated cases was half that calculated for normal controls.

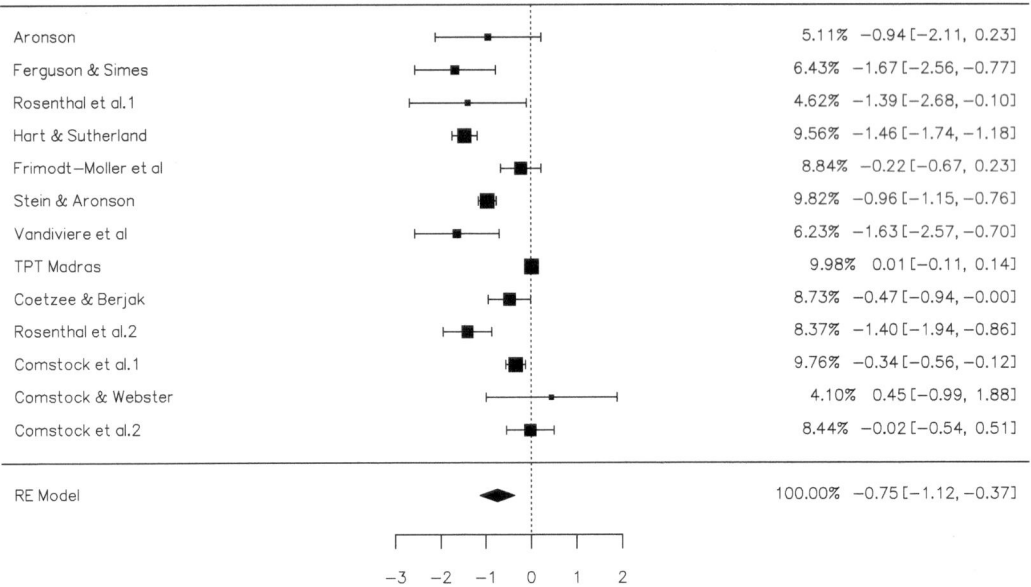

Aronson		5.11% −0.94 [−2.11, 0.23]
Ferguson & Simes		6.43% −1.67 [−2.56, −0.77]
Rosenthal et al.1		4.62% −1.39 [−2.68, −0.10]
Hart & Sutherland		9.56% −1.46 [−1.74, −1.18]
Frimodt−Moller et al		8.84% −0.22 [−0.67, 0.23]
Stein & Aronson		9.82% −0.96 [−1.15, −0.76]
Vandiviere et al		6.23% −1.63 [−2.57, −0.70]
TPT Madras		9.98% 0.01 [−0.11, 0.14]
Coetzee & Berjak		8.73% −0.47 [−0.94, −0.00]
Rosenthal et al.2		8.37% −1.40 [−1.94, −0.86]
Comstock et al.1		9.76% −0.34 [−0.56, −0.12]
Comstock & Webster		4.10% 0.45 [−0.99, 1.88]
Comstock et al.2		8.44% −0.02 [−0.54, 0.51]
RE Model		100.00% −0.75 [−1.12, −0.37]

Fig. 6.11 Forest plot: the relative risk of BCG vaccine, random effect model (RE). Values (95% CI) are presented in the logarithmic scale, Q = 152.2, df = 12, P < 0.001, I^2 = 92.12

$$RR \ (95\% \ CI)_{random \ model} = 0.49 \ (0.35 \ to \ 0.7) \tag{6.132}$$

• Graphic presentation: the forest plot

Figure 6.11 shows the forest plot, with the values being presented in the logarithmic scale as produced by the Jamovi software package [33]. Other software, such as Open meta [35] may present the confidence intervals after being converted into the relative risk itself, which may be more informative. The indices of heterogeneity, such as Q, I^2, df, and P-value, have to be presented on the plot. Those indices' meaning and interpretation will be discussed separately (see Sect. 6.2.7).

The Hazard Ratio

Hazard ratio (HR) is the ratio between 2 hazards: the hazard of developing the event in the treatment group (H_t) to the corresponding hazard in the control group (H_c) "Eq. 6.133". In a time-to-

event study, and assuming that the event rate is constant over time, the hazard ratio can be estimated as the ratio between the median survival in the treatment group (S_t) and the median survival of the control group (S_c) "Eq. 6.134". The hazard ratio is not normally distributed; it must be log-transformed to calculate a proper standard error. The variance of the HR is the sum of the reciprocal values of the number of events in the treatment (E_t) and in the control group (E_c) "Eq. 6.135" and the Se is the square root of the variance, as usual, "Eq. 6.136". Another option is to take the HR and its Se from the software output if a Cox proportional hazard analysis is performed. From the meta-analysis point of view, all other calculations are similar to those performed for the odds ratio and relative risk.

$$HR = \frac{H_T}{H_C}$$
$$= \frac{New \ cases_T / Patients \ remaining \ at \ risk_T}{New \ cases_C / Patients \ remaining \ at \ risk_C} \tag{6.133}$$

$$HR = \frac{S_t}{S_c} \quad (6.134)$$

$$Var_{Log\,HR} = \left(\frac{1}{E_t} + \frac{1}{E_c}\right) \quad (6.135)$$

$$Se(\log HR) = \sqrt{\frac{1}{E_t} + \frac{1}{E_c}} \quad (6.136)$$

- Calculation of the weighted effect size of individual studies

In a fixed-effect model, the weighting factor is the inverse variance of the study (W), to which we add the variance between studies (T^2) in a random effect model (W^R). The weighted effect size (WES) will be the product of the log hazard ratio (log HRi) and either (W) "Eq. 6.137" or (W^R) according to the model type "Eq. 6.138".

$$WES = Log\,HR_i \times \frac{1}{Var_{Log\,HR_i}} \quad (6.137)$$

$$WES^R = Log\,HR_i \times \frac{1}{Var_{Log\,HR_i} + T^2} \quad (6.138)$$

- Calculation of the mean effect size and the standard error

We calculate the mean effect size of the meta-analysis (Mean ES) as the sum of all WES divided by the sum of all weights "Eq. 6.139", its Se is the square root of the reciprocal value of the sum of weights "Eq. 6.140". All calculations are made in the logarithmic scale, using (W) in a fixed-effects model and (W^R) in a random-effects model.

$$\text{Mean ES} = \frac{\sum W_i Log_{HR_i}}{\sum W_i} \quad (6.139)$$

$$\text{Se ES} = \sqrt{\frac{1}{\sum W_i}} \quad (6.140)$$

- Creation of the 95% CI and testing statistical significance

We can create a 95% CI for the mean effect size by placing 1.96 Se on each side of the mean value "Eq. 6.141". In the random-effects model, (W) is substituted with (W^R). We test the significance of the result by a simple Z test. A Z score ≥ 1.96 indicates a statistically significant effect size "Eq. 6.142".

$$95\% \ CI \ (\text{ES}) = \text{Mean ES} \pm 1.96 \ (\text{Se ES}) \quad (6.141)$$

$$Z\,score = \frac{\text{Mean ES}}{\text{Se ES}} \quad (6.142)$$

- Conversion of the log value to the original scale for presentation

The Log HR and the upper and lower borders of the 95% CI of log HR are back-transformed to the original scale for presentation "Eq. 6.143".

$$95\% \ CI(HR) = e^{LL\,95\%\,CI\,(\log HR)} \ to \ e^{UL\,95\%\,CI\,(\log HR)} \quad (6.143)$$

6.2.6.3 Other Methods of Calculation

Hunter and Schmidt classified meta-analysis methods into three categories (see Sect. 6.1.3). The first were purely descriptive and they are rarely used nowadays. The second category represents the many methods that address sampling error from which we have chosen the technique advocated by Hedges and colleagues to be our method of choice. The third is the more complicate psychometric meta-analysis that we will discuss in a separate section (see Sect. 6.3). Among the second category are the methods of: Rosenthal and Rubin, Mantel–Haenszel, the one-step Peto, and the barebone method; which have current indications and hence, they merit to be addressed.

Rosenthal and Rubin Method

Rosenthal and Rubin introduced the binomial effect size display (BESD) to report Pearson's correlation coefficient (r) properly. We expect the reader to know that squaring r (R^2) is the coefficient of determination or the numerical expression of how much one variable is influenced by the other (see Sect. 2.6.1.1). For example, an r-value of 0.32 is usually labelled as being equivalent to modest R^2 of only 10% ($0.32^2 = 0.32 \times 0.32 = 0.1024$). Rosenthal and Rubin have shown that this modest 10% effect of r was the correlation equivalent of a much larger effect, corresponding to an increasing success (or failure) rate from 34 to 66% [9]. Put it this way; the authors gave the mathematical proof that presenting the effect size in terms of BESD is a better estimate than being presented as a correlation coefficient. The reader can refer to the freely available simple original manuscript for the calculation details [9].

Rosenthal and Rubin provided tables to calculate the BESD out of Pearson's r and proposed to directly compute the BESD success rate of the control group as $(0.5 - r/2)$. In contrast, the experimental group success rate is computed as $(0.5 + r/2)$. For example, an r of 0.1 corresponds to 45% and 55% rates, and an r of 0.8 corresponds to success rates of 10% and 90%. As Pearson's correlation coefficient r can be computed with a variety of test statistics, such as Chi-square, Student's (t), and F-statistics; the authors suggested extending the procedure to comparing a quantitative outcome between two groups [21]. The method can adopt either a fixed or random-effects model and was shown to produce similar results as the method of Hedges and colleagues [10], while other reports pointed out that the latter gives distorted results when proportions are away from 50% [11]. The following equations can be used to deduct Pearson's correlation coefficient r from other test statistics such as Chi-square, Student t, and Fisher's F "Eq. 6.144".

$$ r = \sqrt{\frac{\chi^2}{N}}; \quad r = \sqrt{\frac{t^2}{t^2 + df}}; \quad r = \sqrt{\frac{F}{F + df_{error}}} $$

$$ (6.144) $$

The Mantel–Haenszel Method

When data are sparse, either in terms of low event risks or study size being small, the inverse variance method gives poor estimates of the standard errors of the effect size, while the Mantel–Haenszel method was shown to be robust in such cases [12]. We have previously presented the Mantel–Haenszel adjusted Odds ratio (OR_{MH}). Unlike the conventional inverse variance technique, it uses a weighted average odds ratio rather than the log odds ratios (see Sect. 2.9.3.2). The method involves calculating the OR as usual (ad/bc) and the weight (W) is computed as (bc/n); where $n = a + b + c + d$ (Table 6.7). We calculate the weighted odds ratio of each study (i) as the product of its odds ratio (OR_i) by its weight (W_i). The Mantel Haenszel odds ratio (OR_{MH}) is calculated as the sum of the weighted odds ratios ($\sum W_i OR_i$) divided by the sum of weights ($\sum W_i$) "Eq. 6.145".

$$ OR_{MH} = \frac{\sum W_i OR_i}{\sum W_i} \qquad (6.145) $$

While we calculated the (OR_{MH}) without transformation, we have to transform the OR into log units to calculate the variance. However, the calculation is not as straightforward as the variance of the usual OR (sum of reciprocal values) but is quite a long procedure. We thought there was no point in presenting it here since it is calculated by computer software. Once the variance is given, the rest of the procedure runs in the usual sequence. The Se is the square root of the variance, and a simple Z test tests the statistical significance of the effect size. A Z score ≥ 1.96 denotes a statistically significant effect size. As usual, the 95% CI of Mantel–Haenszel OR is calculated by assigning 1.96 (Se) on either side of the mean "Eq. 6.146". The method was further extended to risk ratios (see Sect. 2.9.3.2) and risk differences.

$$ 95\% \ CI \quad OR_{MH} = OR^{1 \pm 1.96/\sqrt{Var \ OR}} \quad (6.146) $$

The Peto One-Step Approach

The method can be used to combine the odds ratios of different studies. The calculation differs from the conventional technique (see Sect. 6.2.6.2.7), yet both methods weight the calculated OR by the inverse variance [13]. We estimate the log OR of each study (i) as the standardized difference between the observed (O_i) and expected values (E_i) "Eq. 6.147". The observed value (O_i) is the value of the (a) cell in each study (see Table 6.7). We compute the expected value (E_i) as in "Eq. 6.148", and the variance as in "Eq. 6.149", where n_i is the number of cases in each study (i).

$$Log\ OR_i = \frac{O_i - E_i}{V_i} \qquad (6.147)$$

$$E_i = \frac{(a_i + b_i)(a_i + c_i)}{n_i} \qquad (6.148)$$

$$V_i = \frac{(a_i + b_i)(c_i + d_i)(a_i + c_i)(b_i + d_i)}{n_i^2(n_i - 1)} \qquad (6.149)$$

We calculate a pooled OR (ORp) as the exponential value of the sum of standardized differences between observed and expected values calculated for each study "Eq. 6.150". We evaluate the statistical significance by the usual simple Z test, "Eq. 6.151," and we calculate the 95% CI as in "Eq. 6.152" [13].

$$OR_p = Exp\left(\frac{\sum(O_i - E_i)}{\sum V_i}\right) \qquad (6.150)$$

$$Z_p = \frac{O - E}{\sqrt{Var_{ORp}}} \qquad (6.151)$$

$$95\%\ CI\ OR_p = (OR_p)^{1 \pm 1.96/\sqrt{Var\ OR}} \qquad (6.152)$$

The Peto method works well when intervention effects are small (odds ratios are close to 1) or when we have an empty cell with equal sample sizes for both groups, provided that the studies have similar numbers in experimental and comparator groups. In other situations, which are the more common, the Peto method has been shown to give biased answers and hence, is not a preferred method by default [31]. The reader can refer to Fleiss for a working example [28].

The Barebones Method

In accordance with the previous methods, the barebones technique only controls for sampling error. Technically, it differs in weighing effect size and estimating variability and heterogeneity. Although advocated by Hunter and colleagues, the authors limit its actual indication to teaching purposes for being simple but not considering the effect of other essential design artifacts [2]. The calculations will be explained as part of the psychometric meta-analysis proposed by the same authors (see Sect. 6.3).

6.2.7 Assessment of Heterogeneity

Each effect size estimate is subject to variability, which may be primarily thought of as being due to variability within the study due to sampling error. However, suppose the variability is above and beyond what can be due to just sampling error. In that case, we can no longer assume that the measurements were made under similar conditions. We can further question whether the observed effect sizes are estimates of the same population? In other words, the question is no longer just about the homogeneity of the included studies. The question is whether the population itself is homogenous or not, is the observed heterogeneity due to an external factor influencing the population or a combination of both [25].

In a fixed-effect model, the different studies are assumed to originate from the same population, and hence, the variability between studies is assumed to be zero. However, the fluctuation due to sampling error can sometimes lead to considerable variability [20]. In other words, we must not just rely on our assumption, and we have to use a statistical test to judge whether the observed variability is above and beyond what can be due to sampling error. Consequently, we should test heterogeneity regardless of the assumptions made for the model type, whether a fixed or a random-effects model. For those adopted the technique advocated by Hedges and colleagues [5–8], the test of choice is a modified Chi-square and is known as the (Q) test, but other tests are available too, such as the likelihood ratio, Wald test, and Rao's score test [38].

As variability is present anyway, Q only tests whether variability is significantly different from zero or not? Q is not a measurement of the amount of variability between studies because it is a statistical test using a standardized scale and not the scale of the effect size itself. Q cannot tell us the reason behind this variability, whether it is due to true differences between the studies or because of an external factor, or just due to sampling error? Other indices, namely I-square (I^2) (see Sect. 6.7.2.2) and Tau-square (T^2) (see Sect. 6.7.2.2), are deducted from Q and may help answer those questions.

6.2.7.1   Testing Heterogeneity: The Cochran Q Test

"Q" tests homogeneity by a modified Chi-square equation. Under the null hypothesis, there should be no difference between the effect size of each study (ES_i) and the average effect size of all studies (ES). In statistical terms, Q calculates the sum of standardized squared differences between the individual weighted effect sizes (WES_i) and the mean weighted effect size (WES) "Eq. 6.153". Another variant of the equation makes it easier to compute "Eq. 6.154"; where $\sum W(ES)^2$ is the sum of weighted squared effect sizes, $(\sum WES)^2$ is the squared value of sum of weighted effect sizes, and $\sum W$ is the sum of all weights.

The forest plot is the graphical presentation of the weighted effect sizes of all studies included in the meta-analysis. The arms of each study represent the span of its 95% CI. Hence, if the arms of any two studies do not overlap, the two studies are significantly different from each other; i.e., the two studies are heterogeneous, and we have to expect a large Q between the two studies. We can get an idea about the value of Q of a meta-analysis by noticing the extent of the overlap of arms among all studies included. The more is the overlap; the smaller is Q and vice versa.

$$Q = \sum W_i(ES_i - ES)^2 \qquad (6.153)$$

$$Q = \sum W(ES)^2 - \frac{(\sum WES)^2}{\sum W} \qquad (6.154)$$

Q follows a Chi-square distribution, and hence, the statistical significance of the test statistics (Q) is checked out in the Chi-square table at a degree of freedom equal to the number of studies minus one (k − 1). The null hypothesis is that all studies are testing the same effect, and hence, there is no variability between the studies (Q = 0), and the alternative hypothesis is that there is variability between studies (Q > 0). The more variability, the larger it will be Q. As the calculation (the play of chance) may sometimes lead to a negative Q value, any such value will be recorded as (0). Unfortunately, *Q tends to be underpowered if the studies included in the meta-analysis have a small number of patients or when the number of included studies themselves (K) is small* [3, 36, 38, 39]. The result is that a non-significant Q test does not exclude heterogeneity, which is why a P value of 0.10, rather than the conventional level of 0.05, is sometimes used to determine statistical significance [39].

In conclusion, Q assesses the null hypothesis that studies are homogeneous or not? It neither explains heterogeneity nor measures its extent. Q is a statistical test that uses a standard scale and not a measurement tool that uses the original scale of effect size. In the case of heterogeneity, Q does not tell us where this variability comes from, but it signals the need for another exploratory measure, such as a subgroup (see Sect. 6.2.8) or moderator analysis (see Sect. 6.2.9). Unfortunately, Q can miss identifying significant heterogeneity in case of the included studies were small or few. Besides sample size, Q is also dependent on the scale of the effect sizes. Consequently, *it can be used to test heterogeneity among subgroups of the same study but not between different meta-analyses* (see Sect. 6.2.8).

A Working Example

We will calculate Q for the example of comparing the duration of hospital stays following minimal invasive versus conventional open-heart surgery (Table 6.5). Note that the results are slightly different from that given by the software (308.7) due to approximations "Eq. 6.155". Comparing Q with the critical limits of Chi-square statistics at five df (number of studies minus one) shows a statically significant heterogeneity between studies (P < 0.001). Another example is the relative risk of the efficacy of the BCG vaccine (Table 6.9) "Eq. 6.156". Checking the critical limits of Chi-square table at 12 df (number of studies minus one) shows a statistically significant heterogeneity among studies; (P < 0.001, exactly 0.00001).

$$Q = \sum W(ES)^2 - \frac{(\sum WES)^2}{\sum W} = 1165 - \frac{(317)^2}{118}$$
$$= 314$$
(6.155)

$$Q = \sum W(ES)^2 - \frac{(\sum WES)^2}{\sum W}$$
$$= 265.1 - \frac{(-262.3)^2}{609.7} = 152.2 \quad (6.156)$$

6.2.7.2 Analyzing Heterogeneity: I^2, H^2 and R^2

The I^2 Index

Let us recall what does Q compare? It compares the weighted squared difference between the effect size of each study and the average of all studies. For a particular study (i), $Q_i = W_i (ES_i - ES)^2$. What is the weighted squared difference? It is the squared difference $(ES_i - ES)^2$ multiplied by its inverse variance: $W_i = 1/(Se_i^2)$. In other words, Q is the squared difference $(ES_i - ES)^2$ divided by the variance of the study (Se_i^2) "Eq. 6.157".

$$W_i(ES_i - ES)^2 = (ES_i - ES)^2 / Se_i^2 \quad (6.157)$$

Under the null hypothesis, there is no difference between the effect size of any study (i) and the average effect size, except what can be due to sampling error (Se_i^2). In other words, under the null hypothesis $(ES_i - ES)^2 = (Se_i^2)$ and the

"Eq. 6.157" produces (1) for each study included in the meta-analysis. Hence, the total amount of variation will be equal to the number of studies (1 × number of studies). If a meta-analysis includes five studies, we have to expect a Q value of 5 − 1 = 4 because, as we have shown before, the probability of a sample of size K is only calculated for the number of studies that are free to vary (df = K − 1) (see Sect. 2.2.2). The question is whether what we did observe in the study (calculated Q) is different from what we expected in the absence of heterogeneity (df)?

The df of the study is the expected amount of heterogeneity due to chance, while Q is the overall heterogeneity observed. Consequently, their difference (Q − df) represents the amount of true heterogeneity between studies, not due to chance. Higgins and collaborators suggested presenting *the proportion of true variation (Q − df) to the overall variation (Q) as a numerical index (I^2)* "Eq. 6.158". The computer software package usually gives the 95% CI of (I^2), and the interested reader can check the detailed equation to calculate the confidence interval elsewhere [3].

$$I^2 = 100\% \; (Q - df)/Q \quad (6.158)$$

As such, I^2 is more a measure of consistency between studies. The larger the test, the more is the proportion of true heterogeneity between studies, and values of 75%, 50% and 25% have been suggested as indicators of large, moderate, and low limits. As in Q, negative values are put equal to zero so that I^2 lies between 0 and 100%. On the other hand, large I^2 indicates true differences across the studies, and hence, it calls upon the meta-analyst to look for the reason behind it, such as subgroups or moderator analysis. On the other hand, a value of 0% indicates that studies are consistent, and most probably, nothing remains to explain or look for [3, 40].

It is important to appreciate the difference between overall testing variation between studies (heterogeneity) by Q test and quantifying true variation that is not due to chance (consistency) by I^2. In other words, I^2 can calculate considerable inconsistency between the studies, but still,

Q may show a statistically-non-significant heterogeneity, which questions the conclusion made by Q in such a case that the studies are homogenous. Consequently, *the researcher is advised to only conclude upon heterogeneity rather than on its absence*. Unlike Q, I^2 is independent of the variable scale, the sample size, or the number of studies, and hence, I^2 *can be calculated and compared across meta-analyses of different sizes, of different types of study, and using different types of outcome data* [3, 40].

A Working Example

We will calculate I^2 for the example of comparing the duration of hospital stays following minimal invasive versus conventional open-heart surgery (see Sect. 6.2.6.2.2) "Eq. 6.159". Another example is the relative risk of the efficacy of the BCG vaccine (see Sect. 6.2.6.2.8) "Eq. 6.160".

$$I^2 = 100\% \frac{Q - df}{Q} = 100\% \frac{314 - 5}{314}$$
$$= 98.4\%$$
(6.159)

$$I^2 = 100\% \frac{Q - df}{Q} = 100\% \frac{152.2 - 12}{152.2}$$
$$= 92.1\%$$
(6.160)

The H^2 Index

Higgie and Thompson suggested another index to express, not the proportion of true variation out of the total variation (I^2), but *the relative excess in Q over what may be due to chance, i.e., what is above the df*. It is just another way to look up to the same thing. Unlike Q, the value of H^2 does not intrinsically depend on the number of studies but with a slight average bias for small numbers of studies. [40]. H^2 can be calculated from Q by a simple equation "Eq. 6.161", provided that Q was calculated from the inverse variance. For the example of testing the efficacy of the BCG vaccine (see Sect. 6.2.6.2.8), H^2 equals 12.68

$$H^2 = \frac{Q}{df}$$
(6.161)

The square root of H can be defined as the residual standard deviation of heterogeneity. Hence, an H value of 2 can be interpreted as the residual amount of heterogeneity is twice what would be expected if the studies were homogenous (Higgins and Thompson 2002). The calculation of the Se of H depends on whether the value of Q is larger than the number of classes (k) "Eq. 6.162", or is equal or smaller than (k) "Eq. 6.163". We can then assign an interval of confidence to H, which means that heterogeneity is real if it does not include the null (i.e., 1) "Eq. 6.164". All calculations are primarily made in the logarithmic scale, and then the values of H and the upper and lower limits of the 95% CI are then converted to the usual scale for presentation "Eq. 6.165".

$$Se_{log\,H} = \frac{1}{2} \times \frac{\log Q - \log(K - 1)}{\sqrt{2Q} - \sqrt{2Q - 3}} \; if\; Q > K$$
(6.162)

$$Se_{log\,H} = \sqrt{\left\{\frac{1}{2(K-2)} \times \left(1 - \frac{1}{3(K-2)^2}\right)\right\}} \; if\; Q \leq K$$
(6.163)

$$95\% \; CI\; Log\, H = Log\, H \pm 1.96 \; Se_{log\,H}$$
(6.164)

$$95\% \; CI\; H = e^{Log\, H \pm 1.96 \; Se_{log\,H}}$$
(6.165)

The R^2 Index

R-squared was proposed to describe the inflation in the confidence interval for an estimate under a random-effects model compared with a fixed-effect model. As the difference between the two models is estimated by the variability between studies (T^2), R^2 can be viewed as a function of T^2. A value of 1 indicates identical inferences under the two models, that is, when treatment effects are homogenous, and the fixed effect model is sufficient. As the sum of weights is the reciprocal value of the variance (inverse variance), R^2 can be the proportion of the sum of weights in a fixed-effect model to that of a random-effects model. The following equation can calculate R^2 "Eq. 6.166" and *its square root R can be interpreted as H*. [40]. The test is similar to H^2, and hence, one of both indices is only necessary to be reported.

$$R^2 = \frac{Var_R}{Var_F} = \frac{\sum W_i}{\sum W_i^R} = \frac{\sum W_i}{\sum (W_i + T^2)} \quad (6.166)$$

6.2.7.3 *Estimation of Variability Between Studies (T^2)*

There is usually a good reason to assume that a random-effects model is most appropriate in most meta-analyses; hence, we have to calculate T^2. There are several methods to calculate the variance between studies in the random effect model, such as the DerSimonian and Laird method [41], Hedges estimator [42], Hunter and Schmidt [2], Sidik-Jonkman [43], empirical Bayes, maximum likelihood and restricted maximum likelihood (REML) [38]. The DerSimonian and Laird method has all the qualities of a popular test. It is simple, understandable and easy to execute; hence, it is the most preferred. Some statisticians favor the (REML) method for the general use [38].

DerSimonian and Laird Method

DerSimonian and Laird's method derives the variability between the studies (T^2) from the same index that is usually used to assess whether this variability is statistically significant, which is Q (see Sect. 6.2.7.1). We have previously shown that the quantity (Q − df) represents the amount of true variation between studies that is not due to chance. However, (Q − df) measures "the weighted" "sum" of true variation between studies, and, what we need, is the "non-weighted" "average" variation between studies. In other words, we need a variance, which by definition should be an "average" and not a

"sum" and should be in the "original" scale and not in the "weighted" scale of the measure. Hence, dividing (Q − df) by the study weights as measured by (C) gives the average variability (variance) between studies in the original (unweighted) scale of effect size (T^2) "Eq. 6.167" [3]. C is the sum of squared differences between the weights of each study and the average weight of all studies "Eq. 6.168" Consequently, (T^2), and not Q, becomes the measure of variability between the studies included in the meta-analysis. The computer software package usually gives the 95% CI of (T^2), and the equations' details can be checked elsewhere [3].

$$T^2 = \frac{Q - df}{C} \quad (6.167)$$

$$C = \sum W_i - \frac{\sum W_i^2}{\sum W_i} \quad (6.168)$$

A Working Example

We will calculate T^2 for the example of comparing the duration of hospital stays following minimal invasive versus conventional open-heart surgery "Eq. 6.169" and "Eq. 6.170" (see Sect. 6.2.6.2.2). The difference noted between our result and the one produced by the software (3.37) is due to approximations. Another example is the calculation of T^2 for a random-effects model evaluating the efficacy of the BCG vaccine in the prevention of new cases of tuberculosis "Eqs. 6.171" and "6.172" (see Sect. 6.2.6.2.8).

$$C = \sum W_i - \frac{\sum W_i^2}{\sum W_i} = 118.2 - \frac{3280}{118.2} = 90.4$$
$$(6.169)$$

$$T^2 = \frac{Q - df}{C} = \frac{314 - 5}{90.4} = 3.4 \quad (6.170)$$

$$C = \sum W_i - \frac{\sum W_i^2}{\sum W_i} = 609.7 - \frac{94804.9}{609.7}$$
$$= 454.2$$
$$(6.171)$$

$$T^2 = \frac{Q - df}{C} = \frac{152.2 - 12}{454.2} = 0.308 \quad (6.172)$$

Variation of effect size

Being an estimate of the variance of the true effects (variations between studies), T^2 is used to assign weights under the random-effects model. The weight assigned to each study (W_i^R) is the reciprocal value of the sum of the variance of the study itself (Se_i^2), to which we add the variance between studies (T^2) "Eq. 6.173". The Se of the effect size (Se^R) is the square root of the reciprocal of the sum of the new random weights "Eq. 6.174".

$$W_i^R = \frac{1}{Se_i^2 + T^2} \quad (6.173)$$

$$Se^R = \sqrt{\frac{1}{\sum W_i^R}} \quad (6.174)$$

Variation of true effects

Being an estimate of the variance of the true effects, we can use T^2 alone and estimate a 95% CI of the true effects only. The standard deviation of the true effect (T) is the square root of T^2. We can assign a 95% CI around the ES by placing 1.96 T on either side of the mean effect "Eq. 6.175". For example, if the ES equals 0.5 and T = 0.1, we will be 95% confident that the true effect size will be between 0.3 and 0.7.

$$95\% \ CI \ ES^R = ES^R \pm 1.96 \ T \quad (6.175)$$

The Prediction Interval of Effect Size at 95%

The 95% CI expresses the width of the interval where there is a 95% probability of finding the mean effect size of the population (ES^R). However, it does not express the diversity of the between-study variance (T^2); which is better expressed by a prediction interval at 95% (95% PI). Put it this way, in order to predict the variability of the range of effects in a random effect model, we have to acknowledge that the summary mean ES^R varies by $(Se^R)^2 = (Se_i^2 + T^2)$ to which we have added the variability of Tau itself (T^2).

Note that we have to apply two rules here. The first is when we have two sources of variability, as in this case (variability of the measure T^2 and variability of the mean itself Se_i^2), we sum both variances. Then we take the square root of the sum "Eq. 6.176". Secondly, it is more prudent to use the t-value at a df that equals the number of studies minus two (K − 2) than the usual Z value of 1.96 because the number of studies in a meta-analysis is usually small [40, 44].

$$95\% \ PI \ ES^R = ES^R \pm t_{K-2}\sqrt{(Se^R)^2} \quad (6.176)$$

Put it this way, in a random-effects model, the 95% CI can be predicted as the summary of "the central distribution" position of the mean of the intervention effects of the included studies. The 95% PI can be interpreted as a summary of "the spread" of those underlying effects. Prediction intervals have proved a popular way of expressing the amount of heterogeneity in a meta-analysis, provided a reasonable number of studies, and the absence of a funnel plot asymmetry [44]. In the case of effect sizes following other distributions than normal, calculations are made in the log scale. The results are back-transformed to the original scale for presentation.

A Running Example

The 95% CI

Assuming a random effects model, the mean effect size (log relative risk) of patients vaccinated with BCG vaccine was −0.71 (95% CI: −1.06 to −0.364), which corresponds to an average relative risk of 0.49 (0.35 − 0.7) (see Sect. 6.2.6.2.8). The result can be interpreted that the average relative risk in the population is expected to be between 0.35 and 0.7.

The 95% PI

We will use the t-distribution instead of Z as suggested by Higgins and colleagues and a Se that is equal to the square root of both within and in-between study variance (0.179 + 0.31). At 11 df, t = 1.79. The prediction interval at 95% shows that although the average outcome is expected to be negative and hence, protective from the disease (-0.71), in some studies the true outcome may be harmful "Eq. 6.177". A log value of 0.33 corresponds to a relative risk of 1.39 "Eq. 6.178". Put it this way, although the use of the vaccine is expected to be associated with about 50% decrease in the risk of developing new cases of TB (relative risk = 0.49), in some studies vaccination may be associated with an increase in the risk of the disease (relative risk > 1).

$$95\% \ PI \ ES^R = -0.71 \pm 1.79\sqrt{0.179^2 + 0.31}$$
$$= -1.75 \ to \ 0.33$$
$$(6.177)$$

$$95\% \ PI \ RR = 0.49 \ (0.17 \ to \ 1.39) \quad (6.178)$$

Maximum Likelihood (ML)

The likelihood is not the probability, which can be defined as the probability of finding a certain value (x) in a given distribution. For example, there is a 5% probability (P = 0.05) of finding a value that is two standard deviations away from the mean in a normal distribution. Changing the data to 1.65 Sd away from the mean changes the probability to 10%, provided that the distribution is the same. In other words, the distribution is fixed (known), and the data is changing.

The likelihood is how much likely a given (x) value that is two standard deviations away from the mean fits a particular distribution, whether being normal or else? In other words, the data is fixed (known), and the distribution is changing; i.e., we are wondering about the distribution that best fits the data. *Maximum likelihood aims to find the optimum way to fit a distribution to a known data set.*

A piece of common knowledge is that a normal distribution is defined by the mean and the standard deviation (see Sect. 1.4). Returning to meta-analysis, if we believe that the effect size observed in the clinical studies included in the meta-analysis (ES_i) is normally distributed, the question would be to locate the population mean effect size (ES) and Sd of the parent distribution. We suggest a certain population mean effect size (ES) and calculate to see whether the effect sizes of individual studies (ES_i) are normally

distributed around it? In other words, whether the majority of (ES_i) has centered around (ES), that two-thirds of (ES_i) is within one standard deviation of (ES), 95% are two standard deviations on either side of (ES), and other criteria of normal distribution.

We keep on shifting the suggested position for the population mean effect size (ES) and repeating all the calculations till we find the optimal value of the population mean effect size (ES) that maximizes the likelihood of our observations being normal. In other words, till we find the best fitting population mean (ES), around which the majority of the (ES_i) of the included studies (i) are present and showing the other desired characteristics of normality just described. The latter is the maximum likelihood. *After finding the best fitting mean (ES), we repeat the same procedure to get the best fitting standard deviation (Sd).* It is evident that the calculations are long, especially compared with the simple DerSimonian equation. However, they are easily performed by computer software.

Restricted Maximum Likelihood (REML)

The maximum likelihood (ML) just described can be thought of as a two-step procedure. We start by estimating the mean effect (ES), and then we estimate the standard deviation (variance) from the estimated mean. But what we really want to do is to estimate the variance from the population mean and not from the observed mean. Another point is that (ML) underestimated the variance, especially in a small sample size [38]. *Unlike the (ML), the restricted maximum likelihood (REML) is not calculated from all data sets but from a set of data contrast created from the original data,* producing less biased estimates of variance and covariances [45]. However, calculations become much more complicated to be executed without a statistical software package.

6.2.7.4 Heterogeneity in Fixed Effect Versus Random Effects Model

We have shown that Q measures and tests the statistical significance of the observed variation between the studies. A challenging question would be why Q is measured under the fixed-effect model, which assumes that there is no variation between the studies? Once more, let us remember what is Q exactly? It is the sum of standardized squared differences between the effect size of individual studies and the average effect size. A Q value of zero indicates that all studies come from the same population, i.e., a theoretically fixed-effect model. Consequently, Q can be seen as the difference between the observed variation and the expected variation in the fixed-effect model. In other words, to calculate Q, we had to challenge our data with the fixed-effect model to see the difference (to see Q).

All other indices of heterogeneity that we have presented are deducted from Q, and hence, *the Q measured under the fixed effect model is the one used to compute I^2, R^2, and T^2*. All indices have to be reported along with the fixed-effect model but not T^2, simply because it must not be used in a fixed model. By definition, a fixed-effect model denies that studies are truly variable. Otherwise, it will turn into a random-effects model, i.e., a model admitting that studies are truly variable. On the other hand, it is this T^2 that is calculated under the fixed effect model that will be added to the within-study variation to weigh the effect size of the random effect model.

Moreover, whenever the researcher believes that a moderator variable interacts with (influences) the effect size, he is tempted to compare subgroups, usually by a random effect model. Consequently, he needs an estimate of T^2 for the whole study and each subgroup. For example, if he has three subgroups, he must calculate four T^2, one for each subgroup and one for the whole study, all being derived (calculated) from the fixed effect model. As T^2 is calculated from Q, C, and df, the meta-analyst has to compute four Q and four C values, too; all being derived from the fixed effect model. A running example will be given in Sect. 6.2.8.2.

Another important question is whether heterogeneity is dependent on the type model? By definition, the variability of a random model is larger than that of a fixed one due to the addition of T^2. Consequently, the relation between studies (heterogeneity) will change too,

which means that we have to calculate a new Q* each time we change the model. Yes, we have to express the changing relation between studies associated with changing the variability or the model, but *this new Q* can only be used to compare the variability between the studies within the new model but must never be used to test the statistical significance of heterogeneity between the studies* (see Sect. 6.2.8.2). The Q calculated under the fixed effect model remains the only one to evaluate and test the statistical significance of heterogeneity between studies, regardless of the model.

6.2.8   Subgroup Analysis

Following the demonstration of significant overall effect size, the meta-analyst is entitled to focus on the variation itself. The result of the meta-analysis is expressed by controlling for the part of variation due to sampling *error*. What remains can be either a *true variation* between studies (internal), an *artificial variation* due to the effect of a moderator variable (external), or both.

In the example of studying the efficacy of the BCG vaccine on the development of new cases of tuberculosis, the vaccine was shown to significantly reduce the risk of new cases, regardless of the model assumed (see Sect. 6.2.6.2.8). On the other hand, the meta-analysis has demonstrated a statistically significant heterogeneity above what can be explained by a random error; i.e., a statistically significant Q (see Sect. 6.2.7.1). The result of I^2 suggested that about 92% of this variation was true, and hence, the meta-analyst wondered whether the effect of moderator variables could explain this variation (see Sect. 6.2.7.2)? He has noticed that studies from warm countries showed a modest protective effect compared to those performed in cold-weather countries, so he decided to test the effect of climate by comparing those two subgroups. If the climate turns out to be a significant risk factor, we can try to change the conditions of vaccination in warm countries to improve the vaccine's protective effect.

As shown in Table 6.8, six studies were carried out in cold-weather countries and seven in warm countries. The usual procedure is to perform a separate mini-analysis for each subgroup. In addition to the main summary of the 13 studies, we will have two additional summary statistics, each including its mean effect size, Se, Q, and I^2. Besides the descriptive benefit of the procedure, we can test whether there is a statistically significant difference between the subgroups, reflecting a significant effect of the moderator variable itself. Each mini meta-analysis follows the same lines as the primary meta-analysis. *The random-effects model is the choice model*, especially since we already admit that subgroups are not the same by doing subgroup analysis. However, for instructive purposes, we will display the results of both models.

6.2.8.1 Fixed Effect Model Within Subgroups

Table 6.11 shows the calculations arranged by subgroups (warm and cold), with the last row showing their combined result. Assuming a fixed-effect model, we will weigh the effect size of each of the 13 studies by its inverse variance and compute three complete independent summary statistics: one for each subgroup and one for both groups combined. As in the primary analysis, we calculate a mean effect size and a standard error, create a 95% confidence interval, test its statistical significance, and analyze heterogeneity. The aim is to show the overall effect of the vaccine (combined effect) and the independent effect in each subgroup. The second step will be to compare the results of both subgroups to test whether there is a significant effect

Table 6.11 The relative risk: evaluation of the efficacy of the BCG vaccine, subgroup analysis, fixed effect model

Study	ES	Var	W	WES	WES²	W²
A—Warm group						
Coetzee 1968	−0.47	0.06	17.72	−8.32	3.90	313.99
Comstock 1969	0.45	0.53	1.88	0.84	0.37	3.53
Comstock 1974	−0.34	0.01	80.57	−27.34	9.28	6491.1
Comstock 1976	−0.02	0.07	14.00	−0.24	0.005	196.13
Frimodt 1973	−0.22	0.05	19.53	−4.25	0.92	381.32
Madras 1980	0.01	0.004	252.4	3.02	0.04	63,705
Vandiviere 1973	−1.62	0.22	4.48	−7.27	11.78	20.11
Total A			390.6	−43.56	26.3	71,110.8
B—Cold group						
Aronson 1948	−0.89	0.33	3.07	−2.73	2.43	9.43
Ferguson 1949	−1.59	0.19	5.14	−8.15	12.92	26.41
Hart 1977	−1.44	0.02	49.98	−72.04	103.85	2497.5
Rosenthal 1960	−1.35	0.42	2.41	−3.25	4.38	5.80
Rosenthal 1961	−1.37	0.07	13.69	−18.78	25.75	187.52
Stein 1953	−0.79	0.01	144.8	−113.8	89.48	20,968
Total B			219.1	−218.8	238.8	23,694.2
C—Combined			609.7	−262.4	265.1	94,805

ES = effect size (Log relative risk), Var = variance within the study, W = weight of the effect size = inverse Var, WES = weighed effect size = W × ES, WES² = WES × ES, W² = W × W of climate on the efficacy of the BCG vaccine or more cautiously a significant interaction between the two variables [46].

Primary Analysis

Since the relative risk (RR) does not follow a normal distribution, all calculations must be made in the log scale. In other words, our effect size (ES) is the Log RR. After we are done with calculations, the final results will be converted back into the usual scale (RR) for presentation. Taking the example of group Warm: we calculate the mean ES "Eq. 6.179", its Se "Eq. 6.180", the 95% CI "Eq. 6.181", the Z value "Eq. 6.182", and the 95% CI "Eq. 6.183"

$$\text{Mean ES} = \frac{\sum W_i Log_{RRi}}{\sum W_i} = \frac{-43.56}{390.6} = -0.111$$
$$(6.179)$$

$$\text{Se ES} = \sqrt{\frac{1}{\sum W_i}} = \sqrt{\frac{1}{390.6}} = 0.05 \quad (6.180)$$

$$95\% \; CI \; (ES) = \text{Mean ES} \pm 1.96(\text{Se ES})$$
$$= -0.111 \pm 1.96(0.05)$$
$$= -0.21 \, to - 0.013$$
$$(6.181)$$

$$Z = \frac{-0.111}{0.05} = -2.23; P = 0.028 \quad (6.182)$$

$$RR \; (95\% \; CI)_{warm\,subgroup} = 0.89 \; (0.81 \, to \, 0.99)$$
$$(6.183)$$

We will not show the details of the calculations made for the subgroup cold and for the two subgroups combined since they are the same. However, Table 6.12 shows the complete results coded serially in 13 rows. These include the effect size (log RR), and the upper and lower limits of its 95% CI (1st, 2nd, and 3rd rows). The effect size was evaluated by dividing each Log RR (1st row) by its Se (4th row) to produce the Z value (5th row). The degree of significance of Z was expressed in terms of P-value (6th row). The following four rows (7th, 8th, 9th and 10th rows) show the heterogeneity statistics namely, T^2, Q, P-value of Q, and I^2. The last three rows show the results as they should be finally reported, in terms of the original scale: RR and the lower and upper limits of its 95% CI (11th, 12th, and 13th row).

There is a statistically significant overall protective effect of the BCG vaccine in both groups combined: relative risk (95% CI) = 0.65 (0.6–

Table 6.12 The relative risk: evaluation of the efficacy of the BCG vaccine, results of subgroup analysis, fixed effect model

Serial		Warm group	Cold group	Combined
	N	7	6	13
1	Log RR	−0.112	−0.999	−0.43
2	UL[a]	−0.21	−1.13	−0.51
3	LL[a]	−0.013	−0.866	−0.35
4	Se	0.05	0.068	0.04
5	Z value	−2.23	−14.78	−10.62
6	P-value	0.028	<0.001	<0.001
7	T^2	0	0	0
8	Q	21.44	20.34	152.2
9	P-value	0.002	0.001	<0.001
10	I^2	72.2%	75.4%	92.1%
11	RR	0.894	0.368	0.65
12	LL[b]	0.81	0.323	0.6
13	UL[b]	0.988	0.421	0.7

N = number of studies, UL and LL = upper and lower limits of the 95% confidence interval, RR = relative risk, T^2 = Tau square, I^2 = I square, a = log value of RR, b = scale of relative risk

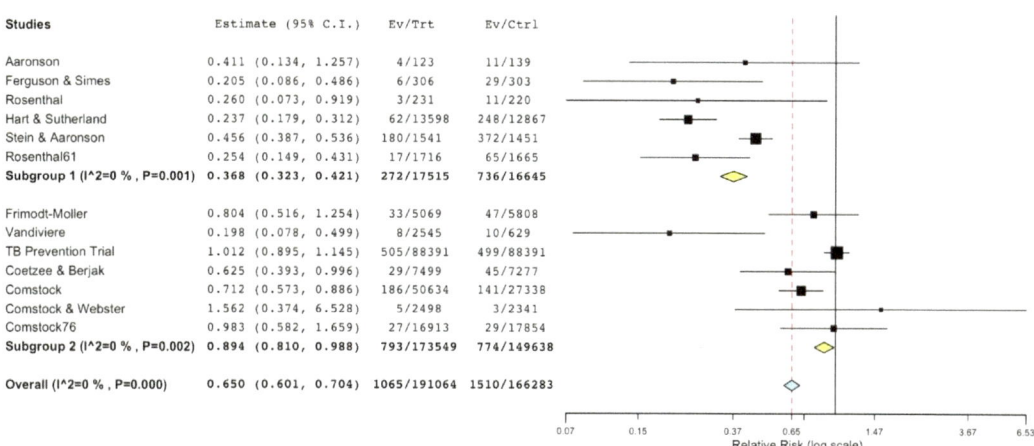

Studies	Estimate (95% C.I.)	Ev/Trt	Ev/Ctrl
Aaronson	0.411 (0.134, 1.257)	4/123	11/139
Ferguson & Simes	0.205 (0.086, 0.486)	6/306	29/303
Rosenthal	0.260 (0.073, 0.919)	3/231	11/220
Hart & Sutherland	0.237 (0.179, 0.312)	62/13598	248/12867
Stein & Aaronson	0.456 (0.387, 0.536)	180/1541	372/1451
Rosenthal61	0.254 (0.149, 0.431)	17/1716	65/1665
Subgroup 1 (I^2=0 % , P=0.001)	0.368 (0.323, 0.421)	272/17515	736/16645
Frimodt-Moller	0.804 (0.516, 1.254)	33/5069	47/5808
Vandiviere	0.198 (0.078, 0.499)	8/2545	10/629
TB Prevention Trial	1.012 (0.895, 1.145)	505/88391	499/88391
Coetzee & Berjak	0.625 (0.393, 0.996)	29/7499	45/7277
Comstock	0.712 (0.573, 0.886)	186/50634	141/27338
Comstock & Webster	1.562 (0.374, 6.528)	5/2498	3/2341
Comstock76	0.983 (0.582, 1.659)	27/16913	29/17854
Subgroup 2 (I^2=0 % , P=0.002)	0.894 (0.810, 0.988)	793/173549	774/149638
Overall (I^2=0 % , P=0.000)	0.650 (0.601, 0.704)	1065/191064	1510/166283

Relative Risk (log scale): 0.07 0.15 0.37 0.65 1.47 3.67 6.53

Fig. 6.12 Forest plot: the relative risk of BCG vaccine, subgroup analysis, fixed effect model (FE). Values are presented as relative risk (95% CI). The average relative risk, I^2%, and Q-test P value are calculated independently and presented for each subgroup

0.7); P < 0.001. Put it this way, the vaccine decreased the risk of developing a new episode of tuberculosis by 35% (30–40%). The subgroup analysis shows that the relative risk in cold weather countries was 0.368 (0.32–0.42); P < 0.001. In other words, the risk of developing new cases decreased by as much as 63% (58–68%) in the vaccinated group compared to non-vaccinated cases; P < 0.001. However, the risk equally decreased significantly in warm countries, with a lower extent of 10.6% (0.1–19%); P = 0.028. There was statistically significant heterogeneity, whether in either group or the combined two groups. To a large extent, heterogeneity seems true, as shown by the high reported I^2 (72–92.1%). Figure 6.12 shows the forest plot of the subgroup analysis assuming a fixed model effect as produced by OpenmetaAnalyst software, which unfortunately does not show the studies' relative weights (Fig. 6.12).

Comparison of Subgroups

We have just shown that the risk of developing new cases was significantly reduced in both subgroups and the question now is whether both relative risks are significantly different from one another or not. Altman and Bland have shown that the best term for such comparison is testing whether there is an interaction between the

climate (warm versus cold) and the estimated effect size (relative risk) rather than comparing subgroup [46]. However, we will proceed with comparing subgroups for their descriptive value and mainly for teaching purposes.

The 95% CI of Log RR was (−0.999 to −0.863) and (−0.212 to −0.012) in the warm and cold countries, respectively. Although both 95% CI do not overlap, we must conduct formal statistical testing. As we have two subgroups only (warm and cold), the mean difference between both effect sizes can be compared by a simple Z test. In the case of multiple groups, the Z test cannot be used, and we have to compare the subgroups by a modified ANOVA. A third approach introduces the final results of the subgroups (the mean effect size and the Se) in a new meta-analysis as if they were the results of individual studies [3]. We will show the three procedures for demonstration.

(A) Z Test

The Z test is simple; we divide the difference between the two logs by the Se of the difference "Eq. 6.184", then we check upon the statistical significance of the result in the Z table. The difference between the two logs is the absolute difference between both values. The Se of the difference is the square root of the sum of both standard errors, and the Z table gives a P-value < 0.001. The 95% CI is calculated as usual: Log RR + 1.96 Se, and then we convert the upper and lower limit of the 95% CI to the original scale for presentation.

$$Z = \frac{|Log_A - Log_B|}{\sqrt{Se_A^2 + Se_B^2}} = \frac{|(-0.112) - (-0.999)|}{\sqrt{0.051^2 + 0.068^2}}$$
$$= \frac{0.089}{0.085} = 10.5$$

(6.184)

Our results showed that there is a statistically significant interaction between the climate and the protection made by the vaccine. The relative risk of a new event in a cold climate is significantly lower than that reported in warm countries. In other words, there is a statistically significant interaction between the climate and the effect size; P < 0.001.

(B) Modified ANOVA

In the case of multiple groups, we can use a modified ANOVA to analyze the variance of the meta-analysis, which is nothing but the Q index. The reader can refer back to the chapter on one-way ANOVA to revise the essential elements of the analysis (see Sect. 2.4.3.1). In brief, One-way ANOVA partitions the total variability into variability between groups and variability within groups. The significance of each part is dependent upon its df. In our subgroup analysis, we have calculated three Q(s): one (Q*) for the warm group, a second (Q*) for the cold group, and a third "Q" for the combined group (the whole study). The variability "within-groups" (cold and warm) is equal to the sum of both within-group variabilities, i.e., the sum of (Q* warm) and (Q* cold) "Eq. 6.185". The variability "between-groups" is the difference between the total variability (Q combined) and the within-groups variabilities (Q* warm + Q* cold) "Eq. 6.186". The degrees of freedom are calculated as usual: the total number of studies minus one for total Q (13 − 2 = 12 df), the number of studies in the

warm group minus one plus the number of studies in the cold group minus one for the within-groups variability [(7 − 1) + (6 − 1) = 11 df], and the number of groups minus one for the between-group's variability (2 − 1 = 1 df). As previously mentioned, and except for the original total Q that is solely used to describe the heterogeneity among the 13 clinical studies, the other Q(s) can only be used for comparison (see Sect. 6.2.7.4). As per the advice of Borenstein and colleagues, those Q(s) were denoted with an Asterix to avoid confusion [3].

$$Q_{within}^* = Q_{warm} + Q_{cold} = 21.44 + 20.34$$
$$= 41.78$$

(6.185)

$$Q_{between}^* = Q_{total} - (Q_{warm} + Q_{within})$$
$$= 152.2 - (21.44 + 20.34) = 110$$

(6.186)

As shown, the within-groups variability = 41.78 and for 11 df, the exact P-value = 0.00018. The between-groups variability = 110.22, and for 1 df, P < 0.0001. The effect of the vaccine is related to the climate being significantly more effective in cold than in warm weather. Note that the two methods produced identical results, and at 1 df (two subgroups), Z is equal to the square root of Q* (10.5 is the square root of 110) [3].

(C) Analysis of heterogeneity among subgroups

We will consider the summary statistics of the two mini meta-analyses (cold and warm subgroups) as the results of two individual studies. We will perform a new meta-analysis for those two studies [3]. As Cochran Q tests the statistical significance of the heterogeneity between the studies included in a meta-analysis, it will test the heterogeneity among our subgroups. Consequently, a statistically significant Q will mean that both groups are significantly heterogeneous (different), which is the aim of the comparison. The meta-analysis follows the same procedure as before (see Sect. 6.2.6.2.8), the calculation details are shown in Table 6.13 and the new produced Q figures in "Eq. 6.187".

Table 6.13 The relative risk: evaluation of the efficacy of the BCG vaccine, analysis of heterogeneity among subgroups, fixed effect model

Study	N	ES	Var	W	WES	WES^2
Warm	7	−0.112	0.0026	384.46	−43.1	4.82
Cold	6	−0.999	0.0046	216.26	−216	215.81
Total				601.22	−259.1	220.65

ES = Log relative risk, Var = variance of log relative risk, W = weighing = inverse variance

In order to prevent confusion, the new Q that is just used for this comparison is also denoted as Q* to differentiate it from the original Q used for testing the significance of heterogeneity. By far, they are not the same and should not be mixed. As our new meta-analysis included only two studies, the statistical significance of Q* will be checked out at the Chi-square table at 1 df (P < 0001). It is clear that the three computational techniques give similar results: the cold significantly reduced the risk of new cases of tuberculosis compared to the warm weather.

$$Q^* = \sum W(ES)^2 - \frac{\left(\sum WES\right)^2}{\sum W}$$
$$= 220.65 - \frac{(-259.1)^2}{601.22} = 110 \quad (6.187)$$

6.2.8.2   Random Effects Model Within Subgroups: Separate Versus Pooled T^2

We will perform two separate mini analyses that consider variability between studies (T^2). We will calculate a mean effect size, a 95% CI, and test its statistical significance for each subgroup and the whole study. Finally, we will compare the subgroups as shown before. However, *the meta-analyst has a decision to make either to calculate a different (T^2) for each subgroup or to use one pooled (T^2) for all.* Keeping separate (T^2) is only adopted when the meta-analyst has reliable evidence that the subgroups have significant variabilities. Moreover, it requires a minimum sample size of five studies in each subgroup. Otherwise, the two calculated standard errors will be unstable and a source of variability

rather than a method to improve precision. Using a pooled standard T^2 is the usual choice and is the default method in Cochran meta-analysis. We will perform both procedures as a demonstration.

Random Effects Model Assuming Separate T^2
In this particular model, we assume that each subgroup has its own pattern of variability; which is of course not the same as the variability between the 13 studies as a whole. As variability is tested by Q, we have to calculate one Q value for each subgroup and a third Q for the whole study (both groups combined). Each Q value is then used to deduct its own T^2 and I^2; i.e., we will end by having three different T^2 and I^2. Afterwards, we will repeat the same calculations three times as in the fixed model: one for each subgroup and one for both subgroups combined. The main difference is that in each of those times, the effect size is not only weighed by the within-study variance (Se^2) but by the reciprocal value of the sum of the latter and the concerned (T^2).

Primary Analysis
(A)   *Computation of separate T^2*

In order to weigh the effect sizes of the 13 studies, we need to compute three T^2 values, one for each subgroup and the third one for both groups combined. Note that we must calculate Q first "Eqs. 6.188 and 6.189," from which we can deduct T^2 "Eq. 6.190" and I^2 "Eq. 6.191". As previously explained (see Sect. 6.2.7.4), the values used for calculation are derived from the data of the fixed-effect model (Table 6.12). As an example, we will show the details of the calculation for the warm group:

$$Q = \sum W(ES)^2 - \frac{(\sum WES)^2}{\sum W}$$
$$= 26.30 - \frac{(43.56)^2}{390.58} = 21.44 \qquad (6.188)$$

$$C = \sum W_i - \frac{\sum W_i^2}{\sum W_i} = 390.58 - \frac{71110.79}{390.58}$$
$$= 208.5$$

$$\qquad (6.189)$$

$$T^2 = \frac{Q - df}{C} = \frac{21.44 - 6}{155} = 0.074 \quad (6.190)$$

$$I^2 = 100\% \frac{Q - df}{Q} = \frac{21.44 - 6}{21.44} = 72\%$$

$$\qquad (6.191)$$

We repeat the same calculations for both the cold and combined groups. Equations are similar, and

the $=T^2$ values calculated for the cold group and both groups combined were: 0.138 and 0.31, respectively. Table 6.14 shows the row and the weighted effect sizes for the 13 studies, using the appropriate T^2 value.

(B) *Calculation of mean effect size, 95% CI and testing its statistical significance*

We can now calculate a mean effect size "Eq. 6.192", a standard error "Eq. 6.193", create a 95% CI "Eq. 6.194" and test its statistical significance "Eq. 6.195". Note that all calculations are made in the logarithmic scale (ES = log RR) but have to be finally converted back into the usual scale for presentation "Eq. 6.196". Taking the example of group Warm:

Table 6.14 The relative risk: evaluation of the efficacy of the BCG vaccine, subgroup analysis, random effects model, assuming separate T^2

Study	ES	Var	Var$_T$	W	WES	WES^2	W^2
A—Warm group							
Coetzee 1968	−0.47	0.06	0.13	7.67	−3.60	1.69	58.78
Comstock 1969	0.45	0.53	0.61	1.65	0.74	0.33	2.72
Comstock 1974	−0.34	0.01	0.09	11.57	−3.93	1.33	133.92
Comstock 1976	−0.02	0.07	0.15	6.88	−0.12	0.00	47.30
Frimodt 1973	−0.22	0.05	0.13	7.99	−1.74	0.38	63.79
Madras 1980	0.01	0.004	0.08	12.83	0.15	0.00	164.53
Vandiviere 1973	−1.62	0.22	0.30	3.37	−5.46	8.85	11.34
Total A				51.95	−13.95	12.58	482.36
B—Cold group							
Aronson 1948	−0.89	0.33	0.46	2.16	−1.92	1.71	4.65
Ferguson 1949	−1.59	0.19	0.33	3.01	−4.77	7.56	9.04
Hart 1977	−1.44	0.02	0.16	6.33	−9.12	13.15	40.05
Rosenthal 1960	−1.35	0.42	0.55	1.81	−2.44	3.28	3.27
Rosenthal 1961	−1.37	0.07	0.21	4.74	−6.50	8.91	22.46
Stein 1953	−0.79	0.01	0.14	6.90	−5.43	4.26	47.62
Total B				24.94	−30.17	38.88	127.9
C—combined				76.88	−44.12	51.45	609.46

ES = effect size (Log relative risk), Var = variance within the study, Var$_T$ = total variance = Var + T^2 = Var + 0.074 in warm group and Var + 0.138 in cold group, W = weight of the effect size = inverse Var$_T$, WES = weighed effect size = W × ES, WES^2 = WES × ES, W^2 = W × W

$$\text{Mean ES}^R = \frac{\sum W_i^R Log_{RRi}}{\sum W_i^R} = \frac{-13.95}{51.95}$$
$$= -0.269 \qquad (6.192)$$

$$\text{Se ES}^R = \sqrt{\frac{1}{51.95}} = \sqrt{\frac{1}{31.36}} = 0.139$$
$$(6.193)$$

$$95\% \ CI \ \text{ES}^R = \text{Mean ES}^R \pm 1.96 \ (Se^R)$$
$$= -0.269 \pm 1.96 \ (0.139)$$
$$= -0.54 \ to \ 0.003$$
$$(6.194)$$

$$Z = \frac{-0.269}{0.139} = -1.93; \ P = 0.053 \qquad (6.195)$$

$$RR \ (95\% \ CI)_{warm \ subgroup} = 0.76 \ (0.58 \ to \ 1) \qquad (6.196)$$

We repeat the same calculations for the cold group and both groups combined. Equations are similar, and the results are shown in Table 6.15. There is a statistically significant overall protective effect of the BCG vaccine. The overall relative risk of vaccinated patients has decreased $(1 - RR\%)$ by as much as 51% (30.5–65.5%),

compared to controls; P < 0.001. In cold weather countries, the risk of developing new cases decreased by 70.2% (56–80%) in the vaccinated group compared to non-vaccinated cases (P = 0.001). On the other hand, the relative risk decrease was less pronounced in warms countries: 24% (0–42%); P = 0.053. The random-effects model makes it harder to conclude upon statistical significance because it considered the variance between studies (T^2). Figure 6.13 shows the forest plot of the subgroup analysis (Fig. 6.13).

Comparison of Subgroups

(A) Z test

As we have two subgroups only (warm and cold), the mean of the difference between both effect sizes can be compared by a simple Z test, as we did in the fixed-effect model. Remember that all calculations are made on the logarithmic scale: the difference between two logs is equal to their absolute difference, and the Se of the difference is the square root of the sum of both

Table 6.15 The relative risk: evaluation of the efficacy of the BCG vaccine, results of subgroup analysis, random effects model, assuming separate T^2

Serial			Warm group	Cold group	Combined
	N		7	6	13
1	Log RR		−0.269	−1.2	−0.714
2	UL[a]		−0.54	−1.6	−1.06
3	LL[a]		0.003	−0.82	−0.36
4	Se		0.139	0.2	0.179
5	Z value		1.935	−6.04	−3.995
6	P-value		0.053	<0.001	<0.001
7	T^2		0.074	0.138	0.31
8	Q		21.44	20.34	152.2
9	P-value		0.002	0.001	<0.001
10	I^2		72%	75.4%	92.1%
11	RR		0.76	0.298	0.49
12	LL[b]		0.58	0.2	0.345
13	UL[b]		1	0.44	0.695

N = number of studies, UL and LL = upper and lower limits of the 95% confidence interval, RR = relative risk, T^2 = Tau square, I^2 = I square, a = log value of RR, b = scale of relative risk

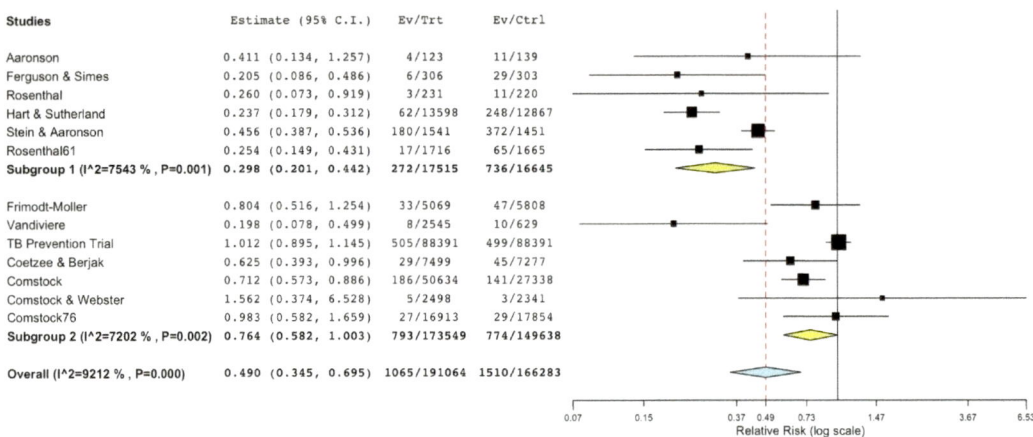

Studies	Estimate (95% C.I.)	Ev/Trt	Ev/Ctrl
Aaronson	0.411 (0.134, 1.257)	4/123	11/139
Ferguson & Simes	0.205 (0.086, 0.486)	6/306	29/303
Rosenthal	0.260 (0.073, 0.919)	3/231	11/220
Hart & Sutherland	0.237 (0.179, 0.312)	62/13598	248/12867
Stein & Aaronson	0.456 (0.387, 0.536)	180/1541	372/1451
Rosenthal61	0.254 (0.149, 0.431)	17/1716	65/1665
Subgroup 1 (I^2=7543 %, P=0.001)	0.298 (0.201, 0.442)	272/17515	736/16645
Frimodt-Moller	0.804 (0.516, 1.254)	33/5069	47/5808
Vandiviere	0.198 (0.078, 0.499)	8/2545	10/629
TB Prevention Trial	1.012 (0.895, 1.145)	505/88391	499/88391
Coetzee & Berjak	0.625 (0.393, 0.996)	29/7499	45/7277
Comstock	0.712 (0.573, 0.886)	186/50634	141/27338
Comstock & Webster	1.562 (0.374, 6.528)	5/2498	3/2341
Comstock76	0.983 (0.582, 1.659)	27/16913	29/17854
Subgroup 2 (I^2=7202 %, P=0.002)	0.764 (0.582, 1.003)	793/173549	774/149638
Overall (I^2=9212 %, P=0.000)	0.490 (0.345, 0.695)	1065/191064	1510/166283

Fig. 6.13 Forest plot: the relative risk of BCG vaccine, subgroup analysis, random effect model (RE). Values are presented as relative risk (95% CI). The average relative risk, $I^2\%$, and Q-test P value are calculated independently and presented for each subgroup

standard errors. The Z score is calculated by dividing the absolute difference by the Se "Eq. 6.197", and the statistical significance of Z is looked for in the Z table (P < 0.001)

$$Z = \frac{|Log_A - Log_B|}{Se_d} = \frac{|Log_A - Log_B|}{\sqrt{Se_A^2 + Se_B^2}}$$

$$= \frac{|(-0.269) - (-1.2)|}{\sqrt{0.139^2 + 0.2^2}} = \frac{0.93}{0.24} = 3.82$$

$$(6.197)$$

We can conclude that there is a statistically significant interaction between the climate and the protection made by the vaccine. The relative risk of a new event in a cold climate is significantly lower than that reported in warm countries.

(B) Modified ANOVA

We have shown that we can compare subgroups by a modified ANOVA (see Sect. 6.2.8.2.1). However, we have to be extremely careful because the Q calculated is not the one used for testing heterogeneity. Its use is limited to this comparative test, so it is better noted as Q* [3]. The data used to calculate Q* are not the fixed

model data used to calculate the original Q but the data derived from the actual model (random model with separate T^2) (Table 6.14).

We have calculated three Q*, one for the warm group "Eq. 6.198", one for the cold group "Eq. 6.199", and the third Q* is calculated for both groups combined "Eq. 6.200". The variability within-groups (cold and warm) is equal to the sum of both within-group variability, i.e., the sum of (Q* warm) and (Q* cold) "Eq. 6.201". The variability between-groups is the difference between the total variability (Q* combined) and the within-groups variability (Q* warm + Q* cold) "Eq. 6.202". The degrees of freedom are calculated as usual: total number of studies minus one for total Q* (13 − 2 = 12 df), number of studies in the warm group minus one plus the number of studies in the cold group minus one for the within-groups variability [(7 − 1) + (6 − 1) = 11 df], and number of groups minus one for the in-between group's variability (2 − 1 = 1 df).

$$Q^*_{warm} = \sum W(ES)^2 - \frac{(\sum WES)^2}{\sum W}$$

$$= 12.58 - \frac{(13.95)^2}{51.95} = 8.76 \qquad (6.198)$$

$$Q^*_{cold} = \sum W(ES)^2 - \frac{(\sum WES)^2}{\sum W}$$
$$= 38.88 - \frac{(30.17)^2}{24.94} = 1.88 \qquad (6.199)$$

$$Q^*_{total} = \sum W(ES)^2 - \frac{(\sum WES)^2}{\sum W}$$
$$= 51.45 - \frac{(44.12)^2}{76.88} = 26.1 \qquad (6.200)$$

$$Q^*_{within} = Q^*_{warm} + Q^*_{cold} = 8.76 + 1.88 = 10.64 \qquad (6.201)$$

$$Q^*_{between} = Q^*_{total} - (Q^*_{warm} + Q^*_{within})$$
$$= 26.1 - (8.76 + 1.88) = 15.46 \qquad (6.202)$$

The corresponding P values for the total variability, variability between groups, and variability within groups are 0.01, <0.001, and 0.011. The overall effect of the vaccine is significantly related to the climate (P = 0.01) being significantly much more effective in cold than in warm weather (P < 0.001); however, there is still a remaining part of residual variability that needs to be explained (P = 0.011).

(C) **Analysis of heterogeneity among subgroups**

We will consider the summary statistics of the two mini meta-analyses (cold and warm subgroups) as the results of two individual studies. We will perform a new meta-analysis just for those two studies and compute Q* "Eq. 6.203"

[3]. A statistically significant Q* means that the subgroups are statistically significantly different from each other. The meta-analysis follows the same procedure as before (see Sect. 6.2.6.2.8), and the details are shown in Table 6.16.

$$Q^* = \sum W(ES)^2 - \frac{(\sum WES)^2}{\sum W}$$
$$= 51.45 - \frac{(-44.12)^2}{76.88} = 26.1 \qquad (6.203)$$

As our new meta-analysis included only two studies, the statistical significance of Q* will be checked out at the Chi-square table at 1 df (P < 0001). It is clear that the three computational techniques give similar results: the cold weather significantly reduced the risk of new tuberculosis cases compared to the warm weather.

Random Effects Model Assuming Pooled T²
In the absence of a strong argument or reliable evidence that subgroups have different patterns of heterogeneity, we have to pool a common T^2 and use it to weigh the effect sizes of all studies, regardless of the assigned subgroup. This is the safest method, especially with a small sample size, such as five studies or less per subgroup. It is the default method in RevMan, while other software, such as comprehensive meta-analysis, allows the researcher to choose whether to pool or not to pool T^2. Consequently, the first step is to compute a common T^2 added to the within-variability calculated for each study. Afterward, computations proceed as routine. We calculate an average effect size, create a 95% CI around the

Table 6.16 The relative risk: evaluation of the efficacy of the BCG vaccine, analysis of heterogeneity among subgroups, random effects model, assuming separate T^2

Study	N	ES	Var	W	WES	WES²
Warm	7	−0.269	0.139	51.95	−13.95	12.58
Cold	6	−1.2	0.2	24.94	−30.17	38.88
Total				76.88	−44.12	51.45

ES = Log relative risk, Var = variance of log relative risk, W = weighing inverse variance mean, test its statistical significance and analyze heterogeneity. The study ends by comparing the means and heterogeneity among subgroups.

Primary Analysis

(A) Computation of pooled T^2

In practice, pooling T^2 should begin by pooling the elements that produce it, namely Q, C, and df [3]. The first step is to calculate C "Eqs. 6.204" and "6.205" and Q "Eqs. 6.206" and "6.207" for both groups. The second step is to calculate the pooled T2 itself from the sums of Q, C, and the df "Eq. 6.208". Note that the data used for all calculations are derived from the fixed-effect model shown in Table 6.11 (see Sect. 6.2.8.2.1).

$$C_{warm} = \sum W_i - \frac{\sum W_i^2}{\sum W_i} = 390.58 - \frac{71110.79}{390.58}$$
$$= 208.5$$
$$(6.204)$$

$$C_{cold} = \sum W_i - \frac{\sum W_i^2}{\sum W_i} = 219.09 - \frac{23694.18}{219.09}$$
$$= 110.94$$
$$(6.205)$$

$$Q_{warm} = \sum W(ES)^2 - \frac{(\sum WES)^2}{\sum W}$$
$$= 26.30 - \frac{(-43.56)^2}{390.58} = 21.44 \quad (6.206)$$

$$Q_{cold} = \sum W(ES)^2 - \frac{(\sum WES)^2}{\sum W}$$
$$= 238 - \frac{(-218.78)^2}{219.09} = 20.34 \quad (6.207)$$

$$T^2_{pooled} = \frac{\sum Q - \sum df}{\sum C}$$
$$= \frac{(21.44 + 20.34) - (6+5)}{(208.5 + 110.94)} = 0.096$$
$$(6.208)$$

Only after calculating pooled T^2, can we weigh the effect size of the 13 studies by the new variance: i.e., the within-study variance plus the pooled T^2, as shown in Table 6.17.

(B) Calculation of average effect size, 95% CI and testing its statistical significance

We calculate the mean effect size "Eq. 6.209", its Se "Eq. 6.210", a 95% CI "Eq. 6.211", and test its statistical significance "Eq. 6.212". Note that all calculations are made in the logarithmic scale but have to be finally converted back into the usual scale for presentation "Eq. 6.213". Taking the example of the subgroup cold:

$$Mean^R_{Log\,RR} = \frac{\sum W_i^R Log_{RRi}}{\sum W_i^R} = \frac{-50.8}{75.3} = -0.67$$
$$(6.209)$$

$$Se^R_{Log\,RR} = \sqrt{\frac{1}{\sum W_i^R}} = \sqrt{\frac{1}{75.3}} = 0.115$$
$$(6.210)$$

$$95\%\ CI = \log RR \pm 1.96(Se_{Log\,RR})$$
$$= -0.67 \pm 1.96\,(0.115)$$
$$= -0.89\ \text{to} -0.44 \quad (6.211)$$

$$Z = \frac{-0.67}{0.115} = -5.8; P<0.001 \quad (6.212)$$

$$RR\ (95\%\ CI)_{\text{cold subgroup}} = 0.51(0.41\ to\ 0.64)$$
$$(6.213)$$

We repeat the same calculations for the subgroup warm and both groups combined. The equations are the same, and the final results are shown in Table 6.18. There was a statistically significant overall protective effect of the vaccination, as shown by a relative risk of 0.51 (0.41–0.64); P < 0.001. In other words, vaccination decreased the overall relative risk of acquiring a new event by 49% (46–59%). The vaccine was even more effective in cold counties achieving a relative risk reduction of 70% (48–79%); P < 0.001. On the other hand, the vaccine's efficacy was less pronounced in warms countries, with an average relative risk reduction of only 24% (P = non-significant). The combined and the subgroup analysis showed a statistically significant heterogeneity that appears to be largely true, with I^2 ranging between 72.2 and 75.4%.

Table 6.17 The relative risk: evaluation of the efficacy of the BCG vaccine, subgroup analysis, random effects model, assuming pooled T^2

Study	ES	Var	Var_T	W	WES	WES^2	W^2
A—Warm group							
Coetzee 1968	−0.47	0.06	0.15	6.56	−3.08	1.45	43.04
Comstock 1969	0.45	0.53	0.63	1.59	0.71	0.32	2.53
Comstock 1974	−0.34	0.01	0.11	9.22	−3.13	1.06	85.08
Comstock 1976	−0.02	0.07	0.17	5.97	−0.10	0.00	35.68
Frimodt 1973	−0.22	0.05	0.15	6.79	−1.48	0.32	46.15
Madras 1980	0.01	0.004	0.10	10.00	0.12	0.001	100.08
Vandiviere 1973	−1.62	0.223	0.32	3.13	−5.08	8.236	9.83
Total				43.28	−12.0	11.38	322.38
B—Cold group							
Aronson 1948	−0.89	0.326	0.42	2.37	−2.11	1.876	5.63
Ferguson 1949	−1.59	0.195	0.29	3.44	−5.46	8.650	11.84
Hart 1977	−1.44	0.020	0.12	8.62	−12.43	17.913	74.30
Rosenthal 1960	−1.35	0.415	0.51	1.96	−2.64	3.554	3.82
Rosenthal 1961	−1.37	0.073	0.17	5.92	−8.11	11.126	35.00
Stein 1953	−0.79	0.007	0.10	9.72	−7.64	6.005	94.43
Total				32.02	−38.38	49.12	225
C—Combined				75.3	−50.8	60.5	547.38

ES = effect size (Log relative risk), Var = variance within the study, Var_T = total variance = Var + pooled T^2 = Var + 0.096, W = weight of the effect size = inverse Var_T, WES = weighed effect size = W × ES, WES^2 = WES × ES, W^2 = W × W

Table 6.18 The relative risk: evaluation of the efficacy of the BCG vaccine, results of subgroup analysis, random effects model, assuming pooled T^2

Serial		Warm group	Cold group	Combined
	N	7	6	13
1	Log RR	−0.277	−1.198	−0.67
2	UL^a	−0.57	−1.55	−0.89
3	LL^a	0.017	−0.85	−0.44
4	Se	0.15	0.177	0.115
5	Z value	−1.84	−6.77	−5.8
6	P-value	0.066	<0.001	<0.001
7	T^2	0.074	0.138	0.31
8	Q	21.44	20.34	152.2
9	P-value	0.002	0.001	<0.001
10	I^2	72%	75.4%	92.1%
11	RR	0.76	0.3	0.51
12	LL^b	0.57	0.21	0.41
13	UL^b	1.017	0.42	0.64

N = number of studies, UL and LL = upper and lower limits of the 95% confidence interval, RR = relative risk, T^2 = Tau square of individual subgroups, I^2 = I square, a = log value of RR, b = scale of relative risk

(C) **R-Squared**

The value of pooled T^2 is like an average T^2, lying in between the T^2 values of both groups (0.074 and 0.163) and is smaller than the total T^2 that was originally calculated for our study (0.31). Using this average pooled T^2 to weigh all effect sizes brings all weighed effect sizes closer together, representing the effect of the grouping variable (climate) on the outcome (effect size). Put it this way, the proportion between the pooled T^2 and total T^2 (T^2 pooled/T^2 total) can be seen as the proportion of variability explained by the moderator (climate) out of the total variability. Consequently, 1—this ratio is the part of variability explained by the predictor (climate). It is the same concept as R^2 of clinical studies but modified for meta-analysis [3]. In our example, climate explains two-thirds of the effectiveness of the BCG vaccine "Eq. 6.214".

$$R^2 = 1 - \frac{explained\ variability}{total\ variability} = 1 - \frac{T^2_{pooled}}{T^2_{total}}$$
$$= 1 - \frac{0.096}{0.31} = 69\%$$

$$(6.214)$$

Comparison of Subgroups

As we have only two subgroups, they can be compared by a simple Z test "Eq. 6.215". We can conclude that there is a statistically significant interaction between the climate and the protection made by the vaccine (P-value = 0.00128). The relative risk of a new event in a cold climate is significantly lower than that reported in warm countries. The other comparison tests (modified ANOVA and Q test of heterogeneity) are not shown. They can be carried out exactly as before and will give the same results (see Sects. 6.2.8.2.1 and 6.2.8.2.2). Just be cautious about calculating Q* from the data of the actual model: the random model with pooled T^2

$$Z = \frac{|\text{Log}_A - \text{Log}_B|}{\text{Se}_d} = \frac{|\text{Log}_A - \text{Log}_B|}{\sqrt{\text{Se}^2_A + \text{Se}^2_B}}$$
$$= \frac{|(-0.277) - (-1.198)|}{\sqrt{0.15^2 + 0.177^2}} = \frac{0.921}{0.232} = 3.97$$

$$(6.215)$$

6.2.9 **Meta Regression**

Meta-regression is the use of regression techniques to evaluate the overall influence and individual contribution of qualitative and quantitative moderator variables on the effect size of meta-analysis. It is like multiple regression used in clinical studies with few differences and modifications. The unit of the analysis is not the patients, but the clinical studies, and the effect size has to be weighted before the calculations. The reader is invited to refer to the chapters on simple (see Sect. 2.6.2) and multiple regression (see Sect. 3.4) to revise the assumptions, the conditions of application, the methods of calculation, and the proper interpretation of the results.

The meta-analyst has to respect the standard meta-regression conditions of application. It is unwise to include large number of covariates (moderator variable in meta regression) particularly if sample size is small, which is unfortunately, the usual case of meta-analysis. In brief, the null hypothesis is that the predictor variable(s) (moderator variable in regression) does not influence the outcome (effect size). Consequently, if their relationship is linear, the series of paired data (predictor-effect size) will form a straight horizontal line; i.e., the effect size remains the same, regardless the value of the moderator variable. Under the alternative hypothesis, the data points will tend to swipe away from the horizon, making a slope that is angled on the horizon (Fig. 2.5). The difference between the two situations (the horizontal line and the slope) expresses the influence of the moderator on the effect size. The more the influence, the more the slope deviates from the horizon (Sect. 2.6.2.1). A simple meta-regression equation is shown below "Eq. 6.216"

$$ES = b_0 + b_1x_1 + b_2x_2 ... b_ix_i \qquad (6.216)$$

The outputs of the analysis include the beta coefficients (b_1, b_2, ... b_i), each expressing the effect of one of the moderator variables (x_1, x_2, ...x_i) on the effect size (ES). The intercept of regression (b_0) can be seen as the residual variation in the effect size, which remains unexplained by the moderators in the model. Take the example of studying the protective effect of the BCG vaccine on the development of a new episode of tuberculosis (Table 6.11). The intercept can be seen as the vaccine's protective effect, regardless of the influence of the climate (moderator). Knowing the intercept and the beta coefficient, we can predict the effect size for a specific value of the moderator variable. Although simple regression is easy to calculate by hand (see Sect. 2.6.2), multiple regression needs a computer software program, which provides several advantages provided we know the correct interpretation of the output. The software also provides the model fit statistics and reports the studentized residuals and Cook distance to detect outliers and influential points (see Sect. 3.4). It produces a modified R-squared, which should not be interpreted as the standard R^2 of regression. The latter is a widely used indicator of the proportion of total variation in outcome by the set of predictors or the model (see Sect. 3.4.6.1). *The R^2 of meta-regression is deducted from one source, which is the variation between studies (T^2), and does not include the variation within the studies themselves (Se^2)* [3].

We have previously discussed the meta-analysis performed by Colditz and colleagues to evaluate the effectiveness of the BCG vaccine in preventing new tuberculosis cases (Sect. 6.2.6.2.8) [37]. We have analyzed the effect of climate on vaccine efficacy by comparing results obtained from two subgroups: cold and warm countries (Sect. 6.2.8). Berkey and colleagues used meta-regression to analyze the

relationship between the absolute distance from the equator and the treatment effect [47]. Although the technique can accommodate multiple quantitative and or qualitative moderators, we will use the data to regress one continuous moderator variable (latitude) on the effect size (log RR). For demonstration, we will start with the simple fixed-effect model and then move to the most commonly used random-effects model.

6.2.9.1 Fixed Effect Model

As the relative risk does not follow a normal distribution, all the calculations will be made on the logarithmic scale. The final results will be converted to the regular scale for proper interpretation.

General output of meta-analysis

The general outputs of this example have been presented before (see Sect. 6.2.6.2.8); the mean log RR (95% CI) was −0.43 (−0.51 to −0.35), which corresponds to an average relative risk of 0.65 (0.6–0.7); P < 0.001. The vaccine was associated with as much 35% (30–40%) reduction in the risk of developing a new event. There was a statistically significant heterogeneity (Q = 152.2; P < 0.001) that seems to be true to a large extent (I^2 = 92.1%), and hence, it needs to be explained, which is a good indicator of moderator analysis.

Output of Meta Regression

(A) *The Regression Table*

Table 6.19 shows the software output of meta-regression: the beta coefficient is the log relative risk (Log RR). It expresses the effect of the moderator variable (climate) on the outcome (−0.029) and the intercept or the amount of variability that remains unexplained (0.344). One unit (degree) increase in latitude decreases the effect size by an average of 0.029. Both moderator variable and intercept were statistically significant, indicating that a significant amount of the protective effect of the vaccine can be explained by the climate (P < 0.001), but yet there is still a significant part remaining unexplained (P < 0.001).

Table 6.19 The relative risk: evaluation of the efficacy of the BCG vaccine, meta regression analysis of a fixed effect model

	Log RR	Se	Z	P value	95% CI
Intercept	0.344	0.08	4.24	<0.001	0.18 to 0.5
Latitude	−0.029	0.0026	−11	<0.001	−0.034 to −0.024

Log RR = log relative risk, Se = standard error, Z = Z value

We can assign a 95% CI for beta by placing a 1.96 standard error on either side of the effect size "Eq. 6.217". The effect size can vary between −0.034 and −0.024, and we can test its statistical significance by a simple Z test "Eq. 6.218". There is a statistically significant negative effect of latitude on the protective effect of the BCG vaccine, meaning that the lower the temperature, the better the protection (P < 0.001).

$$95\% \ CI \ ES = ES \pm 1.96 \ (Se)$$
$$= -0.029 \pm 1.96 \ (0.0026)$$
$$= -0.024 \ to -0.034$$
$$(6.217)$$

$$Z = \frac{beta \ coefficient}{Se} = \frac{-0.029}{0.0026} = -11.1$$
$$(6.218)$$

(B) *Analysis of Q*

In case the investigator wishes to test the effect of other moderator variables besides climates, such as the patient age, he cannot apply the Z test, which limits the comparison to two factors (moderators) only. As Q represents the dispersion of individual studies in terms of the sum of squares, he can use ANOVA to partition Q into its components (see Sect. 2.4.3.1). However, we cannot compute it here by hand as we did in the case of subgroup analysis where we had only two subgroups: cold and warm (see Sect. 6.2.8.1). *In meta-regression, each value of the quantitative moderator variable (each degree of latitude) is one entity.* Hence, computation becomes too complicated to be done by hand and is performed

by a statistical software package. The total variation (Q) is partitioned into (due to) variation related to (can be explained by) the latitude (Q-model) = 121.5; at 1 df; P < 0.0001 and what remained unexplained that is shown in the table as intercept (Q-residual) = 30.7; at 11 df; P < 0.0001. The (Q-model) is analogous to the (Q between groups) in subgroup analysis and has the same df (number of groups minus one). The (Q-residual) is analogous to (Q within groups) of subgroup analysis and has the same df (total sample size minus the number of groups).

(C) *The graphic presentation*

Figure 6.14 shows the regression of effect size (log RR) on the latitude. Each circle represents the magnitude of the effect size of one study. The plot allows to predict the average relative risk for any given latitude, provided it was included in the original study, i.e., between 13 and 55°. It is easily achieved by raising a vertical line at a specific latitude on the x-axis (e.g., point **a**) till it hits the regression line at (e.g., point **b**). A horizontal line from the latter intercepts the y axis at the corresponding log relative risk (e.g., point **c**). The relative risk will be the exponential value of the point (**c**).

(D) *The regression equation*

The regression equation permits predicting the effect size (log relative risk) from the intercept and a known degree of latitude (see Sect. 2.6.2.1). The model is additive and can predict the outcome in the case of multiple quantitative and or qualitative

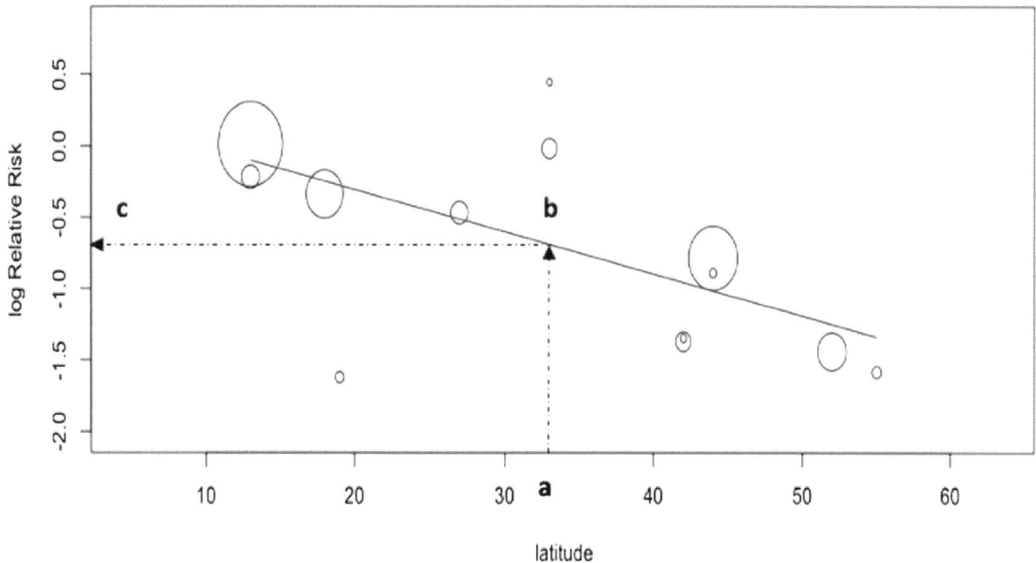

Fig. 6.14 Meta regression: regressing log relative risk on latitude, fixed effect model

moderators (see Sect. 3.4). For example, at a latitude of 30°, the log relative risk is equal to (-0.53) "Eq. 6.219", equivalent to an average relative risk of 0.59 or an average decrease in relative risk of about 41%.

$$ES = b_0 + b_1 x_1 = 0.344 + (-0.029) \times 30$$
$$= -0.53$$

$$(6.219)$$

6.2.9.2 Random Effects Model

General output of meta-analysis

The general outputs of this example have been presented before (see Sect. 6.2.6.2.8); the mean log RR (95% CI) was -0.714 ($-1.06\, to - 0.36$), which corresponds to an average relative risk of 0.49 ($0.35\, to\, 0.7$); P < 0.001. The vaccine was associated with a significant decrease in the risk

of developing the disease: the relative risk of the vaccinated cases was half that calculated for normal controls.

Output of Meta Regression

(A) *The Regression Table*

Table 6.20 shows the software output of the meta-regression of the random effect model. The effect size is about the same as the fixed effect: increasing one unit (one degree of latitude) decreases the effect size (log relative risk) by 0.029. What did change is the standard error due to the addition of the variability between studies (T^2). The result is a much wider 95% CI "Eq. 6.220" and a smaller Z score "Eq. 6.221", making it harder to conclude upon a significant difference. However, we can still conclude that there is a statistically significant negative effect of climate on the protection offered by the BCG

Table 6.20 The relative risk: evaluation of the efficacy of the BCG vaccine, meta regression analysis of a random effects model

	Log RR	Se	Z	P value	95% CI
Intercept	0.259	0.232	1.1	0.26	−0.196 to 0.715
Latitude	−0.029	0.0067	−4.3	<0.001	−0.042 to −0.016

vaccine (P < 0.001). An important difference is the interpretation of the result: the average change in the protective effect is not the same across the levels of the moderator variable (degrees of latitude). Note that this is different from the interpretation of the same test in a fixed model effect, which is that the change in the average protective effect of the BCG vaccine due to altitude is not zero [3].

$$95\% \; CI = Log_{RR} \pm 1.96 \, (Se)$$
$$= -0.029 \pm 1.96 \, (0.0067)$$
$$= -0.042 \; to - 0.016 \qquad (6.220)$$

$$Z = \frac{beta \; coefficient}{Se} = \frac{-0.029}{0.0067} = -4.3$$
$$(6.221)$$

(B)   *Analysis of Q*

Unlike the case of subgroup analysis, the computation of Q cannot be done by hand (see Sect. 6.2.8.1), and we have to use a statistical software package to compute Q and deduct the usual indices, namely T^2 and I^2. The (Q-model) was equal to 18.8, representing the effect of the moderator variable (latitude) on effect size (efficacy of the vaccine). At 1 df, (Q-model) was

statistically significant, indicating that the average effect size at different levels of latitude is not the same (P < 0.001). Note that the interpretation of (Q-model) in a fixed-effect model was different: the effect of latitude on the effect size is significantly different from zero [3].

On the other hand, (Q-residual = 30.7) is the same as in the fixed-effect model. At 11 df, P = 0.001, indicating the presence of a significant amount of unexplained variation. (Q-residual) is used to deduct T^2 (0.0633, Se 0.0548) and I^2 (64.21%). The latter indicates that a considerable part of the variation is true, i.e., due to real differences between studies and not due to random error.

(C)   *The graphic presentation*

Figure 6.15 shows the regression of effect size (log relative risk) on the latitude. Each circle represents the magnitude of the effect size in one study. Compared to the fixed-effect model, and due to the addition of T^2, weights (circles) are more or less similar for more weight is being given to the small studies. The plot (point b) allows predicting the average relative risk (point c) for any given latitude (point a), as shown in the fixed-effect model.

Fig. 6.15 Meta regression: regressing log relative risk on latitude, random effects model

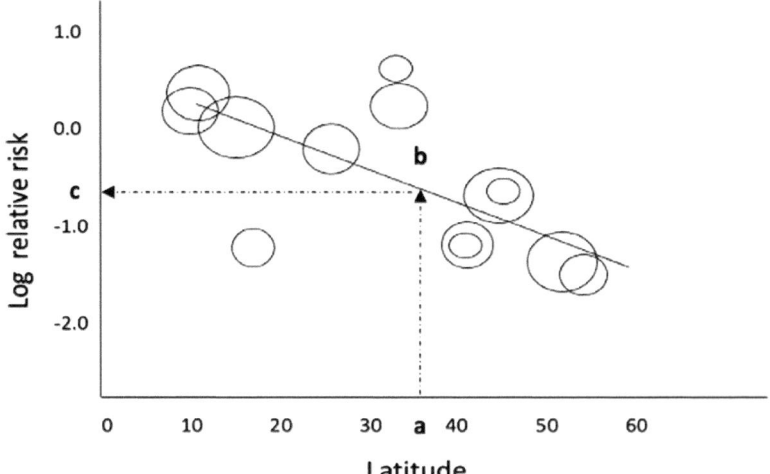

(D) *The regression equation*

The regression equation permits the prediction of outcome (log relative risk) from the intercept and a known value of the moderator variable (see Sect. 2.6.2.1). The model is additive and can predict the outcome in the case of multiple quantitative and or qualitative variables (see Sect. 3.4). Note that the same latitude of 30° is expected to be associated with a log relative risk (−0.61) "Eq. 6.222", equivalent to an average relative risk of 0.54 or an average decrease in relative risk of about 46%.

$$ES = b_0 + b_1 x_1 = 0.259 + (-0.029) \times 30$$
$$= -0.611$$

$$(6.222)$$

(E) *The proportion of variation explained by the model*

The (Q-residual) is used to deduct T^2 (0.0633, Se 0.0548) which expresses the amount of variation in meta-regression, considering the moderator variable. It can be compared to the amount of variation in its absence (T^2 calculated in random effect model = 0.31) to evaluate the role of the moderator variable itself (see Sect. 6.2.6.2.8). The proportion between the two values represents the amount of variation explained by the moderator variable "Eq. 6.223". More straightforwardly, 79.7% of the change in effect size can be explained by the climate, i.e., the latitude. *Remember that the variation explained is the variation between studies (T^2), and it does not include the variation within the studies that cannot be calculated in this model* (see Sect. 6.2.7.2). Put it simpler, the climate (latitude) explains a large part of the variation of effect size between different studies (79.7%), but it cannot explain why patients in a particular study (carried out in the same climate) have different effect sizes; which is logic.

$$R^2 = 1 - \frac{T^2_{meta\ regression}}{T^2_{random\ model}} = \frac{0.063}{0.31} = 0.797$$

$$(6.223)$$

6.2.10 Assessment of Publication Bias and Small-Study Effects

Publication bias has been a central subject of research since the early beginnings of meta-analysis: non-significant results are stored in file drawers without ever being published [18]. In one review, studies with statistically significant or clinically favorable results were estimated to be eight times more likely to be submitted and seven times more likely to be published than non-significant ones [36]. A more extreme situation is selective reporting of favorable results and entirely excluding studies with non-significant or clinically unfavorable data [48]. Besides distorting reality, the file drawer problem inflates the effect size of the meta-analysis simply because the effect size of reported or published studies is large, so they were selectively reported and published in the first place [18].

Trial quality has also been shown to influence the size of treatment effect estimates. On the one hand, small poorly organized studies will most likely show sizeable favorable treatment effects. Small studies have to have large treatment effect in order to be accepted for publication [49]. On the other hand, the more significant investment of money and time in larger studies means that they are more likely to be of high methodological quality, which increases their chance of being published even if their results are negative [49]. The end result is that sample size becomes a ruling factor in publication and the actual models assessing publication bias are based upon this concept [3].

Besides the size, quality and end results of the study, the list is long; extending from expected causes, such as language bias and difficulty in accessing non-English manuscripts and duplicate publications favoring trials named with acronyms than other trials [50]. Moreover, everyone one involved in the publication chain has his own share of bias, starting with researchers arranging for small unorganized studies, to lordly reviewers and up to editors who mainly care about their journals been cited. The meta-analyst has his share of bias, whether by adopting a selective non-systematic approach to the literature, neglecting unpublished data, or failing to complete missing data by directly contacting the original authors [51].

Various techniques have been developed to detect, quantify, and correct publication bias. Each has its advantages and points of weakness. Fortunately, many of those techniques are simple, and hence, they will be explained with running examples, as usual. Other techniques are much more demanding, and hence, they will be explained briefly, with a referral of the interested reader to the appropriate source.

6.2.10.1 The Fail-Safe Methods

The aim of the Fail-Safe methods is to get an estimate of *the number of unpublished clinical studies that would annulate the significant results of the meta-analysis*. The smaller is this number, the more the results of a particular meta-analysis are robust and can still accommodate the few studies that remain in the drawer. In other words, using Fail-Safe numbers is a quick way to estimate whether publication bias is likely to be a problem for a specific study or it can be safely ignored [52].

Fail-Safe N (Rosenthal)

Fail-Safe N is earliest and still a commonly reported statistical analysis of publication bias, aiming to estimate the number of unpublished studies that would need to exist to turn the significant effect size of the meta-analysis into a non-significant one [18]. Rosenthal proposed that the unpublished data remaining in the drawer (X) have zero effect size, with a large P value >0.05, which is why they were not published in the first place. By adding those data to the (K) data of the meta-analysis, which have a significant effect size (>0) and a P-value < 0.05), we can compute a common P-value. Looking the other way round, if we suggest a figure for the common P-value, we can count the number of missing studies (X) that can be added to reach this target.

Suppose the number of those (X) studies is large. In that case, it means that the P-value of

our meta-analysis performed with K studies is robust and can accommodate a large number of non-significant results before the common P becomes non significant. On the other hand, suppose the P-value of the meta-analysis is annulated by just a few missing studies. In that case, it means that the meta-analysis results are very probably due to sampling error (false positive: Type I error), and hence, the drawer theory is the most probable. Although the authors suggested a cut-off value for (X): 5 K plus ten, they equally admitted that it is highly dependent on the data themselves [18].

The approach is appealing but contains many drawbacks; at least two of them are major. First, the authors assumed that the unpublished manuscripts have zero effect size, which is an exaggeration. The studies are not usually published because they have a small or negative effect size but not zero. Second, the idea crossed a red line by summing P-values rather than effect sizes, which is totally against the concept of meta-analysis.

Although the method is not highly recommended, it is reported by many statistical software and publications, which may be due to the simple calculations. The mean difference, the odds ratio, or any other effect size can be standardized by dividing by its standard error, giving the standard normal deviate (SND): ES/Se = Z score. Cochran has shown that we can compute a common Z score (Z_c) for a series of (N) individual studies as the sum of their Z values (εZ_i), divided by the square root of the number of those studies $\sqrt{N}$ "Eq. 6.224" [53]. Squaring both sides of the equation and switching common Z and sample size N, the equation can be rewritten as "Eq. 6.225"

$$Z_c = \frac{\sum Z_i}{\sqrt{N}} \qquad (6.224)$$

$$N = \frac{\left(\sum Z_i\right)^2}{\left(Z_c\right)^2} \qquad (6.225)$$

Returning to meta-analysis and suppose that the number of published studies is (k) and the number of studies in the drawer is (X). Cochran's common Z value of all studies N (K + X) is shown in "Eq. 6.226". Besides the assumption that the effect size of the X studies kept in the drawer is null (0), Rosenthal proposed to target a common Z of 1.65 for all studies "Eq. 6.227" [18]. On the one hand, determining the common Z score $(1.65)^2$, and knowing the effect size of published studies ($\varepsilon\ Z_k$), the effect size of unpublished studies ($\varepsilon\ Z_x = 0$), and the number of published studies (k); will produce the only missing number, which is (X) "Eq. 6.228". On the other hand, the question of why did we target (Z = 1.65) is to calculate the number of missing studies that will annulate the statistical significance of the meta-analysis results.

$$N = K + X = \frac{\left(\sum Z_K + \sum Z_x\right)^2}{(Z_c)^2} \quad (6.226)$$

$$K + X = \frac{\left(\sum Z_K + 0\right)^2}{(1.65)^2} \quad (6.227)$$

$$X = \frac{\left(\sum Z_K\right)^2}{(1.65)^2} - k \quad (6.228)$$

Put it this way, X is the maximum number of unpublished studies that we can tolerate to keep believing that the statistical significance of the K studies is true and not a type I error. The larger is X, the more we believe that the drawer theory is untrue. Suppose a small number of unpublished studies can jeopardize the statistical significance of our results. In that case, we can assume that the drawer theory is true and that the significant result of the meta-analysis is a false positive or just a type I error. Another variant of the equation can calculate (X), knowing the mean effect size and number of K studies only "Eq. 6.229".

$$X = \frac{k}{2.706} \times \left\lceil k(\bar{Z})^2 - 2.706\right\rceil \quad (6.229)$$

Working example

Returning to the example of calculating the relative risk associated with the use of BCG vaccine (Table 6.9), the sum of log relative risk, mean log relative risk and number of studies included in the meta-analysis were (−40.65), (−3.12), and (13), respectively. Using either "Eqs. 6.228" or

"6.229" gives the same number of (X) studies "Eq. 6.230"; P < 0.001.

$$X = \frac{\left(\sum Z_K\right)^2}{(1.65)^2} - k = \frac{(-40.65)^2}{2.706} - 13 = 595$$

$$(6.230)$$

Fail-Safe B (Orwin)

The Fail-Safe N method estimated the number of unpublished studies to those required to annulate the significant results of the meta-analysis. Orwin and colleagues suggested replacing this static zero limit with a predetermined dynamic value that could be more meaningful or clinically relevant, such as the small or the medium Cohen's effect size [54]. Unlike Rosenthal's method, Orwin based his method on Cohen's d, which estimates the standardized difference between treatment and control means (see Sect. 4.2.1.1). Instead of using a predetermined zero effect, the usual minimal effect size chosen using Orwin calculations is the Cohen's small effect of 0.2 [55]. The number of studies left in the drawers is calculated as the proportion between two differences in means: the difference between the mean of the original (n) articles (E_o) and the desired minimal mean of effect size ($E_m = 0.2$), and the difference between the latter (m = 0.2) and the mean of the additional studies (E_n). It is clear that "Eq. 6.231" is just a variation of "Eq. 6.225" and, the remaining calculations are the same. The method can be applied to any other effect size measure.

$$N = \frac{n(E_o - E_m)}{(E_m - E_n)} \quad (6.231)$$

Applying the technique on the previous example brings down the number of missing studies from 595 to only 13 studies.

The Rosenberg Weighting Effect Size Method

Unlike the two previous methods based on unweighted calculation of effect size, Rosenberg suggested a weighted Fail-Safe calculations applicable to both fixed and random effects models [52]. In other words, the calculations focused on the weights of the (n) studies included in the meta-analysis and looked for the weights of the additional unpublished studies (W′) that would bring the sum of weights of a particular meta-analysis (ΣW$_i$) to the desired level of significance, e.g., 0.05. Note that, unlike the previous two method, we summed and compare weighted values rather than Z score [18] or unweighted standardized differences [54], which is in concordance with the concept of meta-analysis "Eq. 6.232".

$$N = \frac{nW'}{\sum W_i} \quad (6.232)$$

Applying "Eq. 6.232" to our example, a significant number of 370 studies are needed to render our effect size to a minimum value of 0.2, as proposed by Cohen [55]; P < 0.001.

6.2.10.2 The Funnel Plot and Correcting Asymmetry

The funnel plot is based on knowing what is missing by plotting the effect size (x-axis), such as the odds ratio or the mean difference, against a measure of precision (y-axis), such as the sample size, the variance, or the standard error [56]. Note that this is the reverse of a usual scatter plot, in which the outcome (effect size in meta-analysis) is plotted on the y-axis and the predictor (sample size in meta-analysis) is plotted on the x-axis. As

shown in Fig. 6.16a, studies tend to accumulate around the mean effect size, which is (0) in our example. The smaller is the sample, the more it is dispersed away from the mean. Consequently, in an unbiased sample, the distribution of the studies will take the form of a symmetrical inverted funnel or a pyramid. The larger sample are few and have small variations around the mean, and hence, they tend to be on the narrow top. The smaller samples are usually many and have a wider variation, hence, the tendency to go down near the wide base of the funnel.

However, the sample size is not the favored estimate of precision because the variance and the standard deviation accumulate two important pieces of information in a single number: sample size and variability, and hence, they are the most commonly used indicators of precision. As the sample size (n) occupies the denominator of the standard error, the y-axis has to be displayed upside down, with small values at the top end of the scale and large values at the bottom. As such, it keeps the shape of the funnel, has no effect on calculations, and is commonly displayed (Fig. 6.16b). Plotting against precision (1/Se) does not need inversion, of course.

Small studies with significantly large effects have more chance to publish than smaller-effect studies of comparable sample size and quality [36]. Moreover, including such an asymmetric sample of studies in a meta-analysis will overestimate the treatment effect [54]. Figure 6.17 shows

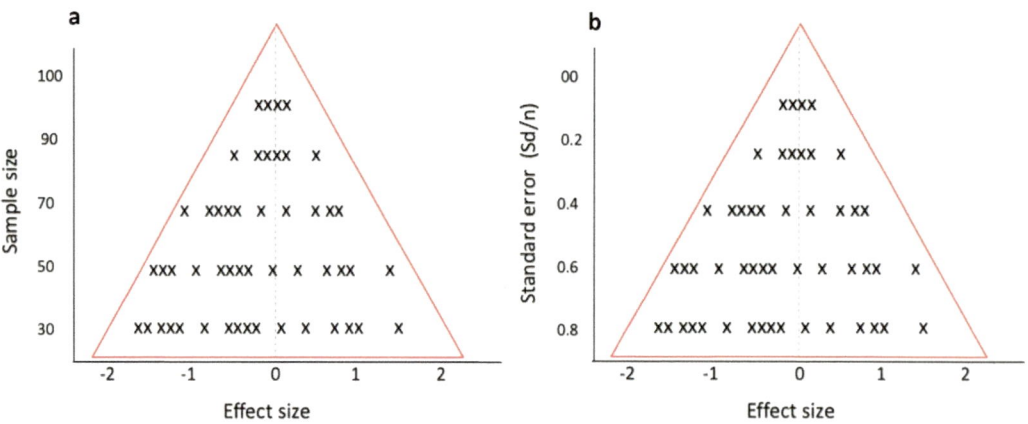

Fig. 6.16 Funnel plot: **a** the method of precision is sample size, **b** the method of precision is the standard error

an empty left side of the pyramid that would have been occupied by many small negative studies that did not find their way to publish. However, asymmetry is not always due to publication bias. Asymmetry can be due to true heterogeneity of effect sizes, studies not precisely measuring the same effect, English language bias, and data irregularities, including fraud and poor study design. Egger and colleagues reported a long list of potential sources of asymmetry, classified into those related to selection bias, true heterogeneity, data irregularities, study artifacts, and just chance [49].

Publication Bias is Only One Reason of Asymmetry

Trials of low quality, which are usually of small size, tend to give more positive results than if they were properly analyzed and hence, will lead to the same asymmetry. They will move from their supposed basal negative side of the plot to the large positive side, leaving the former side empty [49]. In conclusion, the funnel plot displays small-study effects that may be due to the many reasons just mentioned, with publication bias being only one of those reasons [57–59]. Hence, a funnel plot is a good first step to suggest publication bias but needs further analysis.

Trim and Fill Method

Based on the funnel plot, Duval and Tweedy proposed a simple way to correct for publication bias [60]. The two-step procedure starts by omitting the usually small studies with extreme values until the funnel plot is symmetrical (trimming), as shown in Fig. 6.17, on the right side of the figure: A) Trim. If the distribution remains asymmetrical, another iteration is performed. Once the distribution becomes symmetrical, we use the trimmed funnel plot to estimate the true "center" of the funnel.

The next step is to replace the trimmed data and their theoretical counterparts on the other side of the axis of symmetry around the center in Fig. 6.18, as shown on the right side of the figure: B) Fill. Besides estimating the number of missing studies, the method is supposed to adjust effect size based on new recalculations that include the studies that were filled in. *Although the method is easy to apply and can be used in a small sample size, it makes a strong assumption that asymmetry is due to publication bias, which is not always true.* Simulation studies have shown that the method detects missing studies in the absence of asymmetry. Hence, carries the danger of adding non-existing studies and adjusting for non-existing effects [3, 61].

Weight Function Models

Authors have proposed more methods that avoid strong assumptions about the P value and overcorrection. The method used weights to model correction through the likelihood of a study being published varies. However, besides being

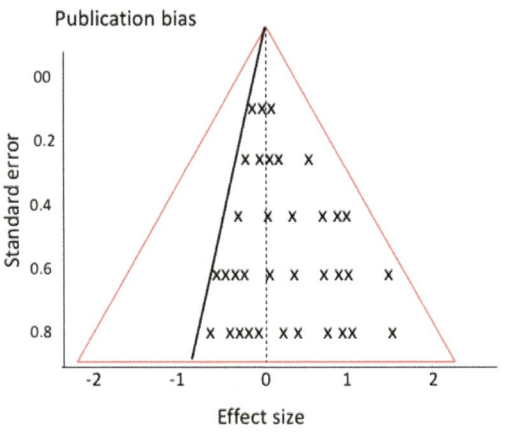
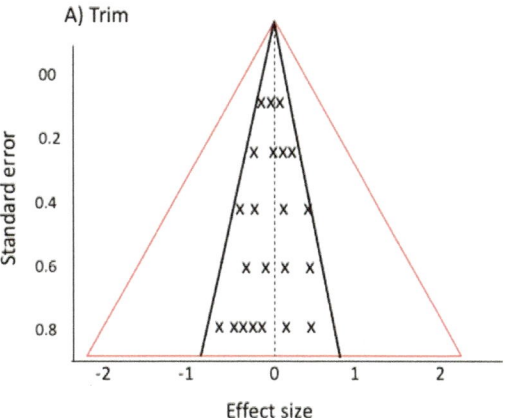

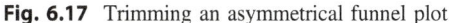

Fig. 6.17 Trimming an asymmetrical funnel plot

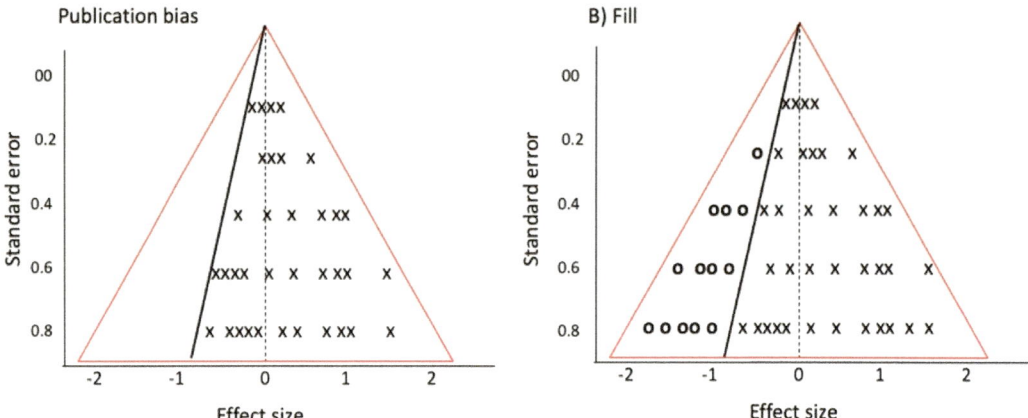

Fig. 6.18 Filling an asymmetrical funnel plot

sophisticated, those methods need a large number of studies, may be over a 100, which is why they are not in common use. The technique suggested by Vevea and Wood's technique is one of those methods designed to avoid the need for a large number of studies [61]. The technique can provide a useful tool for sensitivity analysis by showing the change in effect size estimates under the different selection bias models.

6.2.10.3   Testing the Small-Study Effects

Unsurprisingly, funnel plots have been interpreted differently by a visual examination made by different observers. Hence, there was a need to measure asymmetry numerically and test it formally. Those tests examine whether there is a significant association between effect size and a measure of sample size [59]. *A statistically significant test means a small-sample effect, which may, but does not necessarily, reflect publication bias*. There is a long series of tests that have common rules for application: a minimum sample of ten studies of different sizes, and the results have to be interpreted in light of the visual inspection of the funnel plot. Among the long list of proposed tests [58], two tests are the most suitable for continuous effects: the parametric Egger test and the non-parametric Begg and Mazumdar correlation test. The Egger test was found to give false-positive results in the case of

the odds ratio. Several modifications were made to overcome this, including Peter's test and Harbord's test, which can be produced by STATA software. None of those tests is performed by RevMan, and their use is generally not much considered by Cochrane reviewers for the absence of sufficient studies that give a piece of solid evidence [58].

Begg and Mazumdar Test

Attempts have been made to quantify and test the relationship between the effect size and precision, i.e., the two components of the forest plot. Begg and Mazumdar's suggested testing the correlation between the two components using Kendall's Tau rank correlation test [62]. The latter is a non-parametric alternative to Pearson's correlation and a valid alternative of the non-parametric Spearman's rank test in case of a small sample size. As many effect sizes usually do not follow a normal distribution, the test begins by standardizing the effect size (ES/Se) prior to correlation. The standardized effect sizes of (K) clinical studies (t_1, t_2, t_3,... t_i) and their associated variance (v_1, v_2, v_3, ... v_i) are ranked and, according to the central limit theorem, the mean ranks are expected to follow a normal distribution. Under the null hypothesis, the number of (t, v) pairs of studies that are ranked under the same order (C) is equal to the number of pairs ranked in the reverse order (D). The standardized difference between (C and D) is tested by a simple Z test, using the following equation "Eq. 6.233":

$$Z = \frac{C - D}{\sqrt{k(1 - K)(2K + 5)/18}} \quad (6.233)$$

Remember that the variance is equal to the sum of squares (SS) divided ny the degree of freedom (sample size-1), and hence, the larger is the variance, the smaller the sample size. As the test statistics correlated the effect size with the variance, a strong correlation signifies that small studies produce large effect size; i.e., it indicates small-study effects. In case the latter is thought to be due to publication bias, the presence of the strong correlation may suggest that small and non-significant studies may be missing. *The test is known for the disadvantage of lacking power if the number of studies is small.* In other words, it could fail to cumulate enough differences to reach the limit of statistical significance. Hence, the absence of a statistically significant correlation must not be interpreted as evidence of absence of publication bias or other reasons for small-study effects [36].

A working example

Returning to the example of testing the effect of the BCG vaccine on the risk of developing new cases of tuberculosis (Table 6.9). The correlation between the standardized log risk ratio (ES/√Var) of the 13 studies (ranging from −10.19 to 0.61), and the corresponding 13 (v) variances (ranging from 0.0039 to 0.53) was tested by requesting Kendall Tau correlation in IBM-SPSS software. The program output produced a Kendall-tau correlation coefficient of 0.179, and the P-value was 0.39. Consequently, the test failed to prove a significant correlation between the standardized effect size and variance. Hence, publication bias could not be confirmed but cannot be overruled due to the small power of the test.

Egger Test

Before introducing the equation, we would like to draw the reader's attention that all calculations using effect sizes that follow other distributions than normal, such as odds ratio (OR), are made in the log scale. The null of OR is 1, which is equivalent to a log OR of zero. An OR >1 gives a positive log OR and an OR <1 gives a negative Log OR. The same applies for the relative risk (RR). For simplicity, we will consider the case of the study producing no effect (OR = 1; log OR = 0) or a positive effect (OR > 1; positive log OR). We will not consider the identical other side of the coin (OR < 1; negative log OR) to prevent any confusion for non-statisticians, like myself.

Now joining Egger and his colleagues who proposed a simple linear regression approach in which the standardized log odds ratio (OR/Se), is regressed against an element of precision, which is the reverted standard error (1/Se) [49]. The regression equation is simple: the output is the standardized effect size (ES) and the input is the element of precision (1/Se), plus an error term (b_0) "Eq. 6.234". The reader is invited to refer to chapter two for more information about regression the elements of a simple regression equation (see Sect. 2.6.2).

$$ES = b_0 + b \, (1/Se) \quad (6.234)$$

Figure 6.19a represents the perfect null hypothesis, where precision (1/Se) totally explains the effect size (ES), and hence, there is no other source of variation; i.e., the error term will be equal to zero ($b_0 = 0$). The error term is the area between the (0) scale and the point where the regression line intercepts the (y) axis. As the former intercepts the latter at point (0), the error term equals (0). As precision is inversely related to the standard error, the larger the study, the more the effect size. The regression line passing by the four paired data points (circles) shown in Fig. 6.19a has to pass by the zero of both the x-axis and the y-axis. Put it this way, a zero precision will lead to a zero Log odds ratio (= Odds ratio of 1). Each (I) increment in precision will be reflected on the effect size by exactly similar (I) increment. In statistical terms, the precision explains 100% of effect size. Small studies are expected to have a small effect size, and hence, they will tend to be closer to zero (the bottom) on the y-axis. As they are also expected to be

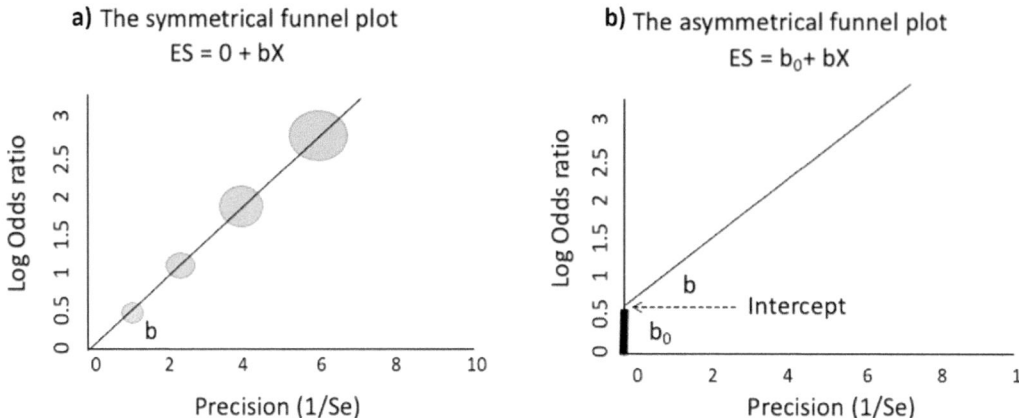

Fig. 6.19 Egger test: analysis of small-study effects: **a)** the case of a symmetrical funnel plot, **b)** the case of an asymmetrical funnel plot. The thick vertical bar on the y-axis of **(b)** represents the intercept (b_0)

unprecise, they tend to be closer to the bottom of the x-axis too due to their significant standard error. In conclusion, small trials remain close to the origin. On the other hand, large studies are more precise; hence, they will tend to move away from the graph origin on the x-axis and, as they are expected to produce positive effect size, they will tend to move away from the origin on the y-axis too. In conclusion, large studies tend to go just in the opposite direction to small studies [49].

Figure 6.19b shows the other side of the coin, where the relationship between the effect size and the sample size is not symmetrical as above. Studies of low precision (small studies) produce a positive effect size. In other words, small studies have an effect unrelated to size, pushing the regression line vertically away from zero to intercept the y-axis at a higher point. The more the small-study effects, the higher the intercept, which now represents the error in the equation (b_0). Hence, *the significance of the small-study effects can be evaluated by testing the statistical significance of the error term.* In the case of a protective small-study effect, as indicated by a negative odds ratio (OR < 1), the regression line will be pushed down to intercept the y-axis below zero [49]. Although the method was first applied in the case of odds ratio, its use was

extended to other effect size measures and is now more recommended for continuous measures [59].

Working example

We are returning to the example of testing the effect of the BCG vaccine on the risk of developing new cases of tuberculosis. We can use the data presented in Table 6.9 to construct the fixed model funnel plot and test the statistical significance of small-study effects by Egger's test (Fig. 6.20). The next step will be to use the calculation data presented in Table 6.10 and apply both procedures in a random-effects model.

Visually, the funnel plot looks to be asymmetrical, missing small studies that could show a higher risk of new cases among those using the vaccine: i.e., a potentially harmful effect for those using the vaccine. Egger's test gave a statistically significant intercept ($Z = -4.8$ and $P < 0.001$) indicating a statistically significant harmful effect in the case of small samples. On the other hand, the test was not significant for a random-model effects. The reason is that we have added the variability between studies (T^2) to the individual variability within each study. The net results are that the influence of small studies is increased in the random effect model, with all studies (small and large) becoming nearer to one another

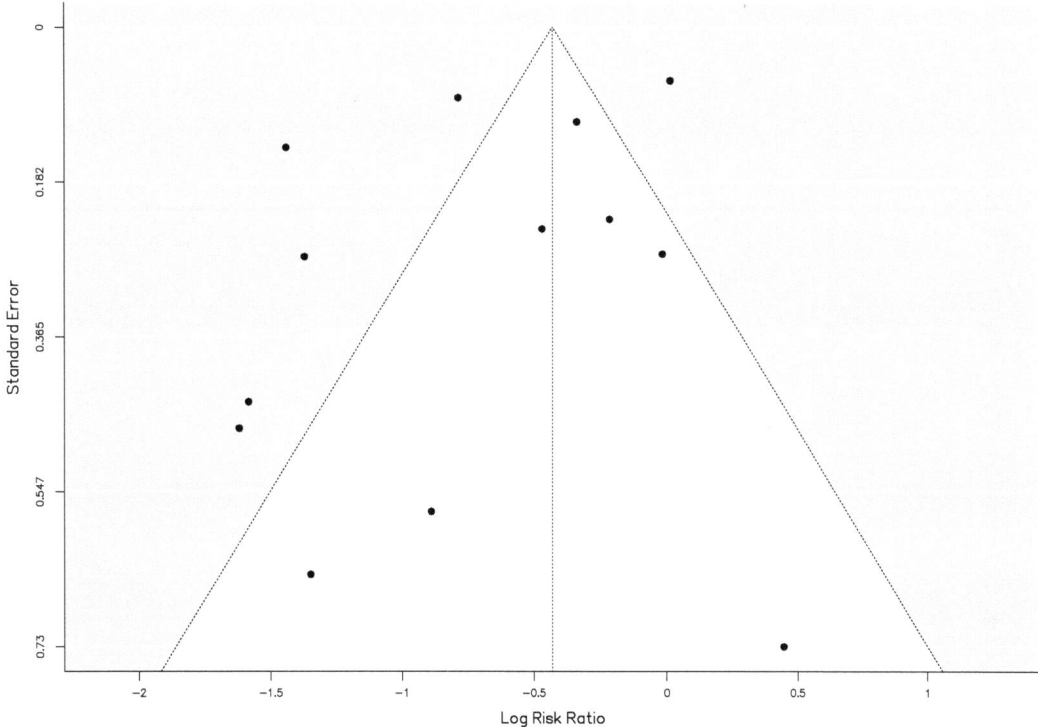

Fig. 6.20 Funnel plot: the efficacy of BCG vaccine in preventing new cases of tuberculosis, fixed effect model

(Fig. 6.21). The net result is that the small-study effects per say is reduced, with a smaller Egger's Z value of only −0.838 and a much larger non-significant P value of 0.4.

Harbord's and Peter's Tests

Although the Egger test was initially proposed to be used with an odds ratio, the authors themselves have noted statistical problems with this approach. The reader is invited to review how we calculated the Se of OR: it is the square root of the sum of the four reciprocal values "Eq. 1.40" and hence, the variability depends on the size and the skewed distribution of the odds ratio. This inherent asymmetry can be visualized on the funnel plot, without true small study effect. In other word, it may lead to a false positive result. Harbord [63], and Peters' tests [64] are two modifications of the Egger test aiming to reduce the correlation between the log odds ratio and its variance and are suggested as better alternatives.

However, none of those tests is used in Cochrane reviews nor included in comprehensive meta-analysis software. STATA software can produce harbor test.

6.2.11 Sensitivity Analysis

There are different statistical methods for meta-analysis, so a thorough sensitivity analysis should always be performed to assess the robustness of the combined estimates [59]. As in any study, the meta-analyst has to rely on certain assumptions and make decisions during the analysis. Some decisions are made a-priori such as model selection; others are made after the data is analyzed, such as subgroup analysis. Those decisions can be based on evidence, while others may be arbitrary. A sensitivity analysis is to test whether or not the results of the meta-analysis are robust to those assumptions and decisions? In

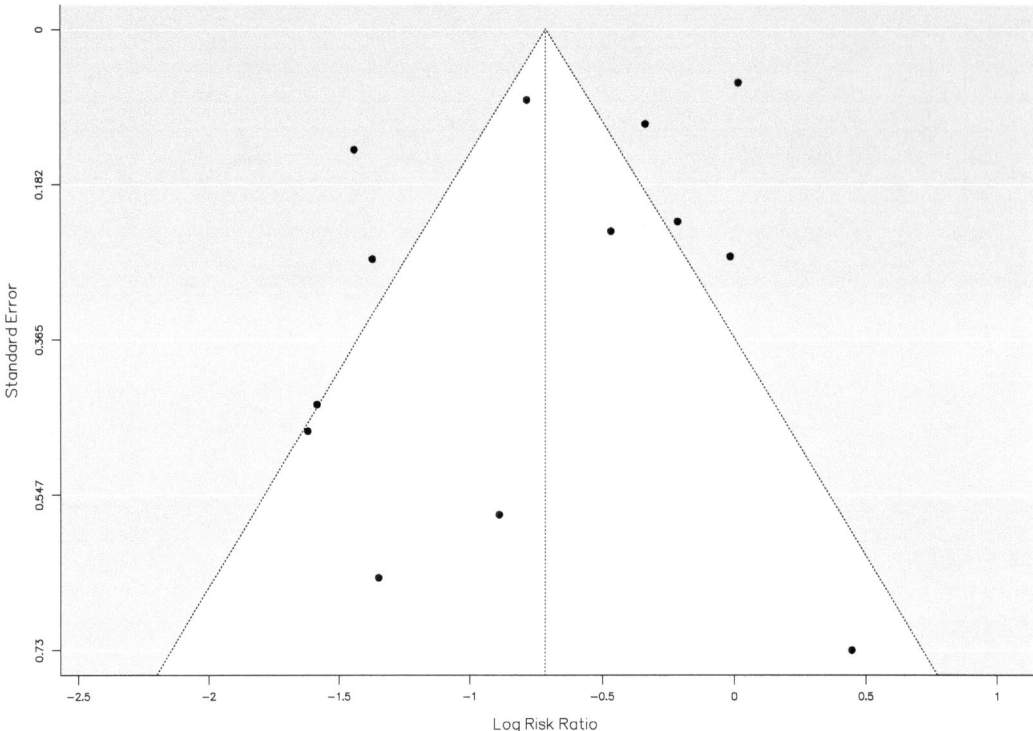

Fig. 6.21 Funnel plot: the efficacy of the BCG vaccine in preventing new cases of tuberculosis, random-effects model

this section, we will give just a few examples, and the interested reader can refer to more specialized resources [59, 61, 65].

6.2.11.1 Reviewing Data

The meta-analyst may wonder if the results will change if one or two of his inclusion or exclusion criteria were different? Especially if any of those criteria were based on debatable cut-off values. Similarly, he has to think about any criterion which has led to the inclusion of an influential or outlier effect. Another example is to review the policy of contacting original authors to complete missing data or to consult the gray literature; failure to perform either procedure may have a similar effect as publication bias.

6.2.11.2 Comparing Fixed to Random Effects Model

The meta-analyst has to study the impact of the adopted methods of analysis. In the case of heterogeneity, with an $I^2 > 0$, comparing fixed to

random-effect model is highly indicated. As the random effect model adds the between-study variability (T^2) to the variability within each study, it weights the studies more or less equally compared to the fixed model. Put this way; a random effect model gives more weight to small studies while a fixed effect model produces the reverse.

If the estimates are similar, then any small-study effects have little influence on the effect estimate. Remember that the small-study effects is the phenomenon in which small studies give a large effect and is one main reason for an asymmetrical funnel plot.

On the other hand, if the random-effects estimate appears to be more beneficial, the meta-analyst may wish to consider concluding with the more effective small studies. However, if the larger studies are more rigorously conducted, as usual, the meta-analysts may choose to report exclusively on the results of larger studies [58].

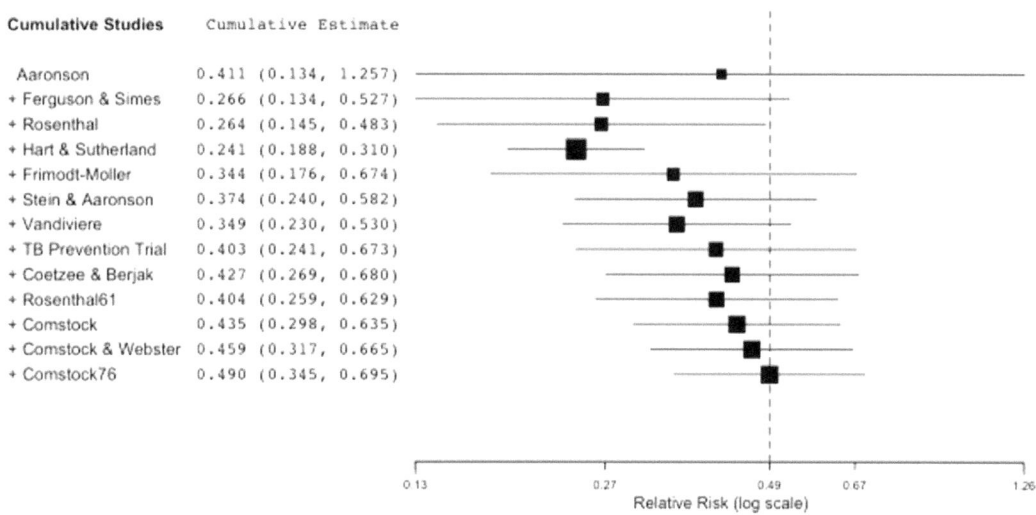

Fig. 6.22 Forrest plot: cumulative meta-analysis. Values are presented as relative risk (95% CI)

Working example

Taking the example of testing the efficacy of the BCG vaccine in the protection of new episodes of tuberculosis. Data are present in Table 6.8, fixed model analysis in Table 6.9, and random model analysis in Table 6.10. There was a statistically significant heterogeneity with $Q = 152.2$; $P < 0.001$ and significant I^2 of 92.2%. The results (relative risk; 95% CI) of the fixed-effect model (0.65; 0.6–0.7) were comparable to those of a random-effects model (0.49; 0.35–0.7), with both showing significant risk reduction in patients receiving the vaccine.

6.2.11.3 Cumulative Meta-Analysis

We have already performed a cumulative meta-analysis by hand (see Sect. 6.2.6.1). We began with one study (Fig. 6.2). We added a second (Fig. 6.3) and a third study (Fig. 6.4), using a fixed model and then random model effects (Fig. 6.5). In case the studies were included chronologically, the procedure can also show how the evidence is cumulated or significantly changed over time.

Working example

Figure 6.22 shows the forest plot of cumulative meta-analysis applied to our previous example on the BCG vaccine. It shows the "play" of meta-

analysis. Adding new results decreases variability and narrows the confidence intervals. As we keep adding studies (moving downwards), the distribution shifts smoothly to the right, stabilizing the results and increasing the study power.

6.2.11.4 Leave One Meta-Analysis

Another technique is to leave one study at a time and analyze the remaining studies. We start with the full meta-analysis, including all studies. Then, we remove one study at a time and see whether the results would change or not? We have to note that subgroup analysis and moderator analysis are not sensitivity analyses but ways to find true differences in the population.

Working example

Figure 6.23 shows the forest plot of leave one technique applied to the same example (Fig. 6.23). It is clear that the results are robust and did not change significantly, regardless of which study has been removed.

6.2.12 Reporting Meta-Analysis

Reporting a meta-analysis has many similarities with reporting primary clinical studies. However, there are particular points that we have to address

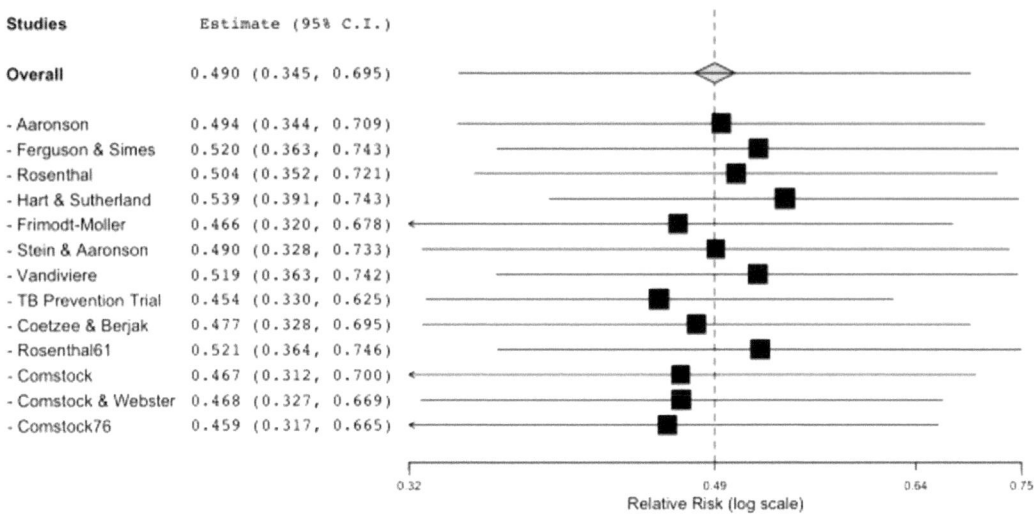

Fig. 6.23 Forest plot: leave one meta-analysis. Values are presented as relative risk (95% CI)

more carefully. There is no one way to perform a meta-analysis, and hence, we have to justify our methods, mainly the chosen effect size and model. There is usually considerable heterogeneity in combining many different studies, which must be analyzed. For the same reason, we have to show if the combined results are robust enough to be generalized to the population by keeping on testing sensitivity throughout the analysis.

Although we have to begin by reporting the systematic review, we will leave this part to the much more specialized resources, such as the Cochran handbook for meta-analysis (Cochran handbook). We are loyal to our main limited aim to simplify the statistical information for the young researcher and the busy clinician. Consequently, we will go directly to discuss the methods and the results of the meta-analysis itself. We will use the same running example that we have been following throughout this chapter: the meta-analysis investigating the efficacy of the BCG vaccine in the prevention of new cases of tuberculosis (see Sect. 6.2.6.2.8).

6.2.12.1 The Effect Size
The starting point of all meta-analyses involves selecting an appropriate effect size, which sometimes requires justification. Concerning a

bivariate effect size, the Odds ratio has many mathematical advantages over the RR. However, we have chosen to report our results regarding the latter for many reasons. The relative risk is easier to understand by the clinicians. The nature of the study permits the assumption of a cause-effect relationship between giving the vaccine and acquiring immunity, which the OR cannot provide. Finally, the low event rate (<10–15%) approximates the numerical values of the two indices and facilitates interchanging the results during the discussion (see Sect. 1.8.2).

6.2.12.2 The Model
We have shown that choosing between a fixed and a random effect had to be made before the analysis. The rule of thumb is that the random-effects model is the model of choice unless we have reliable evidence that the population is exactly the same in all studies. Another indication is that we do not care to propagate the results of our meta-analysis. In this chapter, we have applied the two models for two reasons, the first being for teaching and training. The second purpose was to compare the results of the two models, which is an essential step in analyzing the robustness of the results. In other words, the fixed-effect model has to be always calculated to serve as a benchmark for sensitivity analysis.

6.2.12.3 Analysis of Heterogeneity

Testing the Statistical Significance of Heterogeneity (Q)

The statistical significance of the variability between studies is usually tested by a modified Chi-square test (Q test). While Q is calculated under the assumption of a fixed-effect model, it has to be reported, regardless of the model being used (see Sect. 6.2.7.1). It is important to report the amount of Q, the degree of freedom, and the P-value. Q can be used to calculate the amount of heterogeneity (T^2) and to bread indices to compare heterogeneity among studies, such as I^2 and H^2.

Measuring the Amount of Heterogeneity (T^2)

The meta-analyst has to define the method used to estimate the amount of heterogeneity between the studies (T^2). Tau-square (T^2) measures the variance between the studies, and its square root (T = Tau) is the standard deviation produced on the same scale as the effect size. Defining the method used to measure T^2 may be subsidiary for the clinician for having a limited impact on the results. However, the statisticians need to evaluate and compare their tools. We have chosen the method advocated by DerSimonian and Laird for being in everyday use and, most importantly, for being easy to execute and understand (see Sect. 6.2.7.3). Many statisticians advise the use of the restricted maximum likelihood (REML). It is much more complicated, but most statistical software packages execute it. In a fixed model analysis, the calculated T^2 is not reported because it is assumed to be equal to zero. On the other hand, T^2 has to be reported when we adopt a random-effects model.

Comparing Heterogeneity (I^2 and H^2)

As Q is just the statistic of a modified Chi-square test, it can only be used to indicate whether there is a statistically significant difference between the studies or not? T^2 is dependent upon the scale of the effect size, and hence, statisticians have to breed independent measures to report the extent of variability and compare the variability among studies. I^2 is the proportion of heterogeneity that is above what is due to sampling error. H^2 is another index describing the relative excess in Q over what may be due to chance. We can report either index, but I^2 is the most commonly reported.

6.2.12.4 Reporting the Main Effect

We must present the range, mean, standard error, and 95% confidence interval of the effect size. The presentation must include both the usual scale and the normalized scale for any effect size not following the normal distribution, such as the OR and the RR. We have to report the Z and exact P-value. A P-value smaller than 0.001 can just be given as P < 0.001.

The 95% Prediction Interval

In a fixed-effect model, the 95% CI provides an estimate of the position of a (single) central (mean) distribution of the effect size. In the case of a random effect model, there is no single position of the mean effect size in the population but a summary distribution for the set of possible means. The 95% prediction interval can summarize the spread of these effects and has to be reported. In case any amount of heterogeneity is detected, and regardless of the results of the Q-test, the researcher has to provide a prediction interval for the true outcomes, especially if he has a reasonable number of studies with a symmetrical funnel plot.

Graphic Presentation

Stem-and-leaf and forest plots performed for the main groups and all subgroups.

6.2.12.5 Moderator Analysis

Following the demonstration of significant overall effect size, the meta-analyst is entitled to focus on the variation itself. The meta-analysis result is expressed by controlling for the part of variation due to sampling error. What remains can be either a true variation between studies (internal), an artificial variation due to the effect of a moderator variable (external), or both (see Sect. 6.2.8). Besides a literature review suggesting a significant moderator variable, a statistically significant Q and a high value of I^2 have to draw the attention of the meta-analysis to study the possible effect of the moderator variables, either by subgroup analysis or meta-regression. It would be inconsistent to adopt a fixed model effect the in case we intend to perform moderator analysis.

Analysis by Subgroups

The researcher must indicate whether he has adopted a pooled T^2 or a separate T^2 for each subgroup. He has to report the reasons suggesting a significant difference in the distribution of variability among subgroups, which led to adopting separate T^2. Whether he pooled or did not pool T^2, each subgroup has to be similarly studied and reported as the main group. The next step will be to compare the subgroups, whether by a simple Z test in the case of two subgroups or by a modified ANOVA or analysis of Q in the case of multiple subgroups.

Meta Regression

The researcher has to define the quantitative and the qualitative predictors included in the meta-regression model. Besides reporting the overall significance of the model, he must report the b coefficient and P-value of each predictor, the overall significance of the model, the regression equation, and the regression plot.

R-squared

The R^2 of the moderator variable explains the proportion of the variability of the effect size that the moderator variable can explain. However, unlike the usual R^2, it only explains the part of variability between studies by comparing T^2 calculated in the presence of the moderator variable to T^2 calculated in its absence.

6.2.12.6　Publication Bias and the Small-Study Effects

Since the early beginnings of meta-analysis, publication bias has been a central subject of research: non-significant results are stored in file drawers without ever being published, inflating the published effect size (Rosenthal 1979). On the other hand, large, well-organized studies find their way to publication even if not significant, while small studies have to have a large effect size. The result is what we call the small-study effects, where the effect size is not related to sampling size, as would be expected.

Fail-Safe Methods

The Fail-Safe methods provide a quick way to estimate whether publication bias is likely to be a problem for a specific systematic review by estimating the number of unpublished clinical studies (N) that would annulate the significant results of the meta-analysis. The larger this number (N), the more robust our results are because they can accommodate many missing studies before being reversed. A small (N) means that only a few studies can reverse our conclusion. The statistical software usually allows the researcher to choose between the techniques proposed by Rosenthal, Orwin, or Rosenberg (see Sect. 6.2.10.1).

The Funnel Plot and Correcting Asymmetry

Plotting the effect size on the x-axis and an element of precision on the y-axis is expected to take a funnel's shape. The few large studies with limited variability form the narrow top, and the many small studies with widespread variability will be pushed to the bottom. The funnel plot examines whether the effect size of clinical studies of a particular meta-analysis correlates positively with those studies' size (precision). If this is the case, the funnel plot will be symmetrical, but if the small studies have to have a large effect that is not proportional to their size, in order to be published, the funnel plot will be asymmetrical; this is what the funnel plot is testing.

The common belief that the funnel plot visualizes publication bias is in only one case, where small and non-significant studies are not published and are kept in the drawers, leaving their "expected" position on the funnel empty. Egger and colleagues reported a long list of causes of asymmetry [59].

The researcher has to investigate the cause of asymmetry and report whether he has used one of the methods of correcting asymmetry, such as the Trim and Fill method [60] and the weighted function model, especially the one suggested by Vevea and Wood [61].

Testing the Small-Study Effects

The non-parametric rank correlation test (Begg and Mazumdar) and Egger's regression test were designed to test the small-study effects, which does not necessarily mean publication bias. Both tests perform well in the case of continuous effect size. Harbord (Harbord) and Peter's tests (Peter) are better alternatives if the effect size is the odds ratio (see Sect. 6.2.10.3). The test used has to be reported, with justification.

6.2.12.7 Sensitivity Analysis

Sensitivity analysis is not a single test but an attitude. Any study involves raising assumptions and making decisions which we believe are necessary, objective, and correct. However, we have to expect this is not always the case, so it is better to repeat the meta-analysis while considering different scenarios. The researcher may wonder whether choosing another effect size, adopting a different model, modifying one or two inclusion criteria, completing missing data, or even changing the statistical analysis plan, can significantly change his results or the interpretation of his findings [3].

Consequently, the robustness of data can be tested in many ways but will vary from study to study. A typical sensitivity analysis compares the results of the fixed-effect to the random-effects model. The researcher can evaluate the influence of individual studies by cumulative (see Sect. 6.2.11.3) and leave-one meta-analysis (Sect. 6.2.11.4). Another method is to compare the results of using a pooled or separate (T^2) in subgroup analysis (see Sect. 6.2.7.3). The more the results hold while changing methods, models, variables, and assumptions, the more we have confidence in the results of the meta-analysis. The researcher has to be careful that comparing the results of observational studies to those produced in prospective randomized clinical trials, analyzing the effects of moderator variables on the outcome, and other examples formally comparing the primary effect size across subgroups

are examples of subgroup analysis. They should not be confused with sensitivity analysis.

6.2.12.8 The Example

We will give two reports on our running example on the efficacy of the BCG vaccine in preventing the occurrence of new cases of tuberculosis (see Sect. 6.2.6.2): a brief report based on the fixed-effect model and a detailed report on the more commonly used random-effects model. As moderator analysis (subgroup analysis and meta regression) is performed in the context of a random-effects model, we will omit this part of the study from the report of the fixed-effect model.

The Fixed-Effect Model
Methods

The analysis was carried out using the normalized relative risk (Log RR), weighted by the inverse variance. The significance of heterogeneity was assessed by Cochran Q and reported in $I^2\%$. Outliers and influential points were verified by calculating the studentized residuals and Cook's distance. Small-study effects were evaluated using the non-parametric rank correlation test [62], the Egger regression test [49], and the Fail-Safe N test [18].

Results

A total of 13 studies were included in the analysis. The observed log risk ratios ranged from -1.62 to 0.446, with the majority of estimates being negative; i.e., protective (85%). The estimated average log risk ratio was: -0.43 (95% CI: -0.51 to -0.35). Therefore, the average outcome differed significantly from zero ($z = -10.6$; $P < 0.0001$). According to the Q-test, the true outcomes appear to be heterogeneous (Q at 12 df = 152.2330, $P < 0.0001$, $I^2 = 92.1173\%$). Two studies (Stein & Aaronson; TB Prevention Trial) had relatively large weights compared to the rest of the studies. An examination of the studentized residuals revealed that four studies (Hart & Sutherland; Stein & Aaronson; TB Prevention Trial; Rosenthal 1961) had values larger than ±2.9 and maybe potential outliers in the context of this model. We have performed cumulative analysis as well as leave one sensitivity analysis. Both procedures showed that our results were robust. On the other hand, the regression test indicated funnel plot asymmetry ($Z = -4.8$; $P < 0.001$) but not the rank correlation test ($P = 0.39$). Fail-safe N analysis showed that many studies are expected to remain in the drawer (595 studies; $P < 0.001$). The results of subgroup analysis in a fixed model effect were mainly used for teaching and training purposes, and hence, they will not be reported here.

The Random-Effects Model
Methods

The analysis was carried out using the log risk ratio as the outcome measure. A random-effects model was fitted to the data. The amount of heterogeneity was estimated using the DerSimonian-Laird estimator, tested by the Q test. The amount of true heterogeneity was reported as an I^2 statistic. The Studentized residuals (± 2.9) and Cook's distances were used to examine whether studies may be outliers and/or influential in the context of the model. The rank correlation test and the regression test, using the standard error of the observed outcomes as the predictor, were used to check for funnel plot asymmetry. The researchers noticed a difference between the results achieved in cold weather and those reported in warm countries. They have arranged a subgroup analysis to compare the results obtained in the cold versus warm countries. In addition, they performed a meta-regression to test whether there is a statistically significant interaction between the latitude and effect size.

Main Results

A total of 13 studies were included in the analysis. The observed log risk ratios ranged from -1.62 to 0.446, with the majority of estimates being negative (85%). The estimated average log risk ratio based on the random-effects model was: -0.71 (95% CI: -1.06 to -0.36). Therefore, the

average outcome differed significantly from zero ($z = -4$, $P < 0.000$). In conclusion, there was a statistically significant overall protective effect of the vaccination, as shown by a relative risk of 0.49 (0.35–0.7); $P < 0.001$. In other words, vaccination decreased the overall relative risk of acquiring a new event by 51% (30–65%). The 95% prediction interval for the relative risk was: 0.49 (0.17 to 1.39). The use of the vaccine is expected to be associated with an average 51% risk reduction. However, in some studies, vaccination may be associated with an increase in the risk of the disease (relative risk > 1).

Analysis of Heterogeneity

According to the Q-test, the true outcomes appear to be heterogeneous (Q at 12 df = 152.2330, $P < 0.0001$, $tau^2 = 0.31$, $I^2 = 92.1\%$). A 95% prediction interval for the true outcomes is -1.86 to 0.43. Hence, although the average outcome is estimated to be negative, in some studies, the true outcome may, in fact, be positive. Studentized residuals and Cook's distance did not detect any outliers or influential points.

Moderator analysis

Both subgroup analyses are the two faces of the same coin, and hence, only one out of them had to be executed and reported. We made both analyses for educational and teaching purposes.

Analysis of subgroups

We will report the results of the subgroup analysis assuming the pooled T^2. Subgroup analysis showed that the vaccine was significantly effective in cold weather: Log RR; 95% CI; P-value (-0.67; -0.89 to -0.44; $P < 0.001$) but not in warm countries (-0.277; -0.57 to 0.017; $P = 0.066$).

The vaccine was more effective in cold counties, achieving a relative risk reduction of 70% (48–79%); $P < 0.001$. On the other hand, the vaccine's efficacy was less pronounced in warms countries, with an average relative risk reduction of only 24% (P = non-significant). The weather (cold versus warm) explains 69% of the variability between studies; $R^2 = 0.69$. The results indicate that the conditions associated with the study in warm countries had to be revised. There is still a significant true heterogeneity in both subgroups, with I^2 between 72 and 75.4% in warm and cold subgroups.

Meta regression

Meta-regression showed a statistically significant interaction between latitude and vaccine efficacy; $Z = -4.3$ ($P < 0.001$). A one-unit increase of the predictor (one degree of latitude) decreases the effect size (log relative risk) by 0.029. In other words, there is a statistically significant negative effect of climate on the protection offered by the BCG vaccine.

The (Q-model) was equal to 18.8, representing the effect of the moderator variable (latitude) on effect size (efficacy of the vaccine). At 1 df, (Q-model) was statistically significant, indicating that the average effect size at different levels of latitude is not the same ($P < 0.001$). The R^2 calculated by meta-regression was 79.7%, indicating that the latitude is crucial for explaining such a large amount of the variability between studies.

On the other hand, (Q-residual = 30.7) is the same as in the fixed-effect model. At 11 df, $P = 0.001$, indicating a significant amount of unexplained variation. (Q-residual) is used to deduct T^2 (0.0633, Se 0.0548) and I^2 (64.21%). Finally, the researcher must provide the regression equation, maybe with an example as in "Eq. 6.222".

Assessment of Publication Bias and Small-Study Effects

Both Fail-Safe N and Fail-Safe B analyses showed that a significantly large number of studies are expected to remain in the drawer: 595 studies; $P < 0.001$ and 370 studies; $P < 0.001$. Those results support our study being robust. Neither the rank correlation nor the regression test indicated any funnel plot asymmetry ($P = 0.838$ and $p = 0.40$, respectively).

Sensitivity Analysis

The results of both fixed and random-effects models were comparable. In addition, we have performed cumulative analysis as well as leave one sensitivity analysis. Both procedures showed that our results were robust.

6.3 Psychometric Meta-Analysis (Hunter and Schmidt)

6.3.1 The Basic Concept

No study is methodologically perfect, and hence, studies will always yield unperfect results. For example, studies involving continuous data cannot include the whole range of measurements because of the limited sample size. Hence, their effect size will be smaller (will be attenuated) due to the limited range. Attenuation of effect size can also be produced by dichotomizing the continuous scale or by an error in the measuring instrument itself. Hunter and Schmidt thought of these methodological imperfections as artifacts in the study design and provided a complete list [2].

The other side of the coin is that the variation between observed effects is larger than between any adjustment of effects, such as the adjustment made by considering a moderator variable. Consequently, the increased variability will lead to an inflated moderator effect when moderator analysis is attempted. As we have previously indicated, the increased variability can inflate publication bias assessment (see Sect. 6.2.10). *The net result is that the observed effect size is smaller and of larger variability than it would be. Hence, it has to be adjusted for those two elements before doing the meta-analysis.*

Hunter and Schmidt defined the observed effect size as the attenuated effect size and hence the corrected effect size as the unattenuated effect size. The ratio between the two effects represents the impact of artifacts on the effect size and is called the artifact multiplier or reliability index (a). The aim was to correct those results before doing a meta-analysis. Hence, the estimates of effect size become more valid for generalization on the population, which is why it is called validity generalization. The technique is also called psychometric meta-analysis because it is based on the psychometric principle to correct the attenuated effect size due to measurement errors and other artifacts at the level of the studies before doing the meta-analysis [3].

The ratio between the observed (attenuated) effect size and the expected (unattenuated) effect size of the population (r^u) represents the impact of artifacts on the effect size, and it is called the artifact multiplier or reliability index (a). Provided that Pearson's correlation coefficient (r) is the effect size, and if (a) is known, we can estimate the true effect size (r^u) by dividing the observed attenuated effect size by the artifact "Eq. 6.235". Equally, the true variance: Var (r^u) can be estimated by dividing the observed variance of r by $1/a^2$ "Eq. 6.236". As an example, if the true correlation coefficient between 2 variables is believed to be 0.5 and the reliability index is 0.8, the observed r will be only 0.4 (0.5×0.8). In other words, the observed effect size will be 20% smaller than the true effect size.

$$r^u = \frac{r}{a} \qquad (6.235)$$

$$Var\ (r^u) = \frac{Var\ (r)}{a^2} \qquad (6.236)$$

In case the ES is influenced by multiple artifacts, we can calculate an individual multiplier (a) for each (i) and compute a combined artifact multiplier as the product of all multipliers (= $a_1 \times a_2 \times a_3, \dots a_i$). Once available, we can correct the effect size and its variance and make all calculations with those true values. The net result is the production of an effect size more valid for the population, which was behind the technique's name: generalized validation [2].

We will begin by pointing to the computational differences between the psychometric and the more conventional meta-analysis we followed in this book [5–8]. Addressing those differences is sometimes called barebones meta-

analysis, based on just removing the sampling error variance, without correcting any artifact. The second step correcting the attenuated effect size by the artifact multiplier [2].

6.3.2 The Bare Bones Meta-Analysis

We compute the weighted effect size, which is typically a weighted correlation coefficient in psychometric studies. Unlike the previous method of Hedges and colleagues, the effect size is weighted by the sample size rather than the inverse variance. We calculate the weighted effect size of each study by multiplying its effect size (r_i) by its sample size (n_i). The effect size in the population (r) is estimated as the average of the weighted effect size calculated for all (n_i) studies "Eq. 6.237".

$$r = \frac{\sum n_i r_i}{\sum n_i} \qquad (6.237)$$

We calculate the variability around the observed weighted correlation as the sum of the weighted squared differences between the individual effect size of each study (r_i) and the average effect size (r), divided by the number of studies (n_i) "Eq. 6.238".

$$S_r^2 = \frac{\sum n_i (r_i - r)^2}{\sum n_i} \qquad (6.238)$$

The variability observed in a sample (Sr^2) has two sources of variation: the variability in the population from which the sample was drawn (Sp^2) and the sampling error Se^2. As r-squared (r^2) estimates the amount of variation explained by the sample (see Sect. 2.6.2), then ($1 - r^2$) expresses the part unexplained or sampling error. We calculate the variance of sampling error across all studies, with (N) being the average sample size "Eq. 6.239".

$$S_e^2 = \frac{(1 - r^2)^2}{N - 1} \qquad (6.239)$$

Finally, the amount of variation between studies Sp^2 is what is left after removing the amount of variation due to sampling error "Eq. 6.240".

$$S_P^2 = S_r^2 - S_e^2 \qquad (6.240)$$

If sampling error explains 100% of the variability between the studies, Sp^2 will be null or negative, which is unusual. Commonly, some variability remains between the studies. Part of this can be genuine due to the differences between subgroups or the influence of associated risk factors. The remaining part will be due to artifacts that must be corrected before proceeding to the analysis [2].

6.3.3 Meta-Analysis Corrected for All Artifacts

6.3.3.1 Calculation of the Effect Size

What we have described is called the bare bone meta-analysis and is just not enough for psychometric meta-analysts and what remains is finding the artifact multiplier and use it to estimate the true (unattenuated) effect size and variance to get truer results that can be validated on the population of interest. The analysis is based on the concepts shown before: the observed effect sizes are attenuated and of wider variability than their true counterparts in the population (unattenuated) by a factor (a) or a group of factors due to various reasons explained before. Knowing (a) we can proceed and correct all calculations to by replacing r by (r^u) and n_i by ($n_i a^2$).

Note that Sp^2 as calculated in bare bones analysis is the variability of the population after removing of sampling error only. However, after correcting the effect size by the artifact multiplier and repeated all equations with the corrected values, the calculated $(Sp^u)^2$ becomes the remaining variability in the population after correcting the observed variation (Sr^2) for sampling error as well as other artifacts and hence, the difference between both measures $[(Sr^2) - (Sp^u)^2]$ to the total observed variation (Sr^2) is the proportion of corrected variation by the technique "Eq. 6.241". In other words, the proportion of observed variation

explained by all artifacts can be calculated as the error of variation due to all artifacts

$$\frac{S_r^2 - \left(S_P^u\right)^2}{S_r^2} \qquad (6.241)$$

Correction of artifacts can take two forms. The first is to correct each observed effect size, individually or to correct the entire observed distribution at one time.

The other approach is to perform a bare-bones meta-analysis first, and then to correct the mean and Sd for artifacts rather than sampling error. Applying either method produces identical results [2]. Equations are complicated but can be executed by dedicated software, such as the Source forge [32].

6.3.3.2 Assessment of Heterogeneity

We have previously discussed the sources of heterogeneity in meta-analysis, where variability may be due to variability within the studies (sampling error) and variability between studies. The latter can be either a true variation in the population (internal), an artificial variation produced by an external factor, or a combination of both [25] (see Sect. 6.2.7). In the case of true residual variability, the meta-analyst has to assume heterogeneity, which can be further explained by moderator analysis (see Sect. 6.2.8 and Sect. 6.2.9).

However, from the psychometric meta-analysis point of view, numerous other sources can potentially cause additional artificial variability [66]. Some are simple computational, typographical, and transcription errors [67]. Others are major errors, such as underestimation of the sampling error across studies and the error associated with the sampling process on the aggregate level of meta-analysis, i.e., by combining the studies. Hunter and Schmidt have termed the latter second-order sampling errors [2].

The Hunter and Schmidt Rule of Thumb

Unlike conventional meta-analysis, homogeneity is not usually tested by Cochran Q but evaluated according to Hunter and Schmidt's rule of thumb. The authors assume homogeneity if 75%

or more of the total observed variance is due to a group of errors related to sampling, measuring errors, and selecting a specific effect size range. This rule was based on studies showing that those errors are usually responsible for an average of 72% of the observed variation in meta-analysis studies on employment [2, 67]. Hence, it may need further investigation in other research areas [66].

Formal Statistical Testing (Q Test)
In addition to Hunter and Schmidt's rule of thumb, various statistical tests can be applied in order to assess whether the observed variance is based on artificial variance or true variance. The most frequently used test is the Q test. The statistic is based on the sum of squared errors between each of the (n_i) effect sizes (r_i) and the mean effect size (r), standardized by the error variance $(1 - r)^2$ "Eq. 6.242". The result is checked in the Chi-square table at $n - 1$ df.

$$\chi^2 = \sum \frac{(n_i - 1)(r_i - \bar{r})^2}{(1 - \bar{r})^2} \qquad (6.242)$$

The Prediction Interval (PI)
Unlike the conventional method of Hedges and colleagues, the Hunter and Schmidt method suggests a random model for any meta-analysis. Consequently, the calculated mean effect size is expected to lie within a large spectrum of values and not in a single central point. Put it this way, instead of creating a 95% confidence that may include the population effect size; we produce a wider 95% prediction interval that is expected to include the spectrum of the population effect size.

In other words, instead of trying to locate the mean population effect size, Hunter and Schmidt suggested precision by credibility to generalize the validity of the calculated effect size on the population spectrum. For the usual 5% risk of error, the 95% prediction interval (95% PI)

around (r) can be expressed by the "Eq. 6.243". Note that this amount $(Sp^u)^2$ estimates the variability present in the population, it is calculated after correction of all artifacts, and hence, it does not depend on sampling error.

In case the credibility interval is narrow (tight) and does not include zero, the effect size (r) estimates a single population. On the other hand, large intervals or those including zero reflect heterogeneity or that moderator variables being active. In such a case, (r) can be seen as an estimate of multiple subpopulations [66].

$$95\%PI = r \pm 1.96\sqrt{(S_P^u)^2} \qquad (6.243)$$

6.3.3.3 Interpretation of Results
It is only after validity and reliability have been addressed so that we conclude our results. Reliability refers to the question of whether the meta-analytic results could be based on chance, and validity refers to the question of whether the results of meta-analysis reflect reality [66]. The results are reliable as long as the 95% CI interval excludes zero. On the other hand, the question of validity is not as straightforwards. One point is to conclude upon homogeneity of results, with 75% or more of the variability being due to sampling errors, a non-significant Q and a narrow 95% PI excluding zero. Another point is to exclude publication bias by one of the fail-Safe methods.

The meta-analysis is not a training project on how to collect data and drain conclusion. It requires advanced statistical knowledge and sound reasoning. It cannot a suitable first project for young researchers and medical students unless the leader is a knowledgeable and well-trained primary researcher.

References

1. Page MJ, McKenzie JE, Bossuyt PM, Boutron I, Hoffmann TC, Mulrow CD, et al. The PRISMA 2020 statement: an updated guideline for reporting systematic reviews. Syst Rev. 2021;10:89. https://doi.org/10.1186/s13643-021-01626-4.

2. Hunter JE, Schmidt FL. Methods of meta-analysis. Correcting error and bias in research findings, 2nd ed. Thousand Oaks, CA: Sage publications;2004. https://www.gwern.net/docs/statistics/meta-analysis/2004-hunterschmidt-methodsofmetaanalysis.pdf.

3. Borenstein M, Hedges LV, Higgins JPT, Rothstein HR. Introduction to meta-analysis, 1st ed. Padstow, Cornwall, UK: John Wiley & Sons;2009. https://doi.org/10.1111/j.1751-5823.2009.00095_15.x.

4. Glass GV. Primary, secondary and meta-analysis of research. Educ Res. 1976;5:3–8. https://doi.org/10.2307/1174772.

5. Hedges LV. Estimation of effect size under non-random sampling: the effects of censoring studies yielding statistically insignificant mean differences. J Educ Stat. 1984;9:61–85. https://doi.org/10.2307/1164832.

6. Hedges LV, Olkin I. Statistical methods for meta-analysis. Orlando: FL, Academic Press; 1985.

7. Hedges LV. Meta-analysis. J Educ Stat. 1992;17(4):279–96. https://doi.org/10.2307/1165125.

8. Hedges LV, Vevea JL. Fixed—and random-effects models in meta-analysis. Psychol Methods. 1998;3(4):486–504. https://doi.org/10.1037/1082-989X.3.4.486.

9. Rosenthal R, Rubin DB. A simple general purpose display of magnitude of experimental effect. J Edu Psychol. 1982;74(2):166–9. https://doi.org/10.1037/0022-0663.74.2.166.

10. Johnson BT, Mullen B, Salas E. Comparison of three major meta-analytic approaches. J Appl Psychol. 1995;80(1):94–106. https://doi.org/10.1037/0021-9010.84.1.144.

11. Thompson KN, Schumacker RE. An evaluation of Rosenthal and Rubin's binomial effect size display. J Educ Behav Stat. 1997;22(1):109–17. https://doi.org/10.2307/1165240.

12. Mantel N, Haenszel W. Statistical aspects of the analysis of data from retrospective studies of disease. J Natl Cancer Inst. 1959;22:719–48.

13. Yusuf S, Peto R, Lewis J, Collins R, Sleight P. Beta blockade during and after myocardial infarction: an overview of the randomized trials. Prog Cardiovasc Dis. 1985;27:335–71. https://doi.org/10.1016/s0033-0620(85)80003-7.

14. Cooper H, Hedges LV. The handbook of research synthesis, 1st ed. New York: Russel Sage foundation;1994. https://www.jstor.org/stable/10.7758/9781610441377.

15. Hulley SB, Cummings SR, Browner WS, Grady DG, Newman TB. Designing clinical research. 4th ed. Philadelphia: Lippincott Williams and Wilkins; 2013.

16. Thomas J, Kneale D, McKenzie JE, Brennan SE, Bhaumik S. Determining the scope of the review and the questions it will address. In: Higgins JPT, Thomas J, Chandler J, Cumpston M, Li T, Page MJ, Welch VA, editors. Cochrane Handbook for Systematic Reviews of Interventions version 6.3 (updated February 2022);2022. www.training.cochrane.org/handbook. Accessed April 13, 2022.

17. Prospero international prospective register of systematic review. National institute for health research. York, UK: University of York Centers of review and dissemination. https://www.crd.york.ac.uk/prospero/. Accessed 13 May 2022.

18. Rosenthal R. The file drawer problem and tolerance for null results. Psychol Bull. 1979;86(3):638–41. https://doi.org/10.1037/0033-2909.86.3.638.

19. Higgins JPT, Savović J, Page MJ, Elbers RG, Sterne JAC. Assessing risk of bias in a randomized trial. In: Higgins JPT, Thomas J, Chandler J, Cumpston M, Li T, Page MJ, Welch VA, editors. Cochrane Handbook for Systematic Reviews of Interventions version 6.3 (updated February 2022). Cochrane; 2022. www.training.cochrane.org/handbook. Accessed 20 Feb. 2022.

20. Hunter JE, Schmidt FL. Fixed effects versus random effects meta-analysis models: implications for cumulative research knowledge. Int J Sel Assess. 2000;8(4):275–92. https://doi.org/10.1111/1468-2389.00156.

21. Rosenthal R. Effect sizes: Pearson's correlation, its display via the BESD, and alternative indices. Am Psychol. 1991;46(10):1086–7. https://doi.org/10.1037/0003-066X.46.10.1086.

22. Lenhard W, Lenhard A. Computation of effect sizes. Psychometrica; 2016. https://www.psychometrica.de/effect_size.html. Accessed 7 March 2022.

23. Wilson Db, Mason G. Practical meta-analysis effect size calculator; 2001. https://www.campbellcollaboration.org/escalc/html/EffectSizeCalculator-Home.php. Assessed 9 Apr 2022.

24. Rosenthal R, DiMatteo MR. Meta-analysis: recent developments in quantitative methods for literature reviews. Annu Rev Psychol. 2001;52:59–82. https://doi.org/10.1146/annurev.psych.52.1.59.

25. Lipsey MW, Wilson DB. Practical meta-analysis. Thousand Oaks: CA, Sage Publications; 2001.

26. Peterson RA, Brown SP. On the use of beta coefficients in meta-analysis. J Appl Psychol. 2005;90:175–81. https://doi.org/10.1037/0021-9010.90.1.175.

27. Rosnow RL, Rosenthal R. Effect sizes for experimenting psychologists. Can J Exp Psychol. 2003;57:221–37. https://doi.org/10.1037/h0087427.

28. Fleiss JL. The statistical basis of meta-analysis. Stat Methods Med Res. 1993;2(2):121–45. https://doi.org/10.1177/096228029300200202.

29. Becker LE. Effect size calculator. Colorado Springs: University of Colorado; 1999. https://www.uccs.edu/lbecker/. Accessed 7 March 2022.

30. Fisher RA. On the probable error of a coefficient of correlation deduced from a small sample. Metron. 1921;1:3–32. https://www.jstor.org/stable/2246198.

31. Deeks JJ, Higgins JPT, Altman DG. Analysing data and undertaking meta-analyses. In: Higgins JPT, Thomas J, Chandler J, Cumpston M, Li T, Page MJ, Welch VA, editors. Cochrane handbook for systematic reviews of interventions version 6.3 (updated February 2022). 2022. www.training.cochrane.org/handbook. Accessed 10 Jan. 2022.

32. Viechtbauer W. Conducting meta-analyses in R with the metafor package. J Stat Softw. 2010;36(3):1–48. https://doi.org/10.18637/jss.v036.i03.

33. Jamovi. Stats.Open.Now. Version 2.2.5 for macOS. 2020, https://www.jamovi.org/download.html. Accessed 13 Mar 2022.

34. JASP a fresh way to do statistics. JASP 0.16.2 for macOS. 2018, https://jasp-stats.org/download/. Accessed 5 Apr 2022.

35. OpenMeta[Analyst]. Completely open-source, cross-platform software for advanced meta-analysis. OpenMetaAnalyst for Sierra (10.12). http://www.cebm.brown.edu/openmeta/download.html. Accessed Jul 2021.

36. Field AP, Gillett R. Expert tutorial. How to do a meta-analysis. Br J Math Stat Psychol. 2010;63:665–94. https://doi.org/10.1348/000711010X502733.

37. Colditz GA, Brewer TF, Berkey CS, Wilson ME, Burdick E, Fineberg HV, et al. Efficacy of BCG vaccine in the prevention of tuberculosis. Meta-analysis of the published literature JAMA. 1994;271(9):698–702 PMID: 8309034.

38. Viechtbauer W. Bias and efficiency of meta-analytic variance estimators in the random-effects model. J Educ Behav Stat. 2005;30(3):261–93. http://www.jstor.org/stable/3701379.

39. Hardy RJ, Thompson SG. Detecting and describing heterogeneity in meta-analysis. Stat Med. 1998; 17:841–56. https://doi.org/10.1002/(sici)1097-0258 (19980430)17:8%3C841::aid-sim781%3E3.0.co;2-d.

40. Higgins JPT, Thompson SG. Quantifying heterogeneity in a meta-analysis. Stat Med. 2002;21:1539–58. https://doi.org/10.1002/sim.1186.

41. DerSimonian R, Laird N. Meta-analysis in clinical trials. Control Clin Trials. 1986;7(3):177–88. https://doi.org/10.1016/0197-2456(86)90046-2.

42. Hedges L. Distribution theory for Glass's estimator of effect size and related estimators. J Educ Stat. 1981;6:107–28. https://doi.org/10.2307/1164588.

43. Sidik K, Jonkman N. Simple heterogeneity variance estimation for meta-analysis. J Roy Stat Soc. 2005;54:367–84. https://doi.org/10.1111/j.1467-9876.2005.00489.x.

44. Riley RD, Higgins JPT, Deeks JJ. Interpret Random Eff Meta-Anal BMJ. 2011;342:d549. https://doi.org/10.1136/bmj.d549.

45. Bartlett MS. Properties of sufficiency and statistical test. Proc R Soc A. 1937;160:268–82. https://doi.org/10.1098/rspa.1937.0109.

46. Altman DG, Bland JM. Interaction revisited: the difference between two estimates. BMJ. 2003;326:219. https://doi.org/10.1136/bmj.326.7382.219.

47. Berkey CS, Hoaglin DC, Mosteller F, Colditz GA. A random-effects regression model for meta-analysis. Stat Med. 1995;14(4):395–411. https://doi.org/10.1002/sim.4780140406.

48. Kirkham JJ, Dwan KM, Altman DG, Gamble C, Dodd S, Smyth R, et al. The impact of outcome reporting bias in randomised controlled trials on a cohort of systematic reviews. BMJ. 2010;340:c365. https://doi.org/10.1136/bmj.c365.

49. Egger M, Smith GD, Schneider M, Minder C. Bias in meta-analysis detected by a simple, graphical test. BMJ. 1997;315:629–34. https://doi.org/10.1136/bmj.315.7109.629.

50. Stanbrook MB, Austin PC, Redelmeier DA. Acronym-named randomized trials in medicine—the art in medicine study. N Engl J Med. 2006;355:101–2. https://doi.org/10.1056/NEJMc053420.

51. Ikhlaaq A, Sutton A, Riley RD. Assessment of publication bias, selection bias, and unavailable data in meta-analyses using individual participant data: a database survey. BMJ. 2011;344:d7762. https://doi.org/10.1136/bmj.d7762.

52. Rosenberg MS. The file-drawer problem revisited: A general weighted method for calculating fail-safe numbers in meta-analysis. Evolution. 2005;59(2):464–8. https://doi.org/10.1111/j.0014-3820.2005.tb01004.x.

53. Cochran WG. The combination of estimates from different experiments. Biometrics. 1954;10:101–29. https://doi.org/10.2307/3001666.

54. Orwin RG. A fail-safe N for effect size in meta-analysis. J Educ Stat. 1983;8:157–9. https://doi.org/10.2307/1164923.

55. Cohen J. Statistical power analysis for the behavioral sciences. 1st ed. New York: Academic Press; 1969.

56. Light RJ, Pillemer DB. Summing up: the science of reviewing research. Cambridge, MA: Harvard University Press; 1984. https://doi.org/10.3102/0013189X015008016

57. Sterne JAC, Gavaghan D, Egger M. Publication and related bias in meta-analysis: power of statistical tests and prevalence in the literature. J Clin Epidemiol. 2000;53:1119–29. https://doi.org/10.1016/s0895-4356(00)00242-0.

58. Sterne JAC, Egger M, Moher D, Boutron I. Addressing reporting biases. In: Higgins JPT, Churchill R, Chandler J, Cumpston MS, editors. Cochrane handbook for systematic reviews of interventions version 5.2.0 (updated June 2017); 2017. www.training.cochrane.org/handbook. Accessed 22 Dec 2021.

59. Egger M, Smith GD, Altman DG. Systematic review in health care. Meta-analysis in context, 2nd ed. London: BMJ publishing group; 2001.

60. Duval SJ, Tweedie RL. A nonparametric 'trim and fill' method of accounting for publication bias in meta-analysis. J Am Stat Assoc. 2000;95(449):89–98. https://doi.org/10.1111/j.0006-341X.2000.00455.x.

61. Vevea JL, Woods CM. Publication bias in research synthesis: sensitivity analysis using a priori weight functions. Psychol Methods. 2005;10(4):428–43. https://doi.org/10.1037/1082-989X.10.4.428.

62. Begg CB, Mazumdar M. Operating characteristics of a rank correlation test for publication bias. Biometrics. 1994;50(4):1088–101. https://doi.org/10.2307/2533446.

63. Harbord RM, Egger M, Sterne JA. A modified test for small-study effects in meta-analyses of controlled trials with binary endpoints. Stat Med. 2006;25:3443–57. https://doi.org/10.1002/sim.2380.

64. Peters JL, Sutton AJ, Jones DR, Abrams KR, Rushton L. Comparison of two methods to detect publication bias in meta-analysis. J Am Med Assoc. 2006;295:676–80. https://doi.org/10.1001/jama.295.6.676.

65. Copas J, Shi JQ. Meta-analysis, funnel plots and sensitivity analysis. Biostatistics. 2000;1(3):247–62. https://doi.org/10.1093/biostatistics/1.3.247.

66. Kock A. A guideline to meta-analysis. TIM working paper series, vol. 2;2009. https://www.tim.tu-berlin.de/fileadmin/fg101/TIM_Working_Paper_Series/Volume_2/TIM_WPS_Kock_2009.pdf. Accessed 11 May 2022.

67. Sagie A, Koslowsky M. Detecting moderators with meta-analysis: an evaluation and comparison of techniques. Pers Psychol. 1993;46(3):629–40. https://doi.org/10.1111/j.1744-6570.1993.tb00888.x.

Abstract

This chapter is not a guideline to authors, reviewers, or editors; the literature contains many more valuable resources. I believe that every biologist has the opportunity to participate in research work, one way or another. Some are just following what is published in their specialties, whether as regular or occasional readers. They have to understand the meaning behind numbers and they may need to comment. Others get involved with a research team or participate in a specific research project. Few biologists dedicate part of their time or their entire life to research. Senior researchers are usually requested to review the work of others or to join an evaluating committee. Our book aimed to provide each party with the minimum required statistical knowledge in their language. The following section discusses some pitfalls and common errors encountered when preparing a study, reviewing a manuscript before publication, or reading a research paper.

Keywords

Statistician involvement · Study empowerment · Data management · Statistics software · Online calculators · Data reporting

7.1 Sample Size Calculation

The Unpleasant Surprise

Online power calculators are freely available on the internet, calculating sample size with a click of a button. All that is required is some basic information: the effect size, the direction of the study, and the adopted risks of error (see Sect. 4.1). Many researchers do not appreciate the importance of calculating their sample size before the study. Others only seek calculations after the study when reviewers inquire whether it was computed and request the used formulae and the procedure details. At this point, researchers usually desperately rush to statisticians seeking advice.

In addition to being *no-ethical* to deliver post-hoc calculations as if they were performed before the study, the situation is similar to someone trying to put on his wedding suit 20 years after he got married. He will never fit-in and, and even if he does, it will be by *pure chance*. We have to tailor the sample (the suit) before the beginning of the study (the wedding) and not the reverse; otherwise, we must expect unpleasant surprises.

7.1.1 Empower the Study

A focusing clinician can choose the relevant research outcome measures from the medical point of view, but unfortunately, this is not

enough. The clinician has to have a basic statistical knowledge that helps him "sculpture" the primary outcome of his study to "achieve" a statistically significant result with the help of a professional statistician when necessary.

The primary outcome is the variable used to calculate sample size and finally to judge if the treatment or the procedure was effective, accurate, or, in a more general term, it gave the expected result. The researcher knows that the smaller the treatment effect, the more he must include patients in his study to show it. A common error is to choose the outcome that produces the more prominent effect irrespective of the most crucial property, which is how much it is variable. How much the treatment effect variability interferes with sample size is not as clear to many researchers. We present a simple variant of "Eq. 4.5" used to calculate the sample size for a bilateral study comparing two means or two proportions, with the usual 5% primary risk of error and 80% power "Eq. 7.1". The reader can refer to chapter four to find from where we got the magic number 16 shown in the equation (see Sect. 4.1.5.1).

$$n = \frac{16}{d^2} = 16\left(\frac{Sd}{\Delta}\right)^2 \qquad (7.1)$$

As shown, the sample size (n) is inversely proportional to the target difference between treatments (Δ) and is directly proportional to the variability (Sd). The more variability, the larger (n). If we double variability, it quadruples the sample size, and if we triple variability, the sample size increases as much as nine times. The situation becomes more obscure when the researcher chooses a qualitative primary outcome. Unlike the continuous outcome that is usually presented as mean and Sd, the qualitative outcome is usually expressed as numbers and percentages; hence, the researcher does not "see" a standard deviation to judge the variability of the qualitative variable, which is enormous by default. Unless being able to "imagine or calculate" a standard deviation for the qualitative variable, choosing the latter as a primary outcome is an uncalculated risk. The golden rule is

to choose the primary outcome with the smallest variability (Sd) and reasonably significant effect (Δ), i.e., the outcome with the most significant effect size (Δ/Sd). Section 7.1.2 will outline simple tools that may help the researcher intelligently choose a "statistically promising" primary outcome (see Sect. 7.1.2).

On the other hand, the nature of the primary outcome (the type of variable and its distribution) is not the only source of variability in the study. Many additional sources of variability are related to the design of the study, such as the absence of randomization or the creation of unequal study arms. Those sources must be identified and avoided if unnecessary or controlled before the study. Other designs can empower the study, such as paired or one-tailed analysis and the use of repeated measures. If feasible, the researcher can adopt one of those designs to reduce his sample size (see Sect. 7.1.3).

7.1.2 Sculpture the Primary Outcome

Figure 7.1 shows variables classified in their "increasing natural order" of expected variability (Fig. 7.1). Variability is the main factor that increases sample size, and hence, our primary choice should be towards a quantitative variable, preferably a continuous one. The next best choice is a composite primary outcome (a score), a categorical variable, with the binomial variable being the last resort. The reasons behind this suggested algorithm are summarized below.

7.1.2.1 Choose a Single Outcome
Choosing multiple primary outcomes can be hazardous unless it was pre-planned meticulously. The researcher will be obliged to satisfy all outcomes on the clinical and statistical levels. Let us take the simple example of choosing two outcomes and asking ourselves: how can we accept a study showing that a treatment is safe but ineffective or the reverse? We have to define our primary outcome, whether safety or effectiveness? Of course, we can plan to have both outcomes, but we have to calculate the relevant sample sizes and adopt the largest sample to

Fig. 7.1 Variables classified in the increasing natural order of expected variability

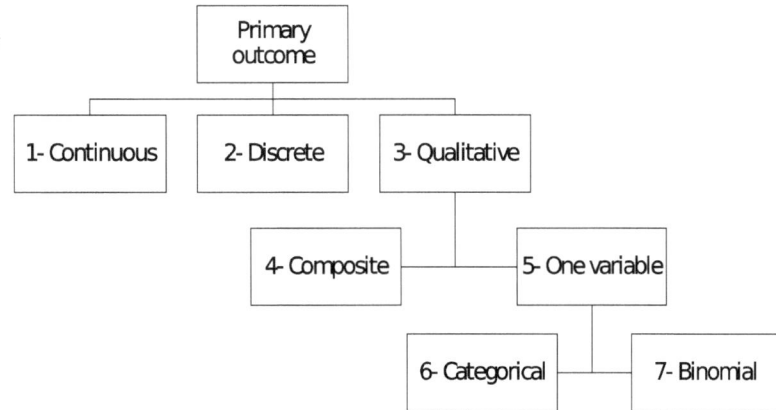

cover both endpoints. Suppose that we are comparing two treatments, A and B. Which treatment would we recommend if treatment A causes significant mortality but fewer cases of stroke. In contrast, treatment B is associated with fewer mortalities but a significantly higher rate of stroke? Which treatment can we recommend to our patients or ourselves? Yes, those are extreme examples, but the perfect treatment does not exist yet, and every treatment will have its advantages and drawbacks. We do not advise against choosing multiple outcomes, but we have to study the issue very carefully before deciding.

7.1.2.2 Choose a Continuous Variable

What is the difference (i.e., the variability) between life and death? It is huge. What is the difference between being healthy and having a cerebrovascular stroke or between being blind and enjoying the beautiful scenes of life? It is substantial. *The inherent variability in a qualitative variable (the difference between its classes, e.g., dead and alive) is not always as evident. We, lay biologists, cannot appreciate it numerically unless calculated.* Let us take the example of a study conducted to evaluate the role of statins in cardiomyopathy. The authors were hesitant to choose the primary outcome between improvement of mortality from 22% with conventional therapy to only 8% with statins or improvement of left ventricle ejection fraction percentage (LVEF%) from 30 to 33% (Sd = 5%). The improvement of mortality per se is an

indisputable treatment outcome. In addition, statins decrease mortality by as much as 60%, compared to a smaller 10% improvement in EF. We must admit that the large difference in mortality will reduce the sample size more than the small difference in LVEF. However, the effect size is not only about the magnitude of the outcome but about the variability too. The variability of the numerical LVEF% is quite evident to any reader, being the Sd of 5% (0.05). On the other hand, the author rarely gives the standard deviation of the qualitative variable (mortality), and the reader has to calculate it himself.

The Variability of a Qualitative Variable is Huge and is Rarely Appreciated

We have previously shown that the variance of a proportion (p) is equal to p $(1 - p)$ and that the common variance for two proportions is the sum of both their variances (Sect. 1.3.4.4). In consequence, the common variance of mortality = 0.22 $(1{-}0.22)$ + 0.08 $(1{-}0.08)$ = 0.172 + 0.074 = 0.25 and, its square root or the standard deviation equals 0.5. *We can now "see" that mortality variability is ten times that of LVEF (0.05), which was not evident looking at the mortality figures.* Now the tradeoff becomes clearer: the appealing large difference in mortality is associated with a very large variability that is ten times that of the smaller difference in LVEF. Table 7.1 shows the effect of this large variability on sample size calculation. Adopting the usual 5 and 20% primary and secondary risks

Table 7.1 Sample size calculation. Evaluation of the role of statins in cardiomyopathy

	Δ	Sd	d	d²	n
LVEF%	0.03	0.05	0.6	0.36	45
Mortality	0.2*	0.5	0.4	0.16	100

LVEF = left ventricular ejection fraction %, Δ = difference between conventional therapy and statins, Sd, standard deviation, d = standardized difference (Δ/Sd), n = sample size per group, * = the difference between 2 proportions a and b = (proportion a-proportion b) × square root of 2 (see Sect. 4.3.1.1)

of error and a bilateral study, we need to include 45 patients per group if we choose LVEF as the primary outcome, compared to 100 patients if we choose mortality (see "Eq. 4.5"). Although a qualitative outcome is usually more attractive than a quantitative one, the inherent variability is usually larger and hidden for the lay biologist unless calculated. In comparison, *the quantitative variable retains information, reduces variability, and offers the possibility of using more powerful and variant statistical tests.*

7.1.2.3 Create a Continuous Endpoint (Composite Score)

If the best solution (a single continuous outcome) is not feasible or not attractive, the researcher may adopt a composite outcome. Unlike the multiple outcomes, which may weaken the study results, *a composite outcome captures the multiple aspects of the study while avoiding competing risks by summarizing the multiple endpoints in one number.* It is most helpful in diseases that affect multiple organs or systems, such as hypertension or those manifesting by multiple related adverse outcomes such as coronary artery disease. It can improve the study efficiency, increase the study's power, and reduce the need for multiple comparisons and allocating of the primary risk of error across the different endpoints. *Robust composite endpoints have to be precise estimates of disease progression and treatment effects and be clinically meaningful to patients and care providers* [1].

The major adverse cardiac events (MACE) represent an excellent example of a composite outcome for patients with ischemic heart disease. It combines mortality, the development of myocardial infarction or cerebrovascular stroke, and the need for revascularization or hospitalization

[2]. As the effect size of each of the individual components is small and necessitates a huge sample to be put into evidence in the study, the composite outcome aims to increase effect size; hence decrease sample size. Only in the case of a statistically significant MACE that can we evaluate the significance of each component separately. Composite endpoints need approval from the medical community and may be more complex if we assign different weights to the different components of the composite. The researcher has to be aware of the probable disadvantages, such as the composite being driven by a particular event or unequilibrated or contradictory treatment effects among the different components [1].

7.1.2.4 Adopt an Ordered Categorical Rather Than a Binomial Variable

We have already shown how variability can be reduced when a binary outcome is transformed into an ordered categorical one (see Sect. 4.4.2.1). In brief, Campbell and colleagues have proposed an equation based upon calculating a cumulative OR, which is calculated as an average of multiple odds ratios calculated between each category and the other categories. The equation is based upon the "pragmatic" assumption that the calculated odds ratios are roughly equal and hence, producing a more or less constant average OR. Their simple equation is valid as long as we have five categories (i.e., a categorical variable with a minimum of five classes).

Interestingly, the sample size per group (n) has to be multiplied by the factors: 1.042, 1.067, 1.125, and 1.333 in the case we have only 5, 4, 3, and 2 categories, respectively [3]. *It is clear that a binomial variable produces the largest variability, and the latter is decreased with* an increasing number of categories. The researcher must weigh between the additional power achieved by the ordered categorical design and the risk associated with the pragmatic assumptions to calculate the cumulative odds ratio.

7.1.2.5 Choose an Optimal Cut-Off Point

A typical analysis technique is to dichotomize a continuous variable by splitting the continuous measurement into two groups, which raises the question: where to pass the knife? Categorization is needed to decide whether to treat or not to treat, to give treatment A or treatment B? *A natural cut-off point or a widely accepted definition are good alternatives.* In the latter case, researchers usually use the guidelines of relevant societies or the results of the meta-analysis and larger randomized controlled studies. *Other suggested cut-off points are highly criticized.* Splitting the data according to the median divides the sample into two equal-size groups. Unlike natural and widely accepted cut-off points, every researcher will have his median value, complicating the comparison of different studies. A more biased approach is to choose the point that makes the groups most different and hence, produces the smallest P-value. The procedure is associated with a high rate of false-positive results and the inflated primary risk of error by multiple comparisons (see Sect. 2.4.3.3).

Let us take an example. In a survey study, sample size required for an expected 5% response (p = 0.05 and q = 0.95) is equal to that calculated for an expected 95% response (p = 0.95 and q = 0.05), provided equality of other parameters such as margin of error, confidence level and population size (see Sect. 4.16). This is because *the power depends not only on the difference but also on the odds*. The odds of the former are just the inverse of the latter and, as sample size n = pq $(1.96/ME)^2$, the sample size will be the same, regardless of which is (p) and which is (q), as long as they have the same distance from the null value of a proportion (0.5). As long the difference between the two proportions is constant, *the lowest power is near the*

50% event rate, and the highest power is at the extremes, near 0 and 100%.

Note that the odds ratio (OR) between 2 proportions (e.g., 80 and 90%; OR = 0.444) is just the inverse of that calculated for their reciprocals (20 and 10%; OR = 2.25) and, in both cases, sample size calculation per group (n) is the same (n = 199; for the usual 5 and 20% primary and secondary risks of error. *As the "same difference" between the 2 proportions moves towards the 50% rate, odds ratio (effect size) decreases and sample size steadily increases*; with n = 294 patients for a difference of 70 versus 80% (OR = 1.71), n = 356 patients for a difference of 60% versus 70% (OR = 1.55). Note that the reciprocal differences (30 versus 20% and 40 versus 30%), will give the reciprocal OR(s) and same (n). Put it this way, *the difference between the two proportions is the magnitude of the effect size, while their distance from the extremes (0 and 100%) is the variability*. Hence, for the same magnitude, the nearer the proportion to the null (50%), the smaller is the variability and the larger is the sample size. This simple statistical information may be helpful in reducing sample size in case the investigator has the luxury of choosing between different clinically relevant cut-off points. The researcher can always verify the calculations using many freely available online calculators [3].

On the other hand, dichotomization has a major disadvantage: the inherent loss of information. For example, being hypertensive or not is based upon dichotomizing the continuous measurement of diastolic blood pressure into being hypertensive (>90 mm Hg) or normotensive (<90 mm Hg). It is clear that the risk in a hypertensive patient whose diastolic blood pressure is 90 mm Hg is different from another hypertensive case whose blood pressure is 180 mm Hg. Dichotomizing throws all the numbers between 90- and 180-mm Hg, reducing the study's statistical power and increasing the need to include more patients in the study. Put it in another way; if we have two patients with a small negligible difference of 1 mm Hg (e.g., 89- and 90-mm Hg), the study will advise treating one and leaving the other untreated. In conclusion, *continuous variables have to be analyzed as such, and dichotomization can be adopted as a post-analysis step to make a decision, provided that it is based on natural or widely accepted standards.*

7.1.2.6　Select the Right Variance

Let us take a simple example. Suppose we compare the mean values (e.g., duration of pain relief) of two analgesics (A and B). Calculating the raw mean of the difference is straightforward: mean A- mean B; e.g., 6 h—4 h = 2 h. The problem is to find the right variance that will weigh the calculated difference. Would it be a *pooled standard error* because we assume that both means came from the same population (see "Eq. 2.20") or the *standard error of the difference* if we assume that both groups issue from different subpopulations (see "Eq. 2.22")? On the other hand, which variance would we choose to calculate the sample size for a future study? Would it be *the variance of a large but unorganized study* or the one calculated in a *small well conducted clinical trial*? No doubt, the latter would be much more informative than the former, despite of the small sample size. Moreover, it is well known that paired design (see Sect. 4.5) and repeated measures reduce variability (see Sect. 4.12). Hence, we cannot adopt their calculated variances if our study compares independent groups or taking a single measurement. Another example, after a statistically significant NOVA, researchers are usually willing to go for a post-hoc analysis and compare groups two-by-two. A better approach to compare subgroups is to *use the residual variance of ANOVA rather than the individual variances of the subgroups themselves.* The former is much more representative than the latter variances. Adopting a smaller variance than the one that should be used in our study, inflates the effect size and underpower the future study. Doing the reverse inflates the calculated sample size unnecessarily. The researcher has to choose the right variance for his study, according to the study design, direction, number of compared groups, numbers of measurements made and all other factors that were shown to influence sample size (see Sect. 4.1).

7.1.2.7　Analyze the Source Study

In defining the primary outcome, a common discussion is a tradeoff between sample size (n) and effect size; for their inverse relationship. Remember the simple equation: sample size per group (n) = $M/(ES)^2$ "Eq. 4.7". Hence, decreasing effect size by 50% approximately quadruples sample size, while doubling ES will tremendously reduce sample size to n/4, for the same value of the constant M (see Sect. 2.1). By definition, all researchers tend to diminish their sample size for being usually short of both patients and financial resources. However, a tendency towards reducing sample size through overestimating effect size may jeopardize the whole research, where effect size becomes "unreachable".

We will take the example of comparing the curative effects of two antibiotics in patients presenting with urinary tract infections. Previous studies carried out on 200 patients equally randomized between the two groups have shown respective cure rates of 75 and 45% in favor of the new treatment (see Sect. 1.4.2.7). Another researcher wished to repeat the study. Adopting a 5% primary and a 20% secondary risk of error and applying the basic sample size calculation formula, sample size per group n = 41 patients (see Sect. 4.3.2.1). The author included a total of 90 patients in the study (2n + 10%), equally split between the two groups. Unfortunately, the study results were not exactly as expected. The cure rate achieved with the classic treatment was 49% (22/45), and that with the new treatment was 60% (27/45). Hence, the difference in cure rates was only 11% (60–49%), which is nearly one-third of what was suggested (75–45%).

Let us now calculate the 95% confidence interval of the difference achieved by the new study: applying the formula presented in Sect. 1.4.2.7 or using an online calculator [5], the 95% CI of this difference = 11 ± 9.7% = (−9.1%) to (+30.1%). In other words, the new study suggests that new treatment can give slightly better results (−9%) and much worse results than the classic treatment (+30%). Of course, no one can draw any meaningful conclusion from such a non-coherent result. Comparing the success rates of both treatments by Chi-square test produces a Chi-square value of 1.12 and a large P-value of 0.29.

Despite using the correct equation to calculate sample size, what brought the study to such a "dead end" was the researcher not considering that the large difference in the cure rates (25%) reported by the previous study had a wide 95% CI ranging between 11.7 and 48.3% (see Sect. 1.4.2.7). Unfortunately, reducing the sample size of his future study by more than 50% (from n = 100 to n = 45) will widen the confidence interval, which may then overlap the null and end by producing a negative study.

The second point is that the researcher neglected checking on the power of the original study. Uploading the sample size of the original study (n = 100) and the two proportions (45 and 75%) to an online calculator shows that the power of the original study was as high as 99%. The researcher has to expect that by reducing the power of the new study to only 80%, the probability of acquiring a statistically significant difference will be reduced too; which brings us to the following section: how to predict his future 95% CI (see Sect. 7.1.2.8)?

7.1.2.8 Predict the Future Confidence Interval

Can we avoid reaching a confusing confidence interval? Yes, we could at least try by predicting the 95% IC, well before the beginning of the study. Goodman and Berlin have shown that *the 95% IC will fluctuate by 60% around the "expected difference" (Δ) for a study power of 80%. It will fluctuate by around 70% for a higher power of 90%* [6].

- Suppose that Δ is the expected difference between 2 means u0 and U1. Under the null hypothesis, Δ = 0 and, the alternative

hypothesis is that $\Delta > 0$. In order to conclude upon a significant difference, (Δ) should be quite large so that the probability that it is just due to chance (primary risk of error or ∝) is 5% or smaller. Provided that our variable is normally distributed and our sample size is large, we consult the Z table to have the equivalent Z value of this small 5% probability. The Z value is the standardized difference between the two means. In other words, how many standard errors should those two means be separated from one another so that the probability that the null hypothesis is still true is only 5% or smaller? In a bilateral study, this probability is equally split between 2 possibilities: U0>U1 or U1>U0. Hence, we consult the Z table for the Z value of ∝/2 = 2.5%. In terms of Z score, the difference between the two means should be at least equivalent to 1.96 standard errors, which we usually approximate to 2 Se. In other words, $\Delta > 1.96$ Se.

- Note that these calculations are based upon the assumption that the sample has 100% power to detect the evidence, which can never be guaranteed. In consequence, and as shown in Fig. 7.2, Δ does not only include the primary risk of error (∝/2) but equally the secondary risk of error (B); which is missing the evidence or lack of power due to small sample size. As this risk is usually set at 10 or 20%, we have to reconsider the Z table to know: how many standard errors should those two means be apart to limit the chance to miss the evidence to either 10 or 20%? The respective Z values are 0.84 Se and 1.28 Se.

- In conclusion, (Δ) has to be at least equal to the combined risks: [Z (∝/2) + Z (B)] Se. Hence, Δ0.80 = 2.8 Se (1.96 + 0.84) for a study power of 80% and, Δ 0.90 = 3.24 Se (1.96 + 1.28) for a study power of 90%. In other words, *the expected Se for studies based upon a specific (Δ), will be equal to (Δ/2.8) and (Δ/3.24) for the respective study powers of 80 and 90%* [6]. The expected Se is our best estimate of the Se of the population.

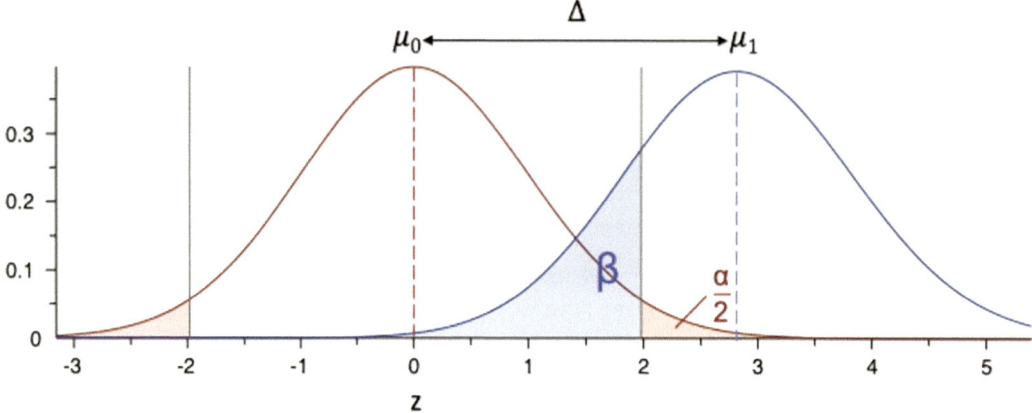

Fig. 7.2 Sample size calculation: predicting the 95%CI of the difference of a future study

- Based on the calculations above, the researcher will study and observe a difference (d_o). The 95% CI of the latter is calculated as routine: observed difference ± 1.96 Se. The question would be: we did predict the observed difference (d_o) before the study as (Δ); couldn't we predict the Se too? Yes, as we already predicted, the Se equals ($\Delta/2.8$) for a study power of 80% and ($\Delta/3.24$) for a study power of 90%. Replacing Se by either $\Delta/2.8$ or $\Delta/3.24$, the 95%CI of the observed difference is expected to be equal to: (d_o) $\pm$ (1.96/2.8) $\Delta = (d_o) \pm 0.7\,\Delta$ for a study power of 80% "Eq. 7.2" and, $d_o \pm$ (1.96/3.24) $\Delta = d_o \pm 0.6$ Δ for a study power of 90% "Eq. 7.3". *The formula is approximative, especially when the sample size is small (<20) or when proportions are outside the 0.25–0.75 range.* For more detailed information, the reader is advised to go back to [6, 7]. Put it this way, what we will get will fluctuate by about two-thirds around what we wish for. *The more we include patients, the less the fluctuation will be.*

$$95\%\ CI\ d_0(80\%\ power) = d_0 \pm 1.96\,Se$$
$$= d_0 \pm 1.96\,\frac{\Delta}{2.8} = d_0 \pm 0.7\Delta$$
$$(7.2)$$

$$95\%\ CI\ d_0(90\%\ power) = d_0 \pm 1.96\,Se$$
$$= d_0 \pm 1.96\,\frac{\Delta}{3.24} = d_0 \pm 0.6\Delta$$
$$(7.3)$$

We are returning to our example in Sect. 7.1.2.7, if the researcher had been aware of this simple formula before the study, he would have discovered that the 95% IC of the results would fluctuate by as much as 17.5% ($0.7 \times \Delta = 0.7 \times 0.25$) around whatever difference achieved by the study. Remember that his study found a 11% difference. According to Goodman and Berlin, the 95%CI will fluctuate between −6.5% and 28.5%, which means the difference cannot favor either procedures? A cleverer researcher would have chosen a modest Δ value of 10% that tightens the fluctuation from 17.5% to only 7% (0.7×0.10). The result would be a meaningful 95% CI between +4 and +18% ($11 \pm 7\%$), instead of the meaningless interval from −6.5 to 28.5%. Targeting a smaller difference (Δ) tightens the interval of confidence and, hence, decreases the latter's chances to become insignificant by including or overlapping zero [6].

7.1.3 Reduce Variability by Ameliorating the Study Design

The following are some tools that can help the researcher reduce the sample size, provided being feasible and suitable for the study.

7.1.3.1 Adopt a Paired or Cross-Over Design

We have previously shown that comparing the patient to himself (or to a matched control), removes (or reduces to a minimum) the variability between subjects) Hence, it empowers the analysis and reduces the required sample size. This gain of power has two sources: arithmetic and statistic. The arithmetic gain is due to the apparent fact that the same patient will be used twice. The statistical gain is based on the variability of one individual's response to the two treatments is theoretically less than when the two treatments are given to 2 different individuals (see Sects. 2.3, 2.4 and 4.5). The ideal situation is the comparison of diagnostic tools such as bedside tests to conventional laboratory analysis. Unfortunately, this is not always feasible in clinical trials, such as those comparing surgery to medical therapy or when serious concerns are raised about drug interaction or the inability to determine a reliable washout period between two treatments given to the same patient.

7.1.3.2 Target Surrogate Endpoints

The researcher must remember that the outcome measure is sometimes the tool and not the core mission. In this setting, surrogates are measurements in the causal pathway of the disease and correlate with the outcome, such as monitoring serum creatinine in the course of renal failure. *Besides being readily available and easier to be measured, surrogates are usually quantitative variables with much smaller variability than the usually qualitative clinical endpoint and can be measured repeatedly*; both reduce variability and eventually sample size. Let us take the example of choosing mortality as an endpoint to compare myocardial preservation techniques during cardiac surgery. Besides its qualitative nature, mortality is not suitable for "the usual small sample size research," which usually reports narrow mortality rates of 1–2% with only a few decimals difference, regardless of the used preservation technique.

Consequently, a large sample will be needed to prove a slight difference between groups. On the other hand, choosing a "more sensitive" biomarker of ischemia, such as troponin I, will reduce the required sample size and increase the chances of unveiling the difference. Compared to mortality, the sensitive biomarker has a much higher probability of delivering a positive message that one method is more protective than the other, even if this was only proved on the biochemical level.

7.1.3.3 Repeat the Measurement

Using a continuous variable is one of the most effective ways to reduce sample size, and repeating its measurements will further reduce variability and sample size. We have previously shown that the means of values are always less variable than the values themselves. The more we add values (measurements), the more variability of their mean decreases. Moreover, the gain in power is proportional to the number of measurements and the correlation (ρ) between measures (see Sects. 2.4.3.4 and 3.2.5.1). If (n) is the number of patients per group, as calculated for a regular Student test, Borm and colleagues have demonstrated that the equivalent number for a repeated measurement ANOVA will be smaller: n $(1 - \rho^2)$ [8]. Kindly refer to the section on sample size calculation for repeated measures of parametric (see Sect. 4.12.1) and non-parametric continuous variables (see Sect. 4.12.2).

7.1.3.4 Make Study Arms Equal

Although unequally sized groups are common in research, it can lead to unequal variances, affecting statistical power and type I error [9]. Variance reflects precision because the smaller the variance, the more precise the study. In other words, variance is indirectly proportional to the power of the study (see Sect. 4.1.1.2). Let us now examine the role of sample size in the case of equality of variances. As a rule of thumb, the larger the sample size, the smaller the variance and the more precise the study. In other words, precision (variance) is directly proportional to the reciprocal sample size $(1/n)$. What about the distribution of the same sample size between the compared groups? What effect will it have on precision? In other words, what would be the effect on precision if we maintain the same sampling effort by keeping the same total number of patients in the study, but we distribute this total number unequally between the compared groups?

Mathematically, suppose any number (e.g., 10) is equally split between two groups (5 and 5). In that case, the sum of the reciprocals of the two equal groups $(1/5 + 1/5 = 2/5 = 0.4)$ will always be smaller than that calculated if the same total number (10) was unequally split between the two groups (e.g., $1/4 + 1/6 = 0.416$, $1/2 + 1/8 = 0.625$, etc…). The unequal splitting is more; the more the deviation from the two equal groups scenario (0.4).

We apply the same rule on our question about splitting the total sample size between two equal or two unequal groups. Provided that both groups have the same variance, the precision of the study is proportional to the sum of the reciprocal of the number of patients in each group, provided the total sample size will be the same. *The sum of the reciprocal values of an equally split sample will always be smaller than any unequal splitting; hence it has the smallest variance and provides the highest precision.*

A Running Example

Suppose that sample size calculation showed that we need to include 32 patients per group (n). The investigator could not collect more than 24 patients in the treatment group (n_0); the question will be how many patients should he include in the control group (Kn_0) to keep the same level of precision in his study?

Provided that the sample size per group was (n), the proportion (K) between the sample sizes of two unequal groups $(n_0$ and $Kn_0) = n/(2n_0 − n)$. The equation can be easily verified if we replace n_0 with n, giving a K value of 1 for the

two equal group scenarios. Applying the equation to our example, $K = 32/(2 × 24 − 32) = 2$, the researcher must include 48 patients in the control group. In other words, a total sample size of 72 patients is needed to maintain the same precision if the study did include 64 patients that were equally distributed between the two groups. In the 2 equal groups scenario, precision $= 1/n + 1/n = 1/32 + 1/32 = 0.0625$.

In the case where the researcher insists on including the same total number of patients calculated for 2 equal groups (2n = 64 patients) in the 2 unequal groups scenario, precision $= 1/24 + 1/40 = 0.042 + 0.025 = 0.067$; reflecting nearly 7% loss in precision $[(0.067 − 0.0625)/0.0625]$. On the other hand, if the researcher increases the size of the control group to Kn_0, he will maintain the same precision: $1/n_0 + 1/Kn_0 = 1/24 + 1/48 = 0.0625$ expense of increasing sample size. In conclusion, making study arms equal offers the highest possible power.

7.1.3.5 Manage Sources of Variability

Block Dispensable Sources

The researcher can *narrow the scope of the study by blocking some sources of variation*, especially when studying a new treatment or technique. The major drawback is the limitation of the application of the results of the study on the excluded subgroups. For example, diabetic patients can be excluded in comparing non-invasive to conventional surgery because diabetes is thought to be a major confounding factor. The drawback is that the results of such study can only be applied on non-diabetic population.

Randomization and Stratification

In the case that the source of variation (e.g., diabetes mellitus) is judged to be indispensable for a particular study, the researcher can dilute this source by two simple tools: randomization and stratification (see Sect. 5.4.2.1). Randomization dilutes those sources of variability between groups. Stratification is another method to reduce variability and increase study power. In short, stratification is considering a prognostic factor during randomization. A common example is stratifying diabetes mellitus in managing patients with ischemic heart disease. Instead of directly randomizing all patients (diabetic and non-diabetics) between two treatment groups, we split patients into two strata: diabetic and non-diabetics. Each stratum is then randomized separately between the treatment groups. The researcher can now be more confident that diabetic patients are equally distributed between the treatment groups instead of leaving this "fair distribution" to hazard play. Later on, during the analysis, stratification may clarify the role of the prognostic factor itself on the study outcome. It is advisable to stratify on the factor center whenever a multicentric trial. Note that stratification creates smaller groups, which may be a source of bias in itself. Consequently, it is advisable to limit stratification to only those factors that are known or highly suspected of having a significant prognostic value.

7.1.3.6 Plan a Tight Study
Although it is advisable to increase the calculated sample size (n) by a minimum of ten percent (1.1n), this will not cover mistakes in design, sloppiness in execution, and mismanagement-related significant or unbalanced dropout rates. Measures to tighten a study are beyond the scope of this chapter, but examples are many, including; training recruitment sites, centralizing laboratory analysis, using the same raters, etc.…. *Regardless of the measures taken, the aim is to empower the study by lowering variability to the minimum.*

7.1.3.7 Choose a One-Tail Design
We have previously shown that a one-tailed study reduces sample size by about 20% for concluding upon a smaller difference than a two-tailed study (see Sect. 4.1.3). Unless treatment is compared to placebo, we have to justify adopting a one-sided test strongly. Otherwise, this may be considered as being cheating.

7.1.4 Prepare the Study to Receive the Selected Tests

Although we have to choose the test that fits the study and best answers the research question, we have to ensure and maintain that the study is well prepared to receive the test once we reach its implementation time. A second common mistake is a researcher postponing the choice of the statistical tests used until he acquires the results. Once more, he has to expect many surprises the idea behind this attitude is to see what he will get and then pick up the most suitable test for the analysis. Unfortunately, this decision is synonymous with jumping into the deep waters without knowing how to swim and then seeing how we would manage to survive. Every statistical test has to verify specific conditions for application well before the beginning of the study. In other words, the study has to be planned and executed to settle the conditions necessary for applying the statistical test when the time comes for the analysis.

Example 1 For example, a multivariable analysis (MVA), such as logistic regression, studies the effect of multiple variables (predictor or explanatory variables) on the outcome variable. A reliable model necessitates, among other things, to have 10–15 patients per predictor (see Sect. 3.3.3). It should be foresighted at the beginning of the study to include a sufficient number of cases. Otherwise, the effect of some of those predictors would not be assessed by the end. Moreover, highly correlated predictors overshadow the results and must be removed during the analysis (see Chap. 3.4.2.3). Although multicollinearity is examined during the final analysis, it can be anticipated early during the literature review. In addition, it can be primarily tested during the study preparation. Unless the researcher has decent statistical knowledge, he has to consult a statistician before the study and not only after it is terminated, when it is sometimes too late.

Example 2 Let us take another small but more detailed example. A study was conducted to compare the prophylactic effect of three anticoagulation regimens (A, B, and C) in preventing anticoagulant-related complications after heart valve replacement. The complications included minor and major bleeding, transient ischemic attacks, cerebrovascular stroke, and peripheral embolism. The authors based their research on a published study carried out on 300 patients, equally distributed between the three regimens (the input study). The input study showed significantly different complication rates between the three groups, A, B, and C: 11, 6, and 1%; Chi-square = 8.87, 4 df, P < 0.012. Table 7.2 shows the results of the published study, with the expected values shown between brackets (see Sect. 2.3.1.2).

Viewing such "convincing" results, the authors decided to repeat the same study, and hence, they were expecting to have the same results. Surprisingly, they got different results, as shown in Table 7.3 (the output study). The new results posed many questions: can they use the Chi-square test of independence to compare the rate of complications among the three groups? If not, what would be the alternatives? If they managed to compare the three groups, what are their chances of recommending one out of the three regimens? Finally, could they expect those pitfalls before the study, and hence, they can be avoided?

Before answering those four questions, we have to note that the authors have just read the literature, but they did not make the necessary effort to understand the meaning behind the numbers. The reported rates of complications (11, 6, and 1%) should be interpreted as follows: whenever we will repeat the same study, we have to expect a complication rate between 6 and 19% for patients following regimen A, a rate between 2 and 13% for regimen B, and a rate between 0.0002% (nearly zero) and 5.4% for those following regimen C. Those are the 95% CI of the input study that had to be constructed by the researchers to appreciate the upper and lower limits of comparable future results (see Sect. 1.4.2.4).

The new study did respect those confidence intervals by producing their lower limits: 6 complications for regimen A (6%), two complications for regimen B (2%), and no complications for regimen C (0%). Yes, the authors can say that we were unlucky to have those numbers, but they had been warned, and they did not listen. They had to expect the possibility of acquiring those figures before the study and had to work on avoiding them, as we will show in a

Table 7.2 Chi-square test of independence: the comparison of the rates of oral anticoagulants-related complications in patients following three anticoagulation regimens: the input study

	Regimen A	Regimen B	Regimen C	Total
Complications	11 (6)	6 (6)	1 (6)	18
No complications	89 (94)	94 (94)	99 (94)	282
Total	100	100	100	300

Values are observed numbers of cases, values between brackets are expected numbers

Table 7.3 Chi-square test of independence: the comparison of the rates of oral anticoagulants-related complications in patients following three anticoagulation regimens: the output study

	Regimen A	Regimen B	Regimen C	Total
Complications	6 (2.7)	2 (2.7)	0 (2.7)	8
No complications	94 (97.3)	98 (97.3)	100 (97.3)	292
Total	100	100	100	300

Values are observed numbers of cases, values between brackets are expected numbers

moment. What can we conclude here? We can conclude that repeating the same study never guarantees the same results but a spectrum of results, i.e., the 95% CI. In other words, the results and P-value of any study are just one incident, and we have to create the 95% CI of any results to visualize the whole spectrum of possible incidents.

- The answer to our first question: Chi-square test cannot be used here for two reasons: first, 50% of the cells (3 out of 6) have expected values less than 5, and one of the cells is empty (no complications were recorded among patients following regimen C).
- To answer the second question about using other tests, we have to revise the conditions of applying the Chi-square test alternatives, namely the corrected Chi-square test by Yates (see Sect. 2.3.1.3) and Fisher's exact test (see Sect. 2.3.1.5). Both tests can only be used to compare two-class qualitative variables, and hence, they cannot be used here to compare the three regimens in one step, which leads us to the third question: how to manage the situation?
- The way to solve this situation is to limit the comparison to two groups and use Fisher's exact test, which will not pose questions, whether about the number of expected values or about the incident that we have one empty cell (2.3.1.5). We have three alternatives: either to combine the results of two groups (e.g., group B and C) and compare them to the third group (group A) or to compare the three groups two by two in a series of repeated comparisons: group A versus group B, group B versus group C, and group A versus group C. The first solution would be highly criticized because it will raise a legitimate question: if the groups B and C can be considered as one group, why regimens B and C were compared in the first place? The problem with the second alternative is that we will make three repeated comparisons, and the inflated

risk of error had to be managed by the Bonferroni correction. Consequently, we will conclude on a significant difference, not at the usual P-value of 0.05, but at a smaller $P = (0.05)/3 = 0.0166$ (see Sect. 2.4.3.3). Consulting an online calculator comparing regimen A to regimen B (6/94 versus 2/98) and regimen B to regimen C (2/98 versus 0/100) produce non-significant P values of 0.28 and 0.49, respectively [10]. Although comparing regimen A to regimen C (6/94 versus 0/100) produces a P value of 0.0289, it is above the corrected limit suggested by Bonferroni, and hence, it should be considered as being statistically non-significant. The answer to the third question is net and clear; we cannot recommend any of the three regimens.

- The answer to the last question is yes, this dilemma could have been avoided by applying the following rules:
  - Create the confidence interval of the published results and take care of the worst-case scenario.
  - Never rely upon the false belief that repeating the same study will produce the same results, which has just been proved unreliable. The new study results will most probably fall within the 95% CI of the results of the input study but will not give the exact figure.
  - Sample size should always be calculated formally. In our example, the authors had to calculate the sample size for comparing the three proportions (11, 6, and 1%). Consulting an online calculator shows that we need to include 500 patients per group to compare regimen A to regimen B at the usual 5% primary risk of error and 80% power. We need 211 patients per group to compare regimen B to regimen C and only 88 patients per group to compare regimen A to regimen C. at the usual risks of error. Knowing that we have to increase the total sample size by 10%, the researchers have

to do their math and revise their resources to decide which regimen would be compared in the first place.

- Finally, comparing multiple groups by the Chi-square test of independence does not provide a final answer to the research question. A statistically significant Chi-square test only tells us that at least one of the three regimens is significantly different from the other two, necessitating a post-hoc analysis and adjustment of the P-values by the number of repeated comparisons made.

- If we included 500 cases per group, in the worst-case scenarios, the number of expected values in groups A, B, and C will be 30 and 10, and 0. Even if we cannot apply a Chi-square test for having one empty cell, the repeated comparison by Fisher's exact test will produce a statistically significant difference between every two groups: group A and group B patients (30/470 versus 10/490; P-value = 0.0018), group B and group C (10/490 versus 0/500; P-value = 0.0019), and group A and group C (30/470 versus 0/500; P < 0.00001); all being smaller than the Bonferroni limit (P = 0.0125).

7.1.5   Account for the Effect of Covariates in Multivariate Analysis

In logistic regression, we have previously shown that the researcher calculates sample size (N), based upon the independent predictor of his choice (see Sect. 4.10.2). The same applies in Cox regression analysis (see Sect. 4.9.2.2). In either case, the effects of other covariates can be considered by calculating a modified larger sample (N') from the equation $N' = N/(1 - R^2)$, where R^2 is the effect of other covariates reported in previous studies. The calculations can be easily made manually or by G*power software.

7.1.6   Manage the Secondary Outcomes

The inclusion of secondary outcomes in the study needs to be justified, such as lending supporting evidence for the primary endpointthe primary endpoint. As an example, if the primary endpoint is the duration of hospital stay after surgery, it will be justifiable to include the total cost of management or the need for hospitalization after discharge as secondary clinical endpoints. Laboratory tests and other surrogate measures are usually reported as secondary outcomes if considered to be of limited importance in informing decisions but helpful in explaining effect or determining intervention integrity. A secondary outcome has to receive the same care given to the primary outcome. It has to be precise, well-defined, indicate how, when and by whom it will be assessed, and adequately reported, precisely as its main variant. *The statistically significant secondary outcome provides solid evidence to justify future studies; however, its value in the actual study is only observational, even in prospective randomized controlled clinical trials.* The young researcher usually raises two questions: should we calculate a different sample size for the secondary outcomes, and do we have the right to conclude on a statistically significant secondary outcome? The two questions are the sides of the same coin. *In order to conclude on any outcome, we have to define the minimal clinically important difference (MID); otherwise, we risk to conclude on something that is clinically not important* [11]. In addition, *the researcher has to specify acceptable levels of power and type I error to reject the null hypothesis.* In other words, he has to calculate the sample size for the secondary outcome he wishes to conclude upon in his study. In case the researcher is short of power (less than 80%), then he may modify the confidence interval, for example, to 90%; i.e., increasing the risk of being wrong about the conclusion made by the secondary outcome from the usual 5–10% [11, 12]. Otherwise, secondary outcomes would be considered as being as exploratory or non-validated [11].

7.2 Data Management

7.2.1 Check on Errors and Data Consistency

We have to check for errors, values that fall outside the range of possible values and for minimum and maximum values, for frequencies on all levels of data. We can check using a spreadsheet such as Excel or statistical software such as IBM-SPSS. In the latter, we can click on "Analyze," then "Descriptive Statistics," then "Explore." We move the variables in question to the "Dependent List:" box and the grouping variables to the "Factor List:" box. We click on "Plots" to request "Histogram" and "Normality Plots and tests." The output displays the mean, 95% CI, median, variance, standard deviation, minimum, maximum, interquartile range, skewness, kurtosis, and the number and percent of missing cases. It draws boxplots, histograms, and stem and leaf plots. It tests normality by Shapiro Wilk and Kolmogorov–Smirnov tests.

On the other hand, we have to check on data consistency; for example, if the study concerns adult males and females managed in a daycare clinic, make sure that none of the males is noted as being pregnant and none of the visit durations exceeded one day. Consistency can be checked by eyeballing or by reviewing the frequencies and the descriptive statistics. We urge the researcher to pay much attention to those two points and not leave them to the statistician unfamiliar with the data set's nature and scale. *For the statistician, data are just numbers, while for the researcher, data are living creatures and he knows them well; hence, he can easily pick up any irregularity or deformity.*

7.2.2 Verify Outliers

Outliers are data points that appear to differ significantly from other data points. They can significantly skew data from a normal distribution, affect how well a sample represents the population, and bias the results of parametric

statistical tests. Outliers can be identified visually in a histogram but, more importantly, by drawing the boundaries of outlier labelling rules. The boundaries will be the difference between the first and third quartiles, and multiply it by 2.2 and either add this value to the third quartile or subtract it from the first quartile value. There are two main simple techniques to deal with outliers: trimming and Winsorizing, each being used in a different situation.

Trimming Illegitimate Outliers

Trimming eliminates the data points from the analysis, usually done when data are out of range, or there is an entry error. Trimming can also be done if we feel that data are biased due to a measurement error. Finally, trimming can be done for subjects who were included in the analysis by mistake. It is essential to report the number of those cases and the reasons behind trimming data.

Winsorizing Legitimate Outliers

The other technique is Winsorizing, where there is a small number of scores that are legitimate outliers but have to be managed to prevent data from being distorted. One method is to assign to them the nearest highest or lowest acceptable value that is not an outlier. We can do this for a limited number of scores, two or three. *Trimming and Winsorizing, more than 5% of the sample, make the sample less representative, reduce the power of the analysis, and may even affect the normality of the data itself.* In such cases, it is better to transform the data, to choose an alternative outcome or another technique for data analysis, such as a non-parametric test [13].

7.2.3 Manage Missing Data

Missing data can lower the study power and affects the precision of the confidence intervals estimated. For example, if we are interested in developing a regression model investigating the effect of age, gender, and duration of symptoms on the outcome of surgery in 100 patients. If each of the three variables had missing data in five cases, the number of listwise cases would drop to 85, which would mean a considerable power loss. Moreover, the average age and duration of surgery and the male-to-female distribution may vary considerably between the sample with missing data and the original sample included in the study.

7.2.3.1 How Much Data is Missing?

If the missing data are as small as 2%, we can remove them from the study after being reported. Other researchers extend this percentage to 5%, as long as those data are unimportant. More extensive data have to be investigated and replaced, if possible, but before doing this, we have to investigate the mechanism of missingness.

7.2.3.2 Mechanisms of Missingness

The critical question is whether missing data have a particular pattern or are just missing at random. If data is missing at random, the researcher has the option of reporting them in the case missing data are few or replacing them with various measures that we will discuss in a short while. The condition becomes more complicated if missing data have a special pattern and are linked to specific variables in the study. In such a case, the researcher must investigate the issue and re-evaluate his results accordingly. We will focus on the case of data being missing at random.

MCAR, MAR, and MNAR

Data can be completely missing at random (MCAR), missing at random (MAR), or not missing at random (MNAR) [14]. MCAR means that missing data of a specific variable, such as y, is related neither to the distribution of (y) nor to other variables in the study. MAR means that the missing data and observed data come from different populations. For example, men are more likely to report their age than women. However, it is not related to other variables in the study, such as occupation. MNAR means that the missing value is dependent on the observed value and other values. For example, most of the missing people at work are the sickest.

Little's MCAR Test

The statistical test known as Little's missing completely at random (MCAR) test differentiates whether data are completely missing at random or not? It is a Chi-square test that investigates whether there is a significant difference between the distribution of missing data and the data available. In IBM-SPSS, the test usually assumes a normal distribution of both types of data, but we can change it to a near-normal or a student distribution. We click on "Analysis" then "Missing Values Analysis" to open a new window. We move the quantitative variables included in the study to the "Quantitative Variables" box and the Categorical Variables" to the Categorical Variables" box. We click on "EM" under "Estimation" and then on "OK". EM means expectation maximization. The output displays the number and percent of missing data in each variable. The P-value of the text is displayed as a footnote under the "EM Means" table. A statistically significant test suggests that the missing and available data are not the same, and hence, we have to discuss with a professional statistician to investigate the problem. The most common situation is that the test shows a non-significant difference (P > 0.05), and we can proceed with our analysis for data being MCAR.

7.2.3.3 Missing Data Statistics

We have to review the statistics of missing data, whether by analyzing the spreadsheet or by a statistical software package.

- In an IBM-SPSS data file, we click on "Analyze", then "Descriptive Statistics", then on "Descriptive", which opens the Descriptive Statistics" window. We move the variables in question to the "Variable(s)" box, and we click "OK". The output shows the number of missing values in each variable. The output also shows the number of values "Valid Listwise", which indicates the number of cases (patients) with complete information in all variables.

- We click on "Analyze", then "Descriptive Statistics", then on "Frequencies", which opens the "Frequencies statistics" window. We move the variables in question to the "Variable(s)" box, and we click "Statistics" to open a new window, where we will request the "Mean", "Median", "Mode", "Minimum", "Maximum", and the "Std. deviation". We click on "Continue" then on "OK". The output shows the number of missing data and other requested information.

- We go to "Transform" and use the function "Compute Variable" to create a target variable for missing data that we will name "missingdata". We go to the "Function group" and choose "Missing Values" and then to the "Functions and Special Variables" box and choose "Nmiss" and click on the blue arrow to move it up to the "Numeric Expression" box. We move all the input variables separated by comma to the "Numeric Expression" box. For example, if our input variables are age, bodyweight, and height, the numeric expression will look like this: NMISS (age, bodyweight, height). We click on "OK" to create a new variable column named "missingdata" that will show in SPSS data file. The latter will show the number of missing data for each row (patient). Running the "Descriptive" on the "missingdata" will show the number of patients missing one variable, two variables, or more.

Creating a Grouping Variable for Missing Data

Suppose that the missing information was the patient's age, and we want to know whether age is missing at random or related to other variables in the study. The first step is to recode the variable "Age" under a new variable name, such as "Age_new". We go to "Transform" and choose "Recode into Different Variables". We move "Age" to the "Numeric Variable-Output Variable," and under the "Output Variable," we type the "Name" of the new variable "Age_new," and we do the same under the "Label," and we click on "Change". We click on the "Old and New Values" button to open a new window named

"Recode into Different Variable: Old and New Values".

Under "Old Value," we click on Value and choose the radio button "System-or user- missing," and under the "New Value," we type (0) and click "Add". The result is that the software is ordered to code any missing value as (0). We choose the last radio button, "All other values," and under the "New value," we type (1) and click "Add". The software will give the code (1) to all non-missing values. As such, we have created two groups of patients: patients with missing values (group 0) and patients with non-missing values (group 1).

Testing a Significant Association with Other Variables

Now we can compare those two groups (0 and 1) for any significant association with other variables in the study. We run a series of unpaired tests of students comparing the 2 groups with and without missing data (group 0 and group 1). Concerning categorical variables, the two groups can be tested for the presence of a significant association with other categorical variables by running a series of Chi-square test or Fisher's exact tests. The absence of a statistically significant difference or association suggests that data are missing at random. Otherwise, the reasons behind such association have to be investigated and analyzed.

7.2.3.4 Replace Missing Data

There is no one way to deal with missing data but several ways depending upon their number, mechanisms, and statistics. We will review some of the common ways and report their advantages and mainly their drawbacks.

Replacing Missing Data with the Mean

If the number of data is below 5%, some researchers suggest replacing missing data with the mean value. In an IBM-SPSS file, we can click on "Transform" and then on "Replace Missing Values," which opens a new window. We shift the variable in question to the "New Variables" box. We click on the "Method," we choose "Series mean," and click on "OK". The software replaces the missing data with the mean value. One important point is to investigate whether this replacement significantly changed the variable. The two variables (the original and the new variable) can be compared by a paired t-test, hoping there will be no significant difference between the two variables. Sometimes the two variables are much alike that SPSS reports that the test cannot be run because the standard error of the difference is zero. Many researchers worn against this method because it dilutes variability and bias representativeness and the results of statistical tests.

Excluding Cases

Statistical software usually offers options to deal with missing data. By clicking on "Options' while performing any statistical test with IBM-SPSS, it offers the option to exclude case analysis by analysis or listwise. The former orders the program to exclude the case with a missing value from this particular analysis, while the latter means that it will be excluded from all analyses.

Expectation-Maximization (EM)

The primary assumption behind EM is that data are missing randomly, and hence, it has to be preceded by a statistically non-significant Little's MCAR test. The EM procedure is a two-step approach: the first is to expect the missing data based on the relations and distribution of available data. The second step is to test the maximum likelihood estimation looking for the model that fits the best. Finally, the filled-in data are saved in a separate data set. Unfortunately, the technique tends to be biased because the error is not added to the newly created data set. Hence, the procedure remains explanatory, and it cannot be used for inferential analysis.

Imputation Methods

In case there is too much data missing, we can use the more advanced techniques of imputations, which places missing values within a reasonable guess based on the distribution and the relationships between the variables in the dataset. It is available for all data, whether they are missing random or non-random. The type of imputation used depends on whether data are missing in a monotone or arbitrary pattern. The procedure runs simulations on patterns on the available data to replace the missing data with data that is most likely similar to the ones available. It is a two-step procedure, the first step is to analyze whether there are patterns of missing data, and the second step is to impute these data [15, 16].

1. *Analysis of Patterns*

The first step is to analyze the patterns of available data. We click on "Analyze," then on 'Multiple Imputations," then on "Analyze Patterns." We select all variables and move them to the "Analyze Across Variables" box. We change the default of "Minimum percentage missing for variable" from 10 to 0.01% to analyze all variables, which is the best choice. The output shows a series of pie charts showing the percentage of missing data in terms of variables, cases, and values. Some researchers may do nothing if the percent of missing values is 5% or smaller. However, we also have to consider the percent of subjects (cases) with missing values. A table will also reveal a list for all variables, with missing percentages, mean, and Sd in descending order. The software output produces the missing chart pattern, and we have to look for whether there is monotonicity, i.e., a rigid pattern of increasing or decreasing sequence. If the figure shows random islands of patterns that are not concentrated in stereotype blocks is a good sign of the absence of a particular pattern. Next, we look at the column chart plotting the various patterns of missing values, including the pattern of no missing value (always coded as 1), versus the percent sum of cases. If the non-missing value column (1) is the highest, it is a good sign.

2. *Imputing Missing Data*

The procedure aims to find the best fitting data by creating multiple iterations based on the distribution and the relationship between observed data. The number of times the software makes those attempts varies from a few to tens or hundreds of times. The researcher has to give the software some instructions by setting the random seed. We go to "Transform" and check on "Random Number Generators" to open a window and select 'Set Active Generator," and choose the radio button "Mersenne Twister". Then, we check on "Set Starting Point" and choose the radio button "Fixed Value" and click on "OK".

We return to the "Analyze" menu, then "Multiple Imputation," then "Impute Missing Data values", which opens a new window. Note that the number of "Imputations" is five by default, which is the number of times the software will produce imputations before taking an average (a pooled) number. We shift the variables with missing values to the "Variables in the Model" box. We click on "create a new dataset" and type a name in the "Data set name".

We click on the "Method" tab and choose the "Automatic" method in which SPSS scans the data and chooses between one of two methods: the Monotone method in case of monotonicity and the Markov chain Monte Carlo method in case of a random pattern. We click on the "Constraints" tab, then the 'Rescan Data" button. The scan results will be shown under the "Variable Summary". We have to go through the minimum and maximum observed data and make sure to have reasonable values, such as minimum and maximum diastolic blood pressure of 60- and 120-mm Hg and. In the case we wish to make changes, we go down and make them in the "Define Covariates" box below. We click on the 'Output" tab and check on the Imputation model", the "Descriptive statistics for variables with imputed values", and "Create iteration history" and type a name for the "Created new dataset". We click on "OK".

The Imputed Data Files

The software ends by producing the final imputation file containing five sets of imputed data, a set of pooled (average) data, and the original data file containing the missing data. The first column in the file allows the researcher to travel through the seven data types. Moreover, each time we request a test, such as the Student test, the software produces seven sets of results. It is the pooled file that we will use at the end. In addition, the researcher can review the iteration history file for documentation.

7.2.4 Normalizing Data

7.2.4.1 Why to Normalize Data?

We need to transform data to enjoy the many advantages of normality, such as the characteristics of the mean and the standard deviation and the intervals of confidence of mean that enables us to assign our results to a group or a population, to compare different groups and to predict future results of comparable studies. Those are three main characteristics descriptive, comparative and predictive values of the 95% CI of the mean of normally distributed data (see Sect. 1.4.2). None of these advantages can be assumed for data following other distribution than normal.

The 95% CI of the difference is the main product of classic meta-analysis. It is calculated for the difference between two normally distributed means or, between the two normalized log values of other indices such as the odds ratio, hazard ratio or relative risk. Moreover, all calculations involving odds ratio in logistic regression and hazard ratio in Cox regression were made possible after normalization of those indices through logarithmic transformation.

The use of powerful parametric tests, such as the test of Student, ANOVA multiple regression and factor analysis necessitates that data are following the normal distribution. However, we should not think about normality as an indispensable necessity. Data following other distributions than normal can be equally described by the median and range and can be compared by non-parametric tests. It is generally known that the loss of information due to ranking increases the risk of type II error of non-parametric tests. However, the associated bias is much more important than analyzing non-parametric data using a parametric test. *In conclusion, data should be normalized when necessary.*

7.2.4.2 Suggested Algorithm

We have previously discussed how to verify normality, whether visually by inspecting a histogram or different plots (see Sect. 1.4.3.1), by calculating skewness and kurtosis (see Sect. 1.4.3.2), or by normality tests, such as the Kolmogorov–Smirnov and the Shapiro–Wilk tests (see Sect. 1.4.3.3). We have equally shown some commonly used simple procedures to normalize data, and, in this section, we will present more variants and practical details.

Check on Normality in Each Group

Normality must be checked out and performed for all categories (classes) of the variable in question and not just the primary variable. For example, if we want to check whether the age is normally distributed among two patient groups, let us say males and females, normality has to be independently checked in each group, whether before or after transformation.

Check on Skewness

Skewness can be checked by statistical software, such as IBM-SPSS, where we can go to "Analyze," then "Descriptive Statistics," then to "Explore". We move the variable in question to the "Dependent List" box, and we click on "Plots" and choose "Histogram". We click on "OK" in the main window. The output shows the test statistics and standard error of Skewness.

Check on Normality

Regardless of the sign, one popular guideline is to accept normality of a particular variable as long as the calculated z values is limited between (+1.96) and (−1.96) (see Sect. 1.4.3.2). The z value is calculated by dividing the test statistics by the standard error, as usual. On the other hand, a test statistic >1 indicates positive or negative skewness, according to the sign. Another way to test skewness is that the test statistic is greater than double the standard error in absolute values.

Positively Skewed Data

Positively skewed data (x) can be normalized by taking the square root of the variable: square root

(x). If moderately skewed, (x) can be normalized by a logarithmic transformation: Log10 (x). In the case of severe Skewness, we can try the reciprocal value (1/x). SPSS can do all three transformations through the "Compute Variable" function. Note that to do log10 (x) transformation, we should not have zero or negative values. In the case of a zero value, a simple remedy is to compute log10 (x + 1), instead of log10 (x). In case of a negative value (e.g., −3), we can add to (x) one plus the value in question, and hence, in our example, we can compute log10 (x + 4). Adding (1) to the zero value or to be on top of the negative value is that the log of (1) is zero; hence, it practically changes nothing to the calculations.

Negatively Skewed Data

Negatively skewed data follow the same procedure of using the square root, then the logarithmic transformation, and finally the reciprocal value in case of highly skewed data. However, we do not make those transformations to the variable (x) itself but its reflection because, as we have just demonstrated, we cannot do log transformation to negative values. The variable reflection (xi) is calculated as $(X + 1 - xi)$, where X is the highest value in the series. For example, if we are trying to normalize the duration of pregnancy and the longest duration is 42 weeks, the transformed value of a patient whose pregnancy duration is 35 weeks = (42 + 1−35 = 8). We calculate the square root of 8 in case the negative skewness was moderate (2.828), log 10 of 8 in case it was strong (0.903), and the reciprocal of 8 in case it was extreme (0.125).

The Two-Step Approach

Data normalization, as described, is not always feasible. Templeton GF suggested a two-step approach to normalize data that is supposed to work well with all continuous variables, regardless of the degree and sign of skewness.

Step One: Statistical Uniformity

The first step involves achieving statistical uniformity by transforming the original variable to a percentile rank score (Pr), as in "Eq. 7.4". For an observation (x_i), the percentile rank is the percent of observations smaller than (x_i).

$$P_r(x_i) = 1 - \left(\frac{rank\, x_i}{n}\right) \qquad (7.4)$$

We were taking the example of a study including 100 patients. If a particular person's age is ranked as being the 30th, his percentile rank = 1 −(30/100) = 0.7, meaning that 70% of the patients in this series are below his age (i.e., younger than him). Note that we are dealing with ranks and not values. Missing data are not allowed, and in case the calculated percentile rank is 0 or 1, it should be replaced by 0.0001 and 0.9999, respectively. In IBM-SPSS, the first part can be achieved by selecting "Transform" and then "Rank Cases," which opens the main window. We move the selected variable to the "Variables box" and keep "the assigned Rank 1" underneath the radio button "Smallest value." We click on the "rank Types" button to open a new window and check on "Fractional rank" only. We click on "Continue" and then on "Ok" in the main window. IBM-SPSS creates the new transformed variable "Pr" in a new column. Statistical uniformity is mandatory to proceed to the second step, and hence, the uniformity of "Pr" must be checked out by the Kolmogorov–Smirnov test (see Sect. 1.4.3.3). In the few times that the test shows a statistically significant result, we should not proceed to step two, and we have to go for a non-parametric analysis [17].

Step Two: Normality

The second step involves the transformation of the (Pr) to normality by calculating its standardized z score. Assuming that the mean and standard deviation of the standard normal distribution are 0 and 1, the Z score of a particular (Pr) value is calculated from the inverse error function (erf^{-1}), as in "Eq. 7.5" [17].

$$Z = \sqrt{2} \times erf^{-1}(-1 + 2P_r) \qquad (7.5)$$

In IBM-SPSS, the second step can be achieved by clicking on "Transform" and then "Compute Variable", which opens the main window. We give a name for the "Target Variable," and then we choose "Inverse DF" from the "Function group", "Idf.Normal" from the "Functions and Special Variables," and we click on the "ascending arrow" to shift the formula to the "Numeric Expression". The formula is IDF. NORMAL(?,?,?). The three interrogation marks are then replaced by the name of the uniform variable, 0 and 1, respectively. By clicking "Ok" in the main window, IBM-SPSS creates the corresponding Z scores in a new column. Personally, every time we tried this two-step approach, it worked well, provided that the variable was continuous, with no missing values.

The procedure is not indicated for coded categorical variables, discrete numerical values of a limited number of levels, such as the 5-point or the 7-point Likert scales, and data showing many influential meaningless mode values, such as zero values in count variables. The author provided a detailed example of how to use the method in excel, SPSS, and SAS [17].

7.3 Tools of the Analysis

7.3.1 The Statistical Software

7.3.1.1 Choose a Statistical Software Program

There is free statistical software, while others offer their services for a charge, which is sometimes beyond the reach of a sector of our target audience. We can usually get around purchasing the (best) paid software by using several free programs that can complement one another to achieve a specific target. An example in this book is when we used Jamovi [18], JASP [19], and OpenMetaAnalyst [20] to perform meta-analysis, which could not be analyzed by our 24th version of IBM-SPSS software (see Chap. 6). Although each one of those programs can execute the basic meta-analysis procedure, none offers the full range of advanced tests or the optimum presentation modalities. JAMOVI and JASP are continuously updating, while the limited financial resources may slow down the development of others and can end their technical support. The OpenMetaAnalyst is a good example. Another example is the excellent G*Power [21] free software that we used for sample size calculation and power analysis. G*power has to be complemented by several free-online calculators to cover a few missing tasks (see Chap. 4).

The (paid) IBM-SPSS was our general use software of choice for the last 15 years, and we used it to execute the remaining bivariate and multivariable analysis (Chaps. 2 and 3). Jamovi [18] and JASP [19] are free alternatives for SPSS users. They share the same interface, and their new versions can execute a good part of the analyses performed by the paid version. Both programs are based on powerful R software, without the need for any background knowledge of R programming.

The main question is, why not use the powerful free, open-source R itself? The answer is straightforward: R can execute all the statistical tests described in this book and much more [22], and it is the perfect solution for students and young researchers. However, unlike the other tests, R is not a plug-and-play program, and hence, it may not suit the busy clinician who usually cannot manage a space in his tight schedule to learn the basic programing language.

7.3.1.2 The Software Does not Ensure the Results' Validity

The statistical software is supposed to use the best method for data analysis. However, the software cannot check whether patients were randomized between treatment groups or they were forced inside those groups by the sole will of the principal investigator. It cannot ensure the correctness of data, that data were collected in the appropriate timing and by the appropriate person. In general, the software will always execute the statistical test as long as we upload the required data, regardless of data is correct or not. *What many of us do not know, and as long as there is no missing data, the software may execute many tests despite of the conditions of application being fulfilled or not; which is a major source of bias for the unexperienced researcher.*

Taking the example of testing the significance of the association of two qualitative variables. In order to apply the Chi-square test, Cochrane have suggested that the expected counts in all cells (or at least 80%) have to be equal or larger than 5 and none is below 1 (see Sect. 2.3.1.2). A naïve researcher would expect that the software will not execute the command if this main condition was not fulfilled, which is not true. IBM-SPSS and other software will execute the command, regardless of the expected values and even if one cell is empty. The legend of the output table will include the following statement: an (x) proportion of cells have expected values smaller than 5. What does this mean? It means that if this proportion is large, let us say 50 or 75%, the results of the test are questionable and, for many researchers, they are not valid. Why did the software execute the command, simply because it was ordered? *The software will execute a given order as long as there are data, regardless of their validity!* The use of such theoretically non-valid results is left to the researcher's own evaluation. Interestingly, some online calculators deny the calculation of a Chi-square test, in case one of the cells is left empty [10]. In conclusion, we have to check for the validity of data ourselves, the software may help on this but will not ensure validity.

7.3.1.3 There Are Many Faces of Reality

The value of the statistical analysis is not measured by the amount of the reported results but by the few ones that we clearly understand, and hence, we can defend. Even in the case of a simple, straightforward bivariate analysis, the statistical software is expected to perform two main procedures: it verifies the conditions of application of the test, and it executes the analysis. We have shown that many times, the software carries both procedures independently. In other words, verifying the application conditions is not always a pre-requisite for the execution of the analysis itself (see Sect. 7.3.1.2). It is up to the researcher to judge which unverified assumption he can accept and which he cannot? On the other hand, we have to admit that many statistical tests can be seen as a pair of sockets that can fit many people of comparable size rather than being a pair of shoes that can fit one size only. Put it in better words, *many statistical tests are robust and can be executed even if the conditions of application are not 100% verified.*

Choosing One Out of Many Valid Results

The software can produce multiple results for the same analysis, which may confuse the young researcher. The multiple results are sometimes due to the fact that there is no single efficient answer to the posed questions and hence, statisticians have produced many alternatives responding to the same need. For example, in logistic regression, residuals cannot be calculated, and hence, a "true" R^2 cannot be computed. Statisticians have invented multiple pseudo-R-squared coefficients to assess how much the variables explain the model, such as Cox and Snell's R^2, Negelkerke's R^2, and McFadden's pseudo R^2. The researcher is free to use and present one of those alternatives, provided that he knows the advantages, limitations, and what a particular alternative means (see Sect. 3.5.1).

Choosing One Out of Different Results

On the other hand, the production of multiple results does not always mean that they are multiple alternatives, but each indicates a special situation or condition, and the researcher has to pick only one from those multiple results. For example, in the case the conditions of application of the Chi-square test were not fulfilled, Yate proposed a correction or some penalty to compensate for the non-fulfilment of those conditions. The penalty is simple and involves the reduction of the test statistics (Chi-square value) by subtracting 0.5 from each cell, provided that the expected value is between 3 and 5 and that both variables are binomial (see Sect. 2.3.1.3). In the case of two binomial variables but with expected values of 2 or smaller, a valid alternative is Fisher's exact test (see Sect. 2.3.1.5). When we request a Chi-square test with two binomial variables, IBM-SPSS software will automatically execute both: the Chi-square test and Fisher's exact test; hence, the researcher will have to choose between both results. In addition, whenever the expected values are between 3 and 5, the software will equally execute the corrected test of Yate, and the researcher will have to choose between the three alternatives. *The condition can be seen like dining in a restaurant, and the waiter presents the menu card, unfortunately without the "plat du jour"; which is the recommended dish (result) for today (your study).*

The results given by Fisher's exact test were found to be more concordant with those given by Pearson's Chi-square compared to the corrected Chi-square test. It is always advisable to use Fisher's exact test when the results of the corrected Chi-square test are borderline. Finally, the difficulty of calculating the test by hand was removed by the development and availability of hand calculators and statistical software packages, which paved the way to replace the corrected Chi-square test practically.

Another typical example is the software output of the results of comparing two means by the unpaired Student t-test. The simple equation of Student is based on the assumption that there is no statistically significant difference between the variances of the two groups, which Levene's test must primarily test. In other words, we have to have a statistically non-significant Levene's test to apply a test of Student. In the case where both variances are significantly different, we cannot calculate a pooled common variance, and we have to use the larger variance of the difference. The latter gives a smaller t-value, a wider interval of confidence, and smaller chances of achieving statistical significance (see Sect. 2.4.1.2). Like in the case of the Chi-square test, the software produces both results, regardless of whether Levene's test was statistically significant or non-significant. In the latter case, the researcher has to pick up the results of the regular student test, while in the latter case, he has to discard those results and adopt the results of the modified test. The software identifies the former as being the results calculated under the assumption of the equality of variances and the latter as being those calculated without this assumption (see Table 2.14).

7.3.1.4 A Bird in the Hand is Worth Two in the Bush

Many research works are simple, and the young researcher should not complicate them by being tempted to use the sophisticated tests provided by the powerful statistical software. Methods are simple when they are based on one or two assumptions, and a common example is the bivariate statistical analysis, such as the Chi-square tests, Students' tests, and Pearson's correlation. Assumptions are not only few, but they can be easily verified by all parties; the researcher, the reviewers, and the readers. For example, the main condition of application of a Chi-square test of independence is a minimum expected value of 5 in 80% of the cells, which can sometimes be verified by reporting the results as numbers and percentages. Let us take one example: "There were 20 cases (50%) of success in the treatment group compared to only four cases (10%) in the control group". The conditions of application and the results of the test were summarized in one phrase. The reader can easily deduce that the total number of cases was 80, equally distributed between the treatment and control groups. The total number of successes and failures were 24 and 56, and, as both groups are equal, the expected values of success and failures are 12 and 28 in each group, and no empty cells, which verify the conditions of application of the test.

The more we develop the analysis, such as introducing a third variable, the more we have to increase the number of posed assumptions and, from the young researcher's point of view, the complexity of verification. *The researcher may reach a point where he does not understand how the analysis is produced, but still, the results are tempting, and the promises are appealing.* The serious researcher has to stop well before reaching this point. We have to be cautious when moving from simple, straightforward bivariate analysis to more complicated tests such as

repeated measures analysis, high-way ANOVA, ANCOVA, and multivariable or multivariate analysis.

An Example: The Logistic Regression Analysis

For example, we do not advise the young researcher to go for multivariable model such as logistic regression when it is not needed or whenever the conditions necessary for its application are not verified. Discussing those conditions before the study with the statistician is always a helpful first step.

Four conditions must be verified before and during the study preparation (see Sect. 3.5.2.1). The second step is to understand what we expect from the software? We expect to verify other assumptions such as linearity between the quantitative predictor and the logit of the outcome (see Sect. 3.5.2.2), the absence of multicollinearity between predictors themselves (see Sect. 3.5.2.3), and the absence of outliers, high leverage, and influential points (see Sect. 3.5.2.4). The researcher has to understand why we have to investigate those points and which part of the software outputs verifies a particular point or a specific assumption. Otherwise, the researcher will not be able to answer to editors, evaluation committees, or reviewers (see Sect. 3.5.5).

The third step is to evaluate the overall model fit (H–L test) and significance (Omnibus test for model coefficients) and the detailed model summary (see Sect. 3.5.6.1). Unless the researcher knows the meaning of the regression coefficients, he will not be able to create a comprehensive discussion. Each unit change in the odds of the predictor changes the outcome by an amount equivalent to the odds ratio of the predictor (see Sect. 3.5.6.2). He must know how to convert the odds to probabilities to simplify his conclusion and to compare his results with his peers when needed (see Sect. 1.8.1). Finally, the researcher is expected to appreciate the points of strength and limitations of his study and how to interpret those points in clear clinical and correct statistical terms. There are much more advanced tests than those explained in this book, and we do not promote against using those tests. On the contrary, we remind our readers and ourselves that *we have to follow the Hippocratic oath of applying (correct) measures according to our ability (limits) and avoiding harm (bias).*

7.3.2 The Complementary Online Calculators

The use of online calculators is a great facility. It allows the researcher to perform what he may consider a difficult task with a simple button push and, most importantly, free of charge. The number of scientific, mathematical, and statistical calculators is more than we can count, and the main question is always: which one to choose? To answer this question, we must know that many calculators are usually based on the same statistical equations; hence, they are expected to produce the same results. As in any business, some providers are serious, and others are not. A trustworthy online calculator must indicate the supporting persons, group, company, or organization, the equations used, and the relevant references. In return, the users must check on all those elements and indicate when the calculator was last assessed online.

7.3.2.1 Check on the Equations and the References' Validity

Before using an online calculator, the researcher has to check that the used equations are cited, and the references are valid, which necessitates familiarity with those equations. If the researcher cannot check by himself, he can seek help from a more experienced colleague or consult one of the many research communities, such as the research gate network. We primarily recommend the online calculators offered by universities, academic sites, and large organizations, whether for sample size calculation [23–25] or for the commonly used statistical tests and indices of clinical outcomes [10, 26, 27]. The reader is requested to review the specific chapter to view our suggested online calculators.

7.3.2.2 Cross-Examine the Results

We have to cross-examine the results of a new calculator with those produced by a trusted one or reliable software. For example, in one study, the incidence of bronchogenic carcinoma among smokers versus non-smokers was 10 versus 3%. The sample size required to put into evidence the carcinogenic effect of smoking using any of the previously verified online calculators was: 153 patients [23], 151 patients [25], and 153 patients per group [4]. Note that the slight differences of 1–2% are due to either an approximative or more exact formula for calculation or due to the rounding of figures, which is why we have to report or refer to those formulas. Still, the calculators produce nearly the same numbers when calculating the sample size per group in the case of a unilateral study.

7.3.2.3 Understand the Equation's Elements

One disadvantage of online calculators is the deficiency of documentation and publications compared to the "classical" statistical software program. Consequently, the researcher sometimes needs a fair statistical background to properly use the calculators.

First Example

We will continue using the same example to show the difference between how different calculators expressed the same element. The equation used to calculate sample size is formed of five basic elements: the primary (α) and the secondary risks of error (β), the target difference that we wish to put into evidence (δ), the outcome variability (Sd) and the direction of the study, whether being bilateral (e.g., comparing two treatments) or unilateral study (e.g., comparing a treatment to a placebo). As shown in "Eq. 7.6", four out of the five elements have symbols (α, β, δ, and Sd), while the direction of the study is not usually symbolized, and the question is why?

$$n_{unilateral} = \frac{2\left[Z_{(1-\alpha)} + Z_{(1-\beta)}\right]^2}{\left(\frac{\delta}{Sd}\right)^2} \qquad (7.6)$$

The answer is simple because this element is not independently calculated as the other four elements, but it is computed from the primary risk of error chosen by the investigator. Let us give more light on this relation. A unilateral study supposes that we are looking for the effect of the treatment (or the risk factor) but not the effect of the placebo (or the absence of the risk factor). Consequently, the whole primary risk of error (the whole α) is confined to the only possible conclusion: treatment is better than placebo (see Sects. 1.5.1 and 4.1.2.1). Compare "Eqs. 7.6" with "7.7" shown below, which is used to calculate the sample size in the case the study was bilateral. The only difference is that (α) used in the former is replaced by (α/2) in the latter. Put it this way; a unilateral study concentrates the whole risk of error ($α = 2 \times α/2$) on the only possible side where it can be committed, i.e., when we conclude that treatment is better than placebo. On the other hand, the bilateral study is designed to reach one out of two possible conclusions and, as it can never reach both conclusions, it can only commit risk of (α/2) (see Sects. 1.7.2 and 1.7.3).

$$n_{bilateral} = \frac{2\left[Z_{(1-\alpha/2)} + Z_{(1-\beta)}\right]^2}{\left(\frac{\delta}{Sd}\right)^2} \qquad (7.7)$$

The universal total primary risk of error of any study (α) is 5% and some calculators will ask the researcher to specify the direction of the study, whether being unilateral or bilateral and then execute "Eq. 7.6" in the first case and "Eq. 7.7" in the second case. The examples are G*power software [21], Epitools epidemiological calculators [24] and the online calculator created by Hylown Consulting Atlanta, GA [25]. Other calculators, such as the sample size calculator offered by the (UCSF) [23], do not pose the question. However, they indicate that the value assigned for (α) is that of a bilateral study, and hence, it is up to the researcher to manually change this value from the usual 0.05 to 0.1 to accommodate for the unilateral design. Note that this does not mean we change the universal primary risk of error from 5 to 10%. The calculator

uses (α/2) in the equation, regardless of the study design. On the other hand, we need to use (α) because our design is unilateral. Consequently, the solution is to provide those calculators by (2α), in case of a unilateral study. Not understanding the direct relation between (α) and the direction of the study may be misinterpreted by the researcher that the calculator gives a different or false result.

Second Example

Some online calculators may give more than one answer (result) for the same question. Although the same situation is observed with the classical software program, the condition is more confusing due to the poor documentation and scarcity of applied publications on many calculators. Take the example of studying the effect of smoking on the development of bronchogenic carcinoma (see Sect.4.3.2.1). The online calculator "sample size net" gives two different results: 153 patients per group (without continuity correction) and a larger sample size of 183 patients per group (with continuity correction) [23]. The researcher has to know the difference between the two results and choose what is best for his study.

In short, and unlike the continuous variable, the binomial variable has no true mean or a true standard error. Hence, we cannot make the usual 95% confidence interval. For example, we can describe the mean age of a group of patients, but what is their mean gender? To calculate a mean, a standard deviation, and a confidence interval for a binomial variable, the statisticians assigned the numbers 0 and 1 to the two classes of the variable. We do not need to know the details of the calculation [28], but we need to know that any approximation necessitates some assumptions, which is, in our case, a sufficiently large sample (see Sects. 1.4.2.4 and 4.3.2.1).

A correction was then made afterward to compensate for the small sample: the continuity correction. The rule is that the smallest np or n (p − 1) should be at least 5. In our example, n (the calculated sample size without the continuity correction = 153) and p is 10% (proportion of patients with carcinoma) and 1 − p is 3%

(proportion of patients without carcinoma); hence, the smallest = 153 × 3% = 4.56, which is smaller than the limit (5). Consequently, it is safer to use the continuity correction (183 patients per group), which is the same result given by the dedicated software G*power (see Sect. 4.3.2.1) [21]. In short, *unless we know what we are looking for, the information produced by online calculators and software can become a source of confusion and bias instead of being an element of precision and correctness*. In conclusion, extra care should be given when consulting an online calculator more than a documented statistical software.

7.3.2.4 Verify the Conditions of Application

As with statistical software, the online calculator cannot check for necessary corners of validity of the results, such as randomization and data correctness, which were collected at the appropriate timing and by the appropriate person. Unlike a statistical software program, many online calculators execute the test without reporting whether the specific conditions of applications were verified or not.

First Example

For example, 20 patients were randomized between two equal groups, one receiving treatment A and the other receiving treatment B. The study showed six successes with treatment A (60%) and only a single case of success with treatment B (10%). Uploading the results to an online calculator, it executes a Chi-square test and produces a statistically significant Chi-square value of 5.49; P = 0.019 [10]. In this example, the conditions of applications of the test are not verified as 2 out of the four expected values (50%) are below 5, but the software did not report this critical information. Another online calculator equally executes the test producing a Chi-square value of 5.22 and a P value of 0.022, without apparent verification of the conditions of applications of the test [27]. Uploading the same data on a classic software package would also execute the non-verified Chi-square test.

However, it will report that 50% of the cells have expected values below 5 (Chi-square = 5.49; P = 0.019). Moreover, it will execute the corrected Chi-square test (Chi-square = 3.51; P = 0.061) and Fisher's exact test (P = 0.057) without being asked to do so. The researcher will now have the opportunity to report the correct answer, the one given by Fisher exact.

Second Example

Equally, the same online calculator can execute an unpaired t-test to compare the means of two samples. However, unlike the classic software, the calculator will not check on the assumption of variance equality by Levene's test, and it will produce only one result based on such an unchecked assumption [10]. Another calculator does not test the equality of variances, producing a single t-value based upon variances being equal [27]. In conclusion, many quick online calculators do not verify the assumptions behind statistical tests, and the researcher has to verify their limits and capabilities more cautiously than in the case of a "classical" statistical software.

Third Example

We can execute One-way ANOVA online [10]. However, the calculator will not offer the many facilities produced by the classic statistical software, such as testing the homogeneity of variances, making a priori contrasts, choosing from a complete armada of post-hoc tests, and offering other variants of ANOVA such as the Welch test and the Brown-Forsythe test and the creation of valuable plots. The output of online calculators is much reduced, compared to statistical software package.

> When consulting an online calculator, the researcher must know what he is looking for and verify the validity of the assumptions and the results. The calculators save us the effort of computation but not evaluation or decision making. We recommend their use in cases where statistical software is deficient.

7.4 Data Reporting in a Manuscript

Forty years ago, listening to a particular musical record had to be well planned. It started with taking time off, traveling downtown, visiting multiple record shops, and, if we were lucky, finding the record hours after searching before making a long trip back home. It took 3–6 weeks in Egypt to receive a requested research paper by express mail through the National Academy of Science. In France, I was amazed by the service of Monsieur Benoit, the librarian of Charles Nichole hospital in Rouen, who managed to get me the manuscripts in two days. Today, we can listen to a record or read a research paper instantaneously, and we can pay online and download it in no time, whenever we need to, any part of day or night. Our wise old consultants are now replaced by substantial, powerful servers working 24/7.

In those days, it was hard to find a written statistical program that could make a complete analysis; results were few, and outputs were poor. The problem now is the overwhelming results generated by the easily available software programs, which often surpass the lay physician and young researcher's limited statistical knowledge. The main concern has changed from finding the information to passing by the useful one among the hundreds provided or reporting statistical results we do not understand. Our advice is to know what we are looking for and report what our peers and reviewers need, provided that we clearly understand and can defend. We encourage the reader to review the guidelines for reporting his study type, and a starting place to look for is the equator website [29]. Once a journal has been chosen, the second landing zone must be the journal's guidelines to authors. In this section, we will go through the main sections of the research work and highlight a few missing points, pitfalls, and common errors in the reported statistical information.

7.4.1 The Introduction

Although the introduction is usually summarized in a few lines, it must point to what is expected to be new in the actual study, based upon previous research findings, all being backed up with numbers, percentages, 95% CIs, and P-values. Unfortunately, many publications usually report a P-value but miss the more meaningful information, which is the 95% CI. In the case of a quantitative outcome, we can easily calculate the confidence interval of one group (see Sect. 1.4.2.2) or the confidence interval of the difference between two groups from the reported means and standard deviations (see Sect. 1.4.2.6). In the case of a qualitative outcome, we can calculate the respective intervals either by hand or by using one of the many available online calculators (see Sect. 1.4.2.7).

Altman and Bland provided simplified equations to calculate the 95% CI of the difference or a proportion from the reported P-value themselves [30] and vice versa [31]. The calculations are based upon the basic formula of standardizing an estimate (Est), whether being a difference (d) or a ratio (r), by dividing the estimate by its standard error, as shown in the "Eq. 7.8".

$$Z = \frac{Est}{Se} = \frac{d}{Se} = \frac{r}{Se} \tag{7.8}$$

Let us take the example of a study that was carried out on two groups of patients with mechanical cardiac valve prostheses. Patients followed one of two regimens: either standard oral anticoagulation (OA) or low-level anticoagulation combined with low-dose antiplatelet therapy (OA + AP). The researchers wish to show which of the two regimens offers the lowest oral anticoagulant-related complications. Previous reports showed that the overall complication rates with the regimen (OA) and (OA + AP) were 9.2% and 2.6%, respectively (P = 0.0044) [32].

Calculation of the 95% CI from a P Value

We will begin by showing how a P-value is calculated? In the usual order of calculations, we start by computing the difference between the two proportions (d), the standard error for the difference (Se), then we divide the difference (d) by the Se to get the standardized difference, which is the Z value. Finally, we check the probability of (z) in the Z table, which is the P-value. What is suggested by Altman and Bland is just to go retrograde by calculating the (z) value from the reported (P-value), as shown in "Eqs. 7.9" and "7.10" The next step is to calculate the Se from the (z) value "Eq. 7.11". Finally, we multiply the Se by (1.96) and place this quantity on either side of the difference to get the 95% CI interval of the difference "Eq. 7.12" [30].

$$Z = -0.862 + \sqrt{\lfloor 0.743 - 2.404 \times \log P_{value} \rfloor} \tag{7.9}$$

$$Z = -0.862 + \sqrt{\lfloor 0.743 - 2.404 \times \log(0.0044) \rfloor} = 2.85 \tag{7.10}$$

$$Se = \frac{d}{Z} = \frac{6.6}{2.85} = 2.315 \tag{7.11}$$

$$95\ CI\ (d) = d \pm 1.96\ Se = 6.6 \pm 1.96\ (2.315)$$
$$= 2.1\% \text{ to } 11.14\%$$
$$\tag{7.12}$$

The same study reported a relative risk reduction of 0.72; P = 0.005. Suppose that we wish to calculate the relative risk and its 95% confidence interval ourselves. We will proceed exactly the same as suggested by Altman and Bland, but we have to remember that the ratio measures, such as relative risk, hazard ratio, and odds ratio, have to be log-transformed first before calculation (see Sect. 1.8.7). In our example, the relative risk = 1- relative risk reduction = 0.28 and its log value = (−1.273). We will apply the same sequence of equations as before. We calculate (z) "Eq. 7.13", then the Se from the ratio (r) "Eq. 7.14". We calculate the 95% CI of the ratio in the log scale "Eq. 7.15", then we back

transform its upper and lower limits into the usual scale "Eq. 7.16". The equation uses the Z value, and hence, they suppose that the sample size is large. Altman and Bland discouraged their use in small samples or whenever a t-test or analysis of variance is used and in case of non-significant P-value [30]. The authors equally provided simple equations to calculate the P-value of a reported 95% CI in another interesting research paper [31].

$$Z = -0.862 + \sqrt{\lfloor 0.743 - 2.404 \times \log(0.005) = 2.81 \rfloor} \tag{7.13}$$

$$Se = \frac{r}{Z} = \frac{-1.273}{2.81} = 0.45 \tag{7.14}$$

$$95\% \text{ CI} \log RR = \log RR \pm 1.96\ (Se)$$
$$= -1.273 \pm 1.96(0.45)$$
$$= -0.38 \text{ to } -2.16$$
$$\tag{7.15}$$

$$\text{RR (95\% CI)} = 0.28(0.11 \text{ to } 0.69) \tag{7.16}$$

7.4.2   The Material and Methods

The material and methods section describes how the study was done so that readers and reviewers can judge the validity of the results while other researchers can repeat the study. The material and methods usually end with the statistical analysis section, which should clearly describe how the study was analyzed descriptively and inferentially.

7.4.2.1   Study Design

The researcher has to specify the study design as a regular superiority, a non-inferiority, or an equivalence study. In the case of a non-inferiority or equivalence study, the researcher has to define the non-inferiority or equivalence margin based upon clinical and statistical evidence with selected references (see Sect. 5.3.4). The researcher has to define whether a superiority study will be bilateral (see Sect. 1.7.3), comparing two treatments, or unilateral, comparing a treatment to a placebo or a standard care therapy (see Sect. 1.7.2). If the control group of a unilateral study is another treatment, the researcher has to justify his choice with selected references. Although many superiority trials have a parallel-group design in which treatment and control are allocated to different individuals, variability can be reduced by the patient serving as his own control or by a matched design. In case of parallel groups, we have to define the number of groups and the number of comparisons made.

7.4.2.2 Population of the Analysis

We have previously shown the three classic populations of the analysis: the intention to treat population, the modified intention to treat and the per-protocol analysis (see Sect. 5.8.1). In brief, most randomized clinical trials follow an intention to treat analysis [8]. The modified intention to treat is criticized for being subjective in removing subgroups of patients. Per-protocol analysis is mainly adopted in the case where the researcher is interested in analyzing treatment-related complications [8] and is recommended in non-inferiority studies, in addition to an intention to treat analysis [33]. Comparing both intention-to-treat and per-protocol strategies is a sensitivity analysis aiming to test the robustness of the results. Regardless of the adopted analysis, the researcher has to report the detailed method, proportions of adherence in both groups, reasons behind deviations, and management strategy. It may be sufficient to report a small percentage (<10%) of overall deviations that are equally distributed between groups; otherwise, its statistical significance must be formally tested.

7.4.2.3 Type of the Analysis

The researchers have to define the type of analysis, whether a single analysis, an analysis adjusted on a factor (subgroup analysis) or covariate, analysis of repeated measures, sequential analysis, or a cluster design. The researcher must be aware of the advantages and possible sources of bias behind each type.

Subgroup Analysis

Unless A priori contrasts were pre-planned before the study, subgroup analysis might become problematic for being underpowered, especially when subgroups are based on variables measured after randomization [34]. The reader is invited to revise the measures of setting a priori contrasts or running a posteriori contrast (post hoc analysis) to control such bias (see Sect. 2.4.3.3).

Adjusted Analysis

An adjusted analysis is sometimes indicated to account for imbalances between study groups or accounts for a known prognostic variable (see Sect. 2.9). The main analysis should be identified when both unadjusted and adjusted analyses are intended. As with subgroup analyses, adjustment variables based on post-randomization data rather than baseline data can be a significant source of bias [35].

Analysis of Repeated Measures

In studies where there are repeated observations done on the same person, whether on different parts of the individual or the same part but repeated over time—sometimes we forget that the individual—and not the parts—is still the unit of analysis [36]. Doing so will lead to two main statistical errors. The violation of the widespread assumption that data should be independent. In other words, as if the two groups of data were taken from two independent groups of persons and not from a single group of persons. The second is sample inflation, like analyzing blood pressure measurement from the two arms of a single patient as being two observations, which may lead to spurious statistical significance [36]. In well-designed studies, the repeated measure ANOVA considers the multiplicity and is provided by most statistical software (see Sects. 2.4.3.4 and 3.2.5.1).

Sequential Analysis

Sequential analysis is indicated whenever the studied disease is rare, e.g., cancer gall bladder. It consists of grouping patients in pairs; each patient receives one of the designed treatments. The difference between treatments (e.g., days of survival) obtained in each pair is cumulated on the following one till a statistically significant result is obtained, and the study can be stopped [37].

Cluster Analysis

Patients may be distributed to either treatments or procedures as groups or clusters. For example, patients can be randomized according to their management hospitals. The unit is no more the individual patient but the group of patients receiving treatment in a particular hospital. Variability will not only be between different hospitals (between clusters) but also between the patients within the same hospital (within the cluster). The intra-cluster correlation coefficient (ricc) can summarize the relationship between the two variance components and express the design effect. Another way to express effect size is by the design effect (N/n), which is the proportion between the always larger sample size calculated in the case of clusters (N) and "regular" sample size (n) (see Sect. 4.3.1.7).

7.4.2.4 Patients' Description, Treatment Allocation and Follow-Up

The researchers must provide a complete description of the population and the sample with inclusion criteria and detailed reasons for exclusion. In case of randomization, the practical steps should be described together with the logistics taken to ensure allocation concealment [38]. In case of follow-up, we have to report our attitude in managing patients who will be lost to follow-up, those who discontinued treatment, withdraw from the study, or cross-over. Would we plan for changes in the allocations, such as by adding, dropping, or combining treatment arms? We may consider downloading a patient flow-chart template, which is mandatory in clinical trials [39] and helpful in large studies.

7.4.2.5 The Statistical Analysis Section

Descriptive Statistics

The statistical analysis should include a summary of how the variables are described. The researchers have to define which of the following common indices has been used in the study.

Numbers and Percentages, Mean and Standard Deviation, Median and Range

Qualitative data are usually described as numbers and percentages, while the description of quantitative variables depends on the variable distribution. The mean and the standard deviation fully describe a normally distributed variable, but they lose their preferential properties in case of variables following other distributions than normal. The mean is no more in the center of the values nor represents their mode, and the standard distribution does not include the same stereotypic number of cases on either side of the mean as in the normal distribution. In quantitative variables following other distributions than normal, the median is a better indicator of the central tendency of the sample, and the dispersion can be reported as the minimum and the maximum or better as the interquartile range (see Sect. 1.3).

The Interval of Confidence at 95%

Reporting the 95% CI of all variables is a must in all randomized controlled studies and in meta-analyses. We encourage reporting the 95% confidence intervals of all variables for their descriptive, predictive, and comparative values (see Sect. 1.4.2). The 95% confidence interval opens a window for the reader "to see", rather than "to imagine", the limits of those values. For example, instead of reporting the patients' mean age and standard deviation as 56 ± 2 years and leaving for the reader the calculation of the upper and lower age limits, we uncover those limits for him by coupling the 95% CI to the mean and the standard deviation: 56 ± 2 (52.8–59.9) years. The upper and lower limits of the 95% CI can be separated by the word "to" (52.8–59.9), by a comma (52.8, 59.9), or by a dash (52.8–59.9), according to the publication type and venue. We discourage the latter form to avoid any confusion when the upper limit is negative. We compute the 95% CI with a z value of 1.96. In the case of a different level of confidence, we compute the 90% CI with a (z) value of 1.65 and the 99% CI with a (z) value of 2.6 (see Sect. 1.4.2). In the case of a small sample, the (z) value is substituted with the t-value at the corresponding df (see Sect. 1.4.2.3).

The Odds, Risk, Hazard and Number Needed to Treat

The researchers can use other indices to describe the relationship between the variables, such as the role of a risk factor in epidemiological studies or the treatment effect in the clinical setting. Among the commonly used indices there is the odds ratio (OR), the relative risk (RR), the number needed to treat (NNT), and the hazard ratio (HR) in case of time-to-event analysis. The risk is the probability of developing the event, while the odds is the proportion between those who developed the event and those who did not. The hazard is the instantaneous risk at a specific time, provided that the patient did not experience the event before that time. The odds ratio (OR), the relative risk (RR), and the hazard ratio (HR) are the odds, the risk, and the hazard in the treatment group to their equivalent values in the control group (see Sect. 1.8). A ratio of (1) means no effect, a ratio (<1) means a negative effect, and a ratio (>1) means a positive effect in the treatment group (group at risk) compared to the control. The researchers choose the indices that describe the relationship between the studied variables, according to the type of the study.

All indices must be reported with the corresponding 95% CI and tested statistically by the usual Z test (see Sect. 1.8.7). The number needed to treat (NNT) is the number of patients we have to treat to prevent one event; hence, it is a significant number for decision-makers (see Sect. 1.8.6). Remember that the NNT and the lower and upper limits of its 95% CI are computed as the reciprocal values of the absolute risk reduction (see Sect. 1.8.7.4). The strength of the OR, RR, HR, and NNT is that they are unaffected by the changes in the baseline references (i.e., the Prevalence), and hence, they are portable.

The Sensitivity, Specificity, Area Under the ROC and Diagnostic Odds Ratio (DOR)

The sensitivity (Sn) describes how many times a test is truly positive when the patient has the disease, while the specificity (Sp) is how many times the test is truly negative when the patient does not have the disease. Graphing all available Sn/Sp pairs through continuously varying the decision threshold over the entire range of observed results is a measure of the overall performance of the test: the area under the ROC. Besides choosing the best Se and Sp thresholds and evaluating the overall discriminative power of the test, we can use ROC plots to compare different tests, different groups of patients, or different observers within studies. Sensitivity and specificity are reported as percentages, and the AUC of a ROC plot is reported in decimals, together with their corresponding 95% CI. Those three discriminative measures are independent of the Prevalence, and hence, they are portable too (see Sects 1.9.1 and 1.9.4).

The Positive and Negative Predictive Values and Likelihood Ratios

The positive predictive value (PPV) and negative predictive values (NPV) provide the patient with the information he needs to know. In short, how many times is he expected to have the disease if the test is positive, and how many times is he expected to be disease-free if the test is negative. Both indices must be reported in percentage with the corresponding 95% CI. The likelihood ratio (LR) provides the doctor with the information he needs. They summarize how many times more (or less) likely patients with the disease are to develop an event or have a particular test result than patients without the disease. A high positive LR > 10 usually rules in the diagnosis, and a negative LR < 0.1 rules out the disease. *Researchers must report Prevalence alongside to be considered in any comparison.* (see Sect. 1.9.2 and 1.9.3).

The Direction of the Study

It must indicate the direction of the study: for example, the study was bilateral comparing treatment A to treatment B, or unilateral comparing treatment A to placebo or standard care therapy. The use of another treatment as a control in a unilateral study has to be justified with references.

Inferential Statistics

Bivariate Analysis

Bivariate analysis tests the statistical significance of the relation between two variables, assuming that other variables are stationary or equally distributed among compared groups. Choosing the appropriate bivariate statistical test is dependent upon many factors, including the study's main hypothesis, study design, and data [40]. Table 2.35 and Fig. 2.15 show the algorithm for choosing a bivariate statistical test in the case of independent groups (see Sect. 2.8.2). Figure 2.16 shows the most commonly used test for a paired design (see Sect. 2.8.3). *Tests or graphs used to check on normality, such as the Shapiro–Wilk test, should be specified, especially in the case of small studies.* Multiple tests are available to compare survival curves. The researcher has to choose the test that best fits the data regarding group size and equality, length of the follow-up period, and possible fluctuation of proportionality of hazard (see Sect. 2.7.4).

Common malpractice is a prêt-a-porter recipe enumerating all the parametric and non-parametric tests used in the study without specifying which test is used to analyze which variable? The same applies to prognostic studies adjusting on bivariate analysis. The researcher has to indicate which test was primarily used to exclude reverse interaction, such as the Z test for a two-class adjustment variable or the Berslow-Day and Tirone tests in case of multiple classes. We have to verify the conditions of applying the tests used for adjustment, whether the Cochran-Mantel–Haenszel test or the Mantel–Haenszel odds or risk ratios, two-way ANOVA, or partial correlation (See Sect. 2.9). *In studies measuring agreement and testing reliability, the researcher has to present the plan of the analysis.* It starts by defining the study material, predictors, and outcome, overruling a systematic bias by the appropriate statistical test. The plan ends by measuring the agreement itself, testing its statistical significance, and interpreting and reporting the findings (see Table 2.41). The researcher has to define which test was used to eliminate a systematic bias (see Sect. 2.10.2.2) and which

test was used to measure agreement. (see Sect. 2.10.2.3).

Multivariable Analysis

Suppose the bivariate analysis has shown that multiple variables are significantly related to the outcome. In that case, the researcher may wish to know how much the set of those variables can explain or predict the outcome? A multivariable model can also test the significance of the contribution of each variable on the outcome, adjusted for the presence of other variables. We have reviewed three commonly used models: logistic regression, multiple regression, and Cox regression analysis. The researcher has to define the number of independent variables introduced in each model and whether they were based upon statistical significance on bivariate analysis, extended to include nearly significant variables such as those with P-value between 0.05 and 0.1, or based upon literature review. He has to specify if variables were sequentially introduced in the model or being weighted by other variables.

Risks of Error

We have to define our primary and secondary risks of error. The usual primary risk of error is 5%, and the usual secondary risk of error is 10 or 20%. In the case of subgroup or repeated analysis, the P-value is inflated per the number of repeated testing. *The researcher has to define whether* a priori *contrasts were pre-planned* or measures were taken to reduce the inflated P-value by *post-hoc analysis.* Increasing the risk of error is unusual but can be justified in special cases, such as the case of a rare disease or advanced malignancy with the absence of known effective treatment.

Sample Size Calculation

The researchers must define *the five main elements* used for sample size calculation, namely, the adopted primary and secondary risks of error, the direction of the study, the targeted difference, and the variability of the primary outcome measure (see Sect. 4.1). Other factors should be identified, and their effect on calculation must be detailed. As an example, *the number of required events and the follow-up duration in Cox regression analysis* (see Sect. 4.9.2.2). We have to get *an estimate of R-squared* to accommodate for the effect of the multiple predictors in logistic or Cox regression analysis (see Sect. 4.11). Researchers have to define *the non-inferiority limit* in a non-inferiority or an equivalence study (see Sect. 4.13). It is crucial to report selected references supporting the main effect size and each one of those factors. Researchers must report *the equations* used for calculation with references, the used *power statistical software* with a version number, or the *online calculator* with the last assessed date. The reader is invited to review our suggestions on how to intelligently reduce the sample size (see Sect. 7.1).

The Interim Analysis

The statistical analysis section should include the details of any suggested interim analysis. In clinical trials, an interim analysis is usually used to compare randomized arms at any time point before the end of recruitment. It provides the opportunity of re-assurance that the trial is going on as pre-planned, the re-evaluation of trial design, or the re-calculation of sample size, the stoppage of trial in case of severe complications, or, on the other hand, in case of achieved statistical significance prematurely. However, every time the data is analyzed, there is a 5% chance of making a Type I error if $\alpha = 0.05$. As the number of analyses increases, the chance of making a Type I also error increases. Hence, (α) is often adjusted by raising its ceiling from the usual 5% to a smaller value. The most common is to include one interim analysis in the middle of the study. Armitage and colleagues suggested that if (N) is the total necessary number of patients, it is decided to carry out an intermediate analysis with a smaller number (n). To maintain the usual risk of error (P = 0.05), the new P* of the intermediate analysis can be calculated according to the proportion N/n. For example, if N/n = 2 (analyzing only half of the necessary number), we should arrive at a P* value of 0.029 to consider that our test was statistically significant at the least accepted degree of significance of 0.05 [41].

However, there is no universally accepted approach, and the researcher must define and justify the approach that best suits his study (Sect. 4.1.4.3). In short, if the primary intention is to stop the trial prematurely for efficacy, the method suggested by Pocock SJ provides a comparatively smaller adjustment for interim analysis [42]. On the other hand, if the primary concern is about the significance of the final analysis, the Haybittle-Peto method will be the procedure of choice for not making any adjustments at the final analysis [43, 44]. A table calculating sample size for different scenarios using the most common methods can be retrieved online [45].

Statistical Software

The statistical analysis section has to report the statistical software used for the analysis with the version and license number.

7.4.3   The Results

We have to expect a gap between the methods displayed in the protocol and their real implementation. It is better to begin the results section by displaying how the researchers managed to apply what was planned for and the difficulties they faced and how they were dealt with. Most of the reviewers will accept some deviations, and the role of the researcher is to keep complete transparency.

7.4.3.1   Verify the Protocol is Being Implemented

Should We Test Randomization?

Randomization, concealment, and blindness aim to create initial comparability. Any observed difference after the study can then be attributed to the treatment effect. An important question is whether to check if randomization was effective in creating comparable groups or not by formal statistical testing of the randomized groups? Some researchers consider it to be an unnecessary step because we cannot repeat randomization. We share the other point of view: test the randomized groups for the differences. In the absence of significant differences, it is well and good. In the presence of one or two significant differences due to chance, it will increase the reader's confidence in the transparency of the work. *The reader has the right to the information, and it will be up to him to judge the validity of the study.* On the other hand, in the absence of randomization, the initial comparison of the study groups is a must. It will significantly affect the readers' judgment of the value of the work.

Report Difficulties in Recruitment and Follow-Up

We have to report patient recruitment problems and any policy changes or delays. The readers must know the detailed reasons behind patients being excluded and the number of cases with incomplete follow-up, those who discontinued treatment, withdrawn from the study, or crossed over. While randomization ensures the initial comparability between the groups, a strict and complete follow-up ensures the maintenance of comparability throughout the study.

Verify the Conditions of Application of the Statistical Tests

The application conditions of bivariate statistical tests are few and easily verified; hence, except for verifying normality, the other conditions of application are not usually reported. On the other hand, multivariable analysis is a combination of regression and ANOVA; hence, it must satisfy the many assumptions behind both techniques. *It is not sufficient to report the results of those tests without indicating that the conditions of their application were verified, even in one or two lines.* For example, in logistic regression, a statistically non-significant Hosmer–Lemeshow (H–L) Goodness of fit shows how well data fit the model. We must report the absence of significant collinearity, outliers, high leverage, or influential points or how the researchers have dealt with them (see Sect. 3.5.5). The reader is requested to check the sections of *what should be reported* in ANOVA, ANCOVA, and multivariable analysis (see Chap. 3).

7.4.3.2 Report the Descriptive Statistics

Report means and standard deviations for continuous variables, the median and interquartile range for variables following other distributions than normal. Report the numbers and the percentages for categorical variables. In the case of time-to-event studies, we have to report the number of events. However, it is meaningless to report their percentage because patients have different participation times [38]. Moreover, we usually report median and not mean survival because the outcome is usually not normally distributed (see Sect. 2.7). All indices of study outcomes (OR, RR, HR, and NNT) and all diagnostic measures (Sn, SP, PPV, NPV, Likelihood ratios, diagnostic OR, and AUC of a ROC plot) must be reported with their corresponding 95% confidence interval.

7.4.3.3 Report the Estimates

Bivariate Analysis

The main estimate of the study depends upon many factors, including the study type, nature, distribution of primary outcome, and the type of analysis. As a rule of thumb, we have to avoid reporting any estimate as a single number but rather as an average value and a 95% confidence interval. *We must indicate the test used to assess the statistical significance, such as the t-test or the Chi-square test, the df, and the corresponding P-value.* It is better to report the exact P-value, even if non-significant unless it is smaller than 0.001, where it is usually reported as $P < 0.001$. *We have to report the appropriate effect size*, increasing the citation probability. The reader is invited to review the statistical test he has used and look for what should be reported by the end of each section (see Chap. 2).

Multivariable Analysis

The reader needs to know how many variables were initially introduced in the model as well as their detailed descriptive statistics. In addition, he needs to know *whether the conditions of application were verified* and *the overall significance of the model and the individual effect of each predictor* on the outcome variable in terms of (B-coefficient) in multiple regression, (OR) in the case of logistic regression, or the (HR) in Cox regression analysis, with the corresponding Wald statistics, 95% CI, and P-value. We have to report *how much the model explains the outcome,* whether in terms of R-square in multiple regression, Negelkerke's R-square, or McFadden R-square in logistic regression or in terms of the deviance between the (-2 log-likelihood ratios) in Cox regression analysis. For more details, the reader can refer to Sects. 3.4.7, 3.5.7, and 3.6.7.

The ANOVA Family

In the case of a two-way ANOVA, we have to report the independent role of each factor on the outcome, as well as any significant interaction, with F ratios, df, and exact P-values (see Sect. 3.2.1.2).

One-way ANCOVA measures the main effect adjusted on the covariate, and hence, the reader expects us to report the non-adjusted as well as the adjusted means, R^2, adjusted R^2, effect size (partial η^2), the statistical significance of the covariate, and treatment effects, with F ratios, df and P-values and, finally, the results of the post-hoc analysis when performed (see Sect. 3.2.3.1).

In the case of two-Way ANCOVA, we have to report the main effects in the absence of a statistically significant dual interaction and simple main effects in its presence. Reporting both effects is confusing, except in the presence of a statistically significant disordinal dual interaction (see Sect. 3.2.3.2). We do not need to repeat what should be reported with other tests, as it was detailed by the end of each section. The reader is invited to review those details in the case of One-way MANOVA (see Sect. 3.2.4.1), two-way RMANOVA (see Sect. 3.2.5.1), and Mixed two-way ANOVA (see Sect. 3.2.5.2).

7.4.3.4 Report the Subgroup and Intermediate Analysis

The Bias Behind Repeated Analysis

In a classic superiority study comparing two treatments, the null hypothesis is that both treatments are equal, and the alternative hypothesis is that they are not. If the alternative hypothesis is true, we can conclude that one treatment is better than the other. However, we know that we can never be 100% sure of our results and that the observed difference can also be acquired under the null hypothesis. The researchers accepted this probability (rejecting a true null hypothesis) as long as it did not exceed an arbitrary value of 5%.

Repeating analyzing the same data cumulates (inflates) this probability; i.e., it increases our chance to conclude upon a true difference between treatments, while it is not (Type I error). Consequently, it was logical and more convincing to correct the inflated P-value by decreasing the accepted conclusion limit from 0.05 to a lower level. In other words, the researcher has to prove that the probability of the observed being untrue is much smaller than 0.05 to compensate for the repeated opportunities he was given to reach such conclusions.

Bonferroni adjustment is a simple and widely used remedy for the inflated P-value due to the repeated comparison. The idea behind the procedure is simple: the universal limit of statistical significance (α) is adjusted by being divided by the number of comparisons made (n), and hence, the adjusted limit of significance is equal to α/n [46]. For example, if n is equal to 2, 3, or 4, we can conclude a statistically significant difference when the calculated P is at least equal to 0.025, 0.0166, or 0.0123. Note that the conclusions will be declared at the original 0.05 value in all those cases.

The Between-Groups Analysis

The need to correct a P-value is more than many researchers expect. The reader is kindly requested to refer to the previously given examples in comparing three regimens of oral anticoagulants by the Chi-square of independence (see Sect. 2.3.1.2 and Table 2.3). Other examples are comparing the fasting blood sugar of three patient groups by one-way ANOVA (see Sect. 2.4.3.3 and Table 2.20) and the cardiac outputs in four groups of patients with the non-parametric Kruskal and Wallace test (see

Sect. 2.5.2.1). In all cases, a statistically signifi-cant test indicates that one of the groups is at least significantly different from the other two but does not tell us which group. Those tests confirm that the compared groups are not all equal, but they do not confirm that they are all different from one another. The researcher has to compare every two groups independently (A versus B, A versus C, and B versus C) to know which group (or groups) is different from the others.

The Case of a Statistical Software Program

A statistical software program provides the researcher with multiple opportunities to execute repeated comparisons. The first is to arrange for a priori contrasts by setting up one of the groups as the reference group (e.g., the placebo) and to compare it to each of the other two treatment groups. The second is to compare all groups using a single post-hoc test designed to consider the inflated P-value, such as Bonferroni, LSD, or Tukey HSD. The third alternative is to compare the three groups two by two (see Sect. 2.4.3.3). Except for the second alternative, where the single test produces a corrected P-value (see Table 2.20), extra work is needed from the researcher to correct the inflated P-value when he reports the results.

The Case of Online Calculators

An online calculator does not usually offer the researcher the opportunity to designate his own (α). However, there are a few exceptions [10]. If this is the case, the researcher can set (α) to (α/n), where n is the number of comparisons made, and the program will directly produce the corrected P-value. The more common is that the program does not give him such an opportunity. The researcher has to correct the P-value himself in two ways. The first is to modify the interpretation of the uncorrected P, and the second is to cal-culate a correct P from the given test statistics.

In the first approach, the researcher will con-clude a statistically significant difference, not at the P-value of 0.05 but at a lower value, depending upon the number of comparisons made (n). He can conclude upon a statistically significant difference at the level of 0.05 if the

given P is at least equal to 0.025, 0.0166, or 0.0123; for the respective numbers of 2, 3, and 4 comparisons.

Alternatively, to get the corrected P-value himself, he disregards the one given by the pro-gram, notes the produced test statistics (such as the t-value or the Chi-square value) and the df, and then checks on the P-value by directly con-sulting the statistical tables. The test statistics must be matched with the critical levels of (α/n) and not the usual (α). For example, in the case where he has made two comparisons, the test statistics must be equal to or larger than the critical values listed under the column of ($\alpha/n = 0.05/2 = 0.025$) to declare a statistically signifi-cant difference at the level of 0.05 (P = 0.05). Hence, if the uncorrected P values of the two comparisons were 0.05 and 0.01, the first com-parison will be non-significant (P = 0.05 × 2 = 0.1), while the second comparison will be sta-tistically significant (P = 0.01 × 2 = 0.02). In the case of (n) comparisons, the test statistics must be equal to or larger than the critical values listed under the column of ($\alpha/n = 0.05/n$) to declare a statistically significant difference at the level of 0.05 (P = 0.05).

Subgroup Analysis Versus Testing Interaction

A common error is to attempt subgroup analysis, where we can test interaction. The bias is using multiple testing by comparing main groups and subgroups instead of using a single test. Let us take the example. A trial was conducted to study the effect of antiplatelet therapy in preventing transient ischemic attacks (TIA) among hyper-tensive patients. Six-hundred cases were equally randomized to either receive treatment or a pla-cebo, and it was suggested that the drug effect has to be verified according to whether the patient had diabetes or not. The results are shown in Table 7.4: the rate of TIA was significantly lower in patients receiving treatment (10%) compared to placebo (16.6%; P = 0.016). This "encouraged" the investigators to test whether this treatment effect was consistent with whether the patient had diabetes or not. The independent analysis of the two subgroups of patients showed a statistically significant effect in non-diabetic

Table 7.4 Testing the efficacy of antiplatelet therapy in hypertensive patients: subgroup analysis		Treatment group	Control group	Chi-square	P value
	All patients	30/300 (10%)	50/300 (16.6%)	5.77	0.016
	–Non-diabetic (540)	24/270 (8.9%)	41/270 (15.2%)	5.1	0.024
	–Diabetic (60)	6/30 (20%)	9/30 (30%)	0.8	0.37

Values are number (%) of transient ischemic attacks

patients (8.9 versus 15.2%; P = 0.024) and a non-significant effect in the diabetic subgroup (20 versus 30%; P = 0.37). The investigators were then tempted to conclude that the difference between the P values establishes a difference between the two subgroups: diabetic and non-diabetic patients; which is not correct.

The Source of Bias (Subgroup Analysis)

The significant P value produced when comparing the nondiabetic patients suggests that the treatment is effective in this subgroup. However, the non-significant P-value produced in the diabetic subgroup does not mean that the treatment is not effective; it just means that we were not able to show its effectiveness. Concluding that treatment is effective in nondiabetic patients and not effective in the diabetic group based on linking both P-values is not correct. Taking a closer look at the numbers shows that the treatment reduced the proportion of TIA in diabetic patients (30 − 20% = 10%) more than in the nondiabetic group (15.2 − 8.9% = 6.3%) compared to placebo. *The difference between both proportions is 3.7%, in favor of the diabetic group, suggesting that treatment may even perform better in diabetic patients.* The limitation of this study was that we were not able to put this information in evidence because of the small proportion of diabetic cases in the sample (10%) compared to nondiabetic patients.

Avoiding the Bias (Testing Interaction)

More precise testing of the interaction between the treatment effect and diabetes is to compare the differences between TIA percentages after

treatment and placebo in diabetic cases (10%) to that observed in nondiabetic patients (6.3%). If there is no interaction between the treatment effect and diabetes, those two differences should be equal (the null hypothesis). In the presence of interaction, both differences will be significantly different. A simple z test tests the significance of interaction by dividing the difference between those two proportions (10 − 6.3% = 3.7%) by the appropriate Se (Se_d) to produce a (z) value. The statistical significance of the latter is directly checked out in the z table, and a value of 1.64 or larger indicates a significant interaction between the treatment effect and diabetes. Note that the limit of significance is 1.64 and not 1.96 because the study is unilateral comparing treatment to placebo.

Calculation of the Se_d

We begin by calculating the Se of the nondiabetic subgroup as in "Eq. 7.17" where (P1) and (P2) are the proportions of TIA in patients receiving treatment and placebo, and n1 and n2 are the respective numbers of patients. The Se in the nondiabetic group will be equal to 2.8%. We repeat the same calculations to find the Se in the diabetic group, equal to 10.5% (equation not shown). Finally, the Se of the difference (Sed) will be the square root of the sum of both variances "Eq. 7.18" (11%). The 95% CI of the difference is calculated as in "Eq. 7.19" (see Sect. 1.4.2.7). The interval of confidence includes (0), and the Z value is non-significant (z = 0.063/0.11 = 0.57). Consequently, we could not find evidence of a significant interaction between the treatment effect and diabetes.

$$Se = \sqrt{\frac{P_1(1 - P_1)}{n1} + \frac{P_2(1 - P_2)}{n2}}$$

$$= \sqrt{\frac{0.089(1 - 0.089)}{270} + \frac{0.152(1 - 0.152)}{270}}$$

$$= 0.028$$

$$(7.17)$$

$$Se_d = \sqrt{(0.028)^2 + (0.105)^2} = 0.11 \quad (7.18)$$

$$p_d \pm Z(Se_d) = 0.063 \pm 1.96\,(0.11)$$
$$= -15.3\% \; to \, 27.8\% \quad (7.19)$$

We have previously presented the example of a multicenter trial conducted to compare the effect of two antihypertensive treatments in two groups of patients (see Sect. 2.9.4.1). Twenty-four patients were recruited from three hospitals (eight patients per hospital) and were equally randomized between the two treatment groups, A and B. The results were shown in Table 2.38. The researcher aimed to find a treatment effect, a hospital effect, and possible interaction. In other words, the researcher had three questions to answer, and the problem will be if he received the bad advice that separate statistical tests can obtain those answers. A two-way ANOVA is a single test used to answer the three questions without the bias of repeated comparison or the bias of subgroup analysis (see Sect. 2.9.4.1).

The Within-Groups Analysis

We often need to analyze data acquired from the same group of patients, whether at different timings or under different conditions. An example of the former is testing whether patients following the same diet regimen progressively lose weight. An example of the latter is comparing the patient losing weight when following a diet regimen alone to when following a diet regimen plus exercise or exercise and medication. The statistical significance of the overall pattern of change can be tested by a single test, such as repeated measures ANOVA, which tells us whether the patient is significantly losing weight over time or that the weight loss is significantly related to the type of regimen. Suppose that weight is observed each month; a statistically

significant overall test does not tell us precisely if the weight loss observed in the third month, for example, is significantly different from the one observed at five months.

We remind the reader of three examples given before. The one-way repeated measures ANOVA analyzes the repeated testing of warfarin doses in one group of patients with DVT (see Sect. 2.4.3.4 and Table 2.21). Another example is the two-way repeated-measures ANOVA compares the effect of low versus high dosing of warfarin on the repeated INR measures in one group of patients (see Sect. 3.2.5.1 and Table 3.26). Finally, a two-way mixed ANOVA makes the same comparison but in two or more different patient groups (see Sect. 3.2.5.2 and Tables 3.29 and 3.33). In the latter, the repeated comparison can be made to detect the difference between independent groups (see Sect. 7.4.1) or to detect the difference between the repeated measures acquired from the same group, which is why the model has been called a mixed model for assessing a mix of within and between in-between variabilities. Friedman's test can be used in the case the quantitative outcome variable follows other distribution than normal (see Sect. 4.12.2). The two-by-two comparisons at different time points can then be made by Wilcoxon-sign (see Sect. 2.5.1.3), with P value adjustment according to the Bonferroni rules.

In case of a qualitative outcome, the McNemar-Bowker test is a modified McNemar that can be used if one of the two variables has more than two classes. An example was given where the patients' symptoms were recorded before and after treatment in a single group of patients as being mild, moderate, or severe. Bowker's test is a test of symmetry, and a statistically significant result tells us that the distribution of the ordinal variable between the two categories of the ordinal variable is not symmetrical; i.e., it is different. It cannot tell us the exact position of this dissymmetry: is it between the mild and the moderate categories, the moderate and the severe categories, or the mild and the severe categories? Only repeated McNemar tests of those classes can answer this question, applying the Bonferroni correction as indicated (see Sect. 2.3.2.2).

The Cochran Q test is another modification, which can be applied to multiple qualitative variables, provided binomial. The test verifies the symmetry of the distribution of a binomial variable, whether measured several times (>3) in a single group of patients or once in (>3) matched groups or experimental conditions (see Sect. 2.3.2.3). Consequently, a statistically significant test measuring over three successive weeks tells us that there was a change across those weeks, but it cannot tell us whether there is a statistically significant difference between the first and the second week, for example? This question can only be answered by applying multiple McNemar tests comparing the timings two-by-two, corrected for the number of comparisons made, according to Bonferroni rules.

7.4.3.5 Create Informative Tables and Figures

Researchers must study the guidelines for authors before sending their manuscripts to a specific journal and pay extreme attention to the tables and the figures. Usually, tables and figures are the next part reviewed in the manuscript, after the title page and the abstract. In short, a table is no more than a set of related data that the researcher decides to put together to draw a complete picture of one face of his study. Consequently, tables have to be complete and independent from one another. A good example is the first table in many manuscripts, which usually describes the patients' demographics and risk factors. It has to show the patients' looks before the study and, most importantly, give the reader sufficient information about which of his patients could have been included in the study that he is about to review. On the other hand, summarizing the most important results in a final table helps the reader see the benefit that his patient can get from adopting the studied treatment or procedure.

Besides visualizing pathological, radiological, or details of other technological outputs, the figures can be used to display multiple or repeated information about one variable or the nature of the relation between a couple of variables. A typical example is to display the pattern of change of a repeated measure, the development of an event over time, and the results of comparing one piece of information among multiple groups. A common error is to repeat the same information between the result lines, inside a table, and sometimes even in a figure. Redundancy is unacceptable in the publishing industry. It distracts the reader, is a source of error while repeating the same information, and can lead to confusion or misinterpretation. The researcher must choose the best place that fits each piece of information.

7.4.4 The Discussion

The results section was where the researcher reported his findings impartial and unbiasedly. *The discussion is not the stage to repeat those results but the arena to defend them.* The researcher is supposed to use this valuable space to show the areas of strength and study limitations, discuss controversies with his peers, and suggest prospects.

7.4.4.1 When Do We Have the Right to Conclude?

Unlike a common erroneous belief, concluding is not based upon a single element, reaching a statistically significant result when the P-value drops to 0.05 or lower. Let us begin by defining what does a P-value tell us? The example is a classical superiority study comparing the effects of two treatments, A and B. Suppose the difference between both treatments is in favor of A, and it is so large that the probability of both treatments being equally effective (P-value) is tiny. In that case, we conclude that treatment A is significantly more effective than treatment B. However, for the sake of honesty and transparency, we couple our conclusion with the small probability that both treatments are equally effective, i.e., the P-value. The reader can refer to Sect. 1.5 (see Sect. 1.5) and, of course, to the statement of the American statistical association for more accurate definitions of the P-value [47]. Nevertheless, what does the P-value tell us, but what does it not? Unfortunately, the P-value does not tell us much about many pillars of concluding upon evidence in clinical research.

What the P-Value Does not Tell?

- The P-value does not tell whether the sample size was adequately calculated. A small underpowered study can still lead to a statistically significant P-value. Consequently, a study power of 80% or more is a prerequisite to making a robust conclusion.
- The P-value does not tell whether the compared groups were initially comparable before the beginning of the study, so the statistically significant P value calculated by the end of the study can be attributed to the treatment effect. Randomization has a substantial role in this matter. In order to conclude, we have to be ascertained that randomization was correctly planned and adequately performed, regardless of the P-value. In order to conclude in non-randomized studies, the authors have to give some evidence that the groups were comparable before the study, at least concerning the main demographics and study-related risk factors.
- The P-value does not tell whether the initial comparability that was created by randomization at the beginning of the study was maintained during the study by close and complete surveillance of all groups, which is a significant source of hidden bias. Examples include the reluctant follow-up of patients receiving placebo or the standard care therapy and the loose surveillance of the intake of associated treatments, whether those being allowed or contraindicated.
- The P-value per se does not tell whether the collected data was adequately managed and checked for errors and outliers. It does not tell us the number of missing observations, the mechanism of missingness, and if missing data were properly replaced (see Sect. 7.2).
- The P-value does not tell whether it was produced by applying the most appropriate statistical test. We have previously shown that the P-value can be inflated by repeating the analysis, which must be corrected before the

interpretation (see Sect. 2.4.3.3). The American Statistical Association warned about basing conclusions solely on whether a p-value passes a specific threshold. They enhanced researchers to bring many contextual factors into play, including the design of a study, the quality of the measurements, the external evidence for the phenomenon under study, and the validity of assumptions that underlie the data analysis [47].

- The P-value does not tell us about the importance of the treatment effect. A large treatment effect can be missed in a small study, while a large study can put into evidence a small treatment effect, which is why researchers must report the effect size.
- The P-value describes a single incident of our results but does not tell us about the set of all possible compatible results, which is why we have to report the 95% CI of treatment effect.

We have the right to conclude when all those assumptions and much more have been verified and not just because of a statistically significant P value.

7.4.4.2 The Absence of Evidence is not Evidence of Absence

A beta error is an erroneous conclusion that there is no treatment effect or difference between two treatment groups when there is one. Committing such an error does not mean that there is no difference but that the researchers failed to show it up [48]. Typically, most investigators adopt a beta error rate of 20%, and hence, they have to expect an equivalent percent of false-negative results, i.e., to miss the evidence. In other words, a common cause of failure to conclude a difference between treatment groups is not because it does not exist but because the study was underpowered to produce the evidence. Note that the power is a factor of both sample size and the number of events in the study; hence, a large study with a limited number of events will be underpowered too. Studies producing statistically non-significant results are usually termed negative studies [48].

Alternatively, a large and well-organized negative study should not be interpreted as an indicator of equality, which does not exist in life. Put another way, the null hypothesis was designed to be disproved and can never be proved. Although some researchers can see a positive side in those studies: the compared treatments are valid alternatives; however, there is no proof for such an assumption. Otherwise, what is the reason for creating non-inferiority and equivalence studies? The non-inferiority and equivalence studies were created to give statistical proof that negative superiority studies failed to provide: the compared treatments are valid alternatives within acceptable limits (see Sect. 5.3.4).

How Should We Interpret Negative Studies?

Statistically non-significant (negative) studies should not be reported as evidence of no difference because they are not. There is no evidence that the treatment has no effect and there is no evidence that it has an effect. If the evidence was to prove that one treatment is superior to the other, the maximum we can say is that the two treatments are comparable but never equal. Pharmaceutical companies have enough large resources to put into evidence the limited effect size of a newly invented treatment, while independent researchers may fail to conclude a large effect because of the limited resources. Two treatments with similar effects will produce significantly different P-values if the estimates have different precisions. In conclusion, the P-value is not a measure of an effect's size or importance [47].

Consequently, the study report should be supported by a measurement of effect size and a justification of the result, such as a wide 95% confidence interval. Unfortunately, authors rarely respect those requirements. For example, in their review of 50 randomized clinical trials with non-statistically significant results, Hemming and collaborators noted that 56% of those studies concluded upon no difference, with only a few providing any justification, such as a wide confidence interval [49].

7.4.5 The Abstract

The abstract is the first and may be the only part read in a manuscript. It is expected to summarize the research paper in about 150–300 words, in no more than a dozen short sentences. The abstract is usually divided into four main parts.

Introduction or Background

The introduction or background shows the actual state of knowledge and the gap the study should fill in one or two short sentences.

Material and Methods

The patients and methods section of a clinical study defines the patients' demographics and risk factors, the study design and direction, and the size and the distribution of the sample among groups. It indicates the methods used to initiate and maintain comparability, such as randomization. It describes the methods by which the treatments were given, and the procedures were implemented, the primary and secondary outcomes, and how data were collected and finally analyzed. Gathering all information in a few sentences is a real art and, often, a tough challenge.

Results

Most readers are usually impatient or not interested in reviewing a sometimes dull or difficult methods section and eventually rush to examine the third section. Unfortunately, those readers sometimes do not find "true results" in their regular scales but mainly P-values, which do not tell us much. Authors are sometimes proud of the statistical significance of their results and forget that readers mainly care about the results themselves and in full detail. What is the benefit for a reader to know that a significantly smaller dose cured patients of treatment A compared to treatment B (P = 0.001) without knowing the average dose and, most importantly, the expected dosing limits, i.e., the confidence interval of the result? *The P-value represents only one incident of testing the treatment effect. The reader is entitled to know the magnitude and the limits of the whole spectrum in terms of means, standard deviations, median and range, numbers and percentages, and, most importantly, effect size and a confidence interval.*

Conclusion

The conclusion section is not the place to repeat the results but to conclude with a short recommendation, pointing to the areas of strength, limitations, and future prospects. Unfortunately, authors may sometimes rush to conclude in their results section and, hence find nothing new to put in the conclusion section than to repeat the results. *We cannot conclude upon negative findings because of the lack of evidence nor the secondary outcomes for the lack of power.* The values of secondary outcomes are observational, even in prospective controlled randomized studies. It is advisable to conclude upon one primary outcome or a score made of a set of related outcomes than on multiple outcomes. It prevents confusion and conflicting results.

Finally, being humble in his conclusions is not only a moral virtue. It is based upon the fact that everything is liable to change over time, even if it once stood on solid scientific ground. Gonon and colleagues selected the ten most echoed publications on attention deficit hyperactivity disorder (ADHD) published in the nineties and collected all their relevant subsequent studies until 2011. Seven of the "top 10" publications were initial studies, and the conclusions in six of them were either refuted or strongly attenuated subsequently. Two were confirmed subsequently among the three remaining studies, and the third was attenuated [50].

7.4.6 Common Pitfalls, Misinterpretations, and Inadequate Reporting

7.4.6.1 Clinical Relevance Must Lead Statistical Significance Statistical

A common error is a researcher letting the statistical findings drive his study because it will end by being drifted. Statistical analysis should be planned before the study, and findings had to be expected rather than being caught by surprise. Unexpected findings should alert the researcher to react, but he should never wait for the finding to decide on the analysis plan. For example, in a meta-analysis, choosing between a fixed-effect model and a random-effects model should be made from the start. It is inappropriate to choose the model based on the results of Q, i.e., choosing a fixed effect if Q is not significant and a random effect if proved to be significant (see Sect. 6.2.7). A common mistake is to decide on the used model based on the test of heterogeneity, which makes no sense. The choice of the model must reflect the goals of the systematic review, which have to be set in advance (see Sect. 6.2.4.4). On the other hand, a significant Q should alert the researcher that it is inappropriate to maintain a fixed-effect model.

Another example is the researcher planning from the start on doing subgroup analysis. He can either arrange for an a-priori contrast or include a sufficient sample to empower any expected post-hoc analysis (see Sect. 2.4.3.3). Waiting for the results to make decisions, whether during or after the analysis, is the worst policy we can follow.

7.4.6.2 Avoid Incomplete and Selective Reporting

In our book, we ended the presentation of each statistical test with a paragraph entitled: what should be reported? We need to report the conditions of application of the test being verified to prepare the reader to accept the produced results. In addition to the "main result", we wish to obtain, the software produces important "collateral results" that must be reported too. Taking the example of a simple unpaired test of Student, besides the produced t- and P-values, the software generates important descriptive statistics for each group (see Sect. 2.4.1.2). Most importantly, we must report effect size, such as Cohen's d (see Sect. 4.2.1.1).and Hedges' g (see Sect. 4.2.1.2), permitting other researchers to calculate their sample sizes. Many software programs report Pearson's correlation coefficient too. Reporting an effect size increases our chances of being cited, while Pearson's correlation helps calculate the sample size of a paired design (see Sect. 4.5.1.2). More information must be reported in multivariable analysis, such as multiple regression. We have to report the verification of the multiple assumptions, such as linearity, homoscedasticity, and the absence of outliers, and the many results, such as R^2, adjusted R^2, and individual b-coefficients. Reporting has to be informative and concise.

On the other hand, reporting has to be complete. In an important statement published in 2016, the American Statistical Association warned against cherry-picking promising findings that lead to a spurious excess of statistically significant results in the published literature [47]. All findings merit having their share of reporting, based upon their relative position in the study, whether a primary or secondary outcome and their clinical relevance, despite the size of the produced P-value.

7.4.6.3 Avoid the Misinterpretation of the Indices of Outcome

The Odds Ratio is Not an Indicator of Causality

The "risk" usually expresses a given event's frequency (probability) among a specific group of patients. The relative risk is the ratio between two probabilities. The probability of developing the event for a patient at risk in the treatment group to the same probability in the control group. It indicates a direct cause-effect relationship: how much can a patient with a risk factor in the treatment group develop more (or fewer) events compared to the control group?

We can calculate the other side of the coin: the probability of having the risk factor for those who already have the event. Calculating the ratio between the risks in the treatment and the control groups produces a different relative risk. The latter describes another direct cause-effect relationship: how much a patient who already has the event in the treatment group can be at higher (or lower) risk than the control group. The two relative risk s are not the same (see Sect. 1.8.2).

The odds are the proportion of patients who developed the event to those who did not. The odds ratio (OR) is the ratio between two odds in the treatment group to that in the control group. Consequently, if we invert the ratios in both treatment and control groups (interchanging the risk factor and the event), their proportion will always be the same. Consequently, unlike having two different relative risks, we have a single OR indicating the tightness between the two variables but never causality. The straightforward interpretation of the RR tempts the researchers to interpret the odds ratio similarly. This approximation is only valid when the probability of the event is rare, with a prevalence of 10% or lower; hence, if the prevalence is high, interpreting the OR as the RR will be false.

The Risk is Not the Hazard

Another false interpretation is not acknowledging the difference between the risk ratio (relative risk) and the hazard ratio. The risk is the probability of developing an event. It is calculated as the number of cases that developed the event to the total number of patients at risk. On the other hand, the hazard is the probability of developing the event, at a specific time (t), provided that the patient was still at risk and did not experience the event before that time. For example, if the outcome event is "cure" and a group of patients were followed up for five years, a RR of 2 means that twice as many patients in the treatment group are expected to be cured after five years as the control group. In other words, the RR is cumulative. An HR of 2 means that twice as many patients in the treatment group are expected to be cured at any time during the five years compared to the control group; i.e., the HR is instantaneous (see Sect. 1.8.3.1).

Pearson's Correlation Coefficient Does Not Indicate Agreement

More than three decades have passed since Bland and Altman have clearly shown that Pearson's correlation coefficient (r) measures the strength of the relation between two variables but not their agreement [53]. Unlike the common belief, Pearson's correlation coefficient, although precise, lacks accuracy and cannot be used to measure agreement. Instead, we can display and measure the extent and limits of an agreement by a Bland and plot. The agreement can then be expressed in a single measure (number), such as Lin's correlation coefficient [54] and the intraclass correlation coefficient [55] (see Sect. 2.10.4).

7.4.6.4 The 95% CI and the P Value Are not Interchangeable

A patient is considered potentially diabetic when his fasting blood sugar lies outside the normal range, which is the 95% CI of normal population. In other words, the 95% CI and statistical significance are interchangeable in the one sample situation. The question is whether it applies on the two-sample situation as well? Assel and colleagues reported event rates of 70 and 50% in 100 patients equally randomized between two groups [38]. The 95% confidence interval of the difference between the two proportions (1.2–38.8%), the OR (1.0272–5.3004), and the RR (1.0052–1.9499) exclude the null (1); which are usually interpreted as statistically significant results (P < 0.05). Although Chi-square test gives an equally significant result (Chi-square value = 4.1667; P 0.041), Fisher's exact test statistics produces a P-value of 0.0656; indicating a statistically non-significant result. Unlike the one sample situation shown at the beginning, the interpretation that two groups are statistically significant based on the 95% confidence interval is not always correct [51].

The other side of the coin is that the confidence intervals of two variables can overlap as much as 29%, and the comparison P-value can be statistically significant [52]. In order to ascertain those two confidence intervals do not overlap, the difference between the two means must be equal to two standard errors of the first mean plus two standard errors of the second mean. For facility, suppose that both standard errors are equal; the difference between the two means must be four standard errors. The ordinary t-test only requires that the difference between the two means is approximately two standard errors of the difference (Sed). In case of the equal standard

error of both means, the Sed will be equal to 2.8 standard errors only and not the four standard errors required for the two CI not to overlap [52]. Put it simpler; the group means only need to differ by about 2.8 standard errors for statistical significance in the t-test, which is smaller than the four standard errors required for the nonoverlapping CI criterion [52]. The statistics of the P-value are not the same as those of the 95% CI and hence, those different pieces of information are not interchangeable.

7.4.6.5 A Smaller P-Value Does not Reflect a Truer or a Larger Effect

P stands for probability, and the P-value can be defined as the probability of obtaining a result equal to or more extreme than the one observed under the null hypothesis, i.e., under the assumption of no treatment effect or no difference between compared treatments (see Sects. 1.5 and 1.6).

A smaller P-value does not mean at all that the effect is "truer" but as being more "credible." Degrees of significance are just probabilities that should never be compared, whether in the same study or other studies [56]. We can put into evidence (get a significant P-value) a tiny effect size if we arrange for a huge sample. On the contrary, we can fail to put into evidence (not significant P-value) a considerable effect size, if we fail to arrange for a sufficient sample.

7.4.6.6 Express the Results with Confidence

We need a confidence interval, usually at 95%, for its valuable descriptive, comparative and predictive values. Those qualities are based on those of the normal distribution, namely the qualities of the mean and the standard error (see Sect. 1.4.1). In the case of variables following a distribution other than normal, the computed CI will not have the desired values. The reader is invited to review the complete section dedicated to the calculations of the different intervals of confidence (see Sect. 1.4.2). We will point to some pitfalls and common errors that should be avoided.

Replace the (z) Value by the Proper Student t-Value in Small Samples

William Sealy Gosset (1876–1937) published his valuable research work under the nickname: "Student". His research mainly focused on the behavior of small samples drawn from a normal population. He noted that the smaller the sample, the more it deviates from normality. Hence, in front of "the one" normal distribution that fits all, he showed that there are "multiple" near-normal distributions, each fitting for a particular sample size [57]. The distribution was later on named after his nickname.

Unfortunately, a common error is to use the (z) value of a (large) normal distribution to create a confidence interval around the mean of a small sample of 30 cases (n) or less per group. We must replace the (z) value with the corresponding (t) value, calculated at n-2 df. For example, suppose that we wish to calculate a 95% CI for a correlation coefficient of (0.89) and Se of (0.16. We check on Student's table at the intersection of the probability column of 5% (P = 0.05) and the df of n-2 to find the corresponding t-value (2.3). The 95% CI = r ± t (Se) = 0.89 ± 2.3 (0.16) = 0.52 to 1.26. If the sample was large, the 95% CI is calculated with the (z) value of 1.96, regardless of the sample size. The 95% CI = r ± z (Se) = 0.89 ± 1.96 (0.16) = 0.58 to 1.2. The studentized CI will always be larger (wider) than the usual CI of a normal distribution because the (t) value is always larger than (z).

Report the 95% CI of a Variable Following Other Distribution than Normal

Some variables encountered in biology, such as the duration of pregnancy or the duration of stay in the intensive care units, follow other distributions than normal. Commonly used indices of clinical outcomes, such as the odds, hazard, and risk ratios, are not normally distributed. Many variables can be normalized by simple logarithmic transformation (see Sect. 7.2.4.2). We are using the odds ratio (OR) example. We transform the OR into log OR, calculate the Se of log OR and the 95% CI of log OR as Log OR ± 1.96 (Se) log OR. Finally, we convert the upper and lower limits of the latter to get the upper and lower limit of the 95% CI of OR in its proper scale (see Sect. 1.8.7.2). We can quickly notice that, in each confidence interval primarily calculated in the log scale, the index (OR) is not centralized in the middle of the interval, unlike when calculations are made directly without passing by the log transformation.

The same applies whenever we use those indices to express the effect of a predictor variable on the outcome in multivariable analysis. All calculations are made in the log scale, as in the case of log OR used to express the effect of each predictor variable in logistic regression analysis. The software produces both: the index in terms of log scale as it was calculated (e.g., log OR) and the back-transformed index in the regular scale for presentation (OR) (see Sect. 3.5.6.2). The hazard ratio in Cox regression analysis is another example (see Sect. 3.6.6.2).

Use the Continuity Correction in Small Sample Size or Small Number of Events

The calculation of the CI of a binomial distribution (p, 1 − p) in a sample of (n) cases approximates the normal distribution, provided that the sample is large. This assumption is verified whenever both (np) and [n(1 − p)] are ≥ 5 and (p) is close to 0.5 [28]. Otherwise, the researcher has to report the continuity correction made to improve those approximations. The correction is made by adding a factor (1/2n) to the upper limit and subtract it from the lower limit of the non-corrected interval. Although the continuity correction version of the CI is wider, it is more accurate, especially in the case of a small sample size. Both the corrected and the uncorrected intervals can be directly assessed online [26].

Calculate the 95% CI of the Median

We have presented the equations that can be used to calculate the 95% confidence interval of the median and the difference between two medians (see Sect. 2.5.1.1). The former can be easily calculated by hand and online [24], but the latter is more complicated but feasible and is provided by few software such as Minitab [58].

Calculate a 95% CI of an Event That Did Not Happen Yet

In case we are studying the effect of a new procedure, it can happen that we do not notice any drawbacks, e.g., failure or complications for a certain period. Any procedure will never be 100% safe or 100% effective, and the question was how to predict a confidence interval for an event that did not happen? In other words, how to predict a 95% IC for a (0%) event rate? The lower limit of the interval is (0-), but what about the upper limit? As an approximation, Henley calculated the upper limit of an event that has never happened as equal to n/3, where (n) is the number of times the procedure was performed (total sample size). The equation gives reasonable estimates as long as n $\geq$ 30 [59]. It follows that the more we experience the procedure, the less is the expected maximum risk of adverse events, which is quite logical. The calculations can equally be easily made online [24, 26, 27].

7.4.6.7 Interpret the Results of the Statistical Analysis Correctly

When do We Have the Right to Compare Subgroups?

Suppose that we are comparing the effect of two treatments, and the result is that one treatment is superior to the other. The researcher wishes to know whether the treatment effect is valid for diabetic as well as non-diabetic cases included in the analysis. We have previously shown that the best approach is to test the interaction between diabetes and treatment effect. Now suppose that the study gave a negative result. Would he think about testing the interaction between diabetes and the treatment effect that he failed to put into evidence? Of course, he would not because it looks to be absurd.

The same logic applies if he thinks comparing subgroups is better than testing interaction. *In the absence of a significant main effect, subgroup comparison would have no sense, and it will be seen as an attempt to get a significant P-value by*

all means. In conclusion, a significant difference between main groups gives the researcher the pretext to go one step further in the analysis and compare subgroups. Otherwise, the researcher will have no right to compare subgroups.

The Interpretation of Tests Excluding a Difference but not Confirming the Required Condition

As we can only prove differences but not equality, the best we can sometimes do is to exclude a statistically significant difference. Tests that examine whether data fit a particular distribution or model are called the goodness of fit tests. They are based upon excluding the presence of a statistically significant difference between data and the distribution or the model of concern. Many are based on the Chi-square equation that tests whether there is a significant difference between an observed (data) and an expected distribution (model) (see Sect. 2.3). An example is testing whether there is a statistically significant difference between an observed and a theoretical distribution by a Chi-square test for goodness-of-fit (see Sect. 2.3.1.1). Hosmer–Lemeshow is a goodness of fit test that examines whether data fit in a logistic regression model (see Sect. 3.5.6.1). Another famous example is the Kolmogorov–Smirnov test of normality. A statistically non-significant test does not confirm normality but indicates the absence of a statistically significant difference between the data and normality (see Sect. 1.4.3.3). The researcher expects a negative result (P > 0.05) to continue suggesting that data are normal. One more example is Beg and Mazumdar test used to test funnel plot asymmetry (see Sect. 6.2.10.3).

Besides not-confirming what we are looking for, another disadvantage of the goodness-of-fit tests based on Chi-square is that they have low power in small studies for not being able to "cumulate" a target difference due to the small sample size. Fortunately, not all tests are based on the Chi-square equation. A good example is Durbin-Watson statistics used in multiple regression to "assume" the absence of autocorrelation between adjacent cases (see Sect. 3.4.2.4). The Shapiro–Wilk test is another example of regression goodness of fit that is used to assess normality. The test is considered to be superior to the Kolmogorov–Smirnov test for being more specific and valid in the case of a small sample (see Sect. 1.4.3.3).

The Fixed and the Random Effects Models of Meta-Analysis Answer Two Different Questions

In a meta-analysis, the different results of the fixed-effect and the random-effects model must not be seen as the two models perform differently simply because each model answers a different question. The fixed-effect model aims to find the mean estimate in the population, while the random-effects model aims to find the range of mean estimates. Hence, they have to produce different results. Kindly refer to Chap. 6 for more details (see Sect. 6.2.4).

The Funnel Plot of Meta-Analysis Measures the Effect of Small Studies and not Necessarily Publication Bias

In a meta-analysis, plotting the effect size on the x-axis and an element of precision on the y-axis is expected to take a funnel's shape. The few large studies with limited variability form the narrow top, and the many small studies with widespread variability will be pushed to the bottom. *The funnel plot examines whether the effect size of clinical studies of a particular meta-analysis correlate positively with those studies' size (precision).* If this is the case, the funnel plot will be symmetrical. However, if the small studies have to have a significant effect that is not proportional to their size, in order to be published, the funnel plot will be asymmetrical; this is what the funnel plot is testing (see Sect. 6.2.10). *The common belief that an asymmetrical funnel plot visualizes publication bias is one case only*, where small and non-significant studies are not published and are kept in the drawers, leaving their "expected" position on the funnel empty. Egger and colleagues reported a long list of causes of asymmetry [60].

7.4.6.8 The Results of the Within-Group Analysis Are not Informative About the Difference Between Groups

Sometimes, researchers are tempted to tie the results of those within-subgroup independent results to inform about the difference between the groups. The reader is invited to review the previous example studying the role of diabetes in studying the efficacy of antiplatelet therapy (see Table 7.4 and Sect. 7.4.3.4). Instead of proceeding to sometimes misinformative subgroup analysis, the researcher can test the interaction between the subgrouping variable (diabetes in our example) and the outcome. Interaction can be determined using the z test in the case of binomial data (see Sect. 2.9.2.1), the Breslow-Day and Tarone tests in the case of categorical data (see Sect. 2.9.2.2), and the two-way ANOVA in the case of continuous data test (see Sect. 2.9.4.1). The reader is invited to review the above sections for more details and informative examples.

7.4.6.9 Whether Placebo is Better Than Treatment is not Tested in a Unilateral Study

A bilateral study's null hypothesis is that the compared treatments are equally effective. The alternative hypothesis (what we want to prove) is that one of the treatments is better than the other. In a unilateral study, the null hypothesis is composed of two parts: treatment and placebo are equally effective, and placebo is better than treatment. The alternative hypothesis is that treatment is better than placebo, which is the only thing we wish to prove. *In a unilateral study, the possibility that the placebo is better than the treatment is part of the null hypothesis we wish to reject but can never prove.* In other words, the unilateral study does not determine if the placebo is better than the treatment; hence, it remains possible. In return, the unilateral design concludes upon a smaller difference (the critical limit of Z changes from 1.96 to 1.64) and empowers the study by reducing the sample size by about

20%. The researcher has to be aware that the effect size reported in a the unilateral study cannot be directly extrapolated on a bilateral design.

7.4.6.10 A Multivariate Test is not More Robust Than a Bivariate Test

Every statistical test is based on some assumptions that must be primarily verified before any result is evaluated. The assumptions of bivariate statistical tests are few and are easily verified, in contrast to the many assumptions that are sometimes hard to verify in the case of multivariate analysis. Moreover, if we have only two independent variables, a simple adjustment is equally effective and less demanding than a multivariable test (see Sect. 2.9). On the other hand, we have suggested five main indications for multivariable analysis (see Sect. 3.3.1). Unless the study is concerned with one of those indications, and the researcher can include a sufficient sample size; he has to satisfy with a robust, simple bivariate or adjusted analysis.

7.4.6.11 The Bias Behind Small Studies

Small Samples Lack Representativeness

By default, the variability in a small sample is much larger than that of the population. Remember how we calculated the variance of a sample (V^2) of size (n). The variance was calculated by dividing the sum of squares (SS) by the df (n-1): $V^2 = SS/(n-1)$. The effect of subtracting the constant number (1) from the denominator will increase the variability calculated for a small study but will have a smaller effect as the sample gets larger. The equation was designed to show the large variability contained in small samples. As the sample grows, the variability is reduced to finally mimic that of the population, where the effect of subtracting (1) from a very large sample becomes minimal (see Sect. 1.3.4.1). For example, subtracting (1) from a small sample of ten cases reduces the variance by 10%. On the other hand, subtracting (1) from a large sample of 1000 cases reduces the variance by 0.01%. The researcher has to be careful when dealing with small samples, especially when representativeness becomes crucial. For example, during stratification, which is mending to distribute key risk factors among randomized groups. Stratification can become a source of bias by creating too small groups for randomization, and hence, it is usually advisable to stratify on a limited number of factors (see Sect. 5.4.2.1).

Small Samples Tend to Exaggerate Effect Size

Large well-organized negative studies can be published for their excellent methodology. On the other hand, small studies have to have significant effect size, in order to be published. Those results are sometimes exaggerated due to their poor methodology. The result is that subsequent larger trials and meta-analysis usually reveal a smaller but truer effect size [61, 62]. Unfortunately, a majority of systematic reviews do not have sufficient power [63, 64].

We May Need to Check on the Results in Special Tables

Most clinical studies are small; however, many researchers follow the rule of including a minimum number of 30 patients per group. A minimum number of 20 patients per group is required to use the test of Student comfortably. In smaller samples, researchers usually use a nonparametric approach, such as the Man and Whitney test, which necessitates a minimum number of cases. As a rule of thumb, a nonparametric test requires a minimum of ten patients per group in a bilateral design and 20 cases in a paired design. If the study is even smaller, the reported equations cannot be used, and the statistical significance of the comparison must be checked in unique tables [65, 66] (see Sect. 2.5.1.1).

7.4.6.12 The Non-parametric Approach is a Benefit

The Non-parametric Tests are not Second Grade Tests

As indicated by their name, parametric tests necessitate the fulfillment of certain parameters (conditions) to be applied, mainly normality and variance equality. In the absence of those parameters, "non–parametric tests" become the tests of choice (see Sect. 2.5). Many researchers will choose a non-parametric test for the difficulty of verifying normality in small samples. Others may be comfortable with them in most situations for the relatively few assumptions to be made.

The non-parametric tests have the advantage of substituting skewed data and outliers, which can produce a major bias if analyzed parametrically by normally distributed ranks. However, the inevitable loss of information due to ranking decreases the power of the test to sense the differences, increasing type II errors or false negative results. Put it this way; a non-parametric test has a low sensitivity to detect the evidence compared to its parametric version, which may be unfavorable for the researcher but not for the reader if the evidence is found already. *However, such loss of power remains negligible compared to the bias of applying a parametric test without reliable verification of the conditions necessary for its use.*

They Come to Our Rescue in Multiple Occasions

We have given the example of using the Chi-square test for trend to analyze the effect of three levels of hypertension (ordinal input) in the development of stroke (binomial outcome: yes or no) (see Sect. 2.3.1.4). However, the Chi-square test for trend cannot be used in case the outcome is ordinal, such as the development of stroke, transient ischemic attack, or none. In this case, we can replace the classes of both variables with ranks and test the significance of the correlation between the classes (ranks) of the input variable and those of the output variable by Spearman's correlation rank test (see Sect. 2.6.1.2). The reader is kindly requested to have a look on Table 2.35 and note how those tests come to our rescue on multiple occasions due to their simplicity and the limited assumptions (see Sect. 2.8).

The Non-parametric Tests Do Not Compare Medians Only

Another misbelief is that non-parametric tests compare the medians of non-normally distributed data, which is an incomplete statement. We have shown the example given by Campbell and Swinscow [40] of two groups having the same median, while the Mann and Whitney test produced a statistically significant difference at the $P < 0.001$. Unlike the parametric t-test, which directly calculates the standardized difference between the two means, the non-parametric version is based on ranking all individual values of the group, with the median being only one of those values. The wider is the distribution of the values of one group; the more significant is the mean of smaller ranks compared to the other group. In other words, besides the median, the distribution matters.

The same results will be obtained if the study was analyzed by another non-parametric test, such as the Wilcoxon rank test. It is only when both groups are assumed to have the "same" distribution then the non-parametric test can be considered as being comparing the medians, and a statistically significant difference can be attributed to a significant difference between medians [40]. Moreover, it can also be assumed that a shift in the central location of similar distributions will move, not only medians but also means by the same amount. Thus, the non-parametric test can also be assumed as a test for the difference in means [67] and spread [68] (see Sect. 2.5.1.1).

7.5 The Role of the Statistician

7.5.1 Include the Statistician in the Research Team

"To consult the statistician after an experiment is finished is often merely to ask him to conduct a post-mortem examination. He can perhaps say what the experiment died of"—Sir Ronald Fisher (1890–1962) in the first session of the Indian Statistical Conference, Calcutta, 1938. "War is too important to be left to the generals"—The French statesman George Clemenceau (1841–1929) [69]. We, researchers, are caught between those two quotations. A common error is to limit and delay the statistical consultation till after the collection of data when it is too late. The other end of the spectrum is to confine the ship rudder to the statistician, which is too dangerous.

The research work is the primary responsibility of the researcher, and the statistician's role is to guide him to the most appropriate statistical tools necessary to plan, conduct, analyze and interpret his research. Statistics may draw the researcher's attention to a certain point but should never have the lead. Concerning the statistician, data are just numbers; for the researcher, they are the living creatures he swore to help. In order to prevent any conflict, we must include the statistician in the research team, as a valuable active member, under the leadership of the primary researcher. In addition, the research team must include a responsible for the finances, an administrator, and a secretariat. According to the type and scope of the study, the team has to include a responsible representative of every involved discipline, such as nursing, pharmacy, radiology, and pathology. The team has to design a plan, meeting schedule, data monitoring, and auditing committee (see Sect. 5.7).

7.5.2 Begin from the Beginning

The statistician has to be included in the team starting on day zero. He must share in discussing the research question formulation and participate in choosing the most appropriate design. Settling on a specific design saves the researcher time by defining the scope of the literature search. For example, suppose the researcher is about to investigate a new treatment, expecting a small difference between it and the reference treatment. The statistician can calculate a "quick" sample size, which shows that a superiority study that can put such a tiny difference into evidence will

require a large sample beyond the available resources, as pointed out by the attending person responsible for finances. Consequently, the researcher may limit his search to non-inferiority studies and, simultaneously, extends his research to studies comparing the classic treatment to placebo to calculate a suitable non-inferiority limit. The role of the statistician in guiding literature search is very important. His coming role in evaluating the outputs of the research will be fundamental, of course.

7.5.3 The Protocol is not a One-Man Show

After completing the literature search, the research team must share almost every main element of the protocol. The team has to reach a common simple language that everyone (researchers, statisticians, responsible for finances, assistants, and other team members) can understand to exchange the relevant clinical, statistical, economic, and logistic information.

Choose the Primary Outcome

The research team needs to settle upon a clinically relevant primary outcome with a good chance of being put into evidence. We have given some clues that may be helpful in this matter (see Sect. 7.1.2). Choosing a quantitative outcome with the most limited variability is advisable, or adopting a score of clinically related outcomes. Categorical clinical hard outcomes are attractive, especially when binomial such as mortality, stroke, and myocardial infarction. However, they are usually multifactorial and are hard to prove. Provided the clinical relevance, the statistician's role in choosing the primary outcome needs no further explanation.

Revise the Expected Predictors

The research team has to revise the expected predictors and remove duplicate recordings. For example, we must not simultaneously record the patient's diastolic blood pressure in mm Hg and as a qualitative variable (hypertensive or not). We have shown that duplicate recording is a source of bias in multivariable analysis for decreasing the tolerance of the variable and increasing the variance inflation factor (see Sect. 3.4.2.3). Revision should also extend to every observed variable in the study. Each variable must be recorded only once and in the most potent statistical form in the following decreasing order: continuous, discrete, ordinal, and finally, binomial. The statistician may have to give short summaries to the whole team about the data properties.

Revise the Conditions of Application of Statistical Tests

The research team has to revise the conditions of applying every statistical test used in the study. The team must indicate which test will be used to execute a particular analysis. Verifying the information before the beginning of the study limits any surprises after collecting the results. We have given multiple examples (see Sect. 7.3.2.4). It will be up to the statistician to explain the required statistical knowledge to all team members in a language they can all understand.

Revise Randomization, Concealment, Stratification, and Blindness

The whole research team is usually involved in implementing those procedures. Hence, they must discuss the details and partition every member's duty and responsibility (see Sects. 5.4.2 and 5.4.3). Rehearsing a complete set of those procedures under the direct supervision of the main researcher and the statistician is the only way to detect the possible sources of bias.

Calculate Sample Size

We have specified a whole chapter on sample size calculation, and we hope we have covered some common study types and designs (see Chap. 4). Although we provided the formula, detailed examples, and links to power software and online calculators, we advise the young researchers to go easy on calculations. We encourage them to compare the results given by different calculators; they should be nearly the same. They must revise their preliminary calculations with more experienced colleagues and, of course, the statistician. The team has to discuss the advantages and disadvantages of repeated measures (see Sects. 4.12.1.2 and 4.12.2.2), subgroup analysis (see Sect. 4.1.4.2), and performing an intermediate analysis (see Sect. 4.1.4.3). Each point has to be discussed from the clinical, statistical, and financial points of view to decide whether it merits being included in sample size calculation or not? The advantage of using power software, such as G*power, is to display a complete scene of probabilities, allowing the researcher to participate in creating his sample size. The role of the statistician is crucial to warn against possible drifts.

7.5.4 Meeting Mid-Way

A momentous meeting occasion(s) is usually arranged in the middle of the study to ensure that the study is going on as pre-planned, re-evaluate the study design, or re-calculate the sample size if necessary. It may end by stopping the trial for futility. The reader can refer to chapter four for more details on the types of interim analysis (see Sect. 4.1.4.3).

7.5.5 Data Management

Once data collection is complete, the research team has to meet to review the spreadsheet. Incomplete data may need to be reassessed in the original patient files or contact the patients or their treating physicians whenever possible. Aberrant data must be checked for mistyping, measurement, or recording errors. As shown before, missing data have to be counted and analyzed (see Sect. 7.2.3.2). The team has to decide whether they can be removed or replaced (see Sect. 7.2.3.4). If normality is required for a particular analysis, data can be verified for normality and transformed if necessary (see Sect. 7.2.4). Transformation usually involves a scale change, such as using the logarithmic value. The team has to revise the final plan of statistical analysis. The role of the statistician is crucial in every one of those procedures.

7.5.6 Statistical Analysis

Although this is usually the only meeting that every researcher is keen to attend with his statistician, a considerable loss would be to focus on exchanging numbers rather than the proper interpretation of each result.

- The team has to start by reviewing the global history of the research and decide whether they managed to conduct it properly, as designed or not. There will always be some flaws and mistakes, but the team must answer the main question: can they still conclude on the primary outcome and to what extent (see Sect. 7.4.4.1)?
- The next step is to review the main and the secondary outcomes and decide on the tables and figures, knowing that for every statistical analysis, there is a most suitable figure. The statistician will be of great help in this matter.
- Following the correct interpretation, the most delicate point would be how to express each piece of information easily but correctly, especially in the discussion section. For example, if the primary outcome is expressed in odds ratio, it would be easier for the reader to have it in proportion rather than as odds. We have previously shown how to exchange the odds and the risk "Eq. 1.23" or directly interpret the odds as a proportion in case of low prevalence (see Sect. 1.8.2).
- Finally, the team has to discuss the points of strength and the study limitations. The statistician has to display any point of weakness in the analysis. It is up to the team to decide whether those points merit being mentioned in the manuscript. It is up to the statistician to choose the appropriate wording.

7.5.7 Publication

The research team, including the statistician, has to review the manuscript before being submitted to a publisher. The statistician will be responsible for reviewing the statistical analysis section and all reported data throughout the manuscript. He is also expected to revise the interpretation and conclusion and to suggest rephrasing if required. Finally, the statistician will be needed to reply to statistical comments raised by the reviewers or the judiciary committee members.

In conclusion: As statistics is not external to medicine but rather an integral fundamental part, the statistician must be an omnipresent valuable member of every serious research team.

References

1. Anker SD, Schroeder S, Atar D, Bax JJ, Ceconi C, Cowie MR, et al. Traditional and new composite endpoints in heart failure clinical trials: facilitating comprehensive efficacy assessments and improving trial efficiency. Eur J Heart Fail. 2016;18(5):482–9. https://doi.org/10.1002/ejhf.516.
2. Choi BG, Rha S-W, Yoon SG, Choi CU, Lee MW, Kim SW. Association of major adverse cardiac events up to 5 years in patients with chest pain without significant coronary artery disease in the Korean population. JAHA. 2019;8:e010541. https://doi.org/10.1161/JAHA.118.010541.
3. Campbell MJ, Julious SD, Altman G. Estimating sample sizes for binary, ordered categorical, and continuous outcomes in two group comparisons. BMJ. 1995;311:1145. https://doi.org/10.1136/bmj.311.7013.1145.
4. Rollin B. Inferences for proportions: comparing two independent samples. In: Department of statistics. Faculty of Science. The University of British Columbia. https://www.stat.ubc.ca/~rollin/stats/ssize/index.html. Accessed 7 Mar 2022.
5. Confidence interval for the difference between proportions calculator. In: Math cracker. 2021 https://mathcracker.com/confidence-interval-for-the-difference-between-proportions-calculator#results. Accessed 8 March 2022.
6. Sn G, Berlin JA. The use of predicted confidence intervals when planning experiments and the misuse

of power when interpreting results. Ann Intern Med. 1994;121:200–6. https://doi.org/10.7326/0003-4819-121-3-199408010-00008.

7. Bristol DR. Sample sizes for constructing confidence intervals and testing hypotheses. Stat Med. 1989;8:803–11. https://doi.org/10.1002/sim.4780080705.

8. Borm GF, Fransen J, Lemmens AJG. A simple sample size formula for analysis of covariance in randomized clinical trials. J Clin Epidemiol. 2007; 60:1234–8. https://doi.org/10.1016/j.jclinepi.2007.02.006.

9. Rusticus SA, Lovato CY. Impact of sample size and variability on the power and type I error rates of equivalence tests: a simulation study. PARE. 2014; 19:11. https://doi.org/10.7275/4s9m-4e81.

10. Statistics calculators. In: Social science statistics 2018. https://www.socscistatistics.com/tests/. Accessed 27 Oct 2021.

11. Jakobsen JC, Ovesen C, Winkel P, Hilden J, Gluud Ch, Wetterslev J. Power estimations for non-primary outcomes in randomised clinical trials. BMJ Open 2019;9:e027092. https://doi.org/10.1136/bmjopen-2018-027092.

12. Gordon Lan KK, DeMets DL. Discrete sequential boundaries for clinical trials. Biometrika. 1983; 70:659–63. https://doi.org/10.2307/2336502.

13. Hawkins DM. Identification of outliers. 1st ed. London: Chapman & Hall; 1980.

14. Bland M. An Introduction to Medical Statistics. 4th ed. New York: Oxford University Press; 2015.

15. Schafer JL. Multiple imputation: a primer. Statistical methods in medical research. 1999;8(1):3–15. https://doi.org/10.1177/2F096228029900800102.

16. Sterne JAC, et al. Multiple imputation for missing data in epidemiological and clinical research: potential and pitfalls. BMJ. 2009;338:b2393. https://doi.org/10.1136/bmj.b2393.

17. Templeton GF. A two-step approach for transforming continuous variables to normal: implications and recommendations for IS research. Commun Assoc Inf Syst. 2011;28:41–58. https://doi.org/10.17705/1CAIS.02804.

18. Jamovi. Stats.Open.Now. Version 2.2.5 for macOS. 2020. https://www.jamovi.org/download.html. Accessed 13 Mar 2022.

19. JASP a fresh way to do statistics. JASP 0.16.2 for macOS. 2018. https://jasp-stats.org/download/. Accessed 5 Apr 2022.

20. OpenMeta[Analyst]. Completely open-source, cross-platform software for advanced meta-analysis. Open MetaAnalyst for Sierra (10.12). http://www.cebm.brown.edu/openmeta/download.html. Accessed Jul 2021.

21. Faul F, Erdfelder E, Lang A-G, Buchner A. G*power 3.1.9.3. Statistical power analysis for MAC and Windows. Heinrich Heine Dusseldorf University, 2009. https://www.psychologie.hhu.de/arbeitsgruppen/allgemeine-psychologie-und-arbeitspsychologie/gpower.html. Accessed March 2022.

22. Viechtbauer W. Conducting meta-analyses in R with the metafor package. J Stat Softw. 2010;36(3):1–48. https://doi.org/10.18637/jss.v036.i03.

23. Kohn MA, Senyak J. Sample Size Calculators [website]. UCSF CTSI. 20 December 2021. https://www.sample-size.net/.Accessed 07 March 2022.

24. Sergeant, ESG. Epitools Epidemiological Calculators. Ausvet. https://epitools.ausvet.com.au/sample size?page=SampleSize (2018). Accessed 7 March 2022.

25. HyLown Consulting LLC, Atlanta, GA. Overview of power and sample size.com calculators. 2013–2021. http://powerandsamplesize.com/Calculators/. Accessed March 2022.

26. Lowry, R. VassarStats: Website for statistical computation. 1998. http://vassarstats.net/. Accessed 23 Oct 2021.

27. MedCalc software Lt. SciStat.com online; (2021). https://www.scistat.com. Accessed 9 Oct 2021.

28. Schwartz D. Méthodes statistiques a l'usage des médecins et des biologistes. 3rd ed. Paris: Médecines-Sciences Flammarion; 1969. http://bdsp-ehesp.inist.fr/vibad/index.php?action=getRecordDetail&idt=194892.

29. The equator network. Centre for Statistics in Medicine (CSM), NDORMS, University of Oxford. https://www.equator-network.org. Accessed 25 June 2022.

30. Altman DG, Bland JM. How to obtain the confidence interval from a P value. BMJ. 2011;343: d2090. https://doi.org/10.1136/bmj.d2090.

31. Altman DG, Bland JM. How to obtain the P value from a confidence interval. BMJ. 2011;343: d2304. https://doi.org/10.1136/bmj.d2304.

32. Hassouna A, Allam H, Awad A, Hassaballah F. Standard versus low-level anticoagulation combined to low-dose dipyridamole after mitral valve replacement. Cardiovasc Surg. 2000;8(6):491–8. https://doi.org/10.1016/S0967-2109(00)00069-7.

33. Pocock SJ. Clinical trials: a practical approach. 6th ed. Chichester: Wiley; 2013.

34. Hirji KF, Fagerland MW. Outcome based subgroup analysis: a neglected concern. Trials. 2009;10:33. https://doi.org/10.1186/1745-6215-10-33.

35. Rochon J. Issues in adjusting for covariates arising postrandomization in clinical trials. Drug Inf J. 1999;33:1219–28. https://doi.org/10.1177/2F009286159903300425.

36. Altman DG, Bland JM. Statistics notes: units of analysis. BMJ. 1997;314:1874. https://doi.org/10.1136/bmj.314.7098.1874.

37. Armitage P. Sequential medical trials: some comments on F.J. Anscombe's paper. JASA 1963; 58:384–7. https://doi.org/10.1080/01621459.1963.10500852.

38. Assel M, Sjoberg D, Elders A, Wang X, Huo D, Botchway A. Guidelines for reporting of statistics for clinical research in urology. BJU Int. 2019;123 (3):401–10. https://doi.org/10.1111/bju.14640.

39. CONSORT. Consort transparent reporting of trials 1993. http://www.consort-statement.org. Accessed 26 June 2022.

40. Campbell MJ, Swinscow TDV. Statistics at square one. 11th ed. Singapore: Wiley-Blackwell, BMJ books; 2009.

41. Armitage P, McPherson K, Rowe BC. Repeated significance tests on accumulative data. JRSS 1969;132:235–44. https://dokumen.tips/documents/repeated-significance-tests-on-accumulating-data.html.

42. Pocock SJ. Clinical trials: a practical approach, 1st ed. Padstow Cornwall: Wiley;1983. https://doi.org/10.1002/bimj.4710270604.

43. Haybittle JL. Repeated assessment of results in clinical trials of cancer treatment. Br J Radiol. 1971;44(526):793–7. https://doi.org/10.1259/0007-1285-44-526-793.

44. Peto R, Pike MC, Armitage P, Breslow NE, Cox DR, Howard SV, et al. Design and analysis of randomized clinical trials requiring prolonged observation of each patient. I. Introduction and design. Br J Cancer. 1976;34 (6):585–612. https://doi.org/10.1038/bjc.1977.1.

45. Frequentist Methods: O'Brien-Fleming, Pocock, Haybittle-Peto. Design and analysis of clinical trials. In: Penn State Eberly college of science 2022. https://online.stat.psu.edu/stat509/lesson/9/9.5. Accessed 2 Feb 2022.

46. Armstrong RA. When to use Bonferroni correction. Ophthalmic Physiol Opt. 2014;34:502–8.

47. Wasserstein Ronald L, Lazar NA. The ASA statement on p–values: context, process, and purpose. Am Stat. 2016;70(2):129–33. https://doi.org/10.1080/00031305.2016.1154108.

48. Altman DG, Bland JM. Absence of evidence is not evidence of absence. BMJ. 1995;311:485. https://doi.org/10.1111/opo.12131.

49. Hemming K, Javid I, Taljaard M. A review of high impact journals found that misinterpretation of non-statistically significant results from randomized trials was common. J Clin Epidemiol. 2022;145:112–20. https://doi.org/10.1016/j.jclinepi.2022.01.014.

50. Gonon F, Konsman J, Cohen D, Boraud T. Why most biomedical findings echoed by newspapers turn out to be false: the case of at- tention deficit hyperactivity disorder. PLoS ONE. 2012;7(9): e44275. https://doi.org/10.1371/journal.pone.0044275.

51. Wolfe R, Hanley J. If we're so different, why do we make overlapping? When 1 plus 1 doesn't make 2. CMAJ. 2002;166(1):65–6. PMCID: PMC99228.

52. Cumming G, Finch S. Inference by eye: confidence intervals and how to read pictures of data. Am Psychol. 2005;60(2):170–80. https://doi.org/10.1037/0003-066X.60.2.170.

53. Bland JM, Altman DG. Statistical methods for assessing agreement between two methods of clinical measurement. Lancet. 1986;327:307–10. https://doi.org/10.1016/S0140-6736(86)90837-8.

54. Lin L. A concordance correlation coefficient to evaluate reproducibility. Biometrics. 1989;45:255–68. https://doi.org/10.2307/2532051.

55. McGraw KO, Wong SP. Forming inferences about some intraclass correlation coefficients. Psychol Methods. 1996;1:30–46. https://doi.org/10.1037/1082-989X.1.1.30.

56. Laplanche A, Com-Nougue C, Flamant R. Methodes statistiques appliquées a la recherche Clinique. Paris: Flammarion-Medecine-Sciences;1987. http://bdsp-ehesp.inist.fr/vibad/index.php?action=getRecordDetail&idt=52329.

57. Student. The probable error of a mean. Biometrika. 1908;6:1–25. https://doi.org/10.2307/2331554.

58. Minitab. Minitab Statistical Software, 2022. https://www.minitab.com/en-us/products/minitab/. Accessed 26 June 2022.

59. Hanley JA, Lippman-Hand A. If nothing goes wrong, is everything alright? JAMA. 1983;259:1743–5 PMID: 6827763.

60. Egger M, Smith GD, Altman DG. Systematic review in health care. Meta-analysis in context, 2nd ed. London: BMJ publishing group;2001. https://doi.org/10.1093/ije/31.3.697.

61. Jakobsen JC, Gluud C, Winkel P, Lange T, Wetterslev J. The thresholds for statistical and clinical significance—a five-step procedure for evaluation of intervention effects in randomised clinical trials. BMC Med Res Methodol. 2014;14:34. https://doi.org/10.1186/1471-2288-14-34.

62. Levin GP, Emerson SC, Emerson SS. Adaptive clinical trial designs with pre-specified rules for modifying the sample size: understanding efficient types of adaptation. Stat Med. 2013;32:1259–75. https://doi.org/10.1002/sim.5662.

63. Turner RM, Bird SM, Higgins JP. The impact of study size on meta- analyses: examination of underpowered studies in Cochrane reviews. PLoS ONE. 2013;8: e59202. https://doi.org/10.1371/journal.pone.0059202.

64. Jackson D, Turner R. Power analysis for random-effects meta-analysis. Res Synth Methods. 2017; 8:290–302. https://doi.org/10.1002/jrsm.1240.

65. Lee PM. Statistical Tables. Department of mathematics. The University of York. 2005. https://www.york.ac.uk/depts/maths/tables/. Accessed 13 Nov 2021.

66. Dugard P. Appendix 1. Statistical tables. In: Online library Wiley. Wiley and Sons. Inc. https://doi.org/10.1002/9780470776124.app1. Accessed 12 Nov 2021.

67. Altman DG. Practical statistics for medical research, 1st ed. London: Chapman and Hall;1991. https://doi.org/10.1201/9780429258589.

68. Hart A. Mann-Whitney test is not just a test of medians: differences in spread can be important. BMJ. 2001;323:391–3. https://doi.org/10.1136/bmj.323.7309.391.

69. Ratcliffe S. Oxford essential quotations, 6th ed. Oxford University Press;2018. https://www.oxfordreference.com/view/https://doi.org/10.1093/acref/9780191866692.001.0001/acref-9780191866692. Accessed 26 June 2022.

List of Equations

Chapter 1 (Descriptive, testing hypothesis)		Number	Page
Mean of values ($\bar{x}$)	$\bar{x} = \dfrac{\sum x_i}{n}$	1.1	7
Sum of differences (example)	$\sum (x_i - \bar{x}) = (49 - 50) + (50 - 50) + (51 - 50) = 0$	1.2	8
Sum of squares (SS)	$SS = \sum (x_i - \bar{x})^2$	1.3	8
SS (example)	$SS = (49 - 50)^2 + (49 - 50)^2 + (49 - 50)^2 = 2$	1.4	8
Variance (S^2)	$S^2 = \dfrac{SS}{n-1} = \dfrac{SS}{df}$	1.5	8
Standard deviation (Sd)	$Sd = \sqrt{S^2}$	1.6	9
Standard error of mean (SEM, Se)	$Se = \sqrt{\dfrac{S^2}{n}} = \dfrac{Sd}{\sqrt{n}}$	1.7	10
Sd and Se of a proportion (p)	$Sd = \sqrt{p(1-p)} \qquad Se = \sqrt{\dfrac{p(1-p)}{n}}$	1.8	10
Z value	$Z = \dfrac{(x_i - \bar{x})}{Sd}$	1.9	13
95% confidence interval (CI) of a proportion (P_0)	$p_0 \pm 1.96 \sqrt{\dfrac{p_0(1-p_0)}{n}}$	1.10	18
95% CI of a proportion (example)	$= 0.25 \pm 1.96 \sqrt{\dfrac{(0.25 \times 0.75)}{100}} = 0.17 - 0.33$	1.11	19
95% CI of the difference between 2 means (m_d)	$m_d \pm 1.96 \sqrt{\dfrac{S_a^2}{n_a} + \dfrac{S_b^2}{n_b}} \qquad m_d \pm (t) \sqrt{\dfrac{S_a^2}{n_a} + \dfrac{S_b^2}{n_b}}$	1.12	21
95% CI of the difference between 2 means (example)	$3186 - 3210 \pm 1.96 \sqrt{\dfrac{262144}{50} + \dfrac{321489}{52}} = -236 \, to + 189 gm$	1.13	21
95% CI of the difference between 2 proportions (p_d): (example)	$p_d \pm Z \sqrt{\dfrac{p_a(1-p_a)}{n_a} + \dfrac{p_b(1-p_b)}{n_b}} = 0.30 \pm 1.96\sqrt{0.0087} = 30 \pm 18.3\%$ $= 11.7 - 48.3\%$	1.14	21
95% CI of the variance	$S^2 \pm 1.96 Se\sqrt{2}$	1.15	24
Adding and subtracting logs	$\log ab = \log a + \log b \qquad \log a - \log b = \log(a/b)$	1.16	30
Null hypothesis (unilateral study)	$H_0 : (A = B) + (A < B)$	1.17	34
Alternative hypothesis (unilateral study)	$H_1 : A > B$	1.18	34
Comparison of 2 means (Z test)	$Z = \dfrac{(\bar{x}_A - \bar{x}_B)}{Se}$	1.19	35
Z test (example)	$Z = \dfrac{(127 - 132)}{16/\sqrt{30}} = -1.71$	1.20	35
Null hypothesis (bilateral study)	$H_0 : A = B$	1,21	36
Alternative hypothesis (bilateral study)	$H_1 : A > B \, or \, A < B$	1.22	36
Chapter 1 (Outcome indices)			
Risks and Odds	$Risk = \dfrac{odds}{(1 + odds)} \qquad Odds = \dfrac{risk}{(1 - risk)}$	1.23	39
Relative risk (RR)	$The \ relative \ risk = RR = \dfrac{a/(a+b)}{c/(c+d)} = \dfrac{a/n_t}{c/n_c} = \dfrac{p_t}{P_c}$	1.24	41

(continued)

Odds ratio (OR)	$The\ Odds\ ratio = OR = \dfrac{a/b}{c/d} = \dfrac{ad}{cb}$	1.25	41
Interpretation of RR from OR and prevalence	$RR = \dfrac{OR}{(1 - P_c) + (P_c \times OR)}$	1.26	41
Interpretation of RR from OR and prevalence (example)	$RR = \dfrac{0.33}{(1 - 0.5) + (0.5 \times 0.33)} = 0.5$	1.27	41
Hazard ratio (HR)	$HR = \dfrac{H_T}{H_C} = \dfrac{New\ cases_T / Patients\ remaining\ at\ risk_T}{New\ cases_C / Patients\ remaining\ at\ risk_C}$	1.28	43
Exponential hazard	$Exponential\ hazard = H_e(<t) = 1 - e^{-\lambda t}$	1.29	46
Exponential event free hazard	$Event-free\ cumulative\ probability(S_t) = 1 - \left(1 - e^{-\lambda t}\right)$	1.30	46
Weibull model	$Weibull\ basic\ hazard = \log(h_0) + \log(\alpha) * \log(t)$	1.31	48
Se of log RR	$Se(\log RR) = \sqrt{\dfrac{1}{a} + \dfrac{1}{c} + \dfrac{1}{a+b} + \dfrac{1}{c+d}}$	1.32	51
Z value (log RR)	$Z = \dfrac{(\log RR)}{Se(\log RR)}$	1.33	51
95% CI log RR	$95\%\ CI(\log RR) = (\log RR) \pm 1.96\,Se(\log RR)$	1.34	51
95% CI of RR	$95\%CI(RR) = e^{LL95\%CI\ (\log RR)}\ to\ e^{UL95\%CI\ (\log RR)}$	1.35	51
Se of log RR (example moderate aortic stenosis: AS)	$Se(\log RR) = \sqrt{\dfrac{1}{10} + \dfrac{1}{30} + \dfrac{1}{200} + \dfrac{1}{200}} = 0.38$	1.36	52
Z value log RR (example moderate AS)	$Z = \dfrac{-1.099}{0.38} = 2.9;\quad P = 0.012$	1.37	52
95% CI log RR (example moderate AS)	$95\%\ CI(\log RR) = -1.099 \pm 1.96(0.38) = -1.84\ to\ -0.35$	1.38	52
95% CI RR (example moderate AS)	$95\%\ CI(RR) = e^{(-1.84)}\ to\ e^{(-0.35)} = 0.16\ to\ 0.7$	1.39	52
Se log OR	$Se(\log OR) = \sqrt{\dfrac{1}{a} + \dfrac{1}{b} + \dfrac{1}{c} + \dfrac{1}{d}}$	1.40	52
Z value log OR	$Z = \dfrac{(\log\ OR)}{Se(\log\ OR)}$	1.41	52
95% CI log OR	$95\%\ CI(\log\ OR) = (\log\ OR) \pm 1.96\,Se\,(\log\ OR)$	1.42	52
95% CI OR	$95\%\ CI\ (OR) = e^{LL\ 95\%\ CI\ (\log\ OR)}\ to\ e^{UL\ 95\%\ CI\ (\log\ OR)}$	1.43	52
Hazard ratio (HR)	$HR = \dfrac{S_t}{S_c}$	1.44	53
Se Log HR	$Se(\log\ HR) = \sqrt{\dfrac{1}{E_t} + \dfrac{1}{E_c}}$	1.45	53
95% CI log HR	$95\%\ CI\ (\log\ HR) = (\log\ HR) \pm 1.96\,Se\,(Log\ HR)$	1.46	53
95% CI HR	$95\%\ CI\ (HR) = e^{LL\ 95\%\ CI\ (\log\ HR)}\ to\ e^{UL\ 95\%CI\ (\log\ HR)}$	1.47	53
95% CI Absolute Risk Reduction (ARR)	$95\%\ CI\ (ARR) = ARR \pm 1.96\sqrt{\dfrac{P_t(1 - P_t)}{n_t} + \dfrac{P_c(1 - P_c)}{n_c}}$	1.48	53
95% CI ARR (example: moderate AS)	$95\%\ CI\ (ARR)moderate\ AS = -0.1 \pm 1.96\sqrt{\dfrac{0.05(0.95)}{200} + \dfrac{0.15(0.85)}{200}}$ $= -0.158\ to\ -0.042$	1.49	53
95% CI ARR (example): severe AS	$95\%\ CI(ARR)severe\ AS = -0.15 \pm 1.96\sqrt{\dfrac{0.05(0.95)}{200} + \dfrac{0.3(0.7)}{200}}$ $= -0.18\ to\ -0.32$	1.50	53
95% CI ARR (example): moderate AS, small sample	$95\%\ CI(ARR)moderate\ AS\ in\ a\ small\ sample$ $= -0.1 \pm 1.96\sqrt{\dfrac{0.05(0.95)}{10} + \dfrac{0.15(0.85)}{10}} = -0.283\ to + 0.083$	1.51	54
Number Needed to Treat: NNT (meta-analysis)	$NNT = \dfrac{1}{(RR \times P_c)}$	1.52	55
NNT benefit (NNTB)	$NNT_{Benefit} = \dfrac{1 - P_c(1 - OR)}{P_c(1 - OR) \times (1 - P_c)}$	1.53	55
NNT harm (NNTH)	$NNT_{Harm} = \dfrac{P_c(OR - 1) + 1}{P_c(OR - 1) \times (1 - P_c)}$	1.54	55
NNT (time-to-event)	$NNT(t_2) = NNT(t_1) \times \dfrac{t_1}{t_2}$	1.55	55
ARR time to event	$ARR = S_t - S_c$	1.56	56
Se ARR	$Se(ARR) = \sqrt{(S_t^2) + (S_C^2)}$	1.57	56

(continued)

Se ARR (variant)	$Se(ARR) = \sqrt{\dfrac{S_t^2(1-S_t)}{n_t} + \dfrac{S_c^2(1-S_c)}{n_c}}$	1.58	56
95% CI ARR	$95\% \, CI(ARR) = ARR \pm 1.96 Se(ARR)$	1.59	56
95% CI NNT	$95\% \, CI(NNT) = \dfrac{1}{UL95\% \, CI(ARR)} \, to \, \dfrac{1}{LL95\% \, CI(ARR)}$	1.60	56
NNT, time to event	$NNT = \dfrac{1}{(S_c)^{HR} - (S_c)}$	1.61	56
95% CI of NNT, time to event	$NNT = \dfrac{1}{(S_c)^{UL \, of \, the \, 95\% \, CI \, of \, HR} - (S_c)} \, to \, \dfrac{1}{(S_c)^{LL \, of \, the \, 95\% \, CI \, of \, HR} - (S_c)}$	1.62	56
Chapter 1 (Diagnostic accuracy)			
Positive predictive value (PPV)	$PPV = \dfrac{SeP}{SeP + (1-Sp)(1-P)}$	1.63	64
Negative predictive value (NPV)	$NPV = \dfrac{Sp(1-P)}{Sp(1-P) + P(1-Se)}$	1.64	64
One-minus specificity (1-Sp) is false positive (FP)	$(1-Sp) = 1 - \dfrac{TN}{(TN+FP)} = \dfrac{(TN+FP)}{(TN+FP)} - \dfrac{TN}{(TN+FP)} = FP$	1.65	66
One-minus sensitivity (1-Sn) is false negative (FN)	$1 - Sn = \dfrac{TP+FN}{TP+FN} - \dfrac{TP}{TP+FN} = FN$	1.66	67
Se Log likelihood ratio (Log LR)	$Se(\log LR) = \sqrt{\dfrac{1-p_1}{n_1 \times p_1} + \dfrac{1-p_2}{n_2 \times p_2}}$	1.67	71
95% CI Log LR	$95\% \, CI(\log LR) = \log LR \pm 1.96 \, Se \log LR$	1.68	71
95% CI LR	$95\% \, CI \, (LR) = e^{LL \, 95\% \, CI \, (\log LR)} \, to \, e^{UL \, 95\% \, CI \, (\log LR)}$	1.69	71
Z value of LR	$Z \, for \, LR = \dfrac{Log \, LR}{Log \, Se}$	1.70	71
P value of LR	$P \, value = \text{Exp}^{(-0.717 \times Z - 0.416 \times Z^2)}$	1.71	71
Diagnostic odds ratio (DOR)	$DOR = \dfrac{TP/FN}{FP/TN}$	1.72	72
DOR (variant)	$DOR = \dfrac{Sn/(1-Sn)}{(1-Sp)/Sp}$	1.73	72
DOR (variant)	$DOR = \dfrac{positive \, LR}{negative \, LR}$	1.74	72
SE log DOR	$Se \, (\log DOR) = \sqrt{\dfrac{1}{TP} + \dfrac{1}{FP} + \dfrac{1}{TN} + \dfrac{1}{FN}}$	1.75	72
Z value of log DOR	$Z = \dfrac{(\log DOR)}{Se(\log DOR)}$	1.76	72
95% CI log DOR	$95\% \, CI(\log DOR) = \log DOR \pm 1.96 \, Se \log DOR$	1.77	72
95% CI DOR	$95\% \, CI(DOR) = e^{LL \, 95\% \, CI \, (\log DOR)} \, to \, e^{UL \, 95\% \, CI \, (\log DOR)}$	1.78	72
DOR (example)	$DOR = \dfrac{80/20}{20/380} = \dfrac{0.8/(1-0.8)}{(1-0.95)/0.95} = \dfrac{4}{0.053} = 76$	1.79	73
Se log DOR (example)	$Se(\log DOR) = \sqrt{\dfrac{1}{80} + \dfrac{1}{20} + \dfrac{1}{380} + \dfrac{1}{20}} = 0.339$	1.80	73
Z value of log DOR (example)	$Z = \dfrac{(\log DOR)}{(Se \log DOR)} = \dfrac{4.33}{0.339} = 12.77; \quad P < 0.001$	1.81	73
95% CI log DOR (example)	$95\% \, CI(\log 76) = 4.33 \pm 1.96(0.339) = 3.65 \, to \, 5$	1.82	73
95% CI DOR (example)	$95\% \, CI(DOR) = e^{3.65} \, to \, e^5 = 39 - 148$	1.83	73
FP = (1-Sp)	$(1-Sp) = 1 - \dfrac{TN}{(TN+FP)} = \dfrac{(TN+FP)}{(TN+FP)} - \dfrac{TN}{(TN+FP)} = FP$	1.84	73
Z value of area under the receiver operating curve (AUC - ROC)	$Z = \dfrac{(AUC - 0.5)}{Se}$	1.85	78
The slope (m) for ROC	$m = \dfrac{FP_c - TN_c}{FN_c - TP_c} \times \dfrac{1-P}{P}$	1.86	79
Standardized partial AUC (AUCp)	$AUCps = 0.5\left(1 + \dfrac{AUCp - AUCp_{min}}{AUCp_{max} - AUCp_{min}}\right)$	1.87	81
Weighted comparison	$WC = \Delta Sn + \left(\dfrac{1-P}{P}\right) \times relative \, cost \left(\dfrac{FP}{TP}\right) \times \Delta Sp$	1.88	84
Chapter 2 (Comparison of 2 proportions)			
Chi-square equation	$\chi^2 = \sum \dfrac{(O_i - E_i)^2}{E_i}$	2.1	98

(continued)

Chi-square (example 1)	$$\chi^2 = \sum \frac{(O_i - E_i)^2}{E_i}$$ $$= \frac{(40 - 25)^2}{25} + \frac{(10 - 25)^2}{25} + \frac{(60 - 75)^2}{75} + \frac{(90 - 75)^2}{75} = 24$$	2.2	99
Chi-square (example 2)	$$\chi^2 = \sum \frac{(O_i - E_i)^2}{E_i}$$ $$= \frac{(28 - 24.5)^2}{24.5} + \frac{(2 - 5.5)^2}{5.5} + \frac{(17 - 20.5)^2}{20.5} + \frac{(8 - 4.5)^2}{4.1}$$ $$= 5.88$$	2.3	102
Chi-square (example 3)	$$\chi^2 = \sum \frac{(O_i - E_i)^2}{E_i}$$ $$= \frac{(19 - 16.5)^2}{16.5} + \frac{(1 - 3.5)^2}{3.5} + \frac{(14 - 16.5)^2}{16.5} + \frac{(6 - 3.5)^2}{3.5}$$ $$= 4.3$$	2.4	103
Yates's chi-square	$$\chi_C^2 = \sum \frac{(O_i - E_i - \mathbf{0.5})^2}{E_i}$$	2.5	103
Yates's chi-square (example)	$$\chi_C^2 = \frac{(16 - 19.1 - \mathbf{0.5})^2}{19.1} + \frac{(9 - 5.9 - \mathbf{0.5})^2}{5.9} + \frac{(26 - 22.9 - \mathbf{0.5})^2}{22.9}$$ $$+ \frac{(4 - 7.1 - \mathbf{0.5})^2}{7.1} = 2.7$$	2.6	103
Chi-square for trend	$$\chi_{trend}^2 = \frac{(\sum r_i x_i - R\bar{x})^2}{p(1 - p)(\sum n_i x_i^2 - N\bar{x}^2)}$$	2.7	105
Chi-square for trend (example)	$$X_{trend}^2 = \frac{(51 - 17 \times 2.5)^2}{0.425(0.575) \ (300 - 40 \times 2.5^2)} = 5.91$$	2.8	105
Fisher's exact test	$$P = \frac{R_1! + R_2! + S_1! + S_2!}{a! + b! + c! + d! + N!}$$	2.9	108
Fisher's exact (example)	$$P = \frac{35! + 5! + 21! + 19!}{17! + 18! + 4! + 1! + 40!} + \frac{35! + 5! + 21! + 19!!}{16! + 19! + 5! + 0! + 40!} = 0.173 + 0.031$$ $$= 0.204$$	2.10	108
McNemar test	$$\chi^2 = \sum \frac{(O_i - E_i)^2}{E_i} = \frac{\left(a - \frac{a+b}{2}\right)^2}{\frac{a+b}{2}} + \frac{\left(b - \frac{a+b}{2}\right)^2}{\frac{a+b}{2}} = \frac{(a-b)^2}{(a+b)}$$	2.11	109
McNemar-Bowker test	$$\chi^2 = \frac{\sum (a_i - b_i)^2}{\sum (a_i + b_i)}$$	2.12	111
McNemar-Bowker test (example)	$$B = \frac{(15 - 9)^2 + (7 - 0)^2 + (17 - 11)^2}{(15 + 9) + (7 + 0) + (17 + 11)} = 9.8$$	2.13	111
Cochran Q test	$$Q = k(1 - k) \frac{\sum_{j=1}^{k} \left(x_j - \frac{N}{k}\right)^2}{\sum_{i=1}^{b} x_i(k - x_i)}$$	2.14	112
Chapter 2 (Comparison of 2 means)			
95% CI of mean for small sample size (Student)	95% CI of mean $(\bar{x}) = \bar{x} \pm (t)Se$	2.15	117
Student test (one sample)	$$t = \frac{(\bar{x} - \mu)}{Se}$$	2.16	117
95% CI of the difference (Student)	95% CI of the difference $= \overline{x_d} \pm t \ Se = -23.2 \pm 2.093 \times 3.1 = -29.7 \ to \ -16.7 \ mm \ Hg$	2.17	118
Unpaired Student test	$$t = \frac{(\bar{x}_a - \bar{x}_b)}{Se}$$	2.18	118
S^2 pooled	$$S_{pooled}^2 = \frac{(n_a - 1)S_a^2 + (n_b - 1)S_b^2}{n_a + n_b - 2} = \frac{(31 - 1)\mathbf{11.5^2} + (33 - 1)\mathbf{7^2}}{\mathbf{31 + 33 - 2}} = 89.3$$	2.19	119
Se pooled	$$Se_{pooled} = \sqrt{\frac{Se_{pooled}^2}{n_a} + \frac{Se_{pooled}^2}{n_b}} = \sqrt{\frac{89.3}{31} + \frac{89.3}{33}} = 2.37$$	2.20	119
t-value	$$t = \frac{(\bar{x}_a - \bar{x}_b)}{Se_{pooled}} = \frac{(94.8 - 60.6)}{2.37} = 14.45$$	2.21	119
Se difference	$$Se_{difference} = \sqrt{\frac{Se_a^2}{n_a} + \frac{Se_b^2}{n_b}} = \sqrt{\frac{11.5^2}{31} + \frac{7^2}{33}} = 2.4$$	2.22	119
df revised	$$df = \frac{(S_a^2/n_a + S_b^2/n_b)^2}{(S_a^2/n_a)^2/(n_a - 1) + (S_b^2/n_b)^2/(n_b - 1)}$$	2.23	119
Cohens ds	$$Cohen \ ds = t\sqrt{\frac{1}{n_a} + \frac{1}{n_b}} = 14.234 \times 0.25 = 3.56$$	2.24	120

(continued)

Hedges g	$Hedges\ g = Cohen\ ds\left(1 - \dfrac{3}{4(n_a + n_b) - 9}\right) = 3.5$	2.25	120
Paired t test	$t = \dfrac{(\overline{x}_{Di} - 0)}{Se_{Di}} = \dfrac{\overline{x}_{Di}}{Se_{Di}}$	2.26	121
Chapter 2 (Comparison of multiple means, post-hoc tests, repeated measures)			
Analysis of variance (ANOVA): total sum of squares (SS)	$SS_{total} = (2-4)^2 + (3-4)^2 + (1-4)^2 + (6-4)^2 + (7-4)^2 + (5-4)^2 = 28$	2.27	126
SS within group a	$SS_{within\ a} = (1-2)^2 + (2-2)^2 + (3-2)^2 = 2$	2.28	126
SS within group b	$SS_{within\ b} = (5-6)^2 + (6-6)^2 + (7-6)^2 = 2$	2.29	126
SS within both groups (a + b)	$SS_{within-groups} = 2 + 2 = 4$	2.30	126
SS within group a	$SS_{within\ a} = (1-2)^2 + (2-2)^2 + (3-2)^2 = 2$	2.31	127
SS within group c	$SS_{within\ c} = (9-10)^2 + (10-10)^2 + (11-10)^2 = 2$	2.32	127
SS within both groups (a + c)	$SS_{within-groups} = 2 + 2 = 4$	2.33	127
SS between group a and group b	$SS_{total\ ab} - SS_{within-groups\ ab} = SS_{between-groups\ ab} = 28 - 4 = 24$	2.34	127
SS between group a and group c	$SS_{total\ ac} - SS_{within-groups\ ac} = SS_{between-groups\ ac} = 100 - 4 = 96$	2.35	127
Variance between group a and group b	$Variance_{between-groups\ ab} = 24/1 = 24$	2.36	127
Variance within group a and group b	$Variance_{within-groups\ ab} = 4/4 = 1$	2.37	127
Variance between group a and group c	$Variance_{between-groups\ ac} = 96/1 = 96$	2.38	127
Variance within group a and group c	$Variance_{within-groups\ ab} = 4/4 = 1$	2.39	127
One-way ANOVA: total SS	$SS_{total} = \sum \dfrac{(x - \overline{x})^2}{N - 1} = \sum x^2 - TG^2/N$	2.40	128
One-way ANOVA: SS within groups	$SS_{within-groups} = \sum x^2 - \sum \left(\dfrac{Ti^2}{n_i}\right)$	2.41	128
One-way ANOVA: SS between groups	$SS_{between-groups} = \sum \left(\dfrac{Ti^2}{n_i}\right) - TG^2/N$	2.42	128
One-way ANOVA: F ratio	$F\ ratio = \dfrac{SS_{between-groups}/df_{between-groups}}{SS_{within-groups}/df_{within-groups}} = \dfrac{Effect\ variance}{Residual\ variance}$	2.43	129
Welch ANOVA, weighted means	$W_K x_K = \dfrac{n x_K}{S^2}$	2.44	130
Welch ANOVA grand mean	$X_{Welch\ grand} = \dfrac{\sum W_K x_K}{\sum W_K}$	2.45	130
Welch ANOVA: Variance (MS)	$MS_{Welch} = \dfrac{SS_{welch\ M}}{df} = \dfrac{\sum W_K \left(x_K - X_{Welch\ grand}\right)}{K - 1}$	2.46	131
Welch ANOVA: Variance (λ)	$\lambda = \dfrac{3 \sum \dfrac{\left(1 - \dfrac{W_K}{\sum W_K}\right)^2}{n_K - 1}}{K^2 - 1}$	2.47	131
Welch ANOVA: F ratio	$F_{Welch} = \dfrac{MS_{Welch\ M}}{1 + 2\lambda(K - 2)/3}$	2.48	131
Post-hoc tests: Tukey HSD	$HSD = q_{crit}\sqrt{\dfrac{MS_w}{n_k}}$	2.49	134
Post-hoc tests: Games Howell test	$GH = q_{crit}\sqrt{\dfrac{1}{2} \times \left(\dfrac{S_a^2}{n_a} + \dfrac{S_b^2}{n_b}\right)}$	2.50	134
Post-hoc tests: Dunnett test	$D_{Dunnett} = t_{Dunnett}\sqrt{\dfrac{2\ MS_w}{n_k}}$	2.51	135
Post-hoc tests: Bonferroni basis	$1 - \alpha^K = 1^K + \alpha^K - (k \times 1 \times \alpha) \approx 1 - \alpha^K$	2.52	135
Post-hoc tests: FEWER	$FWER < 1 - (1 - \alpha)^c$	2.53	136
Post-hoc tests: HB test	$HB = \dfrac{target \propto (usually\ 0.05)}{n_C - rank\ of\ pairs(by\ degree\ of\ significance + 1)}$	2.54	136
One-way RMANOVA: MS error	$MS_{error} = MS_{within\ groups} - MS_{subjects}$	2.55	139
One-way RMANOVA: F ratio	$F_{RM-ANOVA} = \dfrac{MS_{repeated\ measures}}{MS_{error}}$	2.56	139
One-way RMANOVA: SS repeated measures (example)	$SS_{repeated\ measures} = \sum n_i(\overline{x}_i - \overline{x})^2$ $= 10\left[(3.9 - 5.3)^2 + (3.9 - 5.3)^2 + (3.9 - 5.3)^2\right] = 42.1$	2.57	140

(continued)

One-way RMANOVA: SS within-groups	$SS_{within-groups} = \sum_1 (x_i - \bar{x}_1)^2 + \sum_2 (x_i - \bar{x}_2)^2 + \cdots + \sum_k (x_i - \bar{x}_k)^2$	2.58	140
One-way RMANOVA: SS within-groups (example)	$SS_{within-groups} = (5 - 3.9)^2 + (2 - 3.9)^2 + (3 - 3.9)^2 + (5 - 3.9)^2$ $+ (3 - 3.9)^2 + (5 - 3.9)^2 + (4 - 3.9)^2 + (5 - 3.9)^2$ $+ (4 - 3.9)^2 + (3 - 3.9)^2 + (5 - 5.3)^2 + (7 - 5.3)^2$ $+ (4 - 5.3)^2 + (7 - 5.3)^2 + (5 - 5.3)^2 + (6 - 5.3)^2$ $+ (5 - 5.3)^2 + (5 - 5.3)^2 + (6 - 5.3)^2 + (3 - 5.3)^2$ $+ (8 - 6.8)^2 + (7 - 6.8)^2 + (7 - 6.8)^2 + (7 - 6.8)^2$ $+ (6 - 6.8)^2 + (6 - 6.8)^2 + (8 - 6.8)^2 + (9 - 6.8)^2$ $+ (8 - 6.8)^2 + (2 - 6.8)^2 = 58.6$	2.59	140
One-way RMANOVA: SS subjects	$SS_{subjects} = k. \sum (\bar{x}_i - \bar{x})^2$	2.60	140
One-way RMANOVA: SS subjects (example)	$SS_{subjects} = 3 \Big[(6 - 5.3)^2 + (5.3 - 5.3)^2 + (4.6 - 5.3)^2 + (6.3 - 5.3)^2$ $+ (4.6 - 5.3)^2 + (5.7 - 5.3)^2 + (5.7 - 5.3)^2 + (6.3 - 5.3)^2$ $+ (6.3 - 5.3)^2 + (2.6 - 5.3)^2 \Big] = 33.3$	2.61	140
One-way RMANOVA: SS error (example)	$SS_{error} = SS_{within-groups} - SS_{subjects} = 58.6 - 33.3 = 25.7$	2.62	140
One-way RMANOVA: MS repeated measures (example)	$MS_{repeated\ measures} = \dfrac{SS_{repeated\ measures}}{df_{repeated\ measures}} = \dfrac{42.1}{2} = 21$	2.63	140
One-way RMANOVA: MS error (example)	$MS_{error} = \dfrac{SS_{error}}{df_{error}} = \dfrac{25.3}{18} = 1.4$	2.64	140
One-way RMANOVA: F ratio (example)	$F_{(2,18)} = \dfrac{MS_{repeated\ measures}}{MS_{error}} = \dfrac{21}{1.4} = 14.98; P < 0.001$	2.65	141
Chapter 2 (Non-parametric tests)			
Mann and Whitney test	$Z = \dfrac{U_{xy} - U_0}{Sd_u} = \dfrac{U_{xy} - (n_1 \times n_2)/2}{\sqrt{n_1 \times n_2(n+1)/12}}$	2.66	144
Mann and Whitney test (example)	$Z = \dfrac{31 - (10 \times 10)/2}{\sqrt{10 \times 10(20+1)/12}} = 1.44$	2.67	144
95% CI of median	$95\% \ CI \ of \ rank = \dfrac{n}{2} \pm 1.96 \dfrac{\sqrt{n}}{2}$	2.68	146
95% CI of median (example)	$95\% \ CI \ of \ rank = \dfrac{10}{2} \pm 1.96 \dfrac{\sqrt{10}}{2} = 5 \pm 3.1 = 1.88 \ to \ 8.1 \approx 2, 9$	2.69	146
95% CI of the difference between 2 medians (unpaired)	$K_{unpaired} = \dfrac{n_1 n_2}{2} \pm \left(1.96 \sqrt{\dfrac{n_1 n_2(n_1 + n_2 + 1)}{12}} \right)$	2.70	146
95% CI of the difference between 2 medians (paired)	$K_{paired} = \dfrac{n(n+1)}{4} \pm \left(1.96 \sqrt{\dfrac{n(n+1)(2n+1)}{24}} \right)$	2.71	146
95% CI of the difference between 2 medians (example unpaired)	$K_{unpaired} = \dfrac{10 \times 10}{2} - \left(1.96 \sqrt{\dfrac{10 \times 10(10 + 10 + 1)}{12}} \right) = 24$	2.72	146
Wilcoxon rank test	$Z = \dfrac{W_x - n_1(n+1)/2}{\sqrt{n_1 \times n_2(n+1)/12}}$	2.73	148
Wilcoxon sign rank test	$Z = \dfrac{P - n(n+1)/4}{\sqrt{n(n+1)(2n+1)/24}}$	2.74	149
Wilcoxon sign rank test (example)	$Z = \dfrac{32 - 8(8+1)/4}{\sqrt{8(8+1)(2 \times 8 + 1)/24}} = \dfrac{14}{7.14} = 1.96$	2.75	149
Kruskal and Wallis test	$H = \dfrac{\sum n_i \left(\dfrac{W_i}{n_i} - \dfrac{W}{n} \right)^2}{n(n+1)/12}$	2.76	151
Kruskal and Wallis test (example)	$H = \dfrac{5(14.4 - 10.5)^2 + 5(15 - 10.5)^2 + 5(8.6 - 10.5)^2 + 5(4 - 10.5)^2}{20(20+1)/12} = 11.6$	2.77	151
Freidman's test	$F_r = \dfrac{12}{nK(K+1)} \sum R_K^2 - 3n(K+1)$	2.78	153
Freidman's test (example)	$F_r = \dfrac{12}{15 \times 3(3+1)} \left(40^2 + 32.5^2 + 11^2 \right) - 3 \times 15(3 - 1) = 17.5$	2.79	153
Chapter 2 (Simple correlation and regression)			
Calculation of the covariance	$Covariance\ (x, y) = \sum (x - m_x) \dfrac{(y - m_y)}{(n - 1)}$	2.80	157

(continued)

Pearson's correlation coefficient r	$r = \dfrac{Covar(x,y)}{S_x S_y}$	2.81	157
Testing the statistical significance of r	$t = \dfrac{r\sqrt{(n-2)}}{\sqrt{1-r^2}}$	2.82	158
The normalized r (Fisher's transformation)	$z_r = \dfrac{1}{2}\log\dfrac{1+r}{1-r} = \dfrac{1}{2}\log\dfrac{1+0.89}{1-0.89} = 1.42$	2.83	159
Back transformation of log r	$r = \dfrac{e^{2z_r}-1}{e^{2z_r}+1} = \dfrac{e^{2\times2.16}-1}{e^{2\times2.16}+1} = 0.97; \dfrac{e^{2\times0.68}-1}{e^{2\times0.68}+1} = 0.56$	2.84	159
The Se of r	$Se\ r = \dfrac{r^2\sqrt{(1-r^2)}}{n-2} = \dfrac{0.79\sqrt{(1-0.79)}}{10-2} = 0.16$	2.85	159
Spearman's rank correlation coefficient rS	$r_s = 1 - \dfrac{6\sum d_i^2}{n(n^2-1)}$	2.86	161
Simple regression	$y = intercept + Po(x)$	2.87	164
The slope of regression	$Po = \dfrac{Covariance(x,y)}{Variance(x)} = \dfrac{\sum(x-m_x)(y-m_y)}{\sum(x-m_x)^2} = r\dfrac{S_y}{S_x}$	2.88	164
Coefficient beta	$Coefficient\ Beta = b\left(\dfrac{S_x}{S_y}\right)$	2.89	165
Simple regression (variant)	$\hat{y} = b_0 + b_1(x)$	2.90	165
Calculation of residuals and model fit	$(y-y_m) = (y-y_{fit}) + (y_{fit}-y_m)$	2.91	167
ANOVA	$SStotal = SSregression + SSerror$	2.92	167
The coefficient of variation and R^2	$R^2 = \dfrac{SSregression}{SStotal} = \dfrac{SStotal - SSerror}{SStotal}$	2.93	168
Testing the significance of the predictor	$t = \dfrac{P_0 - 0}{\sqrt{varianceP_0}}$	2.94	169
The variance of the slope	$Variance\ Po = \dfrac{\left(\dfrac{Sy}{Sx}\right)^2 - Po^2}{(n-2)}$	2.95	169
Calculation of beta coefficient from r	$b_1 = r\dfrac{Sd\ predictor}{Sd\ outcome}$	2.96	171
Sd of regression	$S_{regression} = \sqrt{(S_y)^2 - (P_0)^2(S_x)^2}$	2.97	171
Chapter 2 (Creation and comparison of survival curves)			
Kaplan Meier: survival probability (SP)	$SP_i = \dfrac{n_i - e_i}{n_i}$	2.98	179
Kaplan Meier: cumulative probability (CP)	$CP = \dfrac{n_0 - e_0}{n_0} \times \dfrac{n_1 - e_1}{n_1} \times \dfrac{n_2 - e_2}{n_2} \times \ldots\ldots \dfrac{n_i - e_i}{n_i}$	2.99	179
Variance of cumulative probability	$var\ CP = CP^2\ x\ \sum\left[\dfrac{e_i}{SP_i}\right]$	2.100	179
95% CI of cumulative probability	$95\%\ CI\ of\ CP = CP \pm 1.96\sqrt{var\ CP}$	2.101	179
Actuarial method: variance of cumulative probability	$var\ CP_{actuarial} = CP^2 \times \sum\left[\dfrac{(1-SP_i)}{n_i(SP_i)}\right]$	2.102	183
Log rank test: number of expected events	$E_g = (e)\dfrac{N_g}{N_T}$	2.103	185
Log rank test	$\chi^2_{log-rank} = \sum_g \dfrac{(O_g - E_g)^2}{E_g}$	2.104	187
Log rank test: multiple groups	$\chi^2 = \left[\dfrac{(O_A - E_A)^2}{E_A} + \dfrac{(O_B - E_B)^2}{E_B} + \cdots \dfrac{(O_i - E_i)^2}{E_i}\right]$	2.105	187
Wilcoxon (Gehan, Breslow) test	$\chi^2_{Gehan} = \sum \dfrac{(O_{gt} - E_{gt})^2}{R_t^2 E_{gt}}$	2.106	190
H-F test: weight calculation	$W^{pq} = St^p \times 1 - St^p$	2.107	190
Chapter 2 (Prognostic studies)			
Exclusion of reverse interaction: the Z test	$Z = \dfrac{d_1 - d_{12}}{\sqrt{\dfrac{Pa_1(1-Pa_1)}{na_1} + \dfrac{Pb_1(1-Pb_1)}{nb_1} + \dfrac{Pa_2(1-Pa_2)}{na_2} + \dfrac{Pb_2(1-Pb_2)}{nb_2}}}$	2.108	199
Exclusion of reverse interaction: Berslow-Day test	$\chi^2_{Berslow-Day} = \sum_{i=1}^{Kstrata} \dfrac{(a_i - A_i)^2}{\left(\dfrac{1}{A_i} + \dfrac{1}{B_i} + \dfrac{1}{C_i} + \dfrac{1}{D_i}\right)^{-1}}$	2.109	200
Mantel–Haenszel variance	$Var\ O_a = \dfrac{n_a\ n_b\ O(n-O)}{n^2(n-1)}$	2.110	201

(continued)

Mantel–Haenszel Chi-square	$\chi^2 = \sum \dfrac{\left(\sum O_a - \sum E_a\right)^2}{\sum \text{Var } O_a}$	2.111	202
Mantel Haenszel odds ratio	$OR_{MH} = \dfrac{\sum \left(\dfrac{ad}{n}\right)}{\sum \left(\dfrac{bc}{n}\right)} = \dfrac{\left(\dfrac{24 \times 22}{80} + \dfrac{56 \times 40}{160}\right)}{\dfrac{16 \times 18}{80} + \dfrac{24 \times 40}{160}} = 2.15$	2.112	202
95% CI of the Mantel–Haenszel odds ratio	$95\% \, CI \, OR_{MH} = OR^{1 \pm 1.96/\sqrt{Var \, OR}} = 2.15^{1 \pm 1.96/\sqrt{8.2}} = 1.27 - 3.62$	2.113	202
Mantel–Haenszel relative risk	$RR_{MH} = \dfrac{\sum \left(\dfrac{a(c+d)}{n}\right)}{\sum \left(\dfrac{c(a+b)}{n}\right)} = \dfrac{\left(\dfrac{24 \times 38}{80} + \dfrac{56 \times 64}{160}\right)}{\dfrac{16 \times 42}{80} + \dfrac{24 \times 96}{160}} = 1.48$	2.114	203
Two-way ANOVA: total SS	$SS_{total} = \sum (x - \bar{x})^2 = \sum x^2 - \dfrac{TG^2}{N}$	2.115	205
Total SS (example)	$SS_{total} = 415313 - \dfrac{3133^2}{24} = 6325.9$	2.116	205
SS between columns	$SS_c = mr \sum (\bar{x}_c - \bar{x})^2$	2.117	205
SS between columns (example)	$SS_c = 4x3 \left[(125.4 - 130.5)^2 + (135.7 - 130.5)^2 \right] = 630.4$	2.118	205
SS between rows	$SS_r = mc \sum (\bar{x}_r - \bar{x})^2$	2.119	206
SS between columns (example)	$SS_r = 4x2 [(111.9 - 130.5)^2 + (130.5 - 130.5)^2 + (149.3 - 130.5)^2] = 5587.6$	2.120	206
SS of interaction	$SS_{cr} = m \sum (\bar{x}_{irc} - \bar{x}_{ir} - \bar{x}_{ic} + \bar{x})^2$	2.121	206
SS of interaction (example)	$SS_{cr} = 4[(108 - 111.9 - 125.4 + 130.5)^2$ $+ (115.8 - 111.9 - 135.7 + 130.5)^2$ $+ (125.3 - 130.5 - 125.4 + 130.5)^2$ $+ (135.8 - 135.7 - 130.5 + 130.5)^2$ $+ (143 - 149.3 - 125.4 + 130.5)^2$ $+ (155.5 - 149.3 - 135.7 + 130.5)^2 = 22.7$	2.122	206
Model SS	$SS_{model} = SS_c + SS_r + SS_{icr}$	2.123	206
Residual SS	$SS_{residual} = SS_{total} - SS_{model}$	2.124	206
Partial correlation: the partial correlation coefficient	$r_{xy.z} = \dfrac{(r_{xy} - r_{xz} r_{yz})}{\sqrt{\left(1 - r_{xz}^2\right)\left(1 - r_{yz}^2\right)}}$	2.125	211
Significance of the partial correlation coefficient	$t = \dfrac{r\sqrt{(n-3)}}{\sqrt{1 - r^2}}$	2.126	211
Chapter 2 (Measuring agreement)			
Cohen Kappa (K)	$k = \dfrac{(P_a - P_c)}{(1 - P_c)} = \dfrac{(n_a - n_c)}{(n - n_c)}$	2.127	219
Se of Kappa	$Se_k = \sqrt{\dfrac{P_a(1 - P_a)}{n(1 - P_e)^2}}$	2.128	219
Prevalence index	$Prevalence \, index = \dfrac{(na1 - na2)}{n}$	2.129	220
Bias index	$Bias \, index = \dfrac{(nd1 - nd2)}{n}$	2.130	221
Kappa max	$k_{max} = \dfrac{(n_{am} - n_c)}{(n - n_c)}$	2.131	221
Weighted Kappa: linear weighting	$\sum W_o = (W_o \times 0) + (W_1 \times 1) + (W_2 \times 2) + \cdots (W_i \times i)$	2.132	223
Weighted Kappa (example): sum of weighted observations	$\sum W_o = (10 \times 0) + (4 \times 1) + (1 \times 2) + (6 \times 1) + (16 \times 0) + (2 \times 1) + (0 \times 2)$ $+ (3 \times 1) + (8 \times 0) = 17$	2.133	223
Weighted Kappa (example): sum of weighted expectations	$\sum W_e = (4.8 \times 0) + (6.9 \times 1) + (3.3 \times 2) + (7.7 \times 1) + (11 \times 0) + (5.3 \times 1)$ $+ (3.5 \times 2) + (5.2 \times 1) + (2.4 \times 0) = 38.6$	2.134	223
Weighted kappa: the index Kw	$k_w = 1 - \dfrac{\sum W_o}{\sum W_e}$	2.135	224
Fleiss Kappa: proportion of observed agreement	$P_i = \dfrac{(2^2 + 0^2 + 1^2) - 3}{3(3 - 1)} = 0.333$	2.136	225
Fleiss Kappa: proportion of observed agreement (the case of total agreement)	$P_I = \dfrac{(0^2 + 3^2 + 0^2) - 3}{3(3 - 1)} = 1$	2.137	226

(continued)

Fleiss Kappa: proportion of observed agreement (the case of total disagreement)	$P_I = \dfrac{(1^2 + 1^2 + 1^2) - 3}{3(3 - 1)} = 0$	2.138	226
Fleiss Kappa: proportion of observed agreement (overall)	$P_a = \sum P_i/n = (0.333 + 0.333 + 0.333 + 1 + 1 + 1 + 1 + 1 + 0.333 + 1)/10 = 0.73$	2.139	226
Fleiss Kappa: proportion of agreement due to chance per outcome	$P_J = \left(\dfrac{2 + 0 + 2 + 3 + 0 + 0 + 0 + 0 + 1 + 0}{(3 \times 10)}\right)^2 = (0.266^2) = 0.07$	2.140	226
Fleiss Kappa: proportion of agreement due to chance (overall)	$P_c = \sum P_J = (0.07 + 0.32 + 0.27) = 0.42$	2.141	226
The concordance of 2 quantitative variables (x, y)	$= (\bar{x} - \bar{y})^2 + S_x^2 + S_y^2 - 2rs_x s_y$	2.142	234
Lin's concordance correlation coefficient (Lin's CCC)	$r_c = 1 - \dfrac{(\bar{x} - \bar{y})^2 + S_x^2 + S_y^2 - 2rs_x s_y}{(\bar{x} - \bar{y})^2 + S_x^2 + S_y^2} = \dfrac{2rs_x s_y}{(\bar{x} - \bar{y})^2 + S_x^2 + S_y^2}$	2.143	234
Lin's CCC (normalized)	$r'c = \dfrac{1}{2} \log\dfrac{1 + rc}{1 - rc} = \dfrac{1}{2} \log\dfrac{1 + 0.965}{1 - 0.965} = 2.012$	2.144	234
Se of Lin's CCC	$Se(r'_c) = \sqrt{\dfrac{1}{n - 2}\left[\dfrac{(1 - r^2)r_c^2}{(1 - r_c^2)r^2} + \dfrac{2(1 - r_c)r_c^3 u^2}{(1 - r_c^2)^2 r} - \dfrac{r_c^4 u^4}{2(1 - r_c^2)r^2}\right]}$	2.145	234
95% CI of Lin's CCC	$95\% \ CI \ r'_c = r'_c \pm Z(Se \ r'_c) = 2 \pm 1.96(0.277) = 2 \pm 0.63 = 2.55 - 1.47$	2.146	234
Back transformation of log Lin's CCC	$r = \dfrac{e^{2rc'} - 1}{e^{2rc'} + 1} = \dfrac{e^{2 \times 2.55} - 1}{e^{2 \times 2.55} + 1} = 0.99; \ r = \dfrac{e^{2 \times 1.47} - 1}{e^{2 \times 1.47} + 1} = 0.89$	2.147	234
Intra-class correlation coefficient (ICC)	$ICC = \dfrac{\sigma_{between}^2}{\sigma_{between}^2 + \sigma_{within}^2}$	2.148	237
ICC: two-way mixed effect, absolute agreement, single rater or measurement	$ICC = \dfrac{MS_R - MS_E}{MS_R + (k - 1)MS_E + \dfrac{K}{n}(MS_C - MS_E)}$	2.149	239
ICC: two-way mixed effect, absolute agreement, single measurement: example on 2 instruments	$ICC = \dfrac{734.5 - 13}{734.5 + (2 - 1)13 + \dfrac{2}{15}(1.2 - 13)} = 0.967$	2.150	239
ICC: two-way mixed effect, absolute agreement, single measurement example on 3 instruments	$ICC = \dfrac{1222.4 - 23.3}{1222.4 + (3 - 1)23.3 + \dfrac{3}{15}(2880.6 - 23.3)} = 0.652$	2.151	240
ICC (3,1): two-way mixed effect, consistency, single rater or measurement	$ICC_{(3,1)} = \dfrac{MS_R - MS_E}{MS_R + (k - 1)MS_E} = \dfrac{1222.4 - 23.3}{1222.4 + (3 - 1)23.3} = 0.945$	2.152	241
Kendall W coefficient of concordance	$W = \dfrac{12 \times \sum(R_i - \bar{R})^2}{K^2(n^3 - n)}$	2.153	242
Kendall W (example)	$W = \dfrac{12 \times 1566.5}{5^2(10^3 - 10)} = 0.76$	2.154	242
Kendall W: the case of multiple ties	$W = \dfrac{12 \times \sum D^2}{m^2(n^3 - n) - mT}$	2.155	243
Testing statistical significance of Kendall W	$\chi^2 = K(n - 1)W$	2.156	243
Testing statistical significance of Kendall W in small samples	$F = \dfrac{W(K - 1)}{(1 - W)}$	2.157	243
Effect size: Spearman's correlation coefficient rS	$r_S = \dfrac{(mw - 1)}{(m - 1)}$	2.158	243
Chapter 3 Multivariable analysis			
The general multivariable equation	$G = b_0 + b_1(x_1) + b_2(x_2) + b_3(x_3) \ldots \ldots + b_i(x_i)$	3.1	248
Interaction SS	$SS_{cr} = 4[(108 - 111.9 - 125.4 + 130.5)^2$ $+ (115.8 - 111.9 - 135.7 + 130.5)^2$ $+ (143 - 149.3 - 125.4 + 130.5)^2$ $+ (155.5 - 149.3 - 135.7 + 130.5)^2 = 22.6$	3.2	253
Residual variance	$S_r^2 = S_t^2 - (1 - R^2)$	3.3	256
General multivariable equation (variant)	$G = b_0 + b_1(x_1) + b_2(x_2) + b_3(x_3) \ldots \ldots + b_i(x_i) + epsilon$	3.4	297

(continued)

Multiple linear regression equation	$y = b_0 + b_1\,x_1 + b_2\,x_2 + b_3\,x_3 \ldots + b_i\,x_i$	3.5	300
R^2 coefficient of variation	$R^2 = 1 - \dfrac{Residual\ SS}{Total\ SS} = 1 - \dfrac{3.983}{148.4} = 0.973$	3.6	311
Adjusted R^2	$Adjusted\ R^2 = 1 - \dfrac{Residual\ MS}{Total\ MS} = 1 - \dfrac{Residual\ SS/df_{resdual}}{Total\ SS/df_{total}}$ $= 1 - \dfrac{5.551/56}{148.4/59} = 0.961$	3.7	312
Multiple regression equation (example)	$ICU\ stay = 4.633 + (0.031)\,surgery\ duration$ $+ (0.00007)\,amount\ of\ blood\ loss + (0.183)\,Gender$	3.8	313
Logistic regression: the Logit	$Logit\,(P) = ln\!\left(\dfrac{P}{1-P}\right)$	3.9	316
Transforming the logit to probability	$P = \dfrac{e^{log(odds)}}{1 + e^{log(odds)}}$	3.10	319
McFadden's pseudo R^2	$R^2 = \dfrac{LL_{overall\ probability} - LL_{fit}}{LL_{overall\ probability}}$	3.11	321
The logistic regression equation	$Logit\,(P) = a + b_1 x_1 + b_2 x_2 + b_3 x_3 + \ldots . b_i x_i$	3.12	321
OR in logistic regression	$OR = e^b$	3.13	321
Calculation of probability from logistic regression	$P = \dfrac{e^{(a+bx)}}{1 + e^{(a+bx)}}$	3.14	322
Cox regression analysis equation	$h(t),(x_1, x_2, x_3, \ldots .x_m) = h_0(t) * exp^G$	3.15	332
Cox regression analysis: the outcome (G)	$G = b_1 x_1 + b_2 x_2 + b_3 x_3 + \ldots + b_m x_m$	3.16	332
Cox regression analysis equation (variant)	$h(t),(x_1, x_2, x_3, \ldots .x_m) = h_0(t) * exp^{b_1 x_1, b_2 x_2, b_3 x_3, \ldots b_m x_m}$	3.17	332
The HR in Cox regression analysis	$HR = \dfrac{h_i(t),x}{h_j(t),x} = \dfrac{h_0(t) * e^{x_i}\beta}{h_0(t) * e^{x_j}\beta} = e^{(x_i - x_j)\beta} = e^{(\Delta x)\beta}$	3.18	332
Chapter 4 (Sample size calculation: comparison of 2 means)			
Difference between 2 means	$\delta = Z_{(1-\alpha/2)}Se + Z_{(1-\beta)}Se = Se\left[Z_{(1-\alpha/2)} + Z_{(1-\beta)}\right]$	4.1	346
Difference between 2 means (variant)	$\delta = Sd\sqrt{\dfrac{2}{n}}\left[Z_{(1-\alpha/2)} + Z_{(1-\beta)}\right]$	4.2	346
Sample size per group (n): bilateral study	$n_{bilateral} = \dfrac{2\left[Z_{(1-\alpha/2)} + Z_{(1-\beta)}\right]^2}{\left(\dfrac{\delta}{Sd}\right)^2} = \dfrac{2\left[Z_{(1-\alpha/2)} + Z_{(1-\beta)}\right]^2}{d^2}$	4.3	346
Sample size per group (n): unilateral study	$n_{unilateral} = \dfrac{2\left[Z_{(1-\alpha)} + Z_{(1-\beta)}\right]^2}{\left(\dfrac{\delta}{Sd}\right)^2} = \dfrac{2\left[Z_{(1-\alpha)} + Z_{(1-\beta)}\right]^2}{d^2}$	4.4	347
The magic formula to calculate (n): bilateral study	$n_{bilateral} = \dfrac{16}{(\delta/Sd)^2} = \dfrac{16}{d^2}$	4.5	347
The magic formula to calculate (n): unilateral study	$n_{unilateral} = \dfrac{13}{(\delta/Sd)^2} = \dfrac{13}{d^2}$	4.6	347
The magic formula of (n) simplified	$n = \dfrac{M}{d^2}$	4.7	347
Cohen ds	$Cohen\ ds = \dfrac{(\mu_a - \mu_b)}{\sqrt{S^2_{pooled}}}$	4.8	349
The non-centrality parameter (ncp)	$\lambda = \dfrac{(\mu_a - \mu_b)}{\sqrt{\dfrac{S^2_a}{n_a} + \dfrac{S^2_b}{n_b}}} = d\sqrt{\dfrac{n_a \times n_b}{n_a + n_b}}$	4.9	349
Calculation total sample size (N) to compare 2 means	$N = \dfrac{\lambda^2}{f(1-f)d^2}$	4.10	349
S^2 pooled (example)	$S^2_{pooled} = \dfrac{S^2_1(n_1 - 1) + S^2_2(n_2 - 1)}{(n_1 + n_1 - 2)} = \dfrac{0.6^2(99) + 1.1^2(99)}{(198)} = 0.785$	4.11	350
Cohen ds (example)	$Cohen\ ds = \dfrac{\Delta}{\sqrt{S^2_{pooled}}} = \dfrac{(\mu_1 - \mu_2)}{\sqrt{S^2_{pooled}}} = \dfrac{(4.1 - 3.8)}{\sqrt{0.785}} = 0.339$	4.12	351
Sd of the difference (example)	$Sd(d) = \sqrt{\dfrac{n_1 + n_2}{n_1 \times n_2} + \dfrac{d^2}{2(n_1 + n_2)}} = 0.142$	4.13	351
Cohen ds (variant)	$Cohen\ ds = t\sqrt{\dfrac{1}{n1} + \dfrac{1}{n2}}$	4.14	351

(continued)

Cohen ds (variant)	$r = \dfrac{d_s}{\sqrt{d_s^2 + (N^2 - 2N)/n_1 n_2}}$	4.15	351
Hedges g	$\text{Hedges } g = \text{Cohen } ds \left(1 - \dfrac{3}{4(n_1 + n_2) - 9}\right)$	4.16	351
Hedges g (variant)	$\text{Hedges } g = \dfrac{(\mu_1 - \mu_2)}{\sqrt{\dfrac{S_1^2}{n_1} + \dfrac{S_2^2}{n_2}}}$	4.17	351
Effect size for a Mann–Whitney test: Pab (Grisson and Kim)	$\hat{P}_{ab} = \dfrac{U}{n_1 n_2} = \dfrac{31}{100} = 0.31$	4.18	352
Effect size for a Mann–Whitney test (variant) or Kruskall and Wallis test	$r = \dfrac{z}{\sqrt{N}} = \dfrac{1.44}{\sqrt{20}} = 0.89$	4.19	352
Calculation of (n) for unequal groups	$n_a = \dfrac{n}{2} \times (1 + K); \quad n_b = \dfrac{n}{2} \times \left(1 + \dfrac{1}{K}\right)$	4.20	353
The (ncp) of the input study (example)	$\lambda_{input\ study} = \dfrac{(4.1 - 3.8)}{\sqrt{\dfrac{1.1^2}{100} + \dfrac{0.6^2}{100}}} = 2.4$	4.21	355
The (ncp) of the output study (example)	$\lambda_{output\ study} = \dfrac{(4.1 - 3.8)}{\sqrt{\dfrac{1.1^2}{138} + \dfrac{0.6^2}{138}}} = 2.8$	4.22	355
Sample size per group (ni) for non-parametric quantitative data	$n_i = nW$	4.23	356
Chapter 4 (Sample size calculation: comparison of 2 proportions)			
Cohen d	$d = \dfrac{\Delta}{Sd} = \dfrac{(Pa - Pb)\sqrt{2}}{\sqrt{Pa(1 - Pb) + Pb(1 - Pa)}} = \dfrac{0.099}{0.35} = 0.28$	4.24	357
Cohen h	$\text{Cohen } h = \emptyset_a - \emptyset_b = 2\arcsin(\sqrt{Pa}) - 2\arcsin(\sqrt{Pb}) = 0.293$	4.25	357
Phi	$\varphi = \sqrt{\dfrac{\chi^2}{N}}$	4.26	357
Cramer's V	$\varphi_C = \sqrt{\dfrac{\chi^2}{N(K - 1)}}$	4.27	357
Cluster d^2	$\text{Cluster } d^2 = \dfrac{\Delta^2}{(S_W^2/m + S_C^2)}$	4.28	359
Intra-cluster correlation coefficient (ricc)	$r_{ICC} = \dfrac{S_C^2}{(S_C^2 + S_W^2)}$	4.29	359
Donner (D) cluster design effect	$D = 1 + (m - 1)r_{icc}$	4.30	359
Calculation of (n) from OR: unilateral study, equal groups	$n = \dfrac{2(z_{1-\alpha} + z_{1-\beta})^2}{(logOR)^2 p(1 - p)} = \dfrac{2(1.64 + 0.84)^2}{(1.28)0.065(1 - 0.065)} = 160\ patients$	4.31	361
Calculation of (n) from OR: unilateral study, unequal groups	$n = \dfrac{(z_{1-\alpha} + z_{1-\beta})^2}{(log\ OR)^2}\left(\dfrac{1}{k\ pA(1 - pA)} + \dfrac{1}{pB(1 - pB)}\right)$	4.32	361
Calculation of (n) from the difference between 2 proportions: unilateral study (example)	$n = \dfrac{(1.64 + 0.84)^2}{(log\ 3.6)^2}\left(\dfrac{1}{1 \times 0.1(1 - 0.1)} + \dfrac{1}{0.03(1 - 0.03)}\right) = 172$	4.33	361
Chi-square test of independence (example)	$\chi^2 = \dfrac{(9 - 7.5)^2}{7.5} + \dfrac{(6 - 7.5)^2}{7.5} + \dfrac{(6 - 6)^2}{6} + \dfrac{(6 - 6)^2}{6} + \dfrac{(3 - 4.5)^2}{4.5} + \dfrac{(6 - 4.5)^2}{4.5} = 1.6$	4.34	363
Cramer's V	$\varphi_C = \sqrt{\dfrac{\chi^2}{N(K - 1)}} = \sqrt{\dfrac{1.6}{36(2 - 1)}} = 0.21$	4.35	363
Cohen W	$\text{Cohen } w = \sqrt{\sum \dfrac{(P_o - P_E)^2}{P_E}} = \sqrt{\dfrac{X^2}{N}}$	4.36	364
Cohen W (example)	$\text{Cohen } W$ $= \sqrt{\begin{array}{c}\dfrac{(0.25 - 0.208)^2}{0.208} + \dfrac{(0.167 - 0.208)^2}{0.208} + \dfrac{(0.167 - 0.167)^2}{0.167} + \dfrac{(0.167 - 0.167)^2}{0.167} \\ + \dfrac{(0.083 - 0.125)^2}{0.125} + \dfrac{(0.167 - 0.125)^2}{0.125}\end{array}} = 0.212$	4.37	364
Cumulative OR	$\text{Cumulative } OR = \dfrac{C_1/(1 - C_1)}{C_2/(1 - C_2)}$	4.38	364
Calculation of (n) from cumulative OR	$n = \dfrac{3M}{(log\ OR)^2}$	4.39	365

(continued)

Calculation of total sample size (N) from Cohen W	$N = \dfrac{\lambda}{(Cohen\ W)^2} = \dfrac{9.634}{(0.212)^2} = 214$	4.40	365
Chi-square test (example)	$\chi^2 = \dfrac{(32-39)^2}{39} + \dfrac{(46-39)^2}{39} = 2.51$	4.41	366
Cohen W (example)	$Cohen\ W = \sqrt{\dfrac{X^2}{N}} = \sqrt{\dfrac{2.51}{78}} = \sqrt{\sum \dfrac{(P_o - P_E)^2}{P_E}}$ $= \sqrt{\dfrac{(0.41-0.5)^2}{0.5} + \dfrac{(0.59-0.5)^2}{0.5}} = 0.18$	4.42	366
Chapter 4 (Sample size calculation for a paired design)			
Cohen dz	$Cohen\ d_z = \dfrac{M_{diff}}{Sd_{diff}} = \dfrac{\mu_1 - \mu_2}{\sqrt{Sd_1^2 + Sd_2^2 - 2rSd_1Sd_2}} = \dfrac{4.1-3.8}{\sqrt{1.1^2 + 0.6^2 - 2(0.4) \times 1.1 \times 0.6}} = 0.294$	4.43	368
Cohen dz (variant)	$Cohen\ d_z = \dfrac{t}{\sqrt{N}} = \dfrac{Cohen\ d_s}{\sqrt{2}}$	4.44	368
Calculation of (N) from Cohen dz and the (ncp)	$N = \dfrac{\lambda^2}{(Cohen\ d_Z)^2}$	4.45	368
Effect size for Wilcoxon-Sign-Rank test: PS_{dep} (Grisson and Kim)	$PS_{dep} = \dfrac{n+}{N} = \dfrac{6}{8} = 0.75$	4.46	369
Effect size for Wilcoxon-Sign-Rank test (variant)	$r = \dfrac{z}{\sqrt{N}} = \dfrac{1.96}{\sqrt{8}} = 0.693$	4.47	369
Effect size for McNemar test (OR)	$OR = \dfrac{(P_{diff} + P_{disc})}{(P_{diff} - P_{disc})}$	4.48	371
Calculation of sample size for McNemar test, using OR	$N = \dfrac{\left\{ Z_{1-\alpha/2}(OR+1) + Z_{1-\beta}\sqrt{(OR+1)^2 - (OR-1)^2 P_{disc}} \right\}^2}{(OR-1)^2 \cdot P_{disc}}$	4.49	371
Calculation of sample size for McNemar test, using proportions	$N = \left[\dfrac{Z_{1-\alpha/2}\sqrt{P_{disc}} + Z_{1-\beta}\sqrt{P_{disc} - P_{diff}^2}}{P_{diff}} \right]^2$	4.50	371
Chapter 4 (Sample size calculation: comparison of multiple means)			
Eta-squared	$Eta\ squared\ \eta^2 = \dfrac{SS_{effect}}{SS_{total}}$	4.51	373
Partial Eta-squared	$Partial\ Eta\ squared\ \eta P^2 = \dfrac{SS_{effect}}{SS_{total} + SS_{error}}$	4.52	374
Omega-Squared	$Omega\ squared\ \omega 2 = \dfrac{SS_{effect}(df_{effect} \times MS_{error})}{SS_{total} - MS_{error}}$	4.53	374
Cohen F	$Cohen\ f = \sqrt{\dfrac{(\mu_k - \mu)^2 / k}{S_{pooled}^2}}$	4.54	374
S^2 pooled: multiple means	$S_{pooled}^2 = \dfrac{S_1^2(n_1-1) + S_2^2(n_2-1) + \cdots + S_k^2(n_k-1)}{(n_1 + n_2 + \ldots + n_k) - k}$	4.55	374
S^2 pooled: multiple means (example)	$S^2 pooled = \dfrac{1^2(4) + 0.547^2(4) + 0.547^2(4)}{(5+5+5) - 3} = 0.533$	4.56	374
Cohen F (example)	$Cohen\ f = \dfrac{\sqrt{\left[(7-4)^2 + (3.6-4)^2 + (1.4-4)^2 \right]/3}}{0.533} = 3.16$	4.57	374
Interchange of effect sizes	$Cohen\ f = \sqrt{\eta^2/(1-\eta^2)} = \sqrt{\eta P^2/(1-\eta P^2)};\ \eta^2 = f^2/(1+f^2)$	4.58	374
(ncp) in ANOVA	$\lambda = \dfrac{SS_{effect}}{MS_{error}}$	4.59	376
(ncp) of multiple means	$\lambda = \dfrac{n(\mu_k - \mu)^2}{S_{pooled}^2}$	4.60	376
(ncp) of multiple means (input study)	$\lambda = \dfrac{5\left[(7-4)^2 + (3.6-4)^2 + (1.4-4)^2 \right]}{0.533} = 149$	4.61	376
Calculation of (N) for multiple means	$N = \dfrac{\lambda}{Cohen\ f^2}$	4.62	376
(ncp) of multiple means (output study)	$\lambda = \dfrac{2\left[(7-4)^2 + (3.6-4)^2 + (1.4-4)^2 \right]}{0.533} = 59.75$	4.63	377
Chapter 4 (Sample size calculation: simple correlation and regression)			
The normalized correlation coefficient r	$C = \dfrac{1}{2}\log\left[\dfrac{(1+r)}{(1-r)} \right]$	4.64	378

(continued)

Back transformation of normalized r	$r = \dfrac{\exp 2z - 1}{\exp 2z + 1}$	4.65	378
Calculation of (N) for simple correlation	$N = \left(\dfrac{Z_{1-\alpha/2} + Z_{1-\beta}}{C}\right)^2 + 3$	4.66	378
Calculation of (N) for regression	$N = \left[\dfrac{(Z_{1-\alpha/2} + Z_{1-\beta})\,\mathrm{Sd}_{regression}}{Po\,Sd_x}\right]^2$ $= \left[\dfrac{(Z_{1-\alpha/2} + Z_{1-\beta})\sqrt{(Sd_y)^2 - (P_0)^2(Sd_x)^2}}{Po\,Sd_x}\right]^2$	4.67	380
The Sd of regression (example)	$Sd_{regression} = \sqrt{92^2 - 1.2^2 \times 37.8^2} = 80$	4.68	380
Calculation of (N) for regression (example)	$N = \left[\dfrac{(1.96 + 0.84) \times 80}{37.8 \times 1.2}\right]^2 = 25$	4.69	380
Chapter 4 (Sample size calculation: Log rank test)			
Variance of survival	$\sigma^2(\lambda_i) = \lambda_i^2\left(1 + \dfrac{e^{-\lambda_i T} - e^{-\lambda_i(T-T_0)}}{\lambda_i\,T_0}\right)^{-1}$	4.70	382
Calculation of sample size in group 2	$n_2 = \dfrac{(Z_{(1-\alpha/2)} + Z_{(1-\beta)})^2}{(\lambda_1 - \lambda_2)^2}\left[\dfrac{\sigma^2(\lambda_1)}{k} + \sigma^2(\lambda_2)\right]$	4.71	382
Variance of survival in group 2 (example)	$\sigma^2(\lambda_1) = 1^2\left(1 + \dfrac{e^{-1\times3} - e^{-1(3-1)}}{1\,x\,1}\right)^{-1} = 0.97$	4.72	382
Variance of survival in group 1 (example)	$\sigma^2(\lambda_2) = 2^2\left(1 + \dfrac{e^{-2\times3} - e^{-2(3-1)}}{1\,x\,1}\right)^{-1} = 3.94$	4.73	382
Calculation of sample size in group 2 (example)	$n_2 = \dfrac{(1.96 + 0.84)^2}{(2-1)^2}\left[\dfrac{0.97}{1} + 3.94\right] = 38.5$	4.74	382
Chapter 4 (Sample size calculation: Cox proportional hazard)			
Total number of events (ne)	$n_e = \dfrac{(Z_{(\alpha/2)} + Z_{(\beta)})^2}{P_1 P_2 (\log_{HR})^2(1 - R^2)}$	4.75	382
Total number of patients	$N = \dfrac{n_e}{Pr_e}$	4.76	383
The probability of an event in the first group	$Pr_{e1} = (1 - S_1) = (1 - e^{(-\lambda x)}) = (1 - e^{(-0.1*1)}) = (1 - 0.905) = 9.5\%$	4.77	383
The probability of an event in the second group	$Pr_{e2} = (1 - S_2) = (1 - e^{(-\lambda HR)}) = (1 - e^{(-0.1*0.5)}) = (1 - 0.951) = 4.9\%$	4.78	383
The average probability of events	$Pr_e = (0.5 \times 9.5\%) + (0.5 \times 4.9\%) = 7.2\%$	4.79	383
Calculation of the total sample size (N)	$N = \dfrac{(Z_{(1-\alpha/2)} + Z_{(1-\beta)})^2}{\text{Log } HR^2 p_1 p_2 Pr_e(1 - R^2)}$	4.80	384
Chapter 4 (Sample size calculation: logistic regression)			
Calculation of total sample size (Hsieh and colleagues): quantitative predictor variable	$N = \dfrac{(z_{(1-\alpha/2)} + z_{(1-\beta)})^2}{P_1(1 - P_1)B^2}$	4.81	385
Calculation of total sample size (Hsieh and colleagues): qualitative predictor variable	$N = \dfrac{\left(z_{(1-\alpha/2)}\sqrt{\dfrac{P(1-P)}{R}} + z_{(1-\beta)}\sqrt{P_0(1-P_0) + \dfrac{P_1(1-P_1)(1-R)}{R}}\right)^2}{(P_0 - P_1)^2(1 - R)}$	4.82	385
Modification of (N) by the addition of covariates with an R^2 effect	$N_c = \dfrac{N}{(1 - R^2)}$	4.83	386
Calculation of (n) as suggested by Campbell and colleagues	$n = \dfrac{2(z_{1-\alpha} + z_{1-\beta})^2}{(\log OR)^2 p(1-p)} = \dfrac{2(1.64 + 0.84)^2}{(2.333)^2 0.4(1 - 0.4)} = 92\ patients$	4.84	387
Chapter 4 (Sample size calculation: multiple regression)			
F^2 effect size: conditional fixed factors model	$f^2 = \dfrac{R_{Y-B}^2}{(1 - R_{Y-B}^2)}$	4.85	388
Computing R^2 from F^2	$R_{Y-B}^2 = \dfrac{f^2}{(1 + f^2)}$	4.86	388
Total sample size (N)	$N = \dfrac{\lambda}{f^2}$	4.87	388
The proportion between effect sizes of the fixed- and the random-effect models	$f^2 = \dfrac{\rho_{yx}^2}{(1 - \rho_{yx}^2)}$	4.88	389

(continued)

Chapter 4 (Sample size calculation: repeated measures)			
W^2 effect size: normally distributed repeated measures (RMANOVA)	$W^2 = \dfrac{(K-1)(F-1)}{(K-1)(F-1)nk}$	4.89	392
Kendall W effect size: repeated measures following other distribution than normal (Freidman's test)	$W = \dfrac{Fr_Q}{N(K-1)} = \dfrac{17.5}{15(3-1)} = 0.614$	4.90	396
Calculation of total sample size from normalized Kendall W (C)	$Sample\ size\ for\ Friedman's\ Test = 0.437\left(\dfrac{Z_{1-\alpha/2}+Z_{1-\beta}}{C}\right)^2 + 4$	4.91	397
Chapter 4 (Sample size calculation: non-inferiority (NIF) and equivalence (Eq.) studies)			
Superiority study: null hypothesis	$H_0 = \mu_1 - \mu_2 = 0$	4.92	397
Superiority study: alternative hypothesis	$H_1 = \mu_1 - \mu_2 \neq 0$	4.93	397
NIF study: null hypothesis	$H_0 = \mu_T - \mu_R \geq \delta$	4.94	397
NIF study: alternative hypothesis	$H_1 = \mu_T - \mu_R < \delta$	4.95	397
Eq. study: null hypothesis 1	$H_{01} = \mu_T - \mu_R \leq \delta_1$	4.96	398
Eq. study: alternative hypothesis 1	$H_{11} = \mu_T - \mu_R > \delta_1$	4.97	398
Eq. study: null hypothesis 2	$H_{02} = \mu_T - \mu_{Rr} \geq \delta_2$	4.98	398
Eq. study: alternative hypothesis 2	$H_{12} = \mu_T - \mu_R < \delta_2$	4.99	398
Eq. study: alternative hypothesis (final)	$H_1 = \delta_1 < \mu_T - \mu_R < \delta_2$	4.100	398
Chapter 4 (Sample size calculation: (NIF) and (Eq.) studies: comparison of 2 means)			
Effect size in NIF study (d_{NIF}): comparison of 2 independent means	$d_{NIF} = \dfrac{(\mu_{T_-}\mu_R) - \delta}{\sqrt{S^2_{pooled}}} = \dfrac{\varepsilon - \delta}{\sqrt{S^2_{pooled}}}$	4.101	398
Effect size in Eq. study (d_{Eq}): comparison of 2 independent means	$d_{Eq} = \dfrac{\delta - (\mu_{T_-}\mu_R)}{\sqrt{S^2_{pooled}}} = \dfrac{\delta - \varepsilon}{\sqrt{S^2_{pooled}}}$	4.102	398
Calculation of sample size per group in NIF study (n_{NIF}): comparison of 2 independent means	$n_{NIF} = 2(z_{1-\alpha} + z_{1-\beta})^2 / d^2_{NIF}$	4.103	398
Calculation of sample size per group in equivalence study (n_{Eq}): comparison of 2 independent means	$n_{Eq} = 2(z_{1-\alpha} + z_{1-\beta/2})^2 / d^2_{Eq}$	4.104	399
d_{NIF} comparison of 2 independent means (example 1):	$d_{NIF} = \dfrac{\varepsilon - \delta}{\sqrt{S^2_{pooled}}} = \dfrac{0 - 30}{60} = -0.5$	4.105	399
n_{NIF} comparison of 2 independent means (example 1)	$n_{NIF} = \dfrac{2(z_{1-\alpha} + z_{1-\beta})^2}{d^2_{NIF}} = \dfrac{2(1.65 + 0.84)^2}{-0.5^2} = 50$	4.106	399
d_{NIF} comparison of 2 independent means (example 2)	$d_{NIF} = \dfrac{\varepsilon - \delta}{\sqrt{S^2_{pooled}}} = \dfrac{-10 - 30}{60} = -0.666$	4.107	399
Calculation of n_{NIF} comparison of 2 independent means (example 2)	$n_{NIF} = \dfrac{2(z_{1-\alpha} + z_{1-\beta})^2}{d^2_{NIF}} = \dfrac{2(1.65 + 0.84)^2}{-0.666^2} = 28$	4.108	399
d_{Eq} comparison of 2 independent means (example 1)	$d_{Eq} = \dfrac{\delta - \varepsilon}{\sqrt{S^2_{pooled}}} = \dfrac{-30 - 0}{60} = 0.5$	4.109	399
Calculation of n_{Eq} comparison of 2 independent means (example 1)	$n_{Eq} = \dfrac{2(z_{1-\alpha} + z_{1-\beta/2})^2}{d^2_{Eq}} = \dfrac{2(1.65 + 1.28)^2}{-0.5^2} = 69$	4.110	399
d_{Eq} comparison of 2 independent means (example 2)	$d_{Eq} = \dfrac{\delta - \varepsilon}{\sqrt{S^2_{pooled}}} = \dfrac{-30 - (-10)}{60} = -0.333$	4.111	400
Chapter 4 (Non-inferiority (NIF) and equivalence (Eq.) studies: comparison of 2 proportions)			
d_{NIF} effect size: comparison of 2 proportions	$d_{NIF} = \dfrac{\delta}{\sqrt{p_R(1-p_R)}}$	4.112	400
d_{NIF} effect size: comparison of 2 proportions (variant)	$d_{NIF} = \dfrac{(p_T - p_R) - \delta}{\sqrt{p_T(1-p_T) + p_R(1-p_R)}}$	4.113	400

(continued)

d_{Eq} effect size: comparison of 2 proportions	$d_{Eq} = \dfrac{\delta - (p_T - p_R)}{\sqrt{p_T(1-p_T) + p_R(1-p_R)}}$	4.114	400
Calculation of n_{NIF}: comparison of 2 independent proportions	$n_{NIF} = \left(z_{1-\alpha} + z_{1-\beta}\right)^2 / d_{NIF}^2$	4.115	401
Calculation of n_{Eq}: comparison of 2 independent proportions	$n_{Eq} = \left(z_{1-\alpha} + z_{1-\beta/2}\right)^2 / d_{Eq}^2$	4.116	401
d_{NIF} comparison of 2 independent proportions (example 1)	$d_{NIF} = \dfrac{(0.65 - 0.85) - (0.1)}{\sqrt{0.65(1-0.65) + 0.85(1-0.85)}} = -0.5$	4.117	401
Calculation of n_{NIF} comparison of 2 independent proportions (example 1)	$n_{NIF} = (1.65 + 0.84)^2 / -0.5^2 = 25$	4.118	401
d_{NIF} comparison of 2 independent proportions (example 2)	$d_{NIF} = \dfrac{(-0.1)}{\sqrt{2 \times 0.85(1-0.85)}} = -0.198$	4.119	401
Calculation of n_{NIF} comparison of 2 independent proportions (example 2)	$n_{NIF} = (1.65 + 0.84)^2 / 0.198^2 = 158$	4.120	401
d_{Eq} comparison of 2 independent proportions (example 1)	$d_{Eq} = \dfrac{0.1 - (0.85 - 0.65)}{\sqrt{0.65(1-0.65) + 0.85(1-0.85)}} = \dfrac{-0.1}{0.6} = -0.167$	4.121	401
Calculation of n_{Eq} comparison of 2 independent proportions (example 1)	$n_{Eq} = (1.64 + 1.28)^2 / 0.167^2 = 307$	4.122	401
d_{Eq} comparison of 2 independent proportions (example 2)	$d_{Eq} = \dfrac{\delta}{\sqrt{2p_R(1-p_T)}} = \dfrac{-0.1}{\sqrt{2 \times 0.85(1-0.85)}} = -0.198$	4.123	401
Calculation of n_{Eq} comparison of 2 independent proportions (example 2)	$n_{Eq} = (1.64 + 1.28)^2 / -0.198^2 = 219$	4.124	401
Calculation of n_{NIF}: Odds ratio	$n_{NIF} = \dfrac{\left(z_{1-\alpha} + z_{1-\beta}\right)^2}{(\log OR - \delta)^2} \left(\dfrac{1}{k\, p_T(1-p_T)} + \dfrac{1}{k\, p_R(1-p_R)}\right)$	4.125	402
Calculation of n_{NIF}: Odds ratio (example)	$n_{NIF} = \dfrac{(1.65 + 0.84)^2}{(1.28 - (-0.02))^2} \left(\dfrac{1}{0.1 \times 0.9} + \dfrac{1}{0.03 \times 0.97}\right) = 167$	4.126	402
Calculation of n_{Eq}: Odds ratio	$n_{Eq} = \dfrac{\left(z_{1-\alpha} + z_{1-\beta/2}\right)^2}{(\delta - \log OR)^2} \left(\dfrac{1}{k\, p_T(1-p_T)} + \dfrac{1}{k\, p_R(1-p_R)}\right)$	4.127	402
Calculation of n_{Eq}: Odds ratio (example 1)	$n_{Eq} = \dfrac{(1.65 + 1.28)^2}{(0.02 - 1.28)^2} \left(\dfrac{1}{0.1 \times 0.9} + \dfrac{1}{0.03 \times 0.97}\right) = 246$	4.128	402
Calculation of n_{Eq}: Odds ratio (variant)	$n_{Eq} = \dfrac{\left(z_{1-\alpha} + z_{1-\beta/2}\right)^2}{(0.5)^2} \left(\dfrac{1}{k\, p_T(1-p_T)} + \dfrac{1}{k\, p_R(1-p_R)}\right)$	4.129	402
Calculation of n_{Eq}: Odds ratio (example 2)	$n_{Eq} = \dfrac{(1.65 + 1.28)^2}{(0.5)^2} \left(\dfrac{1}{0.1 \times 0.9} + \dfrac{1}{0.03 \times 0.97}\right) = 761$	4.130	402
(NIF and Eq. studies: time-event analysis (Log rank test))			
Variance of survival	$\sigma^2(\lambda_i) = \lambda_i^2 \left(1 + \dfrac{e^{-\lambda_i T} - e^{-\lambda_i(T - T_0)}}{\lambda_i\, T_0}\right)^{-1}$	4.131	403
Calculation of sample size in group 2 (superiority study)	$n_{2Sup} = \dfrac{\left(Z_{(1-\alpha/2)} + Z_{(1-\beta)}\right)^2}{(\lambda_1 - \lambda_2)^2} \left[\dfrac{\sigma^2(\lambda_1)}{k} + \sigma^2(\lambda_2)\right]$	4.132	403
Calculation of sample size in group 2 (NIF study)	$n_{2NIF} = \dfrac{\left(Z_{(1-\alpha)} + Z_{(1-\beta)}\right)^2}{(\lambda_1 - \lambda_2 - \delta)^2} \left[\dfrac{\sigma^2(\lambda_1)}{k} + \sigma^2(\lambda_2)\right]$	4.133	403
Calculation of sample size in group 2 (Eq. study)	$n_{2Eq} = \dfrac{\left(Z_{(1-\alpha)} + Z_{(1-\beta/2)}\right)^2}{(\delta)^2} \left[\dfrac{\sigma^2(\lambda_1)}{k} + \sigma^2(\lambda_2)\right]$	4.134	403
Calculation of n_{NIF} (example)	$n_{NIF} = \dfrac{(1.65 + 0.84)^2}{(2 - 1 - (-0.2))^2} [0.97 + 3.94] = 22$	4.135	404
Calculation of n_{Eq} (example)	$n_{Eq} = \dfrac{(1.65 + 1.28)^2}{(-0.5 - 0)^2} [0.97 + 0.97] = 67$	4.136	404
(NIF and Eq. studies: time-event analysis (Cox proportional hazard test))			
Calculation of total sample size (superiority study)	$N_{Sup} = \dfrac{\left(Z_{(1-\alpha/2)} + Z_{(1-\beta)}\right)^2}{\log HR^2 p_1 p_2 Pr_e (1 - R^2)}$	4.137	404
Calculation of total sample size (NIF study)	$N_{NIF} = \dfrac{\left(Z_{(1-\alpha)} + Z_{(1-\beta)}\right)^2}{(\log HR - \delta)^2 p_1 p_2 Pr_e (1 - R^2)}$	4.138	404

(continued)

Calculation of total sample size (Eq. study)	$N_{Eq} = \dfrac{\left(Z_{(1-\alpha)} + Z_{(1-\beta/2)}\right)^2}{(\delta)^2 p_1 p_2 Pr_e(1-R^2)}$	4.139	404
Calculation of N_{INF} (example)	$N_{NIF} = \dfrac{(1.65 + 0.84)^2}{[Log\,0.5 - (-0.1)]^2 0.5 \times 0.5 \times 0.072} = 548$	4.140	404
Calculation of N_{Eq} (example 1)	$N_{Eq} = \dfrac{(1.65 + 1.28)^2}{[(-0.1) - Log\,0.5]^2 0.5 \times 0.5 \times 0.072} = 1350$	4.141	404
Calculation of N_{Eq} (example 2)	$N_{Eq} = \dfrac{(1.65 + 1.28)^2}{(-0.5 - 0)^2 0.5 \times 0.5 \times 0.072} = 1900$	4.142	404
Chapter 4 (Sample size calculation: sensitivity (Sn), Specificity (Sp), and ROC analysis)			
Sample size calculation for establishing: a known Sn or Sp	$n_p = \dfrac{\left(Z_{(1-\alpha/2)}\right)^2 p(1-p)}{d^2}$	4.143	406
Sample size calculation for establishing Sn: an unknown disease state	$n_{Sn} = \dfrac{\left(Z_{(1-\alpha/2)}\right)^2 Sn(1-Sn)}{d^2 \times P}$	4.144	406
Sample size calculation for establishing Sp: an unknown disease state	$n_{Sp} = \dfrac{\left(Z_{(1-\alpha/2)}\right)^2 Sp(1-Sp)}{d^2 \times (1-P)}$	4.145	406
Sample size calculation for establishing Sn: unknown disease state (example)	$n_{Sn} = \dfrac{(1.96)^2 0.8(1-0.8)}{0.05^2 \times 0.2} = 1230$	4.146	406
Sample size calculation comparing Sn or Sp to a theoretical value	$n_p = \dfrac{\left[\left(Z_{(1-\alpha/2)}\right)\sqrt{P_0(1-P_0)} + \left(Z_{(1-\beta)}\right)\sqrt{P_1(1-P_1)}\right]^2}{(P_1 - P_0)^2} = \dfrac{\left[1.96\sqrt{0.7 \times 0.3} + 0.84\sqrt{0.8 \times 0.2}\right]^2}{(0.8 - 0.7)^2} = 154$	4.147	407
Sample size calculation comparing Sn or Sp: 2 independent tests	$n_p = \dfrac{\left[\left(Z_{(1-\alpha/2)}\right)\sqrt{2P_c(1-P_c)} + \left(Z_{(1-\beta)}\right)\sqrt{P_1(1-P_1) + P_2(1-P_2)}\right]^2}{(P_1 - P_2)^2} = 293$	4.148	407
Sample size calculation comparing Sn or Sp: paired design (example)	$n = \dfrac{\left[1.96(3+1) + 0.84\sqrt{(3+1)^2 - (3-1)^2 \times 0.2}\right]^2}{(3-1)^2 \times 0.2} = 156$	4.149	407
Variance of AUC (example)	$Var\,AUC = (0.0099 \times e^{\left(-\frac{a^2}{2}\right)}) \times (6a^2 + 16)$ $= (0.0099 \times e^{\left(-\frac{1.895^2}{2}\right)}) \times (6 \times 1.895^2 + 16) = 0.062$	4.150	409
Calculation of total sample size (example)	$N = \dfrac{\left(Z_{(1-\alpha/2)}\right)^2 Var\,AUC}{d^2} = \dfrac{1.96^2 \times 0.062}{0.05^2} = 95$	4.151	409
Sample size calculation comparing a new AUC to a predetermined AUC	$n = \dfrac{\left[\left(Z_{(1-\alpha/2)}\right)\sqrt{Var\,AUC_0} + \left(Z_{(1-\beta)}\right)\sqrt{Var\,AUC_1}\right]^2}{(AUC_1 - AUC_0)^2}$	4.152	409
Sample size calculation to compare 2 independent ROC curves	$n = \dfrac{\left[\left(Z_{(1-\alpha/2)}\right)\sqrt{2\,Var\,AUC_c} + \left(Z_{(1-\beta)}\right)\sqrt{Var\,AUC_1 + Var\,AUC_2}\right]^2}{(AUC_1 - AUC_2)^2}$	4.153	409
Sample size calculation to compare 2 dependent ROC curves	$n = \dfrac{\left[\left(Z_{(1-\alpha/2)}\right)\sqrt{2Var_{H0}(AUC_1 - AUC_2)} + \left(Z_{(1-\beta)}\right)\sqrt{Var\,AUC_1 + Var\,AUC_2}\right]^2}{(AUC_1 - AUC_2)^2}$	4.154	410
Covariance of two AUC	$Var_{H0}(AUC_1 - AUC_2) = nVar(AUC_1) + nVar(AUC_2) - 2nCov(AUC_1, AUC_2)$	4.155	410
Chapter 4 (Sample size calculation: measuring agreement)			
Proportions of agreement and disagreement (example)	$\pi_A = \dfrac{d_{00} + d_{11}}{N} = \dfrac{52 + 18}{80} = 0.875$ and, $\pi_D = \dfrac{d_{10} + d_{10}}{N} = \dfrac{7 + 10}{80}$ $= 0.125$	4.156	410
Sample size calculation to establish a known Kappa	$n_k = \dfrac{4\left(Z_{(1-\alpha/2)}\right)^2(1-k)}{d^2}\left[(1-k)(1-2k) + \dfrac{k(2-K)}{2\,\pi_D(1-\pi_D)}\right]$	4.157	411
Sample size calculation for agreement (unknown Kappa)	$n = \dfrac{4\left(Z_{(1-\alpha/2)}\right)^2 \pi_D(1-\pi_D)}{d^2} = \dfrac{4 \times 1.96^2 \times 0.125(1-0.125)}{0.2^2} = 43$	4.158	411
Sample size calculation to establish an ICC (Machin and colleagues)	$n_{ICC} = 1 + \dfrac{8\left(Z_{(1-\alpha/2)}\right)^2(1-\rho)^2[1+(K-1)\rho]^2}{k(K-1)d^2}$	4.159	412
Sample size calculation to establish an ICC (variant)	$n_{ICC} = 1 + \dfrac{2\left(Z_{(1-\alpha)} + Z_{(1-B)}\right)^2 k}{(\ln C_0)^2(K-1)}$	4.160	412
The value of C^0	$C_0 = \dfrac{1 + k\theta_0}{1 + k\theta_1}; \quad \theta_0 = \dfrac{R_0}{1 - R_0}; \quad \theta_1 = \dfrac{R_1}{1 - R_1}$	4.161	412

(continued)

Sample size calculation to establish an ICC (example)	$n_{ICC} = 1 + \dfrac{2(1.96 + 0.84)^2 2}{(\ln 0.0168)^2 (2 - 1)}$	4.162	412
Chapter 4 (Sample size calculation: survey analysis)			
The 95% CI of a proportion	$95\% \ CI = p \pm 1.96\sqrt{\dfrac{p(1-p)}{n}} = p \pm ME$	4.163	413
Sample size calculation for a survey	$N = p(1-p)\left(\dfrac{1.96}{ME}\right)^2$	4.164	413
Sample size calculation for a survey: qualitative outcome (infinite population)	$N = p(1-p)\left(\dfrac{Z}{ME}\right)^2$	4.165	414
Sample size calculation for a survey: quantitative outcome (infinite population)	$N = \sigma^2\left(\dfrac{Z}{ME}\right)^2$	4.166	414
Sample size calculation for a survey: qualitative outcome (known population size)	$N = \dfrac{Z^2[p(1-p)]\left(N_p/N_p - 1\right)}{(ME + Z^2\sigma^2)(N_p - 1)}$	4.167	414
Sample size calculation for a survey: quantitative outcome (known population size)	$N = \dfrac{Z^2\sigma^2\left(N_p/N_p - 1\right)}{(ME + Z^2\sigma^2)(N_p - 1)}$	4.168	414
Sample size calculation for a survey: qualitative outcome (example)	$n = 0.4 \times (1 - 0.4) \times \left(\dfrac{1.96}{0.05}\right)^2 = 369$	4.169	415
Sample size calculation for a survey: quantitative outcome (example)	$n = 20^2 \times \left(\dfrac{1.96}{10}\right)^2 = 16$	4.170	415
Checking on the level of confidence of a terminated survey	$Z = \sqrt{\dfrac{ME^2 \times n}{\sigma^2}} = \sqrt{\dfrac{5^2 \times 16}{20^2}} = 1$	4.171	416
Chapter 6 (Meta-analysis: general)			
Point biserial correlation	$r_{AB} = \dfrac{d}{\sqrt{1/[1 - (1 - p)] + d^2}}$	6.1	449
Effect size (r) of multivariable analysis	$r = 0.98\,\beta + 0.05\,\lambda$	6.2	450
Weighting ES, fixed-effect model	$WES_i = ES_i \times \dfrac{1}{Se_i^2}$	6.3	451
Weighting ES, random-effects model	$W^R ES_i = ES_i \times \dfrac{1}{Se_i^2 + T^2}$	6.4	452
Meta-analysis by hand: I	$M_{meta} = \dfrac{\sum WES}{\sum W} = \dfrac{12}{6} = 0.5.(6.5)$	6.5	453
95% CI of I	$95\% \ CI = M_{meta} \pm 1.96(Se_{meta}) = 0.5 \pm 1.96(0.29) = -0.07 \ to \ 1.07$	6.6	453
Z value of I	$Z = \dfrac{M_{meta}}{Se_{meta}^2} = \dfrac{0.5}{\sqrt{0.083}} = 1.73$	6.7	453
Meta-analysis by hand: II	$M_{meta} = \dfrac{\sum WES}{\sum W} = \dfrac{6+6}{12+12} = 0.5.$	6.8	453
Variance of II	$Var_{meta} = \dfrac{1}{\sum W} = \dfrac{1}{12+12} = 0.04$	6.9	454
Se of II	$Se_{meta} = \sqrt{Var_{meta}} = \sqrt{0.04} = 0.2$	6.10	454
95% CI of II	$95\% \ CI = M_{meta} \pm 1.96(Se_{meta}) = 0.5 \pm 1.96(0.2) = 0.1 \ to \ 0.9$	6.11	454
Z value of II	$Z = \dfrac{M_{meta}}{Se_{meta}} = \dfrac{0.5}{0.2} = 2.5.$	6.12	454
Meta-analysis by hand: III	$M_{meta} = \dfrac{\sum WES}{\sum W} = \dfrac{6+6+6}{12+12+12} = 0.5.$	6.13	455
Variance of III	$Var_{meta} = \dfrac{1}{\sum W} = \dfrac{1}{12+12+12} = 0.028$	6.14	455
Se of III	$Se_{meta} = \sqrt{Var_{meta}} = \sqrt{0.08} = 0.17$	6.15	455
95% CI of III	$95\% \ CI = M_{meta} \pm 1.96(Se_{meta}) = 0.5 \pm 1.96(0.17) = 0.16 \ to \ 0.84$	6.16	455
Z value of III	$Z = \dfrac{M_{meta}}{Se_{meta}} = \dfrac{0.5}{0.17} = 2.94.$	6.17	455
Meta-analysis by hand: variance of random-effects model	$Var_i = Se^2 + T^2 = 0.083 + 0.083 = 0.166$	6.18	456
Weight of random-effects model	$W_i = \dfrac{1}{Se^2 + T^2} = \dfrac{1}{0.166} = 6$	6.19	456
Weighted effect size, random-effects model	$WES_i = ES \times \dfrac{1}{Se^2 + T^2} = 0.5 \times \dfrac{1}{0.166} = 3$	6.20	456

(continued)

Main effect, random-effects model	$M_{meta} = \dfrac{\sum WES}{\sum W} = \dfrac{3+3+3}{6+6+6} = 0.5$	6.21	456
Variance, random-effects model	$Var_{meta} = \dfrac{1}{\sum W} = \dfrac{1}{6+6+6} = 0.055$	6.22	456
Se of random-effects model	$Se_{meta} = \sqrt{Var_{meta}} = \sqrt{0.055} = 0.234$	6.23	456
95% CI, random-effects model	$95\% \; CI = M_{meta} \pm 1.96(Se_{meta}) = 0.5 \pm 1.96(0.234) = 0.04 \; to \; 0.96$	6.24	457
Z value, random-effects model	$Z = \dfrac{M_{meta}}{Se_{meta}} = \dfrac{0.5}{0.234} = 2.13.$	6.25	457
Chapter 6 (Meta-analysis: calculation of individual effect sizes: correlation coefficient)			
Correcting r	$r_c = r - \left[\dfrac{r - (1 - r^2)}{2(n-3)} \right]$	6.26	458
Fisher's transformation	$Z = \dfrac{1}{2} \log \dfrac{1 + r_c}{1 - r_c}$	6.27	458
Variance of normalized r	$Var\, Z = \dfrac{1}{n-3}$	6.28	458
Weighted normalized r, fixed-effect model	$WZ_i = Z_i \times \dfrac{1}{Var_{zi}}$	6.29	458
Weighted normalized r, random-effects model	$W^R Z_i = Z_i \times \dfrac{1}{Var_{zi} + T^2}$	6.30	458
Mean weighted normalized r	$Mean\, Z = \dfrac{\sum W_i Z_i}{\sum W_i}$	6.31	458
Se of weighted normalized r	$Se\, Z = \sqrt{\dfrac{1}{\sum W_i}}$	6.32	458
95% CI of the weighted normalized r	$95\% \; CI = Mean\, Z \pm 1.96(Se\, Z)$	6.33	459
Z value of weighted normalized r	$z\, score = \dfrac{Mean\, Z}{Se\, Z}$	6.34	459
Back transformation of normalized r	$r = \dfrac{e^{2z} - 1}{e^{2z} + 1}$	6.35	459
Fisher's normalized r (example)	$Z_i = \dfrac{1}{2} \log \dfrac{1+r}{1-r} = \dfrac{1}{2} \log \dfrac{1+0.1}{1-0.1} = 0.1$	6.36	459
Variance of normalized r (example)	$Var\, Z_i = \dfrac{1}{n_i - 3} = \dfrac{1}{50 - 3} = 0.021$	6.37	459
Weighted r, fixed-effect model (example)	$W_i Z_i = Z_i \times \dfrac{1}{Var\, Z_i} = 0.1 \times \dfrac{1}{0.021} = 4.7$	6.38	459
Mean weighted r, fixed-effect model (example)	$Mean\, Z = \dfrac{\sum W_i Z_i}{\sum W_i} = \dfrac{238}{465} = 0.51$	6.39	459
Se weighted r, fixed-effect model (example)	$Se\, Z = \sqrt{\dfrac{1}{\sum W_i}} = \sqrt{\dfrac{1}{465}} = 0.046$	6.40	459
95% CI weighted r, fixed-effect model (example)	$95\% \; CI = Mean\, Z \pm 1.96(Se\, Z) = 0.51 \pm 1.96(0.046) = 0.423 - 0.604$	6.41	459
Z score and P value of weighted r, fixed-effect model (example)	$z\, score = \dfrac{0.51}{0.046} = 11.1; P < 0.001$	6.42	459
Back transformation of r, fixed-effect model (example)	$r = \dfrac{e^{2z} - 1}{e^{2z} + 1} = \dfrac{e^{2 \times 0.51} - 1}{e^{2 \times 0.51} + 1} = \dfrac{2.77 - 1}{2.77 + 1} = \dfrac{1.77}{3.77} = 0.47$	6.43	460
Weighted r, random-effects model (example)	$W_i^R Z_i = Z_i \times \dfrac{1}{Var_{zi} + T^2} = 0.1 \times \dfrac{1}{0.021 + 0.072} = 10.75$	6.44	460
Mean weighted r, random-effects model (example)	$Mean\, Z^R = \dfrac{\sum W_i^R Z_i}{\sum W_i^R} = \dfrac{26.7}{58.46} = 0.46$	6.45	460
Se weighted r, random-effects model (example)	$Se\, Z^R = \sqrt{\dfrac{1}{\sum W_i^R}} = \sqrt{\dfrac{1}{58.46}} = 0.13$	6.46	461
95% CI weighted r, random-effects model (example)	$95\% \; CI\, Z^R = Mean\, Z^R \pm 1.96(Se\, Z^R) = 0.46 \pm 1.96(0.13) = 0.204 - 0.718$	6.47	461
Z score and P value of weighted r, random-effects model (example)	$z\, score = \dfrac{0.46}{0.13} = 3.52; \; P < 0.001$	6.48	461
Back transformation of r, random-effects model (example)	$r = \dfrac{e^{2z} - 1}{e^{2z} + 1} = \dfrac{e^{2 \times 0.46} - 1}{e^{2 \times 0.46} + 1} = \dfrac{2.51 - 1}{2.51 + 1} = \dfrac{1.51}{3.51} = 0.43$	6.49	462
Chapter 6 (Meta-analysis: calculation of individual effect sizes: unstandardized mean difference)			
Unstandardized mean of the difference (bilateral study)	$d = \mu_a - \mu_b$	6.50	462
Pooled variance	$S_{pooled}^2 = \dfrac{S_a^2(n_a - 1) + S_b^2(n_b - 1)}{(n_a + n_b - 2)}$	6.51	462

(continued)

Variance of the difference (pooled variance)	$\text{Var d} = S^2_{pooled} \dfrac{n_a + n_b}{n_a \times n_b}$	6.52	463
Variance of the difference (significantly different variances)	$\text{Var d} = \dfrac{S_a^2}{n_a} + \dfrac{S_b^2}{n_b}$	6.53	463
Se of the difference	$Se\ d = \sqrt{\text{Var d}}$	6.54	463
Weighted difference, fixed-effect model	$Wd_i = d_i \times \dfrac{1}{\text{Var d}}$	6.55	463
Weighted difference, random-effects model	$W^R d_i = d_i \times \dfrac{1}{\text{Var d} + T^2}$	6.56	463
Mean weighted difference	$Mean\ d = \dfrac{\sum W_i d_i}{\sum W_i}$	6.57	463
Se of the weighted difference	$Se\ d = \sqrt{\dfrac{1}{\sum W_i}}$	6.58	463
95% CI of the mean difference	$95\%\ CI = Mean\ d \pm 1.96\,(Se\ d)$	6.59	463
Z score of the mean difference	$z\ score = \dfrac{Mean\ d}{Se\ d}$	6.60	463
Weighted difference, fixed-effect model (example)	$W_i d_i = d_i \times \dfrac{1}{Var_{di}} = -5 \times \dfrac{1}{17.4} = -86.96$	6.61	464
Mean of the difference, fixed-effect model (example)	$Mean\ d = \dfrac{\sum W_i d_i}{\sum W_i} = \dfrac{-317}{118.16} = -2.69$	6.62	464
Se of the difference, fixed-effect model (example)	$Se\ d = \sqrt{\dfrac{1}{\sum W_i}} = \sqrt{\dfrac{1}{118.16}} = 0.092$	6.63	464
95% CI of the mean difference, fixed-effect model (example)	$95\%\ CI = Mean\ d \pm 1.96(Se\ d) = -2.69 \pm 1.96(0.092) = -2.867\ to\ -2.51$	6.64	464
Z score of the mean difference, fixed-effect model (example)	$Z\ score = \dfrac{-2.69}{0.092} = -29.2$	6.65	464
Weighted difference, random-effects model (example)	$W_i^R d_i = d_i \times \dfrac{1}{Var\ d_i + T^2} = -5 \times \dfrac{1}{3.42} = -1.46$	6.66	464
Mean of the difference, random-effects model (example)	$Mean\ d^R = \dfrac{\sum W_i^R d_i}{\sum W_i^R} = \dfrac{-4.62}{1.72} = -2.68$	6.67	465
Se of the difference random-effects model (example)	$Se\ d^R = \sqrt{\dfrac{1}{\sum W_i}} = \sqrt{\dfrac{1}{1.72}} = 0.76$	6.68	465
95% CI of the mean difference, random-effects (example)	$95\%\ CI = Mean\ d^R \pm 1.96\big(Se\ d^R\big) = -2.68 \pm 1.96(0.76) = -4.17\ to\ -1.19$	6.69	466
Z score of the mean difference, random-effects (example)	$Z\ score = \dfrac{-2.68}{0.76} = -3.54$	6.70	466
Unstandardized mean of the difference paired design	$Mean\ d_p = \mu_a - \mu_b$	6.71	466
Variance of unstandardized difference paired design	$Var\ d_p = \big(S_a^2 + S_b^2\big) - 2 \times r \times S_a S_b$	6.72	466
Se of unstandardized difference paired design	$Se\ d_p = \sqrt{Var\ d_p}$	6.73	466
95% CI of unstandardized mean difference paired design	$95\%\ CI = Mean\ d_p \pm 1.96\big(Se\ d_p\big)$	6.74	466
Chapter 6 (Meta-analysis: calculation of individual effect sizes: standardized mean difference)			
Standardized mean difference (SMD): Cohen ds effect size	$Cohen\ ds = \dfrac{(\mu_1 - \mu_2)}{\sqrt{S^2_{pooled}}}$	6.75	467
SMD: pooled variance	$S^2_{pooled} = \dfrac{S_1^2(n_1 - 1) + S_2^2(n_2 - 1)}{(n_1 + n_2 - 2)}$	6.76	467
SMD: variance of the difference, fixed-effect model	$Var\ d_i = \dfrac{n_1 + n_2}{n_1 n_2} + \dfrac{d^2}{2(n_1 + n_2)}$	6.77	467
Weighted SMD, fixed-effect model	$Wd_i = d_i \times \dfrac{1}{Var\ d_i}$	6.78	467
Weighted SMD, random-effects model	$W^R d_i = d_i \times \dfrac{1}{Var\ d_i + T^2}$	6.79	467
Mean weighted SMD	$Mean\ d = \dfrac{\sum W_i d_i}{\sum W_i}$	6.80	467
Se of weighted SMD	$Se\ d = \sqrt{\dfrac{1}{\sum W_i}}$	6.81	467

(continued)

95% CI of weighted SMD	$95\% \ CI = Mean \ d \pm 1.96(Se \ d)$	6.82	467
Z score of weighted SMD	$z \ score = \dfrac{Mean \ d}{Se \ d}$	6.83	467
SMD: Hedges g effect size	$Hedges \ g = Cohen \ ds \times J = ds\left(1 - \dfrac{3}{4(n_1 + n_2) - 9}\right)$	6.84	468
SMD: Variance Hedges g	$Var \ g = Var_d \times J^2 = Var_d\left(1 - \dfrac{3}{4(n_1 + n_2) - 9}\right)^2$	6.85	468
Chapter 6 (Meta-analysis: calculation of individual effect sizes: standardized mean difference, paired design)			
SMD paired design: Cohen dz effect size	$Cohen \ d_z = \dfrac{M_{diff}}{Sd_{diff}} = \dfrac{\mu_1 - \mu_2}{\sqrt{Sd_1^2 + Sd_2^2 - 2r \ Sd_1 Sd_2}}$	6.86	468
SMD paired design: Variance of Cohen dz	$Var \ d_z = \left(\dfrac{1}{n} + \dfrac{d_z^2}{2n}\right)2(1 - r)$	6.87	468
Weighted SMD, paired design, fixed-effect model	$Wd_z = d_z \times \dfrac{1}{Var \ d_z}$	6.88	468
Weighted SMD, paired design, random-effects model	$W^R d_i = d_i \times \dfrac{1}{Var \ d_z + T^2}$	6.89	468
Hedges g paired design	$Hedges \ g = d_z \times J = d_z\left(1 - \dfrac{3}{4(n - 1)}\right)$	6.90	468
SMD: Variance Hedges g, paired design	$Var \ g = Var \ d_z \times J^2 = Var \ d_z\left(1 - \dfrac{3}{4(n - 1)}\right)^2$	6.91	468
Chapter 6 (Meta-analysis: calculation of individual effect sizes: odds ratio)			
Odds ratio (OR)	$OR = \dfrac{ad}{cb}$	6.92	469
Variance of odds ratio	$Var_i = \dfrac{1}{a} + \dfrac{1}{b} + \dfrac{1}{c} + \dfrac{1}{d}$	6.93	469
Weighted OR, fixed-effect model	$WES_i = Log_{OR} \times \dfrac{1}{Var \ Log_{OR}}$	6.94	469
Weighted OR, random-effects model	$WES_i^R = Log_{OR} \times \dfrac{1}{Var \ Log_{OR} + T^2}$	6.95	469
Mean effect size of meta-analysis (Log OR)	$Mean \ ES = \dfrac{\sum W_i Log_{ORi}}{\sum W_i}$	6.96	469
Se of effect size	$Se \ ES = \sqrt{\dfrac{1}{\sum W_i}}$	6.97	469
95% CI effect size	$95\% \ CI \ ES = Mean \ ES \pm 1.96(Se \ ES)$	6.98	469
Z score of effect size	$Z \ score = \dfrac{Mean \ ES}{Se \ ES}$	6.99	469
95% CI of OR	$95\% \ CI(OR) = e^{LL \ 95\% \ CI \ (\log OR)} \ to \ e^{UL \ 95\% \ CI \ (\log OR)}$	6.100	470
Chapter 6 (Meta-analysis: calculation of individual effect sizes: relative risk)			
Relative risk (RR)	$RR_i = \dfrac{a}{n_t} / \dfrac{c}{n_c}$	6.101	470
Variance of RR	$Var_i = \dfrac{1}{a} + \dfrac{1}{c} + \dfrac{1}{a + b} + \dfrac{1}{c + d}$	6.102	470
Weighted Log RR, fixed-effect model	$WES_i = Log \ RR_i \times \dfrac{1}{Var \ Log_{RRi}}$	6.103	470
Weighted Log RR, random-effects model	$WES_i^R = Log \ RR_i \times \dfrac{1}{Var \ Log_{RRi} + T^2}$	6.104	470
Mean Effect size of meta-analysis (Log RR)	$Mean \ ES = \dfrac{\sum W_i Log_{RRi}}{\sum W_i}$	6.105	470
Variance of effect size	$Var \ ES = \dfrac{1}{\sum W_i}$	6.106	470
Se of effect size	$Se \ ES = \sqrt{\dfrac{1}{\sum W_i}}$	6.107	470
95% CI effect size	$95\% \ CI(ES) = (Mean \ ES) \pm 1.96(Se \ ES)$	6.108	470
Z score of effect size	$Z = \dfrac{Mean \ ES}{Se \ ES}$	6.109	470
95% CI of RR	$95\% CI \ (RR) = e^{LL \ 95\% CI \ (\log RR)} \ to \ e^{UL \ 95\% CI \ (\log RR)}$	6.110	471
RR (example)	$RRi = \dfrac{na}{Na} / \dfrac{nc}{Nc} = \dfrac{4}{123} / \dfrac{11}{139} = 0.41$	6.111	471
Effect size log RR (example)	$ES_i = \log 0.411 = -0.89$	6.112	472
Variance log RR (example)	$Var \ ES_i = \dfrac{1}{na} + \dfrac{1}{nc} + \dfrac{1}{Na} + \dfrac{1}{Nb} = \dfrac{1}{4} + \dfrac{1}{11} + \dfrac{1}{123} + \dfrac{1}{139} = 0.356$	6.113	472

(continued)

Weighted log RR, fixed-effect model (example)	$WES_i = Log\ RR_i \times \dfrac{1}{Var_{Log\ RRi}} = -0.89 \times \dfrac{1}{0.356} = -2.49$	6.114	472
Se weighted log RR, fixed-effect model (example)	$Se\ ES_i = \sqrt{Var\ ES_i} = \sqrt{0.356} = 0.597$	6.115	472
95% CI weighted log RR, fixed-effect model (example)	$95\%\ CI\ ES_i = ES_i \pm 1.96(Se\ ES_i) = -0.89 \pm 1.96(0.597) = -2\ to\ 0.23$	6.116	472
95% CI of RR, fixed-effect model (example)	$RRi(95\%\ CI) = 0.41(0.13\ to\ 1.26)$	6.117	472
Mean weighted Log RR, fixed-effect model (example)	$Mean\ ES = \dfrac{\sum W_i Log_{RRi}}{\sum W_i} = \dfrac{-269}{625} = -0.43$	6.118	473
Se of mean weighted Log RR, fixed effect model (example)	$Se\ ES = \sqrt{\dfrac{1}{\sum W_i}} = \sqrt{\dfrac{1}{625}} = 0.04$	6.119	473
95% CI of mean weighted Log RR, fixed effect model (example)	$95\%\ CI(ES) = MeanES \pm 1.96(SE\ ES) = -0.43 \pm 1.96(0.04)$ $= -0.51\ to -0.35$	6.120	473
Z score and P value of mean weighted Log RR, fixed effect model (example)	$Z = \dfrac{Mean\ ES}{Se\ ES} = \dfrac{-0.43}{0.04} = -10.6;\ \ P < 0.001$	6.121	473
95% CI of mean RR, fixed-effect model (example)	$RR(95\%\ CI)_{fixed\ model} = 0.65(0.6\ to\ 0.7)$	6.122	473
Variance log RR, random-effects model (example)	$Var_i^R = Var\ log_{RRi} + T^2 = 0.33 + 0.31 = 0.63$	6.123	474
Weighted log RR, random-effects model (example)	$WES_i^R = Log\ RR_i \times \dfrac{1}{Var^R} = -0.89 \times \dfrac{1}{0.33 + 0.31} = -1.39$	6.124	474
Standard error log RR, random-effects model (example)	$Se\ ES_i^R = \sqrt{Var_i^R} = \sqrt{0.64} = 0.8$	6.125	474
95% CI log RR, random-effects model (example)	$95\%\ CI\ ES_i = ES_i \pm 1.96\left(Se\ ES_i^R\right) = -0.89 \pm 1.96(0.8) = -2.46\ to\ 0.68$	6.126	474
95% CI RR, random-effects model (example)	$95\%\ CI(RR_i)^R = 0.41(0.08\ to\ 1.97)$	6.127	474
Mean weighted Log RR, random-effects model (example)	$Mean\ ES^R = \dfrac{\sum W_i^R Log_{RRi}}{\sum W_i^R} = \dfrac{-22.28}{31.36} = -0.71$	6.128	474
Se of mean weighted Log RR, random-effects model (example)	$Se\ ES^R = \sqrt{\dfrac{1}{\sum W_i^R}} = \sqrt{\dfrac{1}{31.36}} = 0.179$	6.129	475
95% CI of mean weighted Log RR, random-effects model (example)	$95\%\ CI\ ES = Mean\ ES^R \pm q.96(Se\ ES^R) = -0.714 \pm 1.96(0.179) = -1.06\ to\ -0.36$	6.130	475
Z score and P value of mean weighted Log RR, random-effects model (example)	$Z = \dfrac{-0.71}{0.179} = -4;\ \ P < 0.001$	6.131	475
95% CI of mean RR, random-effects model (example)	$RR(95\%\ CI)_{random\ model} = 0.49(0.35\ to\ 0.7)$	6.132	476
Chapter 6 (Meta-analysis: calculation of individual effect sizes: hazard ratio)			
Hazard ratio (HR) calculation	$HR = \dfrac{H_T}{H_C} = \dfrac{New\ cases_T / Patients\ remaining\ at\ risk_T}{New\ cases_C / Patients\ remaining\ at\ risk_C}$	6.133	476
HR calculated from survival rates	$HR = \dfrac{S_t}{S_c}$	6.134	477
Variance log of HR	$Var_{Log\ HR} = \left(\dfrac{1}{E_t} + \dfrac{1}{E_c}\right)$	6.135	477
Standard error of log HR	$Se(\log\ HR) = \sqrt{\dfrac{1}{E_t} + \dfrac{1}{E_c}}$	6.136	477
Weighted log HR, fixed-effect model	$WES = Log\ HR_i \times \dfrac{1}{Var_{Log\ HRi}}$	6.137	477
Weighted log HR, random-effects model	$WES^R = Log\ HR_i \times \dfrac{1}{Var_{Log\ HRi} + T^2}$	6.138	477
Mean weighted log HR	$Mean\ ES = \dfrac{\sum W_i Log_{HRi}}{\sum W_i}$	6.139	477
Se of the effect size	$Se\ ES = \sqrt{\dfrac{1}{\sum W_i}}$	6.140	477

(continued)

95% CI of effect size	$95\% \; CI \; (ES) = \text{Mean ES} \; \pm 1.96 \; (\text{Se ES})$	6.141	477
Z score of effect size	$Z \; score = \dfrac{\text{Mean ES}}{\text{Se ES}}$	6.142	477
95% CI of HR	$95\% \; CI(HR) = e^{LL \; 95\% \; CI(\log HR)} \; to \; e^{UL \; 95\% \; CI \; (\log HR)}$	6.143	477
Deduction of Pearson r from other statistics	$r = \sqrt{\dfrac{\chi^2}{N}}; \quad r = \sqrt{\dfrac{t^2}{t^2 + df}}; \quad r = \sqrt{\dfrac{F}{F + df_{error}}}$	6.144	478
Mantel–Haenszel odds ratio	$OR_{MH} = \dfrac{\sum W_i OR_i}{\sum W_i}$	6.145	478
95% CI of Mantel–Haenszel odds ratio	$95\% \; CI \; OR_{MH} = OR^{1 \pm 1.96/\sqrt{Var \; OR}}$	6.146	478
Peto one-step approach: Log OR	$Log \; OR_i = \dfrac{O_i - E_i}{V_i}$	6.147	479
Peto one-step approach: expected values	$E_i = \dfrac{(a_i + b_i)(a_i + c_i)}{n_i}$	6.148	479
Peto one-step approach: variance	$V_i = \dfrac{(a_i + b_i)(c_i + d_i)(a_i + c_i)(b_i + d_i)}{n_i^2(n_i - 1)}$	6.149	479
Peto one-step approach: pooled OR	$OR_p = Exp\left(\dfrac{\sum (O_i - E_i)}{\sum V_i}\right)$	6.150	479
Peto one-step approach: z value	$Z_p = \dfrac{O - E}{\sqrt{Var_{OR_p}}}$	6.151	479
Peto one-step approach: 95% CI	$95\% \; CI \; OR_p = (OR_p)^{1 \pm 1.96/\sqrt{Var \; OR}}$	6.152	479
Chapter 6 (Meta-analysis: assessment of heterogeneity)			
Q statistics	$Q = \sum W_i(ES_i - ES)^2$	6.153	480
Q statistics (variant 1)	$Q = \sum W(ES)^2 - \dfrac{(\sum WES)^2}{\sum W}$	6.154	480
Q statistics (example 1)	$Q = \sum W(ES)^2 - \dfrac{(\sum WES)^2}{\sum W} = 1165 - \dfrac{(317)^2}{118} = 314$	6.155	481
Q statistics (example 2)	$Q = \sum W(ES)^2 - \dfrac{(\sum WES)^2}{\sum W} = 265.1 - \dfrac{(-262.3)^2}{609.7} = 152.2$	6.156	481
Q statistics (variant 2)	$W_i(ES_i - ES)^2 = (ES_i - ES)^2/Se_i^2$	6.157	481
I^2 index	$I^2 = 100\%(Q - df)/Q$	6.158	481
I^2 index (example 1)	$I^2 = 100\%\dfrac{Q - df}{Q} = 100\%\dfrac{314 - 5}{314} = 98.4\%$	6.159	482
I^2 index (example 2)	$I^2 = 100\%\dfrac{Q - df}{Q} = 100\%\dfrac{152.2 - 12}{152.2} = 92.1\%$	6.160	482
H^2 index	$H^2 = \dfrac{Q}{df}$	6.161	482
Se of H (Q > K)	$Se_{\log H} = \dfrac{1}{2} \times \dfrac{\log Q - \log(K - 1)}{\sqrt{2Q} - \sqrt{2Q - 3}} \; if \; Q > K$	6.162	482
Standard error of H (Q $\leq$ K)	$Se_{\log H} = \sqrt{\left\{\dfrac{1}{2(K - 2)} \times \left(1 - \dfrac{1}{3(K - 2)^2}\right)\right\}} \; if \; Q \leq K$	6.163	482
95% CI of Log H	$95\% \; CI \; Log \; H = Log \; H \pm 1.96 \; Se_{\log H}$	6.164	482
95% CI of H	$95\% \; CI \; H = e^{Log \; H \pm 1.96 \; Se_{\log H}}$	6.165	482
R^2 index	$R^2 = \dfrac{Var_R}{Var_F} = \dfrac{\sum W_i}{\sum W_i^R} = \dfrac{\sum W_i}{\sum (W_i + T^2)}$	6.166	483
T^2 variance of random-effects model	$T^2 = \dfrac{Q - df}{C}$	6.167	483
Calculation of C of T^2	$C = \sum W_i - \dfrac{\sum W_i^2}{\sum W_i}$	6.168	483
Calculation of C of T^2 (example 1)	$C = \sum W_i - \dfrac{\sum W_i^2}{\sum W_i} = 118.2 - \dfrac{3280}{118.2} = 90.4$	6.169	483
T^2 (example 1)	$T^2 = \dfrac{Q - df}{C} = \dfrac{314 - 5}{90.4} = 3.4$	6.170	483
Calculation of C of T^2 (example 2)	$C = \sum W_i - \dfrac{\sum W_i^2}{\sum W_i} = 609.7 - \dfrac{94804.9}{609.7} = 454.2$	6.171	483
T^2 (example 2)	$T^2 = \dfrac{Q - df}{C} = \dfrac{152.2 - 12}{454.2} = 0.308$	6.172	484

(continued)

Weighted of effect size, random-effects model	$W_i^R = \dfrac{1}{Se_i^2 + T^2}$	6.173	484
Se of effect size, random-effects model	$Se^R = \sqrt{\dfrac{1}{\sum W_i^R}}$	6.174	484
95% CI of effect size, random-effects model	$95\%\ CI\ ES^R = ES^R \pm 1.96\,T$	6.175	484
95% predictive interval (PI) of effect size, random-effects model	$95\%\ PI\ ES^R = ES^R \pm t_{K-2}\sqrt{(Se^R)^2}$	6.176	484
95% predictive interval (PI) of effect size, random-effects model (example)	$95\%\ PI\ ES^R = -0.71 \pm 1.79\sqrt{0.179^2 + 0.31} = -1.75\ to\ 0.33$	6.177	485
95% PI of RR, random-effects model (example)	$95\%\ PI\ RR = 0.49\,(0.17\ to\ 1.39)$	6.178	485
Chapter 6 (Meta-analysis: subgroup analysis, fixed-effect model)			
Mean log RR, fixed-effect model (subgroup warm)	$Mean_{Log\ RR} = \dfrac{\sum W_i Log_{RRi}}{\sum W_i} = \dfrac{-43.56}{390.6} = -0.1112$	6.179	488
Se of log RR, fixed-effect model (subgroup warm)	$Se_{Log\ RR} = \sqrt{\dfrac{1}{\sum W_i}} = \sqrt{\dfrac{1}{390.6}} = 0.051$	6.180	488
95% CI of log RR, fixed-effect model (subgroup warm)	$95\%\ CI = \log RR \pm 1.96(Se_{Log\ RR}) = -0.111 \pm 1.96(0.05) = -0.21\ to\ 0.012$	6.181	488
Z value of log RR, fixed-effect model (subgroup warm)	$Z = \dfrac{-0.1112}{0.051} = -2.2;\ P = 0.028$	6.182	488
95% CI of RR, fixed-effect model (subgroup warm)	$RR(95\%\ CI)_{warm\ subgroup} = 0.89(0.81\ to\ 0.98)$	6.183	488
Z test comparing 2 subgroups, fixed-effect model (example)	$Z = \dfrac{|Log_A - Log_B|}{\sqrt{Se_A^2 + Se_B^2}} = \dfrac{|(-0.112)-(-0.999)|}{\sqrt{0.051^2 + 0.068^2}} = \dfrac{0.089}{0.085} = 10.5$	6.184	490
Modified ANOVA comparing subgroups, fixed-effect model: Q-within (example)	$Q_{within}^* = Q_{warm} + Q_{cold} = 21.44 + 20.34 = 41.78$	6.185	490
Modified ANOVA comparing subgroups, fixed-effect model: Q-between (example)	$Q_{between}^* = Q_{total} - (Q_{warm} + Q_{within}) = 152.2 - (21.44 + 20.34) = 110$	6.186	490
Analysis of heterogeneity among subgroups, fixed-effect model	$Q^* = \sum W(ES)^2 - \dfrac{(\sum WES)^2}{\sum W} = 220.65 - \dfrac{(-259.1)^2}{601.22} = 110$	6.187	491
Chapter 6 (Meta-analysis: subgroup analysis, random-effects model, separate T^2)			
Random-effect model, separate T^2: computation of Q (subgroup warm)	$Q = \sum W(ES)^2 - \dfrac{(\sum WES)^2}{\sum W} = 26.30 - \dfrac{(43.56)^2}{390.58} = 21.44$	6.188	492
Random-effect model, separate T^2: computation of C (subgroup warm)	$C = \sum W_i - \dfrac{\sum W_i^2}{\sum W_i} = 390.58 - \dfrac{71110.79}{390.58} = 208.5$	6.189	492
Random-effect model, separate T^2 (subgroup warm)	$T^2 = \dfrac{Q - df}{C} = \dfrac{21.44 - 6}{155} = 0.074$	6.190	492
Random-effect model, separate T^2: I^2 (subgroup warm)	$I^2 = 100\%\dfrac{Q - df}{Q} = \dfrac{21.44 - 6}{21.44} = 72\%$	6.191	492
Random-effect model: separate T^2, mean log RR (subgroup warm)	$Mean_{Log\ RR}^R = \dfrac{\sum W_i^R Log_{RRi}}{\sum W_i^R} = \dfrac{-13.95}{51.95} = -0.269$	6.192	493
Random-effect model: separate T^2, standard error log RR (subgroup warm)	$Se_{Log\ RR}^R = \sqrt{\dfrac{1}{51.95}} = \sqrt{\dfrac{1}{31.36}} = 0.139$	6.193	493
Random-effect model: separate T^2, 95% CI of log RR (subgroup warm)	$95\%\ CI = \log RR \pm 1.96(Se_{Log\ RR}) = -0.269 \pm 1.96(0.139)$ $= -0.54\ to\ 0.003$	6.194	493
Random-effect model: separate T^2, Z value of log RR (subgroup warm)	$Z = \dfrac{-0.269}{0.139} = -1.93;\ P = 0.053$	6.195	493
Random-effect model: separate T^2, 95% CI of RR (subgroup warm)	$RR(95\%\ CI)_{warm\ subgroup} = 0.76(0.58\ to\ 1)$	6.196	493

(continued)

Z test comparing 2 subgroups, random-effects model, separate T^2 (example)	$Z = \dfrac{\lvert Log_A - Log_B \rvert}{Se_d} = \dfrac{\lvert Log_A - Log_B \rvert}{\sqrt{Se_A^2 + Se_B^2}} = \dfrac{\lvert(-0.269) - (-1.2)\rvert}{\sqrt{0.139^2 + 0.2^2}} = \dfrac{0.93}{0.24} = 3.82$	6.197	494
Modified ANOVA comparing subgroups, random-effects model, separate T^2: (Q-warm subgroup)	$Q_{warm}^* = \sum W(ES)^2 - \dfrac{(\sum WES)^2}{\sum W} = 12.58 - \dfrac{(13.95)^2}{51.95} = 8.76$	6.198	494
Modified ANOVA comparing subgroups, random-effects model, separate T^2: (Q-cold subgroup)	$Q_{cold}^* = \sum W(ES)^2 - \dfrac{(\sum WES)^2}{\sum W} = 38.88 - \dfrac{(30.17)^2}{24.94} = 1.88$	6.199	495
Modified ANOVA comparing subgroups, random-effects model, separate T^2: (Q-total)	$Q_{total}^* = \sum W(ES)^2 - \dfrac{(\sum WES)^2}{\sum W} = 51.45 - \dfrac{(44.12)^2}{76.88} = 26.1$	6.200	495
Modified ANOVA comparing subgroups, random-effects model, separate T^2: Q-within	$Q_{within}^* = Q_{warm}^* + Q_{cold}^* = 8.76 + 1.88 = 10.64$	6.201	495
Modified ANOVA comparing subgroups, random-effects model, separate T^2: Q-between	$Q_{between}^* = Q_{total}^* - (Q_{warm}^* + Q_{within}^*) = 26.1 - (8.76 + 1.88) = 15.46$	6.202	495
Analysis of heterogeneity among subgroups, random-effects model, separate T^2	$Q^* = \sum W(ES)^2 - \dfrac{(\sum WES)^2}{\sum W} = 51.45 - \dfrac{(-44.12)^2}{76.88} = 26.1$	6.203	495
Chapter 6 (Meta-analysis: subgroup analysis, random-effects model, pooled T^2)			
Random-effects model, poled T^2, computation of C (subgroup warm example)	$C_{warm} = \sum W_i - \dfrac{\sum W_i^2}{\sum W_i} = 390.58 - \dfrac{71110.79}{390.58} = 208.5$	6.204	496
Random-effects model, poled T^2, computation of C (subgroup cold example	$C_{cold} = \sum W_i - \dfrac{\sum W_i^2}{\sum W_i} = 219.09 - \dfrac{23694.18}{219.09} = 110.94$	6.205	496
Random-effects model, poled T^2, computation of Q (subgroup warm example)	$Q_{warm} = \sum W(ES)^2 - \dfrac{(\sum WES)^2}{\sum W} = 26.30 - \dfrac{(-43.56)^2}{390.58} = 21.44$	6.206	496
Random-effects model, poled T^2, computation of Q (subgroup cold example	$Q_{cold} = \sum W(ES)^2 - \dfrac{(\sum WES)^2}{\sum W} = 238 - \dfrac{(-218.78)^2}{219.09} = 20.34$	6.207	496
Random-effects model, poled T^2 (example)	$T_{pooled}^2 = \dfrac{\sum Q - \sum df}{\sum C} = \dfrac{(21.44 + 20.34) - (6 + 5)}{(208.5 + 110.94)} = 0.096$	6.208	496
Mean log RR, random-effects model pooled T^2	$Mean_{Log\,RR}^R = \dfrac{\sum W_i^R Log_{RRi}}{\sum W_i^R} = \dfrac{-50.8}{75.3} = -0.67$	6.209	496
Se of log RR, random-effects model pooled T^2	$Se_{Log\,RR}^R = \sqrt{\dfrac{1}{\sum W_i^R}} = \sqrt{\dfrac{1}{75.3}} = 0.115$	6.210	496
95% CI log RR, random-effects model pooled T^2	$95\% \; CI = \log RR \pm 1.96(Se_{Log\,RR}) = -0.67 \pm 1.96(0.115)$ $= -0.89 \text{ to } -0.44$	6.211	496
Z value of log RR, random-effects model pooled T^2	$Z = \dfrac{-0.67}{0.115} = -5.8; \; P < 0.001$	6.212	496
95% CI RR, random effects model pooled T^2	$RR(95\% \; CI)_{warm\,subgroup} = 0.51(0.41 \text{ to } 0.64)$	6.213	496
The proportion variability explained by the model R^2	$R^2 = 1 - \dfrac{explained\;variability}{total\;variability} = 1 - \dfrac{T_{pooled}^2}{T_{total}^2} = 1 - \dfrac{0.097}{0.301} = 67.7\%$	6.214	498
Z test comparing 2 subgroups, random-effects model, pooled T^2 (example)	$Z = \dfrac{\lvert Log_A - Log_B \rvert}{Se_d} = \dfrac{\lvert Log_A - Log_B \rvert}{\sqrt{Se_A^2 + Se_B^2}} = \dfrac{\lvert(-0.277) - (-1.198)\rvert}{\sqrt{0.15^2 + 0.177^2}} = \dfrac{0.921}{0.232} = 3.97$	6.215	498
Chapter 6 (Meta-analysis: meta regression)			
Meta regression equation	$ES = b_0 + b_1 x_1 + b_2 x_2 \ldots b_i x_i$	6.216	499
95% CI of beta coefficient, fixed-effect model (example)	$95\% \; CI = Log_{RR} \pm 1.96(Se) = -0.029 \pm 1.96(0.0026) = -0.024 \text{ to } -0.034$	6.217	500
Z value of beta coefficient, fixed-effect model	$Z = \dfrac{beta\;coefficient}{Se} = \dfrac{-0.029}{0.0026} = -11.1$	6.218	500
Meta regression equation, fixed-effect model (example)	$ES = b_0 + b_1 x_1 = 0.344 + (-0.029) \times 30 = -0.53$	6.219	501
95% CI of beta coefficient, random-effects model (example)	$95\% \; CI = Log_{RR} \pm 1.96(Se) = -0.029 \pm 1.96(0.0067) = -0.042 \text{ to } -0.016$	6.220	502

(continued)

Z value of beta coefficient, random-effects model	$Z = \dfrac{beta\ coefficient}{Se} = \dfrac{-0.029}{0.0067} = -4.3$	6.221	502
Meta regression equation, random-effects model (example)	$ES = b_0 + b_1 x_1 = 0.259 + (-0.029) \times 30 = -0.611$	6.222	503
The proportion variability explained by the model R^2	$R^2 = 1 - \dfrac{T^2_{meta\ regression}}{T^2_{random\ model}} = \dfrac{0.063}{0.308} = 0.795$	6.223	503

Chapter 6 (Meta-analysis: Fail-safe methods)

Cochran common Z score	$Z_c = \dfrac{\sum Z_i}{\sqrt{N}}$	6.224	504
Fail-safe N: calculation of total number of studies	$N = \dfrac{\left(\sum Z_i\right)^2}{\left(Z_c\right)^2}$	6.225	504
Fail-safe N: calculation of number of published and missing studies	$N = K + X = \dfrac{\left(\sum Z_K + \sum Z_x\right)^2}{\left(Z_c\right)^2}$	6.226	505
Fail-safe N: calculation of number of published and missing studies (variant)	$K + X = \dfrac{\left(\sum Z_K + 0\right)^2}{\left(1.65\right)^2}$	6.227	505
Fail-safe N: calculation of number of missing studies	$X = \dfrac{\left(\sum Z_K\right)^2}{\left(1.65\right)^2} - k$	6.228	505
Fail-safe N: calculation of number of missing studies (variant)	$X = \dfrac{k}{2.706} \times k \left(\overline{Z}\right)^2 - 2.706$	6.229	505
Fail-safe N: calculation of number of missing studies (example)	$X = \dfrac{\left(\sum Z_K\right)^2}{\left(1.65\right)^2} - k = \dfrac{\left(-40.65\right)^2}{2.706} - 13 = 595$	6.230	505
Fail-safe B: calculation of total number of studies	$N = \dfrac{n(E_o - E_m)}{(E_m - E_n)}$	6.231	505
Rosenberg weighting effect size method: calculation of total number of studies	$N = \dfrac{nW'}{\sum W_i}$	6.232	506

Chapter 6 (Meta-analysis: testing small study effects)

Begg and Mazumdar test	$Z = \dfrac{C - D}{\sqrt{k(1 - K)(2K + 5)/18}}$	6.233	509
Egger regression test	$ES = b_0 + b_1 Se_1$	6.234	509

Chapter 6 (Meta-analysis: Psychometric meta-analysis, Hunter and Schmidt)

The unattenuated (expected) effect size	$r^u = \dfrac{r}{a}$	6.235	520
Variance of unattenuated (expected) effect size	$Var(r^u) = \dfrac{Var(r)}{a^2}$	6.236	520
Estimated effect size in the population (bare bones meta-analysis)	$r = \dfrac{\sum n_i r_i}{\sum n_i}$	6.237	520
Variance observed (bare bones meta-analysis)	$S_r^2 = \dfrac{\sum n_i (r_i - r)^2}{\sum n_i}$	6.238	520
Variance of sampling error (bare bones meta-analysis)	$S_e^2 = \dfrac{(1 - r^2)^2}{N - 1}$	6.239	520
Variance between studies (bare bones meta-analysis)	$S_P^2 = S_r^2 - S_e^2$	6.240	521
Psychometric meta-analysis: proportion of variability corrected for all artifacts	$\dfrac{S_r^2 - \left(S_P^u\right)^2}{S_r^2}$	6.241	521
Psychometric meta-analysis: testing heterogeneity (Q-test)	$\chi^2 = \sum \dfrac{(n_i - 1)(r_i - \overline{r})^2}{(1 - \overline{r})^2}$	6.242	522
Psychometric meta-analysis: the prediction interval (PI) at 95%	$95\%\ PI = r \pm 1.96 \sqrt{\left(S_P^u\right)^2}$	6.243	522

Chapter 7 (Pitfalls and common errors)

The magic number 16	$n = \dfrac{16}{d^2} = 16 \left(\dfrac{Sd}{\Delta}\right)^2$	7.1	528
Predicting the 95% CI (80% power)	$95\%\ CI\ d_0 (80\%\ power) = d_0 \pm 0.7 \Delta_{0.80}$	7.2	534

(continued)

Predicting the 95% CI (90% power)	$95\% \, CI \, d_0 (90\% \, power) = d_0 \pm 0.6\Delta_{0.90}$	7.3	534
Two-step normalization (step 1)	$P_r(x_i) = 1 - \left(\dfrac{rank \, x_i}{n}\right)$	7.4	547
Two-step normalization (step 2)	$Z = \sqrt{2} \times erf^{-1}(-1 + 2P_r)$	7.5	547
Sample size calculation (unilateral study)	$n_{unilateral} = \dfrac{2\left[Z_{(1-\alpha)} + Z_{(1-\beta)}\right]^2}{\left(\dfrac{\delta}{Sd}\right)^2}$	7.6	551
Sample size calculation (bilateral study)	$n_{bilateral} = \dfrac{2\left[Z_{(1-\alpha/2)} + Z_{(1-\beta)}\right]^2}{\left(\dfrac{\delta}{Sd}\right)^2}$	7.7	552
Calculation of (z) from the estimate (Est) and (Se)	$Z = \dfrac{Est}{Se} = \dfrac{d}{Se} = \dfrac{r}{Se}$	7.8	553
Calculation of (z): Altman and Bland formula	$Z = -0.862 + \sqrt{[0.743 - 2.404 \times \log P_{value}]}$	7.9	555
Calculation of (z): Altman and Bland formula (example 1)	$Z = -0.862 + \sqrt{[0.743 - 2.404 \times \log(0.0044)]} = 2.85$	7.10	555
Calculation of the Se from Z (example 1)	$Se = \dfrac{d}{Z} = \dfrac{6.6}{2.85} = 2.315$	7.11	555
The 95% CI (example 1)	$95 \, CI \, (d) = d \pm 1.96 \, Se = 6.6 \pm 1.96(2.315) = 2.1\%$ to 11.14%	7.12	555
Calculation of (z): Altman and Bland formula (example 2)	$Z = -0.862 + \sqrt{[0.743 - 2.404 \times \log(0.005)} = 2.81]$	7.13	555
Calculation of the Se of Z (example 2)	$Se = \dfrac{r}{Z} = \dfrac{-1.273}{2.81} = 0.45$	7.14	555
The 95% CI in logarithmic value (example 2)	$95\% \, CI \, \log RR = \log RR \pm 1.96(Se) = -1.273 \pm 1.96(0.45)$ $= -0.38$ to -2.16	7.15	555
The 95% CI in the usual scale (example 2)	$RR(95\% \, CI) = 0.28(0.11 \text{ to } 0.69)$	7.16	555
Se of the difference of one subgroup (example)	$Se = \sqrt{\dfrac{P_1(1-P_1)}{n1} + \dfrac{P_2(1-P_2)}{n2}} = \sqrt{\dfrac{0.089(1-0.089)}{270} + \dfrac{0.152(1-0.152)}{270}} = 0.028$	7.17	565
Se of the difference of both subgroups (example)	$Se_d = \sqrt{(0.028)^2 + (0.105)^2} = 0.11$	7.18	565
The 95% CI of the difference (example)	$p_d \pm Z(Se_d) = 0.063 \pm 1.96(0.11) = -15.3 \%$ to 27.8%	7.19	565

Index

A

Analysis of Covariance (ANCOVA), 248, 254, 255, 257–272, 550, 561, 562

ANOVA, 25, 87, 90, 91, 95, 125–134, 136–142, 150, 151, 153, 169, 174, 192, 194, 197, 203–206, 208, 213, 217, 236–240, 247–254, 256, 257, 259, 260, 271–273, 276–280, 282–293, 296, 298, 312, 348, 352, 372–375, 377, 389, 391–395, 411, 412, 422, 435, 436, 489, 490, 494, 498, 500, 516, 532, 535, 545, 550, 553, 556, 559, 561, 562, 565, 574, 587, 589, 590, 594, 605, 606

AUC ROC curve, 71

B

Bland-Altman plots, 229

Blinding, 427, 428

C

Confidence intervals, 3, 15–22, 24, 25, 39, 41, 42, 45, 51–55, 63, 65, 70, 71, 78, 81, 87, 116, 122, 123, 135, 145, 146, 159, 180, 219, 227–230, 232, 234, 236, 240, 258, 260, 264, 267, 268, 277, 283, 284, 291–294, 299, 306, 309, 312, 316, 318, 335, 336, 345, 358, 371, 378, 389, 390, 397, 399, 401, 416, 423, 424, 434, 447, 453, 456, 457, 464, 466, 467, 469–478, 480–482, 487, 488, 493, 497, 513, 515, 532, 533, 538–541, 552, 554, 555, 557, 561, 568, 569, 571–573, 583, 599, 601–606, 608

Cox proportional hazard, 44, 45, 53, 247, 296–298, 329, 331, 382, 384, 403, 404, 476, 595, 597

D

Data management, 432, 433, 541, 578

Data reporting, 554

Diagnostic accuracy, 1, 56, 85, 214, 343, 405, 406, 436, 585

E

Effect size, 34, 87, 99, 102, 103, 105, 106, 108, 109, 111, 113, 117, 120, 123, 130, 131, 141–143, 145, 147, 149, 151, 153, 158, 159, 162, 171, 187, 189, 191, 195, 202, 208, 212, 258, 260, 264, 267, 268, 271, 275, 281, 288, 291, 315, 316, 320, 329, 336, 339–341, 344, 345, 347–358, 360, 363, 364, 366–382, 385–396, 398–400, 402–404, 413, 435, 436, 441, 443, 444, 446–460, 463–475, 477–481, 483–493, 495–510, 514–522, 527–532, 557, 560–562, 567–569, 571, 574, 575, 591, 593–597, 599–605, 607

Equivalence studies, 20–22, 24, 25, 38, 343, 350, 397–404, 423, 436, 555, 560, 568, 596

H

Hand meta-analysis

Hazard ratio, 1, 43–45, 49, 53

K

Kappa statistics

L

Linear regression, 25, 104, 192, 247, 254, 274, 298, 300–303, 309, 315, 317–320, 323, 332, 379, 435, 509, 592

Logistic regression, 30, 41, 42, 192, 193, 197, 203, 247, 296–299, 315–328, 331–333, 384, 386, 435, 537, 540, 545, 549, 550, 559, 561, 562, 572, 573, 592, 595

M

Meta -analysis heterogeneity

Meta regression, 498–502, 516, 517, 519, 606, 607

Mixed models, 237, 238, 240, 565

N

Non-inferiority studies, 22, 38, 116, 397–401, 423, 433, 436, 556, 577

Non-parametric tests, 90, 143–145, 147, 150, 152, 153, 160, 161, 184, 194, 369, 396, 436, 541, 545, 559, 575, 576, 588

O

Odds ratio, 1, 30, 37, 39–43, 51, 52, 55, 56, 71, 72, 99, 102, 103, 106, 108, 109, 111, 199, 200, 202, 203, 215, 296, 298, 321, 322, 327, 328, 332, 341, 358, 361, 362, 364, 365, 370, 371, 385, 386, 398, 401, 402, 407, 408, 435, 436, 444, 445, 449–451, 457, 468–471, 476, 478, 479, 504, 506, 508–511, 514, 517, 530, 531, 545, 550, 555, 558, 570–572, 579, 584, 590, 593, 597, 602, 604

Online calculators, 1, 41, 53, 64, 69, 87, 134, 151, 157, 201, 203, 222, 223, 227, 229, 344, 345, 350, 354, 355, 358, 362, 371, 375, 380, 384, 400–402, 404, 408, 412, 416, 450, 531–533, 539, 548, 551–554, 560, 563, 578

P

Parametric tests, 3, 34, 89, 90, 96, 114, 123, 143, 355, 356, 545, 575, 576

Primary endpoints, 540

Prognostic studies, 195, 559, 589

R

Randomization, 175, 195, 196, 249, 358, 359, 362, 425–431, 433, 434, 437, 447, 528, 536, 537, 553, 556, 557, 560, 561, 567, 568, 575, 578

Relative risk, 1, 39–43, 49–54, 102, 103, 106, 108, 187–189, 203, 341, 357, 358, 361, 362, 435,

449–451, 457, 468, 470–476, 481, 482, 484, 485, 487–501, 503, 505, 509, 513, 514, 517, 518, 545, 555, 558, 570, 583, 584, 590, 602, 603, 605, 606

Reliability testing, 237, 238

S

Sample size, 8–10, 17–19, 22, 23, 34, 35, 38, 39, 54, 70, 71, 78, 87, 89, 91, 92, 95, 102, 105, 110, 111, 113–115, 117, 119–121, 123–125, 127–130, 133–135, 137, 141, 143, 144, 146, 147, 149–151, 153, 159, 162, 169–174, 180, 181, 187, 190, 194, 198, 200, 203, 206, 210, 211, 222, 223, 230, 232, 240, 243, 258–260, 272, 276, 277, 286, 295, 299, 305–307, 309, 315, 316, 322, 324, 326, 329, 331, 333, 336, 339, 340, 342–347, 349–357, 359–416, 422–424, 431, 432, 435–437, 444, 451–458, 460–463, 465–467, 469, 479, 480, 482, 485, 491, 495, 498, 500, 503, 504, 506–510, 519, 520, 527–537, 539, 540, 548, 551, 552, 555, 557, 559, 560, 567, 569, 570, 572–575, 577, 578, 586, 592–599, 608

Small-study effects, 503, 507–512, 516, 517, 519

Statistician involvement

Statistics software

Stratification, 189, 195–197, 213, 248, 427, 536, 537, 575, 578

Study designs, 19–22, 24, 32, 34, 36, 37, 87, 90, 94–96, 111, 116, 142, 174, 191, 195, 213, 256, 262, 272, 279–281, 285, 286, 301, 306, 322, 324, 330, 333, 336, 342, 345, 360–362, 371, 372, 378, 388, 422, 435, 437, 444, 446, 447, 507, 519, 532, 535, 552, 555, 559, 568, 578

Study empowerment

Subgroups meta-analysis

Survival analysis, 45, 174, 179, 331, 336, 381